THE NURSE'S
DRUG HANDBOOK

THE NURSE'S DRUG HANDBOOK

SIXTH EDITION

Suzanne Loebl

George R. Spratto, Ph.D.
Professor of Pharmacology and Associate Dean
School of Pharmacy and Pharmacal Sciences
Purdue University
West Lafayette, Indiana

Adrienne L. Woods, R.N., M.S.N.
Nursing Supervisor
Veterans Administration Hospital
Wilmington, Delaware

Myrtle Matejski, Ph.D., R.N.
Professor of Nursing
University of Delaware
Newark, Delaware

Delmar Publishers Inc.®

Notice to the Reader

The publisher and the authors do not warrant or guarantee any of the products described herein or perform any independent analysis in connection with any of the product information contained herein. The publisher and the authors do not assume and expressly disclaim, any obligation to obtain and include information other than that provided by the manufacturer.

The reader is expressly warned to consider and adopt all safety precautions that might be indicated by the activities described herein and to avoid all potential hazards. By following the instructions contained herein the reader willingly assumes all risks in connection with such instructions.

The publisher and the authors make no representations or warranties of any kind, including but not limited to the warranties of fitness for particular purpose or merchantability nor are any such representations implied with respect to the material set forth herein, and the publisher and the authors take no responsibility with respect to such material. The publisher and the authors shall not be liable for any special, consequential or exemplary damages resulting, in whole or in part, from the reader's use of, or reliance upon, this material.

The authors and publisher have made a conscientious effort to ensure that the drug information and recommended dosages in this book are accurate and in accord with accepted standards at the time of publication. However, pharmacology is a rapidly changing science, so readers are advised, before administering any drug, to check the package insert provided by the manufacturer for the recommended dose, for contraindications for administration, and for added warnings and precautions. This recommendation is especially important for new, infrequently used, or highly toxic drugs.

Delmar staff

Cover illustration
by Gabriel Molano

Executive Editor: Barbara E. Norwitz
Managing Editor: Susan B. Simpfenderfer
Development Editor: Marjorie A. Bruce
Project Editor: Mary P. Robinson

Production Coordinator: Helen Yackel
Pronunciations: Ellen Weil, MS, RPh
Design Supervisor: Susan C. Mathews
Design Coordinator: Karen Kunz Kemp

For information, address Delmar Publishers Inc.,
2 Computer Drive West, Box 15-015
Albany, New York 12212

Printed in the United States of Amercica
Published simultaneously in Canada
By Nelson Canada
A division of The Thomson Corporation

10 9 8 7 6 5 4 3 2 1

Library of Congress Catalog Card Number: 88-655125
ISSN 1042-0002
ISBN 0-8273-4737-5   ISE ISBN 0–534–98479–7

Loebl, Suzanne
    The nurse's drug handbook / Suzanne Loebl, George Spratto,
Adrienne L. Woods, Myrtle Matejski. -- 6th ed.
        p.   cm.
    Includes bibliographical references.
    Includes index.
    ISBN 0-8273-4527-5
    1. Chemotherapy--Handbooks, manuals, etc. 2. Drugs--Handbooks,
manuals, etc. 3. Nursing--Handbooks, manuals, etc. I. Spratto,
George. II. Woods, Adrienne L. III. Title.
    [DNLM: 1. Drug Therapy--nurses' instruction. 2. Drugs--nurses'
instruction. QV 55 L824n]
RM262.L63 1990
615.5'8--dc20
DNLM/DLC
for Library of Congress

90-13947
CIP

Preface

The sixth edition of *The Nurse's Drug Handbook* represents some significant changes in the content and format compared with previous editions of the text. We believe that both nursing students and practitioners will find the book more user-friendly.

As in previous editions, up-to-date information has been used to revise the information on the most widely used prescription and over-the-counter drugs, which are presented by therapeutic or chemical drug class. Approximately forty new drugs have been added to the sixth edition. As in the past, trade names of drugs marketed in both Canada and the United States are listed. The trade names of drugs marketed only in Canada are designated by a maple leaf. General information on drug classes appears first in the chapter followed by a listing of individual drugs.

Several new features have been incorporated into this edition. For individual drugs, a new section, titled *Special Concerns,* has been added. Found in this section is information of special concern to the nurse, such as whether the drug is considered safe and effective for use in children, during lactation, during pregnancy, and in the geriatric patient. Also, the FDA pregnancy category to which the drug has been assigned is listed in this section. The most important new feature is the presentation of nursing considerations in a nursing process format. Such information provides the nurse with guidelines for performing assessments of the client before and after prescribed drug therapy; to initiate nursing interventions; to incorporate client/family teaching to ensure proper drug therapy; and to evaluate the effectiveness of drug therapy. Chapter 1 should be consulted for a more thorough discussion of how nursing considerations are presented.

Another feature of the sixth edition is the incorporation of new supplementary information including commonly used normal physiologic values including SI values, a listing of poison control centers in the United States, and information on the Medic Alert Systems. Also, drugs that are controlled either by the U.S. Controlled Substances Act or the Controlled Substances Law (Canada) are listed with the appropriate schedule under which they have been placed. The commonly used equivalents have been revised as have the therapeutic drug levels and ranges. The appendix listing Food-Drug Interactions has been updated and revised. The definitions of FDA pregnancy categories are also presented. A nomogram for calculating the surface area of patients has been retained.

We believe the significant changes incorporated into this edition make *The Nurse's Drug Handbook* an easy-to-use and valuable text for information on drugs and the proper monitoring of drug therapy by the practitioner as well as the student.

Acknowledgments

The preparation of the sixth edition of *The Nurse's Drug Handbook* occurred at a time when we were also preparing *NDR–91*. The assistance of a number of individuals made a nearly impossible job more bearable. We would like to extend our thanks and appreciation to Barbara Norwitz, Executive Editor, Delmar Publishers, for her support and assistance. Special thanks go to Marjorie Bruce, Mary Robinson, and Debra Flis, of Delmar Publishers, each of whom worked especially hard to ensure that the manuscript process flowed smoothly. We would also like to extend appreciation to Séamus McCague, ICPC, Dublin, Ireland, whose willingness to undertake Herculean efforts made it possible to get the book published in record time.

G. Spratto extends appreciation to Charles O. Rutledge, Dean of the Schools of Pharmacy, Nursing, and Health Sciences at Purdue University for his encouragement and for being understanding of the deadlines. Greatest appreciation and love go to my wife Lynne, and sons, Chris and Gregg, who have always been supportive of the project and who had to make many sacrifices.

A. Woods would like to thank her friends and colleagues, especially Marianne Sarason and Sally Marshall, for their support and encouragement during this endeavor. Special thanks to Susan Fanuele for taking such special care of my babies, Kathryn Ann and Nathaniel Bryan. Most important, I salute my husband, Howard. He was a rock who supported and encouraged me while enduring an unbelievable schedule with our new baby.

M. Matejski wishes to acknowledge her husband, Stanley, for his patience and forbearance as she spent hours at the computer working on the book. I also thank my family for their understanding as they waited patiently to hear from me these past months.

Contents

Part 2   Anti-Infectives

Part 3   Antineoplastic Agents

Part 4   Drugs Affecting Blood Formation and Coagulation

Part 5   Cardiovascular Drugs

Part 6   Drugs Affecting the Central Nervous System

Part 12   Miscellaneous Agents

Appendices

Index of Tables

Commonly Used Abbreviations

A, aa	of each		h.s.	at bedtime
a.c.	before meals		IA	intra-arterial
ad	to, up to		IM, im	intramuscular
ad lib	as desired, at pleasure		IV, iv	intravenous
alt. hor.	every other hour		IVPB	IV piggyback, a secondary IV line
A.M., a.m.	morning		kg	kilogram (2.2 lb)
aq	water		KVO	keep vein open
aq dest.	distilled water		L, l	liter (1,000 mL)
a.u.	each ear, both ears		Ⓛ	left
a.d.	right ear		LDH	lactic dehydrogenase
a.l.	left ear		LDL	low density lipoprotein
b.i.d.	two times a day		LH	luteinizing hormone
b.i.n.	two times a night		m., min	minim
BP	blood pressure		min	minute
BUN	blood urea nitrogen		M	mix
c̄	with		M^2, m^2	square meter
CA	cancer		mg	milligram
Caps, caps	capsule(s)		MAO	monoamine oxidase
CHF	congestive heart failure		max	maximum
cm	centimeter		mCi	millicurie
collyr.	eye wash		mcg	microgram
COPD	chronic obstructive pulmonary disease		mEq	milliequivalent
			mist, mixt	mixture
d.	day		mL	milliliter
dc	discontinue		NG	nasogastric
dil.	dilute		ng	nanogram
dL	deciliter (one-tenth of a liter)		noct	at night, during the night
dr.	dram (0.0625 ounce)		non rep	do not repeat
emuls.	emulsion		NPO	nothing by mouth
elix	elixir		NR	do not refill (e.g., a prescription)
ext.	extract		NSAID	nonsteroidal anti-inflammatory drug
FSH	follicle stimulating hormone			
g (gm)	gram (1,000 mg)		O	pint
GI, gi	gastrointestinal		o.d.	every day
gr	grain		O.D.	right eye
gtt	a drop, drops		o.h.	every hour
GU	genitourinary		ol	oil
h, hr	hour		O.L.	left eye
HAL	hyperalimentation		o.m.	every morning
HDL	high density lipoproteins		o.n.	every night
			O.S.	left eye

os	mouth	SGPT	serum glutamic-pyruvic transaminase
O.U.	each eye, both eyes		
oz.	ounce	Sig, S.	mark on the label
p.c.	after meals	SL	sublinqual (beneath the tongue)
PE	pulmonary embolus	s.o.s.	if necessary, once only
per	by, through	sol	solution
PO, po, p.o.	by mouth	sp	spirits
PR	by rectum	stat	immediately, first dose
PRN, p.r.n.	when needed or necessary	syr	syrup
PUD	peptic ulcer disease	tab	tablet
q	every	t.i.d.	three times daily
q.d.	every day	t.i.n.	three times nightly
q.h.	every hour	T.O.	telephone order
qhs	every night	tr, tinct	tincture
q2h	every two hours	μ	micron
q3h	every three hours	μCi	microcurie
q4h	every four hours	μg	microgram
q6h	every six hours	U	unit
q8h	every eight hours	ung	ointment
q.i.d.	four times daily	ut dict	as directed
q.o.d.	every other day	VLDL	very low density lipoproteins
q.s.	as much as is needed or required	vin	wine
®	right	V.O.	verbal order
Rx	take, symbol for a prescription	>	greater than
Rept.	let it be repeated	<	less than
s̄	without	×	times, frequency
ss	one-half	↑	increasing, higher
SC, sc	subcutaneous	↓	decreasing, lower
SGOT	serum glutamic-oxaloacetic transaminase		

PART ONE

Introduction

CHAPTER ONE

How to Use This Handbook

The sixth edition of *The Nurse's Drug Handbook* has been reorganized and streamlined to facilitate use. Realizing that drugs are classified by either their chemical or therapeutic use (and that pharmacology is most often taught by this approach), a format is used that should increase the consistency and clarity of the information presented as well as make the text easy to use.

The first section discusses general information that will provide the necessary background for subsequent sections. Information is presented on mechanism of action and pharmacokinetics (Chapter 2), side effects (Chapter 3), and drug interactions (Chapter 4). In addition, comprehensive nursing considerations for drug therapy (Chapter 5) and administration of medications by different routes (Chapter 6) are listed. These particular sections are of utmost importance for the nurse who administers drugs as well as for the nurse who provides directions to patients on the proper administration of medication.

The pediatric, geriatric, or pregnant patient often reacts differently to drugs; these groups also manifest special problems/concerns with respect to drug therapy. These issues are discussed in Chapter 7; in addition, nursing considerations, as they relate to these special patients, are presented.

One of the most important problems that faces physicians, nurses, pharmacists, and other members of the health care team is patient compliance with the appropriate medication regimen. Helpful approaches in meeting this challenge are detailed in Chapter 8.

The major portion of the book presents information on individual drugs or drug classes. The *Handbook* is intended to be a quick reference for the practicing nurse as well as a simple text in pharmacology. With these objectives in mind, the following format was developed.

Drugs that either belong to closely related families (e.g., penicillins, sulfonamides) or are used for the treatment of a particular disease (e.g., malaria) are grouped together.

Drugs that mainly affect one physiologic system (e.g., cardiovascular) are grouped together in a section; these sections contain chapters that deal with specific conditions to be treated (e.g., hypertension, arrhythmias, angina).

Drugs that affect hormones or that substitute for them (e.g., insulin, thyroid, estrogens) are presented under appropriate headings.

Drugs are arranged alphabetically within each group or subdivision, with the generic name listed in bold type followed by the trade name(s).

This type of arrangement enables the nurse to locate an individual drug quickly and to find concise information about it. In addition, the introduction for specific chapters presents general information about the drugs themselves or the particular condition for which the drugs are intended. Thus, the introduction to each section should be read carefully. Information for individual drugs is presented as follows:

Drug Names

The generic name for the drug is presented first, followed by one or more trade names. If the trade name is available only in Canada, the name will be followed by a maple leaf. Also, if the drug is controlled by the U.S. Federal Controlled Substances Act, the schedule in which the drug has been placed follows the trade name (e.g., C-II, C-III, C-IV).

Classification

The type of drug is defined unless this is self-evident. Use this information to learn how to categorize drugs.

General Statement

Information is presented about the class of drug and/or what might be unusual about a particular group of drugs. In addition, information may be presented about the disease(s) for which the drugs are indicated.

Action/Kinetics

The action portion of this entry describes the mechanism(s) by which a drug is able to achieve its therapeutic effect, (e.g., certain antibiotics interfere with the growth of bacteria). Not all mechanisms of action are known, and some are self-evident, as when a hormone is administered as a replacement. The kinetics entry lists pertinent facts, if known, about rate of drug absorption, minimum effective serum or plasma level, biologic half-life ($t\frac{1}{2}$), duration of action, metabolism, and excretion. The time it takes for half the drug to be excreted or removed from the blood, $t\frac{1}{2}$, is important in determining how often a drug is to be administered and how long to assess for side effects. Therapeutic serum or plasma levels indicate the desired concentration, in serum or plasma, for the drug to exert its beneficial effect. More and more drug therapy is being monitored in this fashion (e.g., antibiotics, theophylline, cardiac glycosides). A new feature for this edition is a listing of commonly accepted therapeutic drug levels on the inside of the back cover. Metabolism and excretion routes may be important for patients with systemic liver disease or kidney disease or both. Again, information is not available for all therapeutic agents.

Uses

Therapeutic application(s) are listed for the particular agent. Investigational uses are also listed for selected drugs.

Contraindications

Disease states or conditions are described in which the drug should not be used. The safe use of many of the newer pharmacologic agents during pregnancy or childhood has not been established. As a general rule, the use of drugs during pregnancy is contraindicated unless specified by a physician.

Special Concerns

This section lists information that is of special concern to the nurse, such as conditions under which the drug should be used with caution. For example, it is noted whether the drug is considered safe and effective for use in children, during lactation, during pregnancy, and in the geriatric patient. Also, the FDA pregnancy category to which the drug has been assigned is listed in this section.

The pregnancy category identifies the FDA-assigned pregnancy categories, described as follows:

A: Adequate and well-controlled studies have failed to demonstrate a risk to the fetus in the first trimester of pregnancy (and there is no evidence of risk in later trimesters).

B: Animal reproduction studies have failed to demonstrate a risk to the fetus and there are no adequate and well-controlled studies in pregnant women.

C: Animal reproduction studies have shown an adverse effect on the fetus and there are no adequate and well-controlled studies in humans, but potential benefits may warrant use of the drug in pregnant women despite potential risks.

D: There is positive evidence of human fetal risk based on adverse reaction data from investigational or marketing experience or studies in humans, but potential benefits may warrant use of the drug in pregnant women despite potential risks.

X: Studies in animals or humans have demonstrated fetal abnormalities and/or there is positive evidence of human fetal risk based on adverse reaction data from investigational or marketing experience and the risks involved in use of the drug in pregnant women clearly outweigh potential benefits.

Side Effects

Unwanted or bothersome effects the patient *may* experience while taking the particular agent are detailed. Side effects are listed by the body organ or system affected. This feature allows easy access to information on side effects of drugs.

Drug Interactions

Drugs that may interact with one another are listed under this entry. The study of drug interactions is a rapidly expanding area of pharmacology. The compilation of such interactions is far from complete; therefore, listings in this manual are to be considered *only* as general cautionary guidelines.

As detailed in Chapter 4, drug interactions may result from a number of different mechanisms (additive effects, interference with degradation of drug, increased speed of elimination). Such interferences may manifest themselves in a variety of ways; however, an attempt has been made throughout the text to describe these interactions whenever possible as an increase (↑) or a decrease (↓) in the effect of the drug, followed by a brief description of the reason for the change.

It is important to realize that any side effects that accompany the administration of a particular agent may be increased also as a result of a drug interaction.

The reader should be aware that the drug interactions are often listed for classes of drugs. Thus, the drug interaction would be likely to occur for all drugs in that particular class.

Laboratory Test Interferences

How a drug may affect the laboratory test values of the patient is described. Some of these interferences are caused by the therapeutic or toxic effects of the drugs; others result from interference with the testing method itself. Interferences are described as false + or (↑) values and as false − or (↓) values. Many of the laboratory test interferences are also listed under the *Nursing Considerations* for each drug.

Dosage

The adult and pediatric doses, as well as the dosage form(s) for which the drug is available, are presented when possible and are so indicated. The listed dosage is to be considered as a general guideline, because the exact amount of the drug to be given is determined by the physician. However, a nurse should question orders from the physician when dosages differ markedly from the accepted norm. We have tried to give complete data for drugs that are prescribed frequently.

Nursing Considerations

These will be presented in a nursing process format. The nursing considerations are designed to assist the nurse in preparing the medications for administration and proper storage, to perform assessments of the client before and after prescribed drug therapy, to initiate nursing interventions appropriate for the prescribed drug therapy, to incorporate client/family teaching related to therapy, and finally, to provide methods to evaluate the effectiveness of the prescribed drug therapy as well as client response. Throughout this text, nursing assessments, interventions, and evaluations may be used interchangeably, dependent on the context in which they are being addressed and utilized. Nursing considerations that include assessments and interventions may contain specifics such as:

1. Assessment of specific physiologic functions that may be affected by the drug.
2. Physiologic, pharmacologic, and psychologic effects of the drug and how these affect the nursing process.
3. Emergency situations that can arise as a result of drug therapy and appropriate nursing interventions for these situations.
4. Specific nursing interventions that relieve a patient's discomfort that may have been precipitated by a particular drug.
5. Nursing interventions that help ensure the safety of the patient when receiving drug therapy.

The nurse must also assess the patient for the Side Effects listed for that drug. Side effects must be documented and reported to the physician. Severe side effects are usually cause for discontinuation of the drug.

Nursing Considerations related to client/family teaching emphasize the nurse's role as he/she applies the nursing process in patient education and in promoting drug compliance. Emphasis is placed on helping the client/family recognize untoward drug reactions, avoiding potentially dangerous situations, and alleviating anxiety that may result from taking a particular drug.

In addition, specific information on client education is provided in the *Nursing Considerations* for each drug. The proper education of clients is one of the most challenging aspects of nursing, but the instructions must be tailored to the needs, awareness, and sophistication of each client. Some drugs and drug therapy require the active participation of clients and/or family. For example, clients who take medication to lower blood pressure should assume responsibility for taking their own blood pressure or identifying someone, a significant other perhaps, who is willing to learn how to take their blood pressure. Clients should be taught to keep a written record of the drugs they take as well as their blood pressure recordings. This can be done in a notebook or on a calendar. They should be instructed to bring these records with them whenever they go for a check-up or seek medical care. These records may also be shared with the pharmacist if there is a question concerning drugs prescribed, if clients are considering taking an over-the-counter(OTC) medication, or if they have to change pharmacies. The records should be shared with the health care provider to assure accurate evaluation of the response to prescribed therapy. The nurse should utilize a return demonstration teaching format to ensure understanding and compliance, and should provide clients with a phone number to call with any questions or concerns about prescribed therapy.

Finally, when taking the nursing history, emphasis should be placed on the client's ability to read and follow directions. The ability to comprehend what is written or said should not be assumed based on the client's level of education or command of language. Given the current rate of illiteracy, it is possible that persons of another era, who had limited education, may not be able to comprehend what is taught concerning their drug therapy. In addition, client lifestyle and income are important factors that may affect compliance with prescribed drug therapy. The potential for a client being/becoming pregnant, and whether or not a mother is breast feeding her infant, should be included in assessments as appropriate. The age of patients and their state of mental acuity, whether learned from personal observation or from discussion with close friends or family members, can be critical in determining potential relationships between drug therapy and/or drug interactions. Including these factors in the nursing assessment will assist all on the health care team to determine the type of therapy and drug delivery system that is best suited to a particular client and will promote the highest level of client compliance.

The previous points are covered for all drugs or drug classes. When drugs are presented as a group rather than individually, the points may be covered only once for each group. In this case the nurse must look for the appropriate entry at the beginning of the group. For example, the *Contraindications, Side Effects, Drug Interactions,* and *Nursing Considerations* for all the penicillins are so similar that they are listed only once at the beginning of the section.

In some chapters, drugs that are not as widely used are presented in tabular form, especially if differences between the drugs relate mainly to dosage or duration of action. The tables are constructed so that specific information for a particular drug can be listed also.

Information relevant to a particular drug, and not to the whole group, is listed under appropriate headings, such as *Additional Contraindications,* or *Additional Side Effects.* Such entries are *in addition to* and not *instead of* the regular entry, which must be consulted also.

The appendices contain additional information to assist the nurse in administering drugs and monitoring drug therapy appropriately.

All nurses should become proficient in the terminology used in writing prescriptions as well as the procedure to be followed in calculating dosages. Information to assist the nurse with this process is in Chapter 7 and the list of abbreviations.

A brief description of the U.S. Federal Controlled Substances Act and Controlled Substances (Canada) are included in the Appendix 3.

A glossary of terms that some readers may find unfamiliar follows the appendices. Finally, a listing of resources and references that gives additional information or more in-depth treatment of a topic has been included.

You are now ready to use *The Nurse's Drug Handbook.* We hope that the text will be useful and assist you in your profession. Even though the material presented might, at first, appear overwhelming, remember that the effective drugs currently at the disposal of the health care team are the key to today's better, more effective, and efficient medical care. Certainly, the administration of drugs, assessment of potential interactions, and the evaluation of their effects on the client are crucial parts of the nursing process.

CHAPTER TWO

Mechanism of Action/ Pharmacokinetics: General Principles

MECHANISM OF ACTION

The mechanisms by which drugs manifest the desired pharmacologic effect are sometimes clear and sometimes obscure. In some cases, the mechanism of action is obvious; for instance, when the drug replaces a missing biochemical substance, such as insulin does in diabetes. In other cases, the mechanism is more complex, but known; for instance, allopurinol inhibits an enzyme necessary for the formation of uric acid. By decreasing the concentration of uric acid in the blood, allopurinol relieves gout. Sometimes the mechanism of action of a drug is unknown, even though the drug has been used for a long time; for example, the role played by phenytoin in decreasing epileptic convulsions, or the precise manner by which digitalis increases the strength of the heartbeat, is not known. In this book, mechanisms of action of drugs are provided when known.

PHARMACOKINETICS

Pharmacokinetics is the study of the fate of drugs in the body. This science concerns itself with:

Drug absorption and distribution
Drug plasma concentration
Therapeutic plasma levels
Toxic plasma levels
Concentration of the active drug at the target site
Rate of metabolism
Rate of excretion

These parameters, in turn, are affected by:

Physicochemical nature of the drug (e.g., lipid solubility)
Formulation of the drug
Route of administration

Binding of the drug to plasma and/or tissue (bioavailability)

Individual characteristics of the patient

Concomitant diseases

Concomitant administration of food or other drugs

Pharmacokinetics is assuming greater importance in medicine, because many patients are currently taking an increasing number of potent drugs, often concomitantly and for prolonged periods of time. Pharmacokinetic concepts that play a major role in the administration of drugs—administration, absorption, onset of action, peak of activity, half-life, first-pass effect, drug distribution, drug elimination, therapeutic serum levels, bioavailability, therapeutic drug delivery systems—are reviewed briefly below.

Some pharmacokinetic data, as well as mechanisms of action of drugs, have been added to the discussions of individual drugs or drug classes in *The Nurse's Drug Handbook*. The information listed for the various drugs is neither complete nor entirely consistent. Pharmacokinetic data are lacking for some of the older drugs still widely used today. Moreover, data obtained from the literature and/or from drug manufacturers are often inconsistent and spotty. Onset of action is given for some drugs; time to attain peak serum levels or therapeutic serum levels is listed for others. Consistency was sacrificed for completeness of information. When available and/or known, we have listed all or some of the following: mechanism of action, onset of action, therapeutic serum levels, duration of action, metabolism/excretion, time to attain peak serum levels, and biologic half-life ($t\frac{1}{2}$).

Administration

The route used to administer drugs (Figure 1) has a profound effect on drug absorption, distribution, metabolism, and elimination.

Oral (Enteral) Administration: Oral administration is the most economical, most widespread, but least standardized route. Drug absorption after oral administration is affected by the presence of food, gastric emptying time, intestinal motility, the pH of the stomach and intestine, the nature of the drug (small, lipid-soluble molecules are absorbed more quickly than others, for example), the rate of disintegration and dissolution of the tablet (affected by physical state and coating), and blood circulation to the gastrointestinal (GI) tract. Importantly, certain drugs cannot be given orally at all (without special protective measures), because they are destroyed by stomach acid. Often orally administered drugs are degraded partially by various enzymes in the GI tract, in the intestinal mucosa, and most of all, in the liver (see *First-Pass Effect,* below). A combination of all or some of these factors could be responsible for only a fraction of orally administered drugs becoming absorbed into the bloodstream and/or reaching their site of action (see also *Onset of Action* and *Peak of Activity* below).

Intramuscular and Subcutaneous Administration: Drugs are absorbed into plasma from intramuscular (IM) or subcutaneous (SC) injection sites by simple diffusion. Larger molecules (proteins, for example) are absorbed through the lymphatic circulation. Absorption is prompt. Duration of action can be increased by the use of repository preparations that decrease the rate of absorption.

Intravenous Administration: Intravenous (IV) administration ensures prompt onset of action and eliminates uncertainty associated with the incompleteness of drug absorption by other routes. Intravenous administration is the only route that can be used for certain irritating drugs or solutions, because the walls of blood vessels are relatively resistant to irritation. IV administration usually

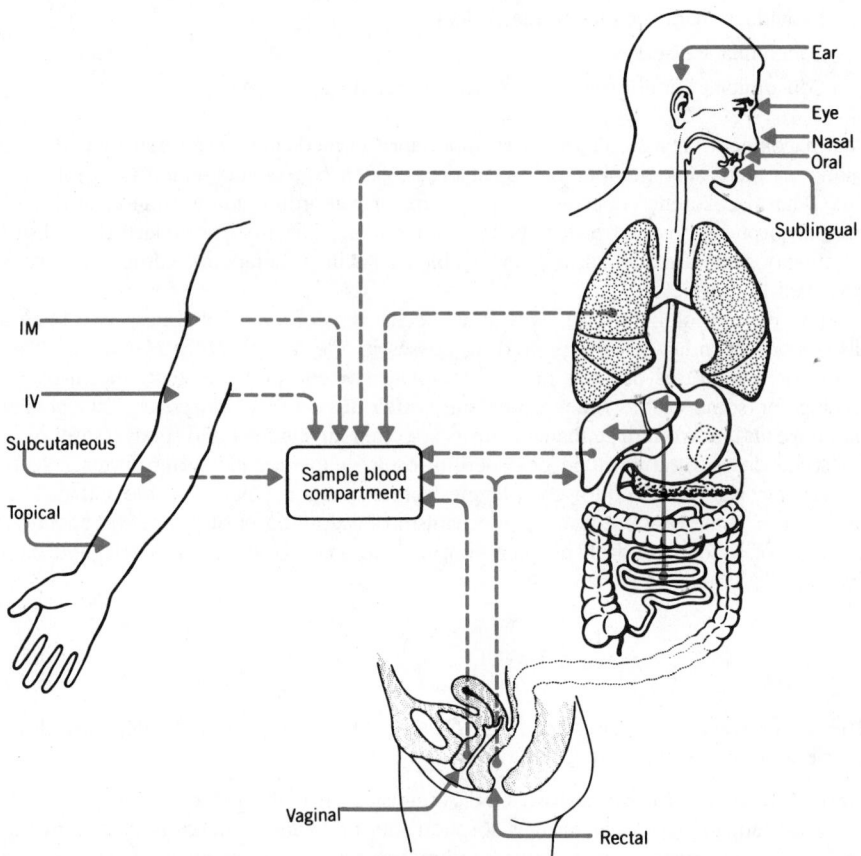

FIGURE 1   Drugs can be administered (input) through a great variety of routes. When given orally, they are absorbed from the stomach and small intestine and must first pass through the liver, the organ chiefly involved in drug metabolism. (See text for a definition of first-pass effects.) Reproduced with permission from Dr. Leslie Benet in E.J. Ariens, ed: *Drug Design, Volume IV*. New York, Academic Press, 1973, p. 5.

requires constant monitoring by a nurse, because this route increases the risk of toxic or untoward reactions.

Sublingual Administration: Drugs placed under the tongue are absorbed rapidly into the vena cava (venous circulation); this method of drug administration avoids the first-pass effect of the liver. This method is only suitable for certain highly active agents, such as nitroglycerin.

Rectal Administration: Rectal administration is used when oral administration is precluded (e.g., in cases of severe vomiting or unconsciousness). However, absorption is slow and uncertain. The drug is absorbed into the GI tract below the portal vein and avoids the first-pass effect of the liver. Also, use of this route is limited, because many drugs are irritating to the rectum.

Intracavitary Administration: Intracavitary administration is useful for certain antineoplastic agents. Intracavitary administration specifically increases the concentration of drug at the site of action.

Intrathecal Administration: The injection of a drug directly into the spinal subarachnoid space is necessary for the administration of certain drugs used for the treatment of meningitis and related disorders; access to their site of action would be precluded or diminished because of the blood-brain barrier. Absorption is rapid.

Mucous Membrane Administration: Mucous membrane administration is usually restricted to localized therapy, although it is used occasionally for systemic administration (antidiuretic hormone, for example). Absorption may be rapid. This route includes intranasal and intravaginal administration.

Skin (Cutaneous) Administration: Intact skin is relatively impermeable to most drugs; therefore, it is a good route for achieving localized results in various skin conditions. Absorption is increased if the skin is abraded or denuded, if the drug is added to a specific solvent, or if medicated skin is covered by occlusive dressing. Also, if a drug is applied over a large surface area of the skin, and for prolonged periods of time, systemic effects may be observed.

Therapeutic Drug-Delivery Systems: In therapeutic drug-delivery systems, a pharmacologic agent is delivered continuously from a reservoir for prolonged periods of time (see *Therapeutic Drug-Delivery Systems* later in this chapter).

Absorption

The rate of absorption of a drug is of paramount importance, because it is reflected in the concentration of the drug in the serum and at the target site. It determines the drug's time of onset of action and the time of peak effect. If absorption is too slow compared with elimination, the drug might never attain the minimum effective therapeutic serum concentration (Figure 2). In addition to being affected by the route of administration, absorption is also affected by:

Formulation of the drug (tablets vs. capsules, inert additives, coatings)
Character of the drug itself (e.g., acidic vs. basic)
Drug solubility
Presence (absence) of food (oral administration only)
Patient characteristics—age, body weight, individual factors, presence of concomitant disease

The customary manner of diagramming drug absorption by plotting serum concentration as a function of time is shown in Figure 2.

Onset of Action

The onset of action refers to the time interval between administration and notation of the first therapeutic effects. It depends on the route of administration, the characteristics of the drug, its rate of absorption through various membranes, and the formulation (how fast the drug is released into the system from the dosage form). The onset of action is especially variable after oral administration, depending on the presence of food in the stomach, the motility of the GI tract, and other factors.

Peak of Activity

The peak of activity—when the drug reaches its maximum effect—coincides often with peak serum concentration (see Figure 2). Many drugs cause this peak to surpass the optimally effective level, but

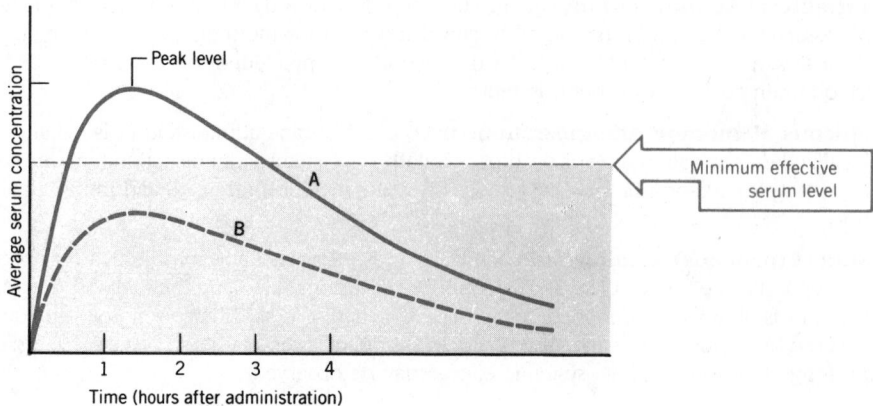

FIGURE 2   Drug absorption curve.

the concentration can fall rapidly below this level as a result of biotransformation and excretion. This drop occurs especially often when a short-acting drug is given initially or intermittently.

In the treatment of diabetes, for example, insulins with various lengths of action are mixed to keep insulin levels at a therapeutically effective level around the clock.

Biologic Half-Life (t$^{1/2}$)

The time in which half the drug has been eliminated is the *biologic half-life,* or t$^{1/2}$. (The concept of half-life was originally introduced in connection with discussion of the decay of radioactive substances.) If no additional drug is administered, it takes *two half-lives* to eliminate 75% of the drug and *four half-lives* to eliminate 93.3% of the drug.

In practice, most drugs are administered more than once; a subsequent dose is administered generally before the previous dose has been eliminated entirely. This overlap can result in drug accumulation.

The biologic half-life is an important concept in establishing dosage frequency. In general, a dosage interval equal to or less than the t$^{1/2}$ is recommended for most drugs. Thus, if t$^{1/2}$ is 4 hr, the drug can be given up to six times per day.

In practice, however, an attempt is made to consider the convenience of the patient in setting dosage schedules.

Most drugs have a short half-life (the effects of short-acting anesthetics often last only a few minutes). Other drugs, the monoamine oxidase (MAO) inhibitors, for example, have exceedingly long half-lives.

The concept of half-life is important in all aspects of drug therapy, including the treatment of drug overdosage. The narcotic antagonist naloxone, for example, has a shorter t$^{1/2}$ than that of morphine; therefore, administration of the antagonist must be repeated until the effects of the narcotic have worn off. The concept of half-life can only be applied to the drugs when they have been absorbed into the blood circulation, and not to those applied topically.

Half-life, as other pharmacokinetic factors, varies with the age of the patient, concomitant diseases (especially renal or hepatic impairment), and the presence of food and/or other drugs. Sometimes a drug (or its active metabolites) is eliminated in two or more stages. In such cases, t$^{1/2}$ is said to be biphasic or multiphasic.

First-Pass Effect

Most toxic substances, including drugs, are degraded by the microsomal enzymes of the liver. Because orally administered drugs are absorbed from the GI tract into the hepatic circulation, they must pass through the liver before they can reach the general circulation and their target. This effect results often in a considerable loss of activity of the administered drug, a phenomenon referred to as the first-pass effect. First-pass effect is measured as hepatic clearance. The first-pass effect is taken into account when drugs are formulated; that is, a higher concentration must be administered orally rather than parenterally. Note that drugs administered sublingually or rectally do not have a first pass through the liver, but enter the general circulation directly (see Figure 1).

Distribution

The distribution of drugs in the body is governed by the physicochemical characteristics of the specific drug. The speed by which a particular agent is absorbed through the various biologic membranes depends on such factors as the size of the molecule, its solubility, and the pH of the tissues.

In general, once the drug has been injected into or has reached the bloodstream, it attains significant concentrations first in such highly perfused organs as the heart, liver, and kidneys (within minutes).

Delivery of the drug to the viscera, skin, and adipose tissue is slower (minutes to hours). Penetration of some tissues is even slower, and the distribution phase can be extremely slow for drugs that bind strongly to serum proteins, because the drug-protein complex is unable to pass out of the plasma.

Distribution of certain pharmacologic agents to the central nervous system (CNS) is often limited, because the blood-brain barrier is selective in admitting compounds.

The ability of a drug to reach the fetus is dependent on its ability to cross the placental barrier (see Chapter 7).

Elimination

A crucial parameter from a therapeutic point of view is the time it takes for a drug to be eliminated from the body.

Elimination rates are determined experimentally on a number of test subjects, and the rate cited in the literature represents an average.

Drug elimination is a composite of drug **metabolism,** which can result in active or inactive metabolites, and drug **excretion.**

Metabolism: Metabolism is the sum total of all the reactions involved in the biotransformation of a pharmacologic agent after it is administered. Most metabolic transformations are enzymatic and take place in the liver, accounting for a decreased rate of drug metabolism in the presence of liver disease, thereby requiring a decrease in dosage.

In contrast, prolonged administration of certain drugs (barbiturates, phenytoin, alcohol) increases the efficacy and/or concentration of drug-metabolizing hepatic enzymes (enzyme induction). This results in an increased rate of metabolism of certain drugs. In such cases, a larger dose of these drugs might be required to attain and/or maintain the drug at effective therapeutic levels.

Metabolism often increases the water solubility of the pharmacologic agent and facilitates its renal excretion.

Sometimes metabolism is required for the drug to become active; in other instances, metabolism might convert the drug to a more toxic compound.

Excretion: The vast majority of drugs and/or their metabolites are excreted through the urine. A number of drugs are excreted by the bile (e.g., chlorpromazine, salicylates, steroid hormones, antibiotics). After entering the intestine in the bile, the drug may be reabsorbed and reenter the blood and again be carried to the liver (called enterohepatic cycle). Drugs excreted in the bile may be eliminated eventually from the body in the feces. A few agents are excreted via the lungs (e.g., volatile anesthetics, such as nitrous oxide, halothane, isoflurane). Small amounts of drugs may appear also in the saliva and sweat and may cause skin rashes. Drugs may find their way also into breast milk and, therefore, will be ingested by the infant. Thus, the benefits versus risks of the mother continuing to nurse when taking a drug known to cause toxic effects should be evaluated carefully.

The rate of renal excretion is determined by the glomerular filtration rate (GFR), tubular reabsorption, and tubular secretion. In general, the more lipid-soluble a substance is, the slower its renal excretion. When elimination is slow or slowed—because of renal disease—the risk of drug accumulation and drug toxicity is increased. Note that dosage is reduced for most drugs in the presence of impaired renal function; in fact, some drugs cannot be given. When available, data on excretion are listed as percentage urinary excretion. Many drugs are excreted unchanged (chemically identical to drug administered) by the kidney (e.g., digoxin).

Therapeutic Serum Levels

This term refers to the concentration of the drug in the serum at which its therapeutic action is manifested. Ideally, the optimal concentration should not be exceeded and should be maintained for prolonged periods of time. In practice, the administration of conventional dosage forms results intermittently in drug concentrations that sometimes exceed the minimal or optimal dosage levels and that sometimes fall below it. Desired serum levels of commonly used drugs are found on the inside back cover of this text.

Consideration of therapeutic serum levels is particularly important for:

1. Certain antibiotics, because growth of most microorganisms is only inhibited above certain serum drug levels (the minimal inhibitory concentration, or MIC).
2. Drugs in which there is a narrow margin between a therapeutic effect and a toxic effect (e.g., digitalis, phenytoin).

Bioavailability

The bioavailability of a drug measures the concentration of the pharmacologically active substance at the target site and/or in the serum.

Bioavailability is a function of:

The drug itself.

The metabolism of the patient.

The rate at which the drug is liberated from its dosage form or from storage in the body proper. For example, many drugs bind to serum protein (plasma albumin in particular), from which they are released gradually; other drugs are stored in specific organs, in adipose tissue (lipid-soluble drugs, such as thiopental), and even in bone (tetracyclines).

Some of these factors are of such magnitude that substitution of one preparation of a specific drug for another can affect bioavailability. For example, the rate of disintegration of tablets of the same drug made by different manufacturers may be significantly different.

A drug is said not to be bioavailable if, or to the extent that, it is:

Bound to protein or to any other substance that renders the drug permanently or temporarily inactive.

Not released from its dosage form or site of administration.

Partially or totally degraded.

Protein binding plays a major role in drug interactions, because when two drugs are administered concomitantly, one drug (drug A) might have a greater affinity for protein than drug B. This action increases the concentration (bioavailability) of drug B, sometimes producing an increase in the duration and/or intensity of effect, necessitating a dosage adjustment.

Bioavailability is taken into account by the manufacturer in establishing dosage levels. To attain the desired therapeutic dosage levels, drugs that bind tightly to serum protein and are released slowly, for example, are given at a higher concentration and less frequently than is a drug that is immediately available and that is degraded or excreted rapidly.

Therapeutic Drug-Delivery Systems

The drug serum concentration that results from drugs administered as conventional preparations (tablets, injections) undergoes wide fluctuations, especially when the pharmacologic agent is metabolized and/or excreted rapidly (i.e., has a short $t^{1/2}$). For drugs with a short $t^{1/2}$, excessively high doses must be given and/or a high frequency of administration must be used to maintain a drug blood concentration at or above the effective therapeutic level. Administration of high levels of medication is undesirable, however, because most drugs have toxic and/or unpleasant side effects at higher dosages. Unfortunately, patients sometimes fail to comply with orders for repeated drug administration (e.g., several times per day for a period of time). However, constant blood levels of drugs may be desired to prevent the occurrence of disease symptoms (e.g., angina, motion sickness).

This difficulty has been partially overcome with the development of sustained-release preparations in which the drug is released in stages. Such preparations often consist of hundreds of small pellets coated with materials that dissolve at different rates, or the drug is incorporated into tablets with varying layers, each layer disintegrating at a different time after oral administration. The development of drugs with long half-lives, which by their nature have to be administered less frequently, may be possible also.

Another mechanism to ensure that adequate therapeutic serum levels are maintained is administration via IV drip. This method is used, for example, when antibiotics are administered to combat life-threatening infections.

A similar principle underlies the therapeutic systems that deliver a drug continuously for a period of hours, weeks, or even months. Small drug reservoirs, enclosed in semipermeable membranes, are inserted into or applied near the target site. Drug diffuses out of these systems into the body; the rate can be adjusted ideally so that input equals output (rate of excretion). Such therapeutic systems are especially suitable for drugs that have a short $t^{1/2}$ and are required at low doses or for maintaining constant blood levels of drugs. Examples of such systems include:

Estraderm, which delivers estradiol for approximately 3 days

Lacrisert, which delivers a moisturizing agent for dry eye syndrome

Ocusert, which delivers pilocarpine into the conjunctival sac for 1 week

Deponit, Nitrocine, Nitrodisc, Nitro-Dur, Transderm-Nitro, all of which deliver nitroglycerin for 24 hr

Progestasert, which delivers progesterone from an intrauterine device (IUD) for about 1 year

Transderm-Scop, which delivers scopolamine for 3 days

For details, see individual agents.

Biotechnology

Techniques are currently available to develop drugs using concepts of molecular biology. Through genetic engineering (e.g., recombinant DNA), a number of drugs have been marketed, including human insulin, interferon alpha, growth hormone, and alteplase (a thrombolytic agent).

The impact of such technology is just beginning to be appreciated. It is now possible to design drugs for specific diseases and to synthesize naturally occurring human hormones (e.g., insulin). Such processes allow for the production of pure products; for example, genetically engineered human insulin is indistinguishable from naturally occurring insulin, thus virtually eliminating the chance of side effects or tolerance.

At the present time all of the drugs developed through genetic engineering must be injected. Thus, it is becoming increasingly important for patients to know how to administer these drugs. Also, it is likely that new methods for administration of drugs will be developed (e.g., nasal sprays, use of antibodies).

Drug Testing

Before a drug can be marketed in the United States, extensive testing is necessary, in both animals and humans, to ensure safety and effectiveness. The Food and Drug Administration (FDA) is the federal agency charged with regulating the testing, marketing, and advertising of drugs in this country.

Testing of a potentially new drug always begins in animals. However, animal studies cannot always predict what effects human patients will manifest. Thus, initial drug testing in humans does carry a certain amount of risk. To protect human subjects in such studies, institutional review boards (IRB) and the informed consent form have been established.

The IRB functions as a body to review proposed drug studies in humans to determine if the studies are sound ethically, medically, and scientifically. Informed consent must be obtained from all humans participating in drug studies. The consent form details, in language easy to understand, the nature of the study; the type of drug to be used; and any potential benefits, risks, or side effects. Subjects should be told that participation is voluntary and that they may withdraw from the study at any time. Opportunities should be made available for subjects to ask questions.

Drug development in humans usually occurs in the following phases:

1. **Phase I (Clinical Pharmacology).** These studies are conducted usually in healthy males between the ages of 18 and 45 years (women who are in their childbearing years are not used, because the drug may affect the fetus if the woman becomes pregnant). The purpose of Phase I studies is to determine the dose level at which symptoms of toxicity occur.
2. **Phase II (Clinical Investigation).** In these studies, the drug is administered to patients with the specific condition for which the drug is intended. The goal is to determine effectiveness of the drug and to establish the optimum dose and dose range.

3. **Phase III (Clinical Trials).** If serious side effects have not occurred during Phase II and if the optimum dose range has been established, the drug is administered to large numbers of patients (hundreds to thousands). The goal is to make sure the drug is effective and to uncover any side effects that were not discovered in Phases I and II.

4. **Phase IV (Postmarketing Studies).** Such studies are undertaken for continuing evaluation of the drug, especially in patients who are usually excluded from Phases II and III (e.g., geriatric patients, children, and women of childbearing age). Also, these studies continue to monitor for the occurrence and frequency of side effects.

CHAPTER THREE

Side Effects and Drug Toxicity

DRUG ALLERGIES

Allergic responses to drugs occur in some patients and not in others. A drug allergy is an adverse response to a drug resulting from previous exposure to that drug or one closely related to it. Drug allergy is exhibited only after a second or subsequent exposure to the drug.

Allergic reactions to drugs differ from drug toxicity in the following ways: (1) the allergic reaction occurs in only a fraction of the population, whereas drug toxicity will occur in all individuals if the dose is high enough; (2) the allergic response is unusual in that a small amount of an otherwise safe dose causes a severe reaction; (3) with allergy, the reaction is *different* from the usual pharmacologic effect of the drug; and (4) for an allergic reaction to occur, the patient must have had a previous exposure to that drug or one closely related to it.

The allergic response may be an *immediate reaction* involving antigen (in this case, the drug or part thereof) and antibody, resulting in the release of histamine. In mild cases the reaction is limited to urticaria, wheals, and itching of the skin. In severe cases, there is an *anaphylactic reaction* characterized by circulatory collapse or asphyxia due to swelling of the larynx and occlusion of the bronchial passages. Many patients are allergic to penicillin, for example. The allergic response may be a *delayed reaction,* occurring several days or even weeks after the drug has been administered. Delayed reactions are characterized by drug fever, swelling of the joints, and reactions involving the blood-forming organs and the kidneys.

Treatment of an anaphylactic reaction may include administration of epinephrine, oxygen, antihistamines, and corticosteroids.

DRUG IDIOSYNCRASIES

Idiosyncratic reactions are defined as those that occur in patients who have a genetically determined abnormal response to a drug. The response may be excessive or unusual. For example, succinylcholine, a muscle relaxant, usually is broken down rapidly by enzymes in the plasma and liver so that the effects of the drug last for only a few minutes. However, in a few patients, a normal dose of succinylcholine produces profound skeletal muscle relaxation and suppression of respiration that may last several hours. Such patients have a genetic defect that produces unusual enzymes, and succinylcholine is not broken down.

DRUG HYPERSENSITIVITY

Drug hypersensitivity occurs when the patient shows extreme sensitivity to an effect of the drug. The response is the usual pharmacologic effect; however, the effect is intense or exaggerated. A simple decrease in the dose may be sufficient to eliminate this type of adverse effect of a drug.

DRUG TOXICITY

Excess dosage of a drug, either accidental or intentional, results in an exaggerated response to that drug. Drug toxicity may be severe and may lead to respiratory depression, cardiovascular collapse, and/or death if the drug is not withdrawn and adequate treatment instituted.

A relative overdose of a drug may be seen in patients who for some reason do not metabolize or excrete a particular drug rapidly enough or who are particularly sensitive to the effects of a drug due to hypersensitivity or idiosyncrasy (see above). This type of overdosage usually can be controlled by reducing the dose or by increasing the interval between doses of the drug.

Note: Elderly or debilitated patients often require smaller doses of drugs.

The nurse is responsible for preventing accidents by teaching the care and storage of drugs, for observing and reporting signs of toxicity, and for providing first aid and emergency drugs and equipment needed for treatment while assisting the physician. A local poison control number should be posted at every nursing station (see Appendix 5, Certified Poison Control Centers). Regardless of whether the poisoning is due to an attempted overdose or is accidental, the family members need emotional support at this time.

GENERAL SIDE EFFECTS

An unpleasant, unwanted, and/or bothersome reaction to a drug is termed a side effect. In some cases, the side effect is predictable and can occur in a large number of patients. For example, an antihistamine administered to reduce symptoms of allergy may cause drowsiness. On the other hand, other side effects are not predictable in all cases and do not occur in a significant number of patients (although such side effects may be quite serious). For example, only a few patients may develop a skin rash from taking thiazide diuretics.

Dermatologic Reactions: The skin is frequently involved in drug reactions. Although all drugs may cause dermatologic disturbances in some patients, certain pharmacologic agents are more prone to do so than others (i.e., penicillin, sulfonamides, bromides, iodides, arsenic, gold, quinine, thiazides, and antimalarials).

The dermatologic manifestations may range from pruritus and mild urticaria to all types of exanthematous eruptions, maculopapular rash, angioedema, pustular eruptions, granulomas, erythema nodosum, photosensitivity reactions, and alopecia.

In general, the administration of a drug is discontinued when the patient manifests even a mild skin reaction. The most serious types of reactions are extensive urticaria, angioedema, and those accompanied by systemic manifestations.

Some of the more serious, drug-induced skin reactions are detailed below.

1. **Exfoliative Dermatitis.** An itchy, scaling of the skin, frequently accompanied by loss of hair and nails. Initial symptoms are a patchy or erythematous eruption accompanied by fever and malaise. Gastrointestinal symptoms are noted occasionally and are possibly caused by a similar lesion of the GI epithelium. Skin color changes from pink to dark red. The characteristic flaking begins after about 1 week. The skin remains smooth and red. New scales form as the old ones peel off. Relapses occur frequently, and death occurs occasionally as a result of secondary infection.

2. **Erythema Multiforme.** An acute or subacute eruption of the skin characterized by macules, papules, wheals, vesicles, and sometimes bullae. The lesions involve mostly the distal portions of the extremities, the face, and the mucous membranes. The condition is accompanied often by generalized malaise, arthralgia, and fever. The condition may recur, and each attack usually lasts 2 to 3 weeks. The most serious type of erythema multiforme is the *Stevens-Johnson syndrome*. The bullous, blistery rash extends to the mucosa of the mouth, pharynx, and anogenital region. The syndrome is accompanied by high fever, severe headache, stomatitis, conjunctivitis, rhinitis, urethritis, and balanitis. It is often fatal, so early detection and treatment is most important.

3. **Photosensitivity.** A wide variety of unusual skin reactions characterized by dermatitis, urticaria, erythema multiforme-like lesions, and thickened and scaling patches may occur in some patients after a few minutes of exposure to sunlight.

Blood Dyscrasias: The bone marrow of certain patients is particularly sensitive to drugs. This may result in the insufficient production of platelets, white blood cells, or red blood cells.

In principle, all drugs may cause blood dyscrasias in a particularly susceptible patient, but drugs such as the antineoplastics, certain antibiotics (including chloramphenicol), and phenylbutazone do so more frequently.

Patients who receive a drug that may cause bone marrow depression are monitored closely by frequent blood counts and for early signs and symptoms of infection.

Some of the frequently observed blood dyscrasias are listed below.

1. **Agranulocytosis.** A complete absence of granulocytes associated with a marked reduction in circulating leukocytes is the most common blood dyscrasia to occur as a side effect of drug therapy. Early clinical signs are symptoms of infection, such as a sore throat, skin rash, fever, or jaundice.

2. **Aplastic Anemia.** When the bone marrow is damaged and blood-forming cells are replaced by fatty tissue, the result is pancytopenia, a reduction in all formed elements of blood. Aplastic anemia is usually fatal. Symptoms include anemia, leukopenia, and thrombocytopenia.

3. **Hemolytic Anemia.** Circulating red blood cells are destroyed either because of an antigen-antibody reaction or when a patient sensitive to certain chemicals has an idiosyncratic reaction. For instance, some black persons or persons originating in certain regions of the Mediterranean

inherit a sex-linked enzyme deficiency (glucose 6-phosphate dehydrogenase deficiency) that makes their red blood cells particularly sensitive to hemolysis by certain "oxidizing" drugs (including aspirin). Ingestion of these agents may cause acute intravascular hemolysis marked by hematuria. Treatment involves withdrawal of drug.

4. **Thrombocytopenia.** Platelet deficiency may result from destruction of the circulating platelets by pharmacologic agents or by depression of the platelet-forming elements of the bone marrow. The latter is the more serious manifestation. Severe thrombocytopenia is characterized by purpura followed by hemorrhage.

Hepatotoxicity (Liver Damage):

1. **Biliary Obstruction.** Some drugs affect the lining of the bile channels, causing them to narrow. Bile may back up into the bloodstream, and the patient appears jaundiced.
2. **Hepatic Necrosis.** Drug-induced damage of liver cells is characterized by nausea, vomiting, and abdominal pain followed by jaundice.

Nephrotoxicity (Kidney Damage): Drug-induced degeneration of renal tubules, which may interfere with further excretion of the drug, results in increased drug toxicity. Nephrotoxicity is characterized by hematuria, anuria, urinary casts, edema, proteinuria, and uremia.

Ototoxicity (Ear Damage): This results in damage to the vestibular and/or auditory portion of the eighth cranial nerve.

1. **Vestibular Damage.** Characterized by vertigo (sensation of turning and falling) and nystagmus (rapid, rhythmic, side-to-side movement of the eyeballs).
2. **Auditory Damage.** Characterized by tinnitus (ringing in the ears or a roaring sound) and progressive hearing loss. This effect may be caused by certain antibiotics (kanamycin, neomycin) and diuretics (ethacrynic acid, furosemide).

CNS Toxicity: Such toxicity is characterized by poor motor coordination, loss of judgment, depression of consciousness, or overstimulation including convulsions. Symptoms of depression are most likely to occur with barbiturates, other sedative-hypnotics, antianxiety agents, and alcohol.

Certain drugs also interfere with the transmission of nerve impulses at the myoneural junction, which causes muscle weakness and reduced ankle and knee reflexes. Gradually this untoward reaction can lead to apnea and cardiac arrest.

Tardive dyskinesia, characterized by the impairment of the power of voluntary movement resulting in fragmentary or incomplete movements, has been observed after long-term administration of antipsychotic drugs.

GI Disturbances: Drug-induced nausea, abdominal pain, diarrhea, and vomiting may result from either local irritation or systemic effects.

Drug Dependence: Although not exactly a side effect, drug dependence is one of the problems associated with the administration of drugs.

The term "drug dependence" was developed to encompass both *psychologic (psychic) dependence*— that is, a drive or craving to take the drug for relief of tensions or discomfort or for pleasure or recreation—and *physical dependence,* characterized by the appearance of physical symptoms when the administration of the drug is discontinued.

1. **Psychological Dependence.** In *mild dependence,* a person is accustomed to taking a drug that gives him/her a sense of well-being—for example, caffeine in coffee or nicotine in cigarettes. Such a person is said to be habituated and will not readily give up the drug. Although

uneasy when deprived of the drug, the habituated person can give up the drug usually without receiving professional help. In *severe dependence* the person craves the feeling that the drug provides and will use compulsive efforts to obtain the drug (e.g., heroin, cocaine, or amphetamines). Severe psychologic dependence on drugs seems to occur in people who, once having experienced a feeling from a drug that is particularly satisfying, will continue to compulsively seek out the drug. Nurses should note patients who are asking for drugs more frequently than most patients with similar conditions. The names of such patients should be brought to the attention of the physician, so that their needs may be evaluated more closely.

2. **Physical Dependence.** The continued ingestion of certain drugs (narcotics and depressants) results in an alteration in the body so that the drug is now required for the individual to function "normally." This is referred to as physical dependence. Discontinuation of a drug on which the patient is physically dependent may lead to *withdrawal symptoms*. Symptoms may vary with the particular drug. The withdrawal from narcotics results in increased autonomic nervous system activity and increased CNS excitability (see general statement on *Narcotic Analgesics,* Chapter 37). Withdrawal from depressants (barbiturates, sedative-hypnotics, antianxiety agents) also results in increased excitability of certain regions of the CNS, notably those controlling motor and mental functions. The patient becomes tremulous and may suffer grand mal seizures, confusion, disorientation, and psychotic reactions.

Sexual Dysfunction: Sexual function may be altered for a time by medication (e.g., tricyclic antidepressants). A change in libido or development of impotence is not necessarily permanent. Adjustment in dosage or substitution of one drug for another may relieve sexual dysfunction.

CHAPTER FOUR

Drug Interactions: General Considerations and Nursing Considerations

4

DRUG-DRUG INTERACTIONS

Because many patients now receive more than one pharmacologic agent, drug interactions are a potentially major clinical problem. Indeed, in addition to having their intended, specific therapeutic effect, drugs may also influence other physiologic systems. The likelihood is high that two concomitantly administered agents influence some of the same pathways.

In most cases it is nevertheless possible to administer two interacting agents concurrently, provided that certain precautions, such as dosage adjustments, are taken. Moreover, drug interactions are not always adverse, and they are sometimes taken advantage of therapeutically. For example, probenecid may be administered with penicillin to decrease the excretion rate of the penicillin and, therefore, result in higher blood level of penicillin.

The study of drug interactions is rapidly becoming a complex subspecialty of pharmacology. An attempt has been made throughout the text to reduce the complex explanation of drug interactions to the simplest possible terms.

A brief review of the major mechanisms that give rise to drug interactions is included in this section. Knowledge of these mechanisms may enable the nurse to anticipate similar situations with other drug combinations.

It is important to remember that interactions apply not only to the intended therapeutic action of the drugs but also to their side effects.

Also the interactant does not have to be a prescription drug. Salicylates (aspirin) are an important interactant, as are common laxatives and constipating agents. Beverages, like alcohol, and foods, like tyramine-rich cheese, may play an important role also.

Drug interactions often require either an adjustment in dosage of one or both agents or a discontinuation of one. Common major drug interactions are described under the drug or drug class.

Drugs with Opposing Pharmacologic Effects: The therapeutic effects of either or both agents may be cancelled, decreased, or abolished. An example is the combination of pilocarpine (a cholinergic drug prescribed for glaucoma) and an anticholinergic or atropine-like drug.

The interaction is usually described as "decreased effect" in the text. Correction could involve administration of only one agent, adjustment in time of administration, or increase in dosage of one or both agents.

Drugs with Similar Pharmacologic Effects: When two drugs have similar pharmacologic effects, their combined use may result in an effect equal to or even larger than the sum of that obtained if either agent were used separately. This interaction is described as "increased effect." The terms "additive" or "potentiation" might be used also to describe this interaction. An example of this interaction is the concomitant use of agents with CNS depressant actions, such as alcohol, antianxiety agents, hypnotics, and antihistamines.

Changes in the Amount of Available Drug:

1. **Change in Absorption from the GI Tract.** The absorption of most drugs from the stomach or GI tract is pH-dependent. The concomitant use of an agent that alters the pH can change the rate of absorption or the amount of drug absorbed, and thus either increase (↑) the effect or decrease (↓) the effect of the drug.

   For example, the use of antacids that increase the pH of the stomach will result in a decrease in the absorption of aspirin, which is more rapidly absorbed at a lower pH.

   The absorption of drugs is affected also by how long drugs reside in the GI tract. Drugs that affect the motility of the GI tract also affect drug absorption. The net effect of a laxative usually is decreased absorption [decreased (↓) effect], because the drug to be absorbed in the GI tract stays there for a shorter period of time. On the other hand, constipating agents, often result in increased absorption [increased (↑) effect].

   The presence of food may affect the rate of absorption of drugs from the GI tract or the total amount of the drug absorbed. For example, the absorption of tetracyclines is inhibited in the presence of dairy products (e.g., milk, cheese), because the calcium present in such foods complexes with the drug.

2. **Alteration of Urinary Excretion.** Closely related to the rate at which drugs are absorbed from the GI tract is the rate at which drugs are eliminated in the urine or reabsorbed from the glomerular filtrate. Drugs that are eliminated more slowly because of another concomitantly administered agent stay in the body longer; thus, the effect of the drug is increased.

   Drugs that are eliminated faster (or are less reabsorbed) because of another concomitantly administered agent result in a decrease in the effect of the drug.

   As in the case of absorption from the GI tract, elimination by the kidney is pH-dependent. The pH of the urine is sometimes altered purposely by the administration of an alkalizing agent (sodium bicarbonate) or an acidifying agent (ammonium chloride). Whether a drug will be excreted faster or slower with a change in pH depends on the drug. The alkalization of the urine, for example, is sometimes undertaken for drugs like the sulfonamides. These agents are more soluble at a higher pH, and thus the possibility of crystallization in the kidney is reduced.

Displacement of Drugs from Protein-Binding Site: Several types of drugs bind to plasma protein; thus, the resulting protein-bound drug is not free to exert a pharmacologic effect.

Protein binding is considered when dosage is established so that a given amount of drug will have the desired pharmacologic effect. However, this relationship may be altered when another agent, which also binds to protein, is added to the therapy. If the attraction of drug B for the protein is greater than that of drug A, drug A will be displaced (or released) from the protein-binding site. This displacement, then, will result in a greater amount of drug A being available, and thus the effect of drug A will be increased. One such example is the coumarin-type anticoagulants, which are bound to protein but can be displaced by a variety of agents. A greater than expected amount of anticoagulant can have severe untoward effects, including fatal hemorrhages.

Changes in Drug Metabolism:

1. Most drugs are degraded in the liver by specific enzymes (drug-metabolizing enzymes). A change in the activity of an enzyme results in a change in the availability of the drug. Often such an interaction results in inhibition of the enzyme, and an increased effect of the drug is observed. However, certain drugs may stimulate the activity of enzymes involved in the breakdown of another pharmacologic agent. For example, the barbiturates appear to stimulate certain drug-metabolizing enzymes in the liver. This results in a more rapid breakdown of the drugs normally degraded by such enzymes (e.g., steroid hormones including estrogen and progesterone, and coumarin-type anticoagulants).

2. The pharmacologic mode of action of certain drugs, such as the MAO inhibitors or disulfiram, consists of inhibiting a particular enzyme. An interaction may occur when this inhibited enzyme system is called upon to degrade another drug or food product. For example, the above mechanism plays a role in the much publicized interaction of the MAO inhibitors and tyramine-rich foods, like cheese. The tyramine cannot be degraded (as usual) by MAO, because the enzyme is inhibited. Tyramine accumulates and may cause severe hypertension. Such an interaction is considered also in the treatment of alcoholics with disulfiram (Antabuse). The latter interferes with the metabolism of alcohol, leading to the accumulation of acetaldehyde, which has such unpleasant physiologic effects that the patient will refrain from alcohol ingestion while on this therapy.

Alteration of Electrolyte Levels: Drugs that promote the loss (e.g., potassium) or retention (e.g., calcium) of electrolytes may cause the heart to become particularly sensitive to the toxic effects of digitalis. Such an interaction has been noted in the concomitant use of thiazide diuretics (which cause potassium loss) and digitalis.

Alteration of GI Flora: Antibiotics and other antimicrobial agents often kill the intestinal flora that synthesize vitamin K. A decrease in the concentration of vitamin K, which is involved in blood coagulation, increases the effect of anticoagulants and may result in hemorrhage.

FOOD-DRUG INTERACTIONS

General Considerations: Although there is increasing knowledge and concern about drug interactions, the effects of food-drug interactions are not as well known. Yet, these interactions can produce dramatic effects; for example, when a food containing tyramine is ingested by a patient on MAO inhibitor therapy, a hypertensive crisis is precipitated. Food-drug interactions can be clinically less significant, as when the absorption of riboflavin is delayed by food ingestion. The mechanisms involved in drug-food interactions are most often attributable to effects on rate and amount of absorption, distribution, metabolism, and excretion. General interference mechanisms are discussed above. See Appendix 2 for specific food-drug interactions.

NURSING CONSIDERATIONS FOR MAXIMIZING THERAPEUTIC EFFECT OF DRUGS

Assessment

1. Assess patients for any ethnic considerations that may interfere with compliance to prescribed drug therapy.
2. Obtain and record a thorough nursing and medication history.
3. Document client age, height, weight, and potential for becoming pregnant.
4. Identify any potential client learning/communication problems concerning prescribed drug therapy.
5. Identify any apparent nutritional or dental problems that may preclude maximizing a client's response to drug therapy.

Interventions

1. Plan to initiate client teaching at a time when there are as few distractions/interruptions as possible.
2. Discuss with client work schedule or other factors that may interfere with taking medication at prescribed times.
3. Identify any ethnic concerns regarding medications, illness, and fluids or foods that should be taken with prescribed drugs and notify physician.

Client/Family Teaching

1. If absorption of prescribed medication is affected by food, explain that the drug should be taken on an empty stomach 1 hr before meals or 2 hr after meals, with a full glass of water.
2. Instruct which foods to include or avoid to promote the maximum therapeutic effect of medication (see Appendix 2).
3. Explain that some foods should be either incorporated into the diet or avoided, if an alkaline or acidic urine promotes or inhibits drug action (see Table 2).

4. *Food reactions in the body*—clarify that the taste of the food does not indicate whether the body will metabolize it to an acid or alkaline ash. The type of ash is determined by the mineral content of the food. Acidic foods, such as coffee or citrus juices, are corrosive because they contain organic acid. They are not metabolized to an acid ash residue and therefore are not urinary acidifiers.

5. Discuss ways by which to follow the recommended diet. Provide written instructions, including a list of foods recommended and/or restricted. Refer for nutritional counseling as needed.

6. Review the appropriate method for ingestion of prescribed medication including not to crush enteric-coated or sustained-release or long-acting medications. Teach client to chew, swallow whole, or let the medication dissolve under the tongue as indicated.

7. Instruct client to report any bothersome side effects to the physician.

DRUGS AND NUTRIENT UTILIZATION

Drugs can affect the way the body uses food by hastening the excretion of certain nutrients, hindering the absorption of nutrients, or interfering with the body's ability to convert nutrients into usable forms. These drug-food interactions lead to vitamin and mineral deficiencies, particularly in children, the elderly, the chronically ill, and those on marginal diets. Therefore, the diets of such patients should be modified to include more foods rich in vitamins and iron.

The psychologic and physical status of the client influences drug action as well. For example, malnutrition reduces the effectiveness of drugs by affecting rates of absorption and elimination of drugs, as well as tissue uptake and response. Depression reduces salivary output, causing changes in nutritional uptake and possibly altering drug action.

Table 1 lists drugs that affect utilization of nutrients; Table 2 presents a compilation of foods that are acid, alkaline, or neutral.

NURSING CONSIDERATIONS FOR MINIMIZING NUTRITIONAL DEFICIENCIES ASSOCIATED WITH DRUG THERAPY

Assessment

1. Obtain a thorough nursing and drug history.

2. *Assess:*
   - Nutritional status of patient before initiating therapy and at periodic intervals during the course of therapy.
   - Subjective and objective data presented by the client for possible negative drug effects.
   - For malabsorption syndrome and nutritional deficiencies in those clients in poor nutritional states who are on a medication regimen with the drugs and foods listed in Tables 1 and 2.

Interventions

1. Consult with physician and dietician regarding the need for diet supplementation.

Client/Family Teaching

1. Emphasize that drugs should **never** be exchanged with others who appear to have the same medical problem or diagnosis.

2. Detail and emphasize possible food-drug interactions that can occur with the medication the client is taking.

3. Explain that OTC medications should not be used before consulting the health care provider.
4. Instruct on how to practice good nutrition and find appropriate resources to ensure compliance.
5. Explain where to apply for dietary funds or services, as needed (e.g., WIC, a supplemental food program for women, infants, and children).
6. Explain that if the patient is or becomes pregnant, this information should be relayed to the physician so he/she can order only the minimum amount of drug necessary to achieve a therapeutic effect.

Table 1   Drugs That Affect Utilization of Nutrients

Drug	Effect
Alcohol	Malabsorption of folic acid and vitamin B_{12}
Antacids	Cause phosphate depletion, muscle weakness, and vitamin D deficiency
Anti-infectives	Decrease utilization of folic acid and malabsorption of vitamin B_{12}, calcium, and magnesium; decrease bacterial synthesis of vitamin K; inactivation of pyridoxine; impair transfer of amino acids
Anticonvulsants	Cause deficiencies of vitamin D, folic acid, and vitamin B_{12} by increasing the turnover rate of vitamins in the body
Antidiabetic agents (oral)	Impair absorption of vitamin B_{12}
Aspirin	Causes folate deficiency
Atropine, cortisone, digitoxin, epinephrine, and ethacrynic acid	Alter pancreatic or intestinal digestive function
Cathartics	Diminish nutrient absorption
Clofibrate	Alter taste sensation; may suppress appetite and reduce nutrient intake; malabsorption of folic acid and vitamin B_{12}, electrolytes, and sugar
Colchicine	Impairs absorption of vitamin B_{12}, fat, lactose, and electrolytes
Contraceptives (oral)	Deplete folic acid and vitamin B_6
Cycloserine	Causes folate deficiency
Diuretics and ganglionic blockers	Cause potassium depletion
Hydralazine and isoniazid	Deplete vitamin B_6 by inhibiting production of enzymes needed to convert it into a form the body can use, or by combining to form a compound that is excreted
Methotrexate	Antagonizes folic acid
Mineral oil	Hinders absorption of vitamins D, E, and K, and carotene
Neomycin	Impairs absorption of vitamin B_{12}; alters pancreatic absorption or digestive function; interferes with bile activity
Phenobarbital	Causes folate deficiency
Phenothiazine, tricyclic antidepressants	Stimulate appetite, results in increased food intake and weight gain
Surface-acting agents	Alter absorption of nutrients by affecting fat dispersion
Thorazine	Induces hypercholesterolemia

Table 2   Acid, Alkaline, and Neutral Foods

Acidifiers: Acid Ash Foods*
Dairy foods: cheeses (all types)
Eggs
Fish (including shellfish)
Fruits: cranberries, plums, and prunes
Gelatin
Macaroni: noodles, spaghetti
Mayonnaise
Meats
Nuts: Brazil nuts, peanuts, walnuts, filberts
Poultry
Vegetables: corn, lentils

Alkalizers: Alkaline Ash Foods
Dairy foods: milk, cream, buttermilk
Fruits (except cranberries, plums, prunes)
Jams, jellies, honey
Molasses
Nuts: almonds, chestnuts, coconuts
Olives
Vegetables (except corn, lentils)

Neutral Foods
Butter or margarine
Beverages: coffee, tea
Cooking oils and fats
Starches: corn, arrowroot
Sugars
Syrup
Tapioca

*Foods yielding an acid ash are urinary acidifiers; foods
yielding an alkaline ash are urinary alkalinizers.

CHAPTER FIVE

Nursing Process and Considerations for Drug Therapy

Caring is the essence of nursing and can best be expressed by the nursing process, the core of nursing practice. The nursing process is central to all nursing actions, applicable to all settings and methods of patient care. Because the nursing process is flexible, it adapts readily to many variables and any conceptual framework a nurse may use in clinical practice. An accurate and systematic application of the nursing process will increase the nurse's expertise and efficiency in assessing clients, their need for drug therapy, and evaluating the results of this therapy. The nurse's knowledge and understanding of a client's medical condition, the use of medication to improve a client's physical and/or emotional health, and determining the extent of the efficacy of this therapy are critical to appropriate nursing care of those who require medication.

Assessment, problem identification, planning, intervention, and evaluation—all components of the nursing process—are important steps in determining if clients need medication and how well they are responding to the prescribed drug therapy. Utilizing the nursing process to record data concerning a client's response to therapy will provide the information necessary to determine how well a client is responding to the prescribed therapy. Consistent adherence to the pattern of the nursing process tends to reduce the possibility of omitting an important finding in the client's overall condition.

It is important to teach clients and/or families to follow a similar format when they are expected to take responsibility for adhering to a drug regimen and accurately reporting the response to therapy.

Assessment involves collecting data systematically concerning the client's current health status. It includes interviewing clients, physically examining them, recording observations, and whenever possible, comparing the information with what is known about the client's prior condition. It includes socioeconomic factors also, because these may have an important bearing on whether a client can be expected to comply with the prescribed drug regimen and what may be essential to promoting compliance.

The nurse identifies the client's physical state, the mental state that may affect the ability to adhere to drug therapy regimens, and possible socioeconomic problems that may need to be addressed to assure the best possible therapeutic outcome. Homelessness, poverty, and lack of adequate health insurance play critical roles in how well a client can be expected to comply with therapy. Assessment should include determining ethnic beliefs concerning illness, nutrition, and drugs that may interfere with client compliance or influence client/family teaching.

Once problems have been identified, goals are set and prioritized, always with client/family input. Prescribed drug therapy is discussed with both the client and family. They are taught the purpose of the drug, signs of physical/mental improvement, and evidence of side effects that should be reported. Finally, the nurse evaluates the client to determine the outcome of the drug therapy, and then documents the results appropriately.

Nursing considerations refer to the actions, precautions, and teaching that must be considered by the nurse when administering a particular drug. The nurse is not merely a drug dispenser blindly following the physician's orders; rather, nurses are professionals who use knowledge of physiology, pathology, sociology, nursing, psychology, and pharmacology as they work with other members of the health care team for disease prevention and drug therapy. Nurses are accountable for their practice and must possess a working knowledge of the medications being dispensed to their clients.

Reports from the client, family, and other health care providers, as well as from the physician, are considered when carrying out the nursing process. Assessing and reporting to the physician both therapeutic and untoward reactions to drugs are critical and essential functions of the professional nurse. The initiation of appropriate nursing interventions significantly influences the success of drug therapy.

The following nursing considerations are related to all types of drug therapy. They will be repeated selectively in the discussion of particular drugs to reinforce the importance of specific nursing interventions related to a classification of drugs or to an individual drug.

GENERAL NURSING CONSIDERATIONS FOR DRUG THERAPY

1. Check the medication card or medication administration record with the physician's written order for client's name, date of order, drug dosage, route, time of administration, and diet. Verify that the order is not outdated by reviewing hospital policy (automatic stop orders).

2. Check whether the client is scheduled for any diagnostic procedures that contraindicate administration of medications (e.g., GI series, FBS). Withhold medication and check with physician if indicated.

3. Check *The Nurse's Drug Handbook* for physiologic action, therapeutic use, side effects, contraindications, drug interactions, nursing considerations, and recommended dosage for those drugs not already known. Use other references such as the *Facts and Comparisons, PDR,* or a formulary service as well as accompanying drug literature if necessary. Consult with the pharmacist and request the drug monograph if the drug is not listed in reference books or is being administered for research purposes.

4. Select the specific drug ordered by the physician. Substitutes are neither acceptable nor legal. Note contraindications to interchange of brands because of potential bioavailability differences among products (e.g., phenytoin sodium).

5. Check that the dosage of the drug is within normal limits. If the dosage is not within normal limits, withhold the drug and discuss the safety of the dosage prescribed with the physician. Request written clarification and administration guidelines if the dosage is not within normal limits. Note also the height, weight, and age of the client. Elderly clients often react differently to standard drug dosages, therefore requiring less medication than other patients.

6. If the client is female and sexually active, there may be a possibility of pregnancy. Not only does pregnancy often alter the effectiveness of some drugs, but because most drugs cross the placental barrier, there is potential for harm to fetal development.

7. Prepare the specific dose ordered by the physician. If the strength of the solution or tablet on hand is not suitable for exact measurement, check with the pharmacist about the availability of another strength. If a more appropriate strength is not available, notify the physician, who may adjust the dosage so that medication can be measured specifically for proper administration.

8. Unless contraindicated, soluble tablets may be crushed and dissolved in a small amount of fluid for clients who are unable to swallow tablets. Alternatively, an elixir may be provided by the pharmacy. Syrups and elixirs should not be given routinely to diabetic patients without physician approval, due to the high sugar alcohol content in these preparations. Tablets may be crushed and administered with a small amount (one teaspoonful) of strained fruit unless contraindicated. Enteric-coated and sustained-released medications should *not* be crushed.

5

9. When preparing and administering drugs, continually assess the client's name, age, sex, ethnic background, religious preferences, diet, allergies, medical history, medical diagnosis, and nursing diagnosis.

10. Ascertain that appropriate diagnostic and baseline tests have been completed before initiating therapy. Review the results of these tests and report any abnormalities.

11. Before drug administration, identify the client by name. If the client is hospitalized or is in an emergency room or similar facility where (name) arm bands are used, the name band should be checked as well.

12. Assess the client's emotional and physical state to determine his/her ability to receive the medication by the prescribed route. If the client (e.g., a child) cannot or will not tolerate the drug by the route indicated, withhold the drug and consult with the physician, who may reduce the dosage, withdraw the drug, change the route of administration, or order another drug. Do not omit therapy unless the physician concurs.

13. Take into consideration laboratory test interferences when selecting a method of testing and when using test results as a guide for administration of medication, for example, urine versus blood (finger sticks) for glucose determinations.

14. Consider the known pharmacokinetics (e.g., absorption, distribution, metabolism, and excretion) of a drug to maximize its therapeutic effect.

15. Administer drugs as close to the designated time as possible. The recommended limits are one-half hour before or one-half hour after the designated time. Drugs ordered a.c. should usually be given 20 min before the meal. Schedule drugs and administer them at times that will maximize their therapeutic effectiveness while minimizing their side effects (e.g., administer diuretics in the morning so that diuresis will be completed before bedtime).

16. Chart fluids taken with drugs if intake and output are being monitored. Provide only liquids allowed on the diet. If working with clients who retain fluids and are being treated at home, teach them or family members to monitor fluid intake and output. Instruct them to weigh themselves daily at the same time (generally before breakfast), wearing the same type of clothing, and to record that weight. This record should be brought to the physician's office or to the clinic when patients come for a follow-up visit. If clients are seen at home or if the nurse is checking patients who reside in retirement/nursing homes, such records should be requested. Also, teach clients to report any symptoms associated with fluid retention, such as increased shortness of breath or swelling of the ankles.

17. Remain with the client until oral drugs have been swallowed.

18. Use your knowledge of desired effects, undesired effects, and drug interactions to assess for positive and negative results. Document and report these observations. Side effects may necessitate withholding the drug or initiating emergency action.

19. Chart the administration of drug and related assessments immediately after administration (or if drug is withheld) to prevent duplication and errors resulting from omissions in communication.

20. After consultation with other members of the health team, the nurse or pharmacist should teach the client and the family the techniques and provide information necessary for successful administration of drugs in the institution or at home. This teaching is essential to promote drug compliance.

21. Many clients have difficulty with vision, hearing, and mobility. Innovative methods to assist them with medication administration may help them to maintain their desired level of independence (e.g., preset insulin syringes; a poster identifying the medication to be taken, including the amount, frequency and route as well as the medication itself; easy-open containers; medications that require less frequent administration, such as sustained-release or long-acting preparations).

22. Understand that ethnic background may alter a client's attitudes and values toward drug therapy and illness and ultimately affect compliance with prescribed regimens.

23. Identify your own attitudes, feelings, inhibitions, and perceptions toward drugs and drug therapy, especially in the areas of pain management and drug dependency.

CHAPTER SIX

Nursing Considerations for the Administration of Medications by Different Routes

The following are general safety precautions that the nurse should observe for the preparation and storage of medications.

GENERAL RULES

1. Double-check all mathematical calculations for preparing and administering medications. Review calculations and verify dosage of highly toxic drugs with another registered professional nurse.

2. Check medication name, dosage, and route of administration with physician's order.

3. Work with adequate lighting.

4. Be attentive; discourage interruptions.

5. Check labels three times: when taking medication from storage; when preparing medication; and when replacing medication in storage.

6. Check expiration date; discard medication if expiration date has passed.

7. Do not use discolored medication or medication with unexpected precipitate unless specifically directed otherwise (e.g., directions for administration may indicate that for a certain medication a change in color does not interfere with the safety of the drug).

8. Never leave medicine cabinets and cart unlocked or medications unattended.

9. At the end of every shift, complete a count of the controlled substances with a professional registered nurse who is starting a tour of duty, as per institutional policy.

10. When working with clients on an outpatient or clinic basis, check the medications they are taking, and if there is a question regarding those medications, consult with the pharmacy filling the prescriptions and/or the physician.

11. When working with elderly patients, determine whether they are taking antacids or other drugs that may reduce the effective absorption of drugs being administered orally.

12. Administer only those medications that you have prepared personally. You are legally liable for all medications you administer.

13. Store drugs as recommended (e.g., tablets should be kept dry and protected from light, some reconstituted injectables should be refrigerated). Medications should be stored at temperatures recommended.

14. Return all containers with damaged labels to pharmacy.

Oral Medications:

1. Hold the medicine cup at eye level to pour medication. The meniscus (the lower curve of the liquid) should be at the calibration line indicating the proper dosage.

2. Pour oral liquids from the bottle on the opposite side from the label.

3. Wipe the bottle after pouring a liquid.

4. Pour tablets or capsules into the cap of the bottle and then empty the cap into the medication cup. Tablets or capsules are not to be poured into the nurse's hand.

5. If giving medications to hospitalized clients, stay with them to assure that the medication has been swallowed. If working with a senile person, be sure to check under the tongue and sides of the mouth to be certain they have swallowed the oral medication.

6. The elderly often have dry oral mucous membranes. Offer fluids before administering tablets or capsules to prevent them from sticking to the sides of the mouth. Also, offer ample fluids after medication administration. Clients who wear dentures may not be aware of the presence of medication in the mouth. Inspect the mouth to ensure all medication has been swallowed.

7. Once poured, do not return medications to the storage container.

Parenteral Medications:

1. Use sterile equipment and sterile technique to prepare parenteral medications.

2. Use recommended diluent for parenteral medications; follow directions for proper concentration and rate of administration of the medication.

3. Discard needles and syringes in appropriate containers; follow specific institutional guidelines for disposal.

4. Discard open ampules with unused portions of medication in designated containers.

THE FIVE RIGHTS OF MEDICATION ADMINISTRATION

1. The RIGHT drug
2. The RIGHT dose
3. The RIGHT patient

4. The RIGHT route
5. The RIGHT time

ADMINISTRATION BY ORAL ROUTE

1. Administer irritating drugs with meals or snacks to minimize their effect on the gastric mucosa, unless contraindicated.
2. If food interferes with the absorption of the drug, or if digestive enzymes destroy a significant portion of the medication, administer between meals or on an empty stomach. (See Appendix 2 for Food-Drug Interactions.)
3. Do not attempt to administer oral medications to a comatose person.
4. If the client is vomiting, withhold medication and report to physician. The client cannot properly absorb what cannot be tolerated.

Tablets/Capsules:

1. Unless a tablet is scored, it should never be broken to adjust dosage. Breaking may cause incorrect dosage, GI irritation, or destruction of drug in an incompatible pH. *Scored tablets* may be broken with a file.
2. *Time-release capsules and enteric-coated tablets* should not be tampered with in any way. Instruct the client to swallow whole and not to chew, crush, or break open.
3. *Sublingual tablets* are to be placed underneath the tongue. Instruct the client not to swallow or chew such tablets and not to drink water, all of which will interfere with the effectiveness of the medication. The medication should be left in place until completely dissolved.
4. *Buccal tablets* should be placed between gum and cheek (next to upper molar). Instruct the client to avoid disturbing tablet until completely dissolved to ensure absorption. Avoid food and liquids until medication is completely dissolved.

Liquids:

1. **Emulsions.** May be diluted with water.
2. **Suspensions.** Shake well until there is no apparent solid material.
3. **Elixirs.** Do not dilute. Diluent may cause precipitation of drug.
4. **Salty solutions.** Unless contraindicated because of client's diet, mix with water or fruit juice to improve taste.

ADMINISTRATION BY NASOGASTRIC TUBE

GENERAL NURSING CONSIDERATIONS

Interventions

1. Place adult client in a sitting position for administration.
2. Position an unconscious client or an infant on the left side, with head of bed in semi-Fowler's position, for administration of medication.

3. *Check for correct placement of tube before initiating administration of medication.*
   - Auscultate for bowel sounds in all four quadrants of the abdomen.
   - Listen to distal end of tube. Normally, no noise should be heard. Remember to turn off or disconnect the gomco or suction apparatus. Place distal end of tube in a glass of water. A few bubbles may occur as the gas in the stomach is released. *Do not administer* medication if bubbles occur with respirations, as this may indicate placement of the tube in the lung.
   - Attempt to withdraw a few mL of fluid with a catheter tip syringe from the distal end of the tube. *Do not administer* if there is an absence of fluid, because this may indicate displacement.
   - Inject 5–10 mL of air or sterile water for an adult (0.5 mL for an infant) into the distal end of the tube and listen over the epigastric area with a stethoscope for a "swooshing" or popping sound, indicating placement in the stomach.
   - If tube is radiolucent and placement cannot be confirmed, request an x-ray to validate placement.
4. *Administration:* Prevent excessive air from entering the stomach by maintaining a flow of fluid from initiation to completion of therapy.
   - Hold or position the tube at a level slightly above the client's nose to prevent reflux.
   - Pour 10–20 mL water into the catheter tip syringe at the distal end of the tubing and permit the fluid to flow in by gravity.
   - Before the syringe is empty, pinch off the tubing and add the medication via the syringe.
   - As the medication is about to flow completely out of the syringe, pinch off the tubing and add 10–20 mL water to ensure that all the medication has reached the stomach; maintain patency of nasogastric tube.
5. After completing administration of medication:
   - Clamp nasogastric tube and remove the attached syringe.
   - Assess for gastric distress demonstrated particularly by distention and regurgitation.
   - Record fluids administered via nasogastric tube.
   - Do not administer enteric-coated or sustained-release tablets through a nasogastric tube, because crushing these tablets destroys their intended therapeutic effect.
6. Cold solutions cause abdominal cramping. Therefore, unless otherwise indicated, bring solutions to room temperature before administering.
7. Avoid oily medications because they may adhere to the tubing and not mix adequately with the irrigating solution.
8. Small-bore feeding tubes, such as the Keyo, do not accommodate crushed medications well. They obstruct easily and should be reserved only for elixirs or solutions. Some of the newer small-bore feeding tubes now have auxiliary medication ports and larger-end exit ports and should facilitate the administration of medications. A syringe smaller than 30 cc should not be used to attempt to dislodge plugs in small-bore feeding tubes. The increased pressure (psi) exerted by small syringes may rupture these tubes.

ADMINISTRATION BY GASTROSTOMY

See also administration guidelines for nasogastric tube.

GENERAL NURSING CONSIDERATIONS

Interventions

1. Select a Fowler's or semi-Fowler's position for nasogastric and gastrostomy tube feedings and

maintain for at least 30 min to aid digestion. This position also facilitates absorption of medications.

2. Determine tube patency by injecting 10 cc air and auscultating abdomen for "swooshing" sound. Also, aspirate for gastric contents.

3. If the clients seem unable to tolerate this position, then place them on their right side with the head of the bed above stomach level. This will help prevent regurgitation yet will facilitate gastric emptying.

4. Position the client on the *left* side with the head of the bed elevated above stomach level for medications such as antacids that should remain in the stomach as long as possible. This position will delay gastric emptying.

5. Assess site around the tube for evidence of leakage of fluids, erythema, and/or skin breakdown and document findings.

6. Administer medications following the instructions for administration by nasogastric tube.

7. When teaching clients self-administration of medication or feedings by nasogastric or gastrostomy tube, utilize a return demonstration teaching format.

8. Assist the client to become comfortable with the altered body image. Your understanding and acceptance may enhance this process.

9. Instructional aids, such as a mirror, may be helpful as the client initially attempts nasogastric self-medication administration.

ADMINISTRATION BY INHALATION

NURSING CONSIDERATIONS FOR ALL METHODS OF ADMINISTRATION BY INHALATION

Assessment

1. Assess the patient both physically and mentally prior to initiating therapy.

Interventions

1. Administer only one medication at a time through a nebulizer, unless specifically ordered otherwise. Several drugs used together may cause undesirable reactions, or they may inactivate each other.

2. Measure medication precisely with a syringe. Dilute medication as ordered and place in nebulizer. For home administration, ascertain that the patient has equipment necessary for preparation of medication and is able to measure accurately. Single-dose, premixed vials may be most useful if available and economically feasible.

3. Seat client comfortably or place in semi-Fowler's position to permit greater diaphragmatic expansion.

4. Discuss the purpose of inhalation therapy with the client.

Client/Family Teaching

1. Teach client how to assemble, disassemble, and clean equipment.

2. Emphasize the importance of cleaning the mouthpiece and nebulizer after each administration.

Any medication left in the nebulizer from the previous treatment should be discarded. Other tubing is to be cleaned each day, as directed.

3. Provide printed instructions for medication treatments and the appropriate steps and methods for cleaning and care of all equipment. Question clients to ensure they can read what is printed and fully understand the instructions.

4. Instruct client and/or designated other to monitor blood pressure and pulse and maintain a written record of these values and to bring this record on each subsequent visit.

Evaluation

1. Have the client do a return demonstration of the procedure to ensure that it is done correctly.
2. Review client record of pulse and blood pressure recordings.

ADDITIONAL NURSING CONSIDERATIONS FOR INHALATION THERAPY BY NEBULIZATION

Types of Systems

1. Commercial metered-dose inhalers (MDI), a self-contained system.
2. Hand nebulizers filled with diluted medication; these include mini-nebulizer or maxi-mist, high flow nebulizers (HFN), etc. These nebulizers are connected by tubing to a source of compressed air or oxygen.
3. Side-stream nebulizers, which include intermittent positive-pressure breathing (IPPB).

Interventions

1. *Test equipment* before initiating therapy.
2. Place prescribed medication in nebulizer.
3. Turn on either compressed air or oxygen as ordered. If the equipment is working properly, a fine mist will be seen leaving the nebulizer.

Client/Family Teaching

1. Teach client/family self-administration of medication by **nebulization,** using the following guidelines:
   - Place prescribed medication in nebulizer cup.
   - First exhale slowly through pursed lips.
   - Position nebulizer in mouth; close lips around the mouthpiece.
   - Take a deep breath through the mouth.
   - Hold breath for 3–4 sec at full inspiration.
   - Exhale slowly through pursed lips to create more pressure in the air passages, which will carry medication through the bronchial tree.
   - Repeat cycle for the number of times ordered to use medication in metered-dose nebulizer, or until all the medication in the misting nebulizer has been dispensed. Written instructions for particular medications and administration techniques should be given to clients. Encourage them to refer to these guidelines as needed.
   - Many medications leave a terrible taste and bad breath following treatment. A rinse or gargle with saline or mouthwash will clear the mouth and throat of medication after the treatment is completed.
   - Warm water should be utilized to rinse out the nebulizer and mouthpiece after each treatment.

2. Teach client/family how to use **metered-dose hand nebulizers** by generally following these guidelines:
   - Shake canister well and remove cap before initiating therapy.
   - Exhale fully and then place mouthpiece into mouth aimed toward the back of the throat. The canister should remain in an upright position.
   - Take a deep breath and press down on the canister concurrently to release one dose.
   - Hold breath as long as comfortable while releasing the canister and removing the mouthpiece from the mouth. Then, exhale slowly.
   - Administer as many doses (puffs) as ordered, following these designated guidelines.
   - Once therapy is completed, remove the mouthpiece from the canister and rinse with warm water. Shake off excess water and replace mouthpiece on canister and cap to protect from dust or other contamination.
   - Refer to written instructions as needed and call health care provider with any additional questions/concerns.

ADDITIONAL NURSING CONSIDERATIONS FOR INHALATION THERAPY BY INTERMITTENT POSITIVE-PRESSURE BREATHING (IPPB)

Interventions

1. Obtain baseline blood pressure and pulse; auscultate chest and document findings.
2. Select the inspiratory flow rate ordered by medical supervision. Initial treatment is often started at 5 cm water pressure to help patient adjust to using the machine correctly; then pressure is increased gradually to the most effective level, which is usually 15–20 cm water pressure for a 15-min treatment 3–4 times a day.
3. Place medication in nebulizer cup.
4. Adjust nebulizer control to dispense medication.
5. Encourage a slow respiratory rate, diaphragmatic breathing, and prolonged expiration through pursed lips.

Client/Family Teaching

1. Instruct client to assume an upright position, which facilitates optimal lung expansion.
2. Advise client to take several deep breaths and to exhale as fully as possible to enhance absorption of medication.
3. Encourage coughing effectively several times during treatment, if clearance of secretions is the goal.
4. Administer at least 1 hr after meals to prevent nausea and vomiting or loss of appetite.
5. Wash mouthpiece or mask and nebulizer cup with warm water, dry thoroughly, and store as directed.
6. Instruct client/family to report any change in respiratory status, including color changes and consistency of secretions.

Evaluation

1. Evaluate the extent of improvement after therapy by having patient breathe after all air has been pushed out. Auscultate chest, assess respiratory rate and effort, and describe any secretions that are produced. Document all findings.

2. Observe clients while they perform therapy to ensure that the correct procedure is being followed.

ADDITIONAL NURSING CONSIDERATIONS AFTER ADMINISTRATION OF MEDICATION BY INHALATION

Interventions
1. Assist patient with postural drainage; perform chest clapping and vibrating as ordered.
2. Auscultate chest, assess respiratory rate and effort, and describe any secretions that are produced. Document all findings.
3. Have tissues and suction equipment readily available.
4. Cleanse equipment thoroughly after each use. At least once daily cleanse equipment by soaking in 1:3 solution of white vinegar and water (or other designated solution), rinsing thoroughly, and air drying, or follow protocol of agency for cleaning equipment.

Client/Family Teaching
1. Teach client/family the appropriate technique for self-administration of medication treatments at home. Provide written guidelines and instructions.
2. Instruct them to report changes in the color, amount, or consistency of secretions.
3. Review the appropriate method for care and maintenance of equipment. Provide written instructions.
4. Teach clients how to protect themselves from infections and recurrent exacerbations of their present illness.

Evaluation
1. Observe self-administration to ensure that treatment is performed correctly.
2. Evaluate the extent of improvement after therapy. Have clients exhale fully and then breathe. Auscultate their chest for any adventitious sounds and/or improvement from initial nursing assessment.
3. Assess respiratory rate and effort and note the color, amount, and consistency of secretions.

ADMINISTRATION BY ORAL IRRIGATIONS AND GARGLES

GENERAL NURSING CONSIDERATIONS
1. Throat irrigations should not be warmer than 120°F in order not to destroy or damage tissue.
2. Warn the client that gargling with full-strength antiseptic solution may destroy normal defenses of the mouth and pharynx.
3. Mouthwashes containing phenol, such as Chloraseptic, may contribute to tissue breakdown after extended use.

ADMINISTRATION BY NASAL APPLICATION

NURSING CONSIDERATIONS FOR ALL METHODS OF NASAL APPLICATION

Interventions

1. Explain goals of therapy to the client/family.
2. Have tissues readily available.
3. Use separate equipment for each client to prevent spread of infection.
4. Instruct client to blow nose gently before initiating therapy. If the client is unable to blow his/her nose, then the nasal passage may be cleared with a bulb-type aspirator.
5. After completing treatment, rinse dropper or tip of spray container (be careful not to introduce water into spray container), and dry with tissue. Wipe the tip of nasal jelly tube with a damp tissue.
6. Replace cap of container as soon as treatment is completed.
7. To prevent cross-contamination, each client should have his/her own dropper and medication container. If only one container is available, use an individual dropper for each client.

Client/Family Teaching

1. Review with the client/family the appropriate technique for nasal administration of drops, spray, or jelly. (See below.) Provide written guidelines and instructions.
2. Explain how to care for medication administration containers before and after treatments to prevent reinfection.
3. Stress the importance of taking medication treatments only as ordered, because overdosage can occur easily.
4. Review the signs and symptoms of overdosage from the prescribed therapy and instruct client to report if evident.
5. Describe the associated side effects to be expected and the side effects that necessitate immediate attention by the physician.
6. Instruct clients/family to follow printed guidelines and instructions during all applications and treatments.
7. Encourage client/family to ask questions if there are any concerns about the procedure or drugs being administered.

ADDITIONAL NURSING CONSIDERATIONS FOR ADMINISTRATION OF NOSE DROPS

Client/Family Teaching

1. Explain intended results of nose drop therapy to client.
2. Instruct client to tilt head back during administration if the sitting or standing position is preferable.
3. Instruct client lying flat in bed to tilt head over the side of the bed, or place a support under the neck so that it is hyperextended.
4. Insert dropper about $\frac{1}{3}$ inch into the nares and instill the drops. Avoid touching the external nares with the dropper, because this may cause sneezing.

5. Do not place more than 3 drops of solution into each nostril unless specifically ordered.
6. Instruct client to maintain this position for 2–5 min after administration so the medication can reach the posterior nares and be absorbed.

ADDITIONAL NURSING CONSIDERATIONS FOR ADMINISTRATION OF NASAL SPRAY

Client/Family Teaching
1. Explain the purpose of using nasal sprays and the intended results.
2. Instruct client to sit upright with head tilted slightly back for administration of spray into nares.
3. To administer, place applicator tip in nostril; cover the opposite nostril with finger pressure to prevent excessive entrance of air.
4. Instruct patient to sniff briskly as spray container is quickly and firmly squeezed.
5. (Optimally) spray once or twice into each nostril, unless otherwise indicated.
6. Allow 3–5 min for medication to be effective; then, instruct client to blow nose gently.
7. Repeat spray if symptoms necessitate and only as ordered by the physician.

ADDITIONAL NURSING CONSIDERATIONS FOR ADMINISTRATION OF NASAL JELLY
Generally, nasal medications should be administered only in the aqueous form.

Client/Family Teaching
1. Review intended goals of therapy with the client.
2. Teach client to finger place jelly (about the size of a pea) into each nostril and then to sniff it well back into nose.

Evaluation
1. Observe self-administration to ensure that the treatment is performed correctly.
2. Assess for evidence of pretreatment symptoms.

ADMINISTRATION OF EYE MEDICATIONS

NURSING CONSIDERATIONS FOR ADMINISTRATION OF EYE DROPS

Interventions
1. Instruct client to lie down or sit with head tilted back.
2. Have a separate tissue available for each eye.
3. If excessive exudate is present, wipe the lids and eyelashes clean before instillation.
4. Use an individual, squeezable plastic container or dropper for each client. If a dropper is used, draw up only the amount of solution needed for administration.
5. Instruct the client to look up toward the ceiling.
6. Hold the applicator close to the eye, but do not touch eyelids or lashes.
7. Expose the lower conjunctival sac by drawing down the skin below the eye with a gauze pad.

8. With the same hand, use a sterile cotton ball and gently press against the lacrimal duct during and for 1–2 min after instillation to prevent excessive systemic absorption of the medication as a result of draining down the lacrimal duct.
9. Place the heel of the hand administering the drops on the hand holding the gauze pad, and instill the number of drops ordered into the center of the exposed conjunctival sac. Avoid dropping medication on the cornea, as this may cause tissue damage and discomfort.
10. Instruct client to keep eye closed for 1–2 min after application to allow for absorption of medication.

Client/Family Teaching

1. Provide written instructions for client/family to follow.
2. Observe self-administration to ensure that treatment is performed correctly and as ordered.

NURSING CONSIDERATIONS FOR ADMINISTRATION OF EYE OINTMENT

Interventions

1. Instruct client to lie down or sit down with head tilted back.
2. Have a separate tissue available for each eye.
3. Expose the lower conjunctival sac as indicated above in administration of eye drops.
4. Squeeze a strip of ointment into the conjunctival pouch (inner edge of lower lid), usually 1 cm (approximately ⅓ inch), unless otherwise ordered.
5. Instruct client to close eyes for 1–2 min after application to permit the warmth of the body to melt the medication and spread medication over area to be treated.
6. A cotton ball may be used (with eyes closed) to lightly rub the lids in a circular motion, to enhance distribution of the medication.
7. Warn client that vision will probably be blurred for a few minutes after application of ointment.

Client/Family Teaching

1. Provide written instructions for client/family to follow.
2. Observe self-administration to ensure that treatment is performed correctly and as ordered.

ADMINISTRATION OF EAR DROPS

GENERAL NURSING CONSIDERATIONS

Interventions

1. Warm drops to body temperature by holding bottle in hand for a few minutes before applying.
2. Have the client lie on his/her side with the ear to be treated facing up.
3. For instillation in adults, pull the cartilaginous part of the pinna (the external part of the ear) back and up; this straightens the ear canal. Point the dropper in the direction of the eardrum and allow the drops to fall in the direction of the external canal.
4. For instillation of drops in children under 3 years of age, pull the pinna back and down; this straightens the ear canal. Point the dropper in the direction of the eardrum and allow the drops to fall on the external canal.

5. Have the client remain on his/her side for a few minutes after instillation to permit the medication to reach the eardrum and be absorbed.
6. Gently massaging the area directly anterior to the ear may facilitate entry of the medication into the canal.
7. Never pack cotton or a wick tightly into the ear. On occasion, a loose cotton wick is inserted into the ear by the physician so that the medication will bathe the eardrum continuously. The wick should be changed when it appears nonabsorbent or soiled.

Client/Family Teaching

1. Review goals of therapy with the client.
2. Describe the appropriate method for medication administration and have client/family demonstrate administration techniques.
3. Provide written guidelines for intended therapy.

Evaluation

1. Observe administration/self-administration to ensure that the medication is administered correctly and as prescribed.
2. Assess for pretreatment symptoms.

ADMINISTRATION OF DERMATOLOGIC PREPARATIONS

Medications can be applied to the skin by rubbing, patting, spraying, painting, or by iontophoresis (medication is driven into skin by means of an electric current).

GENERAL NURSING CONSIDERATIONS

Interventions

1. Assess the client's skin condition and document findings.
2. Explain the intended purpose of the prescribed medication.
3. Use sterile technique if there is a break in the skin.
4. Cleanse skin before medication is applied. The cleansing agent should be specified by the physician.
5. Do not apply medications with bare hands; use gloves, tongue depressors, gauze, cotton, or special applicators.
6. Remove ointment from a jar with a tongue depressor, applicator, or gauze—not with fingers.
7. If medication is to be rubbed in, apply using firm strokes that follow the direction of hair growth.
8. Apply only a thin layer of medication unless specified otherwise.
9. Solutions should be painted on with an applicator.
10. Powders should be administered to clean, dry skin. Instruct client to turn head, or offer gauze to cover mouth, to prevent inhalation of powder particles.
11. If medication stains, cover with sterile gauze and instruct client to take adequate precautions (use old sheets or plastic cloth) to protect clothing and bed linens.

12. Moist dressings or compresses are prepared by soaking sterile towels or dressings in a solution as ordered. Squeeze out excess solution and apply dressings to the area to be treated. The area is then wrapped with a covering such as Kerlix, Kling, towels, or blue pads for a specified amount of time. Sterile gloves should be worn if sterile solution is to be applied.

Client/Family Teaching

1. Demonstrate appropriate technique for medication administration and have client return the demonstration.
2. Review written guidelines with client and explain intended goals of therapy.
3. Address specific adverse medication effects as applicable, such as staining, and the appropriate guidelines for clients to follow.

Evaluation

1. Document pretreatment and posttreatment skin findings.
2. Observe client self-administration to determine ability to follow directions.

RECTAL ADMINISTRATION

Retention Enemas: Retention enemas containing medication should be administered after the client has had a bowel movement to promote maximum absorption of medication in the empty rectum.

NURSING CONSIDERATIONS FOR ADMINISTRATION OF RECTAL ENEMAS

Interventions

1. Explain to the client the purpose of a retention enema.
2. To avoid peristalsis, administer retention enemas slowly, at low pressure, using a small amount of solution (no more than 120 mL) at body temperature, through a small rectal tube or small applicator of a prepackaged enema.
3. Instruct the client to lie on the left side and to breathe through the mouth to relax the rectal sphincter.
4. Apply gloves and gently insert the lubricated tip of the rectal tube (or applicator tip of prepackaged enema) approximately 7–10 cm (3–4 inches) directed toward the umbilicus.
5. When removing the rectal tube or applicator tip, apply finger pressure to the anus for a few seconds until the urge to evacuate passes.
6. Have client remain flat for 30 min after administration of enema. Explain how client should expect to feel.
7. Ensure client privacy throughout procedure.
8. If client is immobile have a bedpan readily available and within easy reach.

Special Concerns

Elderly persons tend to have decreased circulation to the lower bowel and vagina, and a lower body temperature. Therefore, medications administered via this route may not be as readily absorbed. Evaluate the elderly client closely for appropriate response to prescribed drug therapy.

Suppositories: As a rule, suppositories should be refrigerated, because they tend to soften at room temperature.

NURSING CONSIDERATIONS FOR ADMINISTARTION OF SUPPOSITORIES

Interventions

1. Explain to the client the importance of retaining the suppository once it is inserted.
2. Remove the wrapper and coat the suppository with a water-soluble lubricant.
3. Use examination glove or finger cot to protect the finger used for insertion (index finger for adults, fourth finger for infants).
4. Instruct the client to lie on the left side and to breathe slowly through the mouth to relax the rectal sphincter.
5. Spread the buttocks and gently insert the lubricated suppository beyond the internal sphincter (usually about 2 inches).
6. As the suppository enters the rectum, use gentle sideways pressure to direct the medication toward the lateral wall of the mucosa.
7. Have the client remain on his/her side for 20 min after insertion to prevent expulsion. Explain to the client how he/she should expect to feel to assure that the suppository has melted. For the pediatric patient, hold or tape together the buttocks until the impulse to defecate passes.
8. Some suppositories may have difficulty melting and may be expelled. Allow a longer time for these suppositories to melt. Check clients to assure that the suppository has melted before allowing them to resume activities. When there is difficulty in melting, explore alternate routes for medication administration.

Client/Family Teaching

1. Demonstrate appropriate technique for medication administration. Have client return the demonstration as necessary.
2. Review written guidelines with client and explain intended goals of therapy.

VAGINAL ADMINISTRATION

GENERAL NURSING CONSIDERATIONS

Interventions

1. Arrange douche-containing medication so that container hangs just above the client's hip. In this manner the force of the liquid does not drive the solution through the cervical os. Irrigating solution temperatures should be between 105–110°F (40.6–43.3°C) unless otherwise indicated.
2. Vaginal suppositories, creams, gels, and ointments should be administered using an applicator or gloved hand.
3. Instruct client to lie down. A lithotomy position may facilitate medication administration.
4. The medication should be administered high in the vaginal vault.
5. Reusable applicators should be washed with warm soapy water, dried, labeled with client's name, and stored for later use.

Client/Family Teaching

1. Instruct the client how to self-administer vaginal medication. Observe administration technique to ensure that it is done properly.
2. Client should remain with hips elevated for 5 min and then stay in bed for at least 20 min longer to promote absorption of medication and prevent drainage of medication after suppository has melted.
3. Instruct client to wear a sanitary pad to prevent staining and to absorb excess drainage from the medication.
4. Instruct client not to use tampons after inserting medication, as this may absorb medication and alter intended dose.

URETHRAL ADMINISTRATION

GENERAL NURSING CONSIDERATIONS

Interventions

1. Cleanse area around urinary meatus as normally performed for a catheterization.
2. Gently insert lubricated urethral suppository using sterile technique. These suppositories are extremely small and may be compared to the size of lead in a pencil.

ADMINISTRATION BY PARENTERAL ROUTES

Intradermal or Intracutaneous Injections: These injections are made into the dermis and produce local effects. The techniques are used mainly for local anesthesia and sensitivity tests, such as allergy panels and tuberculin tests.

The inner aspect of the forearm is the most common site for intradermal injections because it gives good visualization of the response to test media. The upper aspect of the chest or the back of the client may be used.

NURSING CONSIDERATIONS

Interventions

1. Select a tuberculin-type syringe with a 26–27 gauge needle $1/2$–$5/8$ inch long.
2. Cleanse the site selected for injection with alcohol, using a circular motion moving outward from the projected site of insertion. A dry sterile sponge may be used to dry the area.
3. Stretch the skin and insert the needle with the bevel upward at a 10–15° angle until the bevel of the needle is just under the outer layer of skin. Inject the fluid slowly, usually 0.5 mL or less. Withdraw the needle quickly after injection. A small blister or wheal should have been formed by the solution just below the skin surface. Do not rub the site.
4. After injection, observe the client for local reactions, such as redness and swelling.
5. If a blister or wheal is not present or the site bleeds after the needle is removed, then the needle may have been below the skin layers, and the test results will be invalid.
6. Circle and mark test sites to facilitate interpretation of results.
7. Instruct client to report back in 24–48 hr (or as indicated) to evaluate response.

Intrasynovial and Intra-articular Injection: Used for the relief of joint pain or the local application of medication. Be aware that local discomfort is usually intensified for several hours before palliative effect sets in and may persist for 24–48 hours. Procedure is physician-performed, utilizing sterile technique. Instruct client to avoid excessive use of joint, because medication may mask pain initially.

Intrathecal: This technique permits direct administration of medication (or anesthesia) into the subarachnoid space of the spinal cord. Assist client into the position indicated by the physician. After procedure, instruct client to lie flat and offer fluids to help replace spinal fluid loss and associated spinal headaches. If headaches do not respond to usual therapy and are severe and prolonged, a blood patch may be indicated.

Hypodermoclysis and Clysis: (See also *Subcutaneous Infusions.*) This is the subcutaneous infusion of IV fluids. This technique is used primarily in clients who require parenteral fluids but whose condition or veins do not permit IV infusion.

Because therapy may vary from person to person and institution to institution, it is suggested that you follow your employer's written procedure and physician orders for individualized administration.

NURSING CONSIDERATIONS FOR ADMINISTRATION BY PARENTERAL ROUTES

1. An intramuscular (IM) 20- or 22-gauge needle, 1½ inches long, is recommended for children; a 19-gauge, 2½–3-inch needle is satisfactory for adults.
2. During the procedure, a large amount of fluid is slowly injected subcutaneously into the loose tissues on the outer side of the upper body or, more often, into the anterior aspect of the thighs.
3. If the tissue becomes indurated, clamp the fluid off to allow for fluid absorption. The solution may be restarted after the tissue has become more elastic.
4. Hyaluronidase, an enzyme that breaks down the main constituents of intracellular connective tissue, is sometimes added to the medication so that the fluid will be absorbed rapidly and cause less discomfort.
5. At the completion of the procedure remove the needle and apply pressure; apply a dry sterile dressing to prevent fluid leakage.

Subcutaneous and Intramuscular Injections: *For more detailed instructions about SC and IM injections, see Figure 3 and your textbook on nursing techniques.*

Interventions

1. Always use sterile technique.
2. Assist client into a comfortable position to prevent strain on the muscle.
3. In selecting the proper gauge and length of needle for injection, consider age, weight, condition of client, and physical properties of the medication to be administered.
4. To promote absorption of medication and minimize pain after IM injection, palpate potential site. Choose a site that is not tender to client and where tissue does not become firm on palpation. Alternate the sites of injection, and chart the sites used—for example, RD for right deltoid, RGM for right gluteus medius, or according to institutional guidelines for charting injections (see Figure 3).
5. Cleanse the site selected for injection with alcohol, using a circular motion, moving outward from site of insertion.
6. Generally, for an SC injection, pick up tissue in selected area and hold firmly until needle has been inserted at a 45° angle. If administering injections to elderly clients who have little SC

tissue, spreading the skin may prove most effective. The SC route is appropriate for small doses (0.5–1 mL) of water-soluble drugs.

7. Elderly people have decreased tissue elasticity, muscle mass, and often are less active. As a consequence, when IM and SC injections are administered, medication may ooze from the site resulting in poor absorption of the drug.
   - Use upper, outer quadrant of the buttocks for IM injections.
   - Injection sites should be rotated. To assure the appropriate order of rotation, mark the site of the last injection on the client's chart. If the client is receiving drugs on an outpatient basis, maintain a record in the office or clinic and ensure that the client has a record also.

8. For IM injection, stretch the skin if client is in a normal state of nutrition. If the client is emaciated, pinch the tissue to form a muscle bundle to ensure that the medication is injected into the muscle. Insert needle at a 90° angle. The IM route permits larger volumes (1–5 mL) of more irritating drugs to be administered and produces a more rapid systemic response than the SC route.

9. Leave a margin of needle at least $1/4$–$1/2$ inch from hub to prevent its complete disappearance in case of breakage. Should the needle break, mark the skin at the site and immediately report the incident.

10. When preparing for SC and IM injections, include a small bubble of air in the syringe (0.2–0.3 mL) in addition to medication. The air bubble will help expel all medication from the needle so that irritating solutions will not leak into the tissues as the needle is withdrawn, or leak out of the injection site.

11. Insert the needle quickly to minimize pain. After insertion, aspirate to be sure that the needle is not in a blood vessel. If blood returns into the syringe, withdraw the needle and discard the medication. Prepare another dose using new sterile equipment, select another site, and start the injection procedure again.

12. Administer the medication slowly to allow for absorption, and remove the needle quickly while pressing down at the point of insertion with a sterile sponge to prevent bleeding. Apply an adhesive bandage if necessary.

13. Massage the area after injection to increase circulation and promote absorption of the drug, unless contraindicated. This step is contraindicated in the case of certain drugs, such as penicillin G benzathine, where absorption should be slow.

14. Some irritating drugs may be ordered and administered by the Z-track injection method. This involves placing a clean needle on the syringe after drawing up the medication. Displace the skin, subcutaneous tissue, and fat laterally before inserting the needle. After injecting the medication, release these tissues while withdrawing the needle. When working with elderly clients, use the Z-track injection technique to facilitate sealing. Cleanse skin from any medication that has oozed to the surface to prevent localized irritation.

15. Evaluate client shortly after medication administration and chart effects and/or effectiveness of administered drug.

16. Check injection sites regularly.

Subcutaneous Infusions: These infusions are used usually for chemotherapeutic drugs, morphine, deferoxamine mesylate, or insulin. The route permits certain drugs to be administered generally via a mini-infusion pump over a specified period of time. The clients are taught the appropriate techniques for self-administration of medications at home. Most frequently utilized are insulin infusion pumps for the control of diabetes. Detailed written guidelines should be given for the client to take home, once mastery of the procedure is demonstrated. Extra batteries and a phone number to call for help are a necessity at time of discharge.

Intravenous Injections (Direct or via Continuous Infusion): Responsibilities for IV therapy

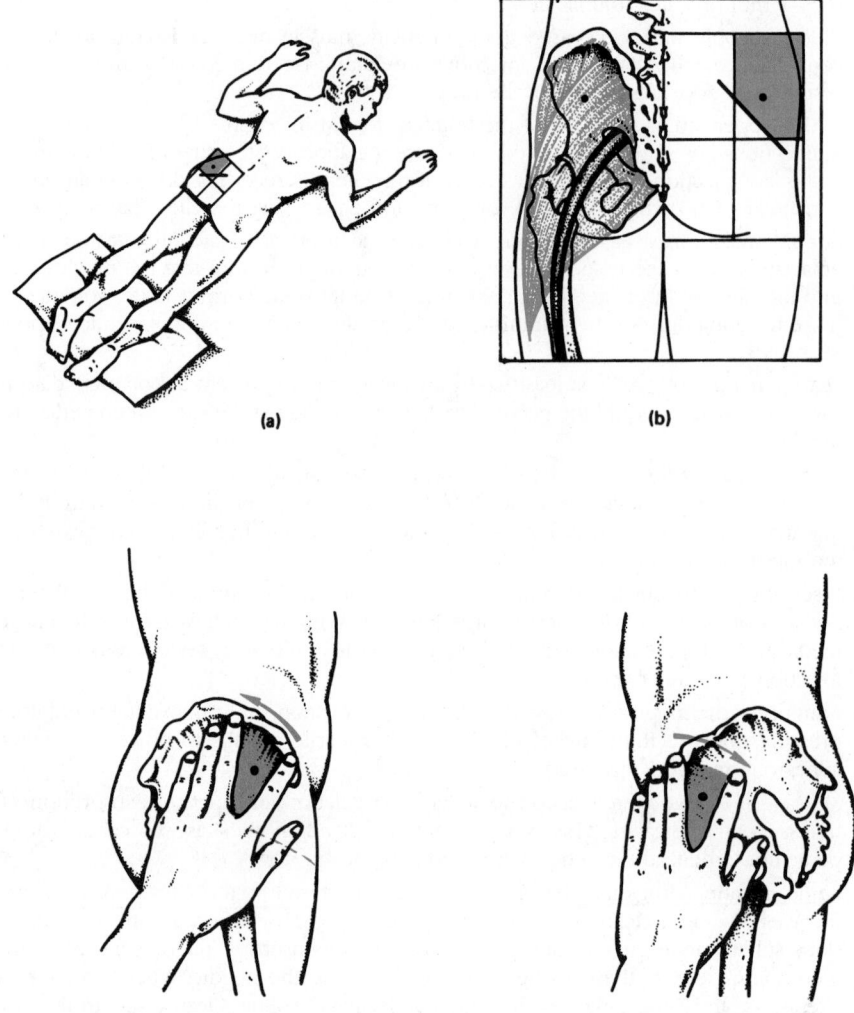

FIGURE 3 Intramuscular (IM) injection sites: (a) position for administration into gluteus maximus area; (b) detailed administration into gluteus maximus; (c) area for IM administration into right ventrogluteal area; (d) area for IM administration into left ventrogluteal area.

vary according to the institution. Follow the appropriate written policies and practices of your employing facility. The following nursing considerations may be generally applied for IV therapy.

NURSING CONSIDERATIONS FOR IV THERAPY

Interventions

1. Review institutional policy concerning procedure for venipuncture and the list of approved solutions and drugs for nurse administration.

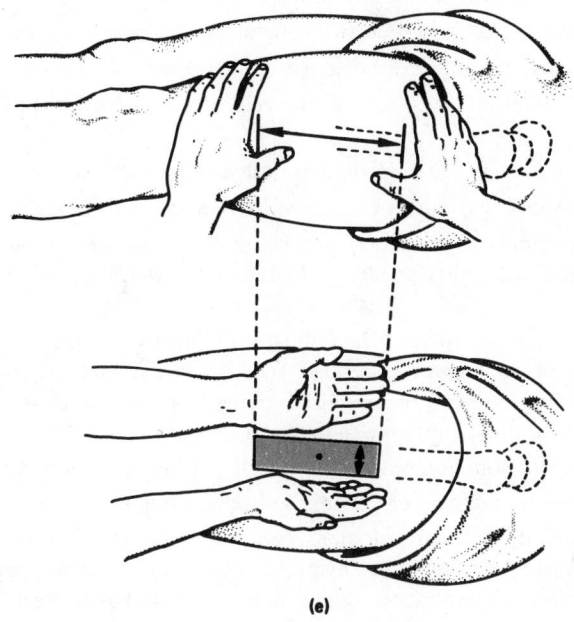

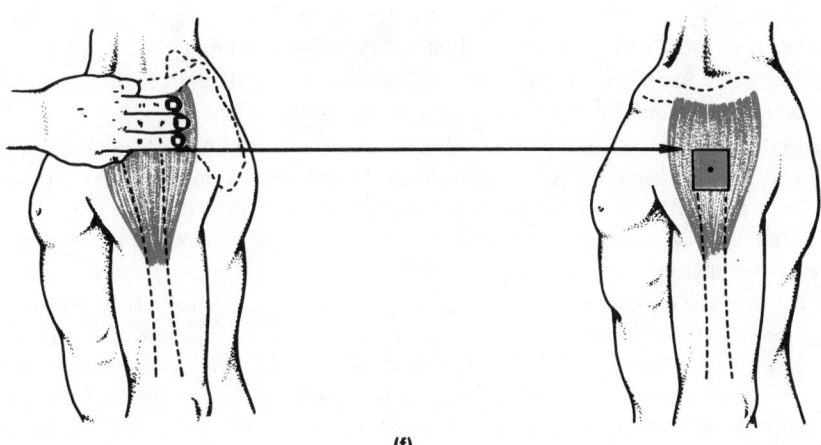

FIGURE 3 (*continued*) (e) area for IM administration into vastus lateralis: top, length of area, bottom, breadth of area; and (f) area for IM administration into the deltoid.

2. Assess client prior to beginning the procedure.
3. Position client as comfortably as possible and explain procedure.
4. If area to be injected is hairy, consider shaving it to prevent adhesive tape from causing discomfort during removal.
5. Select infusion site and place a tourniquet above intended site to dilate the vein.

6. Insertion must be performed using aseptic technique.

7. Prepare the site with povidone-iodine swab and alcohol in a circular, outward motion.

8. Put on disposable nonsterile gloves before inserting catheter.

9. Insert catheter or butterfly, bevel up, into the vein until flashback of blood is noted. Remove tourniquet.

10. Stabilize catheter and dress site according to designated policy.

11. Cap with (heparin) lock and flush or attach to infusion set, whichever is ordered.

12. If administering continuous infusions, attach additional bottles/bags of fluid as ordered; document and label appropriately. IV fluid should be 18–24 inches above the peripheral infusion site.

13. Maintain the rate of flow as ordered. Check the rate of flow by counting drops/min at least every 30 min, or more often if client is restless and moves the limb where the IV is inserted. Periodically count flow rate even if an infusion pump is in use. Check the IV administration set package to determine the drop factor (number of drops/mL or cc).

14. Check amount of fluid administered at least hourly and maintain accurate input and output.

15. Flush IV as required by the type of catheter and other equipment used.

16. Before administering unfamiliar medications, review the drug pharmacology and check hospital policy to ascertain which drugs a nurse may add to an IV on order by a physician. For buretrol, volutrol, or pediatrol administration, dilute as required and regulate the flow according to recommended rate so that the medication will not damage tissue, yet will be absorbed before loss of potency occurs.

17. When medication is added, record the name of the drug, dosage, date and time of addition, and the nurse's signature on a label to be attached to the bottle, bag, or volutrol container. Also, indicate on the client's record that drug has been administered.

18. If flow stops, check that the tubing is not kinked or occluded by the position of the client. If possible, reposition the client's extremity to reestablish flow.

19. Assess for correct placement of needle in the vein and absence of extravasation if the IV rate slows despite clamp or pump adjustment, if the site of injection becomes pale and/or edematous, and/or if the client complains of pain. Remind client to report any "strange" feelings, such as lightheadedness or difficulty in breathing. There are three methods to assess for correct placement of needle in the vein:

    • Lower the container below the level of the vein. If blood flows back into the needle and tubing, most often the needle is in a vein. If blood returns slowly, the needle may have partially slipped out of the vein. If blood does not return, the needle is most likely not in the vein. This procedure is not recommended when the IV contains a drug that may cause necrotic damage to the tissue.
    • Use a transparent dressing so site may be readily evaluated. Observe for swelling, erythema, or pain and instruct client to report these side effects.
    • Try to stop flow by applying a tourniquet 4–6 inches above insertion site and opening roller clamp wide. If IV continues to flow, needle is in SC tissue and IV is infiltrated. Discontinue IV.

20. Prevent air embolism by:

    • Adding additional container of solution ordered before old container is completely emptied.
    • Checking that all connections in IV are tight and taped as necessary.
    • Clamping off the first bottle that is empty in a Y-type set (parallel hookup) to prevent air in the empty bottle from being drawn into the vein.

- Following instructions carefully when blood or any other type of fluid is administered under pressure.
- Positioning the extremity receiving the infusion below the level of the heart to prevent negative pressure, venous collapse, and sucking of air into tubing.
- Positioning the clamp or the infusion pump regulating the flow no lower than the level of the heart and no higher than 4 inches above the level of the heart to prevent the formation of negative pressure in the tubing below.
- Allowing the tubing to fall below the level of the extremity to help prevent air from entering the vein if the infusion bottle empties before the IV is discontinued.
- Checking to make sure pump alarms are turned ON.

21. Recognize an air embolism by the occurrence of respiratory distress, cyanosis, hypotension, weak pulse, elevated central venous pressure, and loss of consciousness.
22. Be prepared to assist with treatment if an air embolism occurs. Stop infusion. Position client on left side and administer oxygen and other supportive measures. Notify physician.
23. Prevent "speed shock" by checking the rate of flow frequently and observing for untoward symptoms associated with the drug being administered.
24. Elderly people tend to have decreased cardiac efficiency. Therefore, there is a danger of circulatory overload during IV administration. Monitor these clients closely for rise in blood pressure, rapid respirations, coughing, and shortness of breath.
25. Assess for symptoms of phlebitis, such as pain, tenderness, and redness along the path of the vein. Clients receiving IV infusions for more than 24 hr are especially susceptible to phlebitis. Alcohol, hypertonic solutions with carbohydrate above 10%, and solutions with high alkaline or acid pH cause phlebitis more frequently. If symptoms of phlebitis appear, restart IV in another limb. Apply warm soaks to the phlebitic area.
26. Do not flush a clogged IV. The flow might have been stopped by an embolus that should not be moved into the circulation. Notify the physician. If an attempt to aspirate the clot with a syringe is unsuccessful, then remove that IV and restart therapy in another area.
27. Schedule incompatible medications to be administered at different times; flush lines thoroughly.
28. Remove the IV when ordered by the physician. Clamp off tubing before removing the IV to prevent extravasation into SC tissues. Press down with a sterile sponge at site of needle or plastic catheter while it is removed to prevent bleeding. Apply bandage to former injection site to prevent bleeding and infection.
29. Chart intake and output. Record all fluids and medications administered.
30. Assess site, and perform dressing and tubing changes according to institutional policy.

CENTRAL VENOUS ADMINISTRATION

GENERAL NURSING CONSIDERATIONS

Interventions

1. Evaluate client's understanding of physician's explanation. Reexplain the procedure for central venous line insertion and fluid/medication administration to the client, as needed.
2. Assemble all necessary equipment.
3. Assist with catheter insertion.
   - Use strict surgical asepsis (gown, mask, and gloves).

- Place client in Trendelenburg's position to raise venous pressure and reduce risk of air embolism.
- Have local anesthetic available if ordered.
- Place a rolled towel lengthwise under client's back to make the subclavian vein more prominent through venous distention.
- Turn client's head away from the insertion site and drape insertion area to prevent airborne contamination. Prepare site according to institutional policy and procedure.
- Instruct the client to bear down (Valsalva's maneuver) when the needle is inserted to prevent air from entering the vein and causing an air embolism.
- Assist as the catheter is sutured to the skin to prevent dislodgement.
- Assist with the application of a sterile dressing at the site of insertion, as per institutional policy. It should be dated, timed, and initialed.
- Run isotonic solution at a keep open rate until an x-ray verifies position of the catheter, before either maintenance infusions or total parenteral nutrition (TPN) is initiated.

4. Control sepsis.
  - Use sterile technique when changing dressings.
  - Frequently assess dressing. If it becomes loose, soiled, or wet, it should be changed immediately. Many institutions use a transparent dressing, which permits direct visualization of the access site. Current research advocates the use of a dry sterile dressing that is secured with occlusive tape as the most effective means to minimize infections.
  - Assess skin at the site of catheter insertion when dressing is changed. Document findings. Notify physician of any increased swelling, leakage, drainage, or erythema at the site.
  - Change infusion tubing and filters q 24–48 hr as per hospital policy. Tape all connections to prevent introduction of air.
  - Refrigerate and discard all TPN solutions as per policy (note expiration dates).
  - Observe solution for clouding, growth, or particulate matter in the bag/bottle. If contamination is observed, hang a new bag/bottle and ensure that contaminated one is cultured.
  - Use 10% dextrose/water if bottle/bag of TPN must be removed and another bottle/bag of TPN is not readily available.
  - Assess body temperature q 4 hr for elevation. After hanging a new bottle/bag, a temperature spike may indicate contamination.
  - If client has chills or fever and other signs of sepsis, notify physician. Replace bottle/bag and tubing and send equipment for culture. Further tests, such as blood, urine, sputum, x-ray films, and physical examination, may be done to locate foci of infection. If the cause of the infection is undetermined and the fever continues for 12–24 hr, assist with removal of catheter and, if indicated, with insertion of catheter on the other side. Send tip for culture.

5. Maintain the rate of flow.
  - Preferably, use an electronic infusion device.
  - Use an infusion pump when a 0.22-μg filter is used. The flow with a 0.45-μg filter will continue by gravity drip so that an infusion pump is not essential.
  - Count the drip rate periodically even if an infusion pump is used.
  - Calculate and maintain a uniform flow rate for 24 hr.
  - Check for kinks and position tube meticulously. Tape all connections to prevent the introduction of air.

6. *Assess:*
  - For evidence of pneumothorax as manifested by: chest pain, dyspnea, cyanosis, diminished breath sounds, and abnormal chest x-ray.
  - For signs of overload such as prominence of neck, arm, and hand veins (early symptoms), elevated central venous pressure, lassitude, headache, nausea, twitching, hypertension, mental fuzziness, somnolence, and convulsions.

- For infiltration by noting pain and swelling in shoulder, neck, or face and x-ray confirmation of displacement of catheter.
- For an improperly placed, slipped, or broken catheter, or a leak at the tubing union, which may be indicated by a wet dressing.
- For catheter blockage by noting occlusion alarms on the infusion pump, inability to administer medication and flush, and inability to withdraw blood. Do NOT forcibly try to flush a blocked catheter; notify physician.
- For evidence of infection such as fever, chills, purulent exudate, elevated white blood cell count. Decrease the incidence of infections by following strict aseptic technique, covering insertion site with appropriate dressing, and changing as indicated.

7. During administration of TPN assess:
- For glycosuria by testing urines q 6 hr. Use Tes-Tape or Diastix to check urine of patient receiving cephalosporin to prevent false-positive results; or perform fingersticks or serum blood sugars for the most reliable indication of blood sugar levels.
- Intake and output and record.
- Weight daily and record.
- Laboratory reports for electrolyte balance and renal and liver function.
- Caloric count of daily oral and parenteral intake and chart as indicated.

IMPLANTED VENOUS ACCESS DEVICES (VADS)

Implantation of these catheters is generally performed by a surgeon, with the client under a local anesthetic. These devices permit the infusion of medications intermittently or continuously, the administration of blood or blood products as well as fluids and TPN, and blood sampling for lab studies in clients generally requiring long-term therapy.

1. Some of the more common implanted SC access devices include:
- Broviac (smaller lumen)
- Hickman
- Hickman/Broviac (double lumen)

These catheters are threaded into the superior vena cava and junction of the right atrium, and tunneled subcutaneously to a distal exit site. Catheter fixation of the Dacron cuff to local tissue usually takes 2–3 weeks. A positive-pressure apparatus (infusion pump) should be used to administer fluids, because these catheters may kink easily and clot. These catheters generally require once a day flushing and/or after each treatment to maintain patency. Follow institutional policy and product literature concerning the gauge and length of needle used to access catheters.

2. Some implanted SC ports include:
- Infuse A-Ports (larger diaphragm)
- Mediport
- Port-A-Cath

These devices consist of a catheter attached to an injection port, which has a self-sealing entry septum (diaphragm). The catheters are threaded through the subclavian vein into the superior vena cava. The port is implanted usually in the right infraclavicular fossa (anterior chest) just below the skin surface. An infusion pump should be used for all continuous fluid administration. Use a noncoring needle (deflected point) to access the port to prevent catheter shear. These ports generally require flushing once a month and/or after each treatment. These ports are easily hidden under clothes and provide the client freedom from the pain of multiple sticks and also from long-term hospitalization.

GENERAL NURSING CONSIDERATIONS

Interventions

1. Inspect site for evidence of hematoma, swelling, excessive accumulation of exudates, infection, and device rotation or erosion after implantation. X-ray confirmation of catheter placement is usually performed after insertion, and always before initial access.
2. Use aseptic technique when accessing all ports. Review product literature and follow institutional policy.
3. Generally, implanted devices may be used 24–48 hr after insertion. Have a trained nurse or physician perform the first access.
4. To prevent blood withdraw occlusion, use a vigorous flush.

Client/Family Teaching

1. Utilize a return demonstration teaching format. A mirror may enhance the client's visualization while the nurse is teaching.
2. Demonstrate the appropriate technique for catheter care and how to access and maintain port.
3. Provide written, step-by-step guidelines for the client/family to follow when using the port at home and explain intended goals of therapy.
4. Discuss and review any signs and symptoms that should be reported immediately.
5. Designate whom to contact with questions or problems.
6. Stress the importance of compliance with prescribed therapy and care guidelines.
7. Closely observe client (or person responsible) during administration of prescribed therapy to ensure procedure is performed safely and properly and to identify any problems.

INFUSION PUMPS

These devices permit the uniform administration and control of fluids and medications with few complications. They do require periodic monitoring, but they save valuable nursing time and may protect the client from potential medication overdosage.

1. The general category of pumps includes:
   - Syringe pump—administers small amounts of medication or fluid (0.01 mL/hr) slowly.
   - Nonvolumetric pump—measures drop rate of fluids; some require special administration tubing.
   - Volumetric pump—measures volume; requires a special cartridge, cassette or tubing for operation.

Because all pumps and manufacturers vary, it is recommended that the product literature and institutional procedures be reviewed prior to initiating therapy.

A variety of compact, lightweight infusers are now available for at home, ambulatory IV chemotherapy. Some in frequent use include:

- Ambulatory Micro Infusers
- Patient-Controlled Analgesic Devices (PCA)
- Auto Syringe Portable Infusion Pumps.

These advanced technological devices all require detailed and thorough inservice for staff and education for the client before application and discharge.

GENERAL NURSING CONSIDERATION

Client/Family Teaching

1. Instruct client/family to wear appropriate protective apparel as necessary.
2. Demonstrate the appropriate technique for pump set-up, medication instillation, and priming of cassette, if applicable. Utilize a return demonstration teaching format.
3. Describe general principles for the correct operation of the specific infusion device.
4. Show client/family how to test and change batteries.
5. Review appropriate corrective actions for each alarm display.
6. Instruct client/family to follow written guidelines provided when using these devices at home.
7. Designate how to contact the health care provider, by phone or otherwise, when clients need assistance.
8. Stress the importance of proper device care and use to ensure proper functioning.
9. Remind clients to report for all scheduled visits, because compliance is of the utmost importance when performing sophisticated therapy at home.
10. Review signs and symptoms that require immediate medical attention.

ADMINISTRATION BY INTRA-ARTERIAL INFUSION

Administration by intra-arterial infusion involves insertion of a catheter by a surgeon under fluoroscopy into the artery leading directly into the area to be treated. The arteries commonly used are the brachial, axillary, carotid, and femoral. The drug is then pumped steadily through the catheter.

Intra-arterial ports may be implanted also. The catheter is inserted usually into the hepatic arterial system. This technique permits direct administration of potent, undiluted chemotherapy to tumors without metabolic breakdown by the liver or kidneys.

The tumor receives a high concentration of the chemotherapeutic agent before the drug is distributed to the rest of the body. The drug may be administered at varying intervals of time. Also, direct arterial infusions of vasopressin may be utilized with severe GI bleeding.

All intra-arterial fluids must be administered with either a positive-pressure device (infusion pump) or a pressure cuff, due to arterial pressure forces. Intra-arterial infusions may be performed on an ambulatory basis with a portable infusion pump, but the client must be taught carefully how to monitor the apparatus.

GENERAL NURSING CONSIDERATIONS

Interventions

1. *Assess:*
   - Tissue in local area for reactions, such as erythema, mild edema, blistering, and petechiae.

- Vital signs periodically (q 15 min) when therapy is instituted initially until BP is stabilized.
- Site of infusion for infection and bleeding.
- Intake and output.
- Complete blood count, bleeding times (prothrombin time/partial thromboplastin time), and renal function studies.
- Client's response to therapy and document.

2. Describe observations completely when charting, and report to physician.

3. Report pain, because it may be indicative of severe injury to normal tissue, vasospasm, or intravasation.

4. Maintain rate of pump as ordered.

5. Do not permit infusion fluid to run through completely, because air will then enter the tubing. Add fluid as needed.

6. Clamp tubing if an air bubble is noted and call physician. *Do not disconnect the tubing between the pump and the client to release the air bubble, because hemorrhage will occur*.

7. Apply direct pressure if hemorrhage occurs from the artery.

8. Check tubing for kinks and prevent compression of tubing.

ADMINISTRATION BY PERFUSION (EXTRACORPOREAL OR ISOLATION PERFUSION)

Administration by perfusion technique involves the administration of large doses of highly toxic drugs to an isolated extremity, organ, or region of the body. For perfusion in the lower extremity, the iliac, femoral, and popliteal arteries and veins are used; for upper extremity perfusion, the axillary artery and vein are injected. The abdominal aorta and vena cava are used for pelvic perfusion. The actual perfusion is accomplished in the operating room where, by means of a pump oxygenator, the client's blood is circulated in a closed system for the part of the body involved. Efforts are made by the use of a tourniquet or ligature to prevent seepage of the concentrated drug into the systemic circulation. Seepage of the drug results in destruction of normal tissue.

GENERAL NURSING CONSIDERATIONS FOR PREOPERATIVE ADMINISTRATION

Interventions

1. Assess client's physical and emotional status.

2. Explain procedure to client and family member. Answer questions in lay terms and provide emotional support throughout procedure.

3. Weigh client, because dosage of chemotherapeutic agent and heparin is calculated on the basis of body weight.

4. Ascertain that hematologic tests, urinalysis, and x-ray films have been done and results are on the chart.

5. Review for potential problems and any contraindications.

6. Explain to client what can be expected in response to drug therapy. Discuss any potential side effects of the prescribed drug therapy.

GENERAL NURSING CONSIDERATIONS FOR POSTOPERATIVE ADMINISTRATION

Interventions

1. Ascertain if hematologic tests have been done and evaluated for depression of bone marrow function, which is due to seepage of concentrated drug into systemic circulation.

2. Assess:
   - Tanning, erythema, or blistering of skin over area perfused—symptoms resemble toxic reaction to radiation.
   - Thrombosis and phlebitis of local tissue.
   - Signs of infection, such as fever and malaise, because septicemia may occur.
   - Color and warmth of extremity perfused and report untoward symptoms.
   - Pain, which may be indicative of severe tissue damage.
   - Hemorrhage, hypotension, fibrillation, arrhythmia, sudden chest pain, and pulmonary edema, all of which may be precipitated by perfusion.

3. Continue to provide comprehensive holistic nursing care, with both physical and emotional support.

CHAPTER SEVEN

Drug Response of the Pediatric, Geriatric, or Pregnant Client

7

DRUG RESPONSE OF THE PEDIATRIC CLIENT

General Considerations: The safe use of many of the newer pharmacologic agents in children has not been established yet. In case of doubt, it is wise to ask the physician whether a particular agent is suitable for pediatric clients.

Pediatric dosages for individual agents are listed whenever relevant and/or available. The safe pediatric dosage can be computed also using the surface area of the child (mg/m^2), or by calculating formulas for recommended pediatric dosage per kilogram body weight (mg/kg). The body weight formula is the most reliable for premature and full-term infants (Table 3).

Table 3   Guidelines For Calculating Dosage For Pediatric Administration

A. Based on child's weight

   1. Augsberger's rule:

$$4 \times (\text{age in years}) + 20\% \text{ of adult dose} = \text{child's approximate dose}$$

   2. Clark's rule:

$$\frac{\text{weight (in pounds)}}{150} \times \text{adult dose} = \text{child's approximate dose}$$

B. Based on child's body surface area

   1. Clark's body area rule:

$$\frac{\text{body surface area (in m}^2)}{1.73} \times \text{adult dose} = \text{child's approximate dose}$$

  Use the body surface area for children – nomogram for determination of body surface area from height and weight (see inside back cover) or the following formulas:

   a. Augsberger's rule:

$$\frac{7 \times (\text{age of child in years}) + 35}{100} = \text{body surface area in m}^2$$

   b. Costeff's rule:

$$\frac{4 \times (\text{weight in kg}) + 7}{(\text{weight in kg}) + 90} = \text{body surface area in m}^2$$

C. Based on child's age (least reliable method)

   1. Fried's rule: for infants under 1 year

$$\frac{\text{child's age (in months)}}{150} \times \text{adult dose} = \text{child's approximate dose}$$

   2. Young's rule:

$$\frac{\text{age (in years)}}{\text{age (in years)} + 12} \times \text{adult dose} = \text{child's approximate dose}$$

The following general considerations apply to the administration of drugs to children. The child has a different pharmacodynamic sensitivity than does the adult. Furthermore, there is often a long delay between the marketing of a drug for adults and the establishment of a rational therapeutic regimen for pediatric clients.

Many of the problems encountered in the pediatric administration of drugs are attributable to age and development and are related to differences in the distribution of drugs in the body and in the rates at which drugs are absorbed and eliminated.

1. **Absorption.** The pH of the GI tract is higher in infants than in adults. Therefore, drugs that are absorbed in an acid environment are absorbed more slowly in children (slower onset of action) than in adults. Conversely, drugs that are destroyed by acid have a longer half-life (longer activity) in children than in adults.

   Topical absorption is usually faster in pediatric clients, because their epidermis is thinner

2. **Distribution Throughout the Body.** Water constitutes a much larger proportion of body weight in children than in adults; the converse is true for fat. Thus, drugs that are water soluble are distributed in a smaller volume (are more concentrated) in adults than in children. Drugs that are fat soluble are more concentrated in children than in adults, because the area for distribution (and dilution) is less.

3. **Plasma Protein Binding.** The plasma protein binding of drugs is usually less extensive in children, especially in neonates, than it is in adults because of a lower percentage of plasma protein. This results in a greater concentration of free drugs (bioavailability) in children than in adults.

4. **Hepatic Degradation and Renal Excretion.** Both the liver and the kidneys of neonates and infants are immature compared with those of adults. The liver of an infant, for instance, has a lower concentration of the enzymes that participate in the degradation of drugs; for example, phenytoin, metabolized by the liver as a rule, is broken down more slowly in infants than in adults.

   Renal excretion, on the other hand, which represents a complex balance between elimination and reabsorption, is often faster in infants than in adults (shorter duration of action).

All these factors are taken into consideration when a pediatric dosage is established. The administration of drugs to pediatric clients also involves many practical considerations detailed below.

An understanding of the various stages of growth and development will help the nurse anticipate and understand the child's response to medication administration.

SPECIAL NURSING CONSIDERATIONS FOR THE ADMINISTRATION OF PEDIATRIC MEDICATIONS

Assessment

1. Assess the child's physical and emotional condition and document.
2. Note child's developmental level and age and record.

Interventions

1. Define goals of drug therapy prescribed and discuss with child and parent.
2. Always wake the child before administering medications (if other than IV). Advise parents to follow this procedure at home as well.
3. Try to gain the child's cooperation by using techniques and an approach appropriate to the level of development derived from the initial nursing assessment.
4. Explain to the parents and child the need for medications to be administered. Indicate to the child in a firm but friendly manner that it is time to take the medication.
5. Explain, in terms the child understands, the purpose and benefits of the medication you administer. If the drug is to be administered by injection, explain that there will be a pin prick. If the drug may cause a stinging sensation, explain to the child that something like a bee sting may be felt at the time of injection.
6. Accept a child's negative feelings and demonstrate empathy. Do not shame the child. Compliment the child on positive aspects of cooperative behavior and demonstrate acceptance and liking even though the child may not have cooperated.

7. Realize that hospitalization and medication are regarded as punishment by some children. Attempt to discourage and disprove this myth.

8. Use diversionary techniques or play therapy appropriate to developmental level when giving medications to a child. For example, suggest that the child count or recite the alphabet while receiving a parenteral injection, or suggest that the child lie on the abdomen and turn his/her toes in (to help relax the gluteal muscles). For a child who is quite young, play a music box or set a toy in motion and talk with the child.

9. Crush pills for infants or children under 5 years of age and dissolve them in syrup, water, or nonessential foods (e.g., applesauce). Do NOT add to their bottle.

10. Do not force oral medications, because aspiration pneumonia is a threat. If the child refuses consistently or spits out the medication, find out if it is taste or consistency of the medication to which the child objects. Consult with the pharmacy to determine if there is another form of the medication or another drug that can be substituted and that is more appealing to the child. Report all incidents of spitting up prescribed medications and your findings to the physician so that another form of medication or different drug can be used.

11. When using a plastic dropper or plastic syringe to administer medication, direct the tip toward the inner aspect of the cheek of the mouth to avoid aspiration and stimulation of the cough reflex. Insert only the amount that can be swallowed at one time.

12. When using a spoon to administer medication to an infant, place the spoon well back on the tongue to prevent stimulating the extrusion reflex.

13. Pouring small amounts of medication into an empty nipple from which the infant will suck may facilitate the administration of medication.

14. When administering *per os* (PO) medication to an infant, hold the child securely against your body with one arm around the child, supporting the head and neck, and with your hand holding the child's free arm while you administer the medication. Elevate the infant's head to prevent aspiration. Cuddle the infant once all medication has been administered to reassure and comfort as well as observe response to therapy.

15. When administering ear drops to a child under 3 years of age, gently pull the pinna of the ear down and back; for a child over 3 years of age, pull the pinna of the ear back and upward.

16. Prepare injections out of sight of the child. If the child cannot, or will not, cooperate so that parenteral medication can be administered, restrain the child with the help of other personnel, as necessary, and then administer medication. Always keep a firm grip on the syringe to prevent dislodgement or contamination.

17. Children under 2 years of age should receive IM injections into the vastus lateralis or rectus femoris (Figure 4), because gluteal muscles are as yet too underdeveloped to be used for IM administration, and damage to the sciatic nerve may occur.

18. After medication, offer juice or water and verbal praise. Try not to offer bribes such as candy, lollipops, or special privileges. These suggest that medications are bad and that reward is necessary for an activity that the child should learn to understand is helpful.

19. After insertion of a suppository, either hold or tape buttocks together until defecation impulse has passed (usually 15 min).

20. An infusion pump should be used for accurate administration of IV infusions to a child. If a pump is not available, adjust rate of flow while the infant is quiet (crying and emotional upset constrict the blood vessels and the rate may then be too rapid when the infant is calm again).

21. Safely and adequately restrain infant and child during IV therapy. Exercise unaffected limbs periodically to maintain circulation. Check that restraints are not inhibiting circulation. Examine insertion site frequently to check for tissue irritation or damage, and check limb for evidence of infiltration or catheter dislodgement.

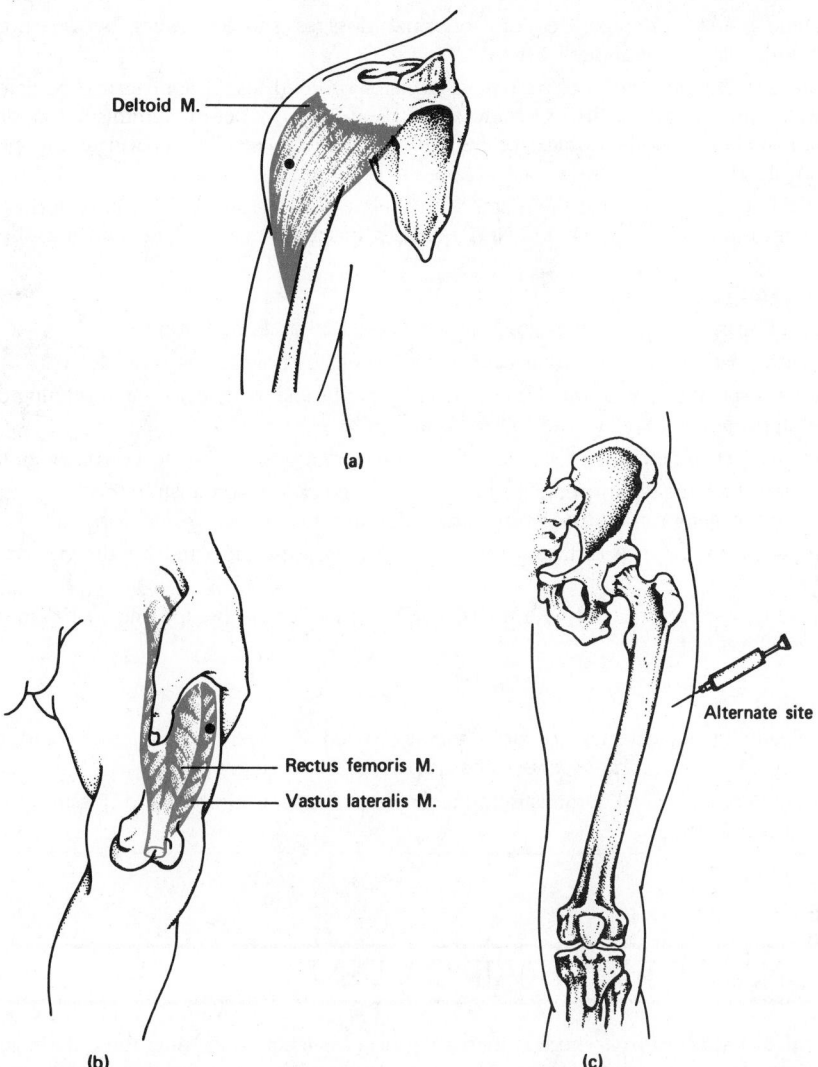

FIGURE 4 Pediatric IM injection sites: (a) deltoid; (b) anterior surface of midlateral thigh; and (c) anterolateral surface of upper thigh.

22. Assess condition of pediatric client, urine output, rate of flow, and amount of IV absorbed at least hourly and record.

23. The medication cart and drugs should be locked and constantly under the eyes of the nurse. The nurse must always be alert to the possibility that children may take medications that are not theirs or may tamper with drugs in some way. Syringes and needles must never be left with a child to use as a toy after the nurse has left.

24. If a child does not have an identification band and/or name tag, identification must be made according to hospital policy before medication is administered.

25. When pouring medications, the nurse should consider the age and weight of the child and

diagnosis. Any discrepancies or abnormal dosages should always be questioned before administering medications.

26. Calculate dosages and check safety of dosages ordered, using appropriate pediatric formulas based on body surface area or body weight (see Table 3). Before administration, double-check with another nurse the dosages of the following: digoxin, insulin, heparin, antineoplastic agents, and blood.

27. Involve parents and have them stay with their child to assist and comfort during medication administration. A parent should NOT be the primary restrainer if the child must be restrained.

Client/Family Teaching

1. Provide parents with written guidelines for medication administration.
2. Review goals of therapy and answer any questions as honestly as possible.
3. Address specific adverse medication effects as applicable, such as iron and staining of teeth, and the appropriate guidelines to follow to minimize side effects.
4. Discuss diet and the need for medication to be administered with food or on an empty stomach.
5. Demonstrate the appropriate technique for medication administration. Have parents/client return the demonstration to ensure that administration is performed correctly.
6. Stress the importance of taking the medication as prescribed and for the correct number of days.
7. Encourage parents to call with questions/concerns during therapy and to report any unusual side effects.

Evaluation

1. Evaluate the effectiveness of drug therapy based on client improvement and response to therapy. Encourage the parents to participate in this evaluation.
2. Observe parent/client administration technique to ensure accuracy and question to assess level of understanding.

DRUG RESPONSE OF THE GERIATRIC CLIENT

General Considerations: There is increasing data available concerning the elderly and how they respond to drug therapy. For example, there is wide variation among the elderly regarding the deterioration in kidney function, sensitivity to drugs, and metabolism of drugs by the liver. Elderly people are more prone to developing infections than are other populations. Not only does age reduce the efficiency of the person's ability to develop antibodies against infections, but many of the elderly are poor and unable to acquire the nutrition that would enable them to develop appropriate resistance against disease, in spite of age. Many elderly people live alone, and this situation is not conducive to promoting good eating habits even when food is available. Finally, many of the illnesses common to the elderly (e.g., diabetes, circulatory diseases) increase the likelihood of their developing bacterial or fungal infections.

A comprehensive discussion of the many factors that may influence the response of the elderly patient to drugs is beyond the scope of this text; however, several points are worthy of consideration.

1. **Chronic Disease States.** Diabetes, heart disease, hypertension, chronic respiratory disease,

and "senility" are diseases that require chronic drug therapy. Some of these diseases may result in an increase, whereas others may result in a decrease in drug response. For example, presence of chronic respiratory disease is known to exaggerate the respiratory depression observed with CNS depressants.

2. **Physiologic and Psychologic Change as a Function of Age.** These changes result in a decrease in the functional capacity of the body leading to an alteration of drug response due to changes in absorption from the GI tract, distribution of the drug in the body (as a result of changes in blood flow or composition of body mass), biotransformation of drugs in the liver (i.e., drug-metabolizing enzymes are decreased), excretion of the drug or its metabolites (due to decreased ability of the kidney to filter or actively secrete drugs), and changes in organ or receptor sensitivity. It also is known that serum albumin decreases with age. Thus, because free drug concentration determines drug distribution and elimination, a decrease in binding of drugs to plasma proteins (or other body tissues) could result in altered responses in the elderly person. For example, a decreased percentage of protein-bound warfarin sodium will lead to a greater pharmacologic effect of the drug. On the other hand, reduced protein binding of phenytoin results in a greater amount of the drug available for excretion, leading to a reduced pharmacologic effect and a shorter duration of action.

3. **Nutrition and Diet.** For many reasons, the elderly population often manifests dietary deficiencies due either to lack of a balanced diet or to low food intake. The resultant vitamin deficiencies or inadequate food intake may alter the response to drugs.

4. **Use of Many Medications.** It is estimated that because of the increased incidence of chronic illness in the elderly, this population uses two and one-half times more medication than the rest of the population. As the number of different drugs used increases, the risk of drug interactions or adverse drug reactions increases.

5. **Lack of Compliance and Medication Errors.** It has been estimated that as much as 60% of the elderly population either fails to take their medication or takes it incorrectly. Reasons for lack of compliance include (1) impaired mental capacity (client forgets to take the medication); (2) problems with sight, hearing, or mobility, which result in failure to take the medication or errors in taking the medication; (3) complicated dosing schedules, which confuse the clients so that they fail to understand what medication to take or when to take it; (4) alteration of drug regimen based on the personal judgment of the client, resulting in overdosage or underdosage; and (5) unavailability of medication because the client is unable to afford it, or because the supply has been used up before the next appointment with the physician.

Thus, it is important for the nurse to ensure that the geriatric client fully understands how and when to take medication and to monitor drug response carefully in the elderly. The nurse must be aware also of specific symptoms caused by an altered drug response.

SPECIAL NURSING CONSIDERATIONS FOR THE ADMINISTRATION OF GERIATRIC MEDICATIONS

Assessment

1. Obtain a complete medication and allergy history from the client and/or family. Include a request to see all the drugs the client takes for any reason to assure that all drugs are included in the history. The pharmacist can provide assistance with taking the history.

2. Many clients are living at home and are more likely to be caring for themselves. Often they take over-the-counter drugs recommended by friends or family and the physician is unaware of their use. Because of the potential for drug interactions and sensitivity, it is important to have clients or their family members aware of the numbers and kinds of drugs the elderly are taking.

3. Query client to evaluate the use of OTC preparations or drugs. Frequently, the elderly misuse laxatives as they become preoccupied with bowel habits and attempt to attain the same regularity they experienced years before when their lifestyle, diet, and physical activity were much different.

4. Assess client's financial status and health insurance coverage. Identify appropriate social service referrals and less expensive alternatives (e.g., generic drugs or clinics/agencies that dispense drugs and are state or federally supported).

5. During medication administration assess:

- If a nonpharmacologic approach could potentially solve the client's problem (e.g., warm milk instead of a sedative; warm soaks instead of an analgesic; change in diet instead of an antacid or laxative).
- Client's baseline weight; assess for signs of fluid overload (e.g., dyspnea, cough, increased respirations, rapid weight gain and edema due to cardiac and renal dysfunction), which is more common in the elderly and alters response to drugs.
- Tongue for signs of dehydration, characterized by furrows. Turgidity or fullness of tongue indicates hydration. Because the mucous membranes of the mouth may be chronically dry because of mouth breathing, an absence of subcutaneous fat, and the presence of atrophic epidermal changes that make checking for elasticity useless, assessment of the tongue is the best indication of the hydration state of the elderly client.
- For adverse drug reactions, recognizing that the earliest manifestation of drug toxicity in the elderly is mental confusion. For example, the initial symptoms of digitalis toxicity in the elderly are not necessarily nausea and vomiting, as in younger clients, but rather are changes in mental status due to decreased cerebral perfusion and decreased cardiac output due to secondary arrhythmias.
- Whether failure to thrive in the elderly (characterized by insidious and progressive physical deterioration, deteriorating social competence, loss of appetite, and diminishing concentration) is the result of adverse drug reactions.
- Whether acute brain syndrome (characterized by disorientation to person, place, or time; memory impairment for both remote and recent past; impairment of intellectual function; and emotional lability) is the result of adverse drug reactions. If so, the syndrome may be reversed by withdrawing medications.
- Whether clients continue to manifest symptoms indicating need for continuous drug therapy or whether they are compensating and may require less medication. Reduction in strength and number of medications, thereby minimizing adverse reactions and interactions, is a major goal of successful drug therapy in the aged.
- Client taking insulin and oral antidiabetics for mild hypoglycemic reactions, characterized by speech disorders, confusion, and disorientation, rather than by the restlessness, tachycardia, and profuse perspiration that occur in the younger client. Because periodic mild hypoglycemic reactions resulting from medication may cause permanent brain damage, and client is unable to ingest recommended dietary intake, confer with physician regarding alternative therapy.
- Client lifestyle. Ask about problems with thirst and if they are related to activity or drug therapy.
- Client's ability to read print, hear, and comprehend what is being said.

Interventions

1. Anticipate that if the half-life of a medication is increased by deficient renal function, the drug may be administered less frequently or in smaller doses.

2. Do not treat the elderly as if they are children. When explaining about the administration of

drugs, inform the client about the purpose of the drug as would be done for any other person unless there is good indication that client may require a different approach. Assess client knowledge of the reasons for taking medications prescribed.

3. Discuss the goals of drug therapy with the client and family.

4. Combine bitter preparations, such as vitamin, mineral, and electrolyte preparations, with foods such as applesauce or juice, to make medication more palatable and to prevent gastric irritation. The geriatric client often loses taste buds for sweetness and may perceive medication as bitter.

5. Inform clients that you are administering medication, even though it may seem that they are only receiving food.

6. Recommend and/or provide, as necessary, good oral hygiene before and after administration of medication to promote ingestion and to prevent an unpleasant aftertaste.

7. Provide sufficient fluids to permit easy swallowing and to help movement of medication through the GI tract. Assist client into a position that prevents aspiration and promotes swallowing of medication.

8. Examine oral cavity of debilitated person to ensure that medication has not adhered to mucous membranes and, in fact, has been swallowed.

9. Administer one dose of medication each day to ensure better drug compliance, unless it is essential to use divided dose schedule.

10. Request doctor to order a slower-acting diuretic for the geriatric client if the stress of a rapid-acting diuretic, such as furosemide, is causing incontinence.

11. Administer tricyclic drugs at bedtime to minimize dry mouth.

12. Discourage continuous use of hypnotics, because they are of little value if taken repeatedly. To promote sleep, provide warm milk and a backrub at bedtime; use relaxation techniques and other forms of relaxation that are effective for the client rather than medication.

13. Take the time to listen to the client's feelings, thoughts, needs, and lifestyle. Consider these and incorporate into the overall therapeutic regimen.

14. Prevent drug-induced immobility, because this leads to perceptual changes, dehydration, and decubitus ulcer formation.

15. Remain with the person receiving a suppository until the drug is absorbed. Because of the reduced body temperature of the elderly client, it may take longer for a suppository to melt in the bowel or vagina than in a younger person. Encourage the client to retain the suppository. The desire to expel the suppository may be strong because of the extended length of time needed to dissolve the medication. If the client has difficulty retaining the suppository, consult with the physician to determine whether another route may be used.

16. Alternate injection sites and apply a small, dry sterile dressing with pressure after an injection, because the geriatric client tends to bleed after an injection due to the loss of elasticity of tissue.

17. Avoid injections into an immobile limb, if possible, because inactivity of limb will reduce the rate of drug absorption.

18. Inspect site of injection of medication because reduction in cutaneous sensation may prevent client awareness of pain, infection, intravasation, extravasation or other trauma.

19. Monitor drug compliance in client taking more than five medications, because this increases the number of adverse reactions and interactions (see Chapter 8, *Nursing Process for Teaching and Promoting Compliance with Medication Regimen*.)

Client/Family Teaching

1. Assist client to maintain a nutritious diet to prevent dietary deficiencies that could result in body dysfunction and may alter response to medications. Refer to appropriate agencies for assistance with food preparation and/or procurement.

2. Encourage client/family to discard drugs no longer part of the medication regimen to prevent self-medication and confusion of drugs.

3. Encourage client/family to confer with physician if they feel that the medication is no longer required rather than to discontinue treatment. Many people stop taking medications when improvement of symptoms is noted.

4. Explain that simple home remedies, such as sodium bicarbonate for upset stomach, may be extremely dangerous.

5. When teaching the client who will be taking drugs at home:
   - Determine the best time of day for the drugs to be taken (e.g., diuretics in the early morning) based on client lifestyle and activity.
   - Stress any special precautions that may be necessary. Discuss with the client and family foods or other drugs that may need to be avoided to prevent drug interactions or other untoward reactions.
   - Teach client and family what indicates a good response to medication and what side effects may be the result of therapy.
   - Warn against sharing their drugs with other elderly friends or relatives (especially important when the elderly client lives in an apartment or other similar accommodation for the elderly).
   - If using printed material, be sure the print is large enough, clear, and on paper with a dull finish.

Evaluation

1. Evaluate client knowledge of the reasons for taking prescribed medications.
2. Assess status (presence or absence) of pretreatment symptoms.

DRUG RESPONSE OF THE PREGNANT CLIENT

Just as nurses need to be concerned about the effects of anti-infective drugs on the elderly, so they must be concerned also about whether a client is pregnant. When there is doubt concerning the likelihood of an anti-infective crossing the placental barrier and harming the fetus, it is better to err on the side of caution. Many of the anti-infectives may appear in small quantities in breast milk, but there seems at this time to be little evidence of untoward effects on the infant. An exception may be made in the case of sulfonamides. In this instance, although sulfonamides are present in small amounts in breast milk, it may be well to avoid administering the drug during the first 5 days of life or when the infant is premature, because hyperbilirubinemia may occur.

The philosophy of drug therapy during pregnancy changed abruptly in 1961 in the wake of the thalidomide tragedy. Thalidomide, believed to be a rather innocuous sleeping medication, turned out to be a powerful teratogen that causes phocomelia when taken by women during the first trimester of pregnancy. The teratogenic effect of drugs was again brought to the attention of the general public when it was demonstrated that the administration of diethylstilbestrol (DES) during pregnancy increased the incidence of adenocarcinoma of the vagina in female offspring of mothers who received the drug.

The FDA now requires that new drugs be tested for teratogenicity in animals before drugs can be used in pregnant women, (see *FDA-assigned Pregnancy Categories,* page 3). However, many older drugs, have never been tested or have been minimally tested under such circumstances. Furthermore, there is a great deal of uncertainty about applying animal data to humans.

Therefore, as a rule, a woman who is pregnant, or who is attempting to become pregnant, should not take any pharmacologic agent unless specifically ordered or permitted by her physician, who will determine whether the *benefit of the therapy outweighs the risk of fetal malformation.*

Thus, all drugs are contraindicated in pregnancy. The warning also applies to OTC agents, alcohol, street drugs, insecticides, and other environmental pollutants. Alcohol, when taken in excess, is known to induce fetal alcohol syndrome.

The implications of the effect of drugs, alcohol, street drugs, and cigarette smoking must be explained to every pregnant woman and/or woman of childbearing age. Common sense as to quantity should be used when discussing the effect of social drugs (alcohol, cigarettes); however, it has been reported that the consumption of three ounces of alcohol per day may cause congenital defects and three cigarettes per day may cause a decrease in birth weight. Therefore, any such use should be strongly discouraged.

Some of the data regarding the effect of maternal drug* ingestion on the embryo, fetus, and neonate are open to question because (1) experimental data on humans are often nonexistent and conclusions must be drawn from long-term retrospective assessment, (2) malformations also occur in clients who have not ingested these agents, and (3) malformations have been observed in clients who ingested more than one agent (epileptics, for example). Thus, it is difficult to ascertain the causative agent.

Most drugs taken by a pregnant woman pass the placental barrier and may affect the embryo, fetus, and neonate. The embryo appears to be particularly sensitive to the effect of drugs during the first trimester of pregnancy, when organogenesis is taking place. The drugs that do not cross the placental barrier usually consist of large molecules (e.g., heparin). Therefore, the decision whether to use a particular drug during pregnancy requires an understanding of the pharmacodynamics of a particular agent. Insulin, for example, is known to be teratogenic when administered directly to the fetus, but it does not cross the placental barrier and hence is not teratogenic. However, excess insulin may cause the fetus to develop hypoglycemia, which may be harmful. Insulin passes into breast milk but is destroyed in the GI tract of the nursing infant and is harmless.

Development of the Fetus

A general review of the stages and development of a fetus may assist to demonstrate the importance of taking only those drugs prescribed by a physician.

First Trimester: This consists of the first 3 months of pregnancy. During the first 6 weeks, the baby is referred to as an embryo. The heart, lungs, and brain are beginning to develop, and the heart will begin to beat by the 25th day. During the second month the embryo becomes a fetus. At this time organs are developing as well as arms, fingers, legs, and toes. The brain is developing and growing rapidly, and ears and hair may be evident on the head. By the third month, the fetus is moving hands, legs, and head. Fingernails and toenails are developing, and the mouth opens and closes.

Second trimester: This period marks the 15th week of pregnancy. During this period the fetus grows rapidly, and you may hear the baby's heartbeat and feel movement. The baby is fully formed by the sixth month.

Third Trimester: This period marks the 25th week of pregnancy. During this time the fetus continues to grow and gain weight.

The first trimester is the most critical during a pregnancy. It is at this time that most women may be taking medication already and find out that they are pregnant. Early prenatal care should be stressed. Only those medications prescribed by a physician should be taken. Many women use OTC

*The term is used here in a broad sense and includes street drugs, alcohol, nicotine, and certain pollutants.

medicines, such as cold medicines, laxatives, aspirin, and nose-sprays, without realizing the impact on the fetus. This practice should be discouraged, and the pregnant mother should be educated concerning the potential effects of any medication during pregnancy.

LACTATION

The rate of transfer of drugs into breast milk depends on whether or not the drug is lipid soluble, its molecular weight, the degree of protein binding, degree of ionization, and the presence or absence of active secretion.

   As a rule, a woman who is breast feeding should not take any pharmacologic agent unless specifically ordered or permitted by her physician. This warning also applies to both prescription and OTC drugs. If drug therapy is required, nursing mothers should take only the prescribed minimum amount of drug necessary to be effective in treating the condition. The nurse should explain this information to nursing mothers.

CHAPTER EIGHT

Nursing Process for Teaching and Promoting Compliance with Medication Regimen

ASSESSMENT

The assessment phase is the first step of the nursing process and begins with taking the nursing and drug history. This information may be obtained from the client, a family member, a significant other, and/or from the client's medical records. Also, assess the client's personality, personal motivation, experiential background, ability to learn, and willingness to change by examining four factors influencing teaching and learning.

1. **Physical.** Appraise weakness, immobility, ability to swallow.
2. **Psychologic.** Discuss understanding and acceptance of condition and therapy.
3. **Sociocultural.** Explore priorities, values, class, economic situation, and lifestyle.
4. **Environmental.** Evaluate physical surroundings and family members.

NURSING DIAGNOSIS

A nursing diagnosis can usually be formulated once all the assessment data have been collected and analyzed. A variety of physical, psychosocial, and environmental factors may have an impact on clients and their support systems; therefore, more than one nursing diagnosis may be generated and applicable. Some potential nursing diagnosis related to medication administration may include areas related to knowledge deficit, noncompliance, anxiety, pain, and altered body image.

PLANNING

The planning phase of the nursing process involves setting clear, specific goals with the client/family and jointly identifying appropriate methods or strategies for achieving these goals. Use assessment in all planning to promote drug compliance.

1. Set up mutually agreeable goals with the client/family. For example, if the physician's order is for Lente insulin 30 units o.d. before breakfast, a mutual goal might be for the client to be able to self-administer insulin.
2. Develop a teaching plan to promote compliance.
   - Identify behavioral objectives for the teaching-learning process. State what the client should be able to do after the teaching-learning process (e.g., "after the teaching-learning process the client will be able to self-administer insulin").
   - Select appropriate methodology for teaching and promoting compliance (e.g., one-to-one, hands-on, return demonstration, lecture, discussion, movies, slides).
   - Always provide for client/family observation times during self-administration. This is to ensure that the intended procedure is performed correctly, and also to identify and answer any questions or problems that may arise before the client is sent home.

8

IMPLEMENTATION

The implementation phase of the nursing process involves initiating actions necessary to attain goals (i.e., teaching and promoting compliance).

1. *Do not rush clients.* Allow them to learn at their rate.
2. Select an area without distractions, where teaching can be effective.

3. Emphasize the reward of maintained health status or improved health status to be achieved by taking medications as ordered, because motivation is of primary importance in achieving drug compliance.

4. Explain the rationale for using the specific medication regimen and rationale for route(s) of administration.

5. Provide client/family with clear, simple verbal and written directions. (Written directions must be large enough to be legible for client.)

6. Determine if client can read and at what level. Provide clear, legible cards with information about name of drug, reason for use, untoward reactions, dosage, frequency of administration, and appropriate action to be taken for untoward reactions; write at a level that the client can understand. If client cannot read, perhaps an audiotape with step-by-step verbal instructions would be a safe alternative.

7. Provide a check-off calendar for client indicating day and time medication is to be taken.

8. Encourage client to associate taking medication with daily events; for example, medication after meals.

9. Provide small containers and label for hours of day client is to take medications. Teach client to stock each container with appropriate medication once a day so that medications will be organized for the entire day. This technique is particularly helpful for clients with poor memory.

10. Provide containers for each day of the week, and put in medications to be taken on specific days for client who has difficulty organizing or handling medications.

11. Arrange for financial assistance if client is financially unable to purchase medication or equipment needed.

12. Use equipment that may be purchased and replaced easily.

13. Use equipment that is easy to handle and adaptable to home use.

14. Note number of tablets/capsules or amount of solution that client receives from pharmacist.

15. Teach appropriate technique for administration of medication.

16. Observe return demonstration by client. Preferably, a family member or significant other should be present during this return demonstration. Have client and/or family member repeat as necessary until performed correctly and all questions are answered.

17. Include a family member or significant other as part of the support system for helping a client achieve compliance with medication regimen.

EVALUATION

The evaluation phase of the nursing process involves evaluating the attainment of goals and the outcome of teaching and drug therapies.

1. Arrange for follow-up care at appropriate intervals.

2. Evaluate:
   - Client's attitude toward self, illness, medication regimen, and compliance by assessing verbal and nonverbal communication.
   - For possible therapeutic effects.
   - For possible side effects.
   - For knowledge of medication regimen and ability to administer medication correctly.

- For correct dosage utilization by counting the number of tablets/capsules or amount of solution remaining and comparing results to the amount issued by pharmacist.
- The effectiveness of your teaching. Request a demonstration of what and how the patient has been doing with prescribed therapy at home. Preferably have a family member or significant other present at this return demonstration. Identify any problems and correct as necessary.

3. Praise client for compliance with medication/treatment regimen when success is demonstrated.

4. Refer those clients who appear to lack motivation or ability to carry out regimen as prescribed to a home health agency for further intervention by a community health nurse.

PART TWO
Anti-Infectives

INTRODUCTION

General Statement: The beginning of modern medicine is generally related to two events: the proof by Pasteur that many diseases are caused by microorganisms and the discovery of effective anti-infective drugs. The first of these drugs were the sulfonamides (1938), followed by penicillin during the early 1940s. Since then, dozens of anti-infectives have been added to the list. Moreover, significant progress has been made in the development of antiviral drugs.

Unfortunately, the advent of the anti-infectives has not been a pure panacea. Some of the bacteria and other microorganisms have adapted to the anti-infectives, and there has been a gradual emergence of bacteria resistant to certain anti-infectives, especially the antibiotics. Fortunately, most resistant strains can be eradicated by new and/or different antibiotics, antibiotic combinations, or higher dosages. Nevertheless, awareness of the problem has prompted somewhat greater scrutiny by the physician as to when and how to prescribe antibiotics.

The following general guidelines apply to the use of most anti-infective drugs:

1. Anti-infective drugs can be divided into those that are *bacteriostatic*—arrest the multiplication and further development of the infectious agent—or *bactericidal*—eradicate all living microorganisms. Both time of administration and length of therapy may be affected by this difference.
2. Some anti-infectives halt the growth of or eradicate many different microorganisms and are termed *broad-spectrum antibiotics*. Others affect only certain specific organisms and are termed *narrow-spectrum antibiotics*.
3. Some of the anti-infectives elicit a hypersensitivity reaction in some persons. Penicillins cause more severe and more frequent hypersensitivity reactions than any other drug.
4. Because of differences in susceptibility of infectious agents to anti-infectives, the sensitivity of the microorganism to the drug ordered should be determined before treatment is initiated. Several sensitivity tests are commonly used for this purpose. The most widely used test—the Kirby-Bauer or disk-diffusion test—gives qualitative results; there are also various quantitative tests aimed at determining the minimal inhibitory concentration (MIC).

2

5. Certain anti-infective agents have marked side effects; some of the more serious of which are neurotoxicity, including ototoxicity, and nephrotoxicity. Care must be taken not to administer two anti-infectives with similar side effects concomitantly, or to administer these drugs to clients in whom the side effects might be damaging (e.g., a nephrotoxic drug to a client suffering from kidney disease). The choice of anti-infective depends also on its distribution in the body (i.e., whether it passes the blood-brain barrier).

6. Another difficulty associated with anti-infective therapy is that these drugs can eradicate the normal intestinal flora necessary for proper digestion, synthesis of vitamin K, and control of fungi that may gain access to the GI tract (superinfection).

Action/Kinetics: The mechanism of action of the anti-infectives varies. The following modes of action have been identified.* Note that there is considerable overlap among these mechanisms:

1. Interference with bacterial cell wall.
   - Inhibition of an enzyme necessary for formation of the cell wall, resulting in cell wall lysis.
   - Activation of an enzyme interfering with formation of the cell wall, resulting in cell wall lysis.
   - Direct action on the cell wall affecting permeability of the cell wall.
2. Interference with intracellular ribosomes, and therefore with protein synthesis.
3. Binding of the drug to a specific ribosomal subunit, which initiates the formation of abnormal polypeptides and proteins.
4. Interference with nucleic acid metabolism, and therefore with protein synthesis.
5. Interference with specific metabolic steps essential to the survival of microorganisms.

Uses: Antibiotics as a group are effective against most bacterial pathogens, as well as against some of the rickettsias and a few of the larger viruses. They are ineffective against viruses that cause influenza, hepatitis, and the common cold. Other anti-infectives are effective against a number of parasites, including helminths, the malarial parasite, fungi, trichomonas, and others.

The choice of the anti-infective depends on the nature of the illness to be treated, the sensitivity of the infecting agent, and the client's previous experience with the drug. Hypersensitivity and allergic reactions may preclude the use of the agent of choice.

In addition to their use in acute infections, anti-infectives may be given prophylactically in the following instances:

1. To protect persons exposed to a known specific organism.
2. To prevent secondary bacterial infections in acutely ill clients suffering from infections unresponsive to antibiotics.
3. To reduce risk of infection in clients suffering from various chronic illnesses.
4. To inhibit spread of infection from a clearly defined focus, as after accidents or surgery.
5. To "sterilize" the bowel or other areas of the body in preparation for extensive surgery.

Instead of using a single agent, the physician may sometimes prefer to prescribe a combination of anti-infective agents.

Contraindications: Hypersensitivity or allergic reaction to certain anti-infectives is common and may preclude the use of a particular agent.

* Sande MA, Mandell GL: Antimicrobial agents. In *The Pharmacological Basis of Therapeutics, 7th ed*. Edited by Gilman AG, Goodman LS, Rau TW. New York, Macmillan, 1985, p. 1067.

Untoward Reactions: The antibiotics and anti-infective agents have few direct toxic effects. Kidney and liver damage, deafness, and blood dyscrasias are observed occasionally.

However, the following undesirable manifestations occur frequently:

1. Antibiotic therapy often suppresses the normal flora of the body, which in turn keeps certain pathogenic microorganisms, such as *Candida albicans, Proteus,* or *Pseudomonas,* from causing infections. If the flora is altered, *superinfections* (monilial vaginitis, enteritis, urinary tract infections), which necessitate the discontinuation of therapy or the use of other antibiotics, can result.

2. Incomplete eradication of an infectious organism can occur. Casual use of anti-infectives favors the emergence of *resistant* strains insensitive to a particular drug. Often, resistant strains are either mutants of the original infectious agents that have developed a slightly different metabolic pathway and can exist in spite of the antibiotic, or are variants that have developed the ability to release a chemical substance—for instance, the enzyme penicillinase—that can destroy the antibiotic.

In order to minimize the chances for the development of resistant strains, anti-infectives are given usually for a prescribed length of time after acute symptoms have subsided. Casual use of antibiotics is discouraged for the same reasons.

Laboratory Tests: The bacteriologic sensitivity of the infectious organism to the anti-infective (especially the antibiotic) should be tested by the laboratory before initiation of therapy and during treatment.

NURSING CONSIDERATIONS

See *General Nursing Considerations For All Anti-Infectives* under *Penicillins,* p. 140.

Administration/Storage

1. Check expiration date on container.
2. Check for recommended method of storage for the drug and store accordingly.
3. Clearly mark the date and time of reconstitution, your initials, and the strength of solutions of all drugs. Note the length of time that the drug may be stored after dilution and store under appropriate conditions.
4. Complete the administration of anti-infective agents by Volutrol (or as ordered) before the drug loses potency.

CHAPTER NINE

Antibiotics

Penicillins

Polymyxins

Tetracyclines

9

AMINOGLYCOSIDES

General Statement: The aminoglycosides are broad-spectrum antibiotics, primarily used for the treatment of serious gram-negative infections caused by *Pseudomonas, Escherichia coli, Proteus, Klebsiella,* and *Enterobacter.* Aminoglycoside antibiotics are distributed in the extracellular fluid, and cross the placental barrier, but not the blood-brain barrier. Penetration of the cerebro-spinal fluid (CSF) is increased when the meninges are inflamed.

The aminoglycosides are excreted, largely unchanged, in the urine. This makes the drugs suitable for urinary tract infections. Concomitant administration of bicarbonate (alkalization of urine) improves the treatment of such infections. There is considerable cross-allergenicity among the aminoglycosides. These drugs are powerful antibiotics that can induce serious side effects. They should not be used for minor infections. Except for streptomycin, resistance of the organisms to aminoglycosides develops slowly. Whenever possible, the sensitivity of the infectious agent should be determined before instituting therapy.

Action/Kinetics: Aminoglycosides are believed to inhibit protein synthesis by binding irreversibly to ribosomes (30S subunit), thereby interfering with an initiation complex between messenger RNA and the 30S subunit. This leads to production of nonfunctional proteins; polyribosomes are split apart and are unable to synthesize protein. The aminoglycosides are usually bactericidal as a result of disruption of the bacterial cytoplasmic membrane.

The aminoglycosides are poorly absorbed from the GI tract and, therefore, are usually administered parenterally, the only occasional exceptions being some enteric infections of the GI tract and prior to surgery. They are absorbed also from the peritoneum, bronchial tree, wounds, denuded skin, and joints.

The aminoglycosides are absorbed rapidly after IM injection. **Peak plasma levels:** Are attained usually ½–2 hr after IM administration. Measurable levels persist for 8–12 hr after a single administration. **t½:** 2–3 hr. This value increases sharply in patients with impaired kidney function. Ranges of t½ from 24 to 110 hr have been observed. The drug is excreted mainly unchanged in urine.

Uses: Gram-negative bacteria causing bone and joint infections, septicemia (including neonatal sepsis), skin and soft tissue infections (including those from burns), respiratory tract infections, postoperative infections, intra-abdominal infections (including peritonitis), urinary tract infections. In combination with clindamycin for mixed aerobic-anaerobic infections. Also, see individual drugs.

They should be used for gram-positive bacteria only when other less toxic drugs are either ineffective or contraindicated. Their use in CNS *Pseudomonas* infections such as meningitis or ventriculitis is questionable.

Contraindications: Hypersensitivity to aminoglycosides, long-term therapy (except streptomycin for tuberculosis). Use with extreme caution in patients with impaired renal function or preexisting hearing impairment. Safe use in pregnancy and during lactation not established.

Special Concerns

Premature infants, neonates, and older clients receiving aminoglycosides should be assessed closely as they are particularly sensitive to their toxic effects.

Side Effects: *Ototoxicity:* Both auditory and vestibular damage have been noted. The risk of ototoxicity and vestibular impairment is increased in patients with poor renal function and in the elderly. Auditory symptoms include tinnitus and hearing impairment, while vestibular symptoms include dizziness, nystagmus, vertigo, and ataxia.

Renal Impairment: This may be characterized by cylindruria, oliguria, proteinuria, azotemia, hematuria, increase or decrease in frequency of urination; increased BUN, nonprotein nitrogen, or creatinine; and increased thirst. *Neurotoxicity:* Neuromuscular blockade, headache, tremor, lethargy, paresthesia, peripheral neuritis (numbness, tingling, or burning of face/mouth), arachnoiditis, encephalopathy, acute organic brain syndrome. CNS depression, characterized by stupor, flaccidity, and, rarely, coma, and respiratory depression in infants. Optic neuritis with blurred vision or loss of vision. *GI:* Nausea, vomiting, diarrhea, increased salivation, anorexia, weight loss. *Allergic:* Rash, urticaria, pruritus, burning, fever, stomatitis, eosinophilia. Rarely, agranulocytosis and anaphylaxis. Cross-allergy among aminoglycosides has been observed. *Miscellaneous:* Joint pain, laryngeal edema, pulmonary fibrosis, superinfection.

Drug Interactions

Bumetanide	↑ Risk of ototoxicity
Capreomycin	↑ Muscle relaxation
Cephalosporins	↑ Risk of renal toxicity
Ciprofloxacin HCl	Additive antibacterial activity
Cisplatin	Additive renal toxicity
Colistimethate	↑ Muscle relaxation
Digoxin	Possible ↑ or ↓ effect of digoxin
Ethacrynic acid	↑ Risk of ototoxicity
Furosemide	↑ Risk of ototoxicity
Methoxyflurane	↑ Risk of renal toxicity
Penicillins	↓ Effect of aminoglycosides
Polymyxins	↑ Muscle relaxation
Skeletal muscle relaxants (surgical)	↑ Muscle relaxation
Vancomycin	Additive ototoxicity and renal toxicity
Vitamin A	↓ Effect of vitamin A due to ↓ absorption from GI tract

Laboratory Test Interferences: ↑ BUN, Bromsulphalein (BSP) retention, creatinine, serum glutamic-oxaloacetic transaminase (SGOT), serum glutamic-pyruvic transaminase (SGPT), bilirubin. ↓ Cholesterol values.

NURSING CONSIDERATIONS

See also *Nursing Considerations For All Anti-Infectives under Penicillins,* p. 140.

Administration/Storage

1. Check expiration date.
2. Warn the client if the particular drug being administered tends to sting or cause a burning sensation.
3. IM administration.
   - Inject drug deep into muscle mass to minimize transient pain.
   - Use a Z track method for thin, elderly clients.
4. IV administration.
   - Dilute with the appropriate compatible solution.
   - Infuse at the rate ordered to prevent excessive serum concentrations.
5. Administer for only 7–10 days and avoid repeating course of therapy unless serious infection is present that does not respond to other antibiotics.

Assessment

1. Assess for any history of adverse reactions and hypersensitivity to anti-infective medications.
2. Weigh client prior to administering medication to ensure correct calculation of dosage.
3. Assess baseline auditory function.
4. Obtain lab studies for renal function levels.
5. Assess renal, auditory, and vestibular function before and regularly during drug administration.

Interventions

1. Monitor intake and output and ensure adequate fluid intake.
2. During therapy, monitor serum drug levels and if levels are elevated, withhold drug and notify the physician. For example, in clients receiving amikacin, blood levels that exceed 30 mcg/mL are considered toxic.
3. Protect client with vestibular dysfunction by supervising ambulation and providing side rails if necessary. Flag chart with (potential for) fall hazard.
4. Continue to monitor for ototoxicity, because the onset of deafness may occur several weeks after the aminoglycoside has been discontinued.
5. Rotate and document injection sites.
6. Do not administer concurrently or sequentially with a topical or systemic nephrotoxic or ototoxic drug (e.g., potent diuretics such as ethacrynic acid or furosemide) unless physician determines that the benefits outweigh the risks.

Client/Family Teaching

1. Review goals of therapy with client and appropriate method of drug administration.
2. Discuss potential side effects and stress the importance of notifying physician if any of these occur, because drug may need to be discontinued.
3. Teach client/family the importance of following a balanced diet and maintenance of good nutrition.
4. Discuss with client/family the importance of taking medications at the appropriate prescribed time intervals.
5. Stress that any alterations in hearing, vision, and/or ambulation should be reported immediately.

Evaluation

1. Assess
   - Client knowledge and understanding and response to teaching.
   - For signs of ototoxicity; pretreatment audiograms may be helpful in evaluating this problem. Subjective hearing loss or loss of high tones on the audiometer is most common with kanamycin and neomycin. Tinnitus and vertigo are signs of vestibular injury more common with gentamicin and streptomycin.
   - For neuromuscular blockade with muscular weakness leading to apnea, when aminoglycoside is administered together with a muscle relaxant or after anesthesia. Have calcium gluconate or neostigmine available to reverse blockade.
   - For presence of cells or casts in urine, oliguria, proteinuria, lowered specific gravity, or increasing BUN, nonprotein nitrogen, or creatinine, all indicators of altered renal function.
2. Monitor serum drug levels and notify physician if toxic levels are reported. Physician will either reduce dosage or discontinue medication.

AMIKACIN SULFATE   (am-ih-**KAY**-sin)

Amikin (Rx)

See also *Anti-Infectives,* p. 71, and *Aminoglycosides,* p. 75.

Classification: Antibiotic, aminoglycoside.

Action/Kinetics: Amikacin is derived from kanamycin. Its spectrum is somewhat broader than that of other aminoglycosides, including *Serratia* and *Acinetobacter* species, as well as certain staphylococci and streptococci. Amikacin is effective against both penicillinase- and nonpenicillinase-producing organisms. **Therapeutic serum levels: IM,** 8–16 mcg/mL after 45–120 min. **t½:** 2–3 hr.

Special Concerns: Pregnancy category: D. Use with caution in premature infants and neonates.

Dosage: IM (preferred) and **IV, adults, children, and older infants:** 15 mg/kg/day in 2–3 equally divided doses q 8–12 hr for 7–10 days; **maximum daily dose:** 15 mg/kg. *Uncomplicated urinary tract infections:* 250 mg b.i.d.; **newborns:** loading dose of 10 mg/kg followed by 7.5 mg/kg q 12 hr. *Impaired renal function:* normal loading dose of 7.5 mg/kg; **then** administration should be monitored by serum level of amikacin (35 mcg/mL maximum) or creatinine clearance rates. Duration of treatment: **Usual:** 7–10 days.

NURSING CONSIDERATIONS

See also *Nursing Considerations* for *Aminoglycosides,* p. 77.

Administration/Storage (for IV Administration)

1. Add 500-mg vial to 200 mL of sterile diluent, such as normal saline or D₅W.
2. Administer over a 30- to 60-min period for children and adults.
3. Administer to infants in the amount of fluid ordered by the doctor. The IV administration to infants should be over 1–2 hr.
4. Store colorless liquid at room temperature for no longer than 2 years.
5. Potency is not affected if the solution turns a light yellow.

GENTAMICIN SULFATE (jen-tah-MY-sin)

Cidomycin ✸, Garamycin, Garamycin Intrathecal, Garamycin IV Piggyback, Garamycin Ophthalmic, Garamycin Pediatric, Genoptic Ophthalmic, Genoptic S.O.P. Ophthalmic, Gentacidin, Gentafair, Gent-AK, Gentamicin, Gentamicin Ophthalmic, Gentamicin Sulfate IV Piggyback, Jenamicin, Pediatric Gentamicin Sulfate (Rx)

See also *Aminoglycosides,* p. 75.

Classification: Antibiotic, aminoglycoside.

Action/Kinetics: Therapeutic serum levels: IM, 4–8 mcg/mL. Prolonged serum levels above 12 mcg/mL should be avoided **t½:** 2 hr. The drug can be used concurrently with carbenicillin for the treatment of serious *Pseudomonas* infections. However, the drugs should not be mixed in the same flask because carbenicillin will inactivate gentamicin.

Uses: Gentamicin is the drug of choice for hospital-acquired gram-negative sepsis (including neonatal sepsis). In combination with carbenicillin for life-threatening infections caused by *Pseudomonas aeruginosa.* Serious staphylococcal infections.

Special Concerns: Pregnancy category: C. Use with caution in premature infants and neonates.

Additional Side Effects: Muscle twitching, numbness, seizures, increased blood pressure, alopecia, purpura, pseudotumor cerebri.

Additional Drug Interaction: With carbenicillin or ticarcillin, gentamicin may result in increased effect when used for *Pseudomonas* infections.

Dosage: IM (usual), IV. Adults with normal renal function: 1 mg/kg q 8 hr, up to 5 mg/kg daily in life-threatening infections; **children:** 2–2.5 mg/kg q 8 hr; **infants and neonates:** 2.5 mg/kg q 8 hr; **premature infants or neonates less than 1 week of age:** 2.5 mg/kg q 12 hr. *Prevention of bacterial endocarditis, dental or respiratory tract procedures:* **Adults:** 1.5 mg/kg gentamicin (not to exceed 80 mg) plus 1 g ampicillin, each IM or IV, 30–60 min before the procedure; one additional dose of each can be given 8 hr later (alternative: penicillin V, 1 g PO, 6 hr after initial dose). *Prophylaxis of bacterial endocarditis in GI or GU tract procedures or surgery:* **Adults,** 1.5 mg/kg gentamicin (not to exceed 80 mg) plus 2 g ampicillin, each IM or IV, 30–60 min before procedure; dose should be repeated 8 hr later. **Children:** 2 mg/kg gentamicin plus penicillin G, 30,000 units/kg, or ampicillin, 50 mg/kg in same dosage interval as for adults. Pediatric dosage should not exceed single or 24-hr adult doses. *Note:* In patients allergic to penicillin, vancomycin, 1 g IV given slowly over 1 hr, may be substituted; the dose of vancomycin should be repeated 8–12 hr later. **Adults with impaired renal function:** to calculate interval (hr) between doses, multiply serum creatinine level (mg/100 mL) by 8. **IV:** *Septicemia,* **initially,** 1–2 mg/kg infused over 30–60 min; **then,** maintenance doses may be administered. **Intrathecal** (*for meningitis*): **Use only the intrathecal preparation. Adults, usual:** 4–8 mg once daily; **children and infants 3 months and older:** 1–2 mg once daily.

Ophthalmic solution (0.3%): *Acute infections:* **initially,** 1–2 drops in conjunctival sac q 15–30 min; **then,** as infection improves, reduce frequency. *Moderate infections:* 1–2 drops in conjunctival sac 2–6 times daily. *Trachoma:* 2 drops in each eye b.i.d.–q.i.d.; treatment should be continued for up to 1–2 months. **Ophthalmic ointment (0.3%):** Depending on the severity of infection, ½ inch ribbon from q 3–4 hr to 2–3 times daily.

Topical Cream/Ointment (0.1%): Apply 1–5 times daily to affected area. The area may be covered with a sterile bandage.

NURSING CONSIDERATIONS

See also *Nursing Considerations* for *Aminoglycosides,* p. 77.

Administration/Storage

1. For intermittent IV administration, the adult dose should be diluted in 50–200 mL of sterile 5% dextrose in water or isotonic saline and administered over a 30–120 min period. The volume should be less for infants and children.
2. Gentamicin should not be mixed with other drugs for parenteral use.
3. For parenteral use, the duration of treatment is 7–10 days, although a longer course of therapy may be required for severe or complicated infections.
4. When used intrathecally, the usual site is the lumbar area.
5. With topical administration:
   - Remove the crusts of impetigo contagiosa before applying ointment to permit maximum contact between antibiotic and infection.
   - Apply ointment gently and cover with gauze dressing if desirable or as ordered.
   - Avoid further contamination of infected skin.

KANAMYCIN SULFATE   (kan-ah-MY-sin)

Anamid✽, Kantrex, Klebcil (Rx)

See also *Anti-Infectives,* p. 71, and *Aminoglycosides,* p. 75.

Classification: Antibiotic, aminoglycoside, and antitubercular agent (tertiary).

Action/Kinetics: The activity of kanamycin resembles that of neomycin and streptomycin. **Therapeutic serum levels: IM,** 8–16 mcg/mL. **t¹/₂:** 2–3 hr.

Uses: Adjunct in treatment of tuberculosis. Orally for hepatic encephalopathy to inhibit ammonia-forming bacteria in the GI tract. Orally to prepare the intestine prior to surgery. Peritoneally to irrigate infected wounds, cavities, surgical sites. As an aerosol for respiratory tract infections.

Special Concerns: Pregnancy category: D. Use with caution in premature infants and neonates.

Additional Side Effects: Sprue-like syndrome with steatorrhea, malabsorption, and electrolyte imbalance.

Additional Drug Interaction: Procainamide ↑ muscle relaxation.

Dosage: Capsules. *Intestinal bacteria suppression:* 1 g q hr for 4 hr; **then,** 1 g q 6 hr for 36–72 hr. *Hepatic coma:* 8–12 g/day in divided doses. **IM, IV. Adults and children:** 15 mg/kg/day in 2–3 equal doses. Maximum daily dose should not exceed 1.5 g regardless of route of administration. For calculating dosage interval (in hours) in patients with impaired renal function, multiply serum creatinine (mg/100 mL) by 9. **Intraperitoneal:** 500 mg diluted in 20 mL sterile distilled water. **Inhalation:** 250 mg in saline—nebulize b.i.d.–q.i.d. **Irrigation of abscess cavities, pleural space, ventricular cavities:** 0.25% solution.
   Tuberculosis. **IM. Adults:** 15 mg/kg once daily. Not recommended for use in children.

NURSING CONSIDERATIONS

See also *Nursing Considerations* for *Aminoglycosides,* p. 77.

Administration

1. Do not mix with any other medication in IV bottle. Administer IV slowly and at concentrations not exceeding 2.5 mg/mL.
2. Unopened vials may change color, but this does not affect potency of drug. Consult pharmacist if unsure of altered vials.
3. Do not mix with other drugs in same syringe for IM injection.
4. Inject deep into large muscle mass to minimize pain and local irritation. Rotate sites of injection. Local irritation may occur with large doses.
5. IV administration is rarely used and must not be used for clients with renal impairment.
6. Drug should not be administered for more than 12 to 14 days.

NEOMYCIN SULFATE   (nee-oh-MY-sin)

Mycifradin Sulfate, Myciguent, Neobiotic, Neo-IM (Rx)

See also *Anti-Infectives,* p. 71, and *Aminoglycosides,* p. 75.

Classification: Antibiotic, aminoglycoside.

Action/Kinetics: Peak plasma levels: PO, 1–4 hr; **Therapeutic serum level:** 5–10 mcg/mL. **t¹/₂:** 2–3 hr.

Uses: PO: Hepatic coma, sterilization of gut prior to surgery, inhibition of ammonia-forming bacteria in GI tract in hepatic encephalopathy. Therapy of intestinal infections due to pathogenic strains of *Escherichia coli,* primarily in children. *Investigational:* Hypercholesterolemia.
   Topical: Used for itching, burning, inflamed skin conditions that are threatened by, or complicated by, a secondary bacterial infection.

Additional Contraindication: Intestinal obstruction (PO).

Special Concerns: Due to the possibility of toxicity, some experts do not recommend the parenteral use of neomycin for any purpose.

Contraindications: Safe use during pregnancy has not been determined.

Additional Side Effects: Sprue-like syndrome with steatorrhea, malabsorption, and electrolyte imbalance. Skin rashes after topical or parenteral administration.

Additional Drug Interactions

Digoxin	↓ Effect of digoxin due to ↓ absorption from GI tract
Penicillin V	↓ Effect of penicillin due to ↓ absorption from GI tract
Procainamide	↑ Muscle relaxation produced by neomycin

Dosage: Oral solution. *Preoperatively in colorectal surgery:* 1 g each of neomycin and erythromycin base for a total of three doses: the first two doses 1 hr apart the afternoon before surgery and the third dose the night before surgery at bedtime. *Hepatic coma, adjunct:* **Adults,** 4–12 g/day in divided doses for 5–6 days; **children:** 50–100 mg/kg/day in divided doses for 5–6 days.

IM. Adults: 15 mg/kg/day in four equal doses, not to exceed 1 g/day. The IM preparation should not be used in infants and children. Maximum course of therapy is 10 days.

Topical Cream, Ointment. Neomycin alone or in combination with other antibiotics (bacitracin or gramicidin) and/or an anti-inflammatory agent (corticosteroid). Apply ointment (0.5%) or cream (0.5%) 1–5 times daily to affected area. If necessary, a bandage may be used to cover the area.

NURSING CONSIDERATIONS

See also *Nursing Considerations* for *Aminoglycosides,* p. 77.

Administration/Storage

1. For IM use, sterile normal saline should be added to the vial to obtain a concentration of 250 mg/mL.
2. Reconstituted neomycin sulfate for IM use should be refrigerated at 2°–8°C (36°–46°F) and used within 1 week.
3. The recommended procedure should be followed to prepare the GI tract for surgery.

Interventions

1. Monitor intake and output and serum electrolyte levels.
2. Have available neostigmine to counteract renal failure, respiratory depression and arrest, side effects that may occur when neomycin is administered intraperitoneally.
3. Anticipate a slight laxative effect produced by oral neomycin. Withhold the drug and consult with physician in case of suspected intestinal obstruction.
4. Anticipate a low-residue diet for preoperative disinfection and, unless contraindicated, a laxative immediately preceding PO administration of neomycin sulfate.
5. Clean the affected area before applying ointment or solution of neomycin.

NETILMICIN SULFATE   (neh-til-**MY**-sin)

Netromycin (Rx)

Classification: Antibiotic, aminoglycoside.

Action/Kinetics: Netilmicin is a semisynthetic aminoglycoside that may be effective in infections resistant to other aminoglycosides **Peak serum levels after IM:** 30–60 min. **Therapeutic serum levels:** 0.5–10 mcg/mL. **t¹/₂:** 2–3 hr.

Additional Uses: Effective against *Salmonella, Shigella,* and *Serratia* species. In combination with carbenicillin or ticarcillin for life-threatening *Proteus aeruginosa* infections.

Special Concerns: Pregnancy category: D. Use with caution in premature infants and neonates.

Dosage: IM, IV. Adults: *Complicated upper respiratory tract infections:* 1.5–2 mg/kg q 12 hr. *Serious systemic infections:* 1.3–2.2 mg/kg q 8 hr or 2–3.25 mg/kg q 12 hr. **Pediatric, 6 weeks–12 years:** 1.8–2.7 mg/kg q 8 hr or 2.7–4 mg/kg q 12 hr; **neonates, less than 6 weeks:** 2–3.25 mg/kg q 12 hr.
   Patients with impaired renal function: Dose individualized based on creatinine clearance; check package insert carefully.

NURSING CONSIDERATIONS

See also *Nursing Considerations* for *Aminoglycosides,* p. 77.

Administration/Storage

1. For IV administration, the dose can be diluted in 50–200 mL of a parenteral solution and given over a period of 30–120 min. For infants and children, the volume of fluid is less.
2. Diluted netilmicin is stable for 72 hr when stored in glass containers either at room temperature or refrigerated.

Interventions

1. Determine the pretreatment weight of the client. For obese clients, an estimate of the lean body mass should be used in dosage calculation.
2. The usual course of therapy is 7–14 days. If longer therapy is indicated, clients should be monitored carefully for changes in auditory, renal, or vestibular function.
3. Because the drug may cause neuromuscular blockade, check rate and quality of respirations at least every 4 hours around the clock during therapy.
4. Measure blood levels carefully in burn clients as they often have altered pharmacokinetics to netilmicin.

PAROMOMYCIN SULFATE   (par-oh-moh-**MY**-sin)

Humatin (Rx)

See also *Aminoglycosides,* p. 75.

Classification: Antibiotic, aminoglycoside.

Action/Kinetics: Paromomycin is obtained from *Streptomyces rimosus forma paromomycina.* Its spectrum of activity resembles that of neomycin and kanamycin. The drug is poorly absorbed from the GI tract and is ineffective against systemic infections when given orally.

Additional Uses: Inhibition of ammonia-forming bacteria in GI tract in hepatic encephalopathy, intestinal amebiasis, preoperative suppression of intestinal flora. *Investigational:* Anthelmintic, to treat *Dientamoeba fragilis, Diphyllobothrium latum, Taenia saginata, T. solium, Dipylidium caninum,* and *Hymenolepis nana*.

Contraindications: Intestinal obstruction.

Special Concerns: Use during pregnancy only if benefits outweigh risks. To be used with caution in the presence of GI ulceration because of possible systemic absorption.

Additional Side Effects: Diarrhea or loose stools. Heartburn, emesis, and pruritus ani. Superinfections, especially by monilia.

Drug Interaction: Penicillin is inhibited by paromomycin.

Dosage: Capsules. *Hepatic coma:* **Adults:** 4 g daily in divided doses for 5–6 days. *Intestinal amebiasis:* **Adults and children:** 25–35 mg/kg/day administered in three doses with meals for 5–10 days. *D. fragilis:* 25–30 mg/kg daily in three divided doses for 1 week. *H. nana:* 45 mg/kg daily for 5–7 days. *D. latum, T. saginata, T. solium, D. caninum:* **Adults:** 1 g q 15 min for a total of four doses; **pediatric:** 11 mg/kg q 15 min for four doses.

NURSING CONSIDERATIONS

See also *Nursing Considerations* for *Aminoglycosides,* p. 77.

Administration/Storage

Do not administer parenterally.

Interventions

1. Administer before or after meals.
2. Report any diarrhea, dehydration and general weakness as drug therapy may need to be interrupted if symptoms are excessive.
3. Monitor serum electrolytes if above symptoms persist.
4. Do not administer concurrently with penicillin.

STREPTOMYCIN SULFATE   (strehp-toe-**MY**-sin)
(Rx)

See also *Aminoglycosides,* p. 75.

Classification: Antibiotic, aminoglycoside.

Action/Kinetics: Like other aminoglycoside antibiotics, streptomycin is distributed rapidly throughout most tissues and body fluids, including necrotic tubercular lesions. **Therapeutic serum levels: IM,** 25 mcg/mL. **t½:** 2–3 hr.

Additional Uses: Tuberculosis in conjunction with other antitubercular agents. Emergence of resistant strains has greatly reduced the usefulness of streptomycin. Also used for tularemia, glanders (*Actinobacillus mallei*), bubonic plague (*Pasteurella pestis*), brucellosis, cholera, and bacterial endocarditis caused by *Hemophilus influenzae*.

Additional Contraindications: Hypersensitivity, contact dermatitis, and exfoliative dermatitis. Do not give to patients with myasthenia gravis.

Special Concerns: Use during pregnancy only if benefits clearly outweigh risks.

Additional Laboratory Test Interference: False + urine glucose determinations with Benedict's solution and Clinitest.

Dosage: IM only. *Tuberculosis (adjunct):* **initial,** 1 g daily with other tuberculostatic drugs; **then,** reduce streptomycin dosage to 1 g 2–3 times/week for minimum of 1 year. **Pediatric:** in combination with other drugs, 20–40 mg/kg once daily (not to exceed 1 g/day). Older, debilitated patients should receive lower dosages. *Bacterial endocarditis due to penicillin-sensitive alpha-hemolytic and nonhemolytic streptococci (with penicillin):* 1 g b.i.d. for 1 week; **then,** 0.5 g b.i.d. for second week. *Enterococcal endocarditis (with penicillin):* 1 g b.i.d. for 2 weeks; **then,** 0.5 g b.i.d. for 4 weeks. *Plague:* 0.5–1 g q 6 hr until patient has no fever for 3 days. *Tularemia:* 0.25–0.5 g q 6 hr for 7–10 days. *Other infections:* **Adults, IM,** 1–4 g/day in divided doses q 6–12 hr, depending on severity of infections; **pediatric:** 20–40 mg/kg/day in divided doses q 6–12 hr.

NURSING CONSIDERATIONS

See also *Nursing Considerations* for *Aminoglycosides,* p. 77.

Administration/Storage

1. Protect hands when preparing drug. Wear gloves if drug is prepared often because it is irritating.
2. In a dry form, the drug is stable for at least 2 years at room temperature.
3. Aqueous solutions prepared without preservatives are stable for at least 1 week at room temperature and for at least 3 months under refrigeration.
4. Use only solutions prepared freshly from dry powder for intrathecal, subarachnoid, and intrapleural administration because commercially prepared solutions contain preservatives harmful to tissues of the CNS and pleural cavity.
5. Commercially prepared, ready-to-inject solutions are for IM use only. These solutions are prepared with phenol and are stable at room temperature for prolonged periods of time.
6. Administer deep into muscle mass to minimize pain and local irritation.
7. Solutions may darken after exposure to light, but this does not necessarily cause a loss in potency. Check with pharmacist if unsure of potency.
8. When injection into the subarachnoid space is required for treatment of meningitis, only solutions made freshly from the dry powder should be used. Commercial solutions may contain preservatives toxic to the CNS.

Interventions

Use Tes-Tape for urine glucose test because Benedict's solution and Fehling's solution can give false + reactions. For more specific results, follow blood sugars with finger sticks.

Client/Family Teaching

Solution is malodorous; inform client that this is normal.

TOBRAMYCIN SULFATE   (toe-brah-MY-sin)

Nebcin, Tobrex Ophthalmic (Rx)

See also *Aminoglycosides,* p. 75

Classification: Antibiotic, aminoglycoside.

Action/Kinetics: This aminoglycoside is similar to gentamicin and can be used concurrently with carbenicillin. **Therapeutic serum levels: IM,** 4–8 mcg/mL. **t½:** 2–2.5 hr.

Additional Uses: Meningitis; neonatal sepsis. **Ophthalmic:** Eye infections, corneal ulcers.

Special Concerns: Pregnancy category: D. Use with caution in premature infants and neonates.

Additional Drug Interactions: With carbenicillin or ticarcillin, tobramycin may have an increased effect when used for *Pseudomonas* infections.

Dosage: IM, IV. Adults: 3 mg/kg/day in 3 equally divided doses q 8 hr; *for life-threatening infections:* up to 5 mg/kg/day in 3 or 4 equal doses. **Pediatric:** Either 2–2.5 mg/kg q 8 hr or 1.5–1.9 mg/kg q 6 hr; **neonates 1 week of age or less:** up to 4 mg/kg/day in 2 equal doses q 12 hr. *Impaired renal function:* **initially,** 1 mg/kg; **then,** maintenance dose calculated according to information supplied by manufacturer.

   Ophthalmic. *Acute infections:* **initial,** 1–2 gtt q 15–30 min until improvement noted; **then,** reduce dosage gradually. *Moderate infections:* 1–2 gtt 2–6 times/day.

NURSING CONSIDERATIONS

See also *Nursing Considerations* for *Aminoglycosides,* p. 77.

Administration/Storage

1. Prepare IV solution by diluting calculated dose of tobramycin with 50–100 mL of IV solution.
2. Infuse over 20–60 min.
3. Use proportionately less diluent for children than for adults.
4. Do not mix with other drugs for parenteral administration.
5. Store drug at room temperature—no longer than 2 years.
6. Discard solution of drug containing up to 1 mg/mL after 24 hr at room temperature.

CEPHALOSPORINS

General Statement: The cephalosporins are semisynthetic antibiotics that resemble the penicillins both chemically and pharmacologically. Some cephalosporins are absorbed rapidly from the GI tract and quickly reach effective concentrations in the urinary, GI, and respiratory tracts except in patients with pernicious anemia or obstructive jaundice. The drugs are eliminated rapidly in patients with normal renal function.

   The cephalosporins are broad-spectrum antibiotics that have been classified as first, second, and third generation drugs. The difference among generations is based on antibacterial spectra; third generation cephalosporins have more activity against gram-negative organisms and resistant organisms and less activity against gram-positive organisms than first generation drugs. Third generation cephalosporins are stable also against beta-lactamases. Cephalosporins can be destroyed by cephalosporinase. Also, the cost increases from first to third generation cephalosporins.

Action/Kinetics: The cephalosporins interfere with a final step in the formation of the bacterial cell wall (inhibition of mucopeptide biosynthesis), resulting in unstable cell membranes that undergo lysis (same mechanism of action as penicillins). Also, cell division and growth are inhibited. The cephalosporins are most effective against young, rapidly dividing organisms. The **t½** ranges from 69 to 132 min, and serum protein binding ranges from 5% to 86%. Cephalosporins are distributed widely to most tissues and fluids. First and second generation drugs do not enter the CSF well, but third generation drugs enter inflamed meninges readily. The cephalosporins are excreted rapidly by the kidneys.

Uses: Cephalosporins are effective against infections of the biliary tract, GI tract, GU system, bones, joints, upper and lower respiratory tract, skin, and skin structures. Also, gynecologic infections, meningitis, osteomyelitis, endocarditis, intra-abdominal infections, peritonitis, otitis media, gonorrhea, septicemia, and prophylaxis prior to surgery. A listing of the organisms against which cephalosporins are effective follows.

First Generation Cephalosporins. Gram-positive cocci including *Staphylococcus aureus, S. epidermidis, S. pyogenes, Streptococcus pneumoniae, S. viridans,* Group A and B streptococci, and anaerobic streptococci. Activity against gram-negative bacteria includes *Escherichia coli, Hemophilus influenzae, Klebsiella,* and *Proteus mirabilis.*

Second Generation Cephalosporins. Spectrum similar to that of first generation cephalosporins. Also active against certain gram-negative bacteria and anaerobes including *Providencia rettgeri, Bacteroides* species, *Peptococcus,* and *Peptostreptococcus* species. Selected second generation cephalosporins are effective against the following species: *Citrobacter, Enterobacter, Providencia, Clostridium, and Fusobacterium,* as well as *Morganella morganii, Neisseria gonorrhoeae,* and *Proteus vulgaris.*

Third Generation Cephalosporins. Less active against gram-positive cocci. Spectrum similar to first and second generation cephalosporins. Most are also active against the following gram-negative and anaerobic species: *Acinetobacter, Citrobacter, Enterobacter, Providencia, Salmonella, Serratia, Shigella, Bacteroides, Clostridium, Fusobacterium, Peptococcus,* and *Peptostreptococcus.* Most are effective against *Morganella morganii, Neisseria gonorrhoeae, Neisseria meningitidis, Proteus vulgaris, Pseudomonas aeruginosa,* and *Bacteroides fragilis.* Selected third generation cephalosporins are effective against *Hemophilus parainfluenzae, Moraxella catarrhalis, Salmonella thypi, Clostridium difficile,* and *Eubacterium* species.

Contraindications: Hypersensitivity to cephalosporins. Patients hypersensitive to penicillin may occasionally cross-react to cephalosporins.

Special Concerns: Safe use in pregnancy and lactation has not been established. Use with caution in the presence of impaired renal or hepatic function or together with other nephrotoxic drugs. Creatinine clearances should be performed on all patients with impaired renal function who receive cephalosporins. Use with caution in patients over 50 years of age.

Side Effects: *GI:* Nausea, vomiting, diarrhea, abdominal cramps or pain, dyspepsia, glossitis, heartburn, sore mouth or tongue, dysgeusia, anorexia, flatulence, cholestasis. Pseudomembranous colitis. *Allergic:* Urticaria, rashes (maculopapular, morbilliform, or erythematous), pruritus (including anal and genital areas), fever, chills, erythema, angioedema, serum sickness, joint pain, exfoliative dermatitis, chest tightness, myalgia, erythema multiforme, edema, itching, numbness, chills, Stevens-Johnson syndrome, anaphylaxis. *Note:* Cross-allergy may be manifested between cephalosporins and penicillins. *Hematologic:* Leukopenia, leukocytosis, lymphocytosis, neutropenia (transient), eosinophilia, thrombocytopenia, thrombocythemia, agranulocytosis, granulocytopenia, bone marrow depression, hemolytic anemia, pancytopenia, decreased platelet function, aplastic anemia, hypoprothrombinemia (may lead to bleeding), thrombocytosis (transient). *CNS:* Headache, malaise, fatigue, vertigo, dizziness, lethargy, confusion, paresthesia. *Hepatic:* Hepatomegaly, hepatitis. Intrathecal use may result in hallucinations, nystagmus, or seizures. *Miscellaneous:* Superinfection including oral candidiasis and enterococcal infections, hypotension, sweating, flushing, dyspnea, interstitial pneumonitis.

IV or IM use may result in local swelling, inflammation, cellulitis, paresthesia, burning, phlebitis, thrombophlebitis. IM use may also cause pain and induration, tenderness, increased temperature. Sterile abscesses have been observed following SC use. Nephrotoxicity (↑ BUN with and without ↑ serum creatinine) may occur in patients over 50 and in young children.

Drug Interactions	
Aminoglycosides	↑ Risk of renal toxicity with certain cephalosporins
Anticoagulants	Certain cephalosporins ↑ prothrombin time
Bacteriostatic agents	↓ Effect of cephalosporins
Bumetanide	↑ Risk of renal toxicity
Colistimethate	↑ Risk of renal toxicity
Colistin	↑ Risk of renal toxicity
Ethacrynic acid	↑ Risk of renal toxicity
Furosemide	↑ Risk of renal toxicity
Polymyxin B	↑ Risk of renal toxicity
Probenecid	↑ Effect of cephalosporins by ↓ excretion by kidneys
Vancomycin	↑ Risk of renal toxicity

Laboratory Test Interferences: False + for urinary glucose with Benedict's solution, Fehling's solution, or Clinitest tablets. Enzyme tests (Clinistix, Tes-Tape) are unaffected. False + Coombs' test and urinary 17-ketosteroids. ↑ AST, ALT, total bilirubin, GGTP, LDH, alkaline phosphatase.

Dosage: See individual drugs.

NURSING CONSIDERATIONS

See also *Nursing Considerations For All Anti-Infectives* under *Penicillins,* p. 140.

Administration/Storage

1. Parenteral solutions infused too rapidly may cause pain and irritation; infuse over 30 minutes unless otherwise indicated.
2. Therapy should be continued for at least 2–3 days after symptoms of infection have disappeared.
3. For Group A beta-hemolytic streptococcal infections, therapy should be continued for at least 10 days to prevent glomerulonephritis or rheumatic fever.

Assessment

1. Assess client with a history of hypersensitivity reaction to penicillin for cross-sensitivity to cephalosporins. Have epinephrine readily available.
2. Assess client's financial status. Many in this group of antibiotics are quite expensive and clients on fixed incomes with limited health benefits may be unable to afford the prescription expense.

Interventions

1. The cephalosporins all have similar sounding and similarly spelled names. Use care when transcribing physician's orders for administration of these drugs and request clarification as needed.
2. Pseudomembranous colitis may occur in clients receiving cephalosporins. If diarrhea develops, report to physician immediately and continue to monitor for signs and laboratory evidence of electrolyte imbalance.
3. Obtain liver and renal function studies and anticipate lower doses for clients with renal impairment. For dialysis clients, administer after treatment.
4. If GI upset occurs, the drug may be administered with meals.
5. Drug may cause a false + Coomb's test. Document appropriately and instruct client.

Client/Family Teaching

1. Emphasize that oral medications should be taken on an empty stomach, unless otherwise directed.
2. Instruct client/family to report any symptoms that may necessitate drug withdrawal, such as vaginal itching or vaginal drainage or diarrhea.
3. Explain that yogurt or buttermilk may be recommended for diarrhea related to intestinal superinfections.
4. Nystatin may be ordered for secondary infections and to take only as directed.
5. Stress the importance of taking medication as ordered and of reporting side effects so that appropriate therapy may be initiated.
6. Explain that medication may cause a false + Coombs' test. This would be of concern if patient is being cross-matched for blood transfusions or in newborns whose mothers have taken cephalosporins during pregnancy.

Evaluation

1. Assess client/family knowledge and understanding of illness, response to therapy and to teaching.
2. Monitor renal and liver function studies to determine if excretion is impaired and function altered.
3. Note status (presence/absence) of pretreatment symptoms and C & S results to determine effectiveness of treatment.

CEFACLOR   (SEF-ah-klor)

Ceclor (Rx)

See also *Anti-Infectives,* p. 71, and *Cephalosporins,* p. 86.

Classification: Antibiotic, cephalosporin (second generation).

Action/Kinetics: Peak serum levels: 5–15 mcg/mL after 1 hr. **t½: PO,** 36–54 min. Well absorbed from GI tract. From 60% to 85% excreted in urine within 8 hr.

Uses: Otitis media. Infections of the upper and lower respiratory tract, urinary tract, skin, and skin structures.

Special Concerns: Pregnancy category: B.

Additional Side Effects: Cholestatic jaundice, lymphocytosis.

Dosage: Capsules, Oral Suspension. Adult: 250 mg q 8 hr. Dose may be doubled in more severe infections or those caused by less susceptible organisms. Total daily dose should not exceed 4 g. **Children:** 20 mg/kg/day in divided doses q 8 hr. Dose may be doubled in more serious infections, otitis media, or for infections caused by less susceptible organisms. Total daily dose should not exceed 1 g. Safety for use in infants less than 1 month of age has not been established.

NURSING CONSIDERATIONS

See *Nursing Considerations* for *Cephalosporins,* p. 88.

Administration/Storage

1. The suspension should be refrigerated after reconstitution and discarded after 2 weeks.
2. The total daily dose for otitis media and pharyngitis can be divided and given q 12 hr.

CEFADROXIL MONOHYDRATE   (sef-ah-**DROX**-ill)

Duricef, Ultracef (Rx)

See also *Anti-Infectives,* p. 71, and *Cephalosporins,* p. 86.

Classification: Antibiotic, cephalosporin (first generation).

Action/Kinetics: Peak serum levels: PO, 15–33 mcg/mL after 90 min. **t½: PO,** 70–80 min. Ninety percent of drug is excreted unchanged in urine within 24 hr.

Uses: Pharyngitis, tonsillitis. Infections of the urinary tract, skin, and skin structures.

Special Concerns: Safe use in children and during pregnancy not established. (Pregnancy category: B.) Creatinine clearance determinations must be carried out in patients with renal impairment.

Dosage: Capsules, Oral Suspension, Tablets. Adults: *Pharyngitis, tonsillitis, skin and skin structure infections:* 1 g daily in single or divided two doses. *Urinary tract infections:* 1–2 g/day in single or two divided doses. **Children:** 30 mg/kg daily in divided doses q 12 hr. **For patients with creatinine clearance rates below 50 mL/min: initial,** 1 g; **maintenance,** 500 mg at following dosage intervals: q 36 hr for creatinine clearance rates of 0–10 mL/min; q 24 hr for creatinine clearance rates of 10–25 mL/min; q 12 hr for creatinine clearance rates of 25–50 mL/min.

NURSING CONSIDERATIONS

See *Nursing Considerations* for *Cephalosporins,* p. 88.

Administration/Storage

1. Cefadroxil can be given without regard to meals.
2. The suspension should be shaken well before using.
3. For beta-hemolytic streptococcal infections, treatment should be continued for 10 days.

CEFAMANDOLE NAFATE   (sef-ah-**MAN**-dole)

Mandol (Rx)

See also *Anti-Infectives,* p. 71, and *Cephalosporins,* p. 86.

Classification: Antibiotic, cephalosporin (second generation).

Action/Kinetics: Cefamandole nafate has a particularly broad spectrum of activity. **Peak serum levels: IM,** 12–36 mcg/mL after 30–120 min. **t½: IM,** 60 min; **IV,** 30 min. From 65% to 85% excreted unchanged in urine.

Uses: Infections of the urinary tract, lower respiratory tract, bones, joints, skin, and skin structures. Mixed infections of the respiratory tract, skin, and in pelvic inflammatory disease. Peritonitis, septicemia, prophylaxis in surgery. Also, with aminoglycosides in gram-positive or gram-negative sepsis.

Special Concerns: Pregnancy category: B. Safety and effectiveness have not been determined in infants less than 1 month of age.

Additional Side Effects: Hypoprothrombinemia leading to bleeding and/or bruising; cholestatic jaundice, decreased creatinine clearance in patients with prior renal impairment.

Additional Drug Interaction: Concomitant use with ethanol produces a disulfiram-type reaction and hypotension.

Dosage: IV or deep IM injection only (in gluteus or lateral thigh to minimize pain). **Adult:** usual, 0.5–1 g q 4–8 hr. *Severe infections:* Up to 2 g q 4 hr. **Infants and children:** 50–100 mg/kg/day in equally divided doses q 4–8 hr. *Severe:* Up to 150 mg/kg/day (not to exceed adult dose) divided as above. *Preoperative:* **Adults: initial,** 1–2 g 30–60 min prior to surgery; **then,** 1–2 g q 6 hr for 1–2 days (3 days for prosthetic arthroplasty). For cesarean section, the first dose should be given just prior to surgery or just after the cord has been clamped. **Pediatric (3 months and older):** 50–100 mg/kg daily in divided doses, using same schedule as for adults. *Impaired renal function:* **initial,** 1–2 g; then a maintenance dosage is given, depending on creatinine clearance, according to schedule provided by manufacturer.

NURSING CONSIDERATIONS

See *Nursing Considerations* for *Cephalosporins,* p. 88.

Administration/Storage

1. Review package insert for details on how to reconstitute drug.
2. Reconstituted solutions of cefamandole nafate are stable for 24 hr at room temperature and for 96 hr when stored in the refrigerator. Cefamandole solutions reconstituted with dextrose or sodium chloride are stable for 6 months when frozen immediately after reconstitution.
3. Carbon dioxide gas forms when reconstituted solutions are kept at room temperature. This gas does not affect the activity of the antibiotic and may be dissipated or used to aid in the withdrawal of the contents of the vial.
4. Use separate IV fluid containers and separate injection sites for each drug when cefamandole is administered concomitantly with another antibiotic such as an aminoglycoside.

CEFAZOLIN SODIUM (seh-FAZ-oh-lin)

Ancef, Kefzol, Zolicef (Rx)

See also *Anti-Infectives,* p. 71, and *Cephalosporins,* p. 86.

Classification: Antibiotic, cephalosporin (first generation).

Action/Kinetics: Peak serum concentration: IM 17–76 mcg/mL after 1 hr. **t½: IM, IV:** 90–130 min. From 80% to 100% excreted unchanged in urine.

Uses: Infections of the urinary tract, biliary tract, respiratory tract, bones, joints, soft tissue, and skin. Endocarditis, septicemia, prophylaxis in surgery.

Special Concerns: Pregnancy category: B.

Additional Side Effects: When high doses are used in renal failure patients: extreme confusion, tonic-clonic seizures, mild hemiparesis.

Dosage: IM, IV only. Adult: *mild infections due to gram-positive cocci:* 250–500 mg q 8 hr; *moderate to severe infections:* 0.5–1 g q 6–8 hr. *Endocarditis, septicemia:* 1–1.5 g q 6 hr (rarely, up to 12 g daily). *Pneumococcal pneumonia:* 0.5 g q 12 hr. *Preoperative:* 1 g 30–60 min prior to surgery. *Acute, uncomplicated urinary tract infections:* 1 g q 12 hr. *Preoperative:* 1 g 30–60 min prior to surgery. *During surgery:* 0.5–1 g. *Postoperative:* 0.5–1 g q 6–8 hr for 24 hr (may be given up to 5 days, especially in open heart surgery or prosthetic arthroplasty). *Impaired renal function:*

initially, 0.5 g; **then,** maintenance doses are given, depending on creatinine clearance, according to schedule provided by manufacturer. **Children over 1 month:** *mild to moderate infections:* 25–50 mg/kg daily in 3–4 doses. *For severe infections,* up to 100 mg/kg daily may be used. Safety in patients under 1 month of age not determined.

NURSING CONSIDERATIONS

See *Nursing Considerations* for *Cephalosporins,* p. 88.

Administration/Storage

1. Dissolve the solute by shaking vial.
2. Discard reconstituted solution after 24 hr at room temperature and after 96 hr when refrigerated.

CEFIXIME, ORAL   (seh-FIX-eem)

Suprax (Rx)

See also *Anti-Infectives,* p. 71, and *Cephalosporins,* p. 86.

Classification: Antibiotic, cephalosporin (third generation).

Action/Kinetics: Stable in the presence of beta-lactamase enzymes. **Peak serum levels:** 2–6 hr. **t½:** averages 3–4 hr. About 50% excreted unchanged in the urine and approximately 10% in the bile. In addition to the microorganisms listed under *Uses* for cephalosporins, cefixime is effective against *Moraxella catarrhalis, Streptococcus agalactiae, Haemophilus parainfluenzae, Pasteurella multocida, Salmonella* species, and *Shigella* species. The following microorganisms are resistant to cefixime: most strains of *Bacteroides fragilis* and clostridia, *Pseudomonas* species, strains of group D *streptococci* including enterococci, *Listeria monocytogenes,* and most strains of staphylococci and *Enterobacter.*

Uses: Uncomplicated urinary tract infections, otitis media, pharyngitis, tonsillitis, acute bronchitis, and acute exacerbations of chronic bronchitis caused by susceptible strains of microorganisms.

Special Concerns: Pregnancy category: B. Safe use in infants less than 6 months has not been established.

Additional Side Effects: *GI:* Flatulence. *Hepatic:* Elevated alkaline phosphatase levels. *Renal:* Transient increases in BUN or creatinine.

Additional Laboratory Test Interference: False + test for ketones using nitroprusside test.

Dosage: Oral Suspension, Tablets. Adults: either 400 mg once daily or 200 mg q 12 hr. **Children:** either 8 mg/kg/day once daily or 4 mg/kg q 12 hr. Patients on renal dialysis or in whom creatinine clearance is between 21 and 60 mL/min, the dose should be 75% of the standard dose (i.e., 300 mg daily). If the creatinine clearance is less than 20 mL/min, the dose should be 50% of the standard dose (i.e., 200 mg daily).

NURSING CONSIDERATIONS

See also *Nursing Considerations* for *Cephalosporins,* p. 88.

Administration/Storage

1. Therapy should be for at least 10 days when treating *S. pyogenes.*
2. Children older than 12 years or weighing more than 50 kg should be given the adult dose.

3. Once reconstituted, the suspension should be kept at room temperature where it maintains potency for 14 days.

Assessment

1. Take drug history, noting any prior sensitivity to cephalosporins or penicillins.
2. Assess client financial status and health care coverage as prescription cost may be prohibitive.

Interventions

1. Anticipate reduced dose with impaired renal function.
2. Use the suspension in children and when treating otitis media.
3. Cefixime may alter results of urine glucose and ketone testing; finger sticks may provide more accurate blood sugar recordings during drug therapy.

Client/Family Teaching

1. Cefixime may cause GI upset; instruct client to report any bothersome side effects, especially persistent diarrhea.
2. Therapy requires only once a day dosing and should be taken at the same time each day.

Evaluation

Note response to therapy, presence/absence of pretreatment symptoms, and results of follow-up C&S.

CEFMETAZOLE SODIUM   (sef-MET-ah-zole)

Zefazone (Rx)

See also *Anti-Infectives,* p. 71, and *Cephalosporins,* p. 86.

Classification: Cephalosporin, (second generation).

Uses: Urinary tract infections, lower respiratory tract infections, skin and skin structure infections, intra-abdominal infections. Preoperatively to decrease incidence of postoperative infections following cesarean section, cholecystectomy (high risk), colorectal surgery, abdominal or vaginal hysterectomy.

Dosage: IV. *Infections:* 2 g q 6–12 hr for 5–14 days. *Prophylaxis, abdominal hysterectomy or high risk cholecystectomy:* 1 g 30–90 min prior to surgery and again 8 and 16 hr following surgery. *Prophylaxis, vaginal hysterectomy:* 2 g 30–90 min prior to surgery or 1 g 30–90 min prior to surgery and again 8 and 16 hr following surgery. *Prophylaxis, cesarean section:* 2 g in a single dose after clamping cord or 1 g after clamping cord and again 8 and 16 hr later. *Prophylaxis, colorectal surgery:* 2 g 30–90 min prior to surgery or 2 g 30–60 min prior to surgery and again 8 and 26 hr following surgery. Dosage and frequency must be reduced in patients with impaired renal function.

NURSING CONSIDERATIONS

See also *Nursing Considerations* for *Cephalosporins,* p. 88.

Administration/Storage:

1. The drug should be reconstituted with sterile water for injection, bacteriostatic water for injection, or 0.9% sodium chloride injection.

2. After reconstitution, the drug is stable for 24 hr at room temperature, for 7 days if refrigerated, and for 6 weeks if frozen.

3. If necessary, the reconstituted solution may be further diluted to concentrations of 1–20 mg/mL with 0.9% sodium chloride injection, 5% dextrose injection, or lactated Ringer's injection. Such solutions are stable as described above.

4. Thawed solutions should not be refrozen.

5. Any unused solutions or frozen material should be discarded.

Interventions

Obtain baseline renal function studies and anticipate reduced dose and frequency of administration of cefmetazole with impaired renal function.

CEFONICID SODIUM   (seh-**FAHN**-ih-sid)

Monocid (Rx)

See also *Anti-Infectives,* p. 71, and *Cephalosporins,* p. 86.

Classification: Antibiotic, cephalosporin (second generation).

Uses: Infections of the lower respiratory tract, urinary tract, bones, joints, skin, and skin structures. Septicemia. Prophylaxis in surgery, especially colorectal surgery, vaginal hysterectomy, cholecystectomy, prosthetic arthroplasty, open heart surgery, cesarean section after the cord has been clamped.

Special Concerns: Pregnancy category: B.

Dosage: IV, Deep IM. Adults. *Uncomplicated urinary tract infections:* 0.5 g once/day. *Mild to moderate infections:* 1 g once/day. *Severe or life-threatening infections:* 2 g once/day. *Prophylaxis in surgery:* **Adults:** 1 g 1 hr prior to surgery; dosage may be repeated for 2 more days if required. In renal impairment: **initial,** 7.5 mg/kg given **IV or IM; then,** follow schedule provided by manufacturer.

NURSING CONSIDERATIONS

See *Nursing Considerations* for *Cephalosporins,* p. 88.

Administration/Storage

1. If 2 g is required IM, half the dose should be given in different large muscle masses.

2. For IV bolus, cefonicid should be given slowly over 3–5 min either through IV tubing or directly, by the physician.

3. For IV infusion, reconstitute in 50–100 mL of appropriate diluent (see package insert). Solutions are stable for 24 hr at room temperature and 72 hr if refrigerated.

CEFOPERAZONE SODIUM   (sef-oh-**PER**-ah-zone)

Cefobid, Cefobine ✿ (Rx)

See also *Anti-Infectives,* p. 71, and *Cephalosporins,* p. 86.

Classification: Antibiotic, cephalosporin (third generation).

Action/Kinetics: Peak serum levels: 73–153 mcg/mL. **t½:** 102–156 min. Approximately 30% excreted unchanged in the urine.

Uses: Infections of skin, skin structures, urinary tract, and respiratory tract. Intra-abdominal infections including peritonitis. Bacterial septicemia, pelvic inflammatory disease, endometritis, other infections of the female genital tract.

Special Concerns: Pregnancy category: B. Use with caution in hepatic disease or biliary obstruction. Safety and effectiveness have not been determined in children.

Additional Side Effects: Hypoprothrombinemia resulting in bleeding and/or bruising.

Additional Drug Interaction: Concomitant use with ethanol may cause an Antabuse-like reaction.

Dosage: IM, IV. Adult, usual: 2–4 g daily in divided doses q 12 hr (up to 12–16 g daily has been used in severe infections or for less sensitive organisms). *Note:* This drug is significantly excreted in the bile; thus, the daily dose should not exceed 4 g in hepatic disease or biliary obstruction.

NURSING CONSIDERATIONS

See also *Nursing Considerations* for *Cephalosporins,* p. 88.

Administration/Storage

1. Following reconstitution, the solution should be allowed to stand for dissipation of any foaming and to determine if complete solubilization has occurred. Vigorous shaking may be necessary to dissolve higher concentrations.
2. Reconstituted drug may be frozen; however, after thawing, any unused portion should be discarded.
3. The unreconstituted powder should be protected from light and stored in the refrigerator.
4. If used for neonates, cefoperazone should not be reconstituted with diluents containing benzyl alcohol.

Assessment

1. Complete nursing history and assess for bruising, hematuria, black stools, or other evidence of bleeding.
2. If client is receiving treatment for skin lesions, inspect lesions closely and note size, location, and extent of involvement.
3. Assess for any evidence/history of excessive use of alcohol.

Client/Family Teaching

1. The client should avoid drinking alcohol for 72 hr after the last dose. An Antabuse-like reaction may occur with the ingestion of alcohol.
2. Review goals of therapy with client/family, note client/family understanding of infection for which client is being treated.
3. Explain the importance of reporting any evidence of bruising or bleeding immediately.

Evaluation

1. Record response to therapy, such as any change in the size of skin lesions.
2. Note client knowledge and understanding of illness and identify any side effects related to therapy.
3. Ensure there is an absence of alcohol intake during therapy.

CEFORANIDE   (seh-FOR-ah-nyd)

Precef (Rx)

See also *Anti-Infectives,* p. 71, and *Cephalosporins,* p. 86.

Classification: Antibiotic, cephalosporin (second generation).

Action/Kinetics: t¹/₂: 2.5–3.5 hr. Over 80% is excreted unchanged in the urine.

Uses: Infections of the lower respiratory tract, urinary tract, bones, joints, skin, and skin structures. Endocarditis, prophylaxis in surgery, septicemia.

Special Concerns: Pregnancy category: B. Safety and effectiveness in children less than 1 year of age have not been determined.

Additional Side Effect: Elevated CPK following IM use.

Dosage: IM, IV. Adults: 0.5–1 g q 12 hr; **pediatric:** 20–40 mg/kg daily in equally divided doses q 12 hr. *Prophylaxis in surgery:* 0.5–1 g 60 min before surgery; may be repeated for 2 days after surgery. For all uses, dosage should be reduced in renal impairment.

NURSING CONSIDERATIONS

See *Nursing Considerations* for *Cephalosporins,* p. 88.

Administration/Storage

1. IM injections should be made into a deep muscle mass.
2. Ceforanide should be used IV in serious or life-threatening infections, such as septicemia.
3. Drug should be administered over 3–5 min if given by direct IV injection or over 30 min if IV infusion is used.

CEFOTAXIME SODIUM   (sef-oh-TAX-eem)

Claforan (Rx)

See also *Anti-Infectives,* p. 71, and *Cephalosporins,* p. 86.

Classification: Antibiotic, cephalosporin (third generation).

Action/Kinetics: Treatment should be continued for a minimum of 10 days for group A beta-hemolytic streptococcal infections to minimize the risk of glomerulonephritis or rheumatic fever. The IV route is preferable for patients with severe or life-threatening infections; for patients after surgery; or for patients manifesting malnutrition, trauma, malignancy, heart failure, or diabetes, especially if shock is present or possible. **t¹/₂:** 1 hr. From 20%–36% is excreted unchanged in the urine.

Uses: Infections of the GU tract, lower respiratory tract (including pneumonia), skin, skin structures, bones, joints, and CNS (including ventriculitis and meningitis). Intra-abdominal infections (including peritonitis), gynecologic infections (including endometritis, pelvic cellulitis, pelvic inflammatory disease), septicemia, bacteremia, and prophylaxis in surgery. Used with aminoglycosides for gram-positive or gram-negative sepsis where the causative agent has not been identified.

Special Concerns: Pregnancy category: B.

Dosage: IV, IM. Adults. *Uncomplicated infections:* 1 g q 12 hr. *Moderate to severe infections:* 1–2 g q 8 hr. *Septicemia:* **IV,** 2 g q 6–8 hr. *Life-threatening infections:* **IV,** 2 g q 4 hr up to 12 g daily.

Gonorrhea: **IM,** single dose of 1 g. *Preoperative prophylaxis:* 1 g 30–90 min prior to surgery. *Cesarean section:* **IV,** 1 g when the umbilical cord is clamped; **then,** give 1 g 6 and 12 hr after the first dose. **Pediatric, 1 month to 12 years, IM, IV:** 50–180 mg/kg daily in 4–6 divided doses; **1–4 weeks, IV:** 50 mg/kg q 8 hr; **0–1 week, IV:** 50 mg/kg q 12 hr. *Note:* Use adult dose in children 50 kg or over. Dosage should be reduced in patients with impaired renal function.

NURSING CONSIDERATIONS

See also *Nursing Considerations* for *Cephalosporins,* p. 88.

Administration/Storage

1. Cefotaxime should not be mixed with aminoglycosides for continuous IV infusion. If they are to be given to the same client, each should be given separately.
2. Cefotaxime is maximally stable at a pH value of 5–7; solutions should not be prepared with diluents having a pH value greater than 7.5 (e.g., sodium bicarbonate injection).
3. Dry cefotaxime should be stored below 30°C and should be protected from excess heat and light to prevent darkening.
4. Add recommended amount of diluent, shake to dissolve, and observe for particles or discoloration of solution. Do not administer if particles are present or if solution is discolored. The normal color of solution ranges from light yellow to amber.
5. For IM use, reconstitute with sterile water for injection or bacteriostatic water for injection. Inject deeply into large muscle. Divide doses of 2 g and administer into different sites.
6. For intermittent IV administration, 1 or 2 g cefotaxime should be mixed with 10 mL sterile water for injection and administered over 3–5 min.
7. Discontinue IV administration of other solutions during administration of cefotaxime.
8. After reconstitution, the drug remains stable for 24 hr at room temperature, 5 days refrigerated, and 13 weeks frozen. Thaw frozen samples at room temperature before use. Do not refreeze unused portions.

Assessment

1. For clients receiving therapy for joint infections, carefully assess the extent of their range of motion and freedom of movement.
2. In clients with gynecological infections, determine how long symptoms have been evident and how extensive the infection is prior to treatment.

Interventions

1. Obtain appropriate lab studies prior to initiating therapy.
2. Maintain careful documentation of the type and extent of infection and subjective complaints.
3. Monitor and record I&O.

Client/Family Teaching

1. Review the drugs that are being prescribed, their side effects, and the expected outcome of therapy.
2. Teach the person administering the drug the appropriate technique for administration and storage.
3. Instruct client/family to monitor and record intake and output and to report any reduction in urinary output to the physician.

4. Diarrhea should be reported to the physician if persistent.

5. Reinforce the need to complete the course of therapy as prescribed despite feeling better.

Evaluation

1. Inspect site of injections for pain and redness. IM administration of these medications may cause thrombophlebitis.

2. Review lab data. Note any evidence of resistance to anti-infective drug therapy.

3. Note client expressions of symptomatic relief.

4. Observe for freedom from complications of drug therapy.

CEFOTETAN DISODIUM   (sef-oh-**TEA**-tan)
Cefotan (Rx)

See also *Anti-Infectives,* p. 71, and *Cephalosporins,* p. 86.

Classification: Antibiotic, cephalosporin (third generation)

Action/Kinetics: Administered parenterally only. **t½:** 3–4.6 hr. From 50% to 80% is excreted unchanged in the urine.

Uses: Infections of the urinary tract, lower respiratory tract, skin and skin structures, bones and joints. Also gynecologic and intra-abdominal infections. Prophylaxis of postoperative infections (e.g., due to abdominal or vaginal hysterectomy, transurethral surgery, GI or biliary tract surgery, cesarean section).

Special Concerns: Pregnancy category: B. Safety and effectiveness have not been determined in children.

Additional Side Effects: Concomitant use with ethanol produces a disulfiram-type reaction and hypotension.

Additional Laboratory Test Interference: The drug may affect measurement of creatinine levels by the Jaffe reaction.

Dosage: Adults, usual IV or IM: 1–2 g q 12 hr for 5–10 days. *Urinary tract infections,* **IV, IM:** Either 0.5 g q 12 hr, or 1–2 g q 12–24 hr. *Severe infections,* **IV:** 2 g q 12 hr. *Life-threatening infections,* **IV:** 3 g q 12 hr. *Prophylaxis of postoperative infection,* **IV:** 1–2 g 30–60 min prior to surgery. Dosage should be reduced in impaired renal function and is dependent on creatinine clearance.

NURSING CONSIDERATIONS

See also *Nursing Considerations* for *Cephalosporins,* p. 88.

Administration/Storage

1. Cefotetan disodium must be administered parenterally, because it is not absorbed from the GI tract.

2. IM injections should be made well within a large muscle (e.g., the gluteus maximus).

3. The IV route is preferred for clients with bacterial septicemia, bacteremia, or other severe or life-threatening infections. The IV route is also preferred for poor-risk clients as the result of malnutrition, surgery, diabetes, trauma, heart failure, malignancy, or if shock is present or impending.

4. Intermittent IV administration may be completed over 3–5 min following reconstitution in sterile water for injection.

5. For IM use, reconstitute with sterile water for injection, normal saline, bacteriostatic water for injection, or 0.5%–1% lidocaine HCl.

6. Reconstituted solutions maintain potency for 24 hr at room temperature, for 96 hr if refrigerated, and for 1 week if frozen.

7. Cefotetan should not be mixed with solutions containing aminoglycosides.

Assessment

Assess for any evidence or history of excessive use of alcohol.

Interventions

1. Anticipate reduced dosage in clients with impaired renal function.

2. Obtain baseline coagulation studies and monitor during therapy.

3. Report any diarrhea to physician and maintain accurate record of intake and output.

Client/Family Teaching

1. Instruct client to avoid alcohol ingestion during and for 72 hr after cefotetan disodium therapy.

2. Have client/family report any side effects, such as diarrhea, bruising/bleeding, or decreased urine output, to the physician.

CEFOXITIN SODIUM   (seh-FOX-ih-tin)

Mefoxin (Rx)

See also *Anti-Infectives,* p. 71, and *Cephalosporins,* p. 86.

Classification: Antibiotic, cephalosporin (second generation).

Action/Kinetics: Broad-spectrum cephalosporin that is penicillinase- and cephalosporinase-resistant and is stable in the presence of beta-lactamases. **Peak serum concentration: IM,** 20–30 min. **t½: IM, IV,** 41–65 min. Eighty-five percent of drug excreted unchanged in urine after 6 hr.

Uses: Infections of the urinary tract (including gonorrhea), bones, joints, lower respiratory tract (including lung abscesses and pneumonia), skin, and skin structures. Intra-abdominal infections (including intra-abdominal abscesses and peritonitis), gynecologic infections (including pelvic inflammatory disease, pelvic cellulitis, and endometritis), septicemia, and prophylaxis in surgery. **Note:** Many gram-negative infections resistant to certain cephalosporins and penicillins respond to cefoxitin.

Special Concerns: Pregnancy category: B.

Additional Side Effects: Higher doses have caused increased incidence of eosinophilia and increased AST in children over 3 months of age.

Additional Laboratory Test Interference: High concentrations may interfere with the measurement of creatinine by the Jaffe method.

Dosage: IM, IV. Adults. *Uncomplicated infections (cutaneous, pneumonia, urinary tract):* **IV, IM,** 1 g q 6–8 hr. *Severe infections:* **IV,** 1 g q 4 hr or 2 g q 6–8 hr. *Gas gangrene:* **IV,** 2 g q 4 hr or 3 g q 6 hr. *Gonorrhea:* 2 g IM with 1 g probenecid PO. *Prophylaxis in surgery:* **IV, IM,** 2 g 30–60 min before surgery followed by 2 g q 6 hr after first dose for 24 hr only (72 hr for prosthetic arthroplasty). *Cesarean section, prophylaxis:* 2 g **IV** when cord is clamped; **then,** give two additional doses IV or IM 4 and 8 hr later. Subsequent doses may be given q 6 hr for no more than 1 day. *Transurethral prostatectomy, prophylaxis:* 1 g before surgery; **then,** 1 g q 8 hr for up to 5 days. *Impaired renal function:* **initial,** 1–2 g; **then,** follow maintenance schedule provided by manufacturer.

Children over 3 months: 80–160 mg/kg daily in 4–6 divided doses. Total daily dosage should not exceed 12 g. *Prophylaxis:* 30–40 mg/kg q 6 hr.

NURSING CONSIDERATIONS

See also *Nursing Considerations* for *Cephalosporins,* p. 88.

Administration/Storage

1. Do not mix with other antibiotics during administration.
2. Reconstituted solutions are stable for 24 hr at room temperature, 1 week in the refrigerator, and 26 weeks when frozen.
3. Store drug vials below 30°C.
4. Reconstituted solutions are white to light amber. Color does not affect potency. Consult pharmacist if unsure of drug potency.
5. For IM injections, lidocaine hydrochloride 0.05% (without epinephrine) may be used as diluent, by physician's order, to reduce pain at injection site.
6. Do not administer cefoxitin rapidly, because it is irritating to veins.

Interventions

1. Monitor intake and output. Upon noting any significant reduction in urinary output, withhold medication, and report to physician.
2. Assess site of infusion for pain and redness, because medication can cause thrombophlebitis.

CEFTAZIDIME   (sef-**TAY**-zih-deem)

Fortaz, Magnacef✸, Tazicef, Tazidime (Rx)

See also *Anti-Infectives,* p. 71, and *Cephalosporins,* p. 86.

Classification: Antibiotic, cephalosporin (third generation).

Action/Kinetics: Only for IM or IV use. **t½:** 2–3 hr. From 80%–90% is excreted unchanged in the urine.

Uses: Bacterial septicemia. Infections of the lower respiratory tract, skin and skin structures, bones and joints, CNS (including meningitis), and urinary tract. Also, intra-abdominal (including peritonitis) and gynecologic infections (including endometritis, pelvic cellulitis). Use with aminoglycosides, clindamycin, or vancomycin in severe or life-threatening infections or in the immunocompromised patient.

Special Concerns: Pregnancy category: B.

Dosage: IM, IV. Adults, usual: 1 g q 8–12 hr. *Urinary tract infections, uncomplicated,* **IM, IV:** 0.25 g q 12 hr. *Urinary tract infections, complicated,* **IM, IV:** 0.5 g q 8–12 hr. *Uncomplicated pneumonia, skin and skin structure infections,* **IM, IV:** 0.5–1 g q 8 hr. *Bone and joint infections,* **IV:** 2 g q 12 hr. *Serious gynecologic or intra-abdominal infections, meningitis, severe or life-threatening infections (especially in immunocompromised patients),* **IV:** 2 g q 8 hr. *Pseudomonal lung infections in cystic fibrosis patients,* **IV:** 30–50 mg/kg q 8 hr, not to exceed 6 g/day. **Neonates,**

0–4 weeks, IV: 30 mg/kg q 12 hr. **Infants and children, 1 month to 12 years, IV:** 30–50 mg/kg q 8 hr not to exceed 6 g/day.

Dosage must be reduced in patients with impaired renal function (see package insert).

NURSING CONSIDERATIONS

See also *Nursing Considerations* for *Cephalosporins,* p. 88.

Administration/Storage

1. Ceftazidime must be administered parenterally, because it is not absorbed from the GI tract.
2. If administering IM, use large muscle mass and inject deeply.
3. The IV route is preferred for clients with bacterial septicemia, peritonitis, bacterial meningitis, or other severe or life-threatening infections. Also, IV should be used for clients considered to be poor risks due to malnutrition, surgery, diabetes, trauma, heart failure, malignancy, or if shock is present or imminent.
4. For direct intermittent IV administration, reconstitute in sterile water for injection and let physician administer over 3–5 min.
5. The drug may be given also via the tubing of an administration set (IVPB) and is compatible with 0.9% sodium chloride injection, Ringer's injection, lactated Ringer's injection, 5% or 10% dextrose injection, M/6 sodium lactate injection, 5% dextrose and 0.25%, 0.45%, or 0.9% sodium chloride injection, 10% invert sugar in water for injection. Sodium bicarbonate injection should not be used for reconstitution.
6. For IM administration, reconstitute in sterile water for injection, bacteriostatic water for injection, or 0.5%–1% lidocaine HCl injection.
7. Ceftazidime should not be added to solutions containing aminoglycosides.

Interventions

1. Anticipate lowered dosage in clients with impaired renal function.
2. Report any diarrhea to the physician.

CEFTIZOXIME SODIUM (sef-tih-**ZOX**-eem)

Cefizox (Rx)

See also *Anti-Infectives,* p. 71, and *Cephalosporins,* p. 86.

Classification: Antibiotic, cephalosporin (third generation).

Action/Kinetics: t½: Approximately 1–2 hr. Approximately 80% excreted unchanged in the urine.

Uses: Infections of the urinary tract, lower respiratory tract, skin, skin structures, bones, and joints. Intra-abdominal infections, septicemia, meningitis (caused by *Hemophilus influenzae* or *Streptococcus pneumoniae),* gonorrhea (including uncomplicated cervical and urethral gonorrhea caused by *Neisseria*).

Special Concerns: Pregnancy category: B.

Additional Side Effects: Transient increased levels of eosinophils, AST, ALT, and CPK have been seen in children greater than 6 months of age.

Dosage: IM, IV. Adults. *Uncomplicated urinary tract and other infections:* 0.5 g q 12 hr. *Severe or resistant infections:* 1 g q 8 hr or 2 g q 8–12 hr. *Life-threatening infections:* up to 3–4 g q 8 hr **IV.**

Uncomplicated gonorrhea: 1 g as a single dose **IM. Pediatric, over 6 months:** 50 mg/kg q 6–8 hr up to 200 mg/kg daily (not to exceed the maximum adult dose). *Impaired renal function:* **initially, IM, IV** 0.5–1 g; **then,** use maintenance schedule in package insert.

NURSING CONSIDERATIONS

See *Nursing Considerations* for *Cephalosporins,* p. 88.

Administration/Storage

1. For IM doses of 2 g, divide the dose equally and give in different large muscle masses.
2. For direct IV administration, give slowly over 3–5 min.
3. Reconstituted solutions are stable at room temperature for 8 hr and, if refrigerated, for 48 hr.

CEFTRIAXONE SODIUM (sef-try-**AX**-ohn)

Rocephin (Rx)

See also *Anti-Infectives,* p. 71, and *Cephalosporins,* p. 86.

Classification: Antibiotic, cephalosporin (third generation).

Action/Kinetics: t½: Approximately 6–8 hr. Significantly protein bound. One third to two thirds excreted unchanged in the urine.

Uses: Infections of the lower respiratory tract, urinary tract, skin, skin structures, bones, joints, abdomen. Also, uncomplicated gonorrhea (cervical, urethral, rectal), pelvic inflammatory disease, meningitis, prophylaxis of infections in surgery, bacterial septicemia. *Investigational:* Lyme disease (infection caused by *Borrelia burgdorferi).*

Special Concerns: Pregnancy category: B.

Additional Side Effects: Increase in serum creatinine, presence of casts in the urine, alteration of prothrombin times (rare).

Dosage: IV, IM. Adults: usual, 1–2 g daily in single or divided doses q 12 hr, not to exceed 4 g/day. Therapy is maintained for 4–14 days, depending on the infection. **Pediatric:** *other than meningitis:* 50–75 mg/kg/day not to exceed total daily dose of 2 g given in divided doses q 12 hr. *Meningitis:* 100 mg/kg/day, not to exceed total daily dose of 4 g given in divided doses q 12 hr. A loading dose of 75 mg/kg may be used. *Prophylaxis of infection in surgery:* 1 g 30–120 min prior to surgery. *Uncomplicated gonorrhea:* **IM,** 250 mg as a single dose. *Lyme disease:* **IV,** 2 g b.i.d. for 14 days. Dosage adjustment is not required for renal or hepatic impairment; however, monitor blood levels in dialysis patients.

NURSING CONSIDERATIONS

See *Nursing Considerations* for *Cephalosporins,* p. 88.

Administration/Storage

1. IM injections should be deep into the body of a large muscle.
2. IV injections should be by infusion of concentrations ranging from 10 to 40 mg/mL.
3. The drug should not be mixed with other antibiotics.
4. Stability of solutions for IM or IV use varies depending on the diluent used; the package insert should be checked carefully.

5. Dosage should be maintained for at least 2 days after symptoms of infection have disappeared (usual course of therapy is 4–14 days, although complicated infections may require longer therapy).
6. Dosage should be continued for at least 10 days when treating *S. pyogenes* infections.

CEFUROXIME AXETIL   (se-fyour-**OX**-eem ax-**EE**-til)

Ceftin (Rx)

CEFUROXIME SODIUM   (se-fyour-**OX**-eem)

Kefurox, Zinacef, Zinnat✹ (Rx)

See also *Anti-Infectives,* p. 71, and *Cephalosporins,* p. 86.

Classification: Antibiotic, cephalosporin (second generation).

Action/Kinetics: Cefuroxime axetil is used orally, whereas cefuroxime sodium is used either IM or IV. **IM, IV: t½:** 1–2 hr; 66%–100% is excreted unchanged in the urine.

Uses: PO. Pharyngitis, tonsillitis, otitis media, bronchitis, urinary tract infections, skin and skin structure infections. **IM, IV.** Infections of the urinary tract, lower respiratory tract (including pneumonia), skin and skin structures, bones joints. Septicemia, meningitis, gonorrhea. Prophylaxis in surgery.

Special Concerns: Pregnancy category: B.

Additional Side Effects: Decrease in hemoglobin and hematocrit.

Additional Laboratory Test Interference: False − reaction in the ferricyanide test for blood glucose.

Dosage: Tablets. Adults and children over 12 years of age: 250 mg q 12 hr, up to 500 mg q 12 hr for severe infections or infections due to less susceptible organisms. *Uncomplicated urinary tract infections:* 125–250 mg q 12 hr. **Infants and children less than 12 years of age:** 125 mg b.i.d. *Otitis media:* **less than 2 years of age:** 125 mg b.i.d.; **greater than 2 years of age:** 250 mg b.i.d.
 IM, IV. Adults. *Uncomplicated infections, including urinary tract, pneumonia, disseminated gonococcal, skin and skin structure:* 0.75 g q 8 hr. *Severe, complicated, or life-threatening infections; bone and joint infections:* 1.5 g q 6–8 hr. *Bacterial meningitis:* Up to 3 g q 8 hr. *Gonorrhea (uncomplicated):* 1.5 g as a single IM dose. *Prophylaxis in surgery:* **IV,** 1.5 g 30–60 min before surgery; if procedure is of long duration, **IM, IV,** 0.75 g q 8 hr. *Open heart surgery, prophylaxis:* **IV,** 1.5 g when anesthesia is initiated; **then,** 1.5 g q 12 hr for a total of 6 g.
 Pediatric, over 3 months. *Uncomplicated infections:* 50–100 mg/kg daily in divided doses q 6–8 hr (not to exceed adult dose for severe infections). *Bacterial meningitis:* **initially, IV,** 200–240 mg/kg daily in divided doses q 6–8 hr; **then,** after clinical improvement, 100 mg/kg daily **IV.** *Bone and joint infections:* 150 mg/kg daily in divided doses q 8 hr (not to exceed adult dose).
 Dosage in adults and children should be reduced in impaired renal function.

NURSING CONSIDERATIONS

See also *Nursing Considerations* for *Cephalosporins,* p. 88.

Administration/Storage

1. Use IV route for severe or life-threatening infections such as septicemia or in poor-risk clients, especially in presence of shock.

2. For direct IV injection, give over 3–5 min; the drug may also be given through the tubing by which other IV solutions are being administered.

3. For IM use, inject deep into a large muscle mass.

4. Prior to reconstitution, protect the drug from light. The powder and reconstituted drug may darken without affecting potency.

5. Cefuroxime sodium should not be added to solutions of aminoglycosides; if both drugs are required, each should be given separately to the client.

6. Cefuroxime axetil for oral use is available only in tablet form. Crushed tablets (even mixed with food) have a strong, persistent, bitter taste; alternative therapy may be required in children who cannot ingest cefuroxime axetil reliably.

7. Therapy should be continued for at least 10 days in infections due to *S. pyogenes*.

8. Food enhances the absorption of cefuroxime axetil.

Assessment

Assess for evidence of anemia.

Interventions

Anticipate reduced dose in clients with impaired renal function.

Client/Family Teaching

1. Report signs of anemia to physician immediately.

2. Take with food to enhance the absorption of the oral medication.

3. Crushed cefuroxime axetil tablets have a distinctive bitter taste even when hidden in foods. If unable to tolerate taste, notify physician so alternative drug therapy may be instituted.

Evaluation

Obtain hemoglobin and hematocrit to ascertain if there is evidence of anemia.

CEPHALEXIN HYDROCHLORIDE MONOHYDRATE (sef-ah-**LEX**-in)

Keftab (Rx)

CEPHALEXIN MONOHYDRATE (sef-ah-**LEX**-in)

Ceporex✸, Keflet, Keflex, Novolexin✸ (Rx)

See also *Anti-Infectives,* p. 71, and *Cephalosporins,* p. 86.

Classification: Antibiotic, cephalosporin (first generation).

Action/Kinetics: Peak serum levels: PO, 9–39 mcg/mL after 1 hr. **t½, PO:** 30–72 min. Absorption delayed in children. The HCl monohydrate does not require conversion in the stomach before absorption. Ninety percent of drug excreted unchanged in urine within 8 hr.

Uses: Infections of the respiratory tract, skin, soft tissues, bones, and GU tract (including acute prostatitis). Otitis media.

Special Concerns: Pregnancy category: B. Safety and effectiveness of the HCl monohydrate have not been determined in children.

Additional Side Effects: Nephrotoxicity, cholestatic jaundice.

Dosage: Capsules, Oral Suspension, Tablets. Adult: Usual, 250 mg q 6 hr up to 4 g daily.

Infections of skin and skin structures, streptococcal pharyngitis, uncomplicated cystitis, over 15 years: 500 mg q 12 hr. **Pediatric:** *monohydrate,* 25–50 mg/kg daily in four equally divided doses. For streptococcal pharyngitis in patients over 1 year and for skin and skin structure infections, the total daily dose should be divided and given q 12 hr. *Otitis media:* 75–100 mg/kg/day in four divided doses. Dosage may have to be reduced in patients with impaired renal function or increased for severe infections. Action of drug can be prolonged by the concurrent administration of oral probenecid.

NURSING CONSIDERATIONS

See *Nursing Considerations* for *Cephalosporins,* p. 88.

Administration/Storage

1. After reconstitution, the drug should be refrigerated and the unused portion discarded after 14 days.
2. Treatment should be continued for at least 10 days for beta-hemolytic streptococcal infections.

CEPHALOTHIN SODIUM (sef-AL-oh-thin)

Ceporacin✹, Keflin✹, Keflin Neutral (Rx)

See also *Anti-Infectives,* p. 71, and *Cephalosporins,* p. 86.

Classification: Antibiotic, cephalosporin (first generation).

Action/Kinetics: Poorly absorbed from GI tract; must be given parenterally. **Peak serum levels: IM,** 6–21 mcg/mL after 30 min. **t½ (IM, IV):** 30–60 min. 55%–90% excreted unchanged in urine. Its low nephrotoxicity, ototoxicity, and neurotoxicity make the drug suitable for patients with impaired renal function.

Uses: Infections of the GU tract, GI tract, respiratory tract, skin, soft tissues, bones, and joints. Meningitis, septicemia (including endocarditis), and prophylaxis in surgery.

Special Concerns: Pregnancy category: B.

Additional Side Effects: Nephrotoxicity, severe phlebitis, hemolytic anemia, increased prothrombin time.

Laboratory Test Interferences: Large doses may produce false + results in urinary protein tests that use sulfosalicylic acid.

Dosage: Deep IM, IV. Adults: usual, 0.5–1 g q 4–6 hr. *Urinary tract infections, uncomplicated pneumonia, furunculosis with cellulitis:* 0.5 g q 6 hr (for severe infections increase the dose to 1 g or give 0.5 g q 4 hr). *Life-threatening infections:* 2 g q 4 hr (up to 12 g daily for bacteremia, septicemia). *Preoperative and during surgery:* 1–2 g 30–60 min prior to surgery and during surgery. *Postoperative:* 1–2 g q 6 hr for 24 hr. *Impaired renal function:* **initially,** 1–2 g; **then,** use manufacturer's guidelines for maintenance doses. **Pediatric:** 80–160 mg/kg daily in divided doses. *Prophylaxis in surgery:* 20–30 mg/kg using adult schedule.

NURSING CONSIDERATIONS

See *Nursing Considerations* for *Cephalosporins,* p. 88.

Administration/Storage

1. Dilute according to directions on package insert.
2. Discard reconstituted solution after 12 hr at room temperature and after 96 hr when refrigerated.

3. Dissolve precipitate by warming vial in hand and shaking. Do not overheat.

4. Replace medication and IV solution after 24 hr.

5. For direct IV administration, add a small needle into larger veins.

CEPHAPIRIN SODIUM   (sef-ah-**PIE**-rin)

Cefadyl (Rx)

See also *Anti-Infectives,* p. 71, and *Cephalosporins,* p. 86.

Classification: Antibiotic, cephalosporin (first generation).

Action/Kinetics: Peak serum levels: IM, 9.4 mcg/mL after 30 min. **t½ (IM, IV):** 21–47 min. Virtually entirely excreted in the urine within 6 hr, with 41%–60% excreted unchanged.

Uses: Infections of the respiratory tract, urinary tract, skin, and skin structures. Septicemia, endocarditis, osteomyelitis, prophylaxis in surgery.

Special Concerns: Pregnancy category: B. Before use in children less than 3 months, assess benefits versus risks.

Additional Side Effects: Increase in serum bilirubin.

Dosage: IM, IV only. Adults: 0.5–1 g q 4–6 hr up to 12 g daily for serious or life-threatening infections. *Preoperatively:* 1–2 g 30–60 min before surgery. *During surgery:* 1–2 g. *Postoperatively:* 1–2 g q 6 hr for 24 hr. **Pediatric, over 3 months:** 40–80 mg/kg daily in four equally divided doses.
In patients with impaired renal function, a dose of 7.5–15 mg/kg q 12 hr may be adequate.

NURSING CONSIDERATIONS

See *Nursing Considerations* for *Cephalosporins,* p. 88.

Administration/Storage

Discard after 12 hr when kept at room temperature and after 10 days, when refrigerated at 4°C.

CEPHRADINE   (**SEF**-rah-deen)

Anspor, Velosef (Rx)

See also *Anti-Infectives,* p. 71, and *Cephalosporins,* p. 86.

Classification: Antibiotic, cephalosporin (first generation).

Action/Kinetics: Similar to that of cephalexin. Rapidly absorbed from GI tract or IM injection site (30 min–2 hr); 60%–90% excreted after 6 hr. **Peak serum levels: PO,** 8–24 mcg/mL after 30–60 min; **IM,** 5.6–13.6 mcg/mL after 1–2 hr. **t½:** 42–120 min. 80%–95% excreted in urine unchanged.

Uses: Infections of the respiratory tract (including lobar pneumonia, tonsillitis, pharyngitis), urinary tract (including prostatitis and enterococcal infections), skin, skin structures, and bone. Otitis media, septicemia, prophylaxis in surgery, following cesarean section to prevent infection. In severe infections, therapy is usually initiated parenterally.

Special Concerns: Pregnancy category: B. Safe use during pregnancy has not been established. Safe use of the parenteral form in infants under 1 month of age and the oral form in children less than 9 months of age has not been established.

Additional Laboratory Test Interference: False + reactions using sulfosalicylic acid for urinary protein tests. High concentrations may interfere with measurement of creatinine by the Jaffe method.

Dosage: Capsules, Oral Suspension. Adults, usual, *Skin and skin structures, respiratory tract infections:* 250 mg q 6 hr or 500 mg q 12 hr. *Lobar pneumonia:* 500 mg q 6 hr or 1 g q 12 hr. *Uncomplicated urinary tract infections:* **usual,** 500 mg q 12 hr; *more serious infections and prostatitis:* 500 mg q 6 hr or 1 g q 12 hr (severe, chronic infections may require up to 1 g q 6 hr). **Pediatric, over 9 months:** 25–50 mg/kg daily in equally divided doses q 6–12 hr (75–100 mg/kg/day for otitis media).

  Deep IM, IV. Adults: 2–4 g daily in equally divided doses q.i.d. *Surgical prophylaxis:* 1 g 30–90 min before surgery; **then,** 1 g q 4–6 hr for 1–2 doses (or up to 24 hr postoperatively). *Cesarean section, prophylaxis:* **IV,** 1 g when the umbilical cord is clamped; **then,** give two additional 1 g doses **IV or IM** 6 and 12 hr after the initial dose. **Pediatric, over 1 year:** 50–100 mg/kg/day in equally divided doses q.i.d.

  Dosage should be reduced in impaired renal function.

NURSING CONSIDERATIONS

See also *Nursing Considerations* for *Cephalosporins,* p. 88.

Administration/Storage

1. Dilute according to directions on package insert.
2. Do not mix with lactated Ringer's solution.
3. Discard reconstituted solution after 10 hr at room temperature and after 48 hr when refrigerated at 5°C.
4. A slightly yellow solution may be retained for use; if unsure of solution potency, consult with pharmacist.
5. Be especially careful to inject into muscle, because sterile abscesses from accidental subcutaneous injection have occurred.
6. Protect before and after reconstitution from excessive heat and light.
7. Replace medication during prolonged IV administration (solution) after 10 hr.
8. Administer PO medication without regard to meals.

Interventions

1. Anticipate reduced dose with impaired renal function.
2. Rotate and document injection sites carefully.

Evaluation

During IM administration assess injection sites for any evidence of abscess formation.

MOXALACTAM DISODIUM   (MOX-ah-lack-tam)

Moxam, Oxalactam ✽ (Rx)

See also *Anti-Infectives,* p. 71, and *Cephalosporins,* p. 86.

Classification: Antibiotic, cephalosporin (third generation).

Action/Kinetics: Broad-spectrum semisynthetic cephalosporin that is stable in the presence of beta-lactamase, penicillinase, and cephalosporinase. Cross-sensitivity with penicillin has not been observed; in selected cases, it can be used instead of chloramphenicol or aminoglycosides.

Well absorbed into pleural, interstitial, and cerebrospinal (both normal and inflamed meninges) fluids, aqueous humor. **Peak serum concentrations (dose-dependent): IM,** 15 mcg/mL 1–2 hr after 500 mg; **IV infusion,** 57 mcg/mL after 500 mg. **t½ [IM]:** 2.1 hr (longer in patients with impaired renal function). From 60% to 90% of the drug is excreted by the kidneys within 24 hr.

Uses: Infections of the urinary tract, CNS (including ventriculitis and meningitis), skin and skin structures, bones, joints, and lower respiratory tract (including pneumonia). Intra-abdominal infections (including endometritis, pelvic cellulitis, peritonitis), bacterial septicemia, *Pseudomonas* infections. Used concomitantly with aminoglycosides in gram-positive or gram-negative sepsis or other serious infections in which the causative organism is not known.

Contraindications: Hypersensitivity to drug.

Special Concerns: Safe use during pregnancy not established (pregnancy category: C). Use with caution in individuals with history of sensitivity to penicillins or other cephalosporins.

Additional Side Effects: Hypoprothrombinemia resulting in bleeding and/or bruising.

Drug Interactions: Moxalactam may induce an Antabuse-like reaction if used with alcohol.

Laboratory Test Interferences: False + test for proteinuria with acid and denaturization-precipitation tests.

Dosage: Deep IM, IV. Adults, usual: 2–4 g daily in divided doses q 8–12 hr for 5–10 days (or up to 14 days). *Mild to moderate infections:* 0.5–2 g q 12 hr. *Mild skin and skin structure infections, uncomplicated pneumonia:* 0.5 g q 8 hr. *Mild, uncomplicated urinary tract infections:* 0.25 g q 12 hr. *Persistent or serious urinary tract infections:* 0.5 g q 8–12 hr. *Life-threatening infections or infections due to less susceptible organisms:* up to 4 g q 8 hr may be required. **Neonates up to 1 week:** 50 mg/kg q 12 hr; **1–4 weeks:** 50 mg/kg q 8 hr. **Infants:** 50 mg/kg q 6 hr. **Children:** 50 mg/kg q 6–8 hr. Pediatric dosage may be increased up to 200 mg/kg but should not exceed the maximum adult dosage. *For pediatric gram-negative meningitis:* initial loading dose, 100 mg/kg; **then,** follow above dosage regimen. *For patients with impaired renal function:* **initially,** 1–2 g; **maintenance:** see recommendations of manufacturer.

NURSING CONSIDERATIONS

See also *Nursing Considerations* for *Cephalosporins,* p. 88.

Administration/Storage

1. *IM:* 1 g moxalactam should be diluted with 3 mL of either sterile water for injection, bacteriostatic water for injection, 0.9% sodium chloride injection, bacteriostatic sodium chloride injection, or 0.5% lidocaine injection.
2. *Intermittent IV:* 1 g moxalactam should be diluted with 10 mL sterile water for injection, 5% dextrose injection, or 0.9% sodium chloride injection. Inject slowly over 3–5 min by physician. (*Note:* IV solutions containing alcohol should be avoided.) If a Y-tube administration set is used, the other solution should be discontinued while moxalactam is being given.
3. *Continuous IV infusion:* 1 g moxalactam should be diluted with 10 mL sterile water for injection and added to appropriate IV solution.
4. Reconstituted moxalactam is stable for 96 hr when refrigerated (5°C) and for 24 hr at room temperature.

Assessment

Assess for bleeding during therapy, caused by eradication of intestinal bacteria that produce vitamin K.

Interventions

1. Rotate sites frequently and observe IV site for phlebitis during IV administration.
2. If drug administered with aminoglycosides, monitor renal function studies for potentiation of nephrotoxic effect.
3. Anticipate that 10 mg/week of vitamin K should be given to clients receiving moxalactam.
4. Anticipate different dosing technique for clients with altered renal function.

Client/Family Teaching

Alcohol should not be ingested while on therapy with moxalactam, because an Antabuse-like reaction may occur.

Evaluation

1. Review PT/PTT for evidence of impairment related to drug therapy and determine if weekly vitamin K dose at effective level.
2. Check for absence of ingestion of alcohol and its associated reaction.
3. Note status of pretreatment symptoms and C&S results to determine effectiveness of therapy.

CHLORAMPHENICOL

CHLORAMPHENICOL   (klor-am-**FEN**-ih-call)

Chloromycetin (Cream, Kapseals, and Otic), Chloroptic✲, Fenicol✲, Mychel, Novochlorocap✲, Pentamycetin✲ (Rx)

CHLORAMPHENICOL OPHTHALMIC   (klor-am-**FEN**-ih-call)

AK Chlor✲, Chlorofair, Chloromycetin Ophthalmic, Chloroptic Ophthalmic, Chloroptic S.O.P. Ophthalmic, Isopto Fenicol✲, Ophthochlor, Pentamycetin✲ (Rx)

CHLORAMPHENICOL PALMITATE   (klor-am-**FEN**-ih-call)

Chloromycetin Palmitate (Rx)

CHLORAMPHENICOL SODIUM SUCCINATE   (klor-am-**FEN**-ih-call)

Chloromycetin Sodium Succinate, Mychel-S (Rx)

See also *Anti-Infectives,* p. 71.

General Statement: This antibiotic was originally isolated from *Streptomyces venezuellae* and is now produced synthetically. The antibiotic can be extremely toxic (due to protein synthesis inhibition in rapidly proliferating cells, as in bone marrow) and should not be used for trivial infections.

Action/Kinetics: Chloramphenicol inhibits protein synthesis in bacteria by binding to ribosomes (50S subunit, an essential link in the protein synthesis machinery of the cell), thus interfering with peptide bond synthesis. Therapeutic serum concentrations: *peak,* 10–20 mcg/mL; *trough:* 5–10 mcg/mL (less for neonates). **Peak serum concentration: IM,** 2 hr. **t½:** 4 hr. Drug is metabolized in the liver; 75%–90% of drug excreted in urine within 24 hr, as parent drug (8%–12%) and inactive metabolites. The drug is mostly bacteriostatic. Chloramphenicol is well absorbed from the

GI tract and is distributed to all parts of the body, including CSF, pleural, and ascitic fluids; saliva; milk; and aqueous and vitreous humors.

Uses: *Not to be used for trivial infections, prophylaxis of bacterial infections, or to treat colds, flu, or throat infections.* Treatment of choice for typhoid fever but not for typhoid carrier state. Serious infections caused by *Salmonella, Rickettsia, Chlamydia,* and lymphogranuloma-psittacosis group. Meningitis due to *Hemophilus influenzae.* Brain abscesses due to *Bacteroides fragilis.* Cystic fibrosis anti-infective. Meningococcal or pneumococcal meningitis. Used topically for bacterial ocular infections, otitis externa, and skin infections.

Contraindications: Hypersensitivity to chloramphenicol; pregnancy, especially near term and during labor; nursing mothers. Avoid simultaneous administration of other drugs that may depress bone marrow.

Special Concerns: Use with caution in patients with intermittent porphyria or glucose-6-phosphate dehydrogenase deficiency.

Side Effects: *Hematologic* (most serious): Aplastic anemia, thrombocytopenia, granulocytopenia, hemolytic anemia, pancytopenia. *Hematologic studies should be undertaken before and every 2 days during therapy. GI:* Nausea, vomiting, diarrhea, glossitis, stomatitis, unpleasant taste, enterocolitis, pruritus ani. *Allergic:* Fever, skin rashes, angioedema, macular and vesicular rashes, hemorrhages of the skin, intestine, bladder, mouth. Anaphylaxis. *CNS:* Headache, delirium, confusion, mental depression. *Neurologic:* Optic neuritis, peripheral neuritis. *Following topical use:* Burning, itching, irritation, redness of skin. *Miscellaneous:* Superinfection. Jaundice (rare). Herxheimer-like reactions when used for typhoid fever (may be due to release of bacterial endotoxins). *Gray syndrome in infants:* Rapid respiration, ashen gray color, failure to feed, abdominal distention with or without vomiting, progressive pallid cyanosis, vasomotor collapse, death. Can be reversed when drug is discontinued. *Note: Neonates should be observed closely, since the drug accumulates in the bloodstream and the infant is thus subject to greater hazards of toxicity.*

Drug Interactions	
Acetaminophen	↑ Effect of chloramphenicol due to ↑ serum levels
Anticoagulants, oral	↑ Effect of anticoagulants due to ↓ breakdown by liver
Antidiabetics, oral	↑ Effect of antidiabetics due to ↓ breakdown by liver
Barbiturates	↑ Effect of barbiturates due to ↓ breakdown by liver
Chlorpropamide	↑ Effect due to ↓ breakdown by liver
Cyclophosphamide	↑ Effect of cyclophosphamide due to ↓ breakdown by liver
Dicumarol	↑ Effect due to ↓ breakdown by liver
Iron preparations	Chloramphenicol ↓ response to iron therapy
Penicillins	Possible ↓ effect of penicillins
Phenobarbital	↑ Effect due to ↓ breakdown by liver
Phenytoin	↑ Effect of phenytoin due to ↓ breakdown by liver
Rifampin	↓ Effect of chloramphenicol due to ↑ breakdown by liver
Tolbutamide	↑ Effect due to ↓ breakdown by liver
Vitamin B$_{12}$	↓ Response to vitamin B$_{12}$ therapy

Dosage: Capsules, Oral Suspension, IV. Chloramphenicol, chloramphenicol palmitate,

Adults: 50 mg/kg daily in four equally divided doses q 6 hr. Can be increased to 100 mg/kg daily in severe infections, but dosage should be reduced as soon as possible. **Neonates and children with immature metabolic function:** 25 mg/kg daily in divided doses q 12 hr. **Pediatric:** 50–75 mg/kg daily in divided doses q 6 hr (50–100 mg/kg daily in divided doses q 6 hr for meningitis). **Newborns:** 25 mg/kg daily in four divided doses (after 2 weeks of life, up to 50 mg/kg daily can be given in four divided doses). **Neonates, less than 2 kg:** 25 mg/kg once daily. **Neonates, over 2 kg, over 7 days of age:** 50 mg/kg daily q 12 hr in divided doses. **Neonates, over 2 kg, from birth to 7 days of age:** 50 mg/kg once daily. *Note:* Carefully follow dosage for premature and newborn infants less than 2 weeks of age, because blood levels differ significantly from those of other age groups.

Chloramphenicol sodium succinate—IV only—same dosage as above; switch to **PO** as soon as possible.

Chloramphenicol Ophthalmic Ointment 1%: 0.5-inch ribbon placed in lower conjunctival sac q 3–4 hr for acute infections and b.i.d.–t.i.d. for mild to moderate infections.

Chloramphenicol Ophthalmic Solution 0.5%: 1–2 drops in lower conjunctival sac 2–6 times daily (or more for acute infections).

Chloramphenicol Otic Solution 0.5%: 2–3 drops in ear t.i.d.

Chloramphenicol Topical Cream 1%: Apply 1–5 times daily.

NURSING CONSIDERATIONS

See also *General Nursing Considerations For All Anti-infectives* under *Penicillins,* p. 140.

Administration/Storage

Administer IV as a 10% solution over at least a 60-sec interval.

Assessment

1. Note any history of hypersensitivity to chloramphenicol.
2. If client is a nursing mother, transmission of the drug to breast milk can result in the infant receiving the drug as well. Infants have underdeveloped capacity to metabolize chloramphenicol.
3. Take a complete client history. Clients who are diabetic and taking oral hypoglycemic agents may have to use insulin during treatment with chloramphenicol.
4. If client is concomitantly receiving drugs that cause bone marrow depression, use of chloramphenicol is contraindicated.
5. Chloramphenicol may produce a false + reaction with Fehling's or Benedict's solutions, both of which contain copper sulfate. In diabetic clients, use Lab-Stix to test the urine or, if available, do finger sticks for enhanced accuracy of glucose determinations.

Interventions

1. Anticipate reduced dosage in clients with impaired renal function and in newborn infants.
2. Be certain that baseline hematologic studies are completed before drug treatment begins.
3. Arrange for further hematologic studies to be conducted every 2 days to detect early signs of bone marrow depression.
4. Become familiar with drugs that enhance the effects of chloramphenicol and monitor closely for evidence of severe toxicity in clients on concurrent therapy.

Client/Family Teaching

1. Advise clients to avoid the use of alcohol during therapy.
2. Review the signs of hypersensitivity, such as rash, and stress the importance of reporting to the physician.

3. Advise clients to report incidents of vaginal or rectal itching or diarrhea.

4. Advise clients to report any incidents of sore throat, unusual fatigue, or bleeding immediately, because drug may need to be discontinued.

5. Client should receive the drug only as necessary; avoid repeated courses of therapy with chloramphenicol, because the drug is highly toxic.

6. The drug should be taken at regularly spaced intervals *around the clock* to be most effective.

7. Chloramphenicol should be taken 1 hr before or 2 hr after meals; however, if GI upset occurs, it can be taken with food.

Evaluation

Evaluate:

- for bone marrow depression characterized by weakness, fatigue, sore throat, and bleeding. Review hematologic studies because discontinuation of the drug may be indicated.
- for optic neuritis, characterized by bilaterally reduced visual acuity, an indication to discontinue the drug immediately.
- for peripheral neuritis, characterized by pain and disturbance of sensation, both of which are indications to discontinue the drug immediately.
- premature and newborn infants for development of gray syndrome, characterized by rapid respiration, failure to feed, abdominal distention with or without vomiting, loose green stools, progressive cyanosis, and vasomotor collapse. Withhold drug and notify physician if any such symptoms are noted.
- for toxic and irritative effects, such as nausea, vomiting, unpleasant taste, diarrhea, and perineal irritation following PO administration. Differentiation of drug-induced diarrhea from that caused by a superinfection is critical and may be accomplished by assessment and analysis of all symptoms presented.

CLINDAMYCIN AND LINCOMYCIN

CLINDAMYCIN HYDROCHLORIDE HYDRATE   (klin-dah-**MY**-sin)
Cleocin Hydrochloride (Rx)

CLINDAMYCIN PALMITATE HYDROCHLORIDE   (klin-dah-**MY**-sin)
Cleocin Pediatric (Rx)

CLINDAMYCIN PHOSPHATE   (klin-dah-**MY**-sin)
Cleocin Phosphate, Cleocin T, Dalacin✣ (Rx)

See also *Anti-Infectives,* p. 71.

Classification: Antibiotic, clindamycin and lincomycin.

General Statement: Clindamycin is a semisynthetic antibiotic. Its spectrum resembles that of the erythromycins and includes a variety of gram-positive organisms, particularly staphylococci, streptococci, and pneumococci, and some gram-negative organisms. Should not be used for trivial infections.

Action/Kinetics: Suppresses protein synthesis by microorganism by binding to ribosomes (50S subunit) and preventing peptide bond formation. Is both bacteriostatic and bactericidal. **Peak serum concentration: PO,** 2.5 mcg/mL after 45 min (**t½:** 2.4 hr). In serious infections the rate of IV administration is adjusted to maintain appropriate serum drug concentrations: 4–6 mcg/mL.

Uses: Serious respiratory tract infections (e.g., empyema, lung abscess, pneumonia) caused by staphylococci, streptococci, and pneumococci. Serious skin and soft-tissue infections, septicemia, intra-abdominal infections, pelvic inflammatory disease, female genital tract infections. May be the drug of choice for *Bacteroides fragilis.* In combination with aminoglycosides for mixed aerobic and anaerobic bacterial infections. Staphylococci-induced acute hematogenous osteomyelitis. Adjunct to surgery for chronic bone/joint infections. Used topically for inflammatory acne vulgaris.

Contraindications: Hypersensitivity to either clindamycin or lincomycin. Not for use in treating viral and minor bacterial infections.

Special Concerns: Safe use during pregnancy has not been established. Use with caution in infants up to 1 month of age. Use with caution in patients with GI disease, liver or renal disease, history of allergy or asthma.

Side Effects: *GI:* Nausea, vomiting, diarrhea, abdominal pain, tenesmus, flatulence, bloating, anorexia, weight loss, esophagitis. Nonspecific colitis, pseudomembranous colitis (may be severe). *Allergic:* Morbilliform rash (most common). Also, maculopapular rash, urticaria, pruritus, fever, hypotension. Rarely, polyarteritis, anaphylaxis, erythema multiforme. *Hematologic:* Leukopenia, neutropenia, eosinophilia, thrombocytopenia, agranulocytosis. *Miscellaneous:* Superinfection. Also sore throat, fatigue, urinary frequency, headache. *Following IV use:* Thrombophlebitis, erythema, pain, swelling. *Following IM use:* Pain, induration, sterile abscesses. *Following topical use:* Erythema, irritation, dryness, peeling, itching, burning, oiliness.
  Note: The injection contains benzyl alcohol which has been associated with a fatal gasping syndrome in infants.

Drug Interactions	
Antiperistaltic antidiarrheals (opiates, Lomotil)	↑ Diarrhea due to ↓ removal of toxins from colon
Ciprofloxacin HCl	Additive antibacterial activity
Erythromycin	Cross-interference → ↓ effect of both drugs
Kaolin (e.g., Kaopectate)	↓ Effect due to ↓ absorption from GI tract
Neuromuscular blocking agents	↑ Effect of blocking agents

Laboratory Test Interferences: ↓ Levels of SGOT, SGPT, nonprotein nitrogen, alkaline phosphatase, bilirubin, BSP retention, and ↓ platelet count.

Dosage: PO only: Capsules, Oral Solution. Adults: Clindamycin HCl hydrate, Clindamycin palmitate HCl: 150–450 mg q 6 hr, depending on severity of infection. **Pediatric:** Clindamycin HCl hydrate: 8–20 mg/kg daily divided into 3–4 equal doses; clindamycin palmitate HCl: 8–25 mg/kg daily divided into 3–4 equal doses. **Children less than 10 kg:** Minimum recommended dose is 37.5 mg t.i.d.
  IV. Clindamycin phosphate. **Adults:** 0.6–2.7 g daily in 2–4 equal doses depending on severity of infection. *Life-threatening infections:* 4.8 g. **Pediatric over 1 month:** 15–40 mg/kg daily in 3–4 equal doses depending on severity of infections. *Severe infections:* Not less than 300 mg daily, regardless of body weight.

Acute pelvic inflammatory disease: **IV,** 600 mg q.i.d. plus gentamicin, 2 mg/kg IV; **then,** gentamicin, 1.5 mg/kg t.i.d. IV. IV therapy should be continued for 2 days after patient improves. The 10- to 14-day treatment cycle should be completed using clindamycin, **PO,** 450 mg q.i.d.

Dosage should be reduced in severe renal impairment.

Topical Gel or Solution: Apply thin film b.i.d. to affected areas.

NURSING CONSIDERATIONS

See also *General Nursing Considerations For All Anti-Infectives* under *Penicillins,* p. 140.

Administration/Storage

1. Give parenteral clindamycin only to hospitalized clients.
2. Dilute IV injections to maximum concentration of 12 mg/mL, with no more than 1,200 mg administered in 1 hr.
3. Single IM injections greater than 600 mg are not advisable. Inject deeply into muscle to prevent induration, pain, and sterile abscesses.
4. Do not refrigerate; otherwise, solution may become thickened.
5. Administer IV over a period of 20–60 min, depending on dose and therapeutic serum concentration to be attained.

Assessment

1. Take full history to determine extensiveness of respiratory tract infections.
2. Note presence of serious skin and soft tissue infections, septicemia, and evidence of infection of the female genital tract.
3. Note any client complaints that are indicative of pelvic inflammatory disease or intra-abdominal infections.
4. Note any client history of liver or renal disease, allergies, or history of GI problems.

Interventions

1. Be prepared to manage colitis, which can occur 2–9 days or several weeks after initiation of therapy, by providing fluids, electrolytes, protein supplements, systemic corticosteroids, and vancomycin as ordered.
2. Do not administer, and caution client against using, antiperistaltic agents if diarrhea occurs, because these can prolong or aggravate the condition.
3. Do not use any acne or topical mercury preparations containing a peeling agent in an area affected by medication, because severe irritation may occur.
4. Do not administer kaolin concomitantly, because this will reduce absorption of antibiotic. If kaolin is required, administer 3 hr before antibiotic.
5. Administer on an empty stomach to ensure optimum absorption. Drug should be administered only as long as necessary.
6. During IV administration observe for hypotension and keep client in bed for 30 min following therapy.
7. Observe for drug interactions caused by concurrent administration of neuromuscular blocking agents. Be alert to hypotension, bronchospasms, cardiac disturbances, hyperthermia, and respiratory depression.
8. Obtain baseline liver and renal function studies.

Client/Family Teaching

1. Take oral medication with a full glass of water to prevent esophageal ulceration.
2. If client has slight GI disturbance, the drug may be taken with food because food does not affect the rate of absorption to any significant extent.
3. Encourage client to report any bothersome side effects such as vomiting, diarrhea, or abdominal pain, and to take only as directed.
4. Teach client/family symptoms of colitis that may be severe and should be reported immediately to the physician, especially when working with the frail elderly.

Evaluation

1. Assess client/family knowledge and understanding of illness, response to therapy, and teaching.
2. Evaluate:
   - for rash, as this is the most frequently reported adverse reaction.
   - clients with renal and/or hepatic impairment and newborns for appropriate organ function.
   - for GI disturbances, such as abdominal pain, diarrhea, anorexia, nausea, vomiting, bloody or tarry stools, and excessive flatulence. Discontinuation of drug may be indicated.
3. Note status (presence/absence) of pretreatment symptoms and C&S results to determine effectiveness of treatment.

LINCOMYCIN HYDROCHLORIDE   (link-oh-**MY**-sin)

Lincocin (Rx)

See also *Anti-Infectives*, p. 71.

Classification: Anti-infective.

Action/Kinetics: Lincomycin is isolated from *Streptomyces lincolnensis*. Its spectrum resembles that of the erythromycins and includes a variety of gram-positive organisms, in particular staphylococci, streptococci, and pneumococci, and some gram-negative organisms. Lincomycin suppresses protein synthesis by microorganisms by binding to ribosomes (50S subunit), which is essential for transmittal of genetic information. It is both bacteriostatic and bactericidal. Lincomycin is absorbed rapidly from the GI tract and is widely distributed. **Peak plasma levels: PO,** 2–4 hr; **IM,** 30 min. **t½:** 5.4 hr. This drug should not be used for trivial infections.

Uses: Not a first-choice drug but useful for patients allergic to penicillin. Used for serious respiratory tract, skin, and soft tissue infections due to staphylococci, streptococci, or pneumococci. Septicemia. In conjunction with diphtheria antitoxin in the treatment of diphtheria.

Contraindications: Hypersensitivity to drugs. Use in infants up to one month of age.

Special Concerns: Safe use during pregnancy has not been established. Use with caution in patients with GI disease, liver or renal disease, or with a history of allergy or asthma. Not for use in treating viral and minor bacteria infections.

Side Effects: *GI:* Nausea, vomiting, diarrhea, abdominal pain, tenesmus, flatulence, bloating, anorexia, weight loss, esophagitis. Nonspecific colitis, pseudomembranous colitis (may be severe). *Allergic:* Morbilliform rash (most common). Also, maculopapular rash, urticaria, pruritus, fever, hypotension. Rarely, polyarteritis, anaphylaxis, erythema multiforme. *Hematologic:* Leukopenia, neutropenia, eosinophilia, thrombocytopenia, agranulocytosis. *Miscellaneous:* Superinfection.

Following IV use: Thrombophlebitis, erythema, pain, swelling. IV lincomycin may cause hypotension, syncope, and cardiac arrest (rare). *Following IM use:* Pain, induration, sterile abscesses. *Following topical use:* Erythema, irritation, dryness, peeling, itching, burning, oiliness. Also, sore throat, fatigue, urinary frequency, headache.

Note: The injection contains benzyl alcohol which has been associated with a fatal gasping syndrome in infants.

Drug Interactions

Antiperistaltic antidiarrheals (opiates, Lomotil)	↑ Diarrhea due to ↓ removal of toxins from colon
Erythromycin	Cross-interference → ↓ effect of both drugs
Kaolin (e.g., Kaopectate)	↓ Effect due to ↓ absorption from GI tract
Neuromuscular blocking agents	↑ Effect of blocking agents

Laboratory Test Interferences: ↓ Levels of SGOT, SGPT, nonprotein nitrogen, alkaline phosphatase, bilirubin, BSP retention, and ↓ platelet count.

Dosage: Capsules, adults: 500 mg t.i.d.–q.i.d.; **children over 1 month of age:** 30–60 mg/kg/day in 3–4 divided doses, depending on severity of infection. **IM, adults:** 600 mg q 12–24 hr; **children over 1 month of age:** 10 mg/kg/day q 12–24 hr, depending on severity of infection. **IV, adults:** 0.6–1.0 g q 8–12 hr up to 8 g daily, depending on severity of infection; **children over 1 month of age:** 10–20 mg/kg/day, depending on severity of infection. **Subconjunctival injection:** 0.75 mg/0.25 mL.

In impaired renal function, reduce dosage by 70%–75%. Total blood counts and liver function tests should be done periodically during long-term therapy.

NURSING CONSIDERATIONS

See also *General Nursing Considerations For All Anti-Infectives* under *Penicillins,* p. 140.

Administration/Storage

1. Prepare drug for administration as directed on package insert.
2. Administer slowly IM to minimize pain.
3. For IV use, carefully follow recommended concentration and rate of administration to prevent severe cardiopulmonary reactions.

Interventions

1. Be prepared to manage colitis, which can occur 2–9 days to several weeks after initiation of therapy, by providing fluids, electrolytes, protein supplements, systemic corticosteroids, and vancomycin.
2. Do not administer, and caution client against using, antiperistaltic agents if diarrhea occurs, because these agents can prolong or aggravate condition.
3. Do not use any acne or topical mercury preparations containing a peeling agent in an area affected by medication, as severe irritation can occur.
4. Do not administer kaolin concomitantly with lincomycin, because kaolin will reduce absorption of antibiotic. If kaolin is required, administer 3 hr before antibiotic.
5. Observe for adverse drug interactions caused by concurrent administration of neuromuscular blocking agents. Be alert to hypotension, bronchospasms, cardiac disturbances, hyperthermia, and respiratory depression.

6. Assess for transient flushing and sensations of warmth, and cardiac disturbances, which may accompany IV infusions. Monitor pulse rate before, during, and after infusion until rate is stable at levels normal for client.

Client/Family Teaching

1. Instruct client to take lincomycin on an empty stomach between meals and not with a sugar substitute.
2. Administer on an empty stomach to ensure optimum absorption. Drug should be taken only as long as directed.

Evaluation

1. Note client response to therapy and teaching.
2. Observe for freedom of complications of drug therapy.
3. Evaluate for GI disturbances, including abdominal pain, diarrhea, anorexia, nausea, vomiting, bloody or tarry stools, and excessive flatulence. Discontinuation of drug may be indicated.

ERYTHROMYCINS

Action/Kinetics: The erythromycins are produced by strains of *Streptomyces erythraeus* and have bacteriostatic and occasionally bactericidal activity (at high concentrations or if microorganism is particularly susceptible).

The erythromycins inhibit protein synthesis of microorganisms by binding reversibly to a ribosomal subunit (50S), thus interfering with the transmission of genetic information and inhibiting protein synthesis. The drugs are effective only against rapidly multiplying organisms. The erythromycins are absorbed from the upper part of the small intestine. Erythromycins for oral use are manufactured in enteric-coated or film-coated forms to prevent destruction by gastric acid. Erythromycin diffuses into body tissues; peritoneal, pleural, ascitic, and amniotic fluids; saliva; through the placental circulation; and across the mucous membrane of the tracheobronchial tree. It diffuses poorly into spinal fluid, although penetration is increased in meningitis.

Peak serum levels: PO, 1–4 hr. **t½:** 1.5–2 hr, *but prolonged in patients with renal impairment.* The drug is metabolized partially by the liver and primarily excreted in bile. Erythromycins are excreted in breast milk also.

Uses: The drug of choice to treat respiratory tract infections due to *Mycoplasma pneumoniae;* intestinal amebiasis due to *Entamoeba histolytica;* Legionnaires' disease due to *Legionella pneumophila;* to eliminate *Bordetella pertussis* from the nasopharynx; and for carriers and erythrasma treatment of infections due to *Corynebacterium diphtheriae* and *C. minutissimum.* Use with sulfonamides to treat upper respiratory tract infections due to *Hemophilus influenzae.*

As an alternate drug to treat the following diseases in patients who are allergic to tetracyclines or penicillin or when these drugs are contraindicated or not tolerated: Upper and lower respiratory tract, soft tissue, or skin infections due to group A beta-hemolytic streptococcus; prior to dental procedures to prevent bacterial endocarditis due to alpha-hemolytic streptococcus in patients with a history of congenital heart or rheumatic disease; acute pelvic inflammatory disease due to *Neisseria gonorrhoeae;* primary syphilis due to *Treponema pallidum;* upper or lower respiratory tract infections due to *Streptococcus pneumoniae;* chlamydial infections; and infections due to *Listeria monocytogenes.*

Investigational: Infections due to *N. gonorrhoeae,* including uncomplicated urethral, rectal, or endocervical infections and disseminated gonococcal infections; severe or prolonged diarrhea due to *Campylobacter fetus;* genital, inguinal, or anorectal infections due to *Lymphogranuloma venereum;* chancroid due to *Haemophilus ducreyi.*

Many erythromycins are available in ointments and solutions for ophthalmic, otic, and dermatologic use.

Contraindications: Hypersensitivity to erythromycin; in utero syphilis.

Special Concerns: Most erythromycins are pregnancy category B. Use with caution in liver disease and during lactation.

Side Effects: Erythromycins have a low incidence of untoward reactions (except for the estolate salt). *GI* (most common): Nausea, vomiting, diarrhea, cramping, abdominal pain, stomatitis, anorexia, melena, heartburn, pruritus ani, pseudomembranous colitis. *Allergic:* Skin rashes with or without pruritus, bullous fixed eruptions, urticaria, eczema, anaphylaxis (rare). *CNS:* Fear, confusion, altered thinking, uncontrollable crying or hysterical laughter, feeling of impending loss of consciousness. *Miscellaneous:* Superinfection, hepatotoxicity. *Following topical use:* Itching, burning, irritation, or stinging of skin. Dry, scaly skin.

IV use may result in venous irritation and thrombophlebitis; IM use produces pain at the injection site, with development of necrosis or sterile abscesses.

Drug Interactions	
Carbamazepine	↑ Effect of carbamazepine due to ↓ breakdown by liver
Cyclosporine	↑ Effect of cyclosporine due to ↓ excretion
Digoxin	Erythromycin ↑ bioavailability of digoxin
Methylprednisolone	↑ Effect of methylprednisolone due to ↓ breakdown by liver
Penicillin	Erythromycins ↓ effect of penicillins
Sodium bicarbonate	↑ Effect of erythromycin in urine due to alkalinization
Theophylline	↑ Effect of theophylline due to ↓ breakdown in liver
Warfarin	Erythromycin ↑ effect of warfarin

Laboratory Test Interferences: False + or ↑ values of urinary catecholamines, urinary steroids, and SGOT and SGPT.

Dosage: PO and **IM** (painful); some preparations can be given **IV.** See individual drugs.

NURSING CONSIDERATIONS

See also *General Nursing Considerations For All Anti-Infectives* under *Penicillins,* p. 140.

Administration/Storage

Inject deep into muscle mass. Injections are painful and irritating.

Assessment

1. Note if client is allergic to any other antibiotic drugs.
2. Determine infection for which client is being treated.
3. Assess for skin reactions when using erythromycin ointment. Discontinue use and report to physician.

4. When using ophthalmic solutions, assess for mild reaction which, although usually transient, should be reported to the physician.

Interventions

1. Do not administer with or immediately prior to ingestion of fruit juice or other acidic drinks because acidity may decrease activity of drug. However, adequate water (up to 8 oz) should be consumed with each dose.
2. Do not routinely administer PO medication with meals because food decreases the absorption of most erythromycins. However, physician may order medication to be given with food to reduce GI irritation.
3. Instill otic solutions at room temperature. Gently pull pinna of ear down and back for children under 3 years of age; pull pinna of ear up and back for clients over 3 years of age.
4. Observe for evidence of impaired liver function, especially among the elderly.

Client/Family Teaching

1. Question clients to ensure they are eating a balanced diet and that fluid intake is adequate.
2. Doses of erythromycins should be evenly spaced throughout a 24-hr period.
3. If clients have difficulty with nausea, have them notify the physician so the prescription can be changed to coated tablets that can be taken with meals.
4. If tablets are not coated, advise client to take them 2 hr after meals.
5. Advise clients not to take erythromycins with juices.
6. Remind client to clean affected area before applying ointment.
7. Instill otic solutions at room temperature. Demonstrate the appropriate method for administration and have client/family return demonstrate.

Evaluation

1. Assess client/family knowledge and understanding of illness, and response to prescribed therapy as well as teaching.
2. Monitor for indications of superinfection, such as furry tongue, vaginal itching, rectal itching, or diarrhea.
3. Evaluate for evidence of reduction of the infection (i.e., client statements on how he/she feels).
4. Note evidence of rash or any complaints of irritation of the mouth or tongue.
5. Note any evidence of hearing loss which is usually temporary.

ERYTHROMYCIN BASE   (eh-rih-throw-**MY**-sin)

Capsules/Tablets: E-Mycin, Eryc, Eryc 125, Ery-Tab, Erythromid✷, Erythromycin Base Film-Tabs, Ilotycin, Novorythro✷, Robimycin. Gel, topical: Erygel. Ointment, topical: Akne-mycin. Ointment, ophthalmic: AK-Mycin, Ilotycin Ophthalmic. Pledgets: Erycette, T-Stat. Solution, topical: Akne-mycin, A/T/S, EryDerm, Erymax, ETS, Mythromycin, Staticin, T-Stat. (Rx)

See also *Erythromycins,* p. 117.

Classification: Antibiotic, erythromycin.

Uses: See *Erythromycins,* p. 117.

Dosage: PO. *Respiratory tract infections due to Mycoplasma pneumoniae:* 500 mg q 6 hr for 5–10 days (up to 3 weeks for severe infections). *Intestinal amebiasis due to Entamoeba histolytica:* **Adults:** 250 mg q.i.d. to 10–14 days; **pediatric:** 30–50 mg/kg daily in divided doses for 10–14 days. *Legionnaire's disease:* 500–1,000 mg q.i.d. for 3 weeks. *Bordetella pertussis:* 500 mg q.i.d. for 10 days. *Infections due to Corynebacterium diphtheriae or C. minutissimum:* 500 mg q.i.d. for 10 days for carriers and 250 mg t.i.d. for 3 wks for erythrasma.

Group A beta-hemolytic streptococcus infections: 250–500 mg q.i.d. for 10 days. *Prior to dental procedures as prophylaxis against bacterial endocarditis:* 1,000 mg 1 hr prior to dental appointment followed by 500 mg in 6 hr. *Primary syphilis:* 30–40 g in divided doses over 10–15 days. *Respiratory tract infections due to Streptococcus pneumoniae:* 250–500 mg q.i.d. *Chlamydial infections:* **Infants:** 50 mg/kg daily in 4 divided doses for 14–21 days; **Adults:** 500 mg q.i.d. for 7 days. *Listeria monocytogenes infections:* 500 mg q 12 hours, up to maximum of 4 g daily.

Nongonococcal urethritis, Campylobacter fetus infections, chancroid, lymphogranuloma venereum: 500 mg q.i.d. for 7 days.

NURSING CONSIDERATIONS
See *Nursing Considerations* for *Erythromycins,* p. 118.

Client/Family Teaching
Food does not affect absorption.

ERYTHROMYCIN ESTOLATE   (eh-rih-throw-**MY**-sin **EH**-stoh-late)
Ilosone, Novorythro✣ (Rx)

See also *Erythromycins,* p. 117.

Classification: Antibiotic, erythromycin.

Action/Kinetics: Most active form of erythromycin, with relatively long-lasting activity.

Uses: See *Erythromycins,* p. 117.

Additional Contraindications: Cholestatic jaundice or preexisting liver dysfunction. Not recommended for treatment of chronic disorders such as acne or furunculosis or for prophylaxis of rheumatic fever.

Additional Side Effects: Hepatotoxicity.

Dosage: Capsules, Drops, Suspension, Tablets, Chewable Tablets. See *Erythromycin base.* Similar blood levels are achieved using erythromycin base, estolate, or stearate.

NURSING CONSIDERATIONS
See also *Nursing Considerations* for *Erythromycins,* p. 118.

Administration/Storage
1. Shake oral suspension well before pouring.
2. Do not store suspension longer than 2 weeks at room temperature.
3. Chewable tablets must be chewed or crushed.

ERYTHROMYCIN ETHYLSUCCINATE   (eh-rih-throw-**MY**-sin eh-thil-**SUCK**-sin-ayt)
E.E.S., E.E.S. 200 and 400, E.E.S. Granules, E-Mycin E, EryPed, Pediamycin, Pediamycin 400, Wyamycin E (Rx)

See also *Erythromycins,* p. 117.

Classification: Antibiotic, erythromycin.

Uses: See *Erythromycins,* p. 117.

Additional Contraindications: The injectable form contains 2% butylbenzocaine; do not use in patients allergic to the "caine" (e.g., procaine, benzocaine) type of local anesthetics. Preexisting liver disease.

Dosage: Oral Suspension, Tablets, Chewable Tablets. See *Erythromycin base.* **Note:** 400 mg of erythromycin ethylsuccinate will achieve the same blood levels of erythromycin as 250 mg of the base, estolate, or stearate forms.

Hemophilus influenzae infections: Erythromycin ethylsuccinate, 50 mg/kg daily with sulfisoxazole, 150 mg/kg daily, both for a total of 10 days.

NURSING CONSIDERATIONS

See also *Nursing Considerations* for *Erythromycins,* p. 118.

Administration/Storage

1. Refrigerate aqueous suspensions and store for maximum of 1 week.
2. Chewable tablets must be chewed or crushed.

ERYTHROMYCIN GLUCEPTATE   (eh-rih-throw-**MY**-sin **GLUE**-sep-tayt)
Ilotycin Gluceptate (Rx)

See also *Erythromycins,* p. 117.

Classification: Antibiotic, erythromycin.

Uses: Primarily for unconscious, vomiting, or gravely ill patients with serious infections of gram-positive bacteria, especially hemolytic streptococci, pneumococci, staphylococci, and gonococci. Legionnaire's disease.

Drug Interactions: Drug for IV administration is incompatible with amikacin, aminophylline, cefazolin, cephalothin, metaraminol, novobiocin, oxytetracycline, pentobarbital, secobarbital, streptomycin, and tetracycline.

Dosage: IV only, Adults and children: 15–20 mg/kg daily (up to 4 g daily may be required for serious infections). *Acute pelvic inflammatory disease caused by gonorrhea:* 500 mg q 6 hr for 3 days, followed by 250 mg erythromycin stearate PO q 6 hr for 7 days. *Legionnaire's disease:* 1–4 g/day in divided doses.

NURSING CONSIDERATIONS

See also *Nursing Considerations* for *Erythromycins,* p. 118.

Administration/Storage

1. Follow directions on vial for dilution.

2. Concentrate (which must be diluted further before administration) will remain stable in refrigerator for 7 days.

3. Administer slowly over period of 20–60 min or by continuous IV infusion over 24 hr.

ERYTHROMYCIN LACTOBIONATE   (eh-rih-throw-**MY**-sin lack-toe-**BYE**-oh-nayt)

Erythrocin Lactobionate IV (Rx)

See also *Erythromycins,* p. 117.

Classification: Antibiotic, erythromycin.

Uses: For seriously ill or vomiting patients suffering from infections caused by susceptible organisms; acute pelvic inflammatory disease due to gonorrhea. Legionnaire's disease.

Additional Side Effect: Transient deafness.

Additional Drug Interaction: Some physicians recommend that no drugs be added to IV solutions of erythromycin lactobionate.

Dosage: IV, Adults and children: 15–20 mg/kg/day up to 4 g/day in severe infections. *Acute pelvic inflammatory disease caused by gonorrhea:* 500 mg q 6 hr for 3 days followed by 250 mg erythromycin stearate, **PO,** q 6 hr for 7 days. *Legionnaire's disease:* 1–4 g/day in divided doses. Change to oral therapy as soon as possible.

NURSING CONSIDERATIONS

See *Nursing Considerations* for *Erythromycins,* p. 118.

ERYTHROMYCIN STEARATE   (eh-rih-throw-**MY**-sin **STEER**-ayt)

Apo-Erythro-S✽, Eramycin, Erypar, Erythrocin Stearate, Ethril 250 and 500, Novorythro✽, Wyamycin S (Rx)

See also *Erythromycins,* p. 117.

Classification: Antibiotic, erythromycin.

Uses: See *Erythromycins,* p. 117.

Additional Side Effects: Drug causes more allergic reactions (e.g., skin rash and urticaria) than other erythromycins. Hepatotoxicity.

Dosage: Tablets. See *Erythromycin base.* Similar blood levels are achieved using erythromycin base, estolate, or stearate forms.

NURSING CONSIDERATIONS

See also *Nursing Considerations* for *Erythromycins,* p. 118.

Administration/Storage

Do not administer with meals because food decreases absorption.

MISCELLANEOUS ANTIBIOTICS

AZTREONAM FOR INJECTION   (az-TREE-oh-nam)

Azactam for Injection (Rx)

See also *Anti-Infectives,* p. 71.

Classification: Monobactam antibiotic.

Action/Kinetics: Aztreonam belongs to a new class of antibiotics called *monobactams.* It is a synthetic drug that is bactericidal against gram-negative aerobic pathogens. The drug acts by inhibiting cell wall synthesis. It is effective against *Escherichia coli, Klebsiella, Enterobacter, Pseudomonas, Proteus, Citrobacter, Serratia marcescens,* and *Hemophilus influenzae.* **t½:** 1.5–2 hr. The t½ is prolonged in patients with impaired renal function.

Uses: The following infections due to gram-negative aerobic organisms may be treated: urinary tract, lower respiratory tract, skin and skin structures, intra-abdominal, gynecologic, and septicemia.

Contraindications: Allergy to aztreonam.

Special Concerns: Pregnancy category B: use in pregnancy only if clearly needed. Safety and effectiveness have not been determined in children and infants. Use with caution in patients allergic to penicillins or cephalosporins and in patients with impaired hepatic or renal function.

Side Effects: *GI:* Nausea, vomiting, abdominal cramps, *Clostridium difficile*-associated diarrhea or GI bleeding. *CNS:* Confusion, seizures, vertigo, paresthesia, insomnia, dizziness. *Hematologic:* Anemia, neutropenia, thrombocytopenia, leukocytosis, thrombocytosis, pancytopenia. *Dermatologic:* Rash, purpura, erythema multiforme, urticaria, petechiae, pruritus, diaphoresis, exfoliative dermatitis. *CV:* Hypotension, transient ECG changes. *Miscellaneous:* Anaphylaxis, headache, weakness, fever, malaise, hepatitis, jaundice, muscle aches, tinnitus, diplopia, nasal congestion, halitosis, altered taste, mouth ulcers, sneezing, vaginal candidiasis, vaginitis, breast tenderness.

Drug Interactions: Antibiotics that increase levels of β-lactamase (e.g., cefoxitin, imipenem) may inhibit the activity of aztreonam.

Laboratory Test Interferences: ↑ SGOT (AST), SGPT (ALT), alkaline phosphatase, serum creatinine, prothrombin time. Positive Coombs' test.

Dosage: IM, IV. *Urinary tract infections:* 0.5–1 g q 8–12 hr, not to exceed 8 g daily. *Moderate to severe systemic infections:* 1–2 g q 8–12 hr, not to exceed 8 g daily. *Severe systemic or life-threatening infections:* 2 g q 6–8 hr, not to exceed 8 g daily. Dosage should be decreased in patients with impaired renal function (see package insert).

NURSING CONSIDERATIONS

See also *General Nursing Considerations For All Anti-Infectives* under *Penicillins,* p. 140.

Administration/Storage

1. The IV route should be used for doses greater than 1 g or in clients with septicemia.
2. Therapy should be continued for at least 48 hr after the client becomes asymptomatic or until laboratory tests indicate that the infection has been eradicated.

3. An IV bolus injected slowly over 3–5 min may be used to initiate therapy.

4. For IM use, the drug should be given in a large muscle mass.

5. For use as a bolus, the 15-mL vial should be diluted with 6–10 mL sterile water for injection. For IM use, the 15-mL vial should be diluted with at least 3 mL of either sterile water for injection, sodium chloride injection, bacteriostatic water for injection, or bacteriostatic sodium chloride injection.

6. Aztreonam is incompatible with cephradine, nafcillin sodium, and metronidazole. Data for other drugs are not available.

Interventions

Obtain baseline liver and renal function studies and anticipate reduced dosage if function is impaired.

Client/Family Teaching

Reassure client that during therapy a slightly itchy, red rash and nasal congestion may occur, but report to physician if symptoms intensify.

BACITRACIN INTRAMUSCULAR   (bass-ih-**TRAY**-sin)

Bacitin ✽, Bacitracin Sterile (Rx)

BACITRACIN OINTMENT   (bass-ih-**TRAY**-sin)

Baciguent (OTC)

BACITRACIN OPHTHALMIC   (bass-ih-**TRAY**-sin)

AK-Tracin, Bacitracin Ophthalmic (Rx)

See also *Anti-Infectives,* p. 71.

Classification: Antibiotic, miscellaneous.

Action/Kinetics: This antibiotic is produced by *Bacillus subtilis.* The drug interferes with synthesis of the cell wall, preventing incorporation of amino acids and nucleotides. Bacitracin is bactericidal, bacteriostatic, and active against protoplasts. It is not absorbed from the GI tract. When given parenterally, drug is well distributed in pleural and ascitic fluids.

Bacitracin has high nephrotoxicity. Its systemic use is restricted to infants (see *Uses*). Renal function must be carefully evaluated prior to, and daily, during use. **Peak plasma levels: IM,** 0.2–2 mcg/mL after 2 hr. From 10%–40% is excreted in the urine after IM administration.

Uses: Bacitracin is used locally during surgery for cranial and neurosurgical infections caused by susceptible organisms.

As an ointment (preferred) or solution, bacitracin is prescribed for superficial pyoderma-like impetigo and infectious eczematoid dermatitis, for secondary infected dermatoses (atopic dermatitis, contact dermatitis), and for superficial infections of the eye, ear, nose, and throat by susceptible organisms.

Parenteral use is limited to the treatment of staphylococcal pneumonia and staphylococcus-induced empyema in infants.

Contraindications: Hypersensitivity or toxic reaction to bacitracin. Pregnancy.

Side Effects: Nephrotoxicity due to tubular and glomerular necrosis, renal failure; toxic reactions; nausea, vomiting.

Drug Interactions	
Aminoglycosides	Additive nephrotoxicity and neuromuscular blocking activity
Anesthetics	↑ Neuromuscular blockade → possible muscle paralysis
Neuromuscular blocking agents	Additive neuromuscular blockade → possible muscle paralysis

Dosage: IM only. Infants, 2.5 kg and below: 900 units/kg/day in 2–3 divided doses; **infants over 2.5 kg:** 1,000 units/kg/day in 2–3 divided doses. **Ophthalmic ointment (500 units/g):** *Acute infections:* ½ inch in lower conjunctival sac q 3–4 hr. *Mild to moderate infections:* ½ inch b.i.d.–t.i.d. **Topical ointment (500 units/g):** Apply 1–5 times daily to affected area.

NURSING CONSIDERATIONS

See also *General Nursing Considerations For All Anti-Infectives* under *Penicillins,* p. 140.

Administration/Storage

Do not mix bacitracin with glycerin or other polyalcohols that cause drug to deteriorate. Bacitracin unguentin base is anhydrous, consisting of liquid and white petrolatum.

Interventions

1. Monitor and maintain adequate fluid intake and output with parenteral use of drug.
2. Withhold drug and consult with physician when fluid output is inadequate. Monitor renal function studies.
3. Test pH of urine daily, because it should be kept at 6 or greater to decrease renal irritation.
4. Have sodium bicarbonate or another alkali available to administer if pH drops below 6.
5. Do not administer concurrently or sequentially with a topical or systemic nephrotoxic drug.
6. Cleanse area before applying bacitracin as a wet dressing or ointment.

Evaluation

1. Note status (presence/absence) of pretreatment symptoms and C&S results to determine effectiveness of treatment.
2. Assess for evidence of toxicity or hypersensitivity.
3. Check urine to determine pH and review I&O during parenteral therapy.

CIPROFLOXACIN HYDROCHLORIDE   (sip-row-**FLOX**-ah-sin)

Cipro (Rx)

Classification: Antibacterial, quinolone derivative.

Action/Kinetics: Ciprofloxacin is a synthetic quinolone with broad-spectrum bactericidal activity. It inhibits the synthesis of bacterial DNA by inhibiting the enzyme DNA gyrase. The drug also inhibits relaxation of supercoiled DNA and promotes double-stranded DNA breakage. Ciprofloxacin is effective against the following gram-positive organisms: *Staphylococcus aureus, Streptococcus pyogenes, S. pneumoniae, S. faecalis, Mycobacterium tuberculosis,* and *Chlamydia trachomatis.* Also, ciprofloxacin is effective against a large number of gram-negative organisms, including: *Escherichia coli, Klebsiella, Proteus mirabilis, P. vulgaris, Enterobacter, Citrobacter, Salmonella, Shigella, Providencia stuartii, P. rettgeri, Serratia, Morganella morganii, Acinetobacter, Pseudomonas aeruginosa, Hemophilus influenzae, Neisseria gonorrhoeae, N. meningitidis, Brucella, Pasturella, Legionella,* and others. **Maximum serum levels:** 1–2 hr. **t½:** 4 hr. Peak serum levels above 5 mcg/mL should be avoided. About 40%–50% of an oral dose is excreted unchanged in the urine.

Uses: Susceptible strains (see above) of organisms causing infections of the urinary tract, lower respiratory tract, bones, joints, skin and skin structures, and infectious diarrhea.

Contraindications: Hypersensitivity to quinolones. Use in children. During lactation, consideration should be given either to discontinuing nursing or the drug.

Special Concerns: Pregnancy category: C.

Side Effects: *GI:* Nausea, vomiting, diarrhea, oral candidiasis, dysphagia, intestinal perforation, anorexia, abdominal discomfort, GI bleeding, oral mucosal pain, bad taste. *CNS:* Headache, restlessness, insomnia, nightmares, hallucinations, tremor, lightheadedness, confusion, seizures, ataxia, mania, weakness, drowsiness, malaise, depression, depersonalization, paresthesia. *GU:* Nephritis, crystalluria, hematuria, cylindruria, renal failure, urinary retention, polyuria, vaginitis, urethral bleeding, acidosis. *Skin:* Rashes, urticaria, photosensitivity, flushing, pruritus, erythema nodosum, cutaneous candidiasis, hyperpigmentation, edema (of lips, neck, face, conjunctivae, hands), angioedema. *Ophthalmic:* Blurred or disturbed vision, double vision, eye pain. *CV:* Hypertension, syncope, angina pectoris, palpitations, atrial flutter, myocardial infarction, cerebral thrombosis, ventricular ectopy, cardiopulmonary arrest. *Respiratory:* Dyspnea, bronchospasm, pulmonary embolism, edema of larynx or lungs, hemoptysis, hiccoughs. *Hematologic:* Eosinophilia, pancytopenia, leukopenia, anemia, leukocytosis, bleeding diathesis. *Miscellaneous:* Superinfections; fever; tinnitus; joint pain or stiffness; back, neck or chest pain; flare-up of gout.

Drug Interactions	
Aminoglycosides	Additive antibacterial activity
Antacids	↓ Rate of absorption of ciprofloxacin
Beta-lactam antibiotics	Additive antibacterial activity
Clindamycin	Additive antibacterial activity
Metronidazole	Additive antibacterial activity
Probenecid	50% ↑ in systemic levels of ciprofloxacin
Theophylline	↑ Plasma levels of theophylline with ↑ possibility of untoward reactions

Laboratory Test Interferences: ↑ SGPT (ALT), SGOT (AST), alkaline phosphatase, serum bilirubin, LDH, serum creatinine, BUN, serum gamma-glutamyltransferase, serum amylase, uric acid, blood monocytes. ↓ Blood glucose, hemoglobin.

Dosage: Tablets. *Urinary tract infections:* 250 mg (mild) to 500 mg (severe) q 12 hr for 7–14 days. *Infectious diarrhea:* 500 mg q 12 hr for 5–7 days. *Skin, skin structures, respiratory tract, bone and joint infections:* 500 mg (mild) to 750 mg (severe) q 12 hr for 7–14 days. Treatment may be required for 4–6 weeks in bone and joint infections. Dose must be reduced in patients with a creatinine clearance less than 50 mL/min.

NURSING CONSIDERATIONS

See also *General Nursing Considerations for All Anti-Infectives* under *Penicillins,* p. 140.

Administration/Storage

Although food delays the absorption of the drug, it may be taken with or without meals. The recommended time for dosing is 2 hr after a meal.

Client/Family Teaching

1. Take medication 2 hr after meals as food may delay absorption.
2. Avoid ingestion of antacids containing magnesium or aluminum within 2 hr of taking drug as antacids may interfere with absorption.
3. Stress the importance of drinking increased amounts of fluids and to keep the urine acidic to minimize the risk of crystalluria.
4. The medication may cause dizziness; use caution in any activity that requires mental alertness or coordination.
5. To report any persistent GI symptoms such as diarrhea, vomiting, or abdominal pain to the physician.

Evaluation

1. Observe for freedom from complications from drug therapy.
2. Clients on theophylline or probenecid require close observation and potential medication adjustments.

FURAZOLIDONE   (fyour-ah-**ZOH**-lih-dohn)

Furoxone (Rx)

Classification: Antibacterial, miscellaneous.

Action/Kinetics: Acts by interfering with crucial enzyme systems. Bactericidal against many pathogens of GI tract, but affects normal flora minimally. Poorly absorbed from and inactivated in intestine.

Uses: Bacterial or protozoal diarrhea; enteritis caused by *Salmonella, Shigella, Staphylococcus, Escherichia, Enterobacter aerogenes, Vibrio cholerae,* and *Giardia lamblia.*

Contraindications: Nursing mothers and infants under 1 month of age.

Special Concerns: Safe use during pregnancy has not been established.

Side Effects: *GI:* Nausea, vomiting, colitis, proctitis, anal pruritus. *Allergic:* Urticaria, rashes, hypotension, fever, arthralgia. *Miscellaneous:* Headache, malaise, Antabuse-like reaction, hemolysis in glucose-6-phosphate dehydrogenase-deficient patients.

Drug Interactions	
Alcohol, ethyl	Antabuse-like reaction possible
Antidepressants, tricyclic	↑ Effects (including toxicity) of furazolidone
Antihistamines	↑ Chance of hypotension and hypoglycemia

Drug Interactions

CNS depressants	Furazolidone ↑ depressant effects
Guanethidine	Hypotensive effect ↓ by furazolidone
Hypoglycemics, oral	↑ Hypoglycemic effect
Insulin	↑ Hypoglycemic effect
Meperidine	Concomitant use may cause unpredictable CNS and cardiovascular effects
Monoamine oxidase inhibitors	↑ Effect due to monoamine oxidase inhibitor activity of furazolidone
Narcotics	↑ Chance of hypotension and hypoglycemia
Sympathomimetics, indirect acting	↑ Effect due to monoamine oxidase inhibitor activity of furazolidone

Laboratory Test Interference: False + urine glucose values.

Dosage: Oral Liquid, Tablets. Adults: 100 mg. q.i.d.; **children 5 years and older:** 25–50 mg q.i.d.; **children, 1–4 years:** 17–25 mg q.i.d. (use liquid); **children, 1 month to 1 year old:** 8–17 mg q.i.d. (use liquid). Daily dosage for all ages should not exceed 8.8 mg/kg.

NURSING CONSIDERATIONS

See also *General Nursing Considerations For All Anti-infectives* under *Penicillins,* p. 140.

Administration/Storage

Store liquid in amber-colored bottles.

Assessment

1. *Assess*
   - for hypersensitivity reactions demonstrated by a drop in BP, arthralgia, fever, and urticaria. Withhold drug if any of these symptoms are observed and notify physician.
   - for GI symptoms, malaise, or headache that subsides when dosage is reduced or drug is withdrawn; document findings.

Client/Family Teaching

1. Client should not eat food containing tyramine (such as broad beans, strong unpasteurized cheeses, yeast extracts, beer, pickled herring, chicken livers, bananas, avocados, or fermented food) because furazolidone is a monoamine oxidase inhibitor. These reactions are more likely to occur in clients receiving doses larger than those usually recommended or who receive the drug for more than 5 days.
2. Instruct not to use sedatives, antihistamines, tranquilizers, or narcotic drugs concurrently with therapy unless their physician specifically prescribes.
3. Do not drink alcohol during therapy or for 4 days after therapy because an Antabuse-like reaction (characterized by flushing, palpitation, dyspnea, hyperventilation, tachycardia, nausea, vomiting, drop in BP, and even profound collapse) may occur.
4. Drug may turn urine a brownish color.
5. Diabetic clients should use finger sticks (or other reliable form) to determine their insulin requirements during therapy.

Evaluation

Anticipate withdrawal of drug if clinical response does not occur within 7 days.

IMIPENEM-CILASTATIN SODIUM   (ih-mih-**PEN**-em-sigh-lah-**STAT**-in)

Primaxin, Zienam ✿ (Rx)

See also *Anti-Infectives,* p. 71.

Classification: Antibiotic combined with inhibitor of dehydropeptidase I.

Action/Kinetics: Imipenem inhibits cell wall synthesis and is thus bactericidal against a wide range of gram-positive and gram-negative organisms. It is stable in the presence of beta-lactamases. Addition of cilastatin prevents the metabolism of imipenem in the kidneys by dehydropeptidase I, thus ensuring high levels of the imipenem in the urinary tract. $t^{1/2}$: 1 hr for each component.

Uses: Serious infections of the lower respiratory tract and urinary tract. Also, serious gynecologic infections, skin and skin structure infections, bacterial septicemia, bone and joint infections, endocarditis, intra-abdominal infections, and infections caused by more than one agent. Infections resistant to aminoglycosides, cephalosporins, or penicillins have responded to imipenem.

Special Concerns: Pregnancy category: C. Use with caution in pregnancy and lactation. Safety and effectiveness have not been determined in children less than 12 years of age.

Side Effects: *GI:* Pseudomembranous colitis, nausea, diarrhea, vomiting, abdominal pain, heartburn, increased salivation, hemorrhagic colitis, gastroenteritis, glossitis, pharyngeal pain. *CNS:* Fever, confusion, seizures, dizziness, sleepiness, myoclonus, headache, vertigo, paresthesia, encephalopathy. *CV:* Hypotension, tachycardia, palpitations. *Dermatologic:* Rash, urticaria, pruritus, flushing, cyanosis, facial edema, erythema multiforme. *Miscellaneous:* Candidiasis, pruritus vulvae, tinnitus, polyuria, increased sweating, joint pain, muscle weakness, anuria/oliguria, chest discomfort, dyspnea, hyperventilation, transient hearing loss in patients with existing hearing impairment.

The following side effects may occur at the injection site: Thrombophlebitis, phlebitis, pain, erythema, induration, infection.

Laboratory Test Interferences: ↑ SGOT, SGPT, alkaline phosphatase, LDH, bilirubin, potassium, chloride, BUN, creatinine. ↓ Sodium. Positive Coombs' test and abnormal prothrombin time.

Dosage: IV. *Gram-positive organisms, highly susceptible gram-negative organisms, anaerobes: Mild,* 250 mg q 6 hr; *moderate,* 500 mg q 6–8 hr; *severe/life-threatening,* 500 mg q 6 hr. *Urinary tract infections:* 250–500 mg q 6 hr, depending on severity.

Gram-negative organisms: Mild, 500 mg q 6 hr; *moderate,* 500–1,000 mg q 6–8 hr; *severe/life-threatening,* 1 g q 6–8 hr. *Urinary tract infections:* 250–500 mg q 6 hr, depending on severity.

The total daily dose should not exceed 50 mg/kg or 4 g, whichever is lower.

The package insert should be consulted for calculation of doses in adults with impaired renal function.

NURSING CONSIDERATIONS

See also *General Nursing Considerations for All Anti-Infectives* under *Penicillins,* p. 140.

Administration/Storage

1. Doses between 250 and 500 mg should be given by IV infusion over 20–30 min; doses of 1 g should be given by IV infusion over 40–60 min. If nausea develops, the infusion rate should be decreased.
2. Reconstituted solutions vary from colorless to yellow.
3. Imipenem-cilastatin should not be physically mixed with other antibiotics; however, the drug may be administered with other antibiotics, if necessary.

4. Most reconstituted solutions can be stored at room temperature for 4 hr and, if refrigerated, for 24 hr. The exception is imipenem-cilastatin reconstituted with 0.9% sodium chloride solution, which is stable at room temperature for 10 hr and, if refrigerated, for 48 hr.

MUPIROCIN   (myou-**PEER**-oh-sin)

Bactroban (Rx)

Classification: Anti-infective, topical.

Action/Kinetics: Mupirocin exerts its antibacterial action by binding to bacterial isoleucyl transfer-RNA synthetase, which results in inhibition of protein synthesis by the organism. The drug is not absorbed into the systemic circulation. Serum present in exudative wounds decreases the antibacterial activity. Mupirocin is metabolized to the inactive monic acid in the skin, and is then removed by normal skin desquamation.

Uses: Topically to treat impetigo due to *Staphylococcus aureus, Streptococcus pyogenes,* and beta-hemolytic streptococcus.

Contraindications: Ophthalmic use. Lactation.

Special Concerns: Pregnancy category: B.

Side Effects: Side effects are all local and include superinfection, itching, rash, burning, stinging, pain, erythema, swelling, dry skin, contact dermatitis, and increased exudate.

Dosage: Topical Ointment. A small amount of ointment is applied to the affected area t.i.d.

NURSING CONSIDERATIONS

Administration/Storage

A gauze dressing may be used if desired.

Interventions

The drug should be discontinued and the client should be reevaluated if symptoms of chemical irritation or hypersensitivity occur. Report all side effects to the physician.

Client/Family Teaching

1. Demonstrate the appropriate technique for applying topical medications.
2. Instruct client/family to report any increased rash, itching, or pain at the site.
3. If no improvement is noted after 5 days of therapy, have client notify physician.

Evaluation

Note if presence/absence of clinical response is observed in 3–5 days.

NITROFURAZONE   (nye-troh-**FYOUR**-ah-zohn)

Furacin (Rx)

See also *Anti-Infectives,* p. 71.

Classification: Antibiotic, miscellaneous (topical germicide).

Action/Kinetics: Nitrofurazone is a broad-spectrum, mostly bactericidal agent for both aerobic and anaerobic gram-positive organisms. Nitrofurazone's activity has been attributed to its interference with enzyme systems necessary for carbohydrate metabolism.

Uses: Adjunctive therapy for patients with second- and third-degree burns or skin grafts. Skin grafting in presence of bacterial contamination may cause rejection of graft or infection of donor site.

Special Concerns: Pregnancy category: C.

Side Effects: Overgrowth by nonsusceptible microorganisms including fungi. Very low incidence of contact dermatitis.

Dosage: Cream, Soluble Ointment, Topical Solution: Apply directly or place on gauze. Used once daily or every few days.

NURSING CONSIDERATIONS

See also *General Nursing Considerations For All Anti-infectives* under *Penicillins,* p. 140.

Administration/Storage

1. Store in light-resistant containers and prevent exposure to light, heat, and/or alkaline materials.
2. Discard cloudy solutions because they suggest microbial contamination of the drug.
3. Discoloration does not indicate a loss in strength of the material, consult with pharmacist if unsure.
4. Reautoclaving may be done at 121°C for 30 min at 15–20 lb of pressure, but discoloration usually occurs and the consistency of the base (particularly an ointment) is changed.
5. To prepare sterile impregnated gauze:
   * Place sterile gauze strips in a tray and cover with Furacin-soluble dressing.
   * Repeat above, adding several layers of gauze for each layer of soluble dressing.
   * To minimize discoloration caused by autoclaving, sprinkle sterile water on each layer of dressing.
   * Cover the tray loosely and autoclave at 121°C for 30 min at 15–20 lb of pressure.
6. Apply soluble dressing directly with a sterile tongue blade or place first on sterile gauze.

Assessment

Note any history of fungus infections and contact dermatitis.

Interventions

1. Protect skin adjacent to chronic stasis ulcers by covering the skin with zinc oxide ointment and using nitrofurazone only on the lesion.
2. Minimize adverse effects by irrigating lesion to remove medication at the first sign of irritation.
3. Flush dressing with sterile saline at time of removal to prevent dressing from adhering to wound.

Interventions for Furacin-Soluble Dressing and Powder

1. Apply directly with a sterile tongue blade or place first on sterile gauze.
2. Impregnate bandage rolls or gauze as described under Administration/Storage.

3. Furacin-soluble powder should be applied directly from the shaker top of a nonmetallic powder insufflator. Protect client from inhalation of powder particles.

Evaluation

Evaluate response to therapy and note rash, pruritus, and/or irritation, which are indications for termination of treatment with nitrofurazone.

NOVOBIOCIN SODIUM (no-voh-**BYE**-oh-sin)
Albamycin (Rx)

Classification: Antibiotic, miscellaneous.

Action/Kinetics: Novobiocin is derived from *Streptomyces niveus* and is primarily bacteriostatic. It inhibits protein and nucleic acid synthesis and interferes with formation of bacterial cell wall, probably affecting its stability. It is readily absorbed from the GI tract and diffuses poorly into pleural, joint, and ascitic fluids. Because of the high incidence of adverse reactions and rapid development of resistance, the drug should be used only for serious infections. **Peak plasma concentration:** 2 hr; higher levels will result if the patient is fasting. Excreted primarily in feces.

Uses: Infections by susceptible strains of staphylococci and *Proteus*. Indicated for the treatment of enteritis, postoperative wound infections, cellulitis, abscesses and ulcers, and resistant urinary tract infections.

Contraindications: Hypersensitivity to drug. Avoid use in newborn or premature infants.

Special Concerns: Pregnancy category: C. Safety during lactation has not been established.

Side Effects: *Allergic:* Skin rash (erythematous, maculopapular, scarlatiniform), urticaria, pruritus. *Hematopoietic:* Eosinophilia, anemia, leukopenia, agranulocytosis, pancytopenia, thrombocytopenia. *GI:* Nausea, vomiting, diarrhea, anorexia, intestinal hemorrhage. *Hepatic:* Jaundice, impaired liver function tests, neonatal hyperbilirubinemia. *Miscellaneous:* Fever, swollen joints, alopecia, light-headedness. The drug may also cause superinfections and favors the emergence of resistant strains, particularly staphylococci.

Drug Interaction: Tetracyclines ↓ effect of novobiocin.

Dosage: Capsules. Adult: 250 mg q 6 hr or 500 mg q 12 hr (in severe infections, can increase dose to maximum of 1 g q 12 hr). **Children:** 15 mg/kg/day in divided doses q 6–12 hr (up to 30–45 mg/kg/day for severe infections).

NURSING CONSIDERATIONS

See also *General Nursing Considerations For All Anti-Infectives* under *Penicillins,* p. 140.

Assessment

1. *Assess*
   - for allergic reactions, since drug is a potent sensitizing agent. Have emergency equipment readily available.
   - for symptoms of blood dyscrasias, such as anemia, purpura, paleness, and bleeding.

2. Determine ability of client to tolerate oral intake of drug so that oral medication can be prescribed as soon as possible.

3. If working with a newborn, assess for presence of jaundice which may lead to kernicterus and subsequent brain damage.

Interventions

1. Frequent total and differential blood counts and liver function tests should be performed during prolonged therapy.

2. Jaundice, hyperbilirubinemia, or sulfobromophthalein retention is an indication to discontinue the drug.

Client/Family Teaching

1. Report any evidence of fever, GI distress, excessive bleeding, or jaundice.

2. Stress the importance of reporting for all scheduled lab studies.

Evaluation

Note response to therapy and any complications of drug therapy such as

- presence of skin rashes, urticaria.
- evidence of GI upset.
- presence of yellow skin and sclera or musty odor which are symptoms of jaundice.
- client complaints of painful joints, swollen joints, lightheadedness.
- presence of fever.
- abnormal lab studies (CBC and liver function studies).

PENTAMIDINE ISETHIONATE   (pen-**TAM**-ih-deen)

NebuPent, Pentam (Rx)

Classification: Antibiotic, miscellaneous (antiprotozoal).

Action/Kinetics: The drug inhibits synthesis of DNA, RNA, phospholipids, and proteins, thereby interfering with cell metabolism. It may interfere also with folate transformation. About one-third of the dose may be excreted unchanged in the urine. Plasma levels following inhalation are significantly lower than after a comparable IV dose.

Uses: Parenteral. Pneumonia caused by *Pneumocystis carinii.* **Inhalation.** Prophylaxis of *Pneumocystis carinii* in high-risk HIV-infected patients defined by one or both of the following: (a) a history of one or more cases of pneumonia caused by *P. carinii* and/or (b) a peripheral CD4 + lymphocyte count less than 200 mm³. *Investigational:* Trypanosomiasis, visceral leishmaniasis.

Contraindications: Patients manifesting anaphylaxis to inhaled or parenteral pentamidine.

Special Concerns: Pregnancy category: C. Use with caution in patients with hepatic or kidney disease, hypertension or hypotension, hyperglycemia or hypoglycemia, hypocalcemia, leukopenia, thrombocytopenia, anemia, ventricular tachycardia, pancreatitis, Stevens-Johnson syndrome.

Side Effects: Parenteral. *CV:* Hypotension, ventricular tachycardia, phlebitis. *GI:* Nausea, anorexia, bad taste in mouth. *Hematologic:* Leukopenia, thrombocytopenia, anemia. *Electrolytes/glucose:* Hypoglycemia, hypocalcemia, hyperkalemia. *CNS:* Dizziness without hypotension, confusion, hallucinations. *Miscellaneous:* Acute renal failure, Stevens-Johnson syndrome, elevated serum creatinine, elevated liver function tests, pain or induration at IM injection site, sterile abscess at injection site, rash, neuralgia.

Inhalation. Most frequent include the following. *GI:* Decreased appetite, nausea, vomiting, metallic taste, diarrhea, abdominal pain. *CNS:* Fatigue, dizziness, headache. *Respiratory:* Shortness of breath, cough, pharyngitis, chest pain, chest congestion, bronchospasm, pneumothorax. *Miscellaneous:* Rash, night sweats, chills, myalgia, headache, anemia, edema.

Dosage: IV, Deep IM. Adults and children: 4 mg/kg once daily for 14 days. Dosage should be reduced in renal disease.

Aerosol. *Prevention of P. carinii pneumonia:* 300 mg q 4 weeks given via the Respirgard II nebulizer.

NURSING CONSIDERATIONS

See also *General Nursing Considerations For All Anti-Infectives* under *Penicillins,* p. 140.

Administration/Storage
1. To prepare IM solution, dissolve one vial in 3 mL of sterile water for injection.
2. To prepare IV solution, dissolve one vial in 3–5 mL of sterile water for injection or 5% dextrose injection. The drug is then further diluted in 50–250 mL of 5% dextrose solution. This solution then can be infused slowly over 60 min.
3. IV solutions in concentrations of 1 and 2.5 mg/mL in 5% dextrose injection are stable for 48 hr at room temperature.
3. The dose using the nebulizer should be delivered until the chamber is empty (30–45 min). The suggested flow rate is 5–7 L/min from a 40–50 pounds per sq inch (psi) air or oxygen source.
4. Reconstitution for use in the nebulizer is accomplished by dissolving the contents of the vial in 6 mL sterile water for injection. Saline solution cannot be used because it causes the drug to precipitate.
6. When used for nebulization, pentamidine should not be mixed with any other drug.
7. The solution for nebulization is stable at room temperature for 48 hr if protected from light.

Assessment
1. Assess extent of infection and document.
2. Determine history of kidney disease, hypertension, and past blood disorders.

Interventions
1. Obtain baseline blood sugar, CBC, renal and liver function studies, and monitor throughout therapy.
2. Monitor and record vital signs and intake and output.
3. Obtain apical pulse, auscultate for any evidence of arrhythmia if client not monitored.

Evaluation
Note response to drug therapy and any adverse effects such as
- bruising, hematuria, blood in stools, or other evidence of bleeding.

- signs and symptoms of hypoglycemia (which may be severe).
- early signs of Stevens-Johnson syndrome (characterized by high fever, severe headaches, stomatitis, conjunctivitis, rhinitis, urethritis, and balanitis), all of which may necessitate the discontinuation of drug therapy.

SPECTINOMYCIN HYDROCHLORIDE   (speck-tin-oh-**MY**-sin)

Trobicin (Rx)

See also *Anti-Infectives,* p. 71.

Classification: Antibiotic, miscellaneous.

Action/Kinetics: Spectinomycin is produced by *Streptomyces spectabilis.* It inhibits bacterial protein synthesis by binding to ribosomes (30S subunit), thereby interfering with transmission of genetic information crucial to life of microorganism. Spectinomycin is mainly bacteriostatic. It is not absorbed from GI tract and is only given IM. **Peak plasma concentration:** 100 mcg/mL after 1 hr. **$t^{1}/_{2}$:** 1.2–2.8 hr. Not significantly bound to protein. Excreted in urine.

Uses: Acute gonorrhea in infections resistant to penicillin or in patients allergic to penicillin. It is ineffective against syphilis, and thus is a poor drug to choose when mixed infections are present.

Contraindications: Sensitivity to drug.

Special Concerns: Safe use during pregnancy has not been established.

Side Effects: A single dose of spectinomycin has caused soreness at the site of injection, urticaria, dizziness, nausea, chills, fever, and insomnia. Multiple doses have caused a decrease in hemoglobin, hematocrit, and creatinine clearance and an increase in alkaline phosphatase, BUN, and SGPT.

Dosage: IM only: 2 g. In areas where antibiotic resistance is known to be prevalent, give 4 g divided between 2 gluteal injection sites.

NURSING CONSIDERATIONS

See also *General Nursing Considerations For All Anti-Infectives* under *Penicillins,* p. 140.

Administration/Storage

1. Powder is stable for 3 years.
2. Use reconstituted solution within 24 hr.
4. Inject deeply into the upper, outer quadrant of the gluteus muscle.
5. Injections may be made in 2 sites for clients requiring 4 g. Rotate and document injection sites.

Client/Family Teaching

1. Advise clients taking spectinomycin, who are suspected to have syphilis, to return for serologic tests monthly for at least 3 months.
2. Refer clients for counseling and encourage sexual partners to seek treatment.

Evaluation

Note response to therapy based on serologic test results.

TROLEANDOMYCIN   (troh-lee-an-doe-MY-sin)
Tao (Rx)

Classification: Antibiotic, miscellaneous.

Action/Kinetics: Troleandomycin is a broad-spectrum antibiotic salt prepared from cultures of *Streptomyces antibioticus*. Its spectrum of activity resembles that of erythromycin in that it is bacteriostatic and effective against gram-negative bacteria. Troleandomycin is widely distributed in body tissues and fluids but not in spinal fluid unless the meninges are inflamed.

It is believed to inhibit protein synthesis of bacteria. **Peak plasma concentration: PO,** 2 mcg/mL within 2 hr. Excreted in urine (20%) and in feces.

Uses: Pneumococcal pneumonia due to *Streptococcus pneumoniae*. Upper respiratory tract infections due to *Streptococcus pyogenes*. Eradication of streptococci from the nasopharynx.

Contraindications: Hypersensitivity to drug. Liver dysfunction or known sensitivity toward hepatotoxic drugs. Not recommended for prophylaxis or therapy for longer than 10 days. Occasional cross-sensitivity with erythromycin.

Special Concerns: Safe use during pregnancy or lactation has not been established.

Side Effects: *Hepatic:* Allergic cholestatic hepatitis, jaundice (accompanied by nausea, vomiting, fever, pain in upper quadrant, leukocytosis, and eosinophilia). *GI:* Abdominal cramps, nausea, vomiting, diarrhea. *Allergic:* Urticaria, skin rashes, anaphylaxis. *Miscellaneous:* Superinfection.

Drug Interactions	
Carbamazepine	↑ Effect of carbamazepine due to ↓ breakdown by liver
Contraceptives, oral	Additive cholestatic jaundice
Corticosteroids	↑ Effect of corticosteroids due to ↓ breakdown by liver
Ergotamine	Ischemic reactions
Theophylline	↑ Effect of theophylline due to ↓ breakdown by liver

Dosage: Capsules. Adults: 250–500 mg q 6 hr; **pediatric:** 6.6–11 mg/kg q 6 hr. Continue therapy for 10 days for streptococcal infections.

NURSING CONSIDERATIONS

See also *General Nursing Considerations For All Anti-Infectives* under *Penicillins,* p. 140.

Interventions

Monitor liver function studies and assess for jaundice, as drug should be discontinued at first signs of hepatotoxicity.

Client/Family Teaching

1. Troleandomycin should be taken on an empty stomach, either 1 hr before or 2 hr after meals.
2. The drug should be taken at regularly spaced intervals around the clock as ordered.

Evaluation

Assess response to therapy based on lab C&S results.

VANCOMYCIN HYDROCHLORIDE (van-koh-MY-sin)

Diatracin✿, Lyphocin, Vancocin, Vancoled (Rx)

See also *Anti-Infectives,* p. 71.

Classification: Antibiotic, miscellaneous.

Action/Kinetics: This antibiotic, derived from *Streptomyces orientalis,* diffuses in pleural, pericardial, ascitic, and synovial fluids after parenteral administration. It appears to bind to bacterial cell wall, arresting its synthesis and lysing the cytoplasmic membrane by a mechanism that is different from that of penicillin. The drug is bactericidal for most organisms and bacteriostatic for enterococci. It is poorly absorbed from GI tract. **Peak plasma levels, IV:** 33 mcg/mL 5 min after 0.5-g dosage. **t½:** 4–8 hr for adults and 2–3 hr for children. The half-life is increased markedly in the presence of renal impairment (240 hr has been noted). Primarily excreted in urine unchanged. Auditory and renal function tests are indicated before and during therapy.

Uses: Agent should be reserved for treatment of life-threatening infections when other treatments have been ineffective. Patients with severe staphylococcal infections resistant to (or patients allergic to) penicillin or cephalosporins (e.g., endocarditis, osteomyelitis, pneumonia, and septicemia). Oral administration is useful in treatment of enterocolitis and pseudomembranous colitis.

Contraindications: Hypersensitivity to drug. Minor infections.

Special Concerns: Pregnancy category: C. Use with extreme caution in the presence of impaired renal function or previous hearing loss. Geriatric patients are at a greater risk of developing ototoxicity.

Side Effects: Ototoxicity (may lead to deafness), nephrotoxicity (may lead to uremia). *Red-neck syndrome:* Chills, erythema of neck and back, fever, paresthesias. *Dermatologic:* Urticaria, macular rashes. *Allergic:* Drug fever, hypersensitivity, anaphylaxis. *Miscellaneous:* Nausea, tinnitus, eosinophilia, neutropenia, hypotension (due to rapid administration). Thrombophlebitis at site of injection. Deafness may progress after drug is discontinued.

Drug Interactions: Never give with other ototoxic or nephrotoxic agents, especially aminoglycosides and polymyxins.

Dosage: Capsules, Oral Solution: Adults, 0.5 g q 6 hr or 1 g q 12 hr. *Pseudomembranous colitis:* **PO: Adults,** 0.5–2 g daily in 3–4 divided doses for 7–10 days; **pediatric,** 40 mg/kg daily in divided doses, not to exceed 2 g daily; **neonates,** 10 mg/kg daily in divided doses. **IV: Adults,** 0.5 g q 6 hr or 1 g q 12 hr; **pediatric,** 40 mg/kg daily in divided doses (add to IV fluids). **Neonates, initial:** 15 mg/kg; **then, up to 1 month of age:** 10 mg/kg q 12 hr and after 1 month of age, 10 mg/kg q 8 hr. *Prophylaxis of bacterial endocarditis, penicillin-sensitive patients undergoing upper respiratory tract surgery/instrumentation or dental procedures:* **IV, Adults and children over 27 kg,** 1 g given slowly over 60 min before procedure; **IV, pediatric, less than 27 kg:** 20 mg/kg given slowly over 60 min before procedure. If patient is at high risk, the dose can be repeated in 8–12 hr. *Prophylaxis of bacterial endocarditis, penicillin-sensitive patients undergoing GI or urinary tract instrumentation/surgery:* **IV, Adults and children over 27 kg,** 1 g given slowly over 60 min concurrently with gentamicin, 1.5 mg/kg, **IV or IM,** 60 min prior to procedure; **IV, pediatric, less than 27 kg:** 20 mg/kg given slowly over 60 min concurrently with gentamicin, 2 mg/kg, **IM or IV,** 60 min prior to procedure. If patient is at high risk, the dose can be repeated in 8–12 hr. Dosage must be reduced in patients with renal disease.

NURSING CONSIDERATIONS

See also *General Nursing Considerations For All Anti-Infectives* under *Penicillins,* p. 140.

Administration/Storage

1. Mix as indicated on package insert.
2. Intermittent infusion is the preferred route, but continuous IV drip may be used.
3. Avoid rapid IV administration, as this may result in nausea, warmth, and generalized tingling.
4. Avoid extravasation during injections.
5. Reduce risk of thrombophlebitis by rotating injection sites or adding additional diluent.
6. Dilute one 500-mg vial in 1 oz of water for oral administration. Client may drink solution or it may be administered by nasogastric tube.
7. Aqueous solution is stable for 2 weeks.
8. Once rubber stopper is punctured, ampule should be refrigerated to maintain stability.

Interventions

1. Anticipate reduced dose with renal dysfunction.
2. Monitor and record vital signs and intake and output.

Evaluation

1. *Evaluate* for evidence of adverse drug effects, such as:
   - ototoxicity, demonstrated by tinnitus, progressive hearing loss, dizziness, and/or nystagmus
   - nephrotoxicity, demonstrated by albuminuria, hematuria, anuria, casts, edema, and uremia
2. Assess response to therapy based on lab results.

PENICILLINS

Classification: Anti-infective.

Action/Kinetics: The bactericidal action of penicillins depends on their ability to bind penicillin-binding proteins (PBP-1 and PBP-3) in the cytoplasmic membranes of bacteria, thus, inhibiting cell wall synthesis. Some penicillins act by acylation of membrane-bound transpeptidase enzymes, thereby preventing cross-linkage of peptidoglycan chains that are necessary for bacterial cell wall strength and rigidity. Cell division and growth are inhibited, and often lysis and elongation of susceptible bacteria occur. Penicillin is most effective against young, rapidly dividing organisms and has little effect on mature resting cells. Depending on the concentration of the drug at the site of infection and the susceptibility of the infectious microorganism, penicillin is either bacteriostatic or bactericidal.

Penicillins are distributed throughout most of the body and pass the placental barrier. They also pass into synovial, pleural, pericardial, intraperitoneal, and spinal fluids and into the fluids of the eye. Although normal meninges are relatively impermeable to penicillins, they are better absorbed by inflamed meninges. **t½:** 30–110 min; protein binding: 20%–98%; (see individual agents).

The renal, cardiac, and hematopoietic functions, as well as the electrolyte balance, of patients receiving penicillin should be monitored at regular intervals.

Uses: Gram-positive cocci including streptococci, meningococci, pneumococci, nonpenicillinase-producing staphylococci, and fusospirochetal infections. Gonococci including uncomplicated gonorrhea, disseminated gonococcal infections, and gonococcal ophthalmia in neonates or adults. Rat-bite fever, anthrax, tetanus, yaws, gas gangrene, and diphtheria (treatment and prophylaxis). Subacute bacterial endocarditis due to group A streptococci and enterococcal endocarditis. Actinomycoses, *Pasteurella,* and clostridial infections (except botulism).

Penicillins are also used for *Listeria*-caused meningitis (in combination with gentamicin or kanamycin). Infections due to *Escherichia coli, Proteus mirabilis, Hemophilus influenzae, Salmonella, Shigella, Proteus aeruginosa*. Syphilis (including primary, secondary, and latent stages, and congenital syphilis). Prophylaxis of rheumatic fever and bacterial endocarditis in patients with congenital or rheumatic heart disease undergoing dental work, instrumentation, or other procedures.

Note: Not all penicillins are used for the above diseases. Specific uses are indicated for each of the individually listed drugs.

Contraindications: Hypersensitivity to penicillins and cephalosporins.

Special Concerns: Most penicillins are pregnancy category B. Use of penicillins during lactation may lead to sensitization, diarrhea, candidiasis, and skin rash in the infant. Use with caution in patients with a history of asthma, hay fever, or urticaria.

Side Effects: Penicillins are potent sensitizing agents; it is estimated that 15% of the U.S. population is allergic to the antibiotic. Hypersensitivity reactions are reported to be on the increase in pediatric populations. Sensitivity reactions may be immediate (within 20 min) or delayed (as long as several days or weeks after initiation of therapy).

Allergic: Skin rashes (including maculopapular and exanthematous), exfoliative dermatitis, erythema, contact dermatitis, hives, pruritus, wheezing, anaphylaxis, fever, eosinophilia. Stevens-Johnson syndrome, angioedema, serum sickness. *GI:* Diarrhea (may be severe), abdominal cramps or pain, nausea, vomiting, bloating, flatulence, increased thirst, bitter/unpleasant taste, dark or discolored tongue, sore mouth or tongue, gastric upset, pseudomembranous colitis. *Hematologic:* Thrombocytopenia, leukopenia, agranulocytosis. *Renal:* Hematuria, pyuria, albuminuria, oliguria. Electrolyte imbalance following IV use. *Miscellaneous:* Hepatotoxicity (cholestatic jaundice), superinfection, swelling of face and ankles, labored breathing, weakness, ecchymoses, hematomas.

IM injection may cause pain and induration at the injection site, while IV use may cause vein irritation and thrombophlebitis.

For **emergency treatment** of severe allergic or anaphylactic reactions, administer epinephrine (0.3–0.5 mL of a 1:1,000 solution SC or IM, or 0.2–0.3 mL diluted in 10 mL saline, given slowly by IV). Corticosteroids should be on hand.

In those instances where penicillin is the drug of choice, the physician may decide to use it even though the patient is allergic, adding a medication to the regimen to control the allergic response.

Drug Interactions

Aminoglycosides	Penicillins ↓ effect of aminoglycosides
Antacids	↓ Effect of penicillins due to ↓ absorption from GI tract
Antibiotics, Chloramphenicol, Erythromycins, Tetracyclines	↓ Effect of penicillins

Drug Interactions

Anticoagulants	Penicillins may potentiate pharmacologic effect
Aspirin	↑ Effect of penicillins by ↓ plasma protein binding
Phenylbutazone	↑ Effect of penicillins by ↓ plasma protein binding
Probenecid	↑ Effect of penicillins by ↓ excretion

Laboratory Test Interferences: Massive doses: False + or ↑ urinary glucose, protein, and turbidity.

Dosage: Penicillins are available in a variety of dosage forms for oral, parenteral, inhalation, and intrathecal administration. Dosages for individual drugs are given in drug entries. Long-acting preparations are frequently used. Oral doses must be higher than IM or SC doses, because a large fraction of penicillin given orally may be destroyed in the stomach.

NURSING CONSIDERATIONS

General Nursing Considerations For All Anti-Infectives, p. 71.

Assessment

1. Determine if client has experienced any unusual reaction or problems associated with penicillin or related drug therapy.
2. Ensure that epinephrine, oxygen, antihistamines, and corticosteroids are immediately available to treat an acute allergic response.

Interventions

1. Report to the physician any history of allergic responses to any anti-infective agents.
2. Conspicuously mark in red, client's chart, medication record, care plan and bed the fact that the client has an allergy and to what. Inform client not to take that drug again unless the physician gives approval after reviewing the history of past allergic reactions to this medication.
3. Once drug therapy is initiated, ask the client about any unusual reactions or problems with the medication. Review with the client possible side effects such as hives, rashes, difficulty breathing, etc. If any of these occur it may indicate a hypersensitivity or allergic response and the drug should be discontinued and the physician notified immediately.
4. Ensure that diagnostic cultures and sensitivity tests have been done before administering the first dose of anti-infective. Use correct procedure for obtaining, storing, and transporting specimen to the laboratory.
5. If the anti-infective is mainly excreted by the kidneys, anticipate reduced dosage in clients with renal dysfunction. Nephrotoxic drugs are usually contraindicated in persons with renal dysfunction, because toxic levels of the drugs are rapidly attained when renal function is impaired.
6. Notify physician when two or more anti-infectives are ordered for the same client, especially if the drugs have similar side effects, such as nephrotoxicity and/or neurotoxicity.
7. Assess client for therapeutic response, such as reduction of fever, increased appetite, and increased sense of well-being.
8. Assess client for superinfections, particularly of fungal origin, characterized by black furred tongue, nausea, and diarrhea.

9. *Prevent superinfections by*
   - limiting client's exposure to persons suffering from an active infectious process.
   - rotating the site of IV administration and by changing IV tubing every 24–48 hr.
   - providing and emphasizing need for good hygiene.
   - instructing care provider to wash own hands carefully before and after contact with the client.
10. Have the order for an anti-infective (administered in the hospital) evaluated at least every 5–7 days for renewal or cancellation.
11. Schedule drug administration throughout 24-hr period to maintain appropriate drug levels. A drug administration schedule is determined by the half-life ($t\frac{1}{2}$) of the drug, the severity of the infection, and the client's need for sleep.
12. Obtain and monitor serum drug levels throughout therapy to ensure that client is receiving the appropriate dose.

Client/Family Teaching

Teach client/family
- to use anti-infectives only under medical supervision.
- the method for taking and time intervals at which to take the anti-infective.
- to report signs and symptoms of allergic reactions and superinfections.
- to prevent recurrence by completing recommended course of therapy, even though they may feel well.
- to discard any drug remaining after course of therapy is completed.
- (for diabetics) to perform finger sticks as opposed to urine testing for the most reliable sugar results.

GENERAL NURSING CONSIDERATIONS FOR PENICILLINS

Administration/Storage

1. IM and IV administration of penicillin causes a great deal of local irritation. These antibiotics should thus be injected slowly.
2. IM injections are made deeply into the gluteal muscle. IV injections are usually made through the tubing of an IV infusion.

Assessment

1. Assess rigorously for allergic reactions, as incidence is higher with penicillin therapy than with other antibiotics. If a reaction occurs, the drug must be discontinued immediately. Epinephrine, oxygen, antihistamines, and corticosteroids must be immediately available.
2. Anticipate that allergic reactions are more likely to occur in clients with a history of asthma, hay fever, urticaria, or allergy to cephalosporins.

Interventions

1. Detain client in an ambulatory care site for at least 20 min after administering a penicillin injection to assess for the onset of anaphylaxis. Be prepared for prompt treatment of anaphylactic reaction.
2. Do not administer long-acting types of penicillin IV, because these types are only for IM use. They may cause emboli or CNS or cardiac pathology if administered IV.
3. Do not massage repository (long-acting) penicillin products after injection, because rate of absorption should not be increased.

4. Prevent rapid administration of IV penicillin, because this method may cause local irritation and may precipitate convulsions.

5. The elderly may be more sensitive to the effects of penicillin than are younger people. Therefore, care should be exerted when calculating the dose based on client weight and height.

6. Most penicillins are excreted in breast milk and should be prescribed cautiously to nursing mothers.

Client/Family Teaching

1. Review the drugs that are being prescribed, their side effects and the expected outcome of therapy.

2. Review the signs and symptoms of allergic reaction, instructing the client to stop medication when noted and to check with medical supervision as soon as possible.

3. Take oral penicillin with a glass of water 1 hr before or 2–3 hr after meals.

4. When to return for repository penicillin injections to complete treatment, if physician orders.

5. To complete entire prescribed course of therapy, even though client may feel well; a person with alpha-hemolytic streptococcus infection must continue with penicillin for a minimum of 10 days, and preferably 14 days, to prevent development of rheumatic fever or glomerulonephritis.

6. Review signs and symptoms of superinfections and instruct client to report to physician.

Evaluation

1. Assess client/family knowledge and understanding of illness, response to therapy and to teaching.

2. Note status (presence/absence) of pretreatment symptoms and C&S results to determine effectiveness of treatment.

3. Inspect injection sites for pain and redness.

4. Observe for freedom from complications of drug therapy.

AMDINOCILLIN   (am-**DEE**-noh-sill-in)

Coactin (Rx)

Classification: Antibiotic, penicillin.

Action/Kinetics: In contrast to other penicillins, amdinocillin binds to penicillin-binding protein-2 (PBP-2), thus preventing bacterial cell elongation. It acts synergistically with other penicillins, because other penicillins bind to PBP-1 and PBP-3.

Uses: Urinary tract infections due to *Escherichia coli, Klebsiella,* and *Enterobacter.* Bacteremia due to *E. coli.* In conjunction with β-lactam antibiotics for severe urinary tract infections.

Dosage: IM, IV. *Serious infections:* 10 mg/kg q 4 hr for 7–10 days. For severe infections, prolonged therapy may be necessary. *As adjunct with β-lactam antibiotic:* 10 mg/kg q 6 hr. In presence of renal dysfunction, reduce dose to 10 mg/kg q 6–8 hr.

NURSING CONSIDERATIONS

See also *Nursing Considerations* for *Penicillins,* p. 141.

Administration/Storage

1. For intermittent IV infusion, dissolve in sterile water for injection and further dilute to 50 mL with 5% dextrose injection. Administer over 15–30 min.

2. When used with a β-lactam antibiotic, the two should be given separately.

3. For IM use, reconstitute with sterile water for injection or 0.9% sodium chloride injection.

4. IM administration should be deep into a large muscle mass in the upper, outer quadrant of the buttocks.

AMOXICILLIN (AMOXYCILLIN) (ah-mox-ih-**SILL**-in)

Amoxil, Amoxil Pediatric Drops, APO-Amoxi✳, Axicillin✳, Larotid, Larotid Pediatric Drops, Novamoxin✳, Polymox, Polymox Drops, Trimox 125, 250, and 500, Utimox, Wymox (Rx)

See also *Anti-Infectives,* p. 71 and *Penicillins,* p. 138.

Classification: Antibiotic, penicillin.

Action/Kinetics: Semisynthetic broad-spectrum penicillin closely related to ampicillin. Destroyed by penicillinase, acid stable, and better absorbed than ampicillin. From 50% to 80% of an oral dose is absorbed from the GI tract. **Peak serum levels: PO:** 4–11 mcg/mL after 1–2 hr. **t½:** 60 min. Mostly excreted unchanged in urine.

Uses: Genitourinary tract infections. Respiratory infections by *Hemophilus influenzae, Streptococcus pneumoniae.* Skin and soft tissue infections by nonpenicillinase-producing staphylococci. Gram-positive streptococci. *Proteus mirabilis, Neisseria gonorrhoeae.*

Dosage: Capsules, Oral Suspension, Tablets. *Susceptible infections of ear, nose, throat, GU tract, skin and soft tissues, lower respiratory tract:* **Adults,** 250–500 mg q 8 hr; **pediatric under 20 kg:** 20–40 (or more) mg/kg daily in three equal doses. *Prophylaxis of endocarditis:* 3 g 60 min prior to procedure and 1.5 g 6 hr later.
  Gonococcal infections: 3 g with probenecid, 1 g given as a single dose. In addition, tetracycline, 0.5 mg, q.i.d. for 7 days. *Gonococcal infection in pregnancy:* 3 g with probenecid, 1 g, given as a single dose. In addition, erythromycin base, 0.5 g q.i.d. for 7 days. *Disseminated gonococcal infections:* 3 g with probenecid, 1 g, given as a single dose; **then,** 0.5 g q.i.d. for 7 days. *Acute pelvic inflammatory disease:* 3 g with probenecid, 1 g, given as a single dose. In addition, doxycycline, 100 mg b.i.d. for 10–14 days. *Sexually transmitted epididymo-orchitis:* 3 g with probenecid, 1 g, given as a single dose. In addition, tetracycline, 0.5 g q.i.d. for 10 days. *Bacterial vaginosis:* 0.5 g q.i.d. for 7 days.

NURSING CONSIDERATIONS

See also *Nursing Considerations* for *Penicillins,* p. 141.

Administration/Storage

1. Dry powder is stable at room temperature for 18–30 months. Reconstituted suspension is stable for 1 week at room temperature and for 2 weeks at 2°–8°C.

2. Chewable tablets are available for pediatric use. These may be administered with food.

AMOXICILLIN AND POTASSIUM CLAVULANATE (ah-mox-ih-**SILL**-in)

Augmentin, Clavulin✳ (Rx)

See also *Anti-Infectives,* p. 71 and *Penicillins,* p. 138.

Classification: Antibiotic, penicillin.

Action/Kinetics: *For details, see amoxicillin.* Potassium clavulanate inactivates lactamase enzymes, which are responsible for resistance to penicillins. Thus, this preparation is effective against microorganisms that have manifested resistance to amoxicillin. For potassium clavulanate: **Peak serum levels:** 1–2 hr. **t½:** 1 hr. **Note:** Both the "250" and "500" tablets contain 125 mg potassium clavulanate.

Uses: For beta-lactamase—producing strains of the following organisms: *Hemophilus influenzae* causing lower respiratory tract infections, otitis media, and sinusitis; *Staphylococcus aureus, Escherichia coli,* and *Klebsiella,* causing skin and skin structure infections; *E. coli, Klebsiella,* and *Enterobacter,* causing urinary tract infections.

Dosage: Oral Suspension, Chewable Tablets, Tablets. Usual: Adults, One "250" tablet q 8 hr; **children less than 40 kg,** 20 mg/kg daily in divided doses q 8 hr. *Respiratory tract and severe infections:* **Adults,** one "500" tablet q 8 hr; **children, less than 40 kg,** 40 mg/kg daily in divided doses q 8 hr (this dose is also used in children for otitis media, lower respiratory tract infections, or sinusitis). *Chancroid:* One "500" tablet t.i.d. for 7 days.

NURSING CONSIDERATIONS

See also *Nursing Considerations* for *Penicillins,* p. 141.

Administration/Storage

1. Both the "250" and "500" tablets contain 125 mg clavulanic acid; therefore, two "250" tablets are not the same as one "500" tablet.
2. The reconstituted suspension should be refrigerated and discarded after 10 days.

AMPICILLIN ORAL   (am-pih-**SILL**-in)

Amcill, APO-Amp✿, D-Amp, Novo-Ampicillin✿, Omnipen, Omnipen Pediatric Drops, Penbritin✿, Polycillin, Polycillin Pediatric Drops, Principen 125, 250, and 500, Totacillin (Rx)

AMPICILLIN SODIUM, PARENTERAL   (am-pih-**SILL**-in)

Ampicin✿, Ampilean✿, Omnipen-N, Penbritin✿, Polycillin-N, Totacillin-N (Rx)

AMPICILLIN WITH PROBENECID   (am-pih-**SILL**-in, proh-**BEN**-eh-sid)

Polycillin-PRB, Principen w/Probenecid, Probampacin (Rx)

See also *Anti-Infectives,* p. 71 and *Penicillins,* p. 138.

Classification: Antibiotic, penicillin.

Action/Kinetics: Synthetic, broad-spectrum antibiotic suitable for gram-negative bacteria. Acid resistant, destroyed by penicillinase. Absorbed more slowly than other penicillins. From 30% to 60% of oral dose absorbed from GI tract. **Peak serum levels: PO:** 1.8–2.9 mcg/mL after 2 hr; **IM,** 4.5–7 mcg/mL. **t½:** 80 min—range 50–110 min. Partially inactivated in liver; 25%–85% excreted unchanged in urine.

Uses: Infections of respiratory, GI, and GU tracts caused by *Shigella, Salmonella, Escherichia coli, Hemophilus influenzae, Proteus* strains, *Neisseria gonorrhoeae, N. meningitidis,* and *Enterococcus.* Also, otitis media in children, bronchitis, rat-bite fever, and whooping cough. Penicillin G-sensitive staphylococci, streptococci, pneumococci.

Additional Drug Interactions

Allopurinol	↑ Incidence of skin rashes
Ampicillin	↓ Effect of oral contraceptives

Dosage: Ampicillin: Capsules, Oral Suspension; Ampicillin sodium: IV, IM. *Respiratory tract and soft tissue infections:* **PO, 20 kg or more:** 250 mg q 6 hr; **less than 20 kg:** 50 mg/kg/day in equally divided doses q 6–8 hr. **IV, IM, 40 kg or more:** 250–500 mg q 6 hr; **less than 40 kg:** 25–50 mg/kg/day in equally divided doses q 6–8 hr.

Gonococcal infections: **PO,** 3.5 g with 1 g probenecid (given SC) simultaneously as a single dose. In addition, tetracycline, 0.5 g q.i.d. is given for 7 days. *Gonococcal infections, in pregnancy:* **PO,** 3.5 g with 1 g probenecid given as a single dose. In addition, erythromycin base, 0.5 mg q.i.d. is given for 7 days. *Disseminated gonococcal infections:* **PO,** 3.5 g with 1 g probenecid given as a single dose. In addition, ampicillin, 0.5 g q.i.d. is given for 7 days.

Bacterial meningitis: **Adults,** A total of 12 g is given in divided doses q 6 hr. **Pediatric:** Up to 400 mg/kg daily in divided doses q 4 hr. *Bacterial endocarditis prophylaxis* (GI or GU tract surgery or instrumentation): **Adult, IM, IV:** 1–2 g plus gentamicin, 1.5 mg/kg IM or IV, or streptomycin, 1 g IM given 30 min before procedure with either 1 g penicillin V 6 hr later, or a parenteral dose of ampicillin is given after 8 hr. **Pediatric:** ampicillin, 50 mg/kg with gentamicin, 2 mg/kg 30 min prior to procedure with either penicillin V, 0.5 g (if child is under 60 lb) after 6 hr or a parenteral dose of ampicillin is given after 8 hr. *Septicemia:* **Adults/children:** 150–200 mg/kg, IV for first 3 days, then IM q 3–4 hr.

Acute pelvic inflammatory disease: **PO,** 3.5 g plus probenecid, 1 g, given as a single dose. In addition, doxycycline, 100 mg, PO, b.i.d. for 10–14 days. *Bacterial vaginosis in pregnancy:* **PO,** 0.5 g q.i.d. for 7 days. *Sexually transmitted epididymo-orchitis:* **PO,** 3.5 g plus probenecid, 1 g, given as a single dose. In addition, either tetracycline, 0.5 g q.i.d., or doxycycline, 100 mg b.i.d., for 10 days.

Ampicillin with Probenecid: Capsules, Oral Suspension. *Gonorrhea:* 3.5 g ampicillin and 1 g probenecid as a single dose.

NURSING CONSIDERATIONS

See also *Nursing Considerations* for *Penicillins,* p. 141.

Administration/Storage

1. After reconstitution for IM or direct IV administration, the solution of sodium ampicillin must be used within the hour.
2. For IM use, dilute only with sterile water for injection or bacteriostatic water for injection.
3. For IV "piggyback," ampicillin may be reconstituted with sodium chloride injection.
4. IV injections of reconstituted sodium ampicillin should be given slowly; 2 mL should be given over a period of at least 3–5 min.
5. Administration by IV drip: Check compatibility and length of time that drug retains potency in a particular solution.

Interventions

1. Obtain and monitor liver and renal function studies. If creatinine clearance is less than 10 mL/min, the dosing interval should be increased to 12 hr.
2. When administering IM, tell the client that it will be painful.
3. Rotate and document injection sites.
4. Monitor urinary output and serum potassium in the elderly.

Client/Family Teaching

1. Teach the person administering the drug the appropriate method for administration and storage.
2. Instruct client to take the drug for the prescribed number of days even if the symptoms subside.
3. If side effects occur, call the physician and refrain from taking the drug until medically cleared.
4. Take the medication 1 hr before or 2 hr after meals.
5. Ampicillin chewable tablets should not be swallowed whole.
6. Not to save any of the drug for future use or to share with family members or friends who may seem to have the same type of infection.

Evaluation

1. Assess client/family knowledge and understanding of illness, response to therapy and to teaching.
2. Observe skin closely for rashes, as they occur more often with this drug than with other penicillins.
3. If clients develop a skin rash, have them tested for mononucleosis as this may be the cause of the rash.
4. Review lab data. Note client response and any development of resistance to anti-infective drug therapy.

AMPICILLIN SODIUM/SULBACTAM SODIUM   (am-pih-**SILL**-in/sull-**BACK**-tam)

Unasyn (Rx)

See also *Anti-Infectives,* p. 71, and *Penicillins,* p. 138.

Classification: Antibiotic, penicillin.

Action/Kinetics: For details, see *Ampicillin oral.* Sulbactam is present in this product because it irreversibly inhibits beta-lactamases, thus ensuring activity of ampicillin against beta-lactamase-producing microorganisms. Thus, sulbactam broadens the antibiotic spectrum of ampicillin to those bacteria normally resistant to it. **Peak serum levels, after IV infusion:** 15 min. **t½, both drugs,** about 1 hr. From 75%–85% of both drugs are excreted unchanged in the urine within 8 hr after administration.

Uses: To treat infections caused by beta-lactamase—producing strains of the following: (a) skin and skin structure infections caused by *Staphylococcus aureus, Escherichia coli, Klebsiella* species (including *K. pneumoniae*), *Proteus mirabilis, Bacteroides fragilis, Enterobacter* species, and *Acinetobacter calcoaceticus;* (b) intra-abdominal infections caused by *E. coli, Klebsiella, Bacteroides* (including *B. fragilis* and *Enterobacter)* (c) gynecological infections caused by *E. coli* and *Bacteroides* (including *B. fragilis).* **Note:** Mixed infections caused by ampicillin-susceptible organisms and beta-lactamase—producing organisms are susceptible to this product; thus, additional antibiotics do not have to be used.

Special Concerns: Safety and efficacy in children less than 12 years of age have not been established.

Additional Side Effects: *At site of injection:* Pain and thrombophlebitis. *GI:* Diarrhea, nausea, vomiting, flatulence, abdominal distention, glossitis. *CNS:* Fatigue, malaise, headache. *GU:* Dysuria, urinary retention. *Miscellaneous:* Itching, chest pain, edema, facial swelling, erythema, chills, tightness in throat, epistaxis, substernal pain, mucosal bleeding.

Laboratory Test Interferences: ↑ AST, ALT, alkaline phosphatase, LDH, creatinine, BUN. ↓ Serum albumin and total proteins. Changes in hemoglobin, red blood cells, white blood cells, and platelets.

Dosage: IV, IM: 1 g ampicillin/0.5 g sulbactam to 2 g ampicillin/1 g sulbactam q 6 hr, not to exceed 4 g sulbactam daily. Doses must be decreased in renal impairment.

NURSING CONSIDERATIONS

See also *Nursing Considerations* for *Penicillins,* p. 141.

Administration/Storage

1. For IV use, drug can be given by slow injection over 10–15 min or, if mixed with 50–100 mL of diluent, can be given over 15–30 min.
2. For IV use, the drug can be reconstituted with any of the following: 5% dextrose injection, 5% dextrose injection in 0.45% saline, 10% invert sugar, lactated Ringer's injection, 0.9% sodium chloride injection, M/6 sodium lactate injection, or sterile water for injection.
3. For IM use, the drug can be reconstituted with sterile water for injection or 0.5% or 2% lidocaine HCl injection.
4. After reconstitution, solutions should stand so that any foaming will dissipate and the vial can be inspected visually to ensure dissolution.
5. Solutions for IM administration must be used within 1 hr after preparation.
6. If aminoglycosides are prescribed concomitantly, administer each separately, because ampicillin will inactivate aminoglycosides.

Assessment

Determine if client has mononucleosis, because drug, in this event, may cause skin rash.

Interventions

1. Anticipate reduced doses in clients with impaired renal function.
2. Intramuscular injections are extremely painful; follow manufacturer's recommendations for IM reconstitution and tell the client to expect some pain.

Evaluation: Monitor culture and sensitivity reports to determine effectiveness of drug therapy.

AZLOCILLIN SODIUM   (az-low-**SILL**-in)

Azlin (Rx)

See also *Anti-Infectives,* p. 71, and *Penicillins,* p. 138.

Classification: Antibiotic, penicillin.

Uses: A broad-spectrum antibiotic used for lower respiratory tract infections caused by *Escherichia coli, Hemophilus influenzae* and *Pseudomonas* infections including those of the respiratory tract, skin, skin structures, bones, joints, and urinary tract. Septicemia caused by *E. coli* or *Pseudomonas.* Used in combination with an aminoglycoside to treat life-threatening *Pseudomonas aeruginosa* infections.

Dosage: IV (slow injection over 5 or more min or infusion over 30 min). *Lower respiratory tract, bone, joint, and skin infections; septicemia:* 3 g q 4 hr or 4 g q 6 hr (not to exceed 24 g/day). If renal clearance is 10–30 mL/min: 2 g q 8 hr; if less than 10 mL/min: 3 g q 12 hr in renal impairment. *Urinary tract infections:* 2 g q 6 hr, up to 3 g q 6 hr for complicated infections. Dosage should be reduced to 1.5 g q 12 hr for uncomplicated infections if creatinine clearance is less than 30 mL/min and 1.5 g q 8 hr for complicated infections. **Pediatric:** *Acute pulmonary worsening of cystic fibrosis:* 75 mg/kg q 4 hr, not to exceed 24 g/day. Not to be used in the newborn.

NURSING CONSIDERATIONS

See also *Nursing Considerations* for *Penicillins,* p. 141.

Administration/Storage

1. If used in combination with other drugs, each drug should be given separately.
2. Azlocillin may be reconstituted by adding 10 mL of sterile water for injection, 0.9% sodium chloride injection, or 5% dextrose injection. This solution may then be diluted with the appropriate IV solution.
3. To minimize vein irritation, the concentration of azlocillin should not exceed 10%.

Evaluation

1. Monitor appropriate lab data to determine effectiveness of drug therapy.
2. Evaluate for side effects such as hypokalemia, muscular weakness, lessening or cessation of peristalsis, postural hypotension, respiratory depression, and cardiac arrhythmias.
3. Note bruising, hematuria, guiac-positive stools, and other signs of bleeding.

BACAMPICILLIN HYDROCHLORIDE   (bah-kamp-ih-**SILL**-in)

Penglobe✸, Spectrobid (Rx)

See also *Anti-Infectives,* p. 71, and *Penicillins,* p. 138.

Classification: Antibiotic, penicillin.

Action/Kinetics: Bacampicillin is a semisynthetic, acid-resistant penicillin that is hydrolyzed to the active ampicillin in the GI tract. Food does not affect absorption of the drug. The drug is 98% absorbed from the GI tract and is approximately 20% plasma protein bound. **Peak serum levels:** obtained in 0.9 hr are approximately 3 times those seen with equivalent doses of ampicillin. Seventy-five percent is excreted in the urine as active ampicillin within 8 hr.

Uses: Upper and lower respiratory tract infections caused by beta-hemolytic streptococcus, *Staphylococcus pyogenes,* pneumococci, nonpenicillinase-producing staphylococci, and *Hemophilus influenzae.* Urinary tract infections caused by *Escherichia coli, Proteus mirabilis,* and enterococci. Skin infections caused by streptococci and susceptible staphylococci. Acute uncomplicated urogenital infections caused by *Neisseria gonorrhoeae.*

Contraindications: History of penicillin allergy. Concomitant use with disulfiram (Antabuse).

Drug Interaction: Bacampicillin should not be used concomitantly with disulfiram.

Laboratory Test Interferences: False + reaction to Clinitest, Benedict's solution, and Fehling's solution. ↑ SGOT.

Dosage: Oral Suspension, Tablets. *Upper respiratory tract infections, urinary tract infections, skin and skin structure infections:* **Adults (25 kg or more),** 400 mg q 12 hr; **pediatric:** 25 mg/kg/day in equally divided doses q 12 hr. Dose may be doubled in lower respiratory tract infections, in cases of severe infection, or in treating less susceptible organisms. *Gonorrhea (males and females):* 1.6 g with 1 g probenecid as a single dose.

NURSING CONSIDERATIONS

See also *General Nursing Considerations For All Anti-Infectives* under *Penicillins,* p. 140.

Interventions

1. Withhold drug and consult with physician if client is receiving disulfiram. Warn client not to start disulfiram therapy while taking bacampicillin.

2. Advise diabetic clients to use Labstix, Clinistix, Tes-Tape, or Diastix for testing urine, as Benedict's and Fehling's solutions result in false + reactions. To enhance accuracy, do finger sticks.

Evaluation

Assess client also on allopurinol for increased incidence of skin rash.

CARBENICILLIN DISODIUM   (kar-ben-ih-**SILL**-in)

Geopen, Pyopen (Rx)

See also *Anti-Infectives,* p. 71, and *Penicillins,* p. 138.

Classification: Antibiotic, penicillin.

Action/Kinetics: Due to high urine levels achieved, carbenicillin is especially suitable for urinary tract infections. It is acid labile and must be injected. **Peak serum levels: IM,** 10–40 mcg/mL after 1 hr. **t½:** 60 min. Rapidly excreted unchanged in urine. Urinary excretion rates can be slowed by concurrent administration of probenecid.

Uses: Urinary tract and systemic infections caused by *Pseudomonas aeruginosa, Proteus, Escherichia coli, Neisseria gonorrhoeae, Streptococcus pneumoniae, Enterobacter,* and *S. faecalis.* Anaerobic bacteria causing septicemia, lung abscess, empyema, pneumonitis, peritonitis, endometritis, pelvic inflammatory disease, pelvic abscess, salpingitis, skin infections.

Additional Contraindications: Pregnancy.

Special Concerns: Use with caution in patients with impaired renal function.

Additional Side Effects: Neurotoxicity in patients with impaired renal function. Vaginitis, increased SGOT levels.

Additional Drug Interactions	
Gentamicin	↑ Effect of carbenicillin when used for *Pseudomonas*
Tobramycin	↑ Effect of carbenicillin when used for *Pseudomonas;* ↑ effect of both drugs when used for *Providencia* strains

Dosage: *Urinary tract infections.* **Adult:** *Uncomplicated,* **IM, IV:** 1–2 g q 6 hr; *severe,* **IV drip:** 200

mg/kg daily. **Pediatric: IM, IV,** 50–200 mg/kg/day in divided doses q 4–6 hr. *Severe systemic infections, septicemia, respiratory infections, soft tissue infections.* **Adult: IV (drip or divided doses):** 15–40 g daily. **Pediatric: IV or IM (divided doses) or IV drip:** 250–500 mg/kg/day. *Meningitis.* **Adult: IV (drip or divided doses):** 30–40 g daily. **Pediatric: IV (drip or divided doses):** 400–500 mg/kg/day. *Proteus or E. coli infections during dialysis or hemodialysis.* **Adult: IV:** 2 g q 4–6 hr. *Gonorrhea (males or females):* **IM:** 4 g as a single dose divided between two sites with probenecid, 1 g **PO,** 30 min before injection. *Note: Severe systemic infections in neonates.* **IM or IV infusion (15 min): over 2 kg, initially,** 100 mg/kg; **then,** for next 3 days, 75 mg/kg q 6 hr. After 3 days of age, 100 mg/kg q 6 hr. **Under 2 kg, initially,** 100 mg/kg; **then,** for next 7 days, 75 mg/kg q 8 hr. After 7 days of age, 100 mg/kg q 6 hr. Reduce all dosages in case of renal insufficiency.

NURSING CONSIDERATIONS

See also *Nursing Considerations* for *Penicillins,* p. 141.

Administration/Storage

1. Minimize pain at site of deep IM injection by reconstituting medication with 0.5% lidocaine (without epinephrine) or bacteriostatic water for injection containing 0.9% benzyl alcohol. Obtain a written order to use lidocaine or benzyl alcohol for dilution.
2. Do not administer more than 2 g in any one IM injection.
3. Read directions carefully on package insert for IM and IV administration, because drug is irritating to tissue.
4. Unused reconstituted drug should be discarded after 24 hr when stored at room temperature, and should be discarded after 72 hr when refrigerated. Label with date, time, and initials when reconstituting drug.

Intervention

Provide frequent mouth care to minimize nausea and unpleasant aftertaste.

Evaluation

1. Assess client with impaired renal function for (a) neurotoxicity, manifested by hallucinations, impaired sensorium, muscular irritability, and seizures, and (b) hemorrhagic manifestations, such as ecchymosis, petechiae, and frank bleeding of gums and/or rectum.
2. Assess client with impaired cardiac function for edema, weight gain, and respiratory distress that may be precipitated by disodium carbenicillin.
3. Assess client for headaches, GI disturbances, or hypersensitivity reactions if probenecid is administered with carbenicillin.

CARBENICILLIN INDANYL SODIUM (kar-ben-ih-**SILL**-in

Geocillin, Geopen Oral✿, (Rx)

See also *Anti-Infectives,* p. 71, and *Penicillins,* p. 138.

Classification: Antibiotic, penicillin.

Action/Kinetics: The drug is acid stable. **Peak serum levels: PO,** 6.5 mcg/mL after 1 hr. **t½:** 60 min. Rapidly excreted unchanged in urine.

Uses: Urinary tract infections or bacteriuria due to *Escherichia coli, Proteus vulgaris, P. mirabilis, Morganella, Providencia, Enterobacter, Pseudomonas,* and enterococci. Prostatitis.

Additional Contraindications: Pregnancy.

Special Concerns: Safe use in children not established. Use with caution in patients with impaired renal function.

Additional Side Effects: Neurotoxicity in patients with impaired renal function.

Additional Drug Interactions: When used in combination with gentamicin or tobramycin for *Pseudomonas* infections, effect of carbenicillin may be enhanced.

Dosage: Tablets: 382–764 mg q.i.d.

NURSING CONSIDERATIONS

See also *Nursing Considerations* for *Penicillins,* p. 141, and *Carbenicillin Disodium,* p. 150.

Administration/Storage

1. Protect from moisture.
2. Store at temperature of 30°C or less.

CLOXACILLIN SODIUM   (klox-ah-**SILL**-in)

Apo-Cloxi❋, Cloxapen, Novocloxin❋, Orbenin❋, Tegopen (Rx)

See also *Anti-Infectives,* p. 71, and *Penicillins,* p. 138.

Classification: Antibiotic, penicillin.

Action/Kinetics: More resistant to penicillinase than is penicillin G. **Peak plasma levels:** 7–15 mcg/mL after 30–60 min. **t½:** 30 min. Protein binding: 88%–96%. Well absorbed from GI tract. Mostly excreted in urine, but some excreted in bile.

Uses: Infections caused by penicillinase-producing staphylococci, streptococci, and pneumococci, excluding enterococci. Osteomyelitis.

Dosage: Capsules, Oral Solution. *Skin and soft tissue infections, mild to moderate upper respiratory tract infections:* **Adults and children over 20 kg:** 250 mg q 6 hr; **pediatric, less than 20 kg:** 50 mg/kg daily in divided doses q 6 hr. *Lower respiratory tract infections or disseminated infections:* **Adults and children over 20 kg:** 0.5–1 g q 6 hr; **pediatric, less than 20 kg:** 100 mg/kg daily in divided doses q 6 hr.

NURSING CONSIDERATIONS

See also *Nursing Considerations* for *Penicillins,* p. 141.

Administration/Storage

1. Add amount of water stated on label in 2 portions; shake well after each addition.
2. Shake well before pouring each dose.
3. Refrigerate reconstituted solution and discard unused portion after 14 days.
4. Administer 1 hr before or 2 hr after meals, because food interferes with absorption of drug.

Evaluation

Assess closely for wheezing and sneezing, because these side effects are more likely to occur with this drug.

ANTI-INFECTIVES

CYCLACILLIN (sye-klah-SILL-in)

Cyclapen-W (Rx)

See also *Anti-Infectives,* p. 71, and *Penicillins,* p. 138.

Classification: Antibiotic, penicillin.

Action/Kinetics: This is a semisynthetic penicillin that is better absorbed from the GI tract than ampicillin and causes less diarrhea.

Uses: Especially indicated for bronchitis, pneumonia, otitis media, tonsillitis, and pharyngitis caused by *Streptococcus pneumoniae, Hemophilus influenzae* and group A beta-hemolytic streptococci. Acute exacerbations of chronic bronchitis. Urinary tract infections caused by *Escherichia coli* and *Proteus mirabilis.* Integumentary infections due to group A beta-hemolytic streptococci and nonpenicillinase-producing staphylococci.

Additional Contraindications: Children under 2 months of age.

Special Concerns: Safe use during pregnancy and lactation not established.

Dosage: Oral Suspension, Tablets. *Tonsillitis/pharyngitis:* **Adults:** 250 mg q 6 hr; **pediatric (over 20 kg):** 250 mg q 8 hr; **pediatric (under 20 kg):** 125 mg q 8 hr. *Otitis media, integumentary infections, bronchitis, and pneumonia:* **Adults:** 250–500 mg q 6 hr; **pediatric:** 50–100 mg/kg/day in equally spaced doses. *GU tract infections:* **Adults:** 500 mg q 6 hr; **pediatric:** 100 mg/kg/day in equally spaced doses.
Dosage should be reduced in presence of renal failure.

NURSING CONSIDERATIONS

See also *Nursing Considerations* for *Penicillins,* p. 141.

Administration/Storage

1. Persistent infections may require therapy for several weeks.
2. The oral suspension should be stored in the refrigerator after reconstitution and any unused portion should be discarded after 14 days (discard after 7 days if stored at room temperature).

DICLOXACILLIN SODIUM (dye-clox-ah-SILL-in)

Dycill, Dynapen, Pathocil (Rx)

See also *Anti-Infectives,* p. 71 and *Penicillins,* p. 138.

Classification: Antibiotic, penicillin.

Action/Kinetics: This drug is penicillinase-resistant. **Peak serum levels: IM, PO,** 4–20 mcg/mL after 1 hr. **t½:** 40 min. Chiefly excreted in urine.

Uses: Resistant staphylococcal infections. To initiate therapy in any suspected staphylococcal infection. Not indicated for meningitis.

Dosage: Capsules, Oral Suspension. *Skin and soft tissue infections, mild to moderate upper respiratory tract infections:* **Adults and children over 40 kg:** 125 mg q 6 hr; **pediatric:** 12.5 mg/kg/day in 4 equal doses. *Lower respiratory tract infections or disseminated infections:* **Adults and children over 40 kg:** 250 mg q 6 hr, up to a maximum of 4 g daily; **pediatric:** 25 mg/kg daily in 4 equal doses. Dosage not established for the newborn.

NURSING CONSIDERATIONS

See also *Nursing Considerations* for *Penicillins,* p. 141.

Administration/Storage

1. To prepare oral suspension, shake container to loosen powder, measure water for reconstitution as indicated on label, add half of the water, and immediately shake vigorously because usual handling may cause lumps. Add the remainder of the water and again shake vigorously.
2. Shake well before pouring each dose.
3. Refrigerate reconstituted solution and discard after 14 days.
4. Give at least 1 hr before meals or no sooner than 2–3 hr after a meal.

METHICILLIN SODIUM (meth-ih-**SILL**-in)

Staphcillin (Rx)

See also *Anti-Infectives,* p. 71, and *Penicillins,* p. 138.

Classification: Antibiotic, penicillin.

Action/Kinetics: This drug is a semisynthetic, penicillinase-resistant salt suitable for soft tissue, penicillin G-resistant, and resistant staphylococcal infections. **Peak plasma levels: IM,** 10–20 mcg/mL after 30–60 min; **IV,** 15 min. **t½:** 30 min. Excreted chiefly in the urine.

Additional Uses: Infections by penicillinase-producing staphylococci, osteomyelitis, septicemia, enterocolitis, bacterial endocarditis.

Special Concerns: Use with caution in patients with renal failure. Safe use in neonates has not been established. Periodic renal function tests are indicated for long-term therapy.

Dosage: IM, continuous IV infusion. Adults: 4–12 g daily, depending on the infection, in divided doses q 4–6 hr. (*Note:* If creatinine clearance is less than 10 mL/min, the dose should not exceed 2 g q 12 hr.) **Pediatric:** 100–300 mg/kg daily in divided doses q 4–6 hr. **Infants over 7 days of age and weighing more than 2 kg:** 100 mg/kg daily in divided doses q 6 hr (*for meningitis:* 150–200 mg/kg daily). **Infants more than 7 days of age and weighing less than 2 kg or less than 7 days of age and weighing more than 2 kg:** 75 mg/kg daily in divided doses q 8 hr (*for meningitis:* 150 mg/kg daily). **Infants under 7 days of age and weighing less than 2 kg:** 50 mg/kg daily in divided doses q 12 hr (*for meningitis:* 100 mg/kg daily).

NURSING CONSIDERATIONS

See also *Nursing Considerations* for *Penicillins,* p. 141.

Administration/Storage

1. Do not use dextrose solutions for diluting methicillin because their low acidity may destroy the antibiotic.
2. For IM administration inject medication slowly. Methicillin injections are particularly painful.
3. Inject deeply into gluteal muscle.
4. To prevent sterile abscesses at injection site, include 0.2–0.3 mL of air in syringe before starting injection so that when the needle is withdrawn the irritating solution will not leak into tissue.
5. Methicillin is sensitive to heat when dissolved. Therefore, solutions for IM administration must

be used within 24 hr if standing at room temperature or within 4 days if refrigerated. Solutions for IV use must be used within 8 hr.

6. For IV administration, dilute 1 mL with 20–25 mL of sterile water for injection or sodium chloride injection USP.

Interventions

1. Do not mix methicillin with any other drug in the same syringe or IV solution.

2. Be sure blood cultures and WBC counts with differential are taken prior to start of, and weekly during, therapy. Many strains of methicillin-resistant staphylococci have been identified. It has been recommended that these clients be isolated until appropriate antibiotic therapy can be instituted to prevent major institutional outbreaks.

Evaluation

Assess

- for pain along course of vein into which the drug is administered, and check for redness or edema at site of injection, because drug is a vesicant.
- for hematuria, casts in urine, BUN, and creatinine levels.
- for pallor, ecchymosis, or bleeding.
- for fever, nausea, and other signs of hepatotoxicity, especially with prolonged therapy.

MEZLOCILLIN SODIUM   (mez-low-SILL-in)

Mezlin (Rx)

See also *Anti-Infectives,* p. 71, and *Penicillins,* p. 138.

Classification: Antibiotic, penicillin.

Action/Kinetics: Mezlocillin is a broad-spectrum (gram-negative and gram-positive organisms, including aerobic and anaerobic strains) antibiotic used parenterally. **Therapeutic serum levels:** 35–45 mcg/mL. $t\frac{1}{2}$: **IV,** 55 min. Excreted mostly unchanged by the kidneys. Penetration to CSF is poor unless meninges are inflamed.

Uses: Septicemia and infections of the lower respiratory tract, urinary tract, abdomen, skin, and female genital tract caused by *Klebsiella, Proteus, Pseudomonas, Escherichia coli, Bacteroides, Peptococcus, Streptococcus faecalis* (enterococcus), *Peptostreptococcus,* and *Enterobacter.* Also, *Neisseria gonorrhoeae* infections of the urinary tract and female genital system. Infections caused by *Streptococcus pneumoniae* and group A beta-hemolytic streptococcus.

Additional Side Effects: Bleeding abnormalities. Decreased hemoglobin or hematocrit values.

Laboratory Test Interferences: ↑ SGOT, SGPT, serum alkaline phosphatase, serum bilirubin, serum creatinine and/or BUN. ↓ Serum potassium.

Dosage: IV, IM. Adults: *Serious infections:* 200–300 mg/kg/day in 4–6 divided doses; **usual:** 3 g q 4 hr or 4 g q 6 hr. *Life-threatening infections:* up to 350 mg/kg/day, not to exceed 24 g daily. *Gonococcal urethritis:* single dose of 1–2 g with probenecid, 1 g. **PO. Infants and children:** *Serious infections:* **1 month–12 years,** 50 mg/kg q 4 hr given **IM** or **IV** over 30 min; **infants more than 2 kg and less than 1 week of age or less than 2 kg and less than 1 week of age:** 75 mg/kg q 12 hr; **infants less than 2 kg and more than 1 week of age:** 75 mg/kg q 8 hr; **infants more than 2 kg and more than 1 week of age:** 75 mg/kg q 6 hr.

Dosage should be reduced in patients with impaired renal function (based on creatinine clearance).

NURSING CONSIDERATIONS

See also *Nursing Considerations* for *Penicillins,* p. 141.

Administration/Storage

1. When given by IV infusion (including piggyback), administration of other drugs should be discontinued during administration of mezlocillin.
2. For pediatric IV administration, infuse over 30 min.
3. Vials and infusion bottles should be stored at temperatures below 30°C.
4. The powder and reconstituted solution may darken slightly, but potency is not affected.
5. IM doses should not exceed 2 g per injection. Mezlocillin should be continued for at least 2 days after symptoms of infection have disappeared.
6. For group A beta-hemolytic streptococcus, therapy should continue for at least 10 days.

Interventions

1. Monitor complete blood count, prothrombin time, partial thromboplastin time, electrolytes, and renal function studies.
2. Anticipate reduced dose with impaired renal function.

Evaluation

Assess for bruising and/or bleeding from any orifice and for drug-induced anemia manifested by fatigue, pallor, weakness, vertigo, headache, dyspnea, and palpitations.

NAFCILLIN SODIUM   (naf-SILL-in)

Nafcil, Nallpen, Unipen (Rx)

See also *Anti-Infectives,* p. 71, and *Penicillins,* p. 138.

Classification: Antibiotic, penicillin.

Action/Kinetics: Used for resistant staphylococcal infections. Parenteral therapy is recommended initially for severe infections. **Peak plasma levels: PO,** 7 mcg/mL after 30–60 min; **IM,** 14–20 mcg/mL after 30–60 min. **t½:** 60 min.

Uses: Infections by penicillinase-producing staphylococci; also certain pneumococci and streptococci.

Additional Side Effects: Sterile abscesses and thrombophlebitis occur frequently, especially in the elderly.

Dosage: IV. Adults: 0.5–1 g q 4 hr. **IM. Adults:** 0.5 g q 4–6 hr. **Children and infants:** 25 mg/kg b.i.d. **Neonates:** 10 mg/kg b.i.d. **Capsules, Oral Solution, Tablets. Adults:** 250–500 mg q 4–6 hr (up to 1 g q 4–6 hr for severe infections). **Pediatric:** *Pneumonia/scarlet fever:* 25 mg/kg/day in 4 divided doses. *Staphylococcal infections:* 50 mg/kg/day in 4 divided doses. **Neonates:** 10 mg/kg t.i.d.–q.i.d. *Streptococcal pharyngitis:* 250 mg t.i.d. IV administration is not recommended for neonates or infants.

NURSING CONSIDERATIONS

See also *Nursing Considerations* for *Penicillins,* p. 141.

Administration/Storage

1. Reconstitute for oral use by adding powder to bottle of diluent. Replace cap tightly. Then *shake* thoroughly until all powder is in solution. Check carefully for undissolved powder at bottom of bottle. Solution must be stored in refrigerator and unused portion discarded after 1 week.
2. Reconstitute for parenteral use by adding required amount of sterile water. Shake vigorously. Date, time and initial bottle. Refrigerate after reconstitution and discard unused portion after 48 hr.
3. For direct IV administration, dissolve powder in 15–30 mL of sterile water for injection or isotonic sodium chloride solution and inject over 5- to 10-min period into the tubing of flowing IV infusion. For IV drip, dissolve the required amount in 100–150 mL of isotonic sodium chloride injection and administer by IV drip over a period of 15–90 min.
4. IV use should be reserved for therapy of 24–48 hr duration due to the possibility of thrombophlebitis, especially in geriatric clients.
5. Administer IM by deep intragluteal injection.

Interventions

1. Do not administer IV to newborn infants.
2. Reduce rate of flow and report any pain, redness, or edema at site of IV administration.

Evaluation

1. Assess client for GI distress after oral administration.
2. Evaluate lab data and assess client for a positive clinical response.

OXACILLIN SODIUM   (ox-ah-**SILL**-in)

Bactocill, Prostaphlin (Rx)

See also *Anti-Infectives,* p. 71, and *Penicillins,* p. 138.

Classification: Antibiotic, penicillin.

Action/Kinetics: This is a penicillinase-resistant, acid-stable drug used for resistant staphylococcal infections. **Peak plasma levels: PO,** 1.6–10 mcg after 30–60 min; **IM,** 5–11 mcg/mL after 30 min. **t½:** 30 min.

Uses: Infections caused by penicillinase-producing staphylococci; also certain pneumococci and streptococci.

Dosage: Capsules, Oral Solution. Adults and children (over 40 kg): *Mild to moderate infections of the upper respiratory tract, skin, soft tissue:* 500 mg q 4–6 hr for at least 5 days. **Children less than 40 kg:** 50 mg/kg daily in equally divided doses q 6 hr for at least 5 days. *Septicemia, deep-seated infections:* Parenteral therapy (see below) followed by oral therapy. **Adults:** 1 g q 4–6 hr; **children:** 100 mg/kg daily in equally divided doses q 4–6 hr.
   IM, IV. Adults and pediatric (over 40 kg): 250–500 mg q 4–6 hr (up to 1 g q 4–6 hr in severe infections of the lower respiratory tract or disseminated infections); **children (less than 40 kg):**

50 mg/kg/day in equally divided doses q 6 hr (up to 100 mg/kg/day in severe infections); **neonates and premature infants:** 25 mg/kg/day. Maximum daily dose: **Adults,** 12 g; **children,** 100–200 mg/kg.

NURSING CONSIDERATIONS

See also *Nursing Considerations* for *Penicillins,* p. 141.

Administration/Storage

1. Administer IM by deep intragluteal injection.
2. Reconstitution: Add sterile water for injection or sodium chloride injection in amount indicated on vial. Shake until solution is clear. For parenteral use, reconstituted solution may be kept for 3 days at room temperature or 1 week in refrigerator. Discard outdated solutions.
3. IV administration (two methods):
   - For rapid, direct administration, add an equal amount of sterile water or isotonic saline to reconstituted dosage and administer over a period of 10 minutes.
   - For IV infusion, add reconstituted solution to either dextrose, saline, or invert sugar solution and administer over a 6-hr period, during which time drug remains potent.
4. Treatment of osteomyelitis may require several months of intensive oral therapy.

Interventions

1. Report all side effects of the drug to the physician.
2. Rotate injection sites and document.

Evaluation

Evaluate for

- effectiveness of drug therapy based on appropriate lab data.
- GI distress after oral administration.
- pain, redness, and edema at the site of IV injection and along the course of the vein.
- pain and swelling at IM injection site.

PENICILLIN G BENZATHINE, ORAL (pen-ih-**SILL**-in, **BEN**-zah-theen)

Bicillin (Rx)

PENICILLIN G BENZATHINE, PARENTERAL (pen-ih-**SILL**-in, **BEN**-zah-theen)

Bicillin L-A, Permapen (Rx)

See also *Anti-Infectives,* p. 71, and *Penicillins,* p. 138.

Classification: Antibiotic, penicillin.

Action/Kinetics: The parenteral product is a long-acting (repository) form of penicillin in an aqueous vehicle; it is administered as a sterile suspension. **Peak plasma levels: PO,** 0.16 unit/mL; **IM,** 0.03–0.05 unit/mL.

Uses: Most gram-positive (streptococci, staphylococci, pneumococci) and some gram-negative (gonococci, meningococci) organisms. Syphilis. Prophylaxis of glomerulonephritis and rheumatic fever. Surgical infections, secondary infections following tooth extraction, tonsillectomy.

Dosage: Tablets. Adults and children over 12 years: 400,000–600,000 units q 4–6 hr. *Prophylaxis of rheumatic fever/chorea:* 200,000 units b.i.d. **Children under 12 years:** 25,000–90,000 units/day in 3–6 divided doses.

Parenteral Suspension (IM only). Adults: *Upper respiratory tract infections, erysipeloid, yaws:* 1,200,000 units as a single dose; **older children:** 900,000 units as a single dose; **pediatric under 27 kg:** 300,000–600,000 units as a single dose. *Early syphilis:* 2,400,000 units as a single dose. *Late syphilis, neurosyphilis:* 2,400,000 units q 7 days for 3 weeks. *Prophylaxis of rheumatic fever:* **Adults and children over 27 kg:** 1,200,000 units; **Children and infants less than 27 kg:** 50,000 units/kg as a single dose.

NURSING CONSIDERATIONS

See also *Nursing Considerations* for *Penicillins,* p. 141.

Administration/Storage

1. Shake multiple-dose vial vigorously before withdrawing the desired dose, because medication tends to clump on standing. Check that all medication is dissolved and that there is no residue at bottom of bottle.
2. Use a 20-gauge needle, and do not allow medication to remain in the syringe and needle for long periods of time before administration, because the needle may become plugged and the syringe "frozen."
3. Inject slowly and steadily into the muscle and *do not massage* injection site.
4. For adults, use the upper outer quadrant of the buttock; for infants and small children, the midlateral aspect of the thigh should be used. Benzathine penicillin should not be administered in the gluteal region in children less than 2 years of age.
5. Before injection of medication, aspirate needle to ascertain that needle is not in a vein.
6. Rotate and chart site of injections.
7. *Do not administer IV.*
8. Divide between two injection sites if dose is large or available muscle mass is small.

Client/Family Teaching

1. Explain to client why it is necessary to return for repository penicillin injections.
2. Evaluate the need for sexual counseling or referral. Stress the importance of the partner undergoing treatment.

PENICILLIN G, BENZATHINE AND PROCAINE COMBINED
(pen-ih-**SILL**-in, **BEN**-zah-theen, **PROH**-caine)

Bicillin C-R, Bicillin C-R 900/300 (Rx)

See also *Anti-Infectives,* p. 71, and *Penicillins,* p. 138.

Classification: Antibiotic, penicillin.

Uses: Streptococcal infections (A, C, G, H, L, and M) without bacteremia, of the upper respiratory tract, skin, and soft tissues. Scarlet fever, erysipelas, pneumococcal infections, and otitis media.

Special Concerns: Pregnancy category: B.

Dosage: IM only. *Streptococcal infections:* **Adults and children over 27 kg:** 2,400,000 units, given at a single session using multiple injection sites or, alternatively, in divided doses on days 1 and 3; **children 13.5–27 kg:** 900,000–1,200,000 units; **infants and children under 13.5 kg:** 600,000 units. *Pneumococcal infections, except meningitis:* **Adults,** 1,200,000 units; **pediatric:** 600,000 units. Give q 2–3 days until temperature is normal for 48 hr.

NURSING CONSIDERATIONS

See *Nursing Considerations* for *Penicillin G Benzathine Oral* and *Penicillin G Benzathine Parenteral,* p. 158, and *Penicillins,* p. 141.

PENICILLIN G POTASSIUM FOR INJECTION   (pen-ih-**SILL**-in, poe-**TASS**-ee-um)
Pfizerpen (Rx)

PENICILLIN G POTASSIUM, ORAL   (pen-ih-**SILL**-in, poe-**TASS**-ee-um)
Megacillin ✻, Novopen-G ✻, P-50 ✻, Pentids, Pentids for Syrup, Pentids 400 Tablets, 400 for Syrup, and 800 Tablets (Rx)

PENICILLIN G SODIUM FOR INJECTION   (pen-ih-**SILL**-in **SO**-dee-um)
Crystapen ✻ (Rx)

See also *Anti-Infectives,* p. 71, and *Penicillins,* p. 138.

Classification: Antibiotic, penicillin.

Action/Kinetics: The low cost of penicillin G still makes it the first choice for treatment of many infections. Rapid onset makes it especially suitable for fulminating infections. Destroyed by acid and penicillinase. **Peak plasma levels: IM or SC,** 6–20 units/mL after 15–30 min. **t½:** 30 min.

Additional Side Effects: Rapid IV administration may cause hyperkalemia and cardiac arrhythmias. Renal damage occurs rarely.

Dosage: Parenteral (IM, continuous IV infusion). Adults: 300,000–30 million units daily, depending on the use. **Pediatric:** 100,000–250,000 units/kg daily (given in divided doses q 4 hr). **Infants over 7 days of age weighing more than 2 kg:** 100,000 units/kg daily (given in divided doses q 6 hr). *For meningitis:* 200,000 units/kg. **Infants over 7 days of age weighing less than 2 kg:** 75,000 units daily (given in divided doses q 8 hr). *For meningitis:* 150,000 units/kg. **Infants less than 7 days of age weighing more than 2 kg:** 50,000 units/kg daily (given in divided doses q 8 hr). *For meningitis:* 150,000 units/kg. **Infants less than 7 days of age weighing less than 2 kg:** 50,000 units/kg daily (given in divided doses q 12 hr). *For meningitis:* 100,000 units/kg daily for 14 days.

 Oral Solution, Tablets. Adults: Depending on the use, 200,000–500,000 units q 6–8 hr; **pediatric under 12 years of age:** 25,000–90,000 units/kg/day in 3–6 divided doses. **Note:** 250 mg Penicillin G potassium, oral, is equivalent to 400,000 units.

NURSING CONSIDERATIONS

See also *Nursing Considerations* for *Penicillins,* p. 141.

Administration/Storage

1. IM administration is preferred; discomfort is minimized by using solutions of up to 100,000 units/mL.

2. Use sterile water, isotonic saline USP, or 5% D₅W and mix drug with volume recommended on label for desired strength.

3. Loosen powder by shaking bottle before adding diluent.

4. Hold vial horizontally and rotate slowly while directing the stream of the diluent against the wall of the vial.

5. Shake vigorously after addition of diluent.

6. Solutions may be stored at room temperature for 24 hr or in refrigerator for 1 week. Discard remaining solution.

7. Use 1%–2% lidocaine solution as diluent for IM, if ordered by physician to lessen pain at injection site. Do not use procaine as diluent for aqueous penicillin.

8. Note the drugs that should *not* be mixed with penicillin during IV administration:

Aminophylline	Metaraminol	Sodium bicarbonate
Amphotericin B	Novobiocin	Sodium salts of barbiturates
Ascorbic acid	Oxytetracycline	Sulfadiazine
Chlorpheniramine	Phenylephrine	Tetracycline
Chlorpromazine	Phenytoin	Tromethamine
Gentamicin	Polymyxin B	Vitamin B complex
Heparin	Prochlorperazine	Vancomycin
Hydroxyzine	Promazine	
Lincomycin	Promethazine	

Interventions

1. Order drug by specifying sodium or potassium salt.

2. Monitor I&O. Dehydration decreases the excretion of the drug by the kidneys and may raise the blood level of penicillin G to dangerously high levels that can cause kidney damage.

Evaluation

Assess client for GI disturbances, which may lead to dehydration.

PENICILLIN G PROCAINE SUSPENSION, STERILE   (pen-ih-**SILL**-in, **PROH**-caine)

Ayercillin✱, Crysticillin 300 A.S. and 600 A.S., Duracillin A.S., Pfizerpen-AS, Wycillin (Rx)

See also *Anti-Infectives,* p. 71, and *Penicillins,* p. 138.

Classification: Antibiotic, penicillin.

Action/Kinetics: Long-acting (repository) form in aqueous or oily vehicle. Destroyed by penicillinase. Because of slow onset, a soluble penicillin is often administered concomitantly for fulminating infections.

Uses: Penicillin-sensitive staphylococci, pneumococci, streptococci, and bacterial endocarditis. Gonorrhea, all stages of syphilis. *Prophylaxis:* Rheumatic fever, pre- and postsurgery. Diphtheria, anthrax, fusospirochetosis (Vincent's infection), erysipeloid, rat-bite fever.

Dosage: IM only. Adults, usual: *Pneumococcal, staphylococcal, streptococcal infections; erysipeloid, rat-bite fever, anthrax, fusospirochetosis:* 600,000–1,200,000 units daily for 10–14 days. **Newborns, usual:** 50,000 units/kg in a single daily dose. *Bacterial endocarditis:* **Adults:** 1,200,000 units penicillin G procaine q.i.d. for 2–4 weeks with streptomycin, 500 mg b.i.d. for the first 14 days.

Diphtheria carrier state: 300,000 units/day for 10 days. *Gonococcal infections:* 4.8 million units given with 1 g PO probenecid. *Neurosyphilis:* 2.4 million units daily for 10 days (given at two sites) with 1 g PO probenecid; **then,** benzathine penicillin G, 2.4 million units/week for 3 weeks. *Congenital syphilis in infants:* 50,000 units/kg daily for at least 10 days. *Acute pelvic inflammatory disease:* Single dose of 4.8 million units (given at two sites) with 1 g PO probenecid; **then,** doxycycline, PO, 100 mg b.i.d. for 10–14 days. *Sexually transmitted epididymo-orchitis, urethritis:* 4.8 million units (given at two sites) with 1 g PO probenecid; **then,** tetracycline, PO, 500 mg q.i.d. for 10 days.

NURSING CONSIDERATIONS

See also *Nursing Considerations* for *Penicillins,* p. 141.

Administration/Storage

1. Note on package whether medication is to be refrigerated, since some brands require this to maintain stability.
2. Shake multiple-dose vial thoroughly to ensure uniform suspension before injection. If the medication is clumped at the bottom of the vial, it must be shaken until clump dissolves.
3. Use a 20-gauge needle and aspirate immediately after withdrawing medication from the vial; otherwise needle may become clogged and syringe may "freeze."
4. Administer into two sites if dose is large or available muscle mass is small.
5. Aspirate to check that the needle is not in a vein.
6. Inject deep into muscle at a slow rate.
7. Do not massage after injection.
8. Rotate and chart injection sites.
9. Drug is for IM use only.

Evaluation

1. Observe for wheal or other skin reactions at site of injection that may indicate a reaction to procaine as well as to penicillin.
2. Evaluate need for sexual counseling/referral. Stress importance of the partner undergoing treatment.

PENICILLIN V POTASSIUM (PHENOXYMETHYLPENICILLIN POTASSIUM) (pen-ih-SILL-in VEE)

Apo-Pen-VK✹, Beepen-VK, Betapen-VK, Ledercillin VK, Nadopen-V✹, Nadopen-VK✹, Novopen-VK✹, Penapar VK, Penicillin VK, Pen-V, Pen-Vee K, Robicillin VK, Suspen, Uticillin VK, V-Cillin K, VC-K✹, Veetids 125, 250, and 500 (Rx)

See also *Anti-Infectives,* p. 71, and *Penicillins,* p. 138.

Classification: Antibiotic, penicillin.

Action/Kinetics: These preparations are related closely to penicillin G. They are acid stable and resist inactivation by gastric secretions. They are well absorbed from the GI tract and are not affected by foods. **Peak plasma levels: PO:** 1–9 mcg/mL after 30–60 min. **t½:** 30 min.

Periodic blood counts and renal function tests are indicated during long-term usage.

Uses: Penicillin-sensitive staphylococci, pneumococci, streptococci, gonococci. Vincent's infection of the oropharynx. *Prophylaxis:* Rheumatic fever, chorea, bacterial endocarditis, pre- and postsurgery. Should *not* be used as prophylaxis for GU instrumentation or surgery, sigmoidoscopy, or childbirth.

Additional Drug Interactions	
Contraceptives, Oral	↓ Effectiveness of oral contraceptives
Neomycin, oral	↓ Absorption of penicillin V

Dosage: Oral Solution, Tablets. Adults and children over 12 years: *Streptococcal infections:* 125–250 mg q 6–8 hr for 10 days. *Pneumococcal or staphylococcal infections, fusospirochetosis of oropharynx:* 250–500 mg q 6–8 hr. *Prophylaxis of rheumatic fever/chorea:* 125–250 mg b.i.d. *Prophylaxis of bacterial endocarditis.* **PO. Adults and children over 27 kg:** 2 g 30–60 min prior to procedure; **then,** 1 g q 6 hr. **Pediatric:** 1 g 30–60 min prior to procedure; **then,** 500 mg q 6 hr. *Anaerobic infections:* 250 mg q.i.d. See also *Penicillin G, Procaine, Aqueous.*

Pediatric, usual: 25–50 mg/kg daily in divided doses q 6–8 hr. *Prophylaxis of septicemia caused by Staphylococcus pneumoniae in children with sickle cell anemia:* 125 mg b.i.d.

Note: 125 mg penicillin V is equivalent to 200,000 units.

NURSING CONSIDERATIONS

See also *Nursing Considerations* for *Penicillins,* p. 141.

Administration/Storage

1. Administer without regard to meals.
2. Do not administer at the same time as neomycin, because malabsorption of penicillin V may occur.

Client/Family Teaching

1. Use an additional form of birth control if taking oral contraceptives, because their effectiveness may be diminished.
2. Report for all scheduled laboratory studies and explain their importance during long-term therapy.

Evaluation

1. Assess client/family knowledge and understanding of illness, response to therapy, and response to teaching.
2. Review appropriate lab data to determine response to therapy.

PIPERACILLIN SODIUM   (pih-per-ah-**SILL**-in)

Pipracil (Rx)

See also *Penicillins,* p. 138.

Classification: Antibiotic, penicillin.

Action/Kinetics: Piperacillin is a semisynthetic, broad-spectrum penicillin for parenteral use. The drug penetrates CSF in the presence of inflamed meninges. **Peak serum level:** 244 mcg/mL. **t½:** 36–72 min. Excreted unchanged in urine and bile.

Additional Uses: Intra-abdominal infections, gynecologic infections, septicemia, skin and skin structure infections, bone and joint infections, mixed infections. Prophylaxis in surgery including GI, biliary, hysterectomy, cesarean section.

Additional Side Effects: Rarely, prolonged muscle relaxation.

Laboratory Test Interference: Positive Comb's test; ↑ (especially in infants) SGOT, SGPT, LDH, bilirubin.

Dosage: IM, IV. *Serious infections,* **IV:** 3–4 g q 4–6 hr (12–18 g/day). *Complicated urinary tract infections,* **IV:** 8–16 g/day in divided doses q 6–8 hr. *Uncomplicated urinary tract infections and most community-acquired pneumonias,* **IM, IV:** 6–8 g/day in divided doses q 6–12 hr. *Uncomplicated gonorrhea infections:* 2 g **IM** with 1 g probenecid **PO** 30 min before injection (both given as single dose). *Prophylaxis in surgery,* **First dose: IV,** 2 g prior to surgery; **second dose:** 2 g either during surgery (abdominal) or 4–6 hr after surgery (hysterectomy, cesarean); **third dose:** 2 g at an interval depending on use. Dosage should be decreased in renal impairment. Dosages have not been established in infants and children under 12 years of age.

NURSING CONSIDERATIONS

See also *Nursing Considerations* for *Penicillins,* p. 141.

Administration/Storage

1. No more than 2 g should be administered IM at any one site.
2. For IM administration, use upper, outer quadrant of gluteus or well-developed deltoid muscle. Do not use lower or mid-third of upper arm.
3. For IV administration reconstitute each gram with at least 5 mL diluent, such as sterile or bacteriostatic water for injection, sodium chloride for injection, or bacteriostatic sodium chloride for injection. Shake until dissolved.
4. Inject IV slowly over a period of 3–5 min to avoid vein irritation.
5. Administer by intermittent IV infusion in at least 50 mL over a period of 20–30 min via "piggyback" or soluset.
6. After reconstitution, solution may be stored at room temperature for 24 hours, refrigerated for 1 week, or frozen for 1 month.

Interventions

1. Monitor complete blood count, liver and renal function studies throughout therapy.
2. Report any diarrhea or other evidence of superinfection.

TICARCILLIN DISODIUM   (tie-kar-**SILL**-in)

Ticar (Rx)

See also *Anti-Infectives,* p. 71, and *Penicillins,* p. 138.

Classification: Antibiotic, penicillin.

Action/Kinetics: This drug is a parenteral, semisynthetic antibiotic with an antibacterial spectrum of activity resembling that of carbenicillin. Primarily suitable for treatment of gram-negative organisms, but also effective for mixed infections. Combined therapy with gentamicin or tobramycin is sometimes indicated for treatment of *Pseudomonas* infections. *The drugs should not be mixed during administration because of gradual mutual inactivation.*

Peak plasma levels: IM, 25–35 mcg/mL after 1 hr; **IV,** 15 min. **t½:** 70 min. Elimination complete after 6 hr.

Uses: Bacterial septicemia, skin and soft tissue infections, acute and chronic respiratory tract infections caused by susceptible strains of *Pseudomonas aeruginosa, Proteus, Escherichia coli,* and other gram-negative organisms. GU tract infections caused by above organisms and by *Enterobacter* and *Streptococcus faecalis.*

Anaerobic bacteria causing empyema, anaerobic pneumonitis, lung abscess, bacterial septicemia, peritonitis, intra-abdominal abscess, skin and soft tissue infections, salpingitis, endometritis, pelvic inflammatory disease, pelvic abscess.

Additional Contraindications: Pregnancy.

Special Concerns: Use with caution in presence of impaired renal function and for patients on restricted salt diets.

Additional Side Effects: Neurotoxicity and neuromuscular excitability, especially in patients with impaired renal function. Elevated alkaline phosphatase, SGOT, and SGPT values.

Additional Drug Interactions: Effect of carbenicillin may be enhanced when used in combination with gentamicin or tobramycin for *Pseudomonas* infections.

Dosage: IV, IM. *Systemic infections.* **IV infusion, adults and children less than 40 kg:** 200–300 mg/kg daily in divided doses q 3–6 hr for adults and q 4–6 hr for children. **IV infusion (10–20 min), IM, neonates over 2 kg, 0–7 days or less than 2 kg, over 7 days:** 75 mg/kg q 8 hr; **neonates over 2 kg, over 7 days:** 100 mg/kg q 8 hr; **neonates, less than 2 kg, 0–7 days:** 75 mg/kg q 12 hr. *Urinary tract infections.* **IV infusion (complicated infections), adults and children (less than 40 kg):** 150–200 mg/kg daily in divided doses q 4–6 hr. **IM or direct IV (uncomplicated infections): Adults,** 1 g q 6 hr; **pediatric (less than 40 kg):** 50–100 mg/kg daily in divided doses q 6–8 hr.

Patients with renal insufficiency should receive a loading dose of 3 g **IV,** and subsequent doses, as indicated by creatinine clearance.

NURSING CONSIDERATIONS

See also *Nursing Considerations* for *Penicillins,* p. 141.

Administration/Storage

1. Discard unused reconstituted solutions after 24 hr when stored at room temperature and after 72 hr when refrigerated.
2. Reconstitute with 1% lidocaine HCl (without epinephrine) or with bacteriostatic water for injection containing 0.9% benzyl alcohol to prevent pain and induration.
3. Use dilute solution of 50 mg/mL or less for IV use, and administer slowly to prevent vein irritation and phlebitis.
4. Do not administer more than 2 g of the drug in each IM site.

Evaluation

1. Evaluate for signs of hemorrhage, such as petechiae, ecchymosis, or frank bleeding.
2. Observe client with cardiac history for edema, weight gain, or respiratory distress precipitated by sodium in the drug.
3. Note client on high doses of drug for signs of electrolyte imbalance, especially in regard to levels of sodium and potassium.
4. Assess bleeding times, liver and renal function studies which should be monitored during therapy.

TICARCILLIN DISODIUM AND CLAVULANATE POTASSIUM

(tie-kar-**SILL**-in, klav-you-**LAN**-ate poe-**TASS**-ee-um)

Timentin (Rx)

See also *Ticarcillin,* p. 163, and *Penicillins,* p. 138.

Classification: Antibiotic, penicillin.

Action/Kinetics: This preparation contains clavulanic acid, which protects the breakdown of ticarcillin by β-lactamase enzymes, thus ensuring appropriate blood levels of ticarcillin.

Uses: Complicated and uncomplicated urinary tract infections; infections of the bones and joints, lower respiratory tract, skin and skin structures; gynecologic infections, bacterial septicemia. In combination with an aminoglycoside for certain *Pseudomonas aeruginosa* infections.

Dosage: IV infusion. *Systemic and urinary tract infections:* **Adults more than 60 kg:** 3 g (containing 0.1 g clavulanic acid) q 4–6 hr for 10–14 days. **Adults less than 60 kg:** 200–300 mg ticarcillin/kg daily in divided doses q 4–6 hr for 10–14 days. *Gynecologic infections:* **Adults more than 60 kg, moderate infections:** 200 mg/kg/day in divided doses q 6 hr; **severe infections:** 300 mg/kg/day in divided doses q 4 hr. *In renal insufficiency,* **initially,** loading dose of 3 g ticarcillin and 0.1 g clavulanic acid; **then,** dose based on creatinine clearance (see package insert).

NURSING CONSIDERATIONS

See also *Nursing Considerations* for *Penicillins,* p. 141, and *Ticarcillin,* p. 164.

Administration/Storage

1. To attain the appropriate dilution for 3 g ticarcillin and 0.1 g clavulanic acid, dilute with 13 mL of either sodium chloride injection or sterile water for injection. Further dilutions, if necessary, can be undertaken with 5% dextrose injection, lactated Ringer's injection, or sodium chloride injection.
2. The drugs should be administered over a period of 30 min, either through a Y-type IV infusion or by direct infusion.
3. This product is incompatible with sodium bicarbonate.
4. Dilutions with sodium chloride injection or lactated Ringer's injection may be stored at room temperature for 24 hr or refrigerated for 7 days. Dilutions with 5% dextrose injection are stable at room temperature for 12 hr or for 3 days if refrigerated.

POLYMYXINS

COLISTIMETHATE SODIUM   (koh-liss-tih-**METH**-ate)

Coly-Mycin M (Rx)

Classification: Antibiotic, polymyxin.

Action/Kinetics: Colistimethate increases the permeability of the plasma cell membrane causing leakage of essential metabolites and, ultimately, inactivation. **Peak blood levels after IM:** 5 mcg/mL after 1–2 hr. **t½, serum:** 2–3 hr

Uses: Acute or chronic infections (e.g., urinary or respiratory tract infections, septicemia, burns) due to gram-negative bacilli including *Enterobacter aerogenes, Escherichia coli, Klebsiella pneumoniae,* and *Pseudomonas aeruginosa.*

Contraindications: Infections due to *Proteus* or *Neisseria.*

Special Concerns: Use during pregnancy only if benefits outweigh risks. Use with caution if renal function is impaired.

Side Effects: *Respiratory:* Respiratory arrest, apnea after IM use. *Renal:* Nephrotoxicity manifested by decreased urine output and increased BUN or serum creatinine. *Musculoskeletal:* Tingling of extremities or tongue, paresthesia. *Other:* GI upset, drug fever, slurred speech, itching, urticaria, vertigo.

Drug Interactions	
Aminoglycosides	Additive nephrotoxicity
Anesthetics, general	Additive neuromuscular blockade and muscle paralysis
Cephalothin	Additive nephrotoxicity
Neuromuscular blocking agents	Additive neuromuscular blockade and muscle paralysis

Dosage: IM, IV: Adults and children, 2.5–5 mg/kg daily in 2–4 divided doses if renal function is normal. Reduce both daily dose and frequency of administration in renal impairment.

NURSING CONSIDERATIONS

See also *General Nursing Considerations For All Anti-Infectives* under *Penicillins,* p. 140.

Administration/Storage

1. For direct, intermittent IV administration, half the daily dose should be given q 12 hr over a period of 3–5 min.
2. For continuous infusion, one-half the total daily dose should be given slowly over 3–5 min. The remaining half-dose should be added to one of the following: 5% dextrose in water, 5% dextrose with 0.9% sodium chloride, 5% dextrose with 0.45% sodium chloride, 5% dextrose with 0.225% sodium chloride, lactated Ringer's solution, 10% invert sugar solution, or 0.9% sodium chloride. The mixture can be given by slow IV infusion beginning 1–2 hr after the initial dose at a rate of 5–6 mg/hr if renal function is normal. In impaired renal function, reduce the rate of infusion.
3. Solutions for infusion should be freshly prepared and used within 24 hr.

Assessment

Note any history of respiratory or kidney dysfunction.

Interventions

1. Anticipate reduced dose with impaired renal function.
2. Monitor intake and output.
3. Have available emergency equipment and calcium chloride for parenteral injection in case of apnea.

Client/Family Teaching

1. Instruct client to report tingling sensation in mouth and tongue, visual and speech disturbances, pruritus, and ototoxic effects.
2. Warn clients to avoid hazardous tasks, since drug may cause dizziness, vertigo, and ataxia.

> **Evaluation**
> Assess for nephrotoxicity demonstrated by albuminuria, hematuria, anuria, casts, edema, and uremia.

COLISTIN SULFATE (POLYMYXIN E)   (koh-**LIS**-tin)
Coly-Mycin S (Rx)

Classification: Antibiotic, polymyxin.

Action/Kinetics: Colistin increases the permeability of the plasma cell membrane of bacteria causing leakage of essential metabolites and ultimately inactivation. Significant amounts are not absorbed into the systemic circulation. Resistance rarely develops to this drug.

Uses: In infants and children for diarrhea caused by *Escherichia coli*. Gastroenteritis due to *Shigella*.

Contraindications: *Proteus* infections.

Side Effects: *Renal:* High doses may result in renal toxicity in patients with azotemia. *GI:* Superinfections.

Dosage: PO: 5–15 mg/kg daily in 3 divided doses (higher doses may be necessary).

NURSING CONSIDERATIONS

See *Nursing Considerations* for *Polymyxin B,* p. 168, and *General Nursing Implications For All Anti-Infectives* under *Penicillins,* p. 140.

Administration/Storage

1. The drug should be reconstituted by adding 18.5 mL distilled water and then shaking well. An additional 18.5 mL of distilled water is then added, followed by additional shaking.
2. The reconstituted solution is stable for 2 weeks if stored below 15°C (59°F).

Intervention

Renal function should be assessed prior to starting therapy.

POLYMYXIN B SULFATE, PARENTERAL   (pol-ih-**MIX**-in)
Aerosporin (Rx)

POLYMYXIN B SULFATE, STERILE OPHTHALMIC   (pol-ih-**MIX**-in)
(Rx)

See also *Anti-Infectives,* p. 71.

Classification: Antibiotic, polymyxin.

Action/Kinetics: Polymyxin B sulfate is derived from the spore-forming soil bacterium *Bacillus polymyxa*. It is bactericidal against most gram-negative organisms and rapidly inactivated by alkali, strong acid, and certain metal ions. Polymyxin increases the permeability of the plasma cell membrane of the bacterium (i.e., similar to detergents), causing leakage of essential metabolites and ultimately inactivation. **Peak serum levels: IM,** 2 hr. **t½:** 4.3–6 hr. Longer in presence of renal impairment. Sixty percent of drug excreted in urine. It is virtually unabsorbed from the GI tract except in newborn infants. After parenteral administration, polymyxin B seems to remain in the plasma.

Uses: Acute infections of the urinary tract and meninges, septicemia caused by *Pseudomonas aeruginosa.* Meningeal infections caused by *Hemophilus influenzae,* urinary tract infections caused by *Escherichia coli,* bacteremia caused by *Enterobacter aerogenes* or *Klebsiella pneumoniae.* Combined with neomycin for irrigation of the urinary bladder to prevent bacteriuria and bacteremia from indwelling catheters.

Topical: Conjunctival and corneal infections. Blepharitis and keratitis due to bacterial infections. Used with systemic agents for anterior intraocular infections and corneal ulcers caused by *Pseudomonas aeruginosa.* Used alone or in combination for ear infections.

Contraindications: Hypersensitivity. Polymyxin B sulfate is a potentially toxic drug to be reserved for the treatment of severe, resistant infections in hospitalized patients. The drug is not indicated for patients with severely impaired renal function or nitrogen retention.

Special Concerns: Safe use during pregnancy has not been established.

Side Effects: *Nephrotoxic:* Albuminuria, cylindruria, azotemia, hematuria, proteinuria, leukocyturia, electrolyte loss. *Neurologic:* Dizziness, flushing of face, mental confusion, irritability, nystagmus, muscle weakness, drowsiness, paresthesias, blurred vision, slurred speech, ataxia, coma, seizures. Neuromuscular blockade may lead to respiratory paralysis. *GI:* Nausea, vomiting, diarrhea, abdominal cramps. *Miscellaneous:* Fever, urticaria, skin exanthemata, eosinophilia, anaphylaxis.

Following intrathecal use: Meningeal irritation with fever, stiff neck, headache, increase in leukocytes and protein in the CSF. Nerve-root irritation may result in neuritic pain and urine retention. *Following IM use:* Irritation, severe pain. *Following IV use:* Thrombophlebitis.

Drug Interactions	
Aminoglycoside antibiotics	Additive nephrotoxic effects
Cephalosporins	↑ Risk of renal toxicity
Phenothiazines	↑ Risk of respiratory depression
Skeletal muscle relaxants (surgical)	Additive muscle relaxation

Laboratory Test Interferences: False + or ↑ levels of urea nitrogen and creatinine. Casts and RBCs in urine.

Dosage: IV: Adults and children, 15,000–25,000 units/kg/day (maximum) in divided doses q 12 hr. **Infants,** up to 40,000 units/kg/day. **IM** (not usually recommended due to pain at injection site): **Adults and children,** 25,000–30,000 units/kg/day in divided doses q 4–6 hr. **Infants,** up to 40,000 units/kg/day. Both IV and IM doses should be reduced in renal impairment. **Intrathecal** (*meningitis*): **Adults and children over 2 years,** 50,000 units once daily for 3–4 days; **then,** 50,000 units every other day until 2 weeks after cultures are negative; **children under 2 years,** 20,000 units once daily for 3–4 days or 25,000 units once every other day; dosage of 25,000 units should be continued every other day for 2 weeks after cultures are negative. **Ophthalmic solution:** 1–2 gtt 2–6 times daily, depending on the infection. Treatment may be necessary for 1–2 months or longer.

NURSING CONSIDERATIONS

See also *General Nursing Considerations* for *All Anti-Infectives* under *Penicillins,* p. 140.

Administration/Storage

1. Store and dilute as directed on package insert.
2. Pain on IM injection can be lessened by reducing drug concentration as much as possible. It is

preferable to give drug more frequently in more dilute doses. If ordered, procaine hydrochloride (2 mL of a 0.5%–1.0% solution per 5 units of dry powder) may be used for mixing the drug for IM injection.

3. *Never use preparations containing procaine hydrochloride for IV or intrathecal use.*

Assessment

1. Determine kidney function and urinary output. Rule out edema or any other evidence of kidney tract problems.
2. Note respiratory function and any history of problems.
3. Utilize assessment information as a baseline against which to measure possible outcomes of the medication therapy.

Interventions

1. Withhold drug when signs of muscle weakness appear. Neuromuscular blockade may respond to calcium chloride. Have emergency equipment readily available.
2. Monitor intake and output.
3. Anticipate reduced dose in clients with impaired renal function.
4. Use safety precautions for ambulatory or bedridden clients with neurologic disturbances.
5. Anticipate a prolonged regimen of topical application of polymyxin B solution, because drug is not toxic when used in wet dressings, and the physician may wish to prevent emergence of resistant strains.

Client/Family Teaching

Advise clients to avoid hazardous tasks as the drug may cause dizziness, vertigo, and ataxia.

Evaluation

1. *Evaluate*
   - for nephrotoxicity, characterized by albuminuria, urinary casts, nitrogen retention, and hematuria
   - for drug fever and neurologic disturbances, demonstrated by dizziness, blurred vision, irritability, circumoral and peripheral numbness and tingling, weakness, and ataxia. These symptoms usually disappear within 24–48 hr after the drug is discontinued.
2. Note any muscle weakness, an early sign of muscle paralysis and impending apnea.
3. Note tolerance and evidence of increased or decreased fatigue.

TETRACYCLINES

Action/Kinetics: The tetracyclines inhibit protein synthesis by microorganisms by binding to a crucial ribosomal subunit (50S), thereby interfering with protein synthesis. The drugs block the binding of aminoacyl transfer RNA to the messenger RNA complex. Cell wall synthesis is not inhibited. The drugs are mostly bacteriostatic and are effective only against multiplying bacteria. Tetracyclines are well absorbed from the stomach and upper small intestine. They are well distributed throughout all tissues and fluids and diffuse through noninflamed meninges and the placental barrier. They become deposited in the fetal skeleton and calcifying teeth. **t¹/₂:** ranges from 7–18.6 hr (see individual agents) and is increased in the presence of renal impairment. The drugs bind to serum protein (range: 20%–93%; see individual agents). The drugs are concentrated in the liver in the bile and are excreted mostly unchanged in the urine and feces.

Uses: Used mainly for infections caused by *Rickettsia, Chlamydia,* and *Mycoplasma.* Due to development of resistance, tetracyclines are usually not used for infections by common gram-negative or gram-positive organisms.

Tetracyclines are the drugs of choice for rickettsial infections such as Rocky Mountain spotted fever, endemic typhus, and others. They are also the drugs of choice for psittacosis, lymphogranuloma venereum, and urethritis due to *Mycoplasma hominis* and *Ureaplasma urealyticum.* Epididymo-orchitis due to *Chlamydia trachomatis* and/or *Neisseria gonorrhoeae.* Atypical pneumonia caused by *Mycoplasma pneumoniae.* Adjunct in the treatment of trachoma.

Tetracyclines are the drugs of choice for gram-negative bacteria causing bartonellosis, brucellosis, granuloma inguinale, cholera. They are used as alternatives for the treatment of plague, tularemia, chancroid, or *Campylobacter fetus* infections. Prophylaxis of plague after exposure. Infections caused by *Acinetobacter, Bacteroides, Enterobacter aerogenes, Escherichia coli, Shigella.* Respiratory and/or urinary tract infections caused by *Hemophilus influenzae* or *Klebsiella pneumoniae.*

As an alternative to penicillin for uncomplicated gonorrhea or disseminated gonococcal infections, especially with penicillin allergy. Acute pelvic inflammatory disease. Tetracyclines are also useful as an alternative to penicillin for early syphilis.

Although not generally used for gram-positive infections, tetracyclines may be beneficial in anthrax, *Listeria* infections, and actinomycosis. They have also been used in conjunction with quinine sulfate for chloroquine-resistant *Plasmodium falciparum* malaria and as an intracavitary injection to control pleural or pericardial effusions caused by metastatic carcinoma. As an adjunct to amebicides in acute intestinal amebiasis. Used orally to treat uncomplicated endocervical, rectal, or urethral *Chlamydia* infections.

Topical uses include skin granulomas caused by *Mycobacterium marinum;* ophthalmic bacterial infections causing blepharitis, conjunctivitis, or keratitis; and as an adjunct in the treatment of ophthalmic chlamydial infections such as trachoma or inclusion conjunctivitis. Tetracyclines are used as an alternative to silver nitrate for prophylaxis of neonatal gonococcal ophthalmia. Vaginitis. Severe acne.

Contraindications: Hypersensitivity; avoid drug during tooth development stage (last trimester of pregnancy, neonatal period, during breast feeding, and during childhood up to 8 years), because tetracyclines interfere with enamel formation and dental pigmentation. Never administer intrathecally.

Special Concerns: Use with caution and at reduced dosage in patients with impaired kidney function.

Side Effects: *GI* (most common): Nausea, vomiting, thirst, diarrhea, anorexia, sore throat, flatulence, epigastric distress, bulky loose stools. Less commonly, stomatitis, dysphagia, black hairy tongue, glossitis, or inflammatory lesions of the anogenital area. Rarely, pseudomembranous colitis. Oral dosage forms may cause esophageal ulcers, especially in patients with esophageal obstructive element or hiatal hernia. *Allergic* (rare): Urticaria, pericarditis, polyarthralgia, fever, rash, pulmonary infiltrates with eosinophilia, angioneurotic edema, worsening of systemic lupus erythematosus, anaphylaxis, purpura. *Skin:* Photosensitivity, maculopapular and erythematous rashes, exfoliative dermatitis (rare), onycholysis, discoloration of nails. *CNS:* Dizziness, lightheadedness, unsteadiness, paresthesias. *Hematologic:* Eosinophilia, hemolytic anemia, neutropenia, thrombocytopenia, thrombocytopenic purpura. *Hepatic:* Fatty liver, increases in liver enzymes; rarely, hepatotoxicity, hepatitis, hepatic cholestasis. *Miscellaneous:* Candidal superinfections including oral and vaginal candidiasis, discoloration of infants' and children's teeth, bone lesions, delayed bone growth, abnormal pigmentation of the conjunctiva, pseudotumor cerebri in adults and bulging fontanels in infants.

IV administration may cause thrombophlebitis; IM injections are painful and may cause induration at the injection site.

The administration of deteriorated tetracyclines may result in Fanconi-like syndrome characterized by nausea, vomiting, acidosis, proteinuria, glycosuria, aminoaciduria, polydipsia, polyuria, hypokalemia.

Drug Interactions

Aluminum salts	↓ Effect of tetracyclines due to ↓ absorption from GI tract
Antacids, oral	↓ Effect of tetracyclines due to ↓ absorption from GI tract
Anticoagulants, oral	IV tetracyclines ↑ hypoprothrombinemia
Bismuth salts	↓ Effect of tetracyclines due to ↓ absorption from GI tract
Bumetanide	↑ Risk of kidney toxicity
Calcium salts	↓ Effect of tetracyclines due to ↓ absorption from GI tract
Cimetidine	↓ Effect of tetracyclines due to ↓ absorption from GI tract
Contraceptives, oral	↓ Effect of oral contraceptives
Digoxin	Tetracyclines ↑ bioavailability of digoxin
Diuretics, thiazide	↑ Risk of kidney toxicity
Ethacrynic acid	↑ Risk of kidney toxicity
Furosemide	↑ Risk of kidney toxicity
Insulin	Tetracyclines may ↓ insulin requirement
Iron preparations	↓ Effect of tetracyclines due to ↓ absorption from GI tract
Lithium	Either ↑ or ↓ levels of lithium
Magnesium salts	↓ Effect of tetracyclines due to ↓ absorption from GI tract
Methoxyflurane	↑ Risk of kidney toxicity
Penicillins	Tetracyclines may mask bactericidal effect of penicillins
Sodium bicarbonate	↓ Effect of tetracyclines due to ↓ absorption from GI tract
Zinc salts	↓ Effect of tetracyclines due to ↓ absorption from GI tract

Laboratory Test Interferences: False + or ↑ urinary catecholamines and urinary protein (degraded); ↑ coagulation time. False − or ↓ urinary urobilinogen, glucose tests (see *Nursing Considerations*). Prolonged use or high doses may change liver function tests and WBC counts.

Dosage: See individual drugs and Table 4.

Table 4   Tetracyclines

Drug	Dosage	Remarks
Chlortetracycline hydrochloride (Aureomycin Ophthalmic Ointment, Aureomycin Topical Ointment) (Rx: Ophthalmic, OTC: Topical.)	**Ophthalmic:** *Acute infections*, ½-inch ribbon in conjuctival sac q 2–4 hr or more frequently until improvement occurs. *Mild to moderate infections*: ½-inch ribbon in conjunctival sac b.i.d.–t.i.d. **Topical, 3%:** Apply to affected area 1–5 times daily.	
Demeclocycline hydrochloride (Declomycin) (Rx)	**PO. Adults:** 150 mg q.i.d. or 300 mg b.i.d. **Children over 8 years:** 3.3–6.6 mg/kg q 12 hr or 1.65–3.3 mg/kg q 6 hr. *Gonorrhea:* **Initial,** 600 mg; **then,** 300 mg q 12 hr for 4 days to a total of 3 g. *SIADH Syndrome:* 3.25–3.72 mg/kg q 6 hr.	**t½:** 10–16 hr; 40%–50% excreted unchanged in urine. Causes photosensitivity more frequently than other tetracyclines. May cause increased pigmentation of skin. Antihistamines and corticosteroids may be useful in treatment of hypersensitivity. Also used to treat chronic inappropriate ADH secretion. *Additional untoward reactions:* Reversible diabetes insipidus syndrome.
Meclocycline sulfosalicylate (Meclan) (Rx)	**Topical use only.** Apply 1% cream to affected areas b.i.d. in AM and PM.	*Use:* Acne vulgaris. *Pregnancy category:* B. *Untoward reactions:* Stinging, burning, yellowing of skin. Rarely, contact dermatitis. *Administration:* To avoid staining of fabrics, do not use excessive amounts. *Additional Nursing Considerations:* 1. Check for history of hypersensitivity. 2. *Teach client:* a. not to allow medication to enter eyes, nose or mouth. b. that stinging or burning after medication is transient. c. that yellow tinge to skin may be removed by washing. d. that cosmetics may be used. e. that fluorescence of treated areas under ultraviolet light may occur.

Table 4   *(continued)*

Drug	Dosage	Remarks
Methacycline hydrochloride (Rondomycin) (Rx)	**PO. Adults:** 150 mg q.i.d. or 300 mg b.i.d. *Severe infections:* **initial,** 300 mg; **then,** 150 mg q 6 hr or 300 mg q 12 hr. **Children over 8 years:** 6–12 mg/kg daily in 2–4 doses. *Gonorrhea:* **initially,** 900 mg; **then,** 300 mg q.i.d. for a total of 5.4 g. *Syphilis:* 18–24 g in divided doses over 10–15 days. *Eaton agent (PPLO) pneumonia:* 900 mg daily for 6 days.	**t½:** 10–16 hr. 40%–50% excreted unchanged in the urine.
Tetracycline hydrochloride and amphotericin B (Mysteclin-F) (Rx)	**PO.** See *Tetracycline.*	**Use:** Candidal infections. See also *Amphotericin B,* p. 179

NURSING CONSIDERATIONS

See also *General Nursing Considerations For All Anti-Infectives* under *Penicillins,* p. 140.

Administration/Storage

1. Do not use outdated or deteriorated drugs, as a Fanconi-like syndrome may occur (see *Side Effects*).
2. Discard unused capsules to prevent use of deteriorated medication.
3. Administer IM into large muscle mass to avoid extravasation into subcutaneous or fatty tissue.
4. Administer on an empty stomach at least 1 hr before or 2 hr after meals. Withhold antacids, iron salts, dairy foods, and other foods high in calcium for at least 2 hr after PO administration. Do not administer milk with tetracyclines.

Assessment

1. Note any evidence of impaired kidney function.
2. Determine if client has any history of colitis or other bowel problems.
3. If the client is female and pregnant, determine what trimester she is in.

Intervention

1. If client experiences gastric distress following administration of medication, report to physician. Suggest that the client be permitted to have a light meal with the medication to reduce distress. An alternative would be to reduce the individual dose of the medication but increase the frequency of administration.
2. Maintain adequate intake and output, because renal dysfunction may result in drug accumulation, leading to toxicity.

3. Prevent or treat pruritus ani by cleansing the anal area with water several times a day and/or after each bowel movement.

4. If GI disturbances occur, avoid antacids that contain calcium, magnesium, or aluminum.

Client/Family Teaching

1. Avoid direct or artificial sunlight, which can cause a severe sunburn-like reaction, and to report erythema if it occurs.

2. Zinc tablets or vitamin preparations containing zinc may interfere with absorption of tetracyclines.

3. Advise clients not to take tetracyclines with milk, cheese, ice cream, or other foods containing calcium. If dose is taken with meals, avoid these foods for 2 hr after the meal.

4. Tetracyclines interfere with formation of tooth enamel and dental pigmentation from pregnancy through age 8.

5. How to prevent or treat pruritus ani by cleansing the anal area with water several times a day and/or after each bowel movement.

Evaluation

Evaluate

- client with impaired kidney function for increased BUN, acidosis, anorexia, nausea, vomiting, weight loss, and dehydration. Continue assessment after cessation of therapy, because symptoms may appear later.
- client on IV therapy for nausea, vomiting, chills, fever, and hypertension resulting from too rapid administration or an excessively high dose. Slow rate of IV infusion and report if symptoms occur.
- infant for bulging fontanelle, which may be caused by a too rapid rate of IV infusion. Slow IV infusion rate and report.
- client with impaired hepatic or renal function for impairment of consciousness or other CNS disturbances.
- for symptoms of enterocolitis, such as diarrhea, pyrexia, abdominal distention, and scanty urine. These symptoms may necessitate discontinuing drug and substituting another antibiotic.
- for indications of an untoward reaction: sore throat, dysphagia, fever, dizziness, hoarseness, and inflammation of mucous membranes of the body.
- for onycholysis (loosening or detachment of the nail from the nail bed).

DOXYCYCLINE CALCIUM   (dox-ih-**SYE**-kleen)
Vibramycin (Rx)

DOXYCYCLINE HYCLATE   (dox-ih-**SYE**-kleen)
Apo-Doxy✿, Doryx, Doxy 100 and 200, Doxy-Caps, Doxychel Hyclate, Vibramycin, Vibramycin IV, Vibra-Tabs, Vivox (Rx)

DOXYCYCLINE MONOHYDRATE   (dox-ih-**SYE**-kleen)
Vibramycin (Rx)

See also *Anti-Infectives*, p. 71 and *Tetracyclines*, p. 169.

Classification: Antibiotic, tetracycline.

Action/Kinetics: More slowly absorbed, and thus more persistent, than other tetracyclines. Preferred for patients with impaired renal function for treating infections outside the urinary tract. From 80%–95% is bound to serum proteins. $t^{1/2}$: 14.5–22 hr; 30%–40% excreted unchanged in urine.

Additional Uses: Orally for uncomplicated gonococcal infections in adults (except anorectal infections in males); acute epididymo-orchitis caused by *N. gonorrhoeae* and *C. trachomatis;* gonococcal arthritis-dermatitis syndrome; nongonococcal urethritis caused by *C. trachomatis* and *Ureaplasma urealyticum.*

Special Concerns: Safety for IV use in children less than 8 years of age has not been established.

Additional Drug Interaction: Carbamazepine, phenytoin, and barbiturates ↓ effect of doxycycline by ↑ breakdown of doxycycline by the liver.

Dosage: Capsules, Delayed-release Capsules, Oral Suspension, Tablets IV. Adult: First day, 100 mg q 12 hr; **maintenance:** 100–200 mg daily, depending on severity of infection. **Children, over 8 years (45 kg or less): First day,** 4.4 mg/kg in 1–2 doses; **then,** 2.2–4.4 mg/kg daily in divided doses depending on severity of infection. Children over 45 kg should receive the adult dose. **PO.** *Acute gonorrhea:* 200 mg at once; **then,** 100 mg h.s. (at bedtime) on first day, followed by 100 mg b.i.d. for 3 days. Alternatively, 300 mg immediately followed in 1 hr with 300 mg. *Syphilis (primary/secondary):* 300 mg daily in divided doses for 10 days. *Chlamydia trachomatis infections:* 100 mg b.i.d. for minimum of 7 days. *Prophylaxis of "traveler's diarrhea":* 100 mg daily.

IV. *Endometritis, parametritis, peritonitis, salpingitis:* 100 mg b.i.d. with 2 g cefoxitin, IV, q.i.d. continued for at least 4 days or 2 days after improvement observed. This is followed by doxycycline, PO, 100 mg b.i.d. for 10–14 days of total therapy.

Note: The Centers for Disease Control have established treatment schedules for sexually transmitted diseases.

NURSING CONSIDERATIONS

See *Nursing Considerations* for *Tetracyclines,* p. 173, and *General Nursing Considerations For All Anti-Infectives* under *Penicillins,* p. 140.

Administration/Storage

1. Powder for suspension has expiration date of 12 months from date of issue.
2. Solution stable for 2 weeks when stored in refrigerator.
3. Follow directions on vial for dilution. Concentrations should be no lower than 0.1 mg/mL and no higher than 1.0 mg/mL.
4. During infusion protect solution from light.
5. Complete administration of solutions diluted with NaCl injection, D_5W, Ringer's injection, and 10% invert sugar within 12 hr.
6. Complete administration of solutions diluted with lactated Ringer's injection or 5% dextrose in lactated Ringer's injection within 6 hr.

MINOCYCLINE HYDROCHLORIDE (mih-no-**SYE**-kleen)

Minocin, Minocin IV (Rx)

See also *Anti-Infectives,* p. 71, and *Tetracyclines,* p. 169.

Classification: Antibiotic, tetracycline.

Action/Kinetics: t½: 11–20 hr. From 5% to 10% excreted unchanged in the urine. From 70%–80% is bound to serum proteins. Absorption less affected by milk or food than for other tetracyclines.

Additional Use: PO. Treat asymptomatic carriers of *Neisseria meningitidis. Mycobacterium marinum* infections. Treatment of uncomplicated endocervical, rectal, or urethral infections caused by *U. urealyticum.* Uncomplicated gonococcal urethritis in males due to *N. gonorrhoeae. Investigational:* Nocardiosis as an alternative to sulfonamides.

Additional Side Effects: Blue-gray pigmentation areas of cutaneous inflammation; vertigo, ataxia, drowsiness, Stevens-Johnson syndrome (rare).

Dosage: Capsules, Oral Suspension, Tablets, IV, adults: initially, 200 mg; **then,** 100 mg q 12 hr or 50 mg q.i.d., not to exceed 400 mg daily. **Pediatric, over 8 years: Initially,** 4 mg/kg; **then,** 2 mg/kg q 12 hr. *Meningococcal carrier state:* 100 mg b.i.d. for 5 days. *Mycobacterium marinum infections:* 100 mg b.i.d. for 6–8 weeks. *GU or rectal Chlamydia trachomatis or Ureaplasma urealyticum infections:* 100 mg b.i.d. for a minimum of 7 days. *Gonococcal urethritis in males:* 100 mg b.i.d. for 5 days. *Gonorrhea, patients sensitive to penicillin:* **Initially,** 200 mg; **then,** 100 mg b.i.d. for at least 4 days, with cultures taken 2–3 days after therapy.

NURSING CONSIDERATIONS

See also *Nursing Considerations* for *Tetracyclines,* p. 173, and *General Nursing Considerations* For *All Anti-Infectives* under *Penicillins,* p. 140.

Administration/Storage

1. When used for syphilis, the drug should be given for at least 10–15 days.
2. Do not dissolve parenteral drug in solutions containing calcium because a precipitate may form.
3. After dissolving medication in vial, it should be further diluted to 500–1,000 mL with any of the following: dextrose injection, dextrose and sodium chloride injection, sodium chloride injection, Ringer's injection, lactated Ringer's injection.
4. Start administration of final dilution immediately.
5. Discard reconstituted solution after 24 hr at room temperature.

Client/Family Teaching

1. Sexual partners should use condoms during therapy, should be medically evaluated, and should have cultures taken.
2. Drug may impair mental alertness.
3. Take medication as ordered and report any bothersome side effects to physician.

OXYTETRACYCLINE   (ox-ee-teh-trah-**SYE**-kleen)

Terramycin IM (Rx)

OXYTETRACYCLINE HYDROCHLORIDE   (ox-ee-**teh**-trah-**SYE**-kleen)

E.P. Mycin, Terramycin, Uri-Tet (Rx)

See also *Anti-Infectives,* p. 71, and *Tetracyclines,* p. 169.

Classification: Antibiotic, tetracycline.

Action/Kinetics: t½: 6–12 hr. 70% excreted unchanged in urine. From 20% to 40% bound to serum proteins.

Dosage: Capsules, Tablets. See oral dosage for tetracycline hydrochloride. **IM. Adults, usual,** 250 mg once daily or 300 mg daily in divided doses q 8–12 hr. Up to 800 mg daily may be used. **Children over 8 years:** 15–25 mg/kg up to maximum of 250 mg in single daily injection or divided and given q 8–12 hr. **IV infusion. Adults:** 250–500 mg (as the base) q 12 hr up to 2 g daily. **Children 8 years of age and older:** 5–10 mg (as the base)/kg q 12 hr.

NURSING CONSIDERATIONS

See *Nursing Considerations* for *Tetracyclines,* p. 173, and *General Nursing Considerations* for *All Anti-Infectives* under *Penicillins,* p. 140.

Administration/Storage

1. Do not give with food or antacids.
2. Pediatric dosage should not be administered with milk or calcium-containing foods.
3. Check dilutions for IV administration.

TETRACYCLINE   (teh-trah-**SYE**-kleen)

Achromycin Ophthalmic (Rx)

TETRACYCLINE HYDROCHLORIDE   (teh-trah-**SYE**-kleen)

Achromycin IM and IV, Achromycin V, Ala-Tet, Apo-Tetra✳, Neo-Tetrine✳, Nor-Tet, Novo-Tetra✳, Panmycin, Robitet, Robicaps, Sumycin 250 and 500, Sumycin Syrup, Teline, Teline-500, Tetracap, Tetralan-250 and -500, Tetralan Syrup, Tetram (Rx)

See also *General Information* on *Tetracyclines,* p. 169.

Classification: Antibiotic, tetracycline.

Action/Kinetics: t½: 7–11 hr. From 40% to 70% excreted unchanged in urine; 65% bound to serum proteins. Dosage is always expressed as the hydrochloride salt.

Additional Uses: Ophthalmic infections, prophylaxis of *Neisseria gonorrhoeae* or *Chlamydia trachomatis* in newborns. **Topical:** Acne vulgaris, prophylaxis or treatment of infection following skin abrasions. *Investigational:* Pleural sclerosing agent in malignant pleural effusions (administered by chest tube); in combination with gentamicin for *V. vulnificus* infections due to wound infection after trauma or by eating contaminated seafood. Mouthwash (use suspension) to treat nonspecific mouth ulcerations, canker sores, aphthous ulcers. Possible drug of choice for stage I Lyme disease.

Dosage: Capsules, Tablets. Adults: usual, *mild to moderate infections:* 500 mg b.i.d. or 250 mg q.i.d.; *severe infections:* 500 mg q.i.d. **Children over 8 years:** 25–50 mg/kg daily in 4 equal doses. *Brucellosis:* 500 mg q.i.d. for 3 weeks with 1 g streptomycin IM b.i.d. for first week and once daily the second week. *Syphilis:* Total of 30–40 g over 10–15 days. *Gonorrhea:* **initially,** 1.5 g; **then,** 500 mg q 6 hr until 9 g has been given. *Gonorrhea sensitive to penicillin:* **initially,** 1.5 g; **then,** 500 mg q 6 hr for 4 days (total: 9 g). *GU or rectal Chlamydia trachomatis infections:* 500 mg q.i.d. for minimum of 7 days. *Severe acne:* **initially,** 1 g daily; **then,** 125–500 mg daily (long-term). **Note:** The Center for Disease Control has established treatment schedules for sexually transmitted diseases.

IM. Adults: usual, 250 mg once daily or 300 mg/day in divided doses q 8–12 hr. Up to 800 mg daily may be used. **Children over 8 years:** 15–25 mg/kg up to maximum of 250 mg in single daily injection. The dose may be divided and given q 8–12 hr.

IV. Adults: 250–500 mg q 12 hr, not to exceed 500 mg q 6 hr. **Children over 8 years:** 12 mg/kg/day in 2 divided doses. Up to 20 mg/kg/day may be given if the disease is severe.

Ophthalmic. *Suspension. Acute infections:* **initially,** 1–2 gtt q 15–30 min; **then,** as infection improves, decrease frequency. *Moderate infections:* 1–2 gtt q 4 hr. *Trachoma:* 2 gtt in each eye b.i.d.–q.i.d. for up to 2 or more months (oral tetracycline may be given concomitantly). *Ointment. Acute infections:* ½ inch q 3–4 hr until improvement noted. *Mild to moderate infections:* ½ inch b.i.d.–t.i.d.

Topical. *Acne:* Apply topical solution to affected areas in the morning and at night, making sure that skin is completely wet after each application. *Infections:* Apply ointment to affected areas 1–5 times daily.

NURSING CONSIDERATIONS

See *Nursing Considerations* for *Tetracyclines,* p. 173, and *General Nursing Considerations For All Anti-Infectives* under *Penicillins,* p. 140.

Administration/Storage

1. To reconstitute solutions for IV use, vials containing 250 or 500 mg should be diluted with 5 or 10 mL, respectively, of sterile water for injection. Further dilution (100–1,000 mL) can be done with sodium chloride injection, 5% dextrose injection, 5% dextrose and sodium chloride, Ringer's injection, and lactated Ringer's injection.

2. Except for Ringer's and lactated Ringer's injections, calcium-containing solutions should not be used to dilute tetracycline HCl.

3. For IM administration, inject into a large muscle mass.

Client/Family Teaching

Transient blurring of vision or stinging may occur when tetracycline is instilled into the eye.

Antifungal Agents

General Statement: Several types of fungi or yeasts are pathogenic for humans. Fungal infections may be systemic; limited to the skin, hair, or nails; or infect moist mucous membranes, including the GI tract and vagina. *Candida* organisms belong to this last group. Drug therapy depends both on the infectious agent and on the type of infection. An accurate diagnosis of the infection, before therapy, is most important for the choice of the therapeutic agents. As in other infections, it is important that drug therapy be continued until the infectious agent has been completely eradicated to avoid the emergence of resistant strains.

10

AMPHOTERICIN B   (am-foe-TEH-rih-sin)

Fungizone, Fungizone IV (Rx)

See also *Anti-Infectives,* p. 71.

Classification: Antibiotic, antifungal.

Action/Kinetics: This antibiotic is produced by *Streptomyces nodosus* and is the drug of choice for deep infections. Amphotericin B binds to specific chemical structures—sterols—of the fungal cellular membrane, increasing cellular permeability and promoting loss of potassium and other substances. Depending on the dose, amphotericin B is fungistatic or fungicidal. Amphotericin B is poorly absorbed from the GI tract although it can be administered IV, used intrathecally, and used topically. It is highly bound to serum protein (90%). **Peak plasma levels:** 2–4 mcg/mL; **t½:** 24 hr. Slowly excreted by kidneys.

Uses: The drug is toxic and should be used only for patients under close medical supervision with a relatively certain diagnosis of deep mycotic infections. IV administration is usually reserved for life-threatening disease. Disseminated North American blastomycosis, cryptococcosis, and other systemic fungal infections, including coccidioidomycosis, paracoccidioidomycosis, histoplasmosis, aspergillosis, disseminated candidiasis, and monilial overgrowth resulting from oral antibiotic therapy. Topical: cutaneous and mucocutaneous infections of *Candida (Monilia)* infections.

Contraindications: Hypersensitivity to drug.

Special Concerns: Pregnancy category: B. The bone-marrow depressant effects may result in increased incidence of microbial infection, delayed healing, and gingival bleeding.

Side Effects: After topical use. Irritation, pruritus, dry skin. **After systemic use.** *GI:* Nausea, vomiting, diarrhea, dyspepsia, anorexia, abdominal cramps, melena, gastroenteritis. *CNS:* Fever, chills, headache, malaise, vertigo, seizures (rare). *CV:* Thrombophlebitis, phlebitis. Rarely, arrhythmias, hyper- or hypotension, ventricular fibrillation, cardiac arrest. *Renal:* Anuria, oliguria, azotemia, hypokalemia, renal tubular acidosis, nephrocalcinosis, hyposthenuria. *Hematologic:* Anemia, thrombocytopenia, leukopenia, agranulocytosis, eosinophilia, leukocytosis. *Miscellaneous:* Muscle and joint pain, weight loss, tinnitus, blurred or double vision, peripheral neuropathy, hearing loss, hepatic failure, pruritus, rashes, flushing, anaphylaxis.

Drug Interactions	
Aminoglycosides	Additive nephrotoxicity and/or ototoxicity
Corticosteroids, Corticotropin	↑ K depletion caused by amphotericin B
Digitalis glycosides	↑ K depletion caused by amphotericin B; ↑ Incidence of digitalis toxicity
Flucytosine	Synergistic antifungal effect
Miconazole	Amphotericin B ↓ effect of miconazole
Rifampin	Synergistic antifungal effect
Skeletal muscle relaxants, surgical *(e.g., succinylcholine, d-tubocurarine)*	↑ Muscle relaxation
Tetracyclines	Synergistic antifungal effect

Laboratory Test Interferences: ↑ SGPT, SGOT, alkaline phosphatase, creatinine, BUN, NPN, BSP retention values.

Dosage: Slow IV infusion, initially: 0.25 mg/kg/day. May be increased gradually by 0.1–0.2 mg/kg/day, up to a maximum dose of 1.0 mg/kg/day to 1.5 mg/kg every other day. A test dose (1 mg) should be given first to assess patient tolerance. Depending on use, treatment may be required for several months. **Topical (lotion, cream, ointment—each 3%):** apply liberally to affected areas b.i.d.–q.i.d. Depending on the type of lesion, up to 4 weeks of therapy may be necessary.

NURSING CONSIDERATIONS

See also *General Nursing Considerations For All Anti-Infectives* under *Penicillins,* p. 140.

Administration/Storage

1. Follow directions on vial for dilution. Use only distilled water without a bacteriostatic agent or 5% dextrose as diluent in order to avoid precipitation of drug.
2. Strict aseptic technique must be used in preparation, as there is no bacteriostatic agent in the medication.
3. Use a sterile 20 gauge needle every time entrance is made into the vial.
4. Do not use saline solution or distilled water with bacteriostatic agent as a diluent, since a precipitate may result.
5. Do not use the initial concentrate if there is any precipitate.
6. An in-line membrane filter with a pore diameter of 1 micron may be used.

7. Protect from light during administration and storage.

8. Minimize local inflammation and danger of thrombophlebitis by administering the solution below the recommended dilution of 0.1 mg.

9. Initiate therapy in the most distal veins.

10. Have on hand 200–400 units of heparin sodium, since it may be ordered for the infusion to prevent thrombophlebitis.

11. Administer IV for 6 hr.

12. Amphotericin may be stored after reconstitution for 24 hr in a dark room or in a refrigerator for 1 week without significant loss of potency.

13. Use dilutions of 0.1 mg/mL immediately after preparation.

14. Rub creams and lotions into lesion.

Assessment

1. Assess for any history of adverse reactions and hypersensitivity to any anti-infectives or drugs in the antifungal category.

2. During nursing and drug history, assess mental status and note client age.

Interventions

1. Ascertain if the physician wants the client to receive antipyretics, antihistamines, and/ or antiemetic drugs during therapy to reduce side effects.

2. Infuse IV slowly and interrupt if client develops any adverse reactions and notify physician.

3. Monitor vital signs frequently during IV administration.

4. Monitor intake and output. Report a reduction in output and blood sediment or cloudiness in the urine.

5. Weigh client twice weekly as a means of determining signs of possible malnutrition or dehydration.

6. Anticipate hypokalemia in clients concomitantly taking digoxin. Observe for toxicity, muscle weakness and monitor serum digoxin levels.

Client/Family Teaching

1. Any incidents of anorexia, nausea, vomiting, headache or chills should be reported.

2. Stress the importance of reporting any decrease in intake and output.

3. Amphotericin therapy usually requires 6–10 weeks to assure an adequate response and to prevent any relapse.

4. If diarrhea develops, try small frequent meals. GI effects may be reduced by administering an antihistamine or antiemetic before drug therapy and by administering the drug before mealtime.

5. Neurological symptoms such as tinnitus, blurred vision or vertigo should be reported immediately.

6. For therapy with creams and lotions:
   - drug does not stain skin when it is rubbed into lesion.
   - any discoloration of fabric caused by cream or lotion may be removed by washing with soap and water.
   - any discoloration of clothing caused by ointment may be removed with a standard cleaning fluid.
   - report any increased itching, burning, or rash at site of local application.

Evaluation

1. Note any alteration in renal function as well as cloudiness or bloody sediment in the urine.
2. Intrathecal administration of amphotericin may cause inflammation of the spinal roots, assess for sensory loss or foot drop in these clients.
3. Assess client/family knowledge and understanding of illness, response to therapy and to teaching.

BUTOCONAZOLE NITRATE   (byou-toe-**KON**-ah-zohl)

Femstat (Rx)

Classification: Antifungal agent.

Action/Kinetics: By permeating chitin in the fungal cell wall, butoconazole increases membrane permeability to intracellular substances, leading to reduced osmotic resistance and viability of the fungus. Approximately 5.5% of drug is absorbed following vaginal administration.

Uses: Vulvovaginal fungal infections caused by *Candida* species.

Contraindications: Use during first trimester of pregnancy.

Special Concerns: Pregnancy category: C (safe use in pregnancy has not been established). Pediatric dosage has not been established. Use with caution during lactation.

Side Effects: *GU:* Vaginal burning, vulvar burning or itching, discharge; soreness, swelling, and itching of the fingers.

Dosage: Vaginal cream. *During pregnancy, second and third trimesters only:* One applicatorful (about 5 g) of the cream intravaginally at bedtime for 6 days. *Nonpregnant:* One applicatorful (about 5 g) intravaginally at bedtime for 3 days (if necessary, may be used for up to 6 days).

NURSING CONSIDERATIONS

Administration/Storage

1. During pregnancy, use of a vaginal applicator may be contraindicated.
2. If there is no response, studies should be repeated to confirm the diagnosis before reinstituting antifungal therapy.

Interventions

1. Determine if client is pregnant.
2. Obtain appropriate lab studies prior to initiating therapy.

Client/Family Teaching

Teach client and/or family

- the appropriate technique for medication administration.
- to continue therapy for prescribed regimen and during menstruation.
- to insert cream high into the vagina.
- to call the physician if irritation or burning occurs.
- that the use of sanitary napkins may prevent soiling and staining of undergarments and clothing.

- that in order to prevent reinfection, the sexual partner should use a condom during intercourse.

Evaluation

Note status (presence/absence) of pretreatment symptoms as well as client's subjective response.

CICLOPIROX OLAMINE   (sye-kloh-**PEER**-ox **OH**-lah-meen)

Loprox (Rx)

Classification: Antifungal, topical.

Action/Kinetics: This broad-spectrum fungicide is effective against dermatophytes, yeast, *Malassezia furfur, Trichophyton rubrum, T. mentagrophytes, Epidermophyton floccosum, Microsporum canis,* and *Candida albicans*. At lower concentrations the drug blocks the transport of amino acids into the cell, whereas at higher concentrations the cell membrane of the fungus is altered so that intracellular material leaks out. The drug may also inhibit synthesis of RNA, DNA, and protein in growing fungal cells. A small amount of drug is absorbed through the skin; it also penetrates to the sebaceous glands and dermis as well as into the hair.

Uses: Tinea pedis, tinea corporis, tinea cruris, tinea versicolor, candidiasis.

Special Concerns: Safety and efficacy in pregnancy (category: B), in lactation, and in children under 10 years of age not established.

Side Effects: *Dermatologic:* Irritation, redness, burning, pain, skin sensitivity.

Dosage: Topical cream. Massage gently into the affected area and surrounding skin morning and evening. If no improvement after 4 weeks, diagnosis should be reevaluated.

NURSING CONSIDERATIONS

Assessment

If drug is used for suspected *Malassezia furfur* infection, assist with establishing diagnosis by describing lesions and obtaining scraping of lesion because a technique for culture of organism does not exist.

Client/Family Teaching

1. The skin should be cleansed with soap and water and dried thoroughly.
2. Occlusive dressings or wrappings should not be used. Also, that adult incontinence pads are an occlusive dressing and should not be used during therapy.
3. Even though symptoms have improved, the drug should be used for the full prescribed time.
4. Shoes and socks should be changed at least once daily. Shoes should be well-fitted and ventilated.
5. Notify care provider if the area of application shows evidence of blistering, burning, itching, oozing, redness or swelling.

Evaluation

Observe infected area for response to treatment.

CLOTRIMAZOLE   (kloh-**TRIM**-ah-zohl)

Canesten✿, Canestin 1✿, Canestin 3✿, Gyne-Lotrimin, Lotrimin, Mycelex, Mycelex-G, Myclo✿ (Rx)

See also *Anti-Infectives,* p. 71.

Classification: Antifungal.

Action/Kinetics: Depending on concentration, this drug may be fungistatic or fungicidal. The drug acts by inhibiting the biosynthesis of sterols resulting in damage to the cell wall and subsequent loss of essential intracellular elements due to altered permeability. Clotrimazole may also inhibit oxidative and peroxidative enzyme activity and inhibit the biosynthesis of triglycerides and phospholipids by fungi. When used for *Candida albicans,* the drug inhibits transformation of blastophores into the invasive mycelial form. It is poorly absorbed from the GI tract and metabolized in the liver to inactive compounds that are excreted through the feces. **Duration:** up to 3 hr.

Uses: Broad-spectrum antifungal effective against *Malassezia furfur, Trichophyton rubrum, T. mentagrophytes, Epidermophyton floccosum, Microsporum canis, Candida albicans.* Used to treat tinea pedis, tinea cruris, tinea corporis, tinea versicolor, and vulvovaginal and oropharyngeal candidiasis.

Contraindications: Hypersensitivity. First trimester of pregnancy.

Special Concerns: Pregnancy category: C for systemic use and B for topical/vaginal use.

Side Effects: *Skin:* Irritation including rash, stinging, pruritus, urticaria, erythema, peeling, blistering, edema. *Vaginal:* Lower abdominal cramps; urinary frequency; bloating; vaginal irritation, itching or burning; dyspareunia. *Hepatic:* Abnormal liver function tests. *GI:* Nausea and vomiting following use of troche.

Dosage: Troche: One troche 5 times daily for 14 consecutive days. **Topical Cream, Lotion, Solution:** Massage into affected skin and surrounding areas b.i.d. in morning and afternoon. Diagnosis should be reevaluated if no improvement occurs in 4 weeks. **Vaginal tablets:** One 100-mg tablet/day at bedtime for 7 days or two 100-mg tablets at bedtime for 3 days. One 500-mg tablet can be inserted once at bedtime. **Vaginal cream:** 5 g (one applicatorful)/day at bedtime for 7–14 consecutive days.

NURSING CONSIDERATIONS

See also *General Nursing Considerations For All Anti-Infectives* under *Penicillins,* p. 140.

Administration/Storage

1. Mycelex-G vaginal cream can be stored between 2° to 30° C (36°–86° F). Mycelex-G, 100-mg vaginal tablets should not be stored above 35° C (95° F), while the 500 mg vaginal tablets should be stored below 30° C (86° F).
2. The troche should be slowly dissolved in the mouth.

Client/family teaching

1. Review goals of therapy and appropriate method for administration.
2. Unless directed by physician to do otherwise, apply after cleaning the affected area.
3. If treating vaginal infections, the client should not engage in intercourse; or, to prevent infection, the partner should wear a condom.
4. To prevent staining of clothes, a sanitary napkin should be used with vaginal tablets or cream.

ECONAZOLE NITRATE   (ee-**KON**-ah-zole)

Ecostatin ✽, Spectazole (Rx)

Classification: Antifungal, topical.

Action/Kinetics: This drug may be fungistatic or fungicidal, depending on concentration. The drug inhibits the synthesis of sterols that damage the cell membrane and increases the permeability, resulting in a loss of essential intracellular elements. It may also inhibit biosynthesis of triglycerides and phospholipids and inhibit oxidative and peroxidative enzyme activity. Effective concentrations are found in the stratum corneum, epidermis, and the dermis. Systemic absorption is low.

Uses: Broad-spectrum fungicide effective against *Microsporum audouinii, M. canis, M. gypseum, Epidermophyton floccosum, Trichophyton mentagrophytes, T. rubrum, T. tonsurans, Candida albicans, Pityrosporum orbiculare,* and some gram-positive bacteria. Used to treat tinea cruris, tinea corporis, tinea pedis, tinea versicolor, cutaneous candidiasis.

Special Concerns: Pregnancy category: C. Use with caution in pregnancy and lactation.

Side Effects: *Topical:* Burning, erythema, itching, stinging.

Dosage: Topical cream. Except for tinea versicolor, apply sufficient cream to cover the affected areas in the morning and evening. *Tinea versicolor:* Apply once daily. If no improvement is noted after recommended treatment period, diagnosis should be reevaluated.

NURSING CONSIDERATIONS

See also *General Nursing Considerations For All Anti-Infectives* under *Penicillins,* p. 140.

Client/Family Teaching

1. Review goals of therapy and the appropriate method for drug administration.
2. The skin should be cleansed with soap and water and dried thoroughly. Unless otherwise directed, cream should be applied after cleaning the affected area.
3. For athlete's foot, the shoes and socks should be changed at least once daily. Shoes should be well-fitted and ventilated.
4. To reduce chance of reinfection, tinea pedis should be treated for 1 month and tinea cruris, tinea corporis, and candidial infections should be treated for 2 weeks.
5. The drug should be used for the full prescribed time even though symptoms have improved.
6. The physician should be notified if condition worsens or symptoms of burning, itching, redness, and stinging occur.

Evaluation

1. Assess client knowledge and understanding of illness, and their response to treatment and teaching.
2. Evaluate status (presence/absence) of pretreatment symptoms.

FLUCONAZOLE   (flew-**KON**-ah-zohl)

Diflucan (Rx)

Classification: Antifungal agent.

Action/Kinetics: Fluconazole inhibits the enzyme cytochrome P-450, which is essential to survival of fungal cells. Inhibition of the enzyme results in a decrease in cell wall integrity and extrusion of intracellular material. Fluconazole apparently does not affect the cytochrome P-450 enzyme in animals or humans. **Peak plasma levels:** 1–2 hr. **t½:** 30 hr which allows for once daily dosing. The drug penetrates all body fluids at steady-state. Bioavailability is not affected by agents that increase gastric pH. Eighty percent of the drug is excreted unchanged by the kidneys.

Uses: Oropharyngeal and esophageal candidiasis. Serious systemic candidal infection (including urinary tract infections, peritonitis, and pneumonia). Cryptococcal meningitis. Maintenance therapy to prevent cryptococcal meningitis in AIDS patients.

Contraindications: Hypersensitivity to fluconazole.

Special Concerns: Use with caution if patient shows hypersensitivity to other azoles. Use during pregnancy (category: C) only if the potential benefit justifies the potential risk to the fetus. Care should be used when fluconazole is prescribed during lactation. The effectiveness of the drug has not been adequately assessed in children.

Side Effects: *Note:* Side effects are more frequently reported in HIV infected patients than in non-HIV infected patients. *GI:* Nausea, vomiting, abdominal pain, diarrhea. *Miscellaneous:* Headache, skin rash, hepatotoxicity, exfoliative skin disorders.

Laboratory Test Interferences: ↑ AST, serum transaminase (especially if used with isoniazid, oral hypoglycemic agents, phenytoin, rifampin, valproic acid).

Drug Interactions

Cimetidine	↓ Plasma levels of fluconazole
Cyclosporine	Fluconazole may ↑ cyclosporine levels in renal transplant patients with or without impaired renal function
Hydrochlorothiazide	↑ Plasma levels of fluconazole due to ↓ renal clearance
Glipizide	↑ Plasma levels of glipizide due to ↓ breakdown by the liver
Glyburide	↑ Plasma levels of glyburide due to ↓ breakdown by the liver
Phenytoin	Fluconazole ↑ plasma levels of phenytoin
Rifampin	↓ Plasma levels of fluconazole due to ↑ breakdown by the liver
Tolbutamide	↑ Plasma levels of tolbutamide due to ↓ breakdown by the liver
Warfarin	↑ Prothrombin time

Dosage: Tablets, IV, Adults: *Oropharyngeal or esophageal candidiasis:* **first day,** 200 mg; **then,** 100 mg once daily for a minimum of 14 days (for oropharyngeal candidiasis) or 21 days (for esophageal candidiasis). Up to 400 mg daily may be required for esophageal candidiasis. *Systemic candidiasis:* **first day,** 400 mg; **then,** 200 mg daily for at least 28 days. *Acute cryptococcal meningitis:* **first day,** 400 mg; **then,** 200 mg daily (up to 400 mg may be required) for 10–12 weeks after CSF culture is negative. *Maintenance to prevent relapse of cryptococcal meningitis:* 200 mg daily. **Pediatric:** 3–6 mg/kg daily. In patients with renal impairment, an initial loading dose of 50–400 mg can be given; daily dose is based then on creatinine clearance.

NURSING CONSIDERATIONS

Administration/Storage

1. The IV solution should not be used if it is cloudy or precipitated or the seal is not intact.
2. The rate of IV infusion of fluconazole should not exceed 200 mg/hr as a continuous infusion.
3. Supplementary medication should not be added to the IV bag.

Assessment

1. Take a thorough nursing and drug history. Note any history of hypersensitivity to azoles or similar class of drugs.
2. Determine if client is HIV infected, (if possible), as this may place client at an increased risk for possible side effects.

Interventions

1. Due to a long half-life, once daily dosing (either IV or PO) is possible.
2. Obtain baseline liver function studies. Clients who develop abnormal liver function tests should be closely monitored for the development of more serious liver toxicity.
3. Observe immunocompromised clients closely for evidence of a rash; if lesions progress, the drug should be discontinued.

Client/Family Teaching

1. Review goals of therapy and appropriate method and schedule for medication administration.
2. Stress the importance of reporting any rash or persistent side effects to the physician.
3. Remind clients to report for all scheduled lab studies.

Evaluation

1. Review liver function studies and CBC for evidence of untoward drug reactions.
2. Note status of pretreatment symptoms as well as client response to therapy.

FLUCYTOSINE (flew-SYE-toe-seen)

Ancobon, Ancotil ✷ (Rx)

Classification: Antibiotic, antifungal.

Action/Kinetics: Fluoytosine is indicated only for serious systemic fungal infections. The drug is less toxic than amphotericin B. Liver, renal system, and hematopoietic system must be monitored closely.

Flucytosine appears to penetrate the fungal cell membrane and then, after metabolism, to act as an antimetabolite interfering with nucleic acid and protein synthesis. It is well absorbed from GI tract. **Peak plasma concentration:** 2–6 hr. **Therapeutic serum concentration:** 20–25 mcg/mL. **t½:** 3–6 hr, higher in presence of impaired renal function. Ninety percent of drug excreted unchanged in urine.

Uses: Serious systemic infections by susceptible strains of *Candida* (e.g., endocarditis, septicemia, urinary tract infections) or *Cryptococcus* (pulmonary or urinary tract infections, meningitis, septicemia).

Contraindications: Hypersensitivity to drug.

Special Concerns: Use with extreme caution in patients with kidney disease or history of bone marrow depression. Use during pregnancy (category: C), lactation, and during childbearing age only if benefits clearly outweigh risks. The bone-marrow depressant effects may cause an increased incidence of microbial infection, gingival bleeding, and delayed healing.

Side Effects: *GI:* Nausea, vomiting, diarrhea. *Hematologic:* Anemia, leukopenia, thrombocytopenia. *CNS:* Headache, vertigo, drowsiness, sedation, confusion, hallucinations. *Other:* Increase in BUN, creatinine, and liver enzymes.

Drug Interaction: Amphotericin B ↑ effect and toxicity of flucytosine due to kidney impairment.

Dosage: Capsules. Adult and children: 50–150 mg/kg daily in four divided doses. Patients with renal impairment receive lower dosages.

NURSING CONSIDERATIONS

See also *General Nursing Considerations For All Anti-Infectives* under *Penicillins,* p. 140.

Administration/Storage

Reduce or avoid nausea by administering capsules a few at a time over a 15-min period.

Assessment

Obtain baseline CBC and liver and renal function studies and monitor throughout therapy.

Interventions

1. Before administering first dose, check that culture has been taken.
2. Ascertain that weekly cultures are taken to determine that strains have not become resistant. A strain is considered resistant if the minimal inhibitory concentration (MIC) value is greater than 100.
3. Monitor input and output. Report reduction in urine output as well as any blood, sediment, or cloudiness in the urine.
4. Anticipate reduced dose with impaired renal function.
5. Hepatic function should be monitored frequently during therapy.

GRISEOFULVIN MICROSIZE   (grih-see-oh-**FULL**-vin)

Fulvicin-U/F, Grifulvin V, Grisactin Grisovin-FP✳ (Rx)

GRISEOFULVIN ULTRAMICROSIZE   (grih-see-oh-**FULL**-vin)

Fulvicin-P/G, Grisactin Ultra, Gris-PEG (Rx)

See also *Anti-Infectives,* p. 71.

Classification: Antibiotic, antifungal.

Action/Kinetics: Griseofulvin is a natural antibiotic derived from a species of *Penicillium*. It is believed to interfere with cell division (metaphase) or DNA replication. When taken systemically, the drug is deposited in the newly formed skin and nails, which are then resistant to reinfection by the tinea. Griseofulvin is absorbed from the duodenum. **Peak plasma concentration:** 0.37–2 mcg/mL after 4 hr. **t½:** 9–24 hr. Levels may be increased by giving the drug with a high-fat diet.

Uses: Tinea (ringworm) infections of skin including athlete's foot, and infections of the scalp, groin, and nails. It is the only oral drug effective against dermatophytic (tinea ringworm) infections. The drug is not effective against *Candida*. Susceptibility of the infectious agent should be established before treatment is begun.

Contraindications: Pregnancy. Porphyria or history thereof, hepatocellular failure, and hypersensitivity to drug. Exposure to artificial light or sunlight.

Side Effects: *Hypersensitivity:* Rashes, urticaria, angioneurotic edema, allergic reactions. *GI:* Nausea, vomiting, diarrhea, epigastric pain. *CNS:* Dizziness, headache, tiredness, confusion, insomnia. *Miscellaneous:* Oral thrush, acute intermittent porphyria, paresthesias of extremities, proteinuria, leukopenia.

Drug Interactions	
Alcohol, ethyl	Tachycardia and flushing
Anticoagulants, oral	↓ Effect of anticoagulants due to ↑ breakdown in liver
Barbiturates	↓ Effect of griseofulvin due to ↓ absorption from GI tract

Laboratory Test Interferences: ↑ SGPT, SGOT, alkaline phosphatase, BUN, and creatinine level values.

Dosage: Capsules, Oral Suspension, Tablets. Adults: *Tinea corporis, cruris, or capitis:* 0.5 g griseofulvin microsize daily in a single dose or divided dose (or 330–375 mg ultramicrosize). *Tinea pedis or unguium:* 0.75–1 g daily of griseofulvin microsize (or 660–750 mg ultramicrosize). After response, decrease dose of microsize to 0.5 g daily.

  PO. Pediatric, 13.6–22.7 kg: 125–250 mg griseofulvin microsize daily (or 82.5–165 mg ultramicrosize); **pediatric, over 22.7 kg:** 250–500 mg microsize daily (or 165–330 mg ultramicrosize). *Note:* Dose has not been determined in children less than 2 years of age.

NURSING CONSIDERATIONS

See also *General Nursing Considerations For All Anti-Infectives* under *Penicillins,* p. 140.

Administration/Storage

Length of treatment varies from 1 month to 1 year.

Client/Family Teaching

Teach client and/or family to
- eat a high-fat diet, since fat enhances the absorption of griseofulvin from the intestines. Refer to dietitian as necessary.
- take all medication as prescribed, to prevent any recurrence.
- practice appropriate hygiene to prevent reinfection.
- avoid exposure to intense natural and artificial light, since photosensitivity reactions may occur.
- report fever, sore throat, and malaise, all symptoms of leukopenia.
- understand that for the client to be considered cured, repeated cultures and scrapings of affected sites must be negative.

Evaluation

1. Note status of pretreatment symptoms and culture and scraping results.
2. Assess client/family knowledge and understanding of illness and their response to therapy and to teaching.

HALOPROGIN   (hal-oh-**PROH**-jin)

Halotex (Rx)

Classification: Antifungal, topical.

Uses: Topical treatment of fungal infections of feet (tinea pedis), male genital region (tinea cruris), smooth skin surfaces (tinea corporis), and hands (tinea manuum) caused by *Trichophyton rubrum, T. tonsurans, T. mentagrophytes, Microsporum canis,* and *Epidermophyton floccosum.* Also, multiple macular patches (tinea versicolor) caused by *Malassezia furfur.*

Contraindications: Hypersensitivity to drug or to any component of preparations. *Avoid contact around eyes.*

Special Concerns: Safe use in children and during pregnancy (pregnancy category: B) or lactation has not been established.

Side Effects: *Topical:* Local irritation, burning sensation, pruritus, erythema, scaling, folliculitis, vesicle formation.

Dosage: Topical Cream, Solution. Apply 1% cream or solution liberally to lesions b.i.d. for 2–3 weeks. Interdigital lesions may require therapy for 4 weeks.

NURSING CONSIDERATIONS

See also *General Nursing Considerations For All Anti-Infectives* under *Penicillins,* p. 140.

Assessment
1. If the drug therapy is not effective after 4 weeks of treatment, reevaluate diagnosis and therapy. Presence of mixed infections or resistant fungi may indicate need for systemic therapy.
2. If irritation or burning occurs or if the condition worsens, the physician should be contacted.

Client/Family Teaching
Teach client and/or family
- to keep the drug out of the eyes.
- to discontinue application of cream and to report to physician if local irritation, burning sensation, or worsening of condition is noted.
- proper technique of application. Observe self-administration to ensure that medication is being applied correctly.
- to continue both haloprogin and additional anti-infective if ordered concomitantly.
- to return to medical supervision if drug is ineffective after 4 weeks.

Evaluation
1. Note status of pretreatment symptoms, and C&S results to determine response to therapy and emergence of resistant strains.
2. Assess client knowledge and understanding of illness and their response to therapy and teaching.

IODOCHLORHYDROXYQUIN (CLIOQUINOL)   (eye-oh-doe-klor-hy-**DROX**-ee-kwin)

Torofor, Vioform (OTC)

Classification: Antibacterial, antifungal.

Action/Kinetics: The drug has both antifungal and antibacterial effects although the precise mechanism is unknown. When used topically, the drug is absorbed rapidly, especially if an occlusive dressing is used.

Uses: Topical fungal infections including athlete's foot and eczema and other fungal infections.

Contraindications: Use in children less than 2 years of age.

Side Effects: Itching, irritation, redness, swelling of skin, painful skin.

Laboratory Test Interference: Interference with thyroid function tests if absorbed through skin. False + ferric chloride test for phenylketonuria is present in urine or diaper of neonate.

Dosage: Apply cream (3%) or ointment (3%) b.i.d.–t.i.d. for not over 1 week.

NURSING CONSIDERATIONS

Client/Family Teaching

1. Instruct client/family to use appropriate protection for clothes, shoes, and bed linens as medication may stain.
2. Not to exceed prescribed treatment times.
3. To report any itching, redness, swelling or pain at the site.

KETOCONAZOLE   (key-toe-**KON**-ah-zohl)

Nizoral (Rx)

Classification: Broad-spectrum antifungal.

Action/Kinetics: Ketoconazole inhibits synthesis of sterols, damaging the cell membrane and resulting in loss of essential intracellular material. It also inhibits biosynthesis of triglycerides and phospholipids and inhibits oxidative and peroxidative enzyme activity. When used to treat *Candida albicans,* it inhibits transformation of blastospores into the invasive mycelial form. **Peak plasma levels:** 3.5 mcg/mL after 1–2 hr. **t½** [biphasic]: first, 2 hr; second, 8 hr. Requires acidity for dissolution. Metabolized in liver and most excreted through feces.

Uses: Candidiasis, chronic mucocutaneous candidiasis, candiduria, histoplasmosis, chromomycosis, oral thrush, coccidioidomycosis, paracoccidioidomycosis. Recalcitrant cutaneous dermatophyte infections. *Investigational:* Onychomycosis due to *Candida* and *Trichophyton.* Tinea versicolor, vaginal candidiasis. Should not be used for fungal meningitis due to poor penetration into the CSF. *Topical:* Tinea corporis, tinea cruris, and tinea versicolor.

Contraindications: Hypersensitivity, fungal meningitis. Topical product not for ophthalmic use. Use during lactation.

Special Concerns: Pregnancy category: C. Use with caution in children less than 2 years of age.

Side Effects: *GI:* Nausea, vomiting, abdominal pain, diarrhea. *CNS:* Headache, dizziness, somnolence, fever, chills. *Miscellaneous:* Hepatotoxicity, photophobia, pruritus, gynecomastia, impotence, thrombocytopenia. *Topical use:* Stinging, irritation, pruritus.

Drug Interactions

Antacids, anticholinergics, cimetidine	↓ Absorption of ketoconazole due to ↑ pH induced by these drugs

Laboratory Test Interference: Transient ↑ serum liver enzymes.

Dosage: Oral Suspension, Tablets. Adults: 200–400 mg as single dose/day. **Pediatric, over 2 years:** 3.3–6.6 mg/kg daily as a single dose. Dosage in children less than 2 years of age not established. *CNS fungal infections:* **PO,** 800–1,200 mg daily. **Topical cream (2%):** Cover the affected and immediate surrounding areas once daily (twice daily for more resistant cases). Duration of treatment is usually 2 weeks.

NURSING CONSIDERATIONS

See also *General Nursing Considerations For All Anti-Infectives* under *Penicillins,* p. 140.

Interventions

1. Minimum duration of treatment for candidiasis is 1–2 weeks, while minimum duration of treatment for other systemic mycoses is 6 months.
2. Ketoconazole should be given a minimum of 2 hr before administration of drugs that increase gastric pH (such as antacids, anticholinergics, or H₂ blockers).

Client/Family Teaching

1. Instruct client to use caution when driving or when performing hazardous tasks because drug can cause headaches, dizziness, and drowsiness.
2. Advise client to report persistent fever, pain, or diarrhea.
3. If client has achlorhydria, instruct him to dissolve each tablet in 4 mL aqueous solution of 0.2 N HCl and to use a straw (glass or plastic) to take this solution to avoid contact with the teeth. This is followed by drinking a glass of tap water.

MICONAZOLE   [my-CON-ah-zohl]

Systemic: Monistat I.V. Topical: Micatin, Monistat-Derm. Vaginal: Monistat✿, Monistat 3, Monistat 5✿, Monistat 7 (Rx except for Micatin, which is OTC)

See also *Anti-Infectives,* p. 71.

Classification: Antifungal agent.

Action/Kinetics: Miconazole may be fungistatic or fungicidal, depending on the concentration. It is a broad-spectrum fungicide that alters the permeability of the fungal membrane by inhibiting synthesis of sterols; thus, essential intracellular materials are lost. The drug also inhibits biosynthesis of triglycerides and phospholipids and also inhibits oxidative and peroxidative enzyme activity. **Peak blood levels:** 1 mcg/mL. The drug is eliminated in three phases. **t½ of each phase:** 0.4, 2.1, and 24 hr. More than 90% of miconazole is bound to serum proteins. Excretion of the drug is unaltered in patients with renal insufficiency, including patients on hemodialysis.

Uses: Systemic fungal infections caused by coccidioidomycosis, candidiasis, cryptococcosis, paracoccidioidomycosis, chronic mucocutaneous candidiasis. When used for the treatment of either fungal meningitis or urinary bladder infection, IV infusion must be supplemented with intrathecal administration or bladder irrigation of the drug. *Investigational:* As ointment for treatment of athlete's foot and vaginal infections.

Contraindications: Hypersensitivity.

Special Concerns: Safe use during pregnancy and in children less than 1 year of age has not been established.

Side Effects: Following topical use: Vulvovaginal symptoms, pelvic cramps, hives, skin rash, headache, burning, irritation, maceration. **Following systemic use.** *GI:* Nausea, vomiting, diarrhea, anorexia. *Hematologic:* Thrombocytopenia, aggregation of erythrocytes, rouleaux formation on blood smears. Transient decrease in hematocrit. *Dermatologic:* Pruritus, rash, flushing. *CV:* Transient tachycardia or arrhythmias following rapid injection of undiluted drug. *Miscellaneous:* Fever, drowsiness, transient decrease in serum sodium values. Hyperlipemia due to the vehicle (PEG 40 and castor oil).

Drug Interactions

Amphotericin B	Amphotericin B ↓ activity of miconazole
Coumarin anticoagulants	Miconazole ↑ anticoagulant effect

Dosage: IV infusion, adults: 200–3,600 mg/day in divided doses depending on the specific organism; **pediatric:** total daily dose, 20–40 mg/kg in divided doses; a dose of 15 mg/kg/infusion should not be exceeded. **Intrathecal:** 20 mg/dose of the undiluted solution as an adjunct to **IV** therapy. **Bladder instillation:** 200 mg of diluted solution as adjunct in treatment of fungal infections of urinary bladder. **Topical, Aerosol Powder, Aerosol Solution, Cream, Lotion, Powder:** Apply to cover affected areas in morning and evening (once daily for tinea versicolor). **Vaginal, Monistat 3:** One suppository daily at bedtime for 3 days. **Vaginal, Monistat 7:** One applicatorful of cream or one suppository at bedtime daily for 7 days. Course may be repeated after presence of other pathogens has been ruled out.

NURSING CONSIDERATIONS

See also *General Nursing Considerations For All Anti-Infectives* under *Penicillins,* p. 140.

Administration/Storage

For IV infusion, the drug should be diluted in at least 200 mL of either 0.9% sodium chloride or 5% dextrose solution and administered over a period of 30–60 min.

Interventions

1. IV therapy may be required for periods ranging from 1 to more than 20 weeks, depending on the organism. Obtain appropriate pretreatment lab studies.
2. Succeeding intrathecal injections should be alternated between lumbar, cervical, and cisternal punctures every 3–7 days. Document sites.

Client/Family Teaching

1. Report any persistent nausea, vomiting, diarrhea, dizziness, and pruritus.
2. Demonstrate appropriate technique for medication administration and instruct client to take medication only as directed.
3. Use sanitary pads with suppositories to protect clothing and linens.
4. When used for vaginal infections, the client should refrain from intercourse; or, to prevent reinfection, the partner should use a condom.
5. When used vaginally, miconazole treatment should be continued during menses.

Evaluation

Review cultures and subjective complaints to evaluate response to therapy and need for continued treatment.

NAFTIFINE HYDROCHLORIDE   (NAF-tih-feen)

Naftin (Rx)

Classification: Antifungal agent.

Action/Kinetics: Naftifine is a synthetic antifungal agent with a broad spectrum of activity. The drug is thought to inhibit squalene 2,3-epoxidase, which is responsible for synthesis of sterols. The decreased levels of sterols (especially ergosterol) and the accumulation of squalene in cells result in fungicidal activity. Although used topically, approximately 6% of the drug is absorbed. Naftifine and its metabolites are excreted via the feces and urine. **t½:** 2–3 days.

Uses: Naftifine is effective against *Candida albicans, Epidermophyton floccosum, Microsporum canis, M. audouinii, M. gypseum, Trichophyton rubrum, T. mentagrophytes,* and *T. tonsurans.* Used to treat tinea cruris and tinea corporis.

Contraindications: Ophthalmic use.

Special Concerns: Pregnancy category: B. Consideration should be given to discontinuing nursing while using naftifine, and for several days after the last application. Safety and efficacy in children have not been determined.

Side Effects: *Topical:* Burning, stinging, dryness, itching, local irritation, erythema.

Dosage: Topical Cream: Massage cream (1%) into affected area and surrounding skin in the morning and evening.

NURSING CONSIDERATIONS

Client/Family Teaching

1. Demonstrate the appropriate technique for topical application.
2. Instruct client/family to wash hands before and after applying medication.
3. Apply carefully so as to avoid contact with the eyes, nose, mouth, or other mucous membranes.
4. Occlusive dressings or wrappings should not be used. Advise not to cover area unless directed by the physician.
5. Beneficial effects are usually observed within 1 week; treatment should be continued as prescribed for 1–2 weeks after symptoms have decreased.
6. Medication is for external use only.
7. Report any excessive itching or burning.

Evaluation

1. Assess client/family knowledge and understanding of illness, their response to therapy and teaching.
2. The client should be reevaluated if beneficial effects are not seen after 4 weeks of treatment.

NATAMYCIN   (nah-tah-MY-sin)

Natacyn (Rx)

See also *Anti-Infectives,* p. 71.

Classification: Antifungal (ophthalmic).

General Statement: Discontinue drug if toxicity is suspected. Review therapy if no improvement noted after 7 to 10 days.

Action/Kinetics: Natamycin is an antifungal antibiotic derived from *Streptomyces natalensis*. The drug binds to the fungal cell membrane, resulting in alteration of permeability and loss of essential intracellular materials. It is fungicidal. After topical administration, the drug reaches therapeutic levels in the corneal stroma but not in the intraocular fluid. It is not absorbed systemically.

Uses: For ophthalmic use only. Drug of choice for *Fusarium solanae* keratitis. For treatment of fungal blepharitis, conjunctivitis, and keratitis caused by susceptible organisms. It is active against a variety of yeasts and filamentous fungi including *Candida, Aspergillus, Cephalosporium, Fusarium,* and *Penicillium*. Before initiating therapy, determine the susceptibility of the infectious organism to drug in smears and cultures of corneal scrapings. Effectiveness of natamycin for use as a single agent in fungal endophthalmitis not established.

Contraindications: Hypersensitivity to drug.

Special Concerns: Safe use during pregnancy not established.

Side Effects: Eye irritation, occasional allergies.

Dosage: Ophthalmic Suspension: *Fungal keratitis:* **Initially,** 1 gtt of 5% suspension in conjunctival sac q 1–2 hr; can be reduced usually, after 3–4 days to 1 gtt 6–8 times/day. Continue therapy for 14–21 days, during which dosage can be reduced gradually at 4- to 7-day intervals. *Blepharitis/conjunctivitis:* 1 gtt 4–6 times daily.

NURSING CONSIDERATIONS

See also *General Nursing Considerations For All Anti-Infectives* under *Penicillins,* p. 140.

Administration/Storage

1. Store natamycin at room temperature or in refrigerator.
2. Shake well before using.
3. Avoid contamination of dropper.

Client/Family Teaching

1. Stress the importance of close medical supervision (initially twice weekly) to regulate dosage.
2. Demonstrate proper administration technique.
3. Instruct client/family to continue therapy for 14–21 days as ordered, even though condition may appear to be under control.

NYSTATIN   (nye-**STAT**-in)

Tablets: Mycostatin, Nilstat Oral. Oral Suspension: Mycostatin, Nadostine✿, Nilstat, Nystex. Troches: Mycostatin Pastilles. Vaginal Tablets: Mycostatin, Nadostine✿, Nilstat, O-V Statin. Topical: Mycostatin, Mykinac, Nadostine✿, Nilstat, Nyaderm✿, Nystex (Rx)

See also *Anti-Infectives,* p. 71.

Classification: Antibiotic, antifungal.

Action/Kinetics: This natural antifungal antibiotic is derived from *Streptomyces noursei* and is both fungistatic and fungicidal against all species of *Candida*. Nystatin binds to fungal cell membranes (sterols), resulting in altered cellular permeability and leakage of potassium and other essential intracellular components. Nystatin is excreted in the feces.

Uses: *Candida* infections of the skin, mucous membranes, GI tract, vagina, and mouth (thrush). The drug is too toxic for systemic infections although it can be given PO for intestinal moniliasis infections as it is not absorbed from the GI tract.

Special Concerns: Pregnancy category: A (for vaginal use). Occlusive dressings should not be used when treating candidiasis. Lozenges should not be used in children less than 5 years of age.

Side Effects: Nystatin has few toxic effects. *GI:* Epigastric distress, nausea, vomiting, diarrhea. *Other:* Rarely, irritation.

Dosage: Lozenge, Oral Suspension, Tablets. *Intestinal candidiasis:* **Tablets,** 500,000–1,000,000 units t.i.d.; continue treatment for 48 hr after cure to prevent relapse. *Oral candidiasis:* **Oral Suspension, adults and children:** 400,000–600,000 units q.i.d. (½ dose in each side of mouth, held as long as possible before swallowing); **infants:** 200,000 units q.i.d. (same procedure as with adults); **premature or low birth weight infants:** 100,000 units q.i.d. **Lozenge, adults and children:** 200,000–400,000 units 4–5 times daily, up to 14 days. *Note:* Lozenges should not be chewed or swallowed. **Vaginal Cream, tablets:** 100,000 units (one tablet) inserted in vagina once or twice each day for 2 weeks. **Topical (ointment, cream, powder**—contains 100,000 units/g): Apply to affected areas b.i.d.–t.i.d., or as indicated, until healing is complete.

NURSING CONSIDERATIONS
See also *General Nursing Considerations* For *All Anti-Infectives* under *Penicillins,* p. 140.

Administration/Storage
1. A powder for extemporaneous compounding of the oral suspension is available. To reconstitute, add ⅛ tsp of the powder (about 500,000 units) to approximately ½–1 cup water and stir well. This product is administered immediately after mixing.
2. Protect drug from heat, light, moisture, and air.
3. The suspension can be stored for 7 days at room temperature or for 10 days in the refrigerator without loss of potency.

Interventions
1. Anticipate that vaginal tablets may be continued in the gravid client for 3 to 6 weeks before term to reduce incidence of thrush in the newborn.
2. Do not mix oral suspension in foods, since the medication will be inactivated.
3. Apply cream or ointment to mycotic lesions with a swab.
4. Drop 1 mL of oral suspension in each side of mouth or apply with a swab to treat oral moniliasis. Instruct client to keep medication in mouth as long as possible before swallowing.
5. For pediatric use, 250,000 units of nystatin has been given frozen in popsicles.
6. Insert vaginal tablets high in vagina with an applicator.
7. For fungal infections of the feet, the powder should be used freely on the feet, as well as in the shoes and socks.
8. For intertriginous areas, the cream should be used; however, for moist lesions, the powder is best.

Client/Family Teaching

1. Review the appropriate method for administration and associated instructions according to area being treated as delineated under *Interventions*.
2. Continue using vaginal tablets even when menstruating since the treatment should be continued for 2 weeks.
3. Report any bothersome symptoms to physician.
4. Discontinue drug and notify physician if vaginal tablets cause irritation.
5. Drug may stain; sanitary pads may help protect clothing and linens.

Evaluation

Assess response to drug therapy based on culture results and client symptoms.

OXICONAZOLE NITRATE   (ox-ih-**KON**-ah-zohl)

Oxistat (Rx)

Classification: Antifungal agent, topical.

Action/Kinetics: Oxiconazole acts by inhibiting ergosterol synthesis, which is required for cytoplasmic membrane integrity of fungi. It is active against a broad range of organisms including many strains of *Trichophyton rubrum* and *T. mentagrophytes*. Systemic absorption of the drug is low.

Uses: Topical treatment of tinea pedis, tinea cruris, and tinea corporis due to *T. rubrum* and *T. mentagrophytes*.

Contraindications: Ophthalmic use.

Special Concerns: Pregnancy category: B. Use with caution during lactation.

Side Effects: *Dermatologic:* Burning, itching, irritation, erythema, fissuring, maceration.

Dosage: Cream, topical: Apply 1% cream to cover affected areas once daily in the evening. To prevent recurrence, treatment should continue for 2 weeks for tinea corporis and tinea cruris and for 1 month for tinea pedis.

NURSING CONSIDERATIONS

Client/Family Teaching

1. Demonstrate how to apply medication and instruct client/family to use medication only as directed.
2. Report any itching and/or burning associated with therapy, as treatment should be discontinued if symptoms appear which suggest sensitivity or chemical irritation.
3. Some infections may require 2 weeks to a month of daily treatments to ensure that there is no recurrence.
4. Oxiconazole is intended for external use only.
5. Oxiconazole should not be introduced into the eye.

Evaluation

Assess client response to therapy. The diagnosis should be reviewed if the client shows no clinical response after the appropriate treatment period.

SULCONAZOLE NITRATE (sul-KON-ah-zohl)

Exelderm (Rx)

Classification: Antifungal, topical.

Action/Kinetics: This broad-spectrum antifungal and antiyeast agent inhibits growth of *Trichophyton mentagrophytes, Epidermophyton floccosum, Microsporum canis,* and *Malassezia fufur* as well as certain gram-positive bacteria.

Uses: Treatment of tinea cruris, tinea corporis, and tinea versicolor. Efficacy has not been demonstrated for tinea pedis (athlete's foot).

Contraindications: Ophthalmic use.

Special Concerns: Pregnancy category: C. Use with caution during lactation. Safety and efficacy have not been demonstrated in children.

Side Effects: *Dermatologic:* Burning, itching, stinging.

Dosage: Solution, topical: A small amount of the 1% solution is gently massaged into the affected area and surrounding skin once or twice daily.

NURSING CONSIDERATIONS

Client/Family Teaching

1. Demonstrate how to apply medication and advise to use only as directed.
2. The drug is for external use only.
3. Contact with the eyes should be avoided.
4. Relief of symptoms usually occurs within a few days of initiating treatment, with clinical improvement occurring within 1 week. If symptoms do not improve after prescribed time interval, notify physician.
5. To reduce the chance of recurrent tinea cruris, tinea corporis, and tinea versicolor client should be treated for 3 weeks.

Evaluation

Assess client response to therapy. An alternate diagnosis should be considered if no improvement is observed after 4 weeks of treatment.

TERCONAZOLE NITRATE (ter-KON-ah-zohl)

Terazol 3, Terazol 7 (Rx)

Classification: Antifungal, vaginal.

Action/Kinetics: Terconazole, a triazole derivative, is thought to exert its antifungal activity by disrupting cell membrane permeability leading to loss of essential intracellular materials. The drug also inhibits synthesis of triglycerides and phospholipids as well as inhibiting oxidative and peroxidative enzyme activity. When used for *Candida,* terconazole inhibits transformation of blastospores into the invasive mycelial form.

Uses: Vulvovaginitis caused by *Candida.* Ineffective in infections due to *Trichomonas* or *Hemophilus vaginalis.*

Special Concerns: Use in pregnancy only on advice of physician (pregnancy category: C). During lactation, consider discontinuing nursing or the drug. Safety and efficacy have not been established in children.

Side Effects: *GU:* Vulvovaginal burning, irritation, or itching. *Miscellaneous:* Headache (most common), body pain, photosensitivity.

Dosage: Topical, vaginal cream: One applicatorful (5 g) intravaginally, once daily at bedtime for 7 days. **Vaginal suppository:** One 80 mg suppository once daily at bedtime for 3 days.

NURSING CONSIDERATIONS

Assessment

1. Obtain a thorough nursing history, as recurrent candidiasis may be caused by oral contraceptives, antibiotics, or diabetes.
2. Intractable candidiasis may be the result of undetected diabetes mellitus or reinfection. The client should be evaluated carefully.

Client/Family Teaching

1. Demonstrate the appropriate method for administration (the cream should be inserted high into the vagina).
2. Discontinue use and report if any burning, irritation, or pain occurs.
3. Medication may stain clothes; use sanitary napkins during therapy and change frequently as damp sanitary napkins may harbor organisms.
4. To avoid reinfection, the client should refrain from sexual intercourse, or the partner should be advised to use a condom.
5. Continue to take medication for prescribed time frame even if symptoms subside.
6. The drug should continue to be used during menses in order to assure a full course of therapy. Effectiveness is not altered by menstruation.

Evaluation

Evaluate response to therapy. Prior to a second course of therapy, the diagnosis should be confirmed to rule out other pathogens associated with vulvovaginitis.

TIOCONAZOLE   (tie-oh-**KON**-ah-zohl)

Vagistat (Rx)

Classification: Antifungal, vaginal.

Action/Kinetics: The antifungal activity of tioconazole is thought to be due to alteration of the permeability of the cell membrane of the fungus, causing leakage of essential intracellular compounds. The systemic absorption of the drug in nonpregnant patients is negligible.

Uses: Local treatment of *Candida albicans* infections of the vulva and vagina. Also effective against *Torulopsis glabrata*.

Contraindications: Use of a vaginal applicator during pregnancy may be contraindicated.

Special Concerns: Pregnancy category: C. Safety and effectiveness have not been determined during lactation or in children.

Side Effects: *GU:* Burning, itching, irritation, vulvar edema and swelling, discharge, vaginal pain, dysuria, dyspareunia, nocturia, desquamation, dryness of vaginal secretions.

Dosage: Vaginal Ointment, 6.5%. One applicatorful (about 5 g) should be inserted intravaginally at bedtime for 3 days. If needed, the treatment period can be extended to 6 days.

NURSING CONSIDERATIONS

Assessment

1. Obtain a thorough nursing history. Clients who do not respond to treatment may have unrecognized diabetes mellitus. Urine and blood glucose studies should be undertaken.
2. An infection which is persistently resistant may be due to reinfection; the sources of infection should be evaluated.

Interventions

Obtain appropriate lab studies as ordered, prior to initiating therapy.

Client/Family Teaching

1. Demonstrate the appropriate method for administration (the cream should be inserted high into the vagina).
2. Report if any burning, irritation, or pain occurs.
3. Medication may stain clothes; use sanitary napkins during therapy and change frequently as damp sanitary napkins may harbor organisms.
4. To avoid reinfection, the client should refrain from sexual intercourse, or the partner should be advised to use a condom.
5. Continue to take medication for prescribed time frame even if symptoms subside.
6. The drug should continue to be used during menses in order to assure a full course of therapy. Effectiveness is not altered by menstruation.
7. Use the medication just prior to bedtime.

Evaluation

Assess client response to therapy, obtain appropriate lab data and note client symptoms. Determine need to extend therapy and notify physician.

TOLNAFTATE   (toll-NAF-tayt)

Aftate for Athlete's Foot, Aftate for Jock Itch, Footwork, Fungatin, Genaspor, NP-27, Pitrex✷, Tinactin, Zeasorb-AF (OTC)

See also *Anti-Infectives,* p. 71.

Classification: Topical antifungal.

Action/Kinetics: The exact mechanism is not known although the drug is thought to stunt mycelial growth causing a fungicidal effect.

Uses: Tinea pedis, tinea cruris, tinea corporis, tinea manuum, and tinea versicolor. Fungal infections of moist skin areas.

Contraindications: Scalp and nail infections. *Avoid getting into eyes.*

Special Concerns: Should not be used in children less than 2 years of age.

Side Effects: Mild skin irritation.

Dosage: Topical: Aerosol Powder, Aerosol Solution, Cream, Gel, Powder, Solution, Spray Solution. Apply b.i.d. for 2–3 weeks, although treatment for 4–6 weeks may be necessary in some instances.

NURSING CONSIDERATIONS

See also *General Nursing Considerations For All Anti-Infectives* under *Penicillins,* p. 140.

Interventions

1. The skin should be thoroughly cleaned and dried before the medication is applied.
2. Carefully inspect the source of infection and document, as the choice of vehicle is important for effective therapy.
   - Powders are used in mild conditions as adjunctive therapy.
   - For primary therapy and prophylaxis, creams, liquids, or ointments are used, especially if the area is moist.
   - Liquids and solutions are used if the area is hairy.
3. Obtain appropriate lab data, as concomitant therapy should be used if bacterial or *Candida* infections are also present.
4. Notify physician and discontinue use if improvement is not noted within 10 days.

Client/Family Teaching

1. Demonstrate the appropriate technique for medication administration.
2. Instruct client/family to use care when administering and not to inadvertently rub medication into eye.
3. Report any bothersome side effects; local relief of symptoms should be evident within the first 24–48 hours of therapy.
4. Continue to use as directed, despite improvement of symptoms.

Evaluation

Assess client response to therapy and any evidence of secondary infections that may necessitate additional treatment.

TRIACETIN   (try-ah-**SEE**-tin)
Enzactin, Fungacetin, Fungoid (Rx: Fungoid; OTC: Enzactin, Fungacetin)

Classification: Antifungal.

Uses: Topical fungal infections including athlete's foot.

Dosage: Apply to affected area b.i.d.

NURSING CONSIDERATIONS

Client/Family Teaching

1. Use dilute alcohol or mild soap and water to clean affected areas prior to use.
2. After symptoms disappear, to continue to use for an additional week.
3. Rayon fabrics should not come in contact with affected areas; use a bandage or clean cloth.

Evaluation

Assess for (presence/absence) of pretreatment symptoms.

UNDECYLENIC ACID AND DERIVATIVES   (un-deh-sill-**ENN**-ick **AH**-sid)

Breezee Mist Aerosol, Caldesene, Cruex, Cruex Aerosol, Decylenes, Desenex, Desenex Aerosol, Kool Foot, Merlenate, Pedi-Dri, Quinsana Plus, Ting Spray, Undoguent (OTC)

Classification: Antibacterial, antifungal.

Action/Kinetics: Undecylenic acid produces a fungistatic effect. One component is zinc undecylenate, which produces an astringent effect in decreasing irritation and rawness.

Uses: Minor skin irritations including diaper rash, burning, prickly heat, chafing, jock itch, excessive perspiration and irritation in the groin. Athlete's foot, ringworm.

Contraindications: Use on pustular, broken skin, raw or oozing areas of skin, over puncture or deep wounds. In diabetics or in impaired circulation unless directed by the physician. *Avoid contact with eyes and mucous membranes.*

Side Effects: Skin irritation.

Dosage: Topical Aerosol Powder, Cream, Ointment, Powder. Rub on or spray as needed to affected area twice daily.

NURSING CONSIDERATIONS

Interventions

Carefully inspect the source of infection and document as the choice of vehicle is important for effective therapy.

- Powders are used in mild conditions as adjunctive therapy.
- For primary therapy and prophylaxis, creams, liquids, or ointments are used, especially if the area is moist.
- Liquids and solutions are used if the area is hairy.

Client/Family Teaching

1. Demonstrate appropriate technique for administration and instruct client to use only as directed.
2. Stress that the affected area should be clean and dry prior to application of medication.
3. Instruct client/family to seek medical attention if symptoms persist as organism may be of yeast origin and alternative therapy would be indicated.

Evaluation

Assess client response to therapy and for any evidence of secondary infections that may necessitate additional treatment.

CHAPTER ELEVEN
Sulfonamides

Action/Kinetics: Sulfonamides are structurally related to para-aminobenzoic acid and, as such, competitively inhibit the enzyme dihydropteroate synthetase that is responsible for incorporating para-aminobenzoic acid into dihydrofolic acid. Thus, the synthesis of dihydrofolic acid is inhibited, resulting in a decrease in the tetrahydrofolic acid that is required for synthesis of DNA, purines, and thymidine. Thus, sulfonamides halt multiplication of bacteria (bacteriostatic) but do not kill fully formed microorganisms.

The various sulfonamides are absorbed and excreted at widely differing rates, which has an important bearing on their therapeutic use. For instance, agents that are poorly absorbed from the GI tract are particularly indicated for intestinal infections, because they remain localized in the intestine for a long time.

Sulfonamides are absorbed into the bloodstream and distributed throughout all tissues, including the CSF, where concentrations attain 50% to 80% of those found in the blood. The sulfonamides are excreted primarily by the kidneys. It is always desirable to determine the susceptibility of the pathogen before, or soon after, initiation of therapy. Sulfonamides have the advantage of being relatively inexpensive.

Uses: The range of usefulness of the sulfonamides has been greatly reduced by the emergence of resistant strains of bacteria and the development of more effective antibiotics.

Acute, nonobstructive urinary tract infections caused by *Escherichia coli, Klebsiella, Enterobacter, Staphylococcus aureus, Proteus mirabilis, P. vulgaris.* Drug of choice for nocardiosis. Elimination of meningococci from the nasopharynx in asymptomatic *Neisseria meningitidis* carriers. As an alternative to penicillin for prophylaxis of rheumatic fever. As an alternative to tetracyclines for chlamydial infections or for trachoma and inclusion conjunctivitis. In conjunction with pyrimethamine for toxoplasmosis. In combination with quinine sulfate and pyrimethamine for chloroquine-resistant *Plasmodium falciparum.* In combination with penicillin for otitis media. See also individual drugs, below and in Table 5.

Contraindications: Except for hypersensitivity reactions, there are few absolute contraindications.

11

Table 5   Sulfonamides

Drug	Main Use	Dosage	Remarks
Silver sulfadiazine (Flammazine ✦, Flint SSD, Silvadene, Thermazine)(Rx)	Topically for prevention and treatment of sepsis in second- and third-degree burns. Minor bacterial skin infections. Dermal ulcers.	**Cream:** Apply 1/16-inch thick film over entire surface of clean and debrided burn with a sterile, gloved hand once or twice daily until healing is progressing satisfactorily or site is ready for grafting.	*Contraindications:* Pregnancy at or near term, premature infants, infants less than 2 months of age. *Special Concerns:.* Use with caution during lactation. Pregnancy category: C. *Untoward Reactions:* Burning, rash, itching, leukopenia. *Drug Interaction:* Silver may inactivate proteolytic enzymes used topically. *Administration:* 1. Dressings are not required. 2. The drug is absorbed from burn areas; thus, plasma levels may reach therapeutic levels. 3. If possible, the patient should be bathed daily to help with debridement.
Sulfapyridine (Dagenan ✦) (Rx)	Dermatitis herpetiformis *Investigational:* Subcorneal pustular dermatosis, pemphigoid, pyoderma gangrenosum.	**PO, initial:** 0.25–1 g q.i.d. (up to 6 g); when improvement is noted, decrease by 500 mg daily at 3-day intervals, until symptom-free maintenance is achieved. Increase dosage if symptoms return. *Subcorneal postular dermatosis:* 0.5 g b.i.d.-0.75 g q.i.d. *Pempbigoid:* 1 g t.i.d.	Intermediate-acting. Slowly and incompletely absorbed from GI tract. **Time to peak levels:** 4–6 hr. *Contraindications:* Pregnancy, lactation, children.

Drug	Indication	Dosage	Remarks
Sulfanilamide (AVC, Vagitrol) (Rx)	Vulvovaginitis due to *Candida albicans*	**Vaginal cream:** 1 applicatorful 1–2 times daily for one complete menstrual cycle. **Vaginal suppositories:** 1 suppository 1–2 times daily for 30 days.	*Contraindication:* Kidney disease. Pregnancy category: C. *Untoward Reactions:* Local irritation, pruritus, urticaria allergic reactions, burning. *Administration:* Insert high into the vagina with the applicator provided.
Triple Sulfa (Sulfathiazole, Sulfacetamide, Sulfabenzamide) Sulfa-Gyn, Sulnac, Sultrin, Trysul, Vagilia, V.V.S.) (Rx)	Vaginitis due to *Haemophilus vaginalis*.	**Vaginal cream:** 1 applicatorful b.i.d. for 4–6 days; then, reduce dosage to 1/4–1/2. **Vaginal tablets:** 1 tablet intravaginally b.i.d. on arising and at bedtime for 10 days; may be repeated.	These products all contain urea. See also *Remarks* for *Sulfanilamide.* The FDA has determined that this combination is probably ineffective.

Sulfonamides, however, are potentially dangerous drugs and cause a 5% overall incidence of major and minor side effects.

Sulfonamides may cause mental retardation and never should be administered during the third term of pregnancy, to nursing mothers, or to infants under 2 months of age, except for the treatment of congenital toxoplasmosis (a serious parasitic disease that can cause brain inflammation) or in life-threatening situations.

Special Concerns: Sulfonamides should be used with caution, and in reduced dosage, in patients with impaired liver or renal function, intestinal or urinary tract obstructions, blood dyscrasias, allergies, asthma, and hereditary glucose-6-phosphate dehydrogenase deficiency.

Side Effects: *GI:* Nausea, vomiting, diarrhea, abdominal pain, glossitis, stomatitis, anorexia, pancreatitis. *Allergic:* Rash, pruritus, photosensitivity, erythema nodosum or multiforme, Stevens-Johnson syndrome, conjunctivitis, rhinitis, balanitis. Serum sickness, disseminated lupus erythematosus, periarteritis nodosa, arteritis. *CNS:* Headaches, dizziness, mental depression, ataxia, confusion, psychoses, drowsiness, restlessness. *Renal:* Renal damage due to precipitation of sulfonamide or its acetyl derivative in the tubules manifested by crystalluria, hematuria, oliguria. *Hematologic:* Acute hemolytic anemia especially in glucose-6-phosphate dehydrogenase deficiency, aplastic anemia, granulocytopenia, leukopenia, eosinophilia, agranulocytosis, thrombocytopenia, methemoglobinemia. *Miscellaneous:* Jaundice, hypoglycemia, arthralgia, acidosis, periorbital edema, purpura, superinfection.

By killing the intestinal flora, the sulfonamides also reduce the bacterial synthesis of vitamin K. This may result in hemorrhage. Administration of vitamin K to patients on long-term sulfonamide therapy is recommended.

Drug Interactions

Anesthetics, local	↓ Effect of sulfonamides
Antacids	↓ Effect of sulfonamides due to ↓ absorption from GI tract
Anticoagulants, oral	↑ Effect of anticoagulants due to ↓ in plasma protein binding
Antidiabetics, oral	↑ Hypoglycemic effect due to ↓ in plasma protein binding
Cyclosporine	↓ Effect of cyclosporine and ↑ nephrotoxicity
Methenamine	↑ Chance of sulfonamide crystalluria due to acid urine
Methotrexate	↑ Effect of methotrexate due to ↓ plasma protein binding and ↓ renal tubular excretion
Oxacillin	↓ Effect of oxacillin due to ↓ absorption from GI tract
Paraldehyde	↑ Chance of sulfonamide crystalluria
Phenylbutazone	↑ Effect of sulfonamides by ↑ blood levels
Phenytoin	↑ Effect of phenytoin due to ↓ breakdown in liver
Probenecid	↑ Effect of sulfonamides by ↓ in plasma protein binding
Salicylates	↑ Effect of sulfonamides by ↑ blood levels

Laboratory Test Interferences: False + or ↑ liver function tests (amino acids, bilirubin, BSP), renal function (BUN, nonprotein nitrogen, creatinine clearance), blood counts, prothrombin time, Coombs' test. False + or ↑ urine glucose (copper reduction methods, such as Benedict's solution or Clinitest), protein, urobilinogen.

Dosage: See drugs listed below as well as Table 5.

Sulfonamides are usually given PO. Dosage is adjusted individually. An initial loading dose is usually recommended. Short-acting compounds must be given every 4–6 hr.

Topical application of sulfonamides is rarely ordered today, except for mafenide acetate, which is used as a 10% ointment to treat burn infections.

Creams of triple sulfa or sulfisoxazole are used for vaginitis.

When sulfonamides are given as adjuncts to GI surgery, medication is usually started 3–5 days before surgery and is given for 1–2 weeks postoperatively after peristalsis has resumed.

NURSING CONSIDERATIONS

See also *General Nursing Considerations For All Anti-Infectives* under *Penicillins*, p. 140.

Assessment

1. Obtain a thorough nursing and drug history.
2. Note if the client has ever received sulfonamide therapy and what response he/she had.
3. Question clients concerning any possible intestinal problems, urinary tract obstructions, or allergies.
4. If the client is pregnant, the physician should be told so that another type of medication not harmful to a developing fetus may be used.

Intervention

1. Ensure that clients have had the appropriate liver and renal function studies prior to initiating therapy.
2. Obtain baseline data such as complete blood counts, blood sugar levels, and bleeding times. Monitor these throughout the therapy.
3. During drug therapy, assess clients for any of the following reactions that may require withdrawal of the drug:
   - skin rashes, abdominal pain, reports of anorexia, irritation of the mouth or tingling of the extremities.
   - blood dyscrasias (characterized by sore throat, fever, pallor, purpura, jaundice, or weakness).
   - serum sickness (characterized by eruptions of purpuric spots and pain in limbs and joints). Serum sickness may develop 7 to 10 days after initiation of therapy.
   - early symptoms of Stevens-Johnson syndrome (characterized by high fever, severe headaches, stomatitis, conjunctivitis, rhinitis, urethritis, and balanitis [inflammation of the tip of the penis]).
   - jaundice, which may indicate hepatic involvement, with onset 3 to 5 days after initiation of therapy.
   - renal involvement (characterized by renal colic, oliguria, anuria, hematuria, and proteinuria).
   - ecchymosis and hemorrhage (caused by decreased synthesis of vitamin K by intestinal bacteria).
   - hemolytic anemia especially in the elderly.
   - behavioral changes or acute mental disturbances.
4. Monitor intake and output and record. Encourage adequate fluid intake to prevent crystalluria. Minimum output of urine should be 1,500 mL daily.
5. If administering long-acting sulfonamides, adequate fluid intake must be maintained for 24–48 hours after the drug has been discontinued.

Client/Family Teaching

1. Report any side effects immediately.
2. Take drug on time and as prescribed and to remain under medical supervision during course of therapy.
3. That certain sulfonamides may color urine orange-red or brown. This should not be cause for alarm but should be reported to the physician.
4. Take medication with 6–8 oz (180–240 mL) of water and to maintain adequate fluid intake for 24–48 hr after discontinuing drug.
5. How to monitor intake and output and to maintain a record during the course of therapy.
6. Demonstrate how to test urine pH daily and to report changes in acidity as additional drug therapy may need to be instituted.
7. Discourage the use of vitamin C while on therapy since it may make the urine more acidic and contribute to crystal formation.
8. If client also taking anticoagulants instruct them to be particularly alert to evidence of an increase in bleeding tendencies (bruising, cuts that bleed for a longer time than usual, etc.).

Evaluation

1. Assess client knowledge and understanding of illness, and their response to therapy and teaching.
2. Test pH level of urine to determine excess acidity.
3. Administration of a particularly insoluble sulfonamide may require alkalinization of urine. The drug of choice for this purpose is sodium bicarbonate.
4. Review lab studies for any evidence of adverse drug effects.
5. Note client's record of intake and output. Observe urinalysis for evidence of crystals.

MAFENIDE ACETATE (MAH-fen-ide AH-seh-tayt)
Sulfamylon (Rx)

See also *Sulfonamides,* p. 203, and *Antacids,* p. 1019.

Classification: Sulfonamide, topical.

Uses: Topical application in the treatment of second- and third-degree burns (prevention of infections).

Contraindication: Not to be used for already established infections.

Special Concerns: Pregnancy category: C. Use with caution during lactation. Use not recommended in infants less than one month of age.

Dosage: Cream: 1/16-inch-thick film applied over entire surface of burn with gloves once or twice daily until healing is progressing satisfactorily or until site is ready for grafting.

NURSING CONSIDERATIONS

See *General Nursing Considerations For All Anti-Infectives* under *Penicillins,* p. 140, and for *Sulfonamides,* p. 207.

Administration

Mafenide, unlike other sulfonamides, is not inhibited by pus or body fluids.

Client/Family Teaching

1. Demonstrate the appropriate method for administration of medication.
2. Burns treated with mafenide are to be covered only with a thin dressing.
3. The drug causes pain upon application.

Evaluation

Assess client response to therapy and evaluate burn site for evidence of infection and readiness for grafting.

PEDIAZOLE   (PEE-dee-ah-zohl)
(Rx)

Classification/Content: This product is available as granules that, when reconstituted, provide an oral suspension.
Antibacterial, antibiotic: Erythromycin ethylsuccinate, 200 mg/5 mL erythromycin activity.
Antibacterial, sulfonamide: Sulfisoxazole, 600 mg/5 mL.
See also information on individual components.

Use: Acute otitis media in children caused by *Haemophilus influenzae*.

Contraindications: Pregnancy at term and in children less than 2 months of age. Use with caution during other times of pregnancy

Dosage: Oral Suspension. Usual: Equivalent of 50 mg/kg daily of erythromycin and 150 mg/kg daily of sulfisoxazole, up to a maximum of 6 g daily. **Over 45 kg:** 10 mL q 6 hr; **24 kg:** 7.5 mL q 6 hr; **16 kg:** 5 mL q 6 hr; **8 kg:** 2.5 mL q 6 hr; **less than 8 kg:** Calculate dose according to body weight.

NURSING CONSIDERATIONS

See *General Nursing Considerations For All Anti-Infectives* under *Penicillins,* p. 140, and *Sulfonamides,* p. 203.

Administration/Storage

The reconstituted suspension should be refrigerated and used within 14 days.

SULFACETAMIDE SODIUM   (sul-fah-SET-ah-myd)
AK-Sulf, Bleph-10, Cetamide, Isopto-Cetamide, I-Sulfacet, Ocu-Sul-10, Ocu-Sul-15, Ocu-Sul-30, Ocusulf-10, Ophthacet, Sodium Sulamyd, Spectro-Sulf, Steri-Units Sulfacetamide, Sulf-10, Sulfair, Sulfair 10, Sulfair 15, Sulfair Forte, Sulfamide, Sulten-10 (Rx)

See also *Sulfonamides,* p. 203.

Classification: Sulfonamide, topical.

Uses: Topically for ophthalmic infections including trachoma, seborrheic dermatitis, and cutaneous bacterial infections.

Special Concerns: Safe use during pregnancy, lactation, or in children has not been established. Use with caution in patients with dry eye syndrome.

Side Effects: *Topical:* Itching, redness, swelling, irritation.

Drug Interactions: Preparations containing silver are incompatible with sulfacetamide sodium.

Dosage: Ophthalmic Solution: 1–3 drops of 10%, 15%, or 30% solution in conjunctival sac q 2–3 hr. **Ophthalmic Ointment (10%):** Apply 1–4 times daily and at bedtime in conjunctival sac. *For cutaneous infections:* Apply **locally** (10%) to affected area b.i.d.–q.i.d. *Seborrheic dermatitis:* Apply 1–2 times daily (for mild cases, apply overnight).

NURSING CONSIDERATIONS

See *General Nursing Considerations For All Anti-Infectives* under *Penicillins,* p. 140, and*Sulfonamides,* p. 207.

Client/Family Teaching

1. When used for seborrheic dermatitis of the scalp, medication should be applied at bedtime and allowed to remain overnight.
2. If hair and scalp are oily or if there is debris, shampoo scalp before application.
3. Ophthalmic use may cause sensitivity to bright light; this can be minimized by wearing sunglasses.

SULFACYTINE   (SUL-fah-SIGH-teen)

Renoquid (Rx)

See also *Sulfonamides,* p. 203.

Classification: Sulfonamide.

Special Concerns: Safe use during pregnancy has not been established. Not recommended for use in children less than 14 years of age. Reduced dosage may be necessary in patients with impaired renal function.

Dosage: Tablets. Adults and children over 14 years, initially: 500 mg; **maintenance:** 250 mg q.i.d. for 10 days. Not indicated for children less than 14 years of age.

NURSING CONSIDERATIONS

See *General Nursing Considerations For All Anti-Infectives* under *Penicillins,* p. 140, and for *Sulfonamides,* p. 207.

SULFADIAZINE   (sul-fah-DYE-ah-zeen)

Microsulfon (Rx)

SULFADIAZINE SODIUM   (sul-fah-DYE-ah-zeen)

(Rx)

See also *Sulfonamides,* p. 203.

Classification: Sulfonamide.

Action/Kinetics: Short-acting, and often combined with other anti-infectives.

Uses: Urinary tract infections, bacillary dysentery, rheumatic fever prophylaxis.

Special Concerns: Safe use during pregnancy has not been established.

Dosage: Tablets. Adults, initial: 2–4 g; **maintenance:** 2–4 g daily in 3–6 divided doses; **infants over 2 months, initial:** 75 mg/kg/day; **maintenance:** 150 mg/kg/day in 4–6 divided doses, not to exceed 6 g daily. *Rheumatic fever prophylaxis,* **under 30 kg:** 0.5 g/day; **over 30 kg:** 1 g daily. *As adjunct with pyrimethamine in congenital toxoplasmosis:* **Infants less than 2 months, initial:** 75–100 mg/kg; **maintenance:** 100–150 mg/kg daily in 4 divided doses.

NURSING CONSIDERATIONS

See *General Nursing Considerations For All Anti-Infectives* under *Penicillins,* p. 140, and for *Sulfonamides,* p. 207.

SULFAMETHIZOLE   (sul-fah-**METH**-ih-zohl)
Proklar (Rx)

See also *Sulfonamides,* p. 203.

Classification: Sulfonamide, short-acting.

Use: Urinary tract infections.

Special Concerns: Safe use during pregnancy has not been established.

Additional Drug Interactions: Sulfamethizone ↑ effects of tolbutamide, phenytoin, and chlorpropamide due to ↓ breakdown by liver.

Dosage: Tablets. Adults, 0.5–1 g t.i.d.–q.i.d.; **infants over 2 months:** 30–45 mg/kg/day in 4 divided doses.

NURSING CONSIDERATIONS

See *General Nursing Considerations For All Anti-Infectives* under *Penicillins,* p. 140, and for *Sulfonamides,* p. 207.

SULFAMETHOXAZOLE   (sul-fah-meh-**THOX**-ah-zohl)
Apo-Sulfamethoxazole✤, Gantanol, Gantanol DS (Rx)

See also *Sulfonamides,* p. 203.

Classification: Sulfonamide, intermediate-acting.

Action/Kinetics: $t^{1/2}$: 8.6 hr. Sulfamethoxazole is also a component of Bactrim, Bactrim DS, Septra, and Septra DS.

Uses: Urinary and upper respiratory tract infections; lymphogranuloma venereum.

Special Concerns: Pregnancy category: C (safe use during pregnancy has not been established). May be an increased risk of severe side effects in elderly patients.

Dosage: Oral Suspension, Tablets. Adults, initially: 2 g; **then,** 1 g in morning and evening (for severe infections, give 2 g initially; then, 1 g t.i.d.). **Infants over 2 months, initial:** 50–60 mg/kg;

then, 25–30 mg/kg in morning and evening, not to exceed 75 mg/kg/day. *Lymphogranuloma venereum:* 1 g b.i.d. for 2 weeks.

NURSING CONSIDERATIONS

See *General Nursing Considerations For All Anti-Infectives* under *Penicillins,* p. 140, and for *Sulfonamides,* p. 207.

SULFAMETHOXAZOLE AND PHENAZOPYRIDINE
(sul-fah-meh-**THOX**-ah-zohl, **FEN**-nay-zoh-**PEER**-ih-deen)

Azo Gantanol, Azo Sulfamethoxazole, Uro Gantanol✳ (Rx)

Classification/Content: *Sulfonamide:* sulfamethoxazole, 500 mg and *urinary analgesic:* phenazopyridine, 100 mg.

See also *Sulfamethoxazole,* p. 211, and *Phenazopyridine,* p. 271.

Uses: Urinary tract infections.

Contraindications: Use in children less than 12 years of age.

Special Concerns: Pregnancy category: C.

Dosage: Tablets. Adults and children over 12 years of age, initially: 2 g sulfamethoxazole and 400 mg phenazopyridine; **then,** 1 g sulfamethoxazole and 200 mg phenazopyridine q 12 hr for up to 3 days. Dose should be decreased in patients with impaired renal function.

NURSING CONSIDERATIONS

See *General Nursing Considerations For All Anti-Infectives* under *Penicillins,* p. 140, and for *Sulfonamides,* p. 203.

Client/Family Teaching

1. Fluid intake must be adequate for urine output to be at least 1,200–1,500 mL daily. Maintain record of intake and output.
2. If GI upset occurs, the drug may be taken with or after meals.

Evaluation

Assess response to therapy and review record of intake and output to determine if dosage should be decreased.

SULFAMETHOXAZOLE AND TRIMETHOPRIM (sul-fah-meh-**THOX**-ah-zohl, try-**METH**-oh-prim)

Apo-Sulfatrim✳, Bactrim, Bactrim DS, Bethaprim, Cheragan w/TMP, Cotrim, Cotrim DS, Novotrimel✳, Novotrimel DS✳, Protrin✳, Protrin DF✳, Roubac✳, Septra, Septra DS, Sulfamethoprim, Sulfamethoprim DS, Sulfaprim, Sulfaprim DS, Sulfatrim, Sulfatrim DS, Sulfoxaprim, Sulfoxaprim DS, Sulmeprim, Triazole, Triazole DS, Trimeth-Sulfa, Trisulfam, Uroplus DS, Urpoplus SS (Rx)

See also *Sulfonamides,* p. 203.

Classification/Content: These products contain the antibacterial agents sulfamethoxazole and trimethoprim.

See also *Sulfamethoxazole,* p. 211.**Oral Suspension:** sulfamethoxazole, 200 mg and trimethoprim, 40 mg/5 mL. **Tablets:** sulfamethoxazole, 400 mg and trimethoprim, 80 mg/tablet. **Double Strength (DS) Tablets:** sulfamethoxazole, 800 mg and trimethoprim, 160 mg/tablet. **Concentrate for injection:** sulfamethoxazole, 80 mg and trimethoprim, 16 mg/mL.

Uses: Urinary tract infections, acute otitis media, acute exacerbation of chronic bronchitis (adults), enteritis caused by *Shigella, Pneumocystis carinii* pneumonia in AIDS patients.

Additional Contraindications: Infants under one month of age. Megaloblastic anemia due to folate deficiency.

Special Concerns: Pregnancy category: C. Use with caution in impaired liver or kidney function.

Dosage: *Urinary tract infections, shigellosis, bronchitis, acute otitis media.* **Adults:** One DS tablet, 2 tablets, or 4 teaspoonfuls of suspension q 12 hr for 10–14 days. **Pediatric:** Total daily dose of 8 mg/kg trimethoprim and 40 mg/kg sulfamethoxazole divided equally and given q 12 hr for 10–14 days (**Note:** For shigellosis, give adult or pediatric dose for 7 days.) *Prostatitis, acute bacterial:* One DS tablet b.i.d. until patient is afebrile for 2 days. *Prostatitis, chronic bacterial:* One DS tablet b.i.d. for 4–6 weeks. *Chancroid:* 1 DS tablet b.i.d. for at least 7 days (alternate therapy: 4 DS tablets in a single dose). *Pharyngeal gonococcal infection due to penicillinase-producing Neisseria gonorrhoeae:* 720 mg trimethoprim and 3,600 mg sulfamethoxazole once daily for 5 days. *P. carinii pneumonia:* **Adults and children:** Total daily dose of 20 mg/kg trimethoprim and 100 mg/kg sulfamethoxazole divided equally and given q 6 hr for 14 days.

NURSING CONSIDERATIONS

See *General Nursing Considerations For All Anti-Infectives* under *Penicillins,* p. 140, and for *Sulfonamides,* p. 207.

Administration/Storage

1. The IV infusion must be administered over a period of 60–90 min.
2. Each 5 mL of the IV infusion must be diluted to 125 mL with 5% dextrose in water and used within 6 hr. If the amount of fluid should be restricted, each 5 mL can be diluted up to 75 mL with 5% dextrose in water and used within 2 hr. The diluted solution should not be refrigerated.
3. The IV infusion should not be mixed with any other drugs or solutions.
4. If the diluted IV infusion is cloudy or precipitates after mixing, it should be discarded and a new solution prepared.

Interventions

1. Obtain baseline lab data to evaluate liver and renal function.
2. Assess for anemia as megaloblastic anemia due to folate deficiency is a contraindication for this drug therapy.

SULFASALAZINE   (sul-fah-**SAL**-ah-zeen)

Azaline, Azulfidine, Azulfidine EN-Tabs, PMS Sulfasalazine ✽, PMS Sulfasalazine E.C.✽, Salazopyrin✽, Salazopyrin-EN Tabs✽, S.A.S.✽. S.A.S. Enteric✽ (Rx)

See also *Sulfonamides,* p. 203.

Action/Kinetics: About one-third of the dose of sulfasalazine passes to the colon, where it is split to 5-aminosalicylic acid and sulfapyridine. The drug does not affect the microflora.

Use: Ulcerative colitis.

Additional Contraindications: Children below 2 years, persons with marked sulfonamide and salicylate hypersensitivity.

Special Concerns: Pregnancy category: B.

Additional Drug Interactions	
Digoxin	Sulfasalazine ↓ effect due to ↓ absorption from GI tract
Ferrous sulfate	Ferrous sulfate ↓ blood levels of sulfasalazine

Dosage: Oral Suspension, Enteric-coated Tablets, Tablets. Adults: initial, 3–4 g daily in divided doses; **maintenance:** 500 mg q.i.d. **Pediatric, initial:** 40–60 mg/kg daily in 3–6 equally divided doses; **maintenance:** 30 mg/kg daily in 4 divided doses. *For desensitization to sulfasalazine:* Reinstitute at level of 50–250 mg daily; **then,** give double dose q 4–7 days until desired therapeutic level reached. Use oral suspension.

NURSING CONSIDERATIONS

See *General Nursing Considerations For All Anti-Infectives* under *Penicillins,* p. 140, and for *Sulfonamides,* p. 207.

Client/Family Teaching

Stress the importance of taking medication exactly as ordered since intermittent therapy (2 weeks on, 2 weeks off) is generally recommended.

SULFISOXAZOLE (sul-fah-**SOX**-ah-zohl)

Gantrisin, Novosoxazole ✦ (Rx)

SULFISOXAZOLE ACETYL (sul-fah-**SOX**-ah-zohl ah-**SEE**-till)

Gantrisin, Lipo Gantrisin (Rx)

SULFISOXAZOLE DIOLAMINE (sul-fah-**SOX**-ah-zohl, dye-**OHL**-ah-meen)

Gantrisin Diolamine (Rx)

See also *Sulfonamides,* p. 203.

Classification: Sulfonamide, short-acting.

Action/Kinetics: $t^{1/2}$: 5.9 hr. Lipo Gantrisin contains sulfisoxazole acetyl in a homogenized vegetable oil mixture.

Uses: Urinary tract infections, topical and ophthalmic infections (including trachoma).

Special Concerns: Pregnancy category: C.

Additional Drug Interaction: Sulfisoxazole may ↑ effects of thiopental due to ↓ plasma protein binding.

Dosage: Oral Suspension, Extended-release Tablets. Adults, initial: 2–4 g; **maintenance:** 4–8 g daily in 4–6 divided doses. **Infants over 2 months, initial:** 75 mg/kg/day; **maintenance:** 150 mg/kg/day in 4–6 doses, up to maximum of 6 g/day. **IM, IV (slow injection or drip), SC: Initially,** 50 mg/kg; **then,** 100 mg/kg in 2–4 divided doses.

Acetyl. **Ophthalmic Solution:** 1–2 gtt in conjunctival sac q 2–3 hr. **Ointment:** Small amount in conjunctival sac 1–3 times during the day and at bedtime.

Diolamine. **Ophthalmic solution (4%):** 1–2 gtt into conjunctival sac several times daily. **Ophthalmic ointment (4%):** Small amount in conjunctival sac 1–3 times daily and at bedtime.

NURSING CONSIDERATIONS

See *General Nursing Considerations For All Anti-Infectives* under *Penicillins,* p. 140, and for *Sulfonamides,* p. 207.

Administration/Storage

For SC administration, dilute commercial solution containing 400 mg/mL with sterile water for injection, to obtain solution containing 50 mg/mL.

SULFISOXAZOLE AND PHENAZOPYRIDINE   (sul-fah-**SOX**-ah-zohl, fen-ay-zoh-**PEER**-ih-deen)

Azo-Cheragan, Azo Gantrisin, Axo-Sulfisoxazole, Azo-Truxazole, Sul-Azo (Rx)

Classification/Content: Each of the products contains sulfisoxazole (antibacterial), 500 mg and phenazopyridine (urinary analgesic), 50 mg.

Also, see information on individual components.

Uses: For the first 2 days in treating uncomplicated urinary tract infections. Sulfisoxazole can be used alone after the first 2 days.

Special Concerns: Pregnancy category: C.

Dosage: Tablets. Adults, initial: 4–6 tablets; **then,** 2 tablets q.i.d. for 2 days.

NURSING CONSIDERATIONS

See *General Nursing Considerations For All Anti-Infectives* under *Penicillins,* p. 140, and for *Sulfonamides,* p. 207.

CHAPTER TWELVE
Anthelmintics

General Statement: Helminthiasis, or infestation of the body by parasites, is a common affliction. Helminths (worms) may infect the intestinal lumen, or the worm also may migrate to a particular tissue. Treatment of helminth infections is complicated by the fact that a worm may have one or more morphological stages. Thus, it is important to ensure that therapy rids the body of eggs and larvae, as well as worms. Also, a patient may be infected by more than one type of worm. Factors such as availability and cost of the drug, toxicity, ease of administration, and how long it takes to complete therapy also have a significant impact on successful treatment of helminths. Accurate diagnosis is extremely important before treatment is started, because its success depends on selecting the drug best suited for the eradication of a specific infestation. Parasites that infest only the intestinal tract can be eradicated by locally acting drugs. Other parasites enter tissues and must be treated by drugs that are absorbed from the GI tract.

Since many parasitic infestations are transmitted by persons sharing bathroom facilities, the physician may wish to examine all members of the household for parasitic infestation. Treatment is often accompanied or followed by repeated laboratory examinations to determine whether the parasite has been eradicated.

Helminths can be divided into three groups: cestodes (flatworms, tapeworms), nematodes (roundworms), and trematodes (flukes). The following is a brief description of the more common helminths and the drug of choice to treat infections by that particular helminth.

Cestodes (Flatworms, Tapeworms)

The more common tapeworms are the beef tapeworm (*Taenia saginata*), pork tapeworm (*T. solium*), dwarf tapeworm (*Hymenolepis nana*), and the fish tapeworm (*Diphyllobothrium latum*). The tapeworm consists of a scolex or head that hooks into a segment of intestine. The body is that of a segmented flatworm, sections of which are found in the stools. Tapeworm infestations are difficult to eradicate but have few side effects. **Drug treatment:** niclosamide and praziquantel.

Nematodes

1. **Filaria (filariasis).** Infections due to *Wuchereria bancrofti, Brugia malayi,* and *B. timori* are transmitted by mosquitoes. These parasites are tiny roundworms that migrate into the lymphatic system and bloodstream. Living and dead worms can obstruct the lymphatic system, causing elephantiasis. Mosquito control is the best means of combating this infestation.

Other filarial infections include *Loa loa,* transmitted by the bite of a horsefly, and *Onchocerca volvulus* (onchocerciasis, river blindness), which is transmitted by the bite of a blackfly.

Drug treatment: Diethylcarbamazine. Suramin sodium (available from Centers for Disease Control) is used to treat onchocerciasis.

2. **Hookworm (uncinariasis).** Intestinal infection caused by *Ancylostoma duodenale* or

Necator americanus, these infections cause debilitation resulting in iron-deficiency anemia, characterized by fatigue, lassitude, and apathy. **Drug treatment:** Mebendazole or pyrantel pamoate.

3. **Pinworm (enterobiasis).** These intestinal infestations are common in school-age children. Complications are rare, although heavy infestations may cause abdominal pain, weight loss, and insomnia. **Drug treatment:** Mebendazole, piperazine, pyrantel pamoate, pyrvinium pamoate, thiabendazole.

4. **Roundworm (ascariasis).** Caused by *Ascaris lumbricoides,* this infection can cause obstruction of the respiratory and GI tracts. **Drug treatment:** Mebendazole, pyrantel pamoate.

5. **Trichinosis.** Caused by *Trichinella spiralis,* these parasites are transmitted by the consumption of raw or inadequately cooked pork. The infection is serious; larvae burrow into the bloodstream and form cysts in skeletal muscle. **Drug treatment:** Corticosteroids to control the inflammation caused by systemic infestation; mebendazole, thiabendazole.

6. **Threadworm (strongyloidiasis).** This parasite (*Strongyloides stercoralis*) infests the upper GI tract. Heavy infestations can result in malabsorption syndrome, diarrhea, and general discomfort. **Drug treatment:** Thiabendazole.

7. **Whipworm (trichuriasis).** This threadlike parasite (*Trichuris trichiura*) lodges in the mucosa of the cecum. **Drug treatment:** Mebendazole.

Trematodes

Schistosomiasis (blood flukes or bilharziasis) can be transmitted by contaminated water supplies. The organisms are *Schistosoma mansoni, S. japonicum, S. haematobium,* and *S. mekongi.* The infection is difficult to eradicate. **Drug treatment:** Praziquantel, oxamniquine (*S. mansoni* only).

Side Effects: Since the anthelmintics do not belong to any one chemical group, their side effects are related to specific compounds. However, nausea, vomiting, cramps, and diarrhea are common to most.

NURSING CONSIDERATIONS

See also *General Nursing Considerations For All Anti-infectives* under *Penicillins,* p. 140.

Client/Family Teaching

1. Provide the client/family with written instructions regarding diet, cathartics, enemas, medications, and follow-up tests when treatment is to be carried out at home.
2. Review these instructions with client/family to be sure they are understood by the person responsible for the client's treatment and care. *Good hygienic practices reduce the incidence of helminthiasis.*
3. Emphasize the need for follow-up examinations to check the results of treatment.
4. Specific practices are as follows:

Pinworms

1. Instruct responsible family member how to prevent infestation with pinworms by:
   • washing hands after toileting and before meals.
   • keeping nails short.
   • washing ova from anal area in the morning.
   • applying antipruritic ointment to anal area to reduce scratching, which transfers pinworms.
2. Alert family that physician may wish all members to be examined for pinworms.
3. After the end of the treatment course, swab the perianal area each morning with transparent tape until no further eggs are found on microscopic examination for 7 consecutive days.

12

Roundworms

Two to 3 weeks after therapy, stools should undergo microscopic examination to determine fecal egg count. Stools must be examined daily until no further roundworm ova are found.

Hookworm/Tapeworm

After administration of medication, cathartics, and enema, examine the results of the enema for the head of the worm, which will appear bright yellow.

Evaluation

1. Assess client/family knowledge and understanding of illness and response to therapy and teaching.
2. Check for evidence of eggs and worms and send specimens for microscopic examination to determine effectiveness of drug therapy.

MEBENDAZOLE   (meh-**BEN**-dah-zohl)

Vermox (Rx)

See also *Anthelmintics,* p. 216.

Classification: Anthelmintic.

Action/Kinetics: Mebendazole exerts its anthelmintic effect by blocking the glucose uptake of the organisms, thereby reducing their energy until death results. **Peak plasma levels:** 2–4 hr. Poorly absorbed from the GI tract. Excreted in feces.

Uses: Whipworm, pinworm, roundworm, common and American hookworm infections; in single or mixed infections.

Contraindications: Hypersensitivity to mebendazole.

Special Concerns: Pregnancy category: C. Use with caution in children under 2 years of age.

Side Effects: Transient abdominal pain and diarrhea.

Dosage: Tablets, Chewable. *Whipworm, roundworm, and hookworm:* **PO, adults and children:** 1 tablet morning and evening on 3 consecutive days. *Pinworms:* one tablet, one time. All treatments can be repeated after 3 weeks.

NURSING CONSIDERATIONS

See *Nursing Considerations* for *Anthelmintics,* p. 217, and *General Nursing Considerations For All Anti-Infectives* under *Penicillins,* p. 140.

Client/Family Teaching

1. Tablet may be chewed, crushed, and/or mixed with food.
2. No prior fasting, purging, or other procedures are required.

NICLOSAMIDE   (nye-**KLOH**-sah-myd)

Niclocide (Rx)

Classification: Anthelmintic.

Action/Kinetics: Niclosamide acts by inhibiting oxidative phosphorylation in the mitochondria of the helminth. Anaerobic metabolism may be inhibited also. The proximal segments and scolex are killed following contact with the drug. The drug is not absorbed from the GI tract, and excreted through the feces.

Uses: Beef tapeworm *(Taenia saginata),* dwarf tapeworm *(Hymenolepsis nana),* fish tapeworm *(Diphyllobothrium latum,)* pork tapeworm *(Taenia solium).*

Special Concerns: Pregnancy category: B. Safety and efficacy in pregnancy, lactation, and in children under 2 years of age have not been established.

Side Effects: *GI:* Nausea and vomiting (most common), loss of appetite, abdominal discomfort, diarrhea, constipation, rectal bleeding, bad taste in mouth, irritation of oral mucosa. *Topical:* Skin rashes, alopecia. *CNS:* Dizziness, drowsiness, headache, weakness. *Miscellaneous:* Backache, irritability, fever, palpitations, sweating.

Dosage: Tablets, Chewable. *Beef and fish tapeworm.* **Adults:** 2 g as single dose. **Pediatric, over 34 kg:** 1.5 g as single dose; **pediatric, 11.4–34 kg:** 1.0 g as single dose. *Dwarf tapeworm:* **Adults,** 2.0 g as single daily dose for 7 days. **Pediatric, over 34 kg:** 1.5 g on first day; **then,** 1.0 g daily for next 6 days. **Pediatric, 11.4–34 kg:** 1.0 g on first day; **then,** 0.5 g daily for next 6 days.

NURSING CONSIDERATIONS

See also *Nursing Considerations* for *Anthelmintics,* p. 217.

Client/Family Teaching

1. Tablets should be chewed thoroughly and swallowed with a little water. For small children, a paste may be made by crushing the tablets with a small amount of water.
2. The drug should be taken after a light meal, as GI upset may occur.
3. If constipation occurs, a mild laxative may be used.
4. The scolex (head) of the tapeworm may be digested in the intestine and thus may not be found in the feces.
5. The stool must be negative for 3 months before the client is considered cured.
6. Stress the importance of taking the medication exactly as ordered and for the specified duration.
7. Report for stool examinations as scheduled to evaluate the effectiveness of drug therapy.
8. Instruct client not to perform activities that require mental alertness, because drug may cause drowsiness and dizziness.

Evaluation

Assess client response to therapy based on stool examinations.

OXAMNIQUINE   (ox-**AM**-nih-kwin)

Vansil (Rx)

Classification: Anthelmintic, antischistosomal.

Action/Kinetics: *S. mansoni* is a trematode parasite found in Egypt, elsewhere in Africa, South America, and the West Indies, including Puerto Rico. The agent is found in water and is transmitted by snails. The drug causes the worms to shift from the mesenteric veins to the liver where, they are destroyed. Oxamniquine is more effective against male than against female schistosomes, but females cease laying eggs following treatment; thus, the infection eventually subsides due to decreased reproduction. **Peak plasma concentration:** 1–1.5 hr. $t^{1}/_{2}$: 1–2.5 hr. The drug is well absorbed after PO administration. Inactive metabolites are excreted in urine.

Uses: All stages of *Schistosoma mansoni* infections (acute and chronic), including involvement of the liver and spleen.

Special Concerns: Pregnancy category: C. Use during pregnancy and lactation only when potential benefits outweigh risks.

Side Effects: Well tolerated. *CNS:* Transient drowsiness and dizziness, headaches. Convulsions have been observed, but mostly in epileptics; therefore, closely monitor patients with history of convulsive disorders. *GI:* Nausea, vomiting, abdominal pain, anorexia. *Dermatologic:* Urticaria.

Dosage: Capsules. Adults: 12–15 mg/kg as single oral dose. **Children (under 30 kg):** 10 mg/kg followed in 2–8 hr with a second 10 mg/kg dose.

NURSING CONSIDERATIONS

See also *Anthelmintics,* p. 216, and *Nursing Considerations For All Anti-Infectives* under *Penicillins,* p. 140.

Client/Family Teaching

1. Inform client not to drive a car or not to operate hazardous machinery, because drug may cause dizziness and/or drowsiness.
2. Administer after food to minimize GI distress.

PIPERAZINE CITRATE   (pip-EHR-ah-zeen)

Vermizine (Rx)

See also *Anthelmintics,* p. 216.

Classification: Anthelmintic.

Action/Kinetics: The drug is believed to paralyze the muscles of parasites; this dislodges the parasites and promotes their elimination. The drug is readily absorbed from the GI tract, is partially metabolized by the liver, and the remainder is excreted in urine. Rate of elimination differs among patients.

Uses: Pinworm (oxyuriasis) and roundworm (ascariasis) infestations. Particularly recommended for pediatric use.

Contraindications: Impaired liver or kidney function, seizure disorders, hypersensitivity.

Special Concerns: Safe use during pregnancy has not been established.

Side Effects: Piperazine has low toxicity. *GI:* Nausea, vomiting, diarrhea, cramps. *CNS:* Tremors, headache, vertigo, decreased reflexes, paresthesias, seizures, ataxia, chorea, memory decrement. *Ophthalmologic:* Nystagmus, blurred vision, cataracts, strabismus. *Allergic:* Urticaria, fever, skin reactions, purpura, lacrimation, rhinorrhea, arthralgia, bronchospasm, cough. *Miscellaneous:* Muscle weakness.

Drug Interactions: Concomitant administration of piperazine and phenothiazines may result in an increase in extrapyramidal effects (including violent convulsions) caused by phenothiazines.

Laboratory Test Interference: False − or ↓ uric acid values.

Dosage: Syrup, Tablets. *Pinworms:* **Adults and children,** 65 mg/kg as a single daily dose for 7 days up to a maximum daily dose of 2.5 g. *Roundworms:* **Adults,** one dose of 3.5 g/day for 2 consecutive days; **pediatric,** one dose of 75 mg/kg/day for 2 consecutive days, not to exceed 3.5 g daily. For severe infections, repeat therapy after 1 week.

NURSING CONSIDERATIONS

See also *Nursing Considerations* for *Anthelmintics,* p. 217.

Client/Family Teaching

1. Keep pleasant-tasting medication out of reach of children.
2. Take medication after breakfast or in 2 divided doses.
3. Report any adverse drug effects to physician immediately.

Evaluation

Assess client response to therapy based on stool examinations.

PRAZIQUANTEL   (pray-zih-**KWON**-tel)

Biltricide (Rx)

Classification: Anthelmintic.

Action/Kinetics: Praziquantel causes increased cell permeability in the helminth, resulting in a loss of intracellular calcium with massive contractions, and paralysis of musculature with breakdown of the integrity of the organism. Thus, phagocytes can attack the parasite and death follows. **Maximum serum levels:** 1–3 hr. **t½:** 0.8–1.5 hr. Significant first-pass effect. Excreted primarily in the urine.

Uses: Schistosomal infections due to *Schistosoma japonicum, S. mansoni, S. mekongi,* and *S. haematobium. Investigational:* Liver flukes, neurocysticercosis.

Contraindications: Ocular cysticercosis. Lactation.

Special Concerns: Pregnancy category: B (use with caution in pregnancy). Safety in children less than 4 years of age not established.

Side Effects: *GI:* Nausea, abdominal discomfort. *CNS:* Malaise, headache, dizziness, drowsiness. *Miscellaneous:* Fever, urticaria (rare). **Note:** These side effects may also be due to the helminth infection itself.

Dosage: Tablets. Three doses of 20 mg/kg, with an interval between doses of not less than 4 hr or more than 6 hr.

NURSING CONSIDERATIONS

See *Nursing Considerations* for *Anthelmintics,* p. 217.

Assessment

The client should be hospitalized for treatment if the schistosomiasis or fluke infection is accompanied by cerebral cysticercosis.

Client/Family Teaching

1. Due to dizziness and drowsiness, caution should be exercised while driving or performing tasks requiring alertness.
2. The tablets should be taken during meals with liquids. The tablets should not be chewed.

PYRANTEL PAMOATE   (pih-**RAN**-tel)

Antiminth, Combantrin ✸ (Rx)

See also *Anthelmintics,* p. 216.

Classification: Anthelmintic.

Action/Kinetics: The anthelmintic effect is attributed to the neuromuscular blocking effect of this agent, which paralyzes the helminth, allowing it to be expelled through the feces. It is poorly absorbed from GI tract. **Peak plasma levels:** 0.05–0.13 mcg/mL after 1–3 hr. Partially metabolized in liver. Fifty percent is excreted unchanged in feces, and less than 15% excreted unchanged in urine.

Uses: Pinworm and roundworm infestations. Multiple helminth infections.

Special Concerns: Use with caution in presence of liver dysfunction. Safe use during pregnancy and in children less than 2 years of age has not been established.

Side Effects: *GI* (most frequent): Anorexia, nausea, vomiting, cramps, diarrhea. *Hepatic:* Transient elevation of SGOT. *CNS:* Headache, dizziness, drowsiness, insomnia. *Miscellaneous:* Skin rashes.

Drug Interactions: Use with piperazine for ascariasis results in antagonism of the effect of both drugs.

Dosage: Oral Suspension, Tablets. Adults and children: 1 dose of 11 mg/kg (maximum). **Maximum total dose:** 1.0 g.

NURSING CONSIDERATIONS

See also *Nursing Considerations* for *Anthelmintics,* p. 217.

Client/Family Teaching

1. Drug may be taken without regard to food intake.
2. Purging is not necessary prior to or during treatment.
3. Drug may be taken with milk or fruit juice.
4. Mix powder with liquid just prior to administering; otherwise, the mixture may become thick and difficult to drink.

THIABENDAZOLE   (thigh-ah-**BEN**-dah-zohl)

Mintezol (Rx)

See also *Anthelmintics,* p. 216.

Classification: Anthelmintic.

Action/Kinetics: The drug interferes with the enzyme fumarate reductase, which is specific to several helminths. It is readily absorbed from the GI tract. **Peak plasma levels:** 1–2 hr. **t½:** 0.9–2 hr. Most of the drug is excreted within 24 hr, mainly through the urine.

Uses: Cutaneous larva migrans, pinworms, threadworms, large roundworms, hookworms, and whipworms. Particularly useful for the treatment of mixed infestations. To reduce symptoms of trichinosis during the invasive phase.

Special Concerns: Pregnancy category: C (safe use during pregnancy has not been established).

Safety and efficacy not established in children less than 13.6 kg. Use with caution in patients with hepatic disease or impaired hepatic function.

Side Effects: *GI:* Nausea, vomiting, anorexia, diarrhea, epigastric distress. *CNS:* Dizziness, drowsiness, headache, irritability, seizures. *Allergic:* Pruritus, angioedema, flushing of face, chills, fever, skin rashes, Stevens-Johnson syndrome, anaphylaxis, lymphadenopathy. *Hepatic:* Jaundice, cholestasis, liver damage, transient increase in SGOT. *Renal:* Crystalluria, hematuria, enuresis, foul odor of urine. *Miscellaneous:* Tinnitus, blurred vision, hypotension, collapse, hyperglycemia, leukopenia, perianal rash.

Dosage: Oral Suspension, Chewable Tablets: 25 mg/kg body weight b.i.d. up to a maximum of 3.0 g/day.

NURSING CONSIDERATIONS

See also *Nursing Considerations* for *Anthelmintics,* p. 217.

Administration/Storage

For strongyloidiasis, cutaneous larva migrans, hookworm, whipworm, or roundworm, 2 doses/day are given for 2 days. For trichinelliasis, give 2 doses/day for 2–4 days. For pinworm, give 2 doses for 1 day, repeat after 7–14 days.

Client/Family Teaching

1. Administer the drug after meals.
2. Decribe CNS disturbances (including muscular weakness and loss of mental alertness) that may be caused by the drug.
3. The client should not operate hazardous machinery after taking the medication.

CHAPTER THIRTEEN

Antitubercular Agents/ Leprostatics

ANTITUBERCULAR AGENTS

General Statement: Tuberculosis is rarely treated by a single drug, because this usually leads to the emergence of resistant strains. Treatment with drugs is usually chronic due to the slow growth rate of mycobacterium. The long duration of drug treatment increases the risk of side effects. Drugs for the treatment of tuberculosis are categorized as either first-line or second-line, depending on their efficacy, activity, and incidence of side effects.

The first-line drugs for the treatment of tuberculosis are ethambutol, isoniazid, rifampin, and streptomycin. Second-line agents include capreomycin, cycloserine, ethionamide, kanamycin, para-aminosalicylic acid, pyrazinamide, and viomycin sulfate. The second-line agents are generally less effective and more toxic than first-line drugs; they are used only when *Mycobacterium tuberculosis* organisms are resistant to first-line therapy. Importantly, drugs with similar toxicity (e.g., ototoxicity or nephrotoxicity) should not be combined.

NURSING CONSIDERATIONS

See also *Nursing Considerations For All Anti-Infectives* under *Penicillins,* p. 140.

Interventions

1. Anticipate that more than one antitubercular agent will be given concomitantly to prevent the emergence of a resistant strain.
2. Do not administer concomitantly antitubercular agents that are highly ototoxic.
3. Obtain appropriate lab data to assess for nephrotoxicity, ototoxicity, and hepatotoxicity, caused by most antitubercular agents.
4. Incorporate safety precautions to protect the client manifesting vestibular difficulties during ambulation to prevent falls and injury.

5. Provide clients with the support necessary to encourage them to complete the long period of therapy for cure.

Client/Family Teaching

1. Explain the nature of tuberculosis infections and how to protect others from contracting the disease.
2. Stress the importance of taking prescribed drugs as ordered and of reporting for monthly check-ups and laboratory studies.
3. Local support groups may assist them to understand and cope with this disease and help them to complete the long period of therapy for cure.

Evaluation

Assess client/family knowledge and understanding of illness, response to therapy based on lab criteria and development of toxic side effects that may interfere with therapy.

AMINOSALICYLATE SODIUM   (ah-meen-oh-sah-**LIH**-sil-ate)

Nemasol Sodium✳, Tubasal(Rx)

Classification: Second-line antitubercular agent.

Action/Kinetics: Aminosalicylic acid interferes with folic acid synthesis of susceptible tubercle microorganisms. The drug is bacteriostatic, readily absorbed from the GI tract, and well distributed in body tissues. **Time to peak serum levels:** 1–2 hr. **t½:** 1 hr. The unchanged (14%–33%) metabolized (50%) drug is excreted in the urine.

Uses: Adjuvant to other tuberculostatic agents in the treatment of pulmonary and extrapulmonary tuberculosis. Often used concurrently with isoniazid and/or streptomycin.

Contraindications: Hypersensitivity to Aminosalyicilate sodium.

Special Concerns: Safe use during pregnancy has not been established. Use with caution in patients with impaired renal or hepatic function, gastric ulcer, or congestive heart failure.

Side Effects: *GI:* Nausea, vomiting, diarrhea, abdominal pain. *Allergic:* Fever, skin rashes, hepatitis. *Hematologic:* Agranulocytosis, thrombocytopenia, hemolytic anemia, leukopenia. *Miscellaneous:* Jaundice, vasculitis, encephalopathy, syndrome resembling infectious mononucleosis, goiter.

13

Drug Interactions	
Ammonium chloride	↑ Chance of aminosalicylic acid crystalluria
Anticoagulants, oral	Additive effect on prothrombin time
Ascorbic acid	↑ Chance of aminosalicylic acid crystalluria
Isoniazid	↑ Effect of isoniazid due to ↓ metabolism
Para-aminobenzoic acid (PABA)	Inhibits activity of aminosalicylic acid
Phenytoin	↑ Effect of phenytoin
Probenecid	↑ Effect of aminosalicylic acid by ↓ excretion by kidneys
Pyrazinamide	↓ Pharmacologic effect of pyrazinamide
Rifampin	↓ Effect of rifampin due to ↓ absorption from GI tract
Salicylates	Possible ↑ effect of Aminosalicylate due to ↓ excretion by kidneys or ↓ plasma protein binding

Laboratory Test Interferences: Discolors urine. False + acetoacetic acid test.

Dosage: Tablets. Adults: 14–16 g/day in 2–3 divided doses. **Pediatric:** 275–420 mg/kg daily in 3–4 divided doses.

NURSING CONSIDERATIONS

See also *Nursing Considerations For All Anti-infectives* under *Penicillins,* p. 140, and *Antitubercular Agents,* p. 224.

Administration/Storage

1. Store in a light-resistant dry jar at a cool temperature.
2. Solutions for oral administration should be used within 24 hr and under no circumstances if color is darker than that of a freshly prepared solution.

Interventions

1. *Assess*
   * for GI distress, which usually disappears after several days of therapy. Persistence may require cessation of therapy.
   * for hypersensitivity reaction characterized by a rise in body temperature (102°F–104°F; 39°F–40°C) in previously afebrile clients.
   * for goiter and hypothyroidism. Anticipate physician ordering thyroid therapy if conditions appear.
   * for electrolyte imbalance in clients with cardiac or renal disease. Monitor electrolyte levels and liver and renal function studies.
2. Use Tes-Tape, Clinistix, or Diastix to evaluate glycosuria because a false-positive reaction may be obtained with Benedict's solution, Clinitest tablets, or Fehling's solution. Finger sticks for blood sugars may prove most accurate.

Client/Family Teaching

1. Administer with meals to minimize GI irritation or with 5–10 mL of aluminum hydroxide, as ordered by the physician.
2. Drug may discolor urine.
3. Report any bothersome side effects to physician before discontinuing therapy.

Evaluation

Assess client response to therapy based on appropriate lab criteria.

CAPREOMYCIN SULFATE (kap-ree-oh-**MY**-sin)

Capastat (Rx)

Classification: Second-line antitubercular agent.

Action/Kinetics: Action unknown. Capreomycin is bactericidal; drug must be administered parenterally. Cross resistance has been noted with kanamycin and neomycin. **Time to peak serum levels:** 1–2 hr after IM. **Peak serum levels, IM:** 20–47 mcg/mL after 1–2 hr. **t½:** 3–6 hr. Primarily excreted unchanged in the urine.

Uses: Resistant-type tubercle bacillus. Should always be given in combination with other antitubercular agents.

Contraindications: Hypersensitivity to drug. Never use together with streptomycin.

Special Concerns: Safe use in pregnancy is not known. Use with caution in renal insufficiency or auditory impairment.

Side Effects: Nephrotoxicity, hepatic toxicity, ototoxicity (tinnitus, vertigo). *Hematologic:* Leukopenia, leukocytosis, eosinophilia. *Allergic:* Urticaria, skin rashes, fever. *Miscellaneous:* Pain at injection site, sterile abscesses, bleeding at injection site. Hypokalemia.

Dosage: IM, deep: 1.0 g daily (not to exceed 20 mg/kg/day) for 60–120 days, followed by 1.0 g every 2–3 weeks. Therapy should be maintained for 18–24 months.

NURSING CONSIDERATIONS

See also *Nursing Considerations For All Anti-Infectives* under *Penicillins,* p. 140, and *Antitubercular Agents,* p. 224.

Administration/Storage

1. Reconstituted solutions are stable for 48 hr at room temperature and for 14 days when refrigerated.
2. Capreomycin sulfate injections may develop a pale straw color and darken, but this does not affect the efficacy of the product.
3. Never use together with streptomycin.

Interventions

1. *Assess*
   * for ototoxicity manifested by damage to vestibular and auditory portion of eighth cranial nerve, tinnitus, deafness, dizziness, and ataxia.
   * for symptoms of nephrotoxicity evidenced by decreasing renal function. If renal function is impaired, client must be evaluated for either reduction of the dose or discontinuation of the drug.
2. Obtain baseline complete blood count and liver and renal function studies; monitor these parameters throughout therapy.
3. Incorporate safety precautions to protect client with vertigo or ataxia during ambulation.
4. With IM therapy, administer deep into large muscle mass to minimize pain, induration, excessive bleeding, and sterile abscesses at site of injection. Rotate and document injection sites.

CYCLOSERINE   (sye-kloh-**SEE**-reen)
Seromycin (Rx)

Classification: Second-line antitubercular agent.

Action/Kinetics: Broad-spectrum antibiotic is produced by a strain of *Streptomyces orchidaceus* or *Garyphalus lavendulae*. Disturbs cell wall synthesis by interfering with the incorporation of the amino acid alanine. The drug is bactericidal and bacteriostatic, well absorbed from the GI tract and widely distributed in body tissues. **Time to peak serum levels:** 3–4 hr. **t½:** 10 hr. From 60% to 70% is excreted unchanged in urine.

Uses: Active pulmonary and extrapulmonary tuberculosis. Indicated only when primary therapy cannot be used. No longer indicated for treatment of urinary tract infections.

Contraindications: Hypersensitivity to cycloserine, epilepsy, depression, severe anxiety, psychosis, severe renal insufficiency, and alcoholism.

Special Concerns: Pregnancy category: C. Safe use during pregnancy and in children has not been established.

Side Effects: *CNS:* Drowsiness, dizziness, headache, mental confusion, tremors, vertigo, loss of memory, psychoses, aggression, increased reflexes, seizures, paresthesias, paresis, dysarthria, coma. Neurotoxic effects depend on blood levels of cycloserine. Hence, frequent determinations of cycloserine blood levels are indicated, especially during the initial period of therapy. *Other:* Skin rashes, increased transaminase.

Drug Interaction: Ethionamide potentiates the CNS toxicity of cycloserine.

Dosage: Capsules. *Tuberculosis:* **initially,** 250 mg q 12 hr for first 2 weeks; **then,** 0.5–1 g daily in divided doses based on blood levels. Dosage should not exceed 1 g daily.

NURSING CONSIDERATIONS

See also *General Nursing Considerations For All Anti-Infectives* under *Penicillins,* p. 140, and *Antitubercular Agents,* p. 224.

Assessment

Obtain thorough nursing and drug history. Note any evidence of depression or alcohol abuse.

Interventions

1. *Assess*
   • for sudden development of congestive heart failure in clients receiving high doses of cycloserine. Monitor serum cycloserine levels throughout therapy.
   • for side effects, especially neurologic reactions, that will necessitate withdrawing the drug, at least for a short period of time. Have available emergency equipment.
2. Obtain baseline parameters and monitor liver and renal function studies throughout therapy.

Client/Family Teaching

Drug causes drowsiness and dizziness; caution against performing tasks that require mental alertness such as driving or operating any machinery.

Evaluation

Assess response to therapy based on appropriate laboratory findings.

ETHAMBUTOL HYDROCHLORIDE   (eh-THAM-byou-tol)

Etibi✳, Myambutol (Rx)

Classification: First-line antitubercular agent.

Action/Kinetics: Tuberculostatic. Arrests multiplication of rapidly dividing tubercle bacilli probably by interfering with RNA synthesis. Readily absorbed after oral administration. Widely distributed in body tissues except CSF. **Peak plasma concentration:** 2–5 mcg/mL after 2–4 hr. **t½:** 3–4 hr. About 65% of metabolized and unchanged drug excreted in urine. Drug accumulates in patients with renal insufficiency.

Uses: Pulmonary tuberculosis in combination with other tuberculostatic drugs.

Contraindications: Hypersensitivity to ethambutol, preexisting optic neuritis, and in children under 13 years of age.

Special Concerns: Should be used with caution and in reduced dosage in patients with gout, impaired renal function, and in pregnant patients.

Side Effects: *Ophthalmologic:* Optic neuritis, decreased visual acuity, loss of color (green) discrimination, temporary loss of vision or blurred vision. *GI:* Nausea, vomiting, anorexia, abdominal pain. *CNS:* Fever, headache, dizziness, confusion, disorientation, malaise, hallucinations. *Allergic:* Pruritus, dermatitis, anaphylaxis. *Miscellaneous:* Peripheral neuropathy (numbness, tingling), precipitation of gout, thrombocytopenia, joint pain, toxic epidermal necrolysis. Renal damage. Also anaphylactic shock, peripheral neuritis (rare), hyperuricemia, and decreased liver function.

Adverse symptoms usually appear during the early months of therapy and disappear thereafter. Periodic renal and hepatic function tests as well as uric acid determinations are recommended.

Dosage: Tablets. Initial treatment: 15 mg/kg/day given once daily until maximal improvement noted; **for retreatment:** 25 mg/kg daily as a single dose with at least one other tuberculostatic drug; **after 60 days:** 15 mg/kg administered once daily.

NURSING CONSIDERATIONS

See also *Nursing Considerations For All Anti-Infectives* under *Penicillins*, p. 140.

Interventions

1. Obtain baseline liver and renal function studies and monitor throughout therapy.
2. Ascertain that client has had visual acuity test before ethambutol therapy and that client does not have preexisting visual problems.

Client/family teaching

1. Stress importance of vision test every 2–4 weeks while on therapy.
2. Reassure client that side effects on eyes generally disappear within several weeks to several months after therapy has been discontinued.
3. Women of childbearing age should practice birth control during therapy. If she should become pregnant, discontinue use of the drug and report immediately to physician.

ETHIONAMIDE (eh-thigh-oh-**NAM**-yd)

Trecator-SC (Rx)

Classification: Second-line antitubercular agent.

Action/Kinetics: Believed to interfere with peptide synthesis of susceptible organisms. Bacteriostatic and bactericidal depending on concentration at the site of infection and susceptibility of the mycobacterium. Well absorbed after oral administration. Widely distributed in body tissues. **Peak plasma concentration:** 3 hr. **t½:** 3 hr. Extensively metabolized by liver. Excreted primarily in urine.

Use: Active tuberculosis (any form). Should be given only with other tuberculostatic drugs after primary therapy has failed.

Contraindications: Children under 12 years of age.

Special Concerns: Use with caution in pregnancy and in children.

Side Effects: *GI:* Nausea, vomiting, anorexia, diarrhea, stomatitis, metallic taste. *CNS:* Asthenia, drowsiness, depression, seizures, dizziness, headache, tremors, restlessness, psychoses. *Ophthalmologic:* Blurred vision, double vision, optic neuritis. *Hepatic:* Jaundice, hepatitis. *Miscellaneous:* Peripheral neuropathy, neuritis, alopecia, acne, skin rashes, postural hypotension, impotence, gynecomastia, menorrhagia, thrombocytopenia, diabetic control more difficult.

Drug Interactions	
Alcohol, ethyl	↑ CNS toxicity of ethionamide
Cycloserine	Ethionamide potentiates CNS toxicity of cycloserine, with possibility of convulsions

Dosage: Tablets. Adults: usual, 0.5–1 g daily in divided doses together with pyridoxine. Given with at least one other tuberculostatic drug.

NURSING CONSIDERATIONS

See also *Nursing Considerations For All Anti-Infectives* under *Penicillins,* p. 140, and *Antitubercular Agents,* p. 224.

Administration

1. Do not administer to children under 12 years of age unless primary therapy has failed.
2. Pyridoxine should be administered with ethionamide.

Interventions

1. *Assess*
   - for toxic effects, particularly severe nausea, that can be treated with antiemetics.
   - for potentiation of toxic effects of cycloserine (congestive heart failure) if given concomitantly.
   - urine or finger sticks of diabetic clients more frequently and also assess for side effects related to diabetes. The latter condition is more difficult to control in clients with tuberculosis.
2. Monitor liver and renal function studies throughout therapy.

Client/Family Teaching

1. Take medication after meals to minimize gastric irritation.
2. Instruct client not to perform any tasks that require mental alertness as drug may cause dizziness and/or drowsiness.

Evaluation

Evaluate response to therapy based on laboratory findings and lack of toxic side effects.

ISONIAZID   (eye-so-NYE-ah-zid)

INH, Isonicotinic Acid Hydrazide, Isotamine❀, Laniazid, Nydrazid, PMS Isoniazid❀, Teebaconin (Rx)

Classification: First-line antitubercular agent.

General Statement: Isoniazid is the most effective tuberculostatic agent. The metabolism of isoniazid is genetically determined and involves the level of a hepatic enzyme. Patients on isoniazid fall into two groups, depending on the manner in which they metabolize isoniazid. As a rule, 50% of whites and blacks inactivate the drug slowly, whereas the majority of American Indians, Eskimos, Japanese, and Chinese are rapid inactivators.

1. **Slow inactivators:** These patients show earlier, favorable response but have more toxic reactions (e.g., neuropathies because of higher blood levels of drug).
2. **Rapid inactivators:** These patients have possible poor clinical response due to rapid inactivation. This group requires an increased daily dose of the drug. They are more likely to develop hepatitis.

Action/Kinetics: Isoniazid probably interferes with lipid and nucleic acid metabolism of growing bacteria, resulting in alteration of the bacterial wall. The drug is tuberculostatic. It is readily absorbed after oral and parenteral (IM) administration and is widely distributed in body tissues. **Peak plasma concentration:** PO, 1–2 hr. $t^{1/2}$, **fast acetylators:** 0.5–6 hr; $t^{1/2}$, **slow acetylators:** 2–5 hr. These values are increased in association with liver and kidney impairment. Drug is metabolized in liver and excreted primarily in urine.

Uses: Tuberculosis caused by human, bovine, and BCG strains of *Mycobacterium tuberculosis*. The drug should not be used as the sole tuberculostatic agent. Prophylaxis of tuberculosis.

Contraindications: Severe hypersensitivity to isoniazid.

Special Concerns: Extreme caution should be exercised in patients with convulsive disorders, in whom the drug should be administered only when the patient is adequately controlled by anticonvulsant medication. Also, use with caution for the treatment of renal tuberculosis and, in the lowest dose possible, in patients with impaired renal function and in alcoholics. Use during pregnancy only if benefits outweigh risks.

Side Effects: Peripheral neuritis, muscle twitches. *CNS:* Ataxia, stupor, seizures, toxic encephalopathy, euphoria, impaired memory, dizziness, toxic psychoses. *GI:* Nausea, vomiting, epigastric distress, xerostomia. *Hypersensitivity:* Fever, skin rashes, vasculitis, lymphadenopathy. *Hepatic:* Liver dysfunction, jaundice, bilirubinemia, hepatitis (especially in patients over 50 years of age). Increases in serum SGOT and SGPT. *Hematologic:* Agranulocytosis, eosinophilia, thrombocytopenia, methemoglobinemia, anemias. *Miscellaneous:* Tinnitus, optic neuritis, optic atrophy, hyperglycemia, metabolic acidosis, urinary retention, gynecomastia in males, lupus-like syndrome, arthralgia.

Note: Pyridoxine, 10–50 mg/day, may be given concomitantly with isoniazid to decrease CNS side effects. Ophthalmologic and liver function tests are recommended periodically.

Drug Interactions	
Aminosalicylic acid	↑ Effect of isoniazid by ↑ blood levels
Atropine	↑ Side effects of isoniazid
Disulfiram	↑ Side effects of isoniazid (especially CNS)
Ethanol	↑ Chance of isoniazid-induced hepatitis
Meperidine	↑ Side effects of isoniazid
Phenytoin	↑ Effect of phenytoin due to ↓ breakdown in liver
Rifampin	Additive liver toxicity

Laboratory Test Interferences: Altered liver function tests. False + or ↑ K, SGOT, SGPT, urine glucose (Benedict's test, Clinitest).

Dosage: Syrup, Tablets. *Active tuberculosis:* **Adults,** 300 mg daily as a single dose; **children and infants:** 10–20 mg/kg/day (up to 300–500 mg total) in a single dose. *Prophylaxis:* **Adults,** 300 mg/day in a single dose; **children and infants:** 10 mg/kg/day (up to 300 mg total) in a single dose. **IM. Adults/adolescents:** *Prophylaxis,* 300 mg daily. *Treatment of tuberculosis:* 5 mg/kg (up to 300 mg) once daily. **Pediatric:** *Prophylaxis,* 10 mg/kg once daily. *Treatment of tuberculosis:* 10–20 mg/kg (up to 300 mg) once daily.

NURSING CONSIDERATIONS
See also *General Nursing Considerations For All Anti-Infectives* under *Penicillins,* p. 140.

Administration/Storage
1. Store in dark, tightly closed containers.
2. Solutions for IM injection may crystallize at low temperature and should be allowed to warm to room temperature if precipitation is evident.
3. Isoniazid should be administered with pyridoxine, 6–50 mg/day, in malnourished, alcoholic, or diabetic clients.

Interventions
1. Obtain baseline liver and renal function studies and monitor throughout therapy.
2. Parenteral sodium phenobarbital is generally used for the control of isoniazid-induced neurotoxic symptoms, particularly convulsions; have readily available.
3. Anticipate that cholinergic drugs, atropine, and certain narcotic analgesics (e.g., meperidine) may aggravate side effects.
4. If there is marked CNS stimulation, withhold the drug and consult with physician.
5. Closely assess diabetic clients because diabetes is more difficult to control when isoniazid is administered.
6. Anticipate reduced dose with renal dysfunction. Monitor intake and output to ascertain that renal output is adequate to prevent systemic accumulation of the drug.
7. Provide client with only a 1-month supply of the drug, because client should be examined and evaluated monthly while on isoniazid.
8. Anticipate a slight local irritation at the site of injection. Rotate and document injection sites.

Client/Family Teaching
1. Instruct client to take drug on an empty stomach 1 hr before or 2 hr after meals.
2. Withhold drug and report fatigue, weakness, malaise, and anorexia immediately, as these may be signs of hepatitis.
3. Advise client of the importance of taking drugs as ordered and of reporting for monthly follow-up and laboratory studies.
4. Explain to client that pyridoxine is given to prevent neurotoxic effects of isoniazid.
5. Advise clients not to use alcohol while on drug therapy.

Evaluation
Assess response to therapy at monthly checkups through lab findings and lack of toxic drug side effects.

KANAMYCIN SULFATE   (kan-ah-**MY**-sin)

Kantrex (Rx)

Classification: Second-line antitubercular agent.
See *Aminoglycosides,* p. 75, for all information on this drug.

PYRAZINAMIDE   (peer-ah-**ZIN**-ah-myd)

PMS Pyrazinamide ✤, Tebrazid ✤ (Rx)

Classification: Second-line antitubercular agent.

Action/Kinetics: Mechanism not known. May be bacteriostatic and bactericidal, depending on concentration and susceptibility of the mycobacterium. Well absorbed from GI tract, widely distributed in tissues. **Peak serum levels:** 2 hr. **t¹/₂:** 9–10 hr, longer in presence of impaired renal and hepatic function. Metabolized in liver; inactive metabolites and unchanged drug (up to 14%) excreted mainly in the urine.

Use: Active tuberculosis in combination with other drugs after failure with first-line drugs.

Contraindications: Preexisting liver malfunction.

Special Concerns: Safety and effectiveness have not been established in children. Use with caution in patients with a history of diabetes mellitus, gout, or acute intermittent porphyria.

Side Effects: *Hepatic:* Cellular damage, hepatomegaly, jaundice, tenderness. Frequent liver function tests are necessary. *GI:* Nausea, vomiting, diarrhea, anorexia. *CNS:* Fever, malaise. *Miscellaneous:* Gout, disturbances in blood clotting, sideroblastic anemia, arthralgia, skin rashes, photosensitivity, splenomegaly.

Drug Interactions	
Aminosalicylic acid	↓ Pharmacologic effect of pyrazinamide
Probenecid	↓ Pharmacologic effect of pyrazinamide
Salicylates	↓ Pharmacologic effect of pyrazinamide

Dosage: Tablets. Adults, usual: 20–35 mg/kg daily in 3–4 divided doses. Maximum daily dose is 3.0 g.

NURSING CONSIDERATIONS

See also *Nursing Considerations For All Anti-Infectives* under *Penicillins,* p. 140, and *Antitubercular Agents,* p. 224.

Interventions

1. Obtain baseline complete blood count and renal and liver function studies and monitor throughout therapy. High doses of pyrazinamide tend to promote hepatic damage.
2. Administer drug to client only under close medical supervision.
3. Evaluate for evidence of jaundice.
4. Observe diabetic clients closely for hypo- or hyperglycemia because drug affects sugar metabolism.

5. Fatigue, poor appetite, weakness, and irritability, may be signs of anemia and prodromal signs of hepatitis; document and report.

6. Monitor uric acid levels and anticipate concomitant administration of uricosuric agents as indicated, except in severe hyperuricemia or if client has acute gouty arthritis; in this case drug should be discontinued.

Client/Family Teaching

1. Report any side effects from drug therapy to physician.

2. Do not take salicylates as these interfere with the intended drug therapy.

3. Stress the importance of reporting for all follow up visits.

Evaluation

Assess response to therapy and lack of toxic organ side effects based on laboratory findings.

RIFAMPIN   (rih-**FAM**-pin)

Rifadin, Rimactane, Rofact✽ (Rx)

Classification: First-line antitubercular agent.

Action/Kinetics: Semisynthetic antibiotic derived from *Streptomyces mediterranei*. Rifampin suppresses RNA synthesis by binding to the beta subunit of DNA-dependent RNA polymerase. This prevents attachment of the enzyme to DNA and blockade of RNA transcription. The drug is both bacteriostatic and bactericidal and is most active against rapidly replicating organisms. The drug is well absorbed from the GI tract and is widely distributed in body tissues. **Peak plasma concentration:** 4–32 mcg/mL after 2–4 hr. **t½:** 1.5–5 hr; higher in patients with hepatic impairment. In normal patients t½ decreases with usage. The drug is metabolized in liver; 60% is excreted in feces.

Uses: Pulmonary tuberculosis. Must be used in conjunction with at least one other tuberculostatic drug (such as isoniazid, ethambutol) but is the drug of choice for retreatment. Also for treatment of asymptomatic meningococcal carriers to eliminate *Neisseria meningitidis. Investigational:* Used in combination for infections due to *Staphylococcus aureus* and *S. epidermidis;* Legionnaire's disease; in combination with dapsone for leprosy; prophylaxis of meningitis due to *Haemophilus influenzae*.

Contraindications: Hypersensitivity; not recommended for intermittent therapy.

Special Concerns: Safe use during lactation has not been established. Use during pregnancy only if benefits clearly outweigh risks. Safety and effectiveness not determined in children less than 5 years of age. Use with extreme caution in patients with hepatic dysfunction.

Side Effects: *GI:* Nausea, vomiting, diarrhea, cramps, heartburn, flatulence. *CNS:* Headache, drowsiness, fatigue, ataxia, dizziness, confusion, fever, difficulty in concentrating. *Hepatic:* Jaundice, hepatitis. Increases in SGOT, SGPT, bilirubin, alkaline phosphatase. *Hematologic:* Thrombocytopenia, leukopenia, hemolytic anemia. *Allergic:* Flu-like symptoms, dyspnea, wheezing, purpura, pruritus, urticaria, skin rashes, sore mouth and tongue, conjunctivitis. *Renal:* Hematuria, hemoglobinuria, renal insufficiency, acute renal failure. *Miscellaneous:* Visual disturbances, muscle weakness or pain, arthralgia, adrenocortical insufficiency, increases in BUN and serum uric acid. **Note:** Body fluids and feces may be red-orange.

Drug Interactions

Aminosalicylic acid	↓ Effect of rifampin due to ↓ absorption from GI tract
Anticoagulants, oral	↓ Effect of anticoagulants due to ↑ breakdown by liver
Barbiturates	↓ Effect of barbiturates due to ↑ breakdown by liver
Contraceptives, oral	↓ Effect of contraceptives due to ↑ breakdown of estrogen by liver
Corticosteroids	↓ Effect of corticosteroids due to ↑ breakdown by liver
Digitoxin	↓ Effect of digitoxin due to ↑ breakdown by liver
Hypoglycemics, oral	↓ Effect of hypoglycemics due to ↑ breakdown by liver
Isoniazid	Additive liver toxicity
Methadone	↑ Chance of methadone withdrawal symptoms due to ↑ breakdown by liver
Quinidine	↓ Effect of quinidine due to ↑ breakdown by liver

Laboratory Test Interferences: ↑ SGOT, SGPT, alkaline phosphatase, BUN, bilirubin, uric acid, BSP retention values. False + Coombs' test.

Dosage: Capsules. *Pulmonary tuberculosis:* **Adults:** single dose of 600 mg daily; **children over 5 years:** 10–20 mg/kg daily, not to exceed 600 mg/day. *Meningococcal carriers:* 600 mg daily for 4 days; **children over 5 years:** 10 mg/kg q 12 hr for 4 doses. Dosage should not exceed 600 mg/day.

NURSING CONSIDERATIONS

See also *General Nursing Considerations For All Anti-Infectives* under *Penicillins,* p. 140.

Administration/Storage

1. Administer once daily 1 hr before or 2 hr after meals to ensure maximum absorption.
2. Check to be sure that there is a desiccant in the bottle containing capsules of rifampin, as these are relatively moisture sensitive.
3. If administered concomitantly with Aminosalicylate Sodium, drugs should be given 8–12 hr apart, as the acid interferes with the absorption of rifampin.

Interventions

1. Obtain appropriate baseline laboratory studies. Evaluate for impaired renal function, blood dyscrasias, and liver dysfunction.
2. Assess for GI disturbance and auditory nerve impairment; document and notify physician.

Client/Family Teaching

1. Rifampin may impart a red-orange color to urine, feces, saliva, sputum, and tears; contact lenses may become *permanently* discolored.

2. Symptoms such as headache, drowsiness, confusion, fever, and muscle and joint aches may occur during the first few weeks of therapy. If symptoms persist or increase in intensity, report to physician.

RIFAMPIN AND ISONIAZID   (rih-FAM-pin, I-SON-ee-ah-zyd)
Rifamate (Rx)

Classification: First-line antitubercular agents.
See also *Isoniazid,* p. 230, and *Rifampin,* p. 234.

Uses: Pulmonary tuberculosis after the patient has been titrated on the individual drugs and the drugs are known to be effective.

Contraindications: This product is not recommended for use in children.

Dosage: Capsules. Adults/adolescents: 600 mg rifampin and 300 mg isoniazid once daily.

NURSING CONSIDERATIONS
See See *Nursing Considerations* for *Rifampin,* p. 235, and *Isoniazid,* p. 232.

STREPTOMYCIN SULFATE   (strep-toe-MY-sin)
(Rx)

Classification: Aminoglycoside, first-line antitubercular agent.
See *Aminoglycoside Antibiotics,* p. 75, for all information on this drug.

LEPROSTATICS

CLOFAZIMINE   (klo-FAZ-ih-meen)
Lamprene (Rx)

Classification: Leprostatic.

Action/Kinetics: This drug is thought to exert a bactericidal effect on the mycobacterium; the drug inhibits mycobacterial growth and binds to mycobacterial DNA. Cross-resistance with rifampin or dapsone is not observed. The drug is concentrated in fatty tissues and the reticuloendothelial system. $t^{1/2}$: 70 days. The drug is excreted in the feces via the bile, as well as in sputum, sweat, and sebum.

Uses: Lepromatous leprosy (including dapsone-resistant leprosy and leprosy complicated by erythema nodosum leprosum). In combination with other drugs to prevent resistance in multibacillary leprosy.

Special Concerns: Pregnancy category: C. Use with caution in patients with abdominal pain or diarrhea. Use during lactation only if benefits outweigh risks. Safety and efficacy have not been determined in children.

Side Effects: *GI:* Nausea, vomiting, diarrhea, abdominal or epigastric pain. Rarely, GI bleeding, intestinal obstruction, anorexia, constipation, liver enlargement. *Dermatologic:* Pink to brownish-black pigmentation of skin, ichthyosis, dryness of skin, pruritus, rash. *Ophthalmologic:* Pigmentation of conjunctiva and cornea (due to clofazimine crystals), phototoxicity, decreased vision, eye irritation, burning, itching, or dryness. *CNS:* Headache, dizziness, drowsiness, neuralgia, fatigue, depression. *Miscellaneous:* Jaundice, weight loss, hepatitis, anemia, thromboembolism, bone pain, edema, cystitis, fever, vascular pain, lymphadenopathy, eosinophilia, hypokalemia. Discoloration of urine, feces, sweat, or sputum.

Laboratory Test Interferences: ↑ SGOT, serum bilirubin, albumin.

Dosage: Capsules. *Leprosy resistant to dapsone:* 100 mg daily together with one or more other leprostatic drugs for a period of 3 years; **maintenance:** clofazimine alone, 100 mg daily. *Erythema nodosum leprosum:* Dosage depends on severity of symptoms, but doses greater than 200 mg daily are not recommended. Goal is 100 mg daily.

NURSING CONSIDERATIONS

Administration/Storage

Clofazimine should be given with one or more other leprostatic agents in order to prevent development of resistance to each drug.

Client/Family Teaching

1. Take medication as ordered and with food to minimize GI irritation.
2. Report any increased GI distress, depression, and/or unusual side effects immediately.
3. Although reversible, clofazimine will cause pink to brownish-black skin discoloration, which may persist after therapy.
4. Not to be alarmed as all body fluids will become discolored during therapy.
5. Oil baths and frequent lotion application may minimize itchy, dry skin formation.

DAPSONE (DDS) [DAP-sohn]
Avlosulfon ✹ (Rx)

Classification: Sulfone, leprostatic.

Action/Kinetics: Dapsone is a synthetic agent with both bacteriostatic and bactericidal activity, especially against *Mycobacterium leprae* (Hansen's bacillus). Although the exact mechanism is not known, dapsone is thought to act similarly to sulfonamides in that it interferes with the metabolism of the infectious organism. Widely distributed throughout the body. **Peak plasma levels:** 4–8 hr. Doses of 200 mg daily for 8 days will lead to a plateau plasma level of 0.1–7 mcg/mL. **t½:** About 28 hr. The drug is acetylated in the liver and metabolites are excreted in the urine.

Uses: Lepromatous and tuberculoid types of leprosy, dermatitis herpetiformis, and for prophylaxis of malaria. *Investigational:* Relapsing polychondritis.

Contraindications: Advanced amyloidosis of kidneys. Lactation.

Special Concerns: Pregnancy category: C.

Side Effects: *Hematologic:* Hemolytic anemia, methemoglobinemia. *GI:* Nausea, vomiting, anorexia, abdominal discomfort. *CNS:* Headache, insomnia, vertigo, paresthesia, psychoses, peripheral neuropathy. *Dermatologic:* Photosensitivity, lupus-like syndrome. *Hypersensitivity:* Severe skin reactions including exfoliative dermatitis, erythema multiforme, urticaria, erythema nodosum, toxic erythema, toxic epidermal necrolysis, morbilliform and scarlatiniform reactions. *Miscellaneous:* Muscle weakness, hypoalbuminemia, albuminuria, nephrotic syndrome, renal papillary necrosis, blurred vision, tinnitus, male infertility, fever, tachycardia, mononucleosis-type syndrome.

A leprosy-reactional state may occur in large numbers of patients during therapy with dapsone. Type 1 occurs soon after therapy is initiated. Patients manifest an enhanced delayed hypersensitivity syndrome, leading to swelling of existing nerve and skin lesions with possible neuritis. However, this is not an indication to discontinue therapy. Steroids, analgesics, and surgical decompression of swollen nerve trunks may be used to reduce symptoms. Type 2 occurs in nearly 50% of patients during the first year of therapy. Symptoms include fever, erythematous skin nodules, joint swelling, neuritis, orchitis, malaise, depression, iritis, or epistaxis. Usually therapy is continued with the use of analgesics, steroids, or clofazimine to suppress the reaction.

Drug Interactions

Para-aminobenzoic acid	↓ Effect of dapsone
Probenecid	↑ Effect of dapsone due to inhibition of renal excretion
Pyrimethamine	↑ Risk of hematologic reactions
Rifampin	↓ Effect of dapsone due to ↑ plasma clearance

Laboratory Test Interference: Altered liver function tests.

Dosage: Tablets. *Leprosy:* **Adults:** 50–100 mg/day. The full dose should be initiated and continued without interruption. *Leprosy, bacteriologically negative tuberculoid and indeterminate type:* **Adults:** 100 mg daily with rifampin, 600 mg daily for 6 months; **then,** continue dapsone for a minimum of 3 years. *Leprosy, lepromatous and borderline patients:* 100 mg daily for at least 10 years. *Dermatitis herpetiformis:* **Adults, initially:** 50 mg/day; dosage may be increased to 300 mg/day or higher, if necessary. **Maintenance:** Reduce dosage to minimum maintenance dose as soon as possible; maintenance dosage may be reduced or eliminated in patients on a gluten-free diet. Dosage should be correspondingly less in children.

NURSING CONSIDERATIONS

See also *Nursing Considerations For All Anti-Infectives* under *Penicillins,* p. 140.

Administration/Storage

1. For tuberculoid and indeterminate clients, dosage should be continued for at least 3 years.
2. For lepromatous clients, full dosage may be necessary for life.
3. Possible resistance to dapsone should be carefully evaluated, especially if lepromatous or borderline lepromatous clients relapse. If there is no response to dapsone therapy within 3–6 months, dapsone resistance can be confirmed.

Interventions

1. Obtain baseline complete blood count, liver and renal function studies, and monitor throughout therapy.
2. Dosage is increased slowly during initiation period.

3. Check whether doctor wishes client to receive hematinics.

4. Use strict medical asepsis, because client may have leukopenia.

5. Document extent and location of lesions.

Client/Family Teaching

1. Instruct lactating mothers to report cyanosis of nursing infant, as this indicates high sulfone levels, and withdrawal of drug may be indicated.

2. To take medication exactly as ordered.

3. The importance of following their diet as prescribed (e.g., gluten-free). Refer to dietitian as needed for additional counseling and instruction.

4. That local support groups may help in understanding and coping with chronic disease.

5. Stress the importance of reporting for scheduled lab studies and follow-up visits to evaluate effectiveness of therapy.

Evaluation

Assess

- for improvement of inflammation and ulceration of the mucous membranes during the first 3–6 months of therapy. Lack of response may indicate need for other therapy.
- for allergic dermatitis, which usually appears before the tenth week of therapy. Allergic dermatitis may develop into fatal exfoliative dermatitis.
- for psychoses, GI disturbances, lepra reaction, headaches, dizziness, lethargy, severe malaise, tinnitus, paresthesias, deep aches, neuralgic pains, and ocular disturbances and report to physician.
- clients in whom there are other concurrent chronic conditions particularly closely and anticipate reduction in dosage of sulfones.
- for symptoms of anemia. Report RBC below 2,500,000/mm^3 or if RBC remains low during first 6 weeks of therapy.
- WBC and report when below 5,000/mm^3.

CHAPTER FOURTEEN

Antimalarials

General Statement: A knowledge of the life cycle of the causative agent is helpful in understanding the mode of action of the antimalarial drugs.

Malaria is transmitted by the *Anopheles* mosquito. The causative organism is a parasite known as *Plasmodium,* of which there are several species infective to humans: *P. falciparum, P. vivax, P. malariae,* and *P. ovale.*

Plasmodia pass through a complex life cycle, part of which takes place in the gut of the mosquito and part of which takes place in humans. In the sporozoite stage of development, the organism is transmitted to humans by a mosquito bite. The sporozoite migrates to the human liver, where it grows and divides (the exoerythrocytic, fixed-tissue stage), emerging as a merozoite. The merozoite enters various tissues, including the red blood cells (the asexual erythrocytic stage), causing them to burst. This results in a rise in body temperature. Some merozoites develop into male parasites and others develop into females. At this stage the plasmodia are known as gametocytes, which infect the mosquito again when it bites a human carrier. The plasmodia then reproduces in the gut of the mosquito and develops to the sporozoite stage to complete the cycle.

Clinical manifestations of malaria are not evident during all stages of the life cycle, and no single drug can eradicate the parasite at all stages. The drug treatment of malaria depends on the end result desired and the stage at which the malaria is being treated. It should be remembered that mixed malarial infections may also be manifested in a patient. Treatment may be approached as follows:

1. *Clinical cure:* Halts further development of erythrocytic stage and terminates a clinical attack. Suitable drugs: chloroquine, amodiaquine, quinine.

2. *Radical cure:* Eradicates erythrocytic and exoerythrocytic forms of the parasite; relieves symptoms. Suitable drugs: chloroquine, amodiaquine, quinine plus primaquine.

3. *Prophylaxis in endemic areas:* Prevents development of malaria in endemic areas. Also called suppressive therapy. Suitable drugs: chloroquine, amodiaquine, pyrimethamine-sulfadoxine.

4. *Prophylaxis and treatment of chloroquine-resistant P. falciparum:* Helps if patient travels to an area where resistant *P. falciparum* is known to occur or if the patient does not respond to chloroquine. Suitable drugs: pyrimethamine-sulfadoxine, quinine sulfate alone or in combination with pyrimethamine or sulfadiazine (to terminate an acute attack).

NURSING CONSIDERATIONS

See *Nursing Considerations For All Anti-Infectives* under *Penicillins*, p. 140.

4-AMINOQUINOLINES

General Statement: Two 4-aminoquinolines—chloroquine (Aralen) and hydroxychloroquine (Plaquenil)—are widely used for the treatment of malaria. They are both synthetic agents that resemble quinine. They are used also as amebicides and in the treatment of rheumatic diseases.

Action/Kinetics: The 4-aminoquinolines are believed to complex with DNA and therefore to interfere with the replication of the infectious organism. The aminoquinolines are absorbed rapidly and almost completely from the GI tract and are widely distributed throughout the body. **Peak serum levels:** 1–2 hr. These agents are excreted extremely slowly, and the presence of some drug has been demonstrated in the bloodstream weeks and even months after the drug has been discontinued. Up to 70% may be excreted unchanged. Urinary excretion is increased by acidifying the urine; excretion is slowed by alkalinization.

Uses: Treatment or prophylaxis of malaria caused by *Plasmodium falciparum, P. vivax, P. ovale,* and *P. malariae.* Will cause a radical cure of falciparum malaria; must be combined with primaquine for a radical cure of *P. vivax* and *P. ovale.* The drugs are effective only against the erythrocytic stages and therefore will not prevent infections.

Extraintestinal amebiasis caused by *Entamoeba histolytica.* Discoid or lupus erythematosus. As an alternative to gold salts or penicillamine in rheumatoid arthritis patients resistant to salicylates or nonsteroidal anti-inflammatory agents.

Contraindications: Unless deemed essential, the drugs should not be used in the presence of psoriasis or porphyria. Not to be used concomitantly with gold or phenylbutazone or in patients receiving drugs that depress blood-forming elements of bone marrow.

Special Concerns: To be used with extreme caution in the presence of hepatic, severe GI, neurologic, and blood disorders. Infants and children are sensitive to the effects of 4-aminoquinolines.

Side Effects: *GI:* Nausea, vomiting, diarrhea, cramps, anorexia, epigastric distress, stomatitis, dry mouth. *CNS:* Headache, fatigue, nervousness, anxiety, irritability, agitation, apathy, confusion, personality changes, depression, psychoses, seizures. *Dermatologic:* Pruritus, changes in pigment of skin and mucous membranes, dermatoses, bleaching of hair. *Hematologic:* Neutropenia, aplastic anemia, thrombocytopenia, agranulocytosis. *Ocular:* Retinopathy that may be permanent and may lead to blindness. Blurred vision, difficulty in focusing or in accommodation; chronic use may lead to corneal deposits or keratopathy. *Miscellaneous:* Hypotension, ECG changes, peripheral neuritis, ototoxicity, neuromyopathy manifested by muscle weakness.

14

Drug Interactions

Acidifying agents, urinary (ammonium chloride, etc.)	↑ Urinary excretion of antimalarial and thus ↓ its effectiveness
Alkalinizing agents, urinary (bicarbonate, etc.)	↓ Excretion of antimalarial and thus ↑ amount of drug in system

Drug Interactions

Antipsoriatics	4-Aminoquinolines inhibit antipsoriatic drugs
MAO inhibitors	↑ Toxicity of 4-aminoquinolines due to ↓ breakdown in liver

Laboratory Test Interference: Colors urine brown.

Dosage: See individual drug entries.

NURSING CONSIDERATIONS

See also *General Nursing Considerations For All Anti-Infectives* under *Penicillins,* p. 140.

Administration/Storage

Store in amber-colored containers.

Assessment

Assess for retinopathy manifested by visual disturbances. Retinal changes are not reversible. Regular ophthalmologic examinations are mandatory during prolonged therapy.

Interventions

1. Observe for acute toxicity, which may occur in accidental overdosage in children or in suicidal clients. Symptoms of acute toxicity develop within 30 min of ingestion. Death may occur within 2 hr.
2. Symptoms of acute toxicity to observe for may include headache, drowsiness, visual disturbances, cardiovascular collapse, convulsions, and cardiac arrest.
3. Have emergency equipment readily available, including setup for gastric lavage, barbiturates, vasopressors, and oxygen. Observe for 6 hours after acute toxicity has been treated.
4. Monitor TPR, blood pressure, intake and output, and state of consciousness at frequent intervals.
5. Anticipate that fluids will have to be forced and ammonium chloride administered for weeks to months to acidify urine and promote renal excretion of the drug.
6. Warn clients to keep drug out of children's reach.
7. Check toxic effects of other drugs being used because the combination with chloroquine may reinforce toxic effects.
8. For suppressive therapy, administer the drug on the same day each week. Give immediately before or after meals to minimize gastric irritation.
9. Administer with the evening meal when managing discoid lupus erythematosus.

Client/Family Teaching

1. Review the method for administration and time intervals at which to take the medication.
2. Instruct client to report any persistent or bothersome side effects. Review the signs and symptoms of toxicity.
3. Stress the importance of reporting for scheduled visits and lab studies.
4. Ensure adequate fluid intake as well as medications prescribed to acidify urine are taken as long as ordered by the physician.
5. Keep medications in child-proof containers and keep out of children's reach.

Evaluation

1. Assess client/family knowledge and understanding of illness, response to therapy and to teaching.

2. Note status of pretreatment symptoms and client subjective response upon questioning of any adverse effects.

3. Observe for freedom from complications of drug therapy.

4. Perform ophthalmologic examination to determine if any retinal damage has occurred.

CHLOROQUINE HYDROCHLORIDE   (KLOR-oh kwin)
Aralen HCl (Rx)

CHLOROQUINE PHOSPHATE   (KLOR-oh-kwin)
Aralen Phosphate (Rx)

See also *4-Aminoquinolines,* p. 241.

Classification: 4-Aminoquinoline, antimalarial, amebecide.

Special Concerns: Use during pregnancy only if benefits outweigh risks.

Additional Untoward Reactions: Chloroquine may exacerbate psoriasis and precipitate an acute attack.

Dosage: Tablets. *Acute malarial attack.* **Adults: initially,** 1 g; **then,** 500 mg after 6–8 hr and 500 mg/day for next 2 days. **Children:** total dose of 41.7 mg/kg given over a 3-day period as follows, **initially:** 16.7 mg/kg (not to exceed a single dose of 1 g); **then,** 8.3 mg/kg (not to exceed a single dose of 500 mg) given 6, 24, and 48 hr after the first dose. *Suppression (prophylaxis) of malaria.* **Adults:** 500 mg per week (on same day each week). If therapy has not been initiated 14 days before exposure, an initial loading dose of 1 g may be given in 500 mg doses 6 hr apart. **Children:** 8.3 mg/kg (not to exceed the adult dose) per week (on same day each week). If therapy has not been initiated 14 days before exposure, an initial loading dose of 16.7 mg/kg may be given in 2 divided doses 6 hr apart.

Amebiasis. **Adults,** 250 mg q.i.d. for 2 days; **then,** 250 mg b.i.d. for 2–3 weeks (combine with an intestinal amebicide). **Children:** 10 mg/kg (not to exceed 500 mg) daily for 3 weeks.

IM. *Acute malarial attack.* **Adults, initially,** 200–250 mg; repeat dosage in 6 hr if necessary. Total daily dose in first 24 hr should not exceed 1 g. Begin PO therapy as soon as possible. **IM, SC. Children and infants:** 6.25 mg/kg repeated in 6 hr; dose should not exceed 12.5 mg/kg/day. **IV infusion, initially:** 16.6 mg/kg over 8 hr; **then,** 8.3 mg/kg q 6–8 hr by continuous infusion.

IM. *Amebiasis:* **Adults,** 200–250 mg daily for 10–12 days. Begin PO therapy as soon as possible. **Children:** 7.5 mg/kg daily for 10–12 days.

NURSING CONSIDERATIONS

See *Nursing Considerations* for *4-Aminoquinolines,* p. 242.

HYDROXYCHLOROQUINE SULFATE   (hi-DROX-ee-KLOH-roh-kwin)
Plaquenil Sulfate (Rx)

See also *4-Aminoquinolines,* p. 241.

Classification: 4-Aminoquinoline, antimalarial, antirheumatic.

Action/Kinetics: Hydroxychloroquine is not a drug of choice for rheumatoid arthritis and should be discontinued after 6 months if no beneficial effects are noted. It is thought to act by suppression of formation of antigens, which leads to hypersensitivity reactions. These reactions cause the symptoms of the disease. **Peak plasma levels:** 1–3 hr. Unchanged drug is excreted in the urine. Excretion may be enhanced by acidifying the urine and decreased by alkalizing the urine.

Patients on long-term therapy should be examined thoroughly at regular intervals for knee and ankle reflexes and hematopoietic studies. *Drug may cause retinopathy;* thus, baseline ophthalmologic examinations, repeated at 3-month intervals, must be performed; the drug should be discontinued in the event of ophthalmic damage, impaired reflexes, and blood dyscrasias.

Treatment of toxic symptoms: Administration of 8 g ammonium chloride in divided doses 3 to 4 times/week for several months to improve residual excretion of drug.

Uses: Antimalarial, antirheumatic, discoid and lupus erythematosus. Not used as a first line of therapy.

Additional Contraindications: Long-term therapy in children, ophthalmologic changes due to 4-aminoquinolines.

Special Concerns: Use with caution in alcoholism or liver disease.

Additional Untoward Reactions: The appearances of skin eruptions or of misty vision and visual halos are indications for withdrawal.

Drug Interactions	
Digoxin	Hydroxychloroquine ↑ serum digoxin levels
Gold salts	Dermatitis and ↑ risk of severe skin reactions
Phenylbutazone	Dermatitis and ↑ risk of severe skin reactions

Dosage: Tablets. *Acute malarial attack:* **Adults, initially,** 800 mg; **then,** 400 mg after 6–8 hr and 400 mg/day for next 2 days. **Children:** A total of 32 mg/kg given over a 3-day period as follows: **initially,** 12.9 mg/kg (not to exceed a single dose of 800 mg); **then,** 6.4 mg/kg (not to exceed a single dose of 400 mg) 6, 24, and 48 hr after the first dose. *Suppression of malaria:* **Adults,** 400 mg q 7 days. If therapy has not been initiated 14 days prior to exposure, an initial loading dose of 800 mg may be given in two divided doses 6 hr apart. **Children:** 6.4 mg/kg (not to exceed the adult dose) q 7 days. If therapy has not been initiated 14 days prior to exposure, an initial loading dose of 12.9 mg/kg may be given in 2 doses 6 hr apart.

Rheumatoid arthritis: **Adults,** 400–600 mg daily taken with milk or meals; *maintenance* (usually after 4–12 weeks): 200–400 mg daily. (*Note:* Several months may be required for a beneficial effect to be seen). *Lupus erythematosus:* **Adults, usual,** 400 mg once or twice daily; **prolonged maintenance:** 200–400 mg daily.

NURSING CONSIDERATIONS

See also *Nursing Considerations* for *4-Aminoquinolines,* p. 242, and *General Nursing Considerations For All Anti-Infectives* under *Penicillins,* p. 140.

Interventions

1. When the drug is given for rheumatoid arthritis:
   - reassure client and indicate that benefits may not occur until 6 to 12 months after therapy has been initiated.
   - anticipate that side effects may necessitate a reduction of therapy. After 5 to 10 days of reduced dosage, it may gradually be increased again to the desired level.

- anticipate that dosage will be reduced when the desired response is attained. Drug will again be effective in case of flare-up.
- reduce GI irritation by administering drug with meal or glass of milk.
- corticosteroids and salicylates may be used concomitantly.

2. When drug is given for lupus erythematosus, administer with evening meal.

3. Suppressive antimalarial therapy should be initiated 2 weeks prior to exposure and should be continued for 6 to 8 weeks after leaving the endemic area. If therapy is not started prior to exposure, the initial loading dose should be doubled (i.e., adults, 620 mg as the base and children 10 mg/kg as the base) and given in 2 doses 6 hr apart.

8-AMINOQUINOLINE

PRIMAQUINE PHOSPHATE (PRIM-ah-kwin)

(Rx)

Classification: 8-aminoquinoline, antimalarial.

Action/Kinetics: Mechanism of action not known but the drug binds to and may alter the properties of DNA leading to decreased protein synthesis. Well absorbed from GI tract. **Peak plasma levels:** 2 hr. Poorly distributed in body tissues.

Uses: Primaquine is active against primary exoerythrocytic forms of vivax and falciparum malaria. It produces radical cure of vivax malaria by eliminating both exoerythrocytic and erythrocytic forms. Primaquine also is active against the sexual forms (gametocytes) of plasmodia resulting in disruption of transmission of the disease by eliminating the reservoir from which the mosquito carrier is infected. It cures suppressed infections after the patient leaves endemic areas and prevents relapse. For this reason, the drug is administered concurrently with quinine or chloroquine.

Contraindications: Very active forms of vivax and falciparum malaria. Use during pregnancy only if benefits outweigh risks.

Side Effects: *GI:* Abdominal cramps, epigastric distress, nausea, vomiting. *Hematologic:* Methemoglobinemia. Blacks and members of certain Mediterranean ethnic groups (Sardinians, Sephardic Jews, Greeks, Iranians) manifest a high incidence of glucose-6-phosphate dehydrogenase deficiency and as a result have a low tolerance for primaquine. These individuals manifest marked hemolytic anemia following primaquine administration. *Miscellaneous:* Headache, pruritus, interference with visual accommodation, cardiac arrhythmias, hypertension.

Drug Interactions	
Bone marrow depressants, hemolytic drugs	Additive side effects
Quinacrine	Quinacrine interferes with metabolic degradation of primaquine and thus enhances its toxic side reactions. **Do not give primaquine** to patients who are receiving or have received quinacrine within the past 3 months.

Dosage: Tablets: *Radical cure of vivax malaria:* 52.6 mg daily for 14 days. *Suppression of malaria:* **Adults,** 26.3 mg daily for 14 days or 78.9 mg once a week for 8 weeks; **children:** 0.68/kg/day for 14 days. *To eliminate gametocytes:* Single dose of 78.9 mg.

NURSING CONSIDERATIONS

See also *General Nursing Considerations For All Anti-Infectives* under *Penicillins,* p. 140.

Administration/Storage

1. Store in tightly closed containers.
2. Therapy is initiated during the last 2 weeks of or after suppressive therapy with chloroquine or a similar drug.

Client/Family Teaching

1. For suppressive therapy, take drug on same day each week.
2. Take medication immediately before or after meal or with antacids, so as to minimize gastric irritation.
3. Monitor color of urine and report immediately any darkening or brown color.

Evaluation

Assess

- for indications to withdraw drug: dark urine that indicates hemolysis, and a marked fall in hemoglobin or erythrocyte count.
- dark-skinned clients. Because of a possible inborn deficiency of glucose-6-phosphate dehydrogenase, these clients are particularly susceptible to hemolytic anemia while on primaquine.

MISCELLANEOUS ANTIMALARIALS

MEFLOQUINE HYDROCHLORIDE   (MEH-floh-kwin)

Lariam (Rx)

Classification: Antimalarial.

Action/Kinetics: Although the precise mechanism of action is not known, mefloquine is related chemically to quinine and acts as a blood schizonticide. Mefloquine is a mixture of enantiomeric molecules that results in differences in the rates of release, absorption, distribution, metabolism, elimination, and activity of the drug. **t½:** 15–33 days (average 3 weeks). The drug is 98% bound to plasma proteins and is concentrated in blood erythrocytes (i.e., the target cells in treatment of malaria).

Uses: Mild to moderate acute malaria caused by mefloquine-susceptible strains of *Plasmodium falciparum* (both chloroquine susceptible and resistant strains) or *P. vivax.* Data are not available regarding effectiveness in treating *P. ovale* or *P. malariae.* Also, prophylaxis of *P. falciparum* and *P. vivax* infections, including prophylaxis of chloroquine-resistant strains of *P. falciparum.*
  Note: Patients with acute *P. vivax* malaria are at a high risk for relapse as mefloquine does not

eliminate the exoerythrocytic (hepatic) parasites. Thus, these patients should also be treated with primaquine.

Contraindications: Hypersensitivity to mefloquine or related compounds.

Special Concerns: Use during pregnancy (pregnancy category: C) only if potential benefits outweigh potential risks. Use with caution during lactation. Safety and effectiveness have not been determined in children.

Side Effects: Note: At the doses used, it is difficult to distinguish side effects due to the drug from symptoms attributable to the disease itself.
   When used for treatment of acute malaria. *GI:* Nausea, vomiting, diarrhea, abdominal pain, loss of appetite. *CNS:* Dizziness, fever, headache, fatigue, emotional problems, seizures. *Miscellaneous:* Myalgia, chills, skin rash, tinnitus, bradycardia, hair loss.
   When used for prophylaxis of malaria. *CNS:* Dizziness, syncope, encephalopathy of unknown etiology. *Miscellaneous:* Vomiting, extrasystoles.
   Postmarketing surveillance: *CNS:* Vertigo, psychoses, confusion, anxiety, depression, hallucinations. *Miscellaneous:* Visual disturbances.

Drug Interactions	
Beta-adrenergic blocking agents	ECG abnormalities or cardiac arrest
Chloroquine	↑ Risk of seizures
Quinidine	↑ Risk of ECG abnormalities or cardiac arrest
Quinine	↑ Risk of seizures, ECG abnormalities, or cardiac arrest
Valproic acid	Loss of seizure control and ↓ blood levels of valproic acid

Laboratory Test Interferences: When used for prophylaxis: Transient ↑ transaminases, leukocytosis, thrombocytopenia. **When used for treatment of acute malaria:** ↓ Hematocrit, transient ↑ transaminases, leukocytosis, thrombocytopenia.

Dosage: Tablets. *Mild to moderate malaria* caused by susceptible strains of *P. falciparum* or *P. vivax:* 1,250 mg (five tablets) as a single dose with at least 8 oz of water. *Prophylaxis of malaria:* 250 mg (1 tablet) once a week for 4 weeks; **then,** 1 tablet every other week.

NURSING CONSIDERATIONS

See also *General Nursing Considerations For All Anti-Infectives* under *Penicillins,* p. 140

Administration

For prophylaxis, therapy with mefloquine should be initiated one week prior to travel to an endemic area and should be continued for 4 additional weeks after return from an endemic area.

Interventions

1. If the client has a life-threatening *P. falciparum* infection, treatment should be initiated with an IV antimalarial drug. This can be followed by mefloquine, orally, to complete therapy.
2. To reduce the potential of cardiotoxic effects, vomiting should be induced in cases of overdose.

Client/Family Teaching

1. Do not take the drug on an empty stomach.
2. Take the medication with at least 8 oz of water.

PYRIMETHAMINE   (peer-ih-**METH**-ah-meen)

Daraprim (Rx)

Classification: Antimalarial, antitoxoplasmotic, folic acid antagonist.

Action/Kinetics: Pyrimethamine inhibits the enzyme dihydrofolate reductase, which is an enzyme catalyzing the conversion of dihydrofolate to tetrahydrofolate. Tetrahydrofolate is essential to the biosynthesis of certain amino acids, purines, and pyrimidines. The drug is selective against plasmodia and stops sporogony in the mosquito. It is not effective against gametocytes. The drug is absorbed from the GI tract and widely distributed throughout the body. $t^{1}/_{2}$: 4 days. Levels to suppress plasmodia are maintained for up to 2 weeks. The drug is excreted slowly in urine; 20–30% excreted unchanged. Drug is detectable in urine 30 or more days after administration.

Uses: In combination with dapsone or sulfadoxine for suppression or prophylaxis of chloroquine-resistant *P. falciparum*. In combination with dapsone and chloroquine in prophylaxis of *P. vivax* malaria. In combination with quinine and a sulfonamide (e.g., sulfadiazine or trisulfapyrimidines) to treat uncomplicated attacks of *P. falciparum*. In combination with a sulfapyrimidine-type sulfonamide to treat toxoplasmosis due to *Toxoplasma gondii*. *Investigational:* In combination with sulfadiazine or sulfadoxine to treat pneumonia caused by *Pneumocystis carinii*.

Special Concerns: Use during pregnancy only if benefits clearly outweigh risks. Safety for use during lactation and in children has not been established.

Side Effects: Few toxic effects at usual dosage. Large doses may cause the following: *GI:* Anorexia, vomiting, atrophic glossitis. *Hematologic:* Megaloblastic anemia, leukopenia, thrombocytopenia, pancytopenia. Anemia in patients with glucose–6-phosphate dehydrogenase deficiency. *CNS:* Very large doses and overdosage may cause convulsions. *Other:* Folic acid deficiency may occur with the large doses used to treat toxoplasmosis.

Drug Interactions	
Folic acid	↓ Effect of pyrimethamine
PABA	↓ Effect of pyrimethamine
Quinine	↑ Effect of quinine due to ↓ in plasma protein binding

Dosage: Tablets. *Acute attack, chloroquine-resistant P. falciparum:* **Adults:** 25 mg b.i.d. for 3 days in combination with a sulfonamide. **Children:** 0.3 mg/kg t.i.d. for 3 days in combination with a sulfonamide. *Prophylaxis or suppressive cure:* **Adults:** 25 mg with 500 mg of sulfadoxine q 7 days. **Children, 1 month to 4 years:** 6.25 mg with 125 mg sulfadoxine q 7 days. **Children, 4–8 years:** 12.5 mg with 250 mg sulfadoxine q 7 days. **Children, 9–14 years:** 18.75 mg with 375 mg sulfadoxine q 7 days. *Toxoplasmosis:* **Adults, initially,** 50–100 mg daily with 1–4 g sulfapyrimidine-type sulfonamide for 1–3 days; **then,** reduce dosage of each drug by one-half and continue treatment for an additional 4–6 weeks. **Pediatric: initially,** 0.5 mg/kg/day b.i.d. with a pediatric dose of a sulfapyrimidine-type sulfonamide for 1–3 days; **then,** reduce dosage of each drug by one-half and continue treatment for 4–6 weeks longer.

NURSING CONSIDERATIONS

See also *Nursing Considerations For All Anti-Infectives* under *Penicillins,* p. 140.

Administration/Storage

1. If folic acid deficiency is noted, leucovorin, 3–9 mg/day IM for 3 or more days, should be administered.

2. Due to its slow onset, pyrimethamine must be combined with another antimalarial to treat acute attacks.

Interventions

1. Anticipate slow onset of action. A faster-acting drug is usually used for an acute malarial attack.
2. Administer for suppressive prophylaxis during the seasons of malarial transmission.
3. Administer at weekly intervals in recommended dosages to avoid interference with blood cell formation and the development of resistance, both of which necessitate changes in therapy.
4. Anticipate that with high doses (as given to clients with toxoplasmosis) signs of folic acid deficiency (e.g., megaloblastic anemia, thrombocytopenia, leukopenia, or GI side effects) may develop. The drug should be discontinued or reduced, and folic acid should be administered.
5. Have available barbiturates and folic acid for emergency treatment for convulsions resulting from ingestion of large overdoses.
6. Assess clients for symptoms of malaria, as resistance to the drug can develop.

QUININE SULFATE   (KWYE-nine)

Novoquinine✳, Quinamm, Quindam, Quiphile, Q-vel, Strema (Rx)

Classification: Antimalarial.

Action/Kinetics: This drug is a natural alkaloid obtained from the bark of the cinchona tree. In addition to its antimalarial properties, it has antipyretic and analgesic properties similar to those of the salicylates. It relieves muscle spasms and is used as a diagnostic agent for myasthenia gravis. Quinine has been used increasingly in the last several years since resistant forms of vivax and falciparum were observed in Southeast Asia. No resistant forms of the parasite have been found for quinine.

The precise antimalarial mechanism of action is not known; quinine does affect DNA replication. The drug eradicates the erythrocytic stages of plasmodia. Quinine also increases the refractory period of skeletal muscle and decreases the excitability of the motor end-plate region, making it useful for nocturnal leg cramps. Quinine is rapidly and completely absorbed from the GI tract, and is widely distributed in body tissues. **t½:** 8.5 hr. The drug is highly bound to protein, and about 10% is excreted unchanged in urine.

Uses: In combination with pyrimethamine and sulfadiazine or sulfadoxine for resistant forms of *Plasmodium falciparum.* Nocturnal leg cramps.

Contraindications: Patients with tinnitus.

Special Concerns: Causes congenital malformations (pregnancy category: X). To be used with caution in patients with optic neuritis.

Side Effects: Use of quinine may result in a syndrome referred to as *cinchonism.* Mild cinchonism is characterized by tinnitus, headache, nausea, slight visual disturbances. Larger doses, however, may cause severe CNS, cardiovascular, GI, or dermatologic effects.

Allergic: Flushing, rashes, fever, facial edema, pruritus, dyspnea, tinnitus, gastric upset. *GI:* Nausea, vomiting, gastric pain. *Ophthalmologic:* Blurred vision, photophobia, diplopia, night blindness, decreased visual fields, impaired color perception. *CNS:* Headache, confusion, restlessness, vertigo, syncope, fever. *Hematologic:* Thrombocytopenia, hypoprothrombinemia. *CV:* Symptoms of angina, ventricular tachycardia, conduction disturbances. *Miscellaneous:* Sweating.

Drug Interactions

Anticoagulants, oral	Additive hypoprothrombinemia
Digoxin	Quinine ↑ effect of digoxin
Heparin	Effect ↓ by quinine
Pyrimethamine	↑ Effect of quinine due to ↓ in plasma protein binding
Skeletal muscle relaxants (surgical)	↑ Respiratory depression and apnea

Dosage: Capsules, Tablets. *Chloroquine-resistant malaria:* **Adults,** 650 mg q 8 hr for at least 3 days (7 days in Southeast Asia) along with pyrimethamine, 25 mg b.i.d. for the first 3 days and sulfadiazine, 2 g daily for the first 5 days. There are two alternative regimens: (1) quinine, 650 mg q 8 hr for at least 3 days (7 days in Southeast Asia) along with a tetracycline, 250 mg q 6 hr for 10 days or (2) quinine, 650 mg q 8 hr for 3 days with sulfadoxine, 1.5 g and pyrimethamine, 75 mg as a single dose. *Nocturnal leg cramps:* 200–300 mg at bedtime; an additional 200–300 mg may be taken after the evening meal.

NURSING CONSIDERATIONS

See *General Nursing Considerations For All Anti-Infectives* under *Penicillins,* p. 140.

Client/Family Teaching

1. Do not take medication with antacids.
2. If also taking cimetidine or digoxin report any side effects immediately, as dosage may need to be adjusted.

Evaluation

Assess for cinchonism (characterized by ringing of ears, blurring of vision, and headache, which may be followed by digestive disturbances, impairment of hearing and sight, confusion, and delirium), which may indicate intolerance or overdosage. Quinine overdosage should be treated by thorough gastric lavage or induced emesis.

SULFADOXINE AND PYRIMETHAMINE   (sul-fah-**DOX**-een, pie-rih-**METH**-ah-meen)

Fansidar (Rx)

See also *Sulfonamides,* p. 203.

Classification: Antimalarial.

Action/Kinetics: Sulfadoxine competes with para-aminobenzoic acid for biosynthesis of folic acid, whereas pyrimethamine inhibits the formation of tetrahydrofolate from dihydrofolate. These reactions are necessary for one-carbon transfer reactions in the synthesis of nucleic acids. Well absorbed following oral use and is widely distributed throughout the body. **Peak plasma levels:** sulfadoxine, 2.5–6 hr; pyrimethamine, 1.5–8 hr. Both drugs are long-acting with a **t½** of 170 hr for sulfadoxine and 110 hr for pyrimethamine. Both drugs are excreted through the urine with about 20%–30% of pyrimethamine excreted unchanged.

Uses: Prophylaxis and treatment of falciparum malaria, especially chloroquine-resistant strains.

Contraindications: Megaloblastic anemia. Infants less than 1 month old. Pregnancy (near term) and lactation. Use with caution in patients with glucose-6-phosphate dehydrogenase deficiency.

Special Concerns: Pregnancy category: C. Use with caution in patients with impaired liver and kidney function, severe allergy, folate deficiency, or bronchial asthma.

Side Effects: See Sulfonamides, p. 203.

Drug Interactions: Sulfonamides, including trimethoprim/sulfamethoxazole, will ↑ risk of folic acid deficiency if used with sulfadoxine and pyrimethamine.

Dosage: Tablets: Contain pyrimethamine, 25 mg, and sulfadoxine, 500 mg. *Acute malaria (in combination with quinine):* **Adults,** 2–3 tablets as a single dose. **Pediatric, 9–14 years of age:** 2 tablets as a single dose; **4–8 years of age:** one tablet as a single dose; **under 4 years of age:** ½ tablet as a single dose. *Prophylaxis:* **Adults,** 1 tablet weekly or 2 tablets biweekly; **Pediatric, 9–14 years of age:** weekly, ¾ tablet; biweekly, 1½ tablets. **4–8 years of age:** weekly, ½ tablet; biweekly, 1 tablet. **Under 4 years of age:** weekly, ¼ tablet; biweekly, ½ tablet.

NURSING CONSIDERATIONS

See also *Nursing Considerations For All Anti-Infectives* under *Penicillins,* p. 140.

Administration

1. High intake of fluid should occur to prevent precipitation in the urine.
2. For prophylaxis, therapy should be initiated 1–2 days before the person enters the endemic area; therapy should continue during stay and for 4–6 weeks after leaving. Primaquine should be given.
3. If folic acid deficiency occurs, leucovorin can be given in a dose of 5–15 mg/day IM for 3 or more days.

Client/Family Teaching

1. Contact the physician immediately if fever, sore throat, purpura, jaundice, pallor, or glossitis is observed.
2. The drug should be discontinued immediately if erythema, rash, pruritus, orogenital lesions, or pharyngitis is noted.
3. Report for lab studies as scheduled since blood counts and urinalyses should be performed periodically if chronic therapy is required.
4. Contraceptive measures should be employed to prevent pregnancy while on this medication.
5. Breast-feeding should not be undertaken while on this medication.
6. Adequate fluids should be taken to prevent crystalluria and stone formation.

CHAPTER FIFTEEN

Amebicides and Trichomonacides

General Statement: Amebiasis is a widely distributed disease caused by the protozoan *Entamoeba histolytica*. The disease has a high incidence in areas with low standards of hygiene. In the United States, the average rate of infestation is generally from 1% to 10% of the population; however, in certain southern localities, the incidence is as high as 40% of the population.

E. histolytica has two forms: (1) an active motile form known as the trophozoite form, and (2) a cystic form that is resistant to destruction and is responsible for the transmission of the disease.

The overt manifestations of amebiasis vary. Some patients manifest violent acute dysentery (characterized by sudden development of severe diarrhea, cramps, and passage of bloody, mucoid stools), whereas others have few overt symptoms or are even completely asymptomatic.

Diagnosis is made on the basis of microscopic examination of fresh, or at least moist, stools by a trained examiner. More than one sample of stool must be negative before amebiasis can be ruled out.

Amebae often migrate from the GI tract to other parts of the body (extraintestinal amebiasis). The spleen, lungs, or liver are frequently affected. The amebae colonize in these organs and form abscesses that may rupture and thereby serve as infectious foci.

At present, no one drug can cure both intestinal and extraintestinal amebic infestations; physicians prefer to use a combination of therapeutic agents. Often the more effective but toxic agents are used initially for a short period of time, whereas long-term eradication or prophylaxis is carried out with less toxic agents.

Because many of the agents used in the treatment of amebiasis are used for trichomoniasis also, nursing implications for both amebicides and trichomonacides are listed below.

Infestation with the parasite *Trichomonas vaginalis* causes vaginitis, characterized by an irritating, profuse, creamy or frothy vaginal discharge associated with severe itching and burning. Diagnosis is made by demonstrating the presence of the trichomonad microscopically in the vaginal secretion.

Vaginitis caused by *T. vaginalis* is treated by various locally applied antitrichomonal agents—often effective amebicides—and also by the oral administration of metronidazole. This drug is usually prescribed for both sexual partners to prevent reinfection. Acid douches (vinegar or lactic acid) are a helpful adjunct to treatment.

Eradication of the infectious agent—which becomes resistant frequently—should be ascertained for 3 months after treatment has ceased. The examination is made after menstruation usually, because trichomonal infections often flare up during menstruation.

The incidence of infections by another protozoan organism, *Giardia lamblia,* is increasing in

North America. The organism is transmitted in the feces. Infections are characterized by mucous diarrhea, abdominal pain, and weight loss. Drugs of choice are metronidazole and quinacrine.

NURSING CONSIDERATIONS

See also *General Nursing Considerations For All Anti-Infectives* under *Penicillins,* p. 140.

Amebicides

Assessment

Closely assess clients on therapy for acute dysentery or extraintestinal amebiasis because the agents of choice are highly toxic.

Interventions

1. Anticipate that clients frequently are on combination-drug therapy for amebiasis; observe for toxic reactions to all drugs.
2. Be prepared to give intensive supportive nursing care to clients having acute dysentery; assist in the effort to control diarrhea, maintain fluid and electrolyte balance, and prevent complications caused by malnutrition. The client's activity may have to be curtailed during the acute phase of the disease.
3. Administer drugs only for the period of time ordered and allow for rest periods between courses of therapy. Advise clients against self-medication.

Client/Family Teaching

1. Carriers must continue with drug therapy. Stress the benefit to themselves, their families, and their co-workers.
2. The necessity for thorough washing of hands, especially in factories, schools, and other institutions where disease is likely to be spread.
3. Strees the need for food handlers to be particularly conscientious about washing hands after toileting. Emphasize the need to use soap, water, and towels.
4. Client and carriers need to have regular stool examinations to check for recurrence.
5. Stress that client and carriers need to report for follow-up visits to ensure eradication of organisms.
6. Instruct clients to have well water tested, as this may be the source of contamination.

Trichomonacides

Client/Family Teaching

1. Review the proper methods for douching and for good feminine hygiene.
2. Demonstrate the methods of insufflation or insertion of vaginal suppository, depending on drug regimen.
3. Wear a sanitary napkin to prevent clothing or bed linen from becoming stained by the medication in vaginal suppositories, especially if they contain iodine (which does stain). Stress that the sanitary pad must be changed frequently and immediately upon staining because it may serve as a growth medium for the infecting organism.
4. The sexual partner may be an asymptomatic carrier and may also require therapy to prevent reinfection of the woman.
5. Use condoms during sexual intercourse while undergoing treatment to prevent reinfections.

15

CHLOROQUINE HYDROCHLORIDE   (KLOR-oh-kwin)

Aralen (Rx)

See *Antimalarials,* p. 240, for all information on this drug.

EMETINE HYDROCHLORIDE   (EM-eh-teen)

(Rx)

Classification: Amebicide.

Action/Kinetics: Emetine is an alkaloid that kills the motile (trophozoite) form of amebae but not amebic cysts. It acts locally on the intestinal wall and in the liver and blocks protein synthesis in the parasite. It tends to accumulate in tissues, especially in the liver, kidneys, spleen, and lungs. The drug is excreted slowly by the kidneys; it is detected in the urine 40–60 days after administration.

Uses: Acute amebic dysentery, amebic hepatitis, amebic abscess, and extraintestinal amebiasis. Also for balantidiasis, fascioliasis, and paragonimiasis.

Contraindications: Emetine is potentially a toxic compound that is not to be used for minor cases, for prophylaxis, or for carriers. Its main toxic effect is on the cardiovascular system. It is contraindicated in patients with cardiac or renal disease (except with amebic abscess or hepatitis not controlled by chloroquine); in aged, debilitated persons; in children (unless severe dysentery is not controlled by other amebicides); and during pregnancy. Not to be used in patients who have received emetine less than 6–8 weeks previously.

Special Concerns: Pregnancy category: X. Safe use has not been established during lactation.

Side Effects: *CV:* Tachycardia, ECG irregularities, congestive heart failure, hypotension, precordial pain, cardiac dilatation, gallop rhythm. *GI:* Nausea, vomiting, diarrhea (common). *CNS:* Headache, dizziness. *Dermatologic:* Urticaria, eczema, purpura. *Miscellaneous:* Dyspnea; muscle weakness, stiffness, and pain.

Dosage: Deep SC or IM (DO NOT USE IV). *Amebiasis.* **Adults:** 65 mg daily in a single dose or two divided doses for 10 days (until acute symptoms subside). Some recommend a dose of 1 mg/kg/day, not to exceed 65 mg/day. Period of treatment should not exceed 10 days, and a rest period of 6 weeks should be observed before treatment is repeated. The dose should be halved in underweight or debilitated patients. **Pediatric (only in severe dysentery not responsive to other amebicides), 8 years and older:** no more than 20 mg/day; **8 years and younger:** no more than 10 mg/day. An alternative dosing schedule in children of 1 mg/kg/day in 2 doses for no more than 5 days has been recommended. *Amebic hepatitis or abscess:* 65 mg/day for 10 days.

   For acute fulminating amebic dysentery, emetine should be administered long enough to control diarrhea or other dysenteric symptoms (usually 3–5 days).

NURSING CONSIDERATIONS

See also *Nursing Considerations For All Anti-Infectives* under *Penicillins,* p. 140, and *Amebecides,* p. 253.

Administration/Storage

Aspirate syringe before injecting because accidental IV administration of emetine is dangerous.

Interventions

1. Maintain client on bed rest during the course of treatment and for several days after therapy has been completed.

2. Assess cardiovascular system (check blood pressure and pulse rate several times daily during the course of therapy). Report a rise in pulse rate above 110 beats/min, tachycardia, and a fall in blood pressure, because such symptoms may require discontinuation of drug therapy.

3. Monitor renal function studies throughout therapy.

4. Injection may cause local irritation, induration and swelling. Keep record of injection site and rotate.

5. Apply heat to relieve pain and hasten absorption of drug.

Client/Family Teaching

1. Review physician's specific recommendations concerning limited activity after a course of therapy so that activities can be planned.

2. Report promptly any unusual symptoms experienced during the posttreatment period.

3. Do not perform any tasks that require mental alertness until drug effects are realized.

ERYTHROMYCINS   (eh-rith-roh-**MY**-sins)

(Rx)

See Chapter 9, *Erythromycins,* p. 117, for all information.

GENTIAN VIOLET   (**JEN**-shun **VYE**-oh-let)

Genapax (Rx)

Classification: Topical and vaginal anti-infective.

Action/Kinetics: This traditional rosaniline dye is effective against some gram-positive bacteria, many fungi (yeasts and dermatophytes), and many strains of *Candida.* Treatment should continue until symptoms subside and cultures are negative.

Uses: Topically for treatment of cutaneous and mucocutaneous *Candida albicans* infections such as thrush, intertriginous and paronychial candidiasis. Vulvovaginal candidiasis.

Contraindications: Hypersensitivity to gentian violet, presence of other vaginal infections, extensive vaginal excoriation, and ulceration. Ulcerative lesions of the face.

Special Concerns: Safe use during pregnancy (category: C) has not been determined. Use with caution in patients suspected of having diabetes mellitus, because vaginal infections often are the first symptoms of this disease.

Side Effects: *Topical:* Irritation, hypersensitivity, ulceration of mucous membranes, permanent staining if applied to granulation tissue. *GI:* Following use for oral candidiasis, esophagitis, laryngitis, tracheitis, laryngeal obstruction. *Vaginal:* Vaginal burning, pain, itching, or other signs of irritation.

Dosage: Vaginal: One tampon (5 mg) inserted for 3–4 hr once or twice daily for 12 consecutive days. An additional tampon may be used overnight in resistant cases. **Topical solution:** Apply 1% or 2% solution to affected areas b.i.d.–t.i.d. for 3 days.

Administration: Tampon should be inserted high into vagina. During last trimester of pregnancy, the suppository should be inserted partially into vagina, preferably by hand.

NURSING CONSIDERATIONS

Client/Family Teaching

1. Review the appropriate method for administration.
2. Stress the importance of good skin care and proper hygiene, to prevent further infection.
3. Keep exposed areas as dry as possible.
4. Wear clean panties with a cotton crotch.
5. Protect skin and clothing from dye.
6. Male partner should wear a condom to prevent re-infection.

IODOQUINOL (DIIODOHYDROXYQUIN)   (eye-OH-doh-KWIN-all)

Diodoquin ✽, Yodoxin (Rx)

Classification: Antiprotozoal.

Action/Kinetics: Mechanism of action is not known. Due to minimal absorption (approximately 8%), high concentrations of the drug are achieved in the intestinal lumen. Drug is eliminated through the feces.

Uses: Acute and chronic intestinal amebiasis.

Contraindications: Hepatic or renal damage or iodine intolerance. Severe thyroid conditions. Nonspecific diarrhea in children. Amebic hepatitis and amebic abscess of the liver.

Special Concerns: Safe use during pregnancy and lactation has not been established. Children may be more likely to develop ophthalmic side effects.

Side Effects: *GI:* Nausea, vomiting, diarrhea, cramps, anal pruritus. *Dermatologic:* Pruritus, urticaria, skin rashes. *Ophthalmologic:* Optic neuritis or atrophy. *CNS:* Fever, chills, headache, vertigo. *Miscellaneous:* Peripheral neuropathy, thyroid enlargement.

Laboratory Test Interferences: Certain thyroid function tests ($\downarrow$ uptake of ^{131}I) for up to 6 months after discontinuance of therapy.

Dosage: Tablets. Adults: 650 mg t.i.d. after meals for 20 days; **pediatric:** 40 mg/kg/day (maximum 650 mg/dose) in three divided doses daily for 20 days. For children, the dose should not exceed 1.95 g in 24 hr for 20 days.

NURSING CONSIDERATIONS

See also *Nursing Considerations For All Anti-Infectives* under *Penicillins,* p. 140.

Interventions

1. Obtain baseline liver and renal function studies and monitor throughout therapy.
2. *For amebiasis, assess* for and report symptoms of iodism, such as furunculosis, dermatitis, sore throat, chills, and fever.

METRONIDAZOLE   (meh-troh-NID-ah-zohl)

Apo-Metronidazole✶, Femazole, Flagyl, Flagyl I.V., Flagyl I.V. RTU, Metizol, Metric 21, MetroGel, Metro I.V., Metryl, Metryl-500, Metryl I.V., Neo-Metric✶, Novonidazole✶, PMS Metronidazole✶, Protostat, Satric, Satric 500 (Rx)

See also *Anti-Infectives,* p. 71.

Classification: Systemic trichomonacide, amebicide.

Action/Kinetics: Effective against anaerobic bacteria and protozoa. Specifically inhibits growth of trichomonae and amebae by binding to DNA resulting in loss of helical structure, strand breakage, inhibition of nucleic acid synthesis, and cell death. Well absorbed from GI tract and widely distributed in body tissues. **Peak serum concentration: PO,** 6–40 mcg/mL, depending on the dose, after 1–2 hr. **t½: PO,** 6–12 hr; average: 8 hr. Eliminated primarily in urine (20% unchanged), which may be red-brown in color following either PO or IV use.

Uses: Systemic. Amebiasis. Symptomatic and asymptomatic trichomoniasis; to treat asymptomatic partner. Amebic dysentery and amebic liver abscess. To reduce postoperative anaerobic infection following colorectal surgery, elective hysterectomy, and emergency appendectomy. Anaerobic bacterial infections of the abdomen, female genital system, skin or skin structures, bones and joints, lower respiratory tract, and CNS. Also, septicemia, endocarditis, hepatic encephalopathy. Orally for Crohn's disease and pseudomembranous colitis. *Investigational:* giardiasis, *Gardnerella vaginalis.* **Topical.** Inflammatory papules, pustules, and erythema of rosacea.

Contraindications: Blood dyscrasias; active organic disease of the CNS. Not recommended for trichomoniasis during the first trimester of pregnancy. During lactation. For topical use: hypersensitivity to parabens or other ingredients of the formulation.

Special Concerns: Pregnancy category: B. Safety and efficacy have not been established in children.

Side Effects: *GI:* Following PO use, nausea, dry mouth, metallic taste, vomiting, diarrhea, abdominal discomfort, constipation. *CNS:* Headache, dizziness, vertigo, incoordination, ataxia, confusion, irritability, depression, weakness, insomnia, syncope, seizures, peripheral neuropathy including paresthesias. *Hematologic:* Leukopenia, bone marrow aplasia. *GU:* Burning, dysuria, cystitis, polyuria, incontinence, dryness of vagina or vulva, dyspareunia, decreased libido. *Allergic:* Urticaria, pruritus, erythematous rash, flushing, nasal congestion, fever, joint pain. *Miscellaneous:* Furry tongue, glossitis, stomatitis (due to overgrowth of *Candida.*) ECG abnormalities, thrombophlebitis.

   Topical Use: Watery eyes if gel applied too closely to this area; transient redness; mild burning, dryness, and skin irritation.

Drug Interactions	
Alcohol, ethyl	Disulfiram-like reaction possible
Anticoagulants, oral	↑ Anticoagulant effect due to ↓ breakdown by liver
Disulfiram	Additive effects

Dosage: Capsules, Tablets. *Amebiasis: Acute amebic dysentery or amebic liver abscess:* **Adult:** 500–750 mg t.i.d. for 5–10 days; **pediatric:** 35–50 mg/kg daily in 3 divided doses for 10 days. *Trichomoniasis, female:* 250 mg t.i.d. for 7 days or 2 g given on 1 day in single or divided doses. **Pediatric:** 5 mg/kg t.i.d. for 7 days. An interval of 4–6 weeks should elapse between courses of therapy. **Note:** Pregnant patients should not be treated during the first trimester. *Male:* Individualize dosage; usual, 250 mg t.i.d. for 7 days. *Giardiasis:* 250 mg t.i.d. for 7 days. *Gardnerella vaginalis:* 500 mg b.i.d. for 7 days. **IV.** *Anaerobic bacterial infections:* **Initially:** 15 mg/kg infused over 1 hr; **then,**

after 6 hr, 7.5 mg/kg q 6 hr for 7–10 days (daily dose should not exceed 4 g). Treatment may be necessary for 2–3 weeks, although PO therapy should be initiated as soon as possible. *Prophylaxis of anaerobic infection during surgery:* **IV,** 15 mg/kg given over a 30- to 60-min period, with completion 1 hr prior to surgery and 7.5 mg/kg infused over 30–60 min 6 and 12 hr after the initial dose.

Topical. *Rosacea:* After washing, apply a thin film and rub in well in the morning and evening for 9 weeks.

NURSING CONSIDERATIONS

See also *General Nursing Considerations For All Anti-Infectives* under *Penicillins,* p. 140.

Administration/Storage

1. If used IV, drug should not be given by IV bolus.
2. Syringes with aluminum needles or hubs should not be used.
3. If a primary IV fluid setup is used, discontinue the primary solution during infusion of metronidazole.
4. The order of mixing to prepare the Powder for Injection is important:
   - Reconstitute.
   - Dilute in IV solutions (in glass or plastic containers).
   - Neutralize pH with sodium bicarbonate solution. Neutralized solutions should not be refrigerated.
5. For topical use, therapeutic results should be seen within 3 weeks with continuing improvement through 9 weeks of therapy.
6. Cosmetics may be used after application of topical metronidazole.

Client/Family Teaching

1. Report any symptoms of CNS toxicity immediately, such as ataxia or tremor, that may necessitate withdrawal of drug.
2. Sexual partners should use a condom throughout therapy.
3. Explain the necessity for the male partner to have therapy also, since organism also may be located in the male urogenital tract.
4. The drug may turn urine brown.
5. Do not drink alcohol when on metronidazole therapy because a disulfiram-like reaction may occur. Symptoms include abdominal cramps, vomiting, flushing, and headache.

PAROMOMYCIN SULFATE   (par-oh-moh-**MY**-sin)

Humatin (Rx)

See Chapter 9, *Aminoglycosides,* p. 75, for all information on this drug.

POVIDONE IODINE   (**POE**-vih-done **EYE**-oh-dyn)

ACU-Dyne, Betadine, Biodine Topical, Bridine✿, Efodine, Frepp, Frepp/Sepp, Iodex Regular, Isodine, Mallisol, Operand, Pharmadine, Polydine, Povadyne, Proviodine✿, Sepp Antiseptic, Surgi-Sep (OTC)

Classification: Antiseptic/germicide.

Action/Kinetics: This product is a nonstinging, nonstaining iodine complex with all of the antiseptic properties of iodine but without skin and mucous membrane irritation. It is bactericidal for gram-positive and gram-negative bacteria, antibiotic-resistant organisms, fungi, viruses, protozoa, and yeasts. It is only used topically. After product application the coloration of skin is an indication of area of antimicrobial activity.

Uses: Topical dressing; degerming of skin; antiseptic for wounds, burns, abrasions; or preoperatively. Treatment of dandruff.

Contraindications: Rare cases of skin sensitivity.

Dosage: All solutions and ointments are used full strength, and all pads, swabs, and other means of application are used only once. Treated area can be bandaged. The following products are available: *Aerosol, Antiseptic Gauze Pads or Solution, Antiseptic Lubricating Gel, Applicators, Helafoam Solution, Iofoam Skin Cleanser, Liquid, Mouthwash/Gargle, Ointment, Perineal Wash Concentrate, Prep Solution, Scrub (including Applicators or Swab Sticks), Shampoo, Skin Cleanser (including foam), Solution (including Prep Pads, Prep Swabs, Swabs, Swab Aid, Swab Sticks, Wipes), Spray, Surgical Scrub (including Sponge/Brush), Whirlpool Concentrate.*

For use as a shampoo for dandruff, 10 mL should be applied to the hair and scalp with warm water. Rinse and repeat application, gently massaging into the scalp and allowing to remain on the scalp for 5 min. Then, rinse scalp thoroughly. Should be repeated twice a week until improvement is observed; then, repeat weekly.

NURSING CONSIDERATIONS

See also *General Nursing Considerations For All Anti-infectives* under *Penicillins,* p. 140.

Client/Family Teaching

1. Assess for skin sensitivity and to report any rash or irritation.
2. Use as directed; drug stains wash off easily.
3. Allow exposed areas to dry before bandaging.

QUINACRINE HYDROCHLORIDE   (KWIN-ah-krin)

Atabrine (Rx)

Classification: Anthelmintic.

Action/Kinetics: Believed to interfere with DNA synthesis of infectious organisms and to release their grip on intestinal wall, allowing parasites to be removed by purging. Well absorbed from GI tract and widely distributed throughout the body. **Peak plasma levels:** 1–3 hr. Highly bound to tissue and plasma proteins. Metabolized and slowly excreted in urine. Remnants of drug are noted 2 months after cessation of therapy.

Uses: Used for giardiasis caused by *Giardia lamblia. Investigational:* Intrapleurally in cystic fibrosis to prevent recurrent pneumothorax.

Contraindications: History of psychosis, in pregnancy, in patients with psoriasis or in those receiving the antimalarial primaquine, porphyria. Use with caution in hepatic disease, alcoholism, and in patients over 60 years of age.

Special Concerns: Children do not tolerate quinacrine as well as adults.

Side Effects:: *CNS:* Headache, dizziness, seizures, vertigo, nervousness, irritability, psychoses, nightmares. *GI:* Nausea, vomiting, diarrhea, anorexia, cramps. *Dermatologic:* Exfoliative dermatitis, contact dermatitis. *Ophthalmologic:* Corneal deposits or edema leading to blurred vision, visual difficulties, halos. Retinopathy. *Miscellaneous:* Aplastic anemia, hepatitis, lichen planus-like eruptions.

Drug Interactions	
Alcohol	Disulfiram-like reaction
Primaquine	↑ Toxicity of primaquine; concomitant use contraindicated

Laboratory Test Interferences: False + or ↑ values for diagenex blue (gastric function test).

Dosage: Tablets. *Giardiasis:* **Adults,** 100 mg t.i.d. for 5 days; **children:** 2 mg/kg t.i.d. after meals for 5 days.

NURSING CONSIDERATIONS

See *Anthelmintics,* p. 216, and *General Nursing Considerations for All Anti-Infectives* under *Penicillins,* p. 140.

Administration/Storage

1. Quinacrine should be taken with a full glass of water, juice, or tea.
2. The drug may be mixed with honey, jam, or chocolate syrup or placed in empty gelatin capsules in order to disguise the bitter taste.

TETRACYCLINES   (teh-trah-**SYE**-kleens)

(Rx)

See Chapter 9, *Tetracyclines,* p. 169, for all information.

CHAPTER SIXTEEN

Urinary Germicides / Analgesics

Urinary tract infections may be treated with one of the sulfonamides, miscellaneous antibiotics, or drugs discussed in this chapter.

ACETOHYDROXAMIC ACID (AHA) (ah-**SEE**-toe-hi-drox-**AM**-ick **AH**-sid)

Lithostat (Rx)

Classification: Antiurolithic, adjunct to treat urinary tract infections.

Action/Kinetics: This drug inhibits the enzyme urease, which decreases the hydrolysis of urea to ammonia. Thus, there is a decrease in both urine alkalinity and ammonia concentration. It is especially useful in urinary tract infections of urea-splitting organisms. Following administration of acetohydroxamic acid, urinary pH decreases, leading to increased efficacy of antibiotics. The drug is not antibacterial itself. Well absorbed from the GI tract and distributed throughout the body. **Peak blood levels:** 15–60 min. **t½:** 5–10 hr. To be effective the drug must be excreted unchanged in the urine (approximately 35%–65%).

Uses: As an adjunct in urinary tract infections due to urea-splitting organisms. Prophylaxis of struvite calculi formation produced by urease-producing bacteria such as *Proteus.*

Contraindications: Should not be used instead of surgery or antibiotic therapy. Renal dysfunction. In females not using contraception. Pregnancy, lactation.

Special Concerns: Pregnancy category: X.

Side Effects: The incidence of adverse effects is high (30%). *GI:* Nausea, vomiting, anorexia. *CNS:* Headaches (common), malaise, depression, tremors, nervousness, anxiety. *Hematologic:* Hemolytic anemia, reticulocytosis without anemia. *Other:* Phlebitis in the legs; nonpruritic, macular skin rash; alopecia.

16

Drug Interactions

| Alcohol | Nonpruritic, macular skin rash within 30–60 min |
| Iron | ↓ Absorption of iron due to chelation by acetohydroxamic acid |

Dosage: Tablets. Adults: 250 mg t.i.d.–q.i.d. up to a maximum of 1.5 g daily. **Pediatric: initially,** 10 mg/kg/day; **then,** adjust dose depending on response and hematologic picture. **Serum creatinine greater than 1.8 mg/dl:** maximum of 1 g/day in divided doses at 12 hr intervals.

NURSING CONSIDERATIONS

Client/Family Teaching

1. Complaints of headaches, especially during the first 2–3 days of therapy, are common and respond well to aspirin.
2. Assure that nausea, vomiting, anorexia, and malaise are usually transient. Drug therapy is rarely terminated because of these symptoms.
3. Demonstrate how to inspect lower legs for redness and tenderness, and pain, which are signs of superficial phlebitis and should be reported to the physician.
4. If loss of body hair is severe, wigs and eye makeup can be utilized.
5. Warn client to forego ingestion of alcohol while on this drug, because a rash may develop.
6. Because drug chelates iron, iron-deficiency anemia may result. Supplemental iron tablets may be recommended.
7. Instruct females of childbearing age to practice some form of birth control.

CINOXACIN (sih-NOX-ah-sin)

Cinobac Pulvules (Rx)

See also *Anti-Infectives,* p. 71.

Classification: Urinary anti-infective.

Action/Kinetics: Cinoxacin acts by inhibiting DNA replication, resulting in a bactericidal action. It is rapidly absorbed after oral administration; a 500-mg dose results in a urine concentration of 300 mcg/mL during the first 4-hr period and 100 mcg/mL during the second 4-hr period. Within 24 hr, 97% is excreted in the urine, 60% unchanged. **Mean serum t½:** 1.5 hr. Food decreases peak serum levels by approximately 30%.

Uses: Initial and recurrent urinary tract infections caused by *Escherichia coli, Proteus mirabilis, P. vulgaris, Klebsiella,* and *Enterobacter* species. *Note:* Cinoxacin is ineffective against *Pseudomonas,* staphylococci, and enterococci infections. Prophylaxis of urinary tract infections.

Contraindications: Hypersensitivity. Infants and prepubertal children. Anuric patients. Lactation.

Special Concerns: Pregnancy category: C. Use with caution in patients with hepatic or kidney disease.

Side Effects: *GI:* Nausea, vomiting, anorexia, cramps, diarrhea. *CNS:* Headache, dizziness, insomnia, confusion, nervousness. *Dermatologic:* Rash, pruritus, urticaria, edema. *Other:* Tingling sensation, photophobia, perineal burning, tinnitus.

Drug Interaction: Probenecid ↓ excretion of cinoxacin → ↓ concentration in the urine.

Laboratory Test Interference: ↑ BUN, SGOT, SGPT, serum creatinine, and alkaline phosphatase.

Dosage: Capsules. Adults: 1 g/day in 2–4 divided doses for 7–14 days. *In patients with impaired renal function:* **Initially,** 500 mg; **then,** dosage schedule based on creatinine clearance (see package insert). *Prophylaxis of infections:* 250 mg at bedtime for up to 5 months.

NURSING CONSIDERATIONS

See also *General Nursing Considerations For All Anti-Infectives* under *Penicillins,* p. 140.

Interventions

1. Ascertain that renal and hepatic function tests are completed before initiating therapy.
2. Do not administer to anuric client.

FLAVOXATE HYDROCHLORIDE   (flay-VOX-ate)

Urispas (Rx)

Classification: Urinary tract antispasmodic.

Action/Kinetics: Flavoxate relieves muscle spasms of the urinary tract by acting directly on the smooth muscle and by cholinergic blockade. The drug has local anesthetic and analgesic effects also. It is well absorbed from GI tract; 10%–30% is excreted in urine.

Uses: Symptomatic relief of urinary tract irritation, dysuria, urgency, nocturia, suprapubic pain, incontinence associated with cystitis, prostatitis, urethritis, urethrocystitis, and other urinary tract disorders. Compatible for use with urinary tract germicides.

Contraindications: Obstructive disorders of urinary tract, including pyloric or duodenal obstructions, intestinal lesions, ileus, achalasia (absence of gastric acid), and GI hemorrhage.

Special Concerns: Use with caution in glaucoma. Safe use in pregnancy (category: B) or in children under 12 years of age not established. Confusion is more likely to occur in geriatric patients.

Side Effects: *GI:* Nausea, vomiting, xerostomia. *CNS:* Drowsiness, headache, vertigo, nervousness, mental confusion (especially in the elderly). *CV:* Tachycardia, palpitations. *Hematologic:* Eosinophilia, leukopenia. *Ophthalmologic:* Blurred vision, increased ocular tension, accommodation disturbances. *Other:* Urticaria, skin rashes, fever, dysuria.

Dosage: Tablets. Adults and children over 12 years: 100 or 200 mg t.i.d.–q.i.d. Dose may be reduced when symptoms decrease.

NURSING CONSIDERATIONS

See also *Nursing Considerations* for *Cholinergic Blocking Agents,* p. 949.

Client/Family Teaching

1. Do not drive a car or operate hazardous machinery as drug may cause drowsiness and blurred vision.
2. Practice good oral hygiene. Relieve dryness of mouth with ice chips or hard candy.
3. Report any persistent, bothersome side effects.

METHENAMINE   (meh-**THEN**-ah-meen)

(OTC)

METHENAMINE HIPPURATE   (meh-**THEN**-ah-meen)

Hip-Rex✳, Hiprex, Urex (Rx)

METHENAMINE MANDELATE   (meh-**THEN**-ah-meen)

Deltamine, Mandelamine, Methendelate (Rx)

Classification: Urinary tract anti-infective.

Action/Kinetics: This drug is converted in an acid medium into ammonia and formaldehyde (the active principle), which denatures protein. Thus it is most effective when the urine has a pH value of 5.5 or less, which is maintained by using the hippurate or mandelate salt. Readily absorbed from GI tract but up to 60% may be hydrolyzed by gastric acid if tablets are not enteric-coated. To be effective, urinary formaldehyde concentration must be greater than 25 mcg/mL. **Peak levels of formaldehyde:** 2 hr if using hippurate and 3–8 hr if using mandelate (if urinary pH is 5.5 or less). **t¹/₂:** 3–6 hr. Seventy to 90% of drug and metabolites excreted in urine within 24 hr.

Uses: Acute, chronic, and recurrent urinary tract infections by susceptible organisms, especially gram-negative organisms including *E. coli*. As a prophylactic before urinary tract instrumentation. Never used as sole agent in the treatment of acute infections.

Contraindications: Renal insufficiency, severe liver damage, or severe dehydration.

Special Concerns: Pregnancy category: C. Use with caution in gout (methenamine may cause urate crystals to precipitate in the urine).

Side Effects: *GI:* Nausea, vomiting, diarrhea, anorexia, cramps, stomatitis. *GU:* Hematuria, albuminuria, crystalluria, dysuria, urinary frequency or urgency, bladder irritation. *Dermatologic:* Skin rashes, urticaria, pruritus. *Other:* Tinnitus, muscle cramps, headache, dyspnea, edema, lipoid pneumonitis.

Drug Interactions	
Acetazolamide	↓ Effect of methenamine due to ↑ alkalinity of urine by acetazolamide
Sodium bicarbonate	↓ Effect of methenamine due to ↑ alkalinity of urine by sodium bicarbonate
Sulfonamides	↑ Chance of sulfonamide crystalluria due to acid urine produced by methenamine
Thiazide diuretics	↓ Effect of methenamine due to ↑ alkalinity of urine produced by thiazides

Laboratory Test Interference: False-positive urinary glucose with Benedict's solution. Drug interferes with determination of urinary catecholamines and estriol levels by acid hydrolysis technique (enzymatic techniques not affected). False + catecholamines, hydroxycorticosteroids, vanillylmandelic acid; false − 5-hydroxyindoleacetic acid.

Dosage: Tablets. *Hippurate:* **Adults and children over 12 years:** 1 g b.i.d. in the morning and evening; **children, 6–12 years:** 0.5 g b.i.d.

Oral Solution, Oral Suspension, Tablets. *Mandelate:* **Adults:** 1 g q.i.d. after meals and at bedtime; **children 6–12 years:** 0.5 g q.i.d.; **children under 6 years:** 0.25 g/30 lb q.i.d.

NURSING CONSIDERATIONS

See also *Nursing Considerations For All Anti-Infectives* under *Penicillins,* p. 140.

Interventions

1. An acidic urine should be maintained, especially when treating *Proteus* or *Pseudomonas* infections.

2. Oral methenamine mandelate suspensions have a vegetable oil base; particular care should thus be taken in the elderly or debilitated to prevent lipid pneumonia.

3. If GI upset occurs, the drug can be taken with food.

4. Alkalinizing foods (e.g., milk products) or medication (e.g., acetazolamide, bicarbonate) should not be taken in excess in order to maintain an acidic urine.

5. *Assess*
   - for skin rash, which is an indication of drug withdrawal.
   - clients on high dosage of drug for bladder irritation, painful and frequent micturition, albuminuria, and hematuria.
   - for idiosyncratic effect (characterized by nausea, vomiting, dermatologic reaction, tinnitus, and muscle cramps).

6. Clearly indicate on chart that client is receiving drug, because drug will interfere with tests to determine urinary estriol, catecholamines, and hydroxyindoleacetic acid.

7. Maintain an adequate fluid intake (between 1,500 and 2,000 mL daily).

8. Monitor intake and output.

9. Use Labstix or Nitrazine paper daily to test that pH of urine is 5.5 or lower.

10. Urine may become turbid and full of sediment when methenamine mandelate is administered concomitantly with sulfamethizole.

METHYLENE BLUE (METH-ih-leen)

Urolene Blue (Rx)

Classification: Urinary germicide, antidote, oxidizing agent.

Action/Kinetics: Methylene blue is a dye possessing bacteriostatic activity. High doses oxidize Fe^2 (ferrous ion) of reduced hemoglobin to Fe^3 (ferric ion), resulting in methemoglobinemia (basis for use in cyanide poisoning). Lower doses increase the conversion of methemoglobin to hemoglobin.

Uses: Mild GU tract antiseptic, drug-induced methemoglobinemia, antidote for cyanide poisoning, treatment of urinary tract calculi (oxalate). *Investigational:* Diagnosis of ruptured amniotic membranes; by its dye effect can determine body structures and fistulas.

Contraindications: Hypersensitivity to drug. Renal insufficiency.

Special Concerns: Use with caution in patients with glucose-6-phosphate dehydrogenase deficiency, as hemolysis may result.

Side Effects: *GI:* Nausea, vomiting, diarrhea. *GU:* Dysuria, bladder irritation, may cause urine or feces to turn blue-green. *Other:* Anemia, fever, cyanosis, CV abnormalities.

Dosage: Tablets. *GU antiseptic:* 55–130 mg t.i.d. after meals with a full glass of water. **IV.** *Antidote:* 1–2 mg/kg slowly over several minutes.

NURSING CONSIDERATIONS

Client/Family Teaching
Stress that medication may turn urine and stools a blue-green color and will stain tissue.

Evaluation
Obtain and review appropriate lab data and assess for symptoms of GI or GU dysfunction.

NALIDIXIC ACID   (nah-lih-**DIX**-ick **AH**-sid)

NegGram (Rx)

Classification: Urinary germicide.

Action/Kinetics: Nalidixic acid is believed to inhibit the DNA synthesis of the microorganism, probably by interfering with DNA polymerization. The drug is either bacteriostatic or bactericidal. Nalidixic acid is rapidly absorbed from the GI tract. **Peak plasma concentration:** 20–40 mcg/mL after 1–2 hr; **peak urine levels:** 150–200 mcg/mL after 3–4 hr. **t½:** 1.1–2.5 hr, increased to 21 hr in anuric patients. The drug is extensively protein bound, partially metabolized in liver, and rapidly excreted in urine.

Sensitivity determinations are recommended before and periodically during prolonged administration of nalidixic acid. Renal and liver function tests are advisable if course of therapy exceeds 2 weeks.

Uses: Acute and chronic urinary tract infections caused by susceptible gram-negative organisms, including *Escherichia coli, Proteus, Enterobacter,* and *Klebsiella.*

Contraindications: To be used with caution in patients with liver disease, severely impaired kidney function, epilepsy, and severe cerebral arteriosclerosis. Lactation. Use not recommended in infants and children.

Special Concerns: Safety in pregnancy has not been established.

Side Effects: *GI:* Nausea, vomiting, diarrhea, pain. *CNS:* Drowsiness, headache, dizziness, weakness, vertigo, toxic psychoses, seizures (rare). *Allergic:* Photosensitivity, skin rashes, arthralgia, pruritus, urticaria, angioedema, eosinophilia. *Hematologic:* Leukopenia, thrombocytopenia, hemolytic anemia (especially in patients with glucose 6-phosphate dehydrogenase deficiency). *Other:* Metabolic acidosis, cholestatic jaundice, paresthesia.

Drug Interactions	
Antacids, oral	↓ Effect of nalidixic acid due to ↓ absorption from GI tract
Anticoagulants, oral	↑ Effect of anticoagulants due to ↓ in plasma protein binding
Nitrofurantoin	↓ Effect of nalidixic acid

Laboratory Test Interferences: False + for urinary glucose with Benedict's solution, Fehling's solution, or Clinitest Reagent tablets. Falsely elevated 17-ketosteroids.

Dosage: Oral Suspension, Tablets. Adults: initially, 1 g q.i.d. for 1–2 weeks; **maintenance,** if necessary, 2 g daily.

NURSING CONSIDERATIONS

See also *Nursing Considerations For All Anti-infectives* under *Penicillins*, p. 140.

Intervention

Use Clinistix Reagent Strips or Tes-Tape for urinary tests because other methods may result in a false-positive reaction. Finger sticks are the most reliable for client glucose determinations.

NITROFURANTOIN   (nye-troh-fyou-**RAN**-toyn)

Apo-Nitrofurantoin✤, Furadantin, Furalan, Furan, Furanite, Furatoin, Furaton, Nephronex✤, Nitrofan, Nitrofor, Nitrofuracot, Novofuran✤, Ro-Antoin (Rx)

NITROFURANTOIN MACROCRYSTALS   (nye-troh-fyou-**RAN**-toyn)

Macrodantin (Rx)

See also *Anti-Infectives*, p. 71.

Classification: Urinary germicide.

Action/Kinetics: Nitrofurantoin interferes with bacterial carbohydrate metabolism by inhibiting acetylcoenzyme A; the drug also interferes with bacterial cell wall synthesis. It is bacteriostatic at low concentrations and bactericidal at high concentrations. Tablets are readily absorbed from the GI tract. **t½:** 20 min. **Urine levels:** 50–250 mcg/mL. From 30% to 50% excreted unchanged in the urine. Nitrofurantoin macrocrystals (Macrodantin) are available; this preparation maintains effectiveness while decreasing GI distress.

Uses: Severe urinary tract infections refractory to other agents. Useful in the treatment of pyelonephritis, pyelitis, or cystitis caused by susceptible organisms, including *Escherichia coli, Staphylococcus aureus,* and *Streptococcus faecalis* and certain strains of *Enterobacter, Proteus,* and *Klebsiella.*

Contraindications: Anuria, oliguria, and patients with impaired renal function (creatinine clearance below 40 mL/min); pregnant women, especially near term; infants less than 1 month of age; and nursing mothers.

Special Concerns: To be used with extreme caution in patients with anemia, diabetes, electrolyte imbalance, avitaminosis B, or a debilitating disease.

Side Effects: Nitrofurantoin is a potentially toxic drug with many side effects. *GI:* Nausea, vomiting, anorexia, diarrhea, abdominal pain, parotitis, pancreatitis. *CNS:* Headache, dizziness, vertigo, drowsiness, nystagmus. *Hematologic:* Leukopenia, thrombocytopenia, eosinophilia, megaloblastic anemia, agranulocytosis, granulocytopenia, hemolytic anemia (especially in patients with glucose-6-phosphate dehydrogenase deficiency). *Allergic:* Drug fever, skin rashes, pruritus, urticaria, angioedema, exfoliative dermatitis, erythema multiforme (rarely, Stevens-Johnson syndrome), anaphylaxis, arthralgia, asthma symptoms in susceptible patients. *Respiratory:* Dyspnea, cough, chest pain, permanent impairment of pulmonary function with chronic therapy. *Hepatic:* Hepatitis, cholestatic jaundice, cholestatic hepatitis, liver dysfunction. *Miscellaneous:* Peripheral neuropathy, alopecia, superinfections of the GU tract, hypotension, muscle pain.

Drug Interactions

Acetazolamide	↓ Effect of nitrofurantoin due to ↑ alkalinity of urine produced by acetazolamide
Antacids, oral	↓ Effect of nitrofurantoin due to ↓ absorption from GI tract
Anticholinergic drugs	↑ Effect of nitrofurantoin due to ↑ absorption from stomach
Magnesium trisilicate	Mg trisilicate ↓ absorption of nitrofurantoin from GI tract
Nalidixic acid	Nitrofurantoin ↓ effect of nalidixic acid
Probenecid	High doses ↓ secretion of nitrofurantoin → toxicity
Sodium bicarbonate	↓ Effect of nitrofurantoin due to ↑ alkalinity of urine produced by sodium bicarbonate

Dosage: Capsules, Oral Suspension, Tablets. Adults: 50–100 mg q.i.d., not to exceed 400 mg/day; **prolonged therapy:** 50–100 mg at bedtime. **Children:** 5–7 mg/kg/day in 4 equal doses; **prolonged therapy:** 1 mg/kg/day in 1–2 doses.

NURSING CONSIDERATIONS

See also *General Nursing Considerations For All Anti-Infectives* under *Penicillins,* p. 140.

Administration/Storage

1. Administer oral medication with meals or milk to reduce gastric irritation.
2. Preferably, administer capsules containing crystals, instead of tablets, because crystals cause less GI intolerance.
3. Store oral medications in amber-colored bottles.
4. The medication should be continued for a minimum of 3 days after obtaining a negative urine culture.

Interventions

1. Observe client for acute or delayed anaphylactic reaction and have emergency equipment readily available.
2. Clearly label chart to show that client is on drug, because it may alter certain laboratory determinations.

Client/Family Teaching

1. Drug may turn urine a brown color.
2. Take as prescribed and complete the full course of therapy.
3. Take with food or milk to minimize GI upset.
4. Report any persistent or bothersome side effects.

Evaluation

Assess

- for peripheral neuropathy, manifested by numbness and tingling in the extremities. These side effects are indications for drug withdrawal, since the condition may worsen and become irreversible.

- for superinfection of the GI tract.
- Blacks and ethnic groups of Mediterranean and Near Eastern origin for symptoms of anemia.

NORFLOXACIN   (nor-**FLOX**-ah-sin)
Noroxin (Rx)

See also *Anti-Infectives,* p. 71.

Classification: Urinary anti-infective.

Action/Kinetics: Norfloxacin manifests activity against gram-positive and gram-negative organisms by inhibiting bacterial DNA synthesis. It is not effective against obligate anaerobes. **Peak plasma levels:** 1.4–1.6 mcg/mL after 1–2 hr following a dose of 400 mg and 2.5 mcg/mL 1–2 hr after a dose of 800 mg. **t½:** 3–4 hr. Approximately 30% excreted unchanged in the urine and 30% through the feces.

Uses: Complicated and uncomplicated urinary tract infections caused by *Escherichia coli, K. pneumoniae, E. cloacae, Proteus mirabilis* and *P. vulgaris. Providencia rettgeri, Pseudomonas aeruginosa, Citrobacter freundii, Morganella morganii, Staphylococcus aureus, S. epidermidis,* and Group D streptococci.

Contraindications: Hypersensitivity to nalidixic acid, cinoxacin, or norfloxacin. Lactation, infants and children.

Special Concerns: Pregnancy category: C. Use with caution in patients with a history of seizures and in impaired renal function.

Side Effects: *GI:* Nausea, abdominal pain, dyspepsia, heartburn, constipation, flatulence, diarrhea, vomiting, dry mouth. *CNS:* Dizziness, headache, fatigue, depression, insomnia, somnolence. *Hematologic:* Decreased hematocrit, eosinophilia, decreased WBC count or neutrophil count. *Other:* Rash, fever, erythema, visual disturbances.

Drug Interactions

Nitrofurantoin	↓ Antibacterial effect of norfloxacin
Probenecid	↓ Urinary excretion of norfloxacin

Laboratory Test Interferences: ↑ SGPT, SGOT, alkaline phosphatase, BUN, serum creatinine, and LDH.

Dosage: Tablets. *Uncomplicated urinary tract infections:* 400 mg b.i.d. for 7–10 days. *Complicated urinary tract infections:* 400 mg b.i.d. for 10–21 days. Maximum dose for urinary tract infections should not exceed 800 mg daily. *Impaired renal function, with creatinine clearance equal to or less than 30 mL/min/1.73 m²:* 400 mg once daily for 7–10 days.

NURSING CONSIDERATIONS
See also *General Nursing Considerations For All Anti-Infectives* under *Penicillins,* p. 140.

Interventions
1. The drug is not for use in pregnant women or in children.
2. Anticipate reduced dosage with impaired renal function.

Client/Family Teaching

1. The medication should be taken 1 hr before or 2 hr after meals, with a glass of water.
2. To prevent crystalluria, clients should be well hydrated.
3. Antacids should not be taken with or for 2 hr after a dose of norfloxacin.
4. Use caution while operating equipment or in driving a motor vehicle as the drug may cause dizziness.

OXYBUTYNIN CHLORIDE (ox-ee-BYOU-tih-nin)

Ditropan (Rx)

Classification: Antispasmodic.

Action/Kinetics: Oxybutynin causes increased vesicle capacity and delay of initial urgency to void by exerting a direct antispasmodic effect. Has no effect at either the neuromuscular junction or autonomic ganglia. Has 4–10 times the antispasmodic effect of atropine but only one-fifth the anticholinergic activity. **Onset:** 30–60 min; **Time to peak effect:** 3–6 hr; **duration:** 6–10 hr. Eliminated through the urine.

Use: Neurogenic bladder disease characterized by urinary retention, urinary overflow, incontinence, nocturia, urinary frequency or urgency, reflex neurogenic bladder.

Contraindications: Glaucoma, GI obstruction, paralytic ileus, intestinal atony, megacolon, severe colitis, myasthenia gravis, obstructive urinary tract disease, massive hemorrhage.

Special Concerns: *Use with caution when increased cholinergic effect is undesirable and in the elderly.* Safe use during pregnancy (pregnancy category: B) and in children less than 5 years of age has not been determined. Use with caution in geriatric patients; in patients with autonomic neuropathy, renal, or hepatic disease; and in patients with hiatal hernia with reflex esophagitis.

Side Effects: *GI:* Nausea, vomiting, constipation, bloated feeling. *CNS:* Drowsiness, insomnia, weakness, dizziness. *EENT:* Dry mouth, blurred vision, dilation of pupil, cycloplegia, increased ocular tension. *CV:* Tachycardia, palpitations. *Miscellaneous:* Decreased sweating, urinary hesitancy and retention, impotence, suppression of lactation, severe allergic reactions, drug idiosyncrasies, urticaria, and other dermal manifestations. **Note:** The drug may aggravate symptoms of prostatic hypertrophy, hypertension, coronary heart disease, congestive heart failure, hyperthyroidism, cardiac arrhythmias, and tachycardia.

Overdosage

Intense CNS disturbances (restlessness, psychoses), circulatory changes (flushing, hypotension) and failure, respiratory failure, paralysis, coma.

Treatment of Overdosage

Stomach lavage, physostigmine (0.5–2 mg IV; repeat as necessary up to maximum of 5 mg). Supportive therapy, if necessary. Counteract excitement with sodium thiopental (2%) or chloral hydrate (100–200 mL of 2% solution) rectally. Artificial respiration may be necessary if respiratory muscles become paralyzed.

Dosage: Syrup, Tablets. Adults: 5 mg b.i.d.–t.i.d.; maximum dosage, 20 mg daily. **Children, over 5 yr:** 5 mg b.i.d.–t.i.d.; maximum dosage, 15 mg daily.

NURSING CONSIDERATIONS

See also *Nursing Considerations* for *Cholinergic Blocking Agents,* p. 949.

Administration/Storage

Store in tight containers at 15°–30°C.

Intervention

Review technique and be prepared to assist with treatment of overdose, as noted under *Treatment of Overdosage.*

Client/Family Teaching

1. Review prescription and instruct client to take only as directed.
2. Report any persistent complications noted under *Side Effects* to physician.
3. Use caution in driving a car or in operating dangerous machinery, as drug may cause drowsiness and blurred vision.
4. Consult with physician before continuing with medication if diarrhea occurs (especially in clients with an ileostomy or colostomy), as diarrhea may be an early symptom of intestinal obstruction.
5. Avoid overexposure to heat and acknowledge the body's need for increased fluids in hot weather, because sweating is inhibited by the drug and heat stroke may occur.
6. Instruct to occasionally rinse mouth with water and to increase fluid intake unless contraindicated, to relieve dryness of mouth.
7. Return as scheduled for cystometry to evaluate response to therapy and to determine the need for continuation of medication.

Evaluation

Note response to therapy and results of cystometry.

PHENAZOPYRIDINE HYDROCHLORIDE   (fen-ay-zoh-**PEER**-ih-deen)

A20–Standard, Baridium, Eridium, Geridium, Phenazo✹, Phenazodine, Phenylazo Diamino Pyridine HCl, Pyrazodine, Pyridate, Pyridin, Pyridium, Pyronium✹, Urodine, Urogesic, Viridium (Rx)

Classification: Urinary analgesic.

Action/Kinetics: Phenazopyridine HCl is an azo dye with local anesthetic effects on the urinary tract. Up to 90% excreted unchanged or as metabolites within 24 hr.

Uses: Pain relief in chronic urinary tract infections or irritation, including cystitis, urethritis and pyelitis, trauma, surgery, or urinary tract instrumentation. May also be used as an adjunct to antibacterial therapy.

Contraindications: Renal insufficiency.

Special Concerns: Pregnancy category: B.

Side Effects: *GI:* Nausea. *Hematologic:* Methemoglobinemia, hemolytic anemia (especially in patients with glucose-6-phosphate dehydrogenase deficiency). *Dermatologic:* Yellowish tinge of the skin or sclerae may indicate accumulation of drug due to renal insufficiency. *Miscellaneous:* Renal and hepatic toxicity.

Laboratory Test Interferences: Clinistix or Tes-Tape, colorimetric laboratory test procedures.

Dosage: Tablets. Adults: 200 mg t.i.d. with or after meals. **Pediatric, 6–12 years:** 4 mg/kg t.i.d. with food.

Treatment of Overdosage: To treat methemoglobinemia, administer methylene blue (IV: 1–2 mg/kg) or ascorbic acid (PO: 100–200 mg).

NURSING CONSIDERATIONS

Assessment

Note any history of liver and/or renal dysfunction.

Client/Family Teaching

1. Take medication with or after meals to prevent GI upset.
2. Should be used for only 2 days when taken together with an antibacterial agent for urinary tract infections.
3. Inform client how to monitor intake and output and record.
4. Utilize finger sticks to evaluate blood sugar in clients with diabetes.
5. Drug turns urine orange-red; may stain fabrics.

CHAPTER SEVENTEEN
Antiviral Drugs

General Statement: Viruses consist of a core of nucleic acid (either DNA or RNA but not both) and a coat of protein or lipoprotein; they are the most elementary of the infectious agents. To replicate, viruses must penetrate suitable cells whose machinery they take over to make copies of themselves. Thus, it has been difficult to discover drugs selective against viruses that do not interfere with host cell function. Most antibiotics are ineffective against viruses, because viruses do not have cell walls whose synthesis is usually interfered with by antibiotics. Several drugs have been developed that are effective against certain viruses. Further development of such drugs promises significant advances in the treatment of virally induced diseases, such as Acquired Immune Deficiency Syndrome (AIDS).

Vaccination has been widely used to prevent certain viral infections. For example, viruses causing measles, small pox, polio, rubella, yellow fever, hepatitis B, and others can be controlled in this manner. However, there are no vaccinations available for viruses causing influenza, upper respiratory tract infections, and cold sores.

ACYCLOVIR (ACYCLOGUANOSINE)   (ay-SYE-kloh-veer, ay-SYE-kloh-gwon-oh-seen)
Zovirax (Rx)

Classification: Antiviral anti-infective.

Action/Kinetics: Acyclovir is converted to acyclovir triphosphate, which interferes with herpes simplex virus DNA polymerase, thereby inhibiting DNA replication. Systemic absorption is minimal from the GI tract (although therapeutic levels are reached) and following topical administration. **Peak levels after PO:** 1.5–2 hr. **t½, PO:** 3.3 hr. Metabolites and unchanged drug (up to 85%) are excreted through the kidney. Dosage should be reduced in patients with impaired renal function.

Uses: PO. Initial and recurrent genital herpes in immunocompromised and nonimmunocompromised patients. Prophylaxis of frequently recurrent genital herpes infections in nonimmunocompromised patients. **Parenteral.** Initial therapy for severe genital herpes; initial and recurrent mucosal and cutaneous HSV-1 and HSV-2 infections in immunocompromised individuals. Varicella zoster infections (shingles) in immunocompromised patients. Herpes simplex encephalitis (HSE). **Topical.** Acyclovir decreases healing time and duration of viral shedding in initial herpes genitalis. Also used for limited nonlife-threatening mucocutaneous herpes simplex virus infections in immunocompromised patients. The drug does not seem to be beneficial in recurrent herpes genitalis or in herpes labialis in nonimmunocompromised patients.

Investigational: Cytomegalovirus and HSV infection following bone marrow or renal transplantation; herpes simplex ocular infections; herpes simplex proctitis; herpes simplex whitlow; herpes zoster encephalitis; disseminated primary eczema herpeticum; herpes simplex-associated erythema multiform; infectious mononucleosis, varicella pneumonia, varicella zoster in immunocompromised patients.

Contraindications: Hypersensitivity to formulation. Use in the eye.

Special Concerns: Pregnancy category: C. Use with caution during lactation. Use with caution with concomitant intrathecal methotrexate or interferon. Safety and efficacy of oral form not established in children.

Side Effects: PO. *Short-term treatment. GI:* Nausea, vomiting, diarrhea, anorexia, sore throat, taste of drug. *CNS:* Headache, dizziness, fatigue. *Miscellaneous:* Edema, skin rashes, leg pain, inguinal adenopathy. *Long-term treatment. GI:* Nausea, vomiting, diarrhea, sore throat. *CNS:* Headache, vertigo, insomnia, fatigue, fever, depression, irritability. *Other:* Arthralgia, rashes, palpitations, superficial thrombophlebitis, muscle cramps, menstrual abnormalities, acne, lymphadenopathy, alopecia.

Parenteral. *At injection site:* Phlebitis, inflammation. *CNS:* Encephalopathic changes, jitters, headache. *Miscellaneous:* Skin rashes, urticaria, sweating, hypotension, nausea, thrombocytosis.

Topical. Transient burning, stinging, pain. Pruritus, rash, vulvitis. *Note:* All of these effects have also been reported with the use of a placebo preparation.

Dosage: Capsules, Tablets. *Initial genital herpes:* 200 mg q 4 hr (while awake) for a total of 5 capsules/day for 10 days. *Chronic genital herpes:* 200 mg t.i.d. for up to 12 months. Up to five 200-mg capsules/day may be required. *Intermittent therapy:* 200 mg q 4 hr (while awake) for a total of 5 capsules/day for 5 days.

IV infusion. *Mucosal and cutaneous herpes simplex:* **Adults,** 5 mg/kg infused at a constant rate

17

over 1 hr, q 8 hr (15 mg/kg/day) for 7 days. **Children:** 250 mg/m^2 infused at a constant rate over 1 hr, q 8 hr for 7 days. *Varicella-zoster infections:* **Adults,** 10 mg/kg infused over a constant rate over 1 hr, q 8 hr for 7 days. **Children:** 500 mg/m^2 infused at a constant rate over at least 1 hr, q 8 hr for 7 days. *Herpes simplex encephalitis:* **Adults,** 10 mg/kg infused at a constant rate over at least 1 hr, q 8 hr for 10 days. **Children:** 500 mg/m^2 infused at a constant rate over at least 1 hr, q 8 hr for 10 days.

   Topical (5% ointment), Adults and children: Lesion should be covered with sufficient amount of ointment (0.5 inch ribbon per 4 sq in. of surface area) every 3 hr 6 times/day for 7 days.

NURSING CONSIDERATIONS

See also *General Nursing Considerations For All Anti-Infectives* under *Penicillins,* p. 140.

Administration/Storage

1. Reconstituted solution should be used within 12 hr.
2. If refrigerated, reconstituted solution may show a precipitate, which dissolves at room temperature.
3. Store ointment in a dry place at room temperature.
4. To prevent spread of infection to other body sites, use a finger cot or rubber glove when applying the cream.

Client/Family Teaching

1. Cover all lesions with acyclovir as ordered, but not to exceed the frequency or length of time that treatment is recommended.
2. Apply acyclovir ointment in the amount directed with a finger cot or rubber glove to prevent transmission of infection.
3. Report any burning, stinging, itching, and rash if they occur due to application of acyclovir.
4. Encourage client to complete the examination and tests to rule out possible presence of other sexually transmitted diseases.
5. Return for medical supervision if there is a recurrence of herpes simplex virus, as acyclovir is ineffective for treatment of reinfection.
6. Acyclovir will not prevent transmission of disease to others or prevent reinfection.
7. The total dose and dosage schedule differ depending on whether the infection is initial or chronic and whether intermittent therapy regimen is being used. Therefore, following prescribed dosage and duration of treatment is extremely important.
8. Use condoms for sexual intercourse to prevent reinfections while undergoing treatment.
9. Abstain from intercourse during acute outbreaks.

Evaluation

1. Assess client/family knowledge and understanding of illness, response to therapy and to teaching.
2. Observe for freedom from complications of drug therapy.

AMANTADINE HYDROCHLORIDE   (ah-**MAN**-tah-deen)

Symadine, Symmetrel (Rx)

Classification: Antiviral and antiparkinson agent.

Action/Kinetics: As an antiviral agent, amantadine is believed to prevent penetration of the virus into cells, possibly by inhibiting uncoating of the RNA virus. Amantadine may also prevent the release of infectious viral nucleic acid into the host cell. The drug reduces symptoms of viral infections if given within 24–48 hr after onset of illness.

For the treatment parkinsonism, the drug causes release of dopamine from synaptosomes or blocks the reuptake of dopamine into presynaptic neurons. Either of these mechanisms results in an increase in the levels of dopamine in dopaminergic synapses in the corpus striatum. Well absorbed from GI tract. **Onset:** 48 hrs. **Peak serum concentration:** 0.2 mcg/mL after 1–4 hr. **t½:** range of 9–37 hr, longer in presence of renal impairment. Ninety percent excreted unchanged in urine.

Use: Influenza A viral infections of the respiratory tract (prophylaxis and treatment of high-risk patients with immunodeficiency, cardiovascular, metabolic, neuromuscular or pulmonary disease).

Symptomatic treatment of idiopathic parkinsonism and parkinsonism syndrome resulting from encephalitis, carbon monoxide intoxication, drugs, or cerebral arteriosclerosis. The drug decreases extrapyramidal symptoms, including akinesia, rigidity, tremors, excessive salivation, gait disturbances, and total functional disability. Favorable results have been obtained in about 50% of the patients. Improvements can last for up to 30 months, although some patients report that the effect of the drug wears off in 1 to 3 months. A rest period or an increased dosage may reestablish effectiveness. For parkinsonism, amantadine hydrochloride is usually used concomitantly with other agents, such as levodopa and anticholinergic agents.

Contraindications: Hypersensitivity to drug.

Special Concerns: Administer with caution to patients with liver and renal disease, history of epilepsy, CHF, peripheral edema, orthostatic hypotension, recurrent eczematoid dermatitis, or severe psychosis, to patients on CNS stimulant drugs, to those exposed to rubella, and to nursing mothers. Safe use for those who may become pregnant (category: C), for lactating mothers, and in children less than one year has not been established.

Side Effects: *GI:* Nausea, vomiting, constipation, anorexia, xerostomia. *CNS:* Depression, psychosis, convulsions, hallucinations, lightheadedness, confusion, ataxia, irritability, anxiety, headache, dizziness, fatigue, insomnia. *CV:* Congestive heart failure, orthostatic hypotension, peripheral edema. *Miscellaneous:* Urinary retention, leukopenia, neutropenia, mottling of skin of the extremities due to poor peripheral circulation (livedo reticularis), skin rashes, visual problems, slurred speech, oculogyric episodes, dyspnea, weakness, eczematoid dermatitis.

Drug Interactions	
Anticholinergics	Additive anticholinergic effects (including hallucinations, confusion), especially with trihexyphenidyl and benztropine
CNS stimulants	May ↑ CNS and psychic effects of amantadine; use cautiously together
Hydrochlorothiazide/triamterene combination	↓ Urinary excretion of amantadine → ↑ plasma levels
Levodopa	Potentiated by amantadine

Dosage: Capsules, Syrup. *Antiviral.* **Adults:** 200 mg daily as a single or divided dose. **Children, 1–9 years:** 4.4–8.8 mg/kg/day up to a maximum of 150 mg/day in 1 or 2 divided doses (use syrup); **9–12 years:** 100 mg b.i.d. *Prophylactic treatment:* institute before or immediately after exposure and continue for 10–21 days if used concurrently with vaccine or for 90 days without vaccine. *Symptomatic management:* initiate as soon as possible and continue for 24–48 hr after disappearance of symptoms. Dose should be decreased in renal impairment (see package insert). *Parkinsonism.* When used as sole agent, usual dose is 100 mg b.i.d.; may be necessary to increase up to 400 mg/day in divided doses. When used with other antiparkinson drugs: 100 mg 1–2 times/day. *Drug-induced extrapyramidal symptoms:* 100 mg b.i.d. (up to 300 mg/day may be required in some). Dosage should be reduced in patients with impaired renal function.

Treatment of Overdosage: Gastric lavage or induction of emesis followed by supportive measures. Ensure that patient is well hydrated; give IV fluids if necessary.

NURSING CONSIDERATIONS

See also *General Nursing Considerations For All Anti-Infectives* under *Penicillins,* p. 140.

Administration/Storage

Protect capsules from moisture.

Assessment

1. Obtain a thorough nursing history and note any history of seizures, CHF and renal insufficiency.
2. Anticipate that following loss of effectiveness of the drug, benefits may be regained by increasing the dosage or discontinuing the drug for several weeks and then reinstituting it.

Client/Family Teaching

1. Do not drive a car or work in a situation where alertness is important, because medication can affect vision, concentration, and coordination.
2. Rise slowly from a prone position, because orthostatic hypotension may occur.
3. Lie down if dizzy or weak, in order to relieve these symptoms of orthostatic hypotension.
4. Report patchy discoloration of the skin, but also that discoloration lessens when legs are elevated and usually fades completely within weeks after discontinuing drug.
5. Report any exposure to rubella, because drug may increase susceptibility to disease.
6. Susceptible individuals should avoid crowds during "flu" season.
7. Notify physician of any persistent or bothersome side effects.
8. Administer last daily dose several hours before retiring to prevent insomnia.

Evaluation

Assess

- clients with a history of epilepsy or other seizures for an increase in seizure activity and take appropriate precautions.
- clients with a history of CHF or peripheral edema for increased edema and/or respiratory distress and report promptly.
- clients with renal impairment for crystalluria, oliguria, and increased BUN or creatinine levels and report promptly.

GANCICLOVIR SODIUM (DHPG)   (gan-**SYE**-Kloh-veer)

Cytovene (Rx)

Classification: Antiviral.

Action/Kinetics: Upon entry into viral cells infected by cytomegalovirus (CMV), ganciclovir is converted to ganciclovir triphosphate by the CMV. Ganciclovir triphosphate inhibits viral DNA synthesis by competitive inhibition of viral DNA polymerases and direct incorporation into viral DNA; this results in eventual termination of viral DNA elongation. Ganciclovir is active against CMV, herpes simplex virus-1 and -2, Epstein-Barr virus, and varicella zoster virus. **t^{1}/$_{2}$:** Approximately 2.9 hr. The drug is believed to cross the blood-brain barrier. Most of the drug is excreted unchanged through the urine. Renal impairment increases the t^{1}/$_{2}$ of the drug.

Uses: At the present time, ganciclovir is indicated only in immunocompromised patients with CMV retinitis, including AIDS patients. Diagnosis may be confirmed by culture of CMV from the blood, urine, or throat; note that a negative CMV culture does not rule out CMV retinitis.

Contraindications: Hypersensitivity to acyclovir or ganciclovir. Lactation.

Special Concerns: Safety and effectiveness of ganciclovir have not been established for non-immunocompromised patients, treatment of other CMV infections such as pneumonitis or colitis, or for congenital or neonatal CMV disease. Use with caution in impaired renal function and in elderly patients. Use during pregnancy (category: C) and in children only if potential benefits outweigh potential risks.

Side Effects: *Hematologic:* Granulocytopenia, thrombocytopenia, neutropenia (may be irreversible), eosinophilia, anemia. *CNS:* Ataxia, coma, confusion, abnormal dreams or thoughts, dizziness, headache, paresthesia, psychosis, nervousness, somnolence, tremor. *GI:* Nausea, vomiting, diarrhea, anorexia, hemorrhage, abdominal pain. *CV:* Hypertension or hypotension, arrhythmias. *Body as a whole:* Fever (most common), chills, edema, infections, malaise. *Dermatologic:* Rash (most common), alopecia, pruritus, urticaria. *Miscellaneous:* Abnormal liver function values; inflammation, pain, or phlebitis at injection site; hematuria, dyspnea, retinal detachment in CMV retinitis patients.

Laboratory Test Interferences: ↑ Serum creatinine, BUN. ↓ Blood glucose.

Drug Interactions	
Adriamycin	Additive cytotoxicity
Amphotericin B	Additive cytotoxicity
Dapsone	Additive cytotoxicity
Flucytosine	Additive cytotoxicity
Imipenem/cilastatin combination	Possibility of seizures
Pentamidine	Additive cytotoxicity
Probenecid	↑ Effect of ganciclovir due to ↓ renal excretion
Sulfamethoxazole/trimethoprim combinations	Additive cytotoxicity
Vinblastine	Additive cytotoxicity
Vincristine	Additive cytotoxicity
Zidovudine	↑ Risk of granulocytopenia

Dosage: IV infusion, induction: 5 mg/kg over 1 hr q 12 hr for 14–21 days in patients with normal renal function. **Maintenance:** 5 mg/kg over 1 hr by IV infusion daily for 7 days or 6 mg/kg daily for 5 days each week. Dosage must be reduced in patients with renal impairment.

NURSING CONSIDERATIONS

Administration/Storage

1. Doses greater than 6 mg/kg infused over 1 hr may result in increased toxicity.
2. Due to the high pH (9–11) of reconstituted ganciclovir, the drug should not be given by IM or SC injection. The drug should not be given by IV bolus or rapid IV injection.

3. To minimize phlebitis or pain at the injection site, ganciclovir should be given into veins with an adequate blood flow to allow rapid dilution and distribution.

4. The dose should not exceed 1.25 mg/kg daily in clients undergoing hemodialysis.

5. The drug should be reconstituted by injecting 10 mL sterile water for injection followed by shaking. The vial should be discarded if particulate matter or discoloration is noted. Since parabens is incompatible with ganciclovir, bacteriostatic water for injection should not be used for reconstitution.

6. The reconstituted solution is stable for 12 hr at room temperature.

7. IV infusion concentrations greater than 10 mg/mL are not recommended.

8. Reconstituted ganciclovir is compatible with the following infusion solutions: 5% dextrose, lactated Ringer's injection, Ringer's injection, 0.9% sodium chloride.

Assessment

Note lab reports for evidence of hematological disorders that could preclude use of the drug.

Interventions

1. Monitor CBC frequently as granulocytopenia and thrombocytopenia are side effects of drug therapy. Ganciclovir should not be administered if neutrophil count drops below 500 cells/mm^3 or the platelet count falls below 25,000/mm^3.

2. Assess intake and output. Ensure that client is adequately hydrated before and during therapy with ganciclovir since drug is excreted through the kidneys.

3. Anticipate reduced dose in clients with impaired renal function; monitor renal function studies throughout therapy.

4. Concomitant therapy with zidovidine may increase neutropenia.

5. Client may experience pain and/or phlebitis at infusion site since pH of *diluted* solution is high (pH 9–11). Follow administration guidelines carefully.

6. Review list of drug interactions as some may induce renal failure and have additive toxicity if given during ganciclovir therapy.

7. Follow guidelines for handling cytotoxic drugs during handling and disposal of drug. Avoid inhalation and contact with skin. Latex gloves and safety glasses should be used when handling drug. Ideally, ganciclovir should be mixed under a laminar flow hood.

8. Hemodialysis and hydration may reduce plasma levels in cases of overdosage.

Client/Family Teaching

1. Drug therapy should not be interrupted unless deemed necessary by physician, since a relapse may occur.

2. Report any dizziness, confusion, and/or seizures immediately.

3. Stress the importance of reporting for scheduled lab studies as results may require adjustment of dose or even discontinuation of therapy.

4. Stress the importance of regular ophthalmologic examinations as retinitis may progress to blindness.

5. Ganciclovir may impair fertility.

6. During and for 90 days following drug therapy, women of childbearing age should use safe contraception and men should practice barrier contraception.

Evaluation

1. Assess client/family knowledge and understanding of illness, response to therapy and to teaching.

2. Review lab data closely as drug may need to be discontinued.

3. Observe for freedom from complications of drug therapy.

4. Follow ophthalmologic exams closely to evaluate progression of CMV retinitis.

IDOXURIDINE (IDU) (eye-dox-**YOU**-rih-deen)

Herplex Liquifilm, Stoxil (Rx)

Classification: Antiviral agent, ophthalmic.

Action/Kinetics: Idoxuridine, which resembles thymidine, inhibits thymidylic phosphorylase and specific DNA polymerases that are required for incorporation of thymidine into viral DNA. Idoxuridine, instead of thymidine, is incorporated into viral DNA resulting in faulty DNA and the inability of the virus to infect tissue or reproduce. Idoxuridine may also be incorporated into mammalian cells. The drug does not penetrate the cornea well. It is rapidly inactivated by nucleotidases or deaminases.

Uses: Herpes simplex keratitis, especially for initial epithelial infections characterized by the presence of thread-like extensions. *Note:* Idoxuridine will control infection but will not prevent scarring, loss of vision, or vascularization. Alternative form of therapy must be instituted if no improvement is noted after 7 days or if complete reepithelialization fails to occur after 21 days of therapy.

Contraindications: Hypersensitivity; deep ulcerations involving stromal layers of cornea. Lactation. Concomitant use of corticosteroids in herpes simplex keratitis.

Special Concerns: Use with caution during pregnancy.

Side Effects: Localized to eye. Temporary visual haze, irritation, pain, pruritus, inflammation, folicular conjunctivitis with preauricular adenopathy, mild edema of eyelids and cornea, allergic reactions (rare), photosensitivity, corneal clouding and stippling, small punctate defects. **Note:** Squamous cell carcinoma has been reported at the site of application.

Drug Interaction: Concurrent use of boric acid may cause irritation.

Dosage: Ophthalmic (0.1%) solution: initially, 1 drop q hr during day and q 2 hr during night; **following improvement:** 1 drop q 2 hr during day and q 4 hr at night. Continue for 3–5 days after healing is complete. **Ophthalmic (0.5%) ointment:** Insert in conjunctival sac 5 times/day q 4 hr, with last dose at bedtime; continue for 3–5 days after healing is complete.

NURSING CONSIDERATIONS

See also *General Nursing Considerations For All Anti-Infectives* under *Penicillins,* p. 140.

Administration/Storage

1. Store idoxuridine solution at 2°C–8°C and protect from light.

2. Do not mix with other medications.

3. Store idoxuridine ointment at 2°C–15°C.

4. Administer ophthalmic medication as scheduled, even during the night.

5. Do not use drug that was improperly stored because of loss of activity and increased toxic effects.

6. Topical corticosteroids may be used with idoxuridine in the treatment of herpes simplex with corneal edema, stromal lesions, or iritis.

7. To control secondary infections, antibiotics may be used with idoxuridine.

8. Atropine may be used concomitantly with idoxuridine, if appropriate.

Interventions

1. *Assess* client for symptoms of vision loss.

2. *Do not* apply boric acid to the eye when client is on idoxuridine therapy because boric acid may cause irritation.

3. Reassure client that hazy vision following instillation of medication will be of short duration.

4. Encourage clients to wear dark glasses if photophobia occurs.

5. Anticipate that if idoxuridine has been used concurrently with corticosteroids, the idoxuridine will be continued longer than the steroid, to prevent reinfection.

RIBAVIRIN   (rye-bah-VYE-rin)

Virazole (Rx)

Classification: Antiviral agent.

Action/Kinetics: Although the precise mechanism is not known, ribavirin may act as a competitive inhibitor of cellular enzymes that act on guanosine and xanthosine. Ribavirin is distributed to the plasma, respiratory tract, and red blood cells and is rapidly taken up by cells. **t½:** 9.5 hr. Eliminated through both the urine and feces.

Uses: Hospitalized pediatric patients (including infants) with severe lower respiratory tract infections (viral pneumonia including bronchiolitis) due to respiratory syncytial virus (RSV). Ribavirin is intended to be used along with standard treatment (including fluid management) for such patients with severe lower respiratory tract infections. *Investigational:* Ribavirin aerosol has been used against influenza A and B. Oral ribavirin has been used against herpes genitalis, acute and chronic hepatitis, measles, and Lassa fever.

Contraindications: Infants requiring artificial respiration (the drug may precipitate in the equipment and interfere with appropriate ventilation of the patient). Children with mild RSV lower respiratory tract infections who require a shorter hospital stay than required for a full course of ribavirin therapy. Pregnancy or women who may become pregnant during drug therapy (the drug may cause fetal harm and is known to be teratogenic). Lactation.

Special Concerns: Pregnancy category: X. Use with caution in adults with asthma or chronic obstructive lung disease (deterioration of respiratory function may occur).

Side Effects: *Pulmonary:* Worsening of respiration, pneumothorax, apnea, bacterial pneumonia, dependence on ventilator. *CV:* Hypotension, cardiac arrest, manifestations of digitalis toxicity. *Other:* Anemia (with IV or oral ribavirin); conjunctivitis and rash (with the aerosol).

Dosage: Aerosol only, to an infant oxygen hood using the Small Particle Aerosol Generator-2 (SPAG-2): The concentration administered is 20 mg/mL and the average aerosol concentration for a 12-hr period is 190 mcg/L of air. *See Administration/Storage.*

NURSING CONSIDERATIONS

Administration/Storage

1. Administration of the drug should be carried out for 12–18 hr/day for 3 (minimum)–7 (maximum) days.

2. Treatment is most effective if initiated within the first 3 days of the respiratory syncytial virus which causes lower respiratory tract infections.

3. Ribavirin aerosol should only be administered using the SPAG-2 aerosol generator.

4. Therapy should not be instituted in clients requiring artificial respiration.

5. No other aerosolized medications should be given if ribavirin aerosol is being used.

6. The drug may be solubilized with sterile water (USP) for injection or inhalation in the 100-mL vial. The solution is then transferred to the SPAG-2 reservoir utilizing a sterilized 500 mL wide mouth Erlenmeyer flask and further diluted to a final volume of 300 mL with sterile water.

7. Solutions in the SPAG-2 reservoir should be replaced daily. Also, if the liquid level is low, it should be discarded before new drug solution is added.

8. Reconstituted solutions of ribavirin may be stored at room temperature for 24 hr.

Interventions

1. It is essential that constant monitoring be undertaken for both the fluid and respiratory status of the client.

2. Assess frequently for evidence of respiratory distress; stop therapy and call physician if distress occurs.

3. Monitor and record vital signs and intake and output.

4. Anticipate limited use in infants and adults with chronic obstructive pulmonary disease or asthma.

5. With prolonged therapy (more than 7 days), observe for signs and symptoms of anemia.

TRIFLURIDINE   (try-**FLEW**-rih-deen)
Viroptic (Rx)

See also *Anti-Infectives,* p. 71.

Classification: Antiviral, ophthalmic.

Action/Kinetics: Trifluridine closely resembles thymidine; the drug inhibits thymidylic phosphorylase and specific DNA polymerases necessary for incorporation of thymidine into viral DNA. Trifluridine, instead of thymidine, is incorporated into viral DNA, resulting in faulty DNA and the inability to infect or reproduce in tissue. Trifluridine is also incorporated into mammalian DNA. $t^{1/2}$: 12–18 min.

Uses: Primary keratoconjunctivitis and recurrent epithelial keratitis caused by herpes simplex virus types 1 and 2. Epithelial keratitis resistant to idoxuridine. Is especially indicated for infections resistant to idoxuridine or vidarabine.

Contraindications: Hypersensitivity or chemical intolerance to drug.

Special Concerns: Safe use during pregnancy not established.

Side Effects: *Ophthalmic:* Local, usually transient; irritation of conjunctiva and cornea, including burning or stinging and edema of eyelids. Increased intraocular pressure. *Other:* Superficial punctate keratopathy, epithelial keratopathy, hypersensitivity, stromal edema, irritation, keratitis sicca, hyperemia.

Dosage: Solution, 1%. One drop of solution q 2 hr onto cornea, up to maximum of 9 drops/eye/day during acute stage (presence of corneal ulcer). Following reepithelialization, decrease dosage to 1 drop q 4 hr (or minimum of 5 drops/eye/day) for 7 days. Do not use for more than 21 days.

NURSING CONSIDERATIONS

See also *General Nursing Considerations For All Anti-Infectives* under *Penicillins,* p. 140.

Administration/Storage

1. May be used concomitantly in the eye with antibiotics (chloramphenicol, bacitracin, polymyxin B sulfate, erythromycin, neomycin, gentamicin, tetracycline, sulfacetamide sodium), corticosteroids, anticholinergics, epinephrine HCl, and sodium chloride.
2. Drug is heat-sensitive. Store in refrigerator at 2°–8°C.

Client/Family Teaching

1. Instill drop onto cornea. Apply finger pressure lightly to lacrimal sac for 1 minute after instillation.
2. A mild, transient burning sensation may occur on instillation.
3. Report any bothersome side effects to physician, but do not stop medication without specific instructions to do so.
4. Arrange for regular examination by an ophthalmologist.
5. Improvement usually occurs within 7 days and healing takes place within 14 days. Thereafter, 7 more days of therapy are necessary to prevent recurrence.
6. Report to physician if no improvement is noted within 7 days.
7. Do not administer drug for more than 21 days, because toxicity may occur (remaining medication should be discarded after 21 days).
8. Keep medication in the refrigerator.

VIDARABINE   (vi-**DAIR**-ah-been)

Vira-A (Rx)

See also *Anti-Infectives,* p. 71.

Classification: Antiviral, ophthalmic.

Action/Kinetics: Vidarabine is phosphorylated in the cell to arabinosyl adenosine monophosphate (ara-AMP) or the triphosphate (ara-ATP). These compounds cause inhibition of viral DNA polymerase, inhibition of virus-induced ribonucleotide reductase, or inhibition of enzymes specific for viruses to synthesis of DNA. These effects prevent lengthening of the DNA chain. Vidarabine is rapidly metabolized to ara-HX, which has decreased antiviral activity. **Peak plasma levels:** Vidarabine, 0.2–0.4 mcg/mL; ara-HX, 3–6 mcg/mL. **t½: IV,** vidarabine, 1.5 hr; ara-HX, 3.3. hr. Drug and metabolites excreted by kidneys.

Uses: *Systemic:* Herpes simplex viral encephalitis. *Topical:* Primary keratoconjunctivitis and recurrent epithelial keratitis caused by herpes simplex virus types 1 and 2. Epithelial keratitis resistant to idoxuridine. It is more effective than idoxuridine for deep recurrent infections.

Contraindications: Hypersensitivity to drug. Concomitant use of adrenocorticosteroids usually contraindicated.

Special Concerns: Safe use during pregnancy not established (pregnancy category: C). *Systemic:* use with caution in patients susceptible to fluid overload, cerebral edema, or with impaired renal or hepatic function.

Side Effects: Systemic. *GI:* Nausea, vomiting, diarrhea, hematemesis. *CNS:* Tremor, dizziness, ataxia, confusion, hallucinations, psychoses, encephalopathy (may be fatal). *Hematologic:* Decrease in reticulocytes, hemoglobin, and hematocrit. *Miscellaneous:* Weight loss, malaise, rash, pruritus, pain at injection site. *Topical:* Photophobia, lacrimation, conjunctival injection, foreign body sensation, temporal visual haze, burning, irritation, superficial punctate keratitis, pain, punctal occlusion, sensitivity.

Laboratory Test Interferences: ↑ Bilirubin, SGOT.

Dosage: IV infusion: 15 mg/kg/day for 10 days. **Ophthalmic ointment:** ½ inch of 3% ointment applied to lower conjunctival sac 5 times daily at 3-hr intervals. Continue therapy for 7 days after complete reepithelialization but at reduced dosage (e.g., twice daily).

NURSING CONSIDERATIONS

See also *General Nursing Considerations For All Anti-Infectives* under *Penicillins,* p. 140.

Administration/Storage

1. Systemic: slowly infuse total daily dose at constant rate over 12–24 hr.
2. A total of 2.2 mL of IV solution is required to dissolve 1 mg of medication. A maximum of 450 mg may be dissolved in 1 L. Should be used within 48 hr after dilution. Do not refrigerate solution.
3. Any carbohydrate or electrolyte solution is suitable as diluent. Do not use biologic or colloidal fluids.
4. Shake vidarabine vial well before withdrawing dosage. Add to prewarmed (35°–40°C) infusion solution. Shake mixture until completely clear.
5. For final filtration use an in-line filter (0.45 μm).
6. Dilute just before administration and use within 48 hr.
7. Topical corticosteroids or antibiotics may be used concomitantly with vidarabine, but benefits and risks must be assessed.
8. Wait 10 min before use of an additional topical ointment.

Client/Family Teaching

1. Ophthalmic ointment will cause a temporary haze after application.
2. Report any bothersome side effects.
3. Take only as directed.
4. Client must remain under close supervision of an ophthalmologist while receiving therapy for ophthalmic problem.

Evaluation

1. Review intake and output and observe client on systemic therapy for fluid overload.
2. Assess client for renal, liver, and hematologic dysfunction precipitated by vidarabine; monitor appropriate laboratory data.

ZIDOVUDINE (AZIDOTHYMIDINE, AZT)   (zye-DOE-vyou-deen, ah-zee-doh-THIGH-mih-deen)

Retrovir (Rx)

See also *Anti-Infectives,* p. 71.

Classification: Antiviral.

Action/Kinetics: The active form of the drug is zidovudine triphosphate, which is derived from zidovudine by cellular enzymes. Zidovudine triphosphate competes with thymidine triphosphate (the natural substrate) for incorporation into growing chains of viral DNA by retroviral reverse transcriptase. Once incorporated, zidovudine triphosphate causes premature termination of the growth of the DNA chain. Low concentrations of zidovudine also inhibit the activity of *Shigella, Kebsiella, Salmonella, Enterobacter, E. coli,* and *Citrobacter,* although resistance develops rapidly. The drug is absorbed rapidly from the GI tract and is distributed to both plasma and CSF. **Peak serum levels:** 0.1–1.5 hr. **t½:** approximately 1 hr. The drug is metabolized rapidly by the liver and excreted through the urine.

Uses: Adults manifesting symptoms due to human immunodeficiency virus (HIV) (i.e., acquired immunodeficiency syndrome [AIDS] or AIDS-related complex [ARC]) and who have confirmed *Pneumocystis carinii* pneumonia or a peripheral blood T_4 helper/inducer lymphocyte count of less than 200/mm³.

Note: Zidovudine syrup has been authorized for use in HIV-infected children from 3 months to 12 years of age who have either HIV-associated symptoms or a CD4 (T_4) cell count of less than 400.

Contraindications: Allergy to zidovudine or its components. Lactation.

Special Concerns: Use with caution in patients who have a hemoglobin level of less than 9.5 g/dL or a granulocyte count less than 1,000/mm³. Use during pregnancy only if benefits clearly outweigh risks (pregnancy category: C).

Side Effects: *Hematologic:* Anemia, granulocytopenia. *GI:* Nausea, vomiting, diarrhea, anorexia, GI pain, dyspepsia. *CNS:* Dizziness, headache, malaise, sleepiness, insomnia, paresthesias. *Other:* Myalgia, asthenia, diaphoresis, dyspnea, rash, change in taste perception.

Drug Interactions

Acetaminophen	↑ Risk of granulocytopenia
Adriamycin	↑ Risk of cytotoxicity, nephrotoxicity, or hematologic toxicity
Amphotericin B	See *Adriamycin*
Dapsone	See *Adriamycin*
Flucytosine	See *Adriamycin*
Interferon	See *Adriamycin*
Pentamidine	See *Adriamycin*
Probenecid	↓ Biotransformation or renal excretion of zidovudine
Vinblastine	See *Adriamycin*
Vincristine	See *Adriamycin*

Dosage: Capsules/Syrup. Initially: 200 mg (capsules) or 20 mL (syrup) q 4 hr around the clock. After 1 month, the dose may be decreased to 100 mg q 4 hr. **IV. Initially:** 1–2 mg/kg infused over 1 hr. The IV dose is given q 4 hr around the clock only until oral therapy can be instituted. Dosage adjustment may be necessary due to hematologic toxicity.

NURSING CONSIDERATIONS

See also *General Nursing Considerations For Anti-Infectives* under *Penicillins,* p. 140.

Administration/Storage

1. The nurse must be aware that zidovudine therapy is not a cure for HIV infections, and clients may continue to develop opportunistic infections and other complications due to AIDS or AIDS-related complex. Thus, the client must be closely observed.

2. Blood counts should be performed at least every 2 weeks. If anemia or granulocytopenia is severe, the dose of zidovudine must be adjusted or discontinued. A blood transfusion may also be required.

3. Safety and effectiveness of chronic zidovudine therapy in adults are not known, especially in clients who have a less advanced form of disease.

Client/Family Teaching

1. Stress the importance of taking the medication around the clock as ordered; sleep must be interrupted to take medication.

2. Report for all laboratory studies, especially complete blood count because drug causes anemia and the client may require a blood transfusion.

3. The early signs and symptoms of anemia, such as shortness of breath, weakness, lightheaded-ness, or palpitations and increased tiredness should be reported to the physician.

4. Avoid acetaminophen and any other nonprescribed drugs that may exacerbate the toxicity of zidovudine.

5. Remind clients/family that the medication is not a cure, but it alleviates the symptoms of HIV infections.

6. Clients should be advised not to share medication and not to exceed the recommended dose of zidovudine.

7. The risk of transmission of HIV to others through blood or sexual contact is not reduced in individuals on zidovudine therapy.

8. Local support groups may help client/family to understand and cope with the disease.

Evaluation

1. Assess client/family knowledge and understanding of illness, response to therapy and to teaching.

2. Observe for freedom from complications from drug therapy.

3. Review lab data (CBC) for evidence of complications that may require dose adjustment or discontinuation of drug therapy.

PART THREE
Antineoplastic Agents

CHAPTER EIGHTEEN
Antineoplastic Agents

3

General Statement: Significant progress continues to be made in the drug therapy of neoplastic diseases. There are types of cancer that can now be considered "curable" by chemotherapy alone. In many other forms of cancer, especially in cases of suspected metastatic disease, chemotherapy is an important adjunct in treatment. Progress can be attributed, in part, to the more judicious use of an increasing number of combination regimens of antineoplastic agents, the composition and time of administration of which are based on a better understanding of the characteristics of a specified neoplastic disease, on the kinetics of the cell cycle (see *Action/Kinetics*), and on the mechanism of action of the drugs used. Some of the principles underlying successful cancer chemotherapy are reviewed below. Extensive nursing considerations to increase the comfort of the patient during cancer therapy are provided.

General Impact of Antineoplastic Agents: There are many antineoplastic agents that slow down the disease process and induce a remission. All antineoplastic agents are cytotoxic (i.e., cell poisons) and therefore interfere with normal as well as neoplastic cells. However, neoplastic cells are much more active and multiply more rapidly than normal cells, and are thus more affected by the antineoplastic agents.

Normal tissue cells, such as those of the bone marrow, the GI mucosal epithelium, and hair follicles are naturally active and particularly susceptible to antineoplastic agents. The margin between the dose of antineoplastic drug needed to destroy the neoplastic cells and that needed to cause bone marrow damage, for example, is narrow. Thus, patients who receive antineoplastic agents are closely watched for signs of bone marrow depression, which is characterized by low blood counts (leukocytes, erythrocytes, platelets). Since white blood cells (WBCs) or platelets show the effect of an overdose more rapidly than do erythrocytes, the platelet and WBC count is often used as a guide to dosage. If a blood or marrow test indicates a precipitous fall in the WBC or platelet count, the antineoplastic agent may have to be discontinued or the dosage modified significantly. Drugs are usually withheld when the WBC count falls below 2,000/mm^3 and the platelet count falls below 100,000/mm^3. Sometimes the effect of the antineoplastic drugs on the bone marrow is cumulative, with the depression of WBCs and platelets occurring weeks or months after initiation of therapy. Thus patients must be followed carefully.

Antineoplastic agents should be administered only by people knowledgeable in their management. Facilities must be available for frequent laboratory evaluations, especially total blood counts and bone marrow tests.

Table 6 Summary of Antineoplastic Agents

Agent	Abbreviation	Type	Disease	Toxicity
Asparaginase	L-ASP	Enzyme (natural product)	Acute lymphocytic leukemia	*Acute:* Nausea, fever, anaphylaxis *Delayed:* Hypersensitivity, abdominal pain, coagulation defects, renal and hepatic damage, pancreatitis, hyperglycemia, CNS depression, others
Bleomycin Sulfate	BLM	Antibiotic	Squamous cell carcinoma of the head and neck; lymphomas (reticulum cell sarcoma, lymphosarcoma, Hodgkin's); testicular carcinoma	*Acute:* Nausea, vomiting, anaphylaxis, hypotension *Delayed:* Pneumonitis, pulmonary fibrosis, skin reactions, alopecia, stomatitis
Busulfan	BUS	Alkylating agent, alkylsulfonate	Chronic myelogenous leukemia (granulocytic, myeloid, myelocytic)	*Acute:* Mild nausea and vomiting *Delayed:* Bone marrow depression, hyperpigmentation, pulmonary fibrosis, acute leukemia
Carboplatin		Alkylating agent	Recurrent ovarian platinum compound	*Acute:* Vomiting, nausea, anaphylaxis *Delayed:* Bone marrow depression, electrolyte disturbances, pain, peripheral and central neurotoxicity
Carmustine	BCNU	Alkylating agent, nitrosourea	Brain tumors, Hodgkin's disease, non-Hodgkin's lymphomas, multiple myeloma	*Acute:* Nausea, vomiting, local phlebitis *Delayed:* Bone marrow depression, pulmonary toxicity, alopecia
Chlorambucil	CHL	Alkylating agent, nitrogen mustard	Chronic lymphocytic leukemia, lymphosarcoma, Hodgkin's disease, giant follicular lymphoma	*Acute:* Nausea, vomiting *Delayed:* Bone marrow depression, carcinogenesis, mutagenic, teratogenic, pulmonary fibrosis, bronchopulmonary dysplasia, sterility, seizures
Chromic Phosphate P 32		Radioactive isotope	Peritoneal or pleural effusions of metastatic cancer; localized disease	*Acute:* Radiation sickness *Delayed:* Bone marrow depression, pleuritis, peritonitis

Table 6 (*Continued*)

Agent	Abbreviation	Type	Disease	Toxicity
Cisplatin	CDDP	Alkylating agent	Metastatic ovarian tumors, metastatic testicular tumors, advanced bladder cancer	*Acute:* Nausea, vomiting, anaphylaxis *Delayed:* Bone marrow depression, renal damage, ototoxicity
Cyclophosphamide	CYC	Alkylating agent, nitrogen mustard	Malignant lymphomas including lymphocytic lymphoma, Hodgkin's disease, mixed-cell type lymphoma, Burkitt's lymphoma, histiocytic lymphoma; multiple myeloma; chronic lymphocytic leukemia; chronic granulocytic leukemia; acute lymphoblastic leukemia in children; acute myelogenous leukemia; acute monocytic leukemia; mycosis fungoides; neuroblastoma; adenocarcinoma of the ovary; breast cancer; retinoblastoma	*Acute:* Nausea, vomiting *Delayed:* Bone marrow depression, alopecia, hemorrhagic cystitis
Cytarabine	Ara-C	Antimetabolite, pyrimidine analog	Acute lymphotic leukemia in adults and children; acute myelotic leukemia; meningeal leukemia; non-Hodgkin's lymphoma in children	*Acute:* Nausea and vomiting *Delayed:* Bone marrow depression, megaloblastosis, diarrhea, hepatic damage
Dacarbazine	DTIC	Miscellaneous	Malignant melanoma (metastatic); Hodgkin's disease	*Acute:* Nausea, vomiting, facial flushing and paresthesia *Delayed:* Bone marrow depression, hepatic necrosis, flu-like syndrome, alopecia
Dactinomycin (Actinomycin D)	ACT	Antibiotic	Metastatic and nonmetastatic choriocarcinoma; rhabdomyosarcoma; nonseminomatous testicular cancer; Ewing's sarcoma; sarcoma botryoides; Wilms' tumor	*Acute:* Nausea, vomiting, cheilitis, ulcerative stomatitis, pharyngitis, corrosive to soft tissue *Delayed:* Bone marrow supression, acne, alopecia, erythema, increased pigmentation in previously irradiated skin

Drug	Abbreviation	Classification	Indications	Toxicity
Daunorubicin	DNR	Antibiotic	Acute nonlymphocytic leukemia (erythroid, monocytic, myelogenous); acute lymphocytic leukemia in children and adults	*Acute:* Nausea, vomiting, local irritation *Delayed:* Cardiotoxicity, bone marrow supression, alopecia
Doxorubicin Hydrochloride	ADR	Antibiotic	Acute lymphoblastic leukemia; acute myeloblastic leukemia; Wilms' tumor; bone and soft tissue sarcomas; breast and ovarian cancer; neuroblastoma; thyroid cancer; Hodgkin's and non-Hodgkin's lymphomas; transitional cell bladder cancer; small cell bronchogenic cancer	*Acute:* Nausea, vomiting, local irritation *Delayed:* Bone marrow depression, cardiotoxicity, stomatitis, diarrhea, erythema in irritated area, local tissue necrosis, alopecia, hyperpigmentation of nailbeds
Estramustine Phosphate Sodium		Hormone, nitrogen mustard	Metastatic or progressive prostate cancer	*Acute:* Nausea, vomiting, GI bleeding *Delayed:* Cardiovascular accident, edema, congestive heart failure, rash, pruritus, breast enlargement
Etoposide	VP-16–213	Inhibitor of mitosis	Refractory testicular tumors; small cell lung cancer	*Acute:* Nausea, vomiting, hypotension, anaphylaxis *Delayed:* Leukopenia, thrombocytopenia, alopecia, peripheral neuropathy
Floxuridine	FUDR	Antimetabolite	GI adrenocarcinoma metastatic to the liver	*Acute:* Nausea, vomiting, diarrhea *Delayed:* Bone marrow supression, dermatitis, alopecia, myocardial ischemia, angina, acute cerebellar syndrome, photosensitivity (erythema or pigmentation)
Fluorouracil	5-FU	Antimetabolite	Cancer of the breast, pancreas, stomach, colon, rectum	See *Floxuridine,* above
Flutamide		Hormone, antiandrogen	Metastatic prostate cancer used in combination with leuprolide	*Acute:* Nausea, vomiting, diarrhea *Delayed:* Hot flashes, impotence, loss of libido, gynecomastia

Table 6 (*Continued*)

Agent	Abbreviation	Type	Disease	Toxicity
Goserelin Acetate		Hormone	Advanced cancer of the prostate (palliation)	*Acute:* Vomiting diarrhea, constipation *Delayed:* Hot flashes, sexual dysfunction, decreased erections, lower urinary tract symptoms, lethargy
Hydroxyurea	HYD	Miscellaneous	Melanoma, resistant chronic myelocytic leukemia, metastatic cancer of ovary, carcinoma of head and neck	*Acute:* Nausea, vomiting, stomatitis *Delayed:* Bone marrow depression, impaired renal function, maculopapular rash, facial edema, fever, chills, malaise
Ifosfamide		Nitrogen mustard	In combination with drugs for germ cell testicular cancer	*Acute:*Nausea, vomiting, hematuria *Delayed:* Hemorrhagic cystitis (use Mesna to minimize), confusion, coma, alopecia
Interferon alfa-2a	IFLrA, rIFN-A	Miscellaneous	Hairy cell leukemia, bladder tumors, chronic myelogenous leukemia, Kaposi's sarcoma, non-Hodgkin's lymphoma, carcinoid tumor, cutaneous T-cell lymphoma	*Acute:* Nausea, diarrhea, vomiting *Delayed:* Flu-like symptoms, dizziness, hypotension, edema, rash, pruritus, alopecia, weight loss, change in taste, impotence, arthralgia, numbness, lethargy
Interferon alfa-2b	IFN-alpha 2, rIFN-α2	Miscellaneous	See *Interferon alpha-2a*, above	See *Interferon alpha-2a*, above
Interferon alfa-n3		Miscellaneous	Condylomata acuminata, many unlabeled uses for certain cancers or viral infections	*Acute:* "Flu-like" symptoms, fever, chills, malaise, myalgias, headache *Delayed:* Hypersensitivity
Leuprolide Acetate		Hormone	Advanced prostatic cancer	*Acute:* Nausea, vomiting, constipation *Delayed:* Congestive heart failure, peripheral edema, hot flashes, dizziness, headache, impotence, bone pain

Drug	Abbreviation	Classification	Indications	Toxicity
Lomustine	CCNU	Alkylating agent, nitrosourea	Primary and metastatic brain tumors; Hodgkin's disease	*Acute:* Nausea, vomiting *Delayed:* Bone marrow depression, hepatotoxicity, renal abnormalities, pulmonary fibrosis, secondary malignancies, alopecia, stomatitis
Mechlorethamine Hydrochloride	HN$_2$	Alkylating agent, nitrogen mustard	Hodgkin's disease; chronic myelotic or lymphocytic leukemia; lymphosarcoma; polycythemia vera; mycosis fungoides; bronchial cancer	*Acute:* Nausea, vomiting, anorexia *Delayed:* Bone marrow depression, thrombosis, thrombophlebitis, dermatoses, delayed menses, amenorrhea, impaired spermatogenesis, azoospermia, vertigo
Medroxy-progesterone Acetate		Hormone	Palliation of endometrial or renal cancer	*Delayed:* Thrombophlebitis, pulmonary embolism, angioneurotic edema, pruritus, urticaria, acne, alopecia, hirsutism, rashes, insomnia, nervousness
Megestrol Acetate		Hormone	Palliation of recurrent, inoperable, or metastatic breast or endometrial cancer	*Delayed:* Deep vein thrombophlebitis, alopecia, carpal tunnel syndrome
Melphalan	MPL	Alkylating agent, nitrogen mustard	Nonresectable epithelial ovarian cancer; multiple myeloma	*Acute:* Nausea, vomiting, diarrhea *Delayed:* Bone marrow depression, alopecia, pulmonary fibrosis, leukemia, amenorrhea, interstitial pneumonitis, vasculitis, hemolytic anemia, allergies
Mercaptopurine	6-MP	Antimetabolite	Acute lymphocytic or lymphoblastic leukemia; acute myelogenous or acute myelomonocytic leukemia	*Acute:* Nausea and vomiting *Delayed:* Bone marrow depression, liver damage, oral ulcers potentiated by allopurinol, hyperuricemia, drug fever, hyperpigmentation, skin rashes

Table 6 (*Continued*)

Agent	Abbreviation	Type	Disease	Toxicity
Methotrexate Sodium	MTX	Antimetabolite, folic acid analog	Acute lymphoblastic leukemia in children; acute lymphocytic leukemia; meningeal leukemia; breast cancer; lung cancer; epidermoid cancer of the head and neck; lymphosarcoma, especially in children; mycosis fungoides	*Acute:* Nausea, vomiting, diarrhea, ulcerative stomatitis, anorexia, death *Delayed:* Bone marrow depression, hepatotoxicity, congenital anomalies, alopecia, skin rashes, renal toxicity, interstitial pneumonitis, menstrual dysfunction, CNS symptoms
Mitomycin	MTC	Antibiotic	Disseminated adenocarcinoma of the pancreas and stomach; superficial bladder cancer	*Acute:* Fever, nausea, vomiting, anorexia *Delayed:* Bone marrow depression, hemolytic uremic syndrome, cellulitis, microangiopathic hemolytic anemia, CNS symptoms, alopecia, stomatitis
Mitotane	o,p'-DDD	Miscellaneous	Functional or nonfunctional adrenal cortical carcinoma	*Acute:* Nausea, vomiting *Delayed:* CNS depression, dermatitis, visual disturbances, adrenal insufficiency, diarrhea
Mitoxantrone Hydrochloride		Antibiotic	Acute leukemias including myelogenous, monocytic, erythroid, or promyelocytic	*Acute:* Nausea, vomiting, diarrhea *Delayed:* GI bleeding, ecchymosis, jaundice, congestive heart failure, arrhythmias; infections including pneumonia, sepsis, urinary tract, and fungal; headache, fever, alopecia, dyspnea, conjunctivitis
Pipobroman		Alkylating agent	Polycythemia vera, chronic granulocytic leukemia	*Acute:* Nausea, vomiting, abdominal cramps *Delayed:* Skin rash, diarrhea, bone marrow depression

Drug	Abbreviation	Classification	Indications	Toxicity
Plicamycin (Mithramycin)	MTH	Antibiotic	Testicular cancer; hypercalcemia and hypercalciuria associated with advanced carcinoma	*Acute:* Nausea, vomiting, local irritation *Delayed:* Bone marrow depression, hemorrhagic diathesis, stomatitis, diarrhea, hepatic damage, hypocalcemia
Polyestradiol Phosphate		Hormone	Palliation of prostatic cancer	*Acute:* Nausea, vomiting, headaches *Delayed:* Edema, thrombophlebitis, coronary thrombosis, pulmonary embolism, cerebral thrombosis, gynecomastia, loss of libido, testicular atrophy
Prednisone	PRED	Corticosteroid	Acute leukemias in children; leukemias and lymphomas in adults	See *Adrenocorticosteroids*, p. 1148
Procarbazine Hydrochloride	MIH	Miscellaneous	Hodgkin's disease	*Acute:* Nausea, vomiting *Delayed:* Bone marrow depression, stomatitis, dermatitis, neuropathy, CNS depression, hypotension, shock, hematuria, urinary frequency, gynecomastia (in prepubertal/pubertal boys), paresthesias, hepatic dysfunction, retinal hemorrhage, ocular problems, nonlymphoid malignancies
Sodium Iodide I 131		Radioactive isotope	Thyroid cancer	*Acute:* Radiation sickness *Delayed:* Bone marrow depression, severe sialoadenitis
Sodium Phosphate P 32		Radioactive isotope	Chronic myelocytic leukemia; chronic lymphocytic leukemia; multiple skeletal metastases; polycythemia vera	*Acute:* Radiation sickness
Streptozocin		Alkylating agent, nitrosourea	Metastatic islet cell pancreatic carcinoma	*Acute:* Nausea, vomiting, confusion, depression, lethargy *Delayed:* Hematologic toxicity, glucose intolerance, renal toxicity

Table 6 (*Continued*)

Agent	Abbreviation	Type	Disease	Toxicity
Tamoxifen		Hormone, antiestrogen	Advanced breast cancer in postmenopausal women	*Acute:* Occasional nausea *Delayed:* Hot flashes, vaginal bleeding, pruritis vulvae
Testolactone		Hormone	Advanced or disseminated breast cancer	*Acute:* Nausea, vomiting, anorexia, glossitis *Delayed:* Paresthesias, alopecia, edema, masculinization, hypercalcemia, maculopapular erythema
Thioguanine	6-TG	Antimetabolite	Acute nonlymphocytic leukemia; chronic myelogenous leukemia	*Acute:* Nausea, vomiting, anorexia, stomatitis *Delayed:* Bone marrow depression, hepatotoxicity, hyperuricemia, intestinal necrosis, intestinal perforation
Thiotepa	Thio	Alkylating agent	Adenocarcinoma of the breast or ovary; superficial papillary carcinoma of the urinary bladder; neoplasms of serosal cavities; Hodgkin's disease; lymphosarcomas	*Acute:* Nausea, vomiting, anorexia, dizziness, headache *Delayed:* Bone marrow depression, amenorrhea, hives, skin rash, fever, interference with spermatogenesis
Uracil Mustard		Alkylating agent, nitrogen mustard	Chronic lymphocytic leukemia; non-Hodgkin's lymphomas; chronic myelogenous leukemia; early treatment of polycythemia vera; mycosis fungoides	*Acute:* Nausea, vomiting, diarrhea, nervousness *Delayed:* Bone marrow depression, pruritus, dermatitis, alopecia, hepatotoxicity, azoospermia, amenorrhea
Vinblastine Sulfate	VLB	Mitotic inhibtor	Hodgkin's disease; mycosis fungoides; lymphocytic lymphoma; histiocytic lymphoma; advanced testicular cancer; Kaposi's sarcoma; choriocarcinoma resistant to other therapy; breast cancer unresponsive to other approaches	*Acute:* Nausea, vomiting, diarrhea, anorexia, abdominal pain, CNS symptoms *Delayed:* Bone marrow depression, hypertension; pharyngitis; vesiculation of the mouth; paresthesias; depression; seizures; alopecia; bone and jaw pain; peripheral neuritis; loss of deep tendon reflexes

| Vincristine Sulfate | LCR, VCR | Mitotic inhibitor | Acute leukemia; Hodgkin's disease; non-Hodgkin's malignant lymphomas; lymphosarcomas; reticulum cell sarcoma; neuroblastoma; Wilm's tumor; rhabdomyosarcoma; breast or bladder cancer; Kaposi's sarcoma | *Acute:* Nausea, vomiting, diarrhea, anorexia, fever, headache
Delayed: Neurologic disorders, inappropriate secretion of antidiuretic hormone; oral ulceration, intestinal necrosis or perforation; bone marrow depression; constipation; paralytic ileus; urinary retention, polyuria; dysuria; optic atrophy; severe bronchospasms; shortness of breath; alopecia; hyper- or hypotension; weight loss |

The toxicity of the antineoplastic agents is manifested in the lining of the GI tract by development of oral ulcers, intestinal bleeding, and diarrhea. Finally, since hair follicles are also rapidly proliferating tissue, alopecia often accompanies the drug treatment of antineoplastic disease.

Antineoplastic agents fall into several broad categories: Alkylating Agents, Antimetabolites, Antibiotics, Natural Products and Miscellaneous Agents, Hormonal and Antihormonal Agents, and Radioactive Isotopes.

The choice of the chemotherapeutic agent(s) depends both on the type of the tumor and on its site of growth. Although it has been said that cancer is not one disease but many, a simpler major subdivision involves separation into solid tumors and hematologic malignancies. The former are confined to a specific tissue or organ site initially and usually involve surgery and/or irradiation. Chemotherapy is used to eradicate remaining cells or metastases, or when primary treatment is insufficient or impossible. Chemotherapy is usually the major form of therapy in hematologic malignancies (i.e., leukemias, lymphomas); some cures have been achieved, notably in Hodgkin's disease and the leukemias of childhood.

General information applying to all antineoplastic agents (action, uses, contraindications, side effects, administration, and extensive nursing considerations) is presented below. For quick reference, agents are also listed alphabetically in Table 6. Also included are the abbreviations by which the antineoplastic agents are known and the combination regimens in which they are often included (Table 7).

Action: During division, cells go through a definite number of stages during which they are more or less susceptible to various chemotherapeutic agents (see *Action/Kinetics* of various agents). Some agents, notably the alkylating agents, have been shown to be effective during all stages of the cycle, while others, the antimetabolites, for example, are effective only during stages of DNA synthesis.

The various cell stages are described in Figure 5.

Uses: Most of the drugs discussed in this section are used exclusively for neoplastic disease. A few are used on an experimental basis for some of the rheumatic diseases. See individual drugs.

Contraindications: Hypersensitivity to drug. Most antineoplastic agents are contraindicated for a period of 4 weeks after radiation therapy or chemotherapy with similar drugs. Use with caution, and at reduced dosages, in patients with preexisting bone marrow depression, malignant infiltration of bone marrow or kidney, or liver dysfunction.

The safe use of these drugs during pregnancy has not been established; they are contraindicated during the first trimester.

Side Effects: *Bone marrow depression* (leukopenia, thrombocytopenia, agranulocytosis, anemia) *is the major danger of antineoplastic therapy. Bone marrow depression can sometimes be irreversible. It is mandatory that the patient have frequent total blood counts and bone marrow examinations. Precipitous falls must be reported to a physician.*

Other side effects include: *GI:* Nausea, vomiting (may be severe), anorexia, diarrhea (may be hemorrhagic), stomatitis, enteritis, abdominal cramps, intestinal ulcers. *Hepatic:* Hepatic toxicity including jaundice and changes in liver enzymes. *Dermatologic:* Dermatitis, erythema, various dermatoses including maculopapular rash, alopecia (reversible), pruritus, urticaria, cheilosis. *Immunologic:* Immunosuppression with increased susceptibility to viral, bacterial, or fungal infections.

CNS: Depression, lethargy, confusion, dizziness, headache, fatigue, malaise, fever, weakness. *Genitourinary:* Acute renal failure, reproductive abnormalities including amenorrhea and azoospermia. **Note:** Alkylating agents, in particular, may be both carcinogenic and mutagenic.

Table 7 Commonly Used Antineoplastic Combinations

Name	Drugs in Regimen	Use
ABDIC	Bleomycin Dacarbazine Doxorubicin Lomustine Prednisone	Hodgin's disease resistant to MOPP therapy
ABVD	Bleomycin Dacarbazine Doxorubicin Vinblastine	Induction of therapy for Hodgkin's disease resistant to MOPP therapy
ACE	Cyclophosphamide Doxorubicin Etoposide	Small cell carcinoma of the lung
ACe	Cyclophosphamide Doxorubicin	Recurrent or metastatic breast cancer
A-COPP	Cyclophosphamide Doxorubicin Prednisone Procarbazine Vincristine	Induction of therapy for Hodgkin's disease in children only
Adria + BCNU	Carmustine Doxorubicin	Multiple myeloma
Ara-C + ADR	Cytarabine Doxorubicin	Induction of therapy for acute myelocytic leukemia
Ara-C + DNR + PRED + MP	Cytarabine Daunorubicin Mercaptopurine Prednisolone	Treatment of acute myelocytic leukemia in children only
Ara-C + 6-TG	Cytarabine Thioguanine	Acute myelocytic leukemia
B-CAVe	Bleomycin Doxorubicin Lomustine Vinblastine	Advanced Hodgkin's disease resistant to MOPP therapy
BCVPP	Carmustine Cyclophosphamide Prednisone Procarbazine Vinblastine	Induction of therapy for Hodgkin's disease
CAF	Cyclophosphamide Doxorubicin Flourouracil	Breast cancer, including metastases
CAMP	Cyclophosphamide Doxorubicin Methotrexate Procarbazine	Lung cancer, non-oat cell cancers

Table 7 *(Continued)*

Name	Drugs in Regimen	Use
CAP	Cisplatin Cyclophosphamide Doxorubicin	Non-small cell carcinoma of the lung
CAV	Cyclyophosphamide Doxorubicin Vincristine	Induction of therapy for small cell lung cancer
CAVe	Doxorubicin Lomustine Vincristine	Induction of therapy for Hodgkin's disease resistant to MOPP therapy
CHL + PRED	Chlorambucil Prednisone	Chronic lymphocytic leukemia
CHOP	Cyclophosphamide Doxorubicin Prednisone Vincristine	Non-Hodgkin's lymphoma
CHOR	Cyclophosphamide Doxorubicin Vincristine	Lung cancer, small cell carcinoma
CISCA	Cisplatin Cyclophosphamide Doxorubicin	Urinary tract, metastatic disease
CISCA$_{II}$/VB$_{IV}$	Bleomycin Cisplatin Cyclophosphamide Doxorubicin Vinblastine	Advanced germ cell tumors
CMC-High Dose	Cyclophosphamide Lomustine Methotrexate	Small cell carcinoma of the lung
CMF	Cyclophosphamide Flourouracil Methotrexate	Recurrent and metastatic breast cancer
CMFP	Cyclophosphamide Flourouracil Methotrexate Prednisone	Breast cancer and metastases
CMFVP (Cooper's Regimen)	Cyclophosphamide Flourouracil Methotrexate Prednisone Vincristine	Recurrent or metastatic breast cancer
COMLA	Cyclophosphamide Cytarabine Leucovorin Methotrexate Vincristine	Non-Hodgkin's lymphoma

Table 7 *(Continued)*

Name	Drugs in Regimen	Use
COP	Cyclophosphamide Prednisone Vincristine	Non-Hodgkin's lymphoma
COP-BLAM	Bleomycin Cyclophosphamide Doxorubicin Prednisone Procarbazine Vincristine	Non-Hodgkin's lymphoma, advanced histiocytic (stage III or IV)
COPP or "C" MOPP	Cyclophosphamide Prednisone Procarbazine Vincristine	Non-Hodgkin's lymphoma, Hodgkin's disease, lymphomas with unfavorable histology
CVP	Cyclophosphamide Prednisone Vincristine	Non-Hodgkin's lymphoma, lymphomas with favorable histology
CY-VA-DIC	Cyclophosphamide Dacarbazine Doxorubicin Vincristine	Adult sarcomas, soft tissue sarcomas
FAC	Cyclophosphamide Doxorubicin Flourouracil	Breast cancer, metastatic disease
FAM	Doxorubicn Flourouracil Mitomycin	Non-oat cell carcinoma of the lung, advanced gastric or pancreatic cancer
FOMi	Flourouracil Mitomycin Vincristine	Non-small cell cancer of the lung
M-2 Protocol	Carmustine Cyclophosphamide Melphalan Prednisone Vincristine	Multiple myeloma
MAC	Cyclophosphamide Doxorubicin Mitomycin	Advanced ovarian cancer
MACC	Cyclophosphamide Doxorubicin Lomustine Methotrexate	Lung cancer, non-oat cell carcinoma
MOPP	Mechlorethamine Prednisone Procarbazine Vincristine	Induction of therapy for Hodgkin's disease

Table 7 *(Continued)*

Name	Drugs in Regimen	Use
MOPP/ABVD	Bleomycin Dacarbazine Doxorubicin Mechlorethamine Prednisone Procarbazine Vinblastine Vincristine	Advanced Hodgkin's disease
MOPP-LO BLEO	Bleomycin Mechlorethamine Prednisone Procarbazine Vincristine	Induction of therapy for Hodgkin's disease
MPL + PRED (MP)	Melphalan Prednisone	Multiple myeloma
MTX + MP	Mercaptopurine Methotrexate	Maintenance therapy for acute lymphocytic leukemia
MTX + MP + CTX	Cyclophosphamide Mercaptopurine Methotrexate	Maintenance therapy for acute lymphocytic leukemia
M-VAC	Cisplatin Doxorubicin Methotrexate Vinblastine	Transitional cell carcinoma of the bladder
POCC	Cyclophosphamide Lomustine Procarbazine Vincristine	Lung cancer, small cell carcinoma
PVB	Bleomycin Cisplatin Vinblastine	Testicular cancer
T-2 Protocol 　Cycle E1	Month 1: Dactinomycin, Doxorubicin, radiation therapy Month 2: Cyclophosphamide, Doxorubicin, Vincristine, radiation therapy Month 3: Cyclophosphamide, Vincristine	Ewing's sarcoma
Cycle E2	Same as Cycle E1 without radiation therapy	
Cycle E3	Month 1: Dactinomycin, Doxorubicin Month 2: Cyclophosphamide, Vincristine Month 3: No drugs for 28 days	
Cycle E4	Repeat Cycle E3	

Table 7   *(Continued)*

Name	Drugs in Regimen	Use
VAB-6	*Induction*: Bleomycin Cisplatin Cyclophosphamide Dactinomycin Vinblastine *Maintenance*: Dactinomycin Vinblastine	Testicular cancer
VAC Pulse	Cyclophosphamide Dactinomycin Vincristine	Rhabdomyosarcoma in children, soft tissue sarcomas
VAC Standard	Cyclophosphamide Dactinomycin Vincristine	Rhabdomyosarcoma, soft tissue sarcomas, undifferentiated sarcoma
VAD	Dexamethasone Doxorubicin Vincristine	Refractory multiple myeloma
VBP	Bleomycin Cisplatin Vinblastine	Disseminated testicular cancer
VP	Prednisone Vincristine	Induction of therapy for acute lymphocytic leukemia
VP-L-Asparaginase	L-Asparaginase Prednisone Vincristine	Induction of therapy for acute lymphocytic leukemia

GENERAL NURSING CONSIDERATIONS FOR ANTINEOPLASTIC AGENTS

Administration

1. Antineoplastic drugs should be prepared only by trained personnel; preparation is contraindicated by pregnant personnel.
2. Antineoplastic drugs should be prepared under a laminar flow hood.
   - If a laminar flow hood is not available, preparation should be done in a work area away from cooling or heating vents and away from other people. The work area should be covered with a disposable plastic liner.
   - Use latex gloves to protect the skin when reconstituting antineoplastic drugs. Do not use gloves made of polyvinyl chloride since these are permeable to some cytotoxic drugs. Use caution in preparation, particularly to prevent skin reactions. Prevent contact of the drugs with skin or mucous membranes. If this occurs, wash the area immediately with copious amounts of water and document accordingly.
   - Wash the hands well both before and after removing the gloves used for drug preparation.

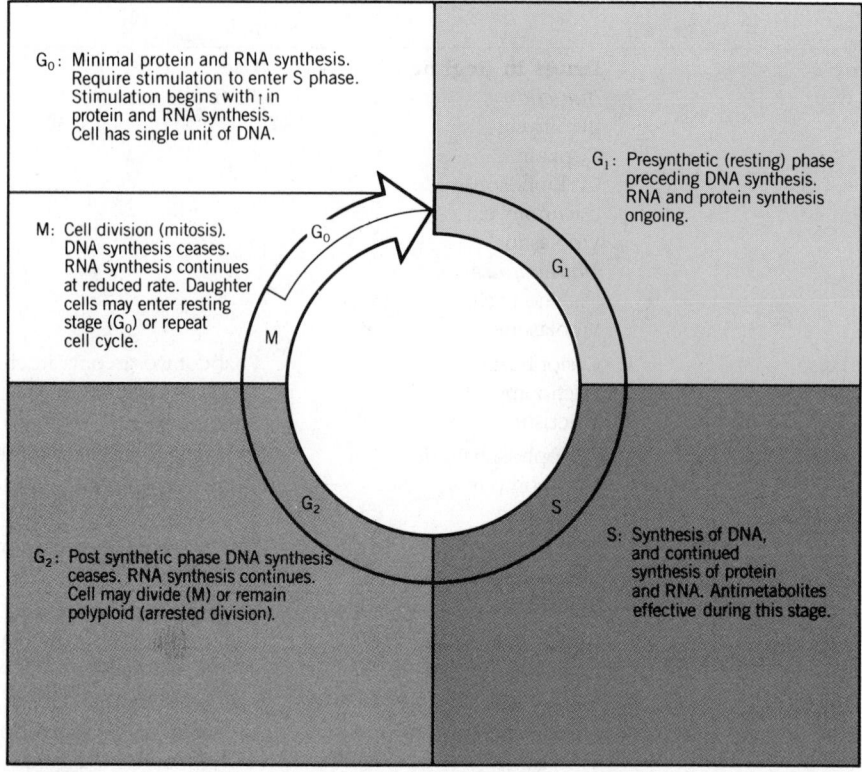

G_0: Minimal protein and RNA synthesis. Require stimulation to enter S phase. Stimulation begins with ↑ in protein and RNA synthesis. Cell has single unit of DNA.

M: Cell division (mitosis). DNA synthesis ceases. RNA synthesis continues at reduced rate. Daughter cells may enter resting stage (G_0) or repeat cell cycle.

G_1: Presynthetic (resting) phase preceding DNA synthesis. RNA and protein synthesis ongoing.

G_2: Post synthetic phase DNA synthesis ceases. RNA synthesis continues. Cell may divide (M) or remain polyploid (arrested division).

S: Synthesis of DNA, and continued synthesis of protein and RNA. Antimetabolites effective during this stage.

FIGURE 5

- Before beginning preparation the nurse should put on a disposable, nonpermeable surgical gown with a closed front, and knit cuffs that completely cover the wrists.
- Should material accidentally enter the eyes, wash eyes out well with isotonic saline eyewash (or water if isotonic saline is unavailable) and immediately see an ophthalmologist for further care.

3. Use piggyback setup with an electronic infusion pump.
4. Start infusion with a solution not containing the vesicant drug.
5. If possible, do not use the dorsum of the hand, wrist, or antecubital fossa as the site of infusion.
6. Avoid administering medication through a previously used site.
7. After IV has been started and unmedicated solution is being infused, check for blood return and for pain, redness, or edema before starting solution containing medication.
8. Luer-Lok fittings should be a part of all syringes and IV equipment used. Equipment should be disposable.
   - If the drug is to be reconstituted from a vial, vent the vial at the beginning of the procedure. This lowers the internal pressure and reduces the risk of spilling or spraying solution when the needle is withdrawn from the diaphragm.
   - Use a sterile alcohol wipe around the needle and vial top when withdrawing the drug.
   - Place a sterile alcohol wipe around the needle when expelling air from the syringe.
9. Once the drug has been prepared the external surfaces of syringes and bottles should be wiped

with an alcohol sponge. All disposable equipment should be placed in a separate disposable plastic bag and marked for incineration.

10. Instruct client to report pain, redness, or edema near the injection site during or after treatment.
11. Due to effects on the reproductive system, client should be advised to practice contraception.
12. Nurses should wear latex gloves when disposing of vomitus, urine or feces from clients receiving cytotoxic drug therapy.

Interventions

1. Establish a team involving the client, family, nurse, physician, pharmacist, social worker, and other health care workers to develop a holistic, therapeutic plan for the client's physical, emotional, social, and spiritual concerns.
2. Initially, identify one family member through which the health care team can direct and receive information and have that person function as a liaison for all family members. This should be someone in whom the client has complete confidence.
3. Whenever possible assure that the members of the health team are people who are committed to a long term relationship with the client. This assures that there will be consistency in follow-through of care and provides the client with the emotional support that will be necessary for treatment in the long months and possibly years ahead.
4. Utilize the nursing process format while working with the client and family. Learn from the client and family what they understand from what the physician has explained to them and clarify any misconceptions they may have.
5. Work closely with the client and family as they experience the effects and problems of chemotherapy associated with cure, remission, or palliation.

NURSING CONSIDERATIONS DURING INITIATION OF CHEMOTHERAPY

Assessment

1. Conduct a complete physical assessment of the client. Determine the client's emotional status, and note any history of hypersensitivity to drugs or foods.
2. Examine the client's mouth for any abnormalities or problems. If possible or indicated, contact the client's dentist to clarify any findings.
3. Determine what experience the client has had concerning surgery, prior radiation therapy, or with chemotherapy.
4. If dealing with someone who has just moved to the area or who is visiting and has experienced problems concerning his illness which necessitate treatment, contact the health professional with whom the client has been working to learn of any potential problems.
5. Assure that the necessary blood work has been completed. This provides important baseline data against which to measure client progress.

Interventions

1. Place client on careful intake and output and record.
2. Instruct client to report any pain, redness or edema that occurs near the site of injection during or after treatment.
3. Report extravasation to the physician and follow the institutional protocol for minimizing the effects.

4. Chart administration of antineoplastic drugs on the medication record and according to the established protocol for the institution.
   - Record client's drug protocol on medication sheet.
   - Day 1 is the first day of the first dose.
   - Number each day after that in sequence, even though client may not receive drug daily.
   - Indicate when the nadir (the time of most severe physiologic depression) is likely to occur so that possible complications, such as infection and bleeding, can be anticipated and treated early.
   - When the drug regimen is repeated, the first day of therapy is charted as day 1.
5. Establish appropriate principles to promote client compliance.
6. Assist the client and family in locating an appropriate support group in their community to assist them in coping with the problems that are caused by the client's illness and associated therapy.

Client/Family Teaching

1. Stress the importance of complying with all aspects of the therapeutic regimen.
2. Supply the client and family with the information and literature appropriate to the particular type of cancer or illness the client has.
3. Outline the types of side effects the client may be expected to experience and identify a means for coping with these problems.
4. That local cancer support groups in their community may assist them to understand and perhaps begin to cope with their illness.
5. That appropriate literature, such as *Chemotherapy and You,* published by the U.S. Department of Health and Human Services, NIH Publication 81–1136, may be useful as a guide during treatment.
6. Identify how and where to contact their health care providers to report any untoward reactions, ask questions, or to request clarification of instructions.
7. Review with the client and family the drugs to be used and the anticipated results.
8. In the event that antineoplastic agents are prepared and administered in the home, families need to be advised as to the proper disposal of urine, feces and vomitus.
9. If solutions are prepared in the home and accidents of spilling the drug occur, medical attention must be sought immediately. The health department should be notified. The name of the drug, and the type and duration of exposure must be recorded and reported.
10. When clients are at home, instruct them to maintain accurate intake and output. Provide them with appropriate conversion charts as necessary.

Evaluation

1. Assess client/family knowledge and understanding of illness, drug side effects and goals of therapy.
2. Evaluate the extent of client complaints of nausea and vomiting, anorexia, or diarrhea.
3. Note evidence of hepatic toxicity or changes in liver enzymes and alert the medical personnel responsible for the client's drug protocol.
4. Note presence of and extent of psychological depression, lethargy or other signs of possible changes in mental status. Document and report these changes to the physician and other members of the treatment team.
5. Note any evidence of acute renal failure. Review appropriate lab data and report to physician.

NURSING CONSIDERATIONS FOR BONE MARROW DEPRESSION

Leukopenia

Assessment

1. Check WBC count (normal values: 5,000–10,000/mm^3).

2. Review differential (normal values: neutrophils 60%–70%, lymphocytes 25%–30%, monocytes 2%–6%, eosinophils 1%–3%, basophils 0.25%–0.5%).

3. Note any sudden sharp drop in WBC count or a reduction below 2,000/mm^3, because these findings might necessitate reduction in dosage or withdrawal of the drug. Withhold drug and report.

4. Check temperature q 4 hr and recheck in 1 hr if there is a slight elevation. Report fever above 38°C (100°F) because client has limited resistance to infection resulting from leukopenia and immunosuppression.

5. Assess skin and orifices of body for signs of infection. Early identification is extremely important, since due to the absence of granulocytes, local abscesses do not form with pus, but infection becomes systemic as a septicemia.

6. Be aware of any signs of infection that may be present. Check the oral cavity for sores or the presence of ulcerated areas.

7. Be alert to any client report of increased weakness or fatigue. These symptoms may indicate anemia or electrolyte imbalance.

8. Continually assess for any changes in client morale.

Interventions

1. *Prevent infection by* using strict medical asepsis.

2. Provide frequent meticulous body care.

3. Use pHisoHex or an antiseptic to wash client who has a tendency to have skin eruptions.

4. Provide mouth care q 4–6 hr, with either normal saline or hydrogen peroxide diluted to half strength with water. Follow with a substrate of milk of magnesia. (Make substrate of milk of magnesia by discarding the clear liquid in the top of the bottle and using the thick white liquid that remains to coat the oral mucosa.) Do not use lemon or glycerin, because they tend to reduce the production of saliva and change the pH of the mouth. Mucosal deterioration occurs if mouth care is not provided at least q 6 hr.

5. Cleanse and dry the rectal area after each bowel movement. Apply A&D ointment if there is irritation.

6. Be prepared to initiate reverse isolation if WBC count falls below 1,500–2,000/mm^3 by

   • maintaining client in private room and explaining reasons for this procedure.
   • practicing universal precautions; use gloves, masks, and gowns as ordered.
   • limiting articles brought into room.
   • providing private bathroom or bedside commode.
   • minimizing unnecessary traffic into and out of room.
   • screening visitors for infection before they enter room.

7. Prevent nosocomial infections from invasive procedures by

   • cleansing skin with an antiseptic before procedure.
   • changing tubing of IV infusion q 24 hr.
   • changing site of IV infusion q 48 hr, if client does not have an implanted venous access device.

Thrombocytopenia

Assessment

1. Obtain platelet count (normal values: 200,000–300,000/mm^3). Client with a platelet count below 150,000/mm^3 should be closely monitored.
2. Check urine for blood cells.
3. Check stool for occult blood.
4. Inspect skin for petechiae or bruising.
5. Assess all orifices for bleeding.
6. Assess blood pressure of hospitalized client q.d. and prn.

Interventions

1. Prevent bleeding by minimizing SC or IM injections. When injections are necessary, apply pressure for 3–5 minutes to prevent leakage or hematoma.
2. Report and document any unusual bleeding after injection.
3. Do not apply a blood pressure cuff or other tourniquet for excessive periods of time.
4. Advise the client to use safety measures to *prevent bleeding* from cuts or bruises by
   - not picking at their nose, as bleeding may result.
   - using an electric razor for shaving rather than a blade.
   - providing a soft-bristled toothbrush or having client massage gums with fingers to limit irritation.
   - rearranging furniture so that area for ambulation is unimpeded (also, to prevent bumping into furniture at nighttime when getting out of bed to go to the bathroom).
   - having a night light to permit visualization in the event client must get up during the night.
5. *Assist with treatment of bleeding*
   - due to epistaxis by pinching nose for 10 min and applying pressure to upper lip to stop nosebleed.
   - with transfusion (usually ordered if platelet count falls below 150,000/mm^3). Take baseline vital signs before start of transfusion and then q 15 min after transfusion is started. Monitor vital signs for at least 2 hr after transfusion is completed. Assess for histoincompatibility, indicated by chills, fever, and urticaria. Stop transfusion, provide supportive care, and follow appropriate institutional protocol.

Anemia

Assessment

1. Check hemoglobin (normal values: 14–16 g/100 mL blood) and hematocrit (normal values: men, 40%–54%; women, 37%–47%).
2. Assess client for pallor, lethargy, or unusual fatigue.

Interventions

1. *Minimize anemia by*
   - providing a nutritious diet that client can tolerate.
   - administering or instructing client to take vitamins and iron supplements as ordered.
2. *Assist with treatment of anemia by*
   - administering diet high in iron that client can tolerate.
   - administering vitamins and iron supplements as ordered.
   - assisting with transfusion, as noted above, for treatment of thrombocytopenia.

NURSING CONSIDERATIONS FOR GI TOXICITY

Nausea/Vomiting

Assessment

1. Determine if the client is refusing food or fluids or just experiencing anorexia.
2. Compare client's nutritional status and weight with the baseline established at the start of therapy and monitor on subsequent visits.
3. Include the family in discussions on nutrition problems as they often supply information the client either forgets to mention or is afraid to talk about.
4. Examine the frequency, character and amount of vomitus. If the client has been vomiting at home be sure the family member in attendance has been taught to follow the procedure and document accordingly.

Interventions

1. *Prevent nausea and vomiting by*
   - premedicating with antiemetic as ordered, before administering antineoplastic drug. Usually the antiemetic is ordered to be administered 30 min before or just after administration of antineoplastic agent.
   - administering antineoplastic on an empty stomach, with meals, or at bedtime, to minimize nausea and vomiting and to produce the most therapeutic effect for the client.
   - teaching client and/or family how to insert an antiemetic suppository.
   - providing ice chips at onset of nausea.
   - providing carbonated beverages to counteract nausea.
   - encouraging ingestion of dry carbohydrates such as toast and dry crackers before initiating activity.
   - waiting for nausea and vomiting to pass before serving food.
   - providing small, nutritious snacks and planning meal schedules to coincide with client's best tolerance time.
   - providing nourishing foods that the client likes.
   - encouraging intake of a high-protein diet.
   - freezing dietary supplements and serving them like ice cream to make them more palatable.
   - avoiding foods with overpowering aroma.
   - encouraging client to chew foods well.
   - providing good oral hygiene both before and after meals.
   - encourage the client to eat favorite foods where possible. Such encouragement tends to assure some nutrition will be provided even though the client feels ill.
   - where possible, encourage clients to eat their meals with others, preferably at a table. Sharing with other clients has been shown to encourage some clients to eat.
2. *Assist with treatment of nausea and vomiting by*
   - administering antiemetic, as ordered, or contacting physician if antiemetic has not been ordered. All vomiting should be reported to physician, as a change in chemotherapeutic regimen or correction of electrolyte balance may be required.
   - providing supportive care to keep client as comfortable, clean, and free from odor as possible.
   - explaining to client that GI discomfort is generally a sign that the drug is also affecting tumor cells.
   - attending to correction of electrolyte balance and providing hyperalimentation as necessary.

Diarrhea/Abdominal Cramping

Assessment

1. Note frequency and severity of cramping caused by hypermotility.
2. Document frequency, color, consistency, and amount of diarrhea, all of which indicate amount of tissue destruction occurring.
3. Assess for signs of dehydration and acidosis indicating electrolyte imbalance, and maintain careful intake and output.

Interventions

1. *Prevent diarrhea/abdominal cramping by*
   - providing a bland low-roughage diet.
   - increasing the use of constipating foods, such as hard cheeses, in the diet.
2. *Assist with the treatment of diarrhea by*
   - administering antidiarrheal, if ordered, or contacting physician if antidiarrheal has not been ordered. Diarrhea or abdominal cramping should be reported, as a change in chemotherapeutic regimen or correction of electrolyte balance may be required.
   - increasing fluids, unless contraindicated.
   - assisting with correction of electrolyte imbalance.
   - providing good skin care, especially to the perianal area to prevent skin breakdown. Apply A&D ointment for perianal tenderness. Change client's gown and bed linens frequently; use room deodorizers as needed.

Stomatitis (Mucosal Ulceration)

Assessment

Assess for dryness of the mouth, erythema, and white patchy areas of the oral mucous membranes that indicate developing stomatitis. Assessment should be done each time the drug/drugs are administered.

Interventions

1. *Prevent stomatitis by*
   - assessing mouth t.i.d. and reporting bleeding gums or burning sensation especially when acid liquids such as fruit juice are ingested.
   - setting up a regular schedule for oral care.
   - providing good mouth care.
   - applying Vaseline to lips at least t.i.d.
2. *Assist with treatment of stomatitis by*
   - continuing to provide good oral care.
   - applying topical viscous anesthetic, such as lidocaine (Xylocaine), before meals, or providing a swish of lidocaine to anesthetize oral mucosa. Client may swallow lidocaine after swishing it around oral cavity but should be encouraged to expectorate it. A physician's order is required for the use of lidocaine.
   - providing bland foods at medium temperatures.

NURSING CONSIDERATIONS FOR NEUROTOXICITY

Assessment

1. Assess for symptoms of minor neuropathies, such as tingling in hands and feet and loss of deep tendon reflexes.

2. Observe for symptoms of serious neuropathies, such as weakness of hands, ataxia, loss of coordination, foot drop or wrist drop, and paralytic ileus.

3. Note what kind of activities the clients liked to do that required using their hands. This could be an important clue when asking clients about changes in sensation or weakness involving the hands.

Interventions

1. *Prevent functional loss due to neurotoxicity by*
   - reporting symptoms of neuropathies to the physician early and discuss findings. The physician may decide to change the medication regimen.
   - practicing and teaching seizure precautions.
2. *Assist with treatment of neuropathies by*
   - using appropriate safety measures in caring for client with a functional loss.
   - maintaining good body alignment by frequent and anatomically correct repositioning.
   - obtaining medical orders for stool softeners and laxatives as needed.

NURSING CONSIDERATIONS FOR OTOTOXICITY

Assessment

Assess for hearing difficulties before initiating therapy.

Interventions

1. Instruct client to report tinnitus or alteration in hearing.
2. Perform audiometry testing if indicated throughout therapy.

NURSING CONSIDERATIONS FOR HEPATOTOXICITY

Assessment

1. Obtain and assess the following liver function tests
   - Serum bilirubin (normal values: 0.3–1.0 mg/dl). An elevation may indicate there is liver disease or an increased rate of RBC hemolysis.
   - SGOT (normal values: 5–40 units/mL). Elevation is indicative of changes in the liver, skeletal muscles, lungs, pancreas, and heart. Hepatitis produces striking elevations in the SGOT.
   - SGPT (normal values: 5–35 units/mL). Elevation may be indicative of conditions leading to hepatic necrosis.
   - LDH (normal values: 100–225 units/mL). Elevation may be indicative of hepatitis, pulmonary infarction, and congestive heart failure.
2. Observe for signs of liver involvement, such as abdominal pain, high fever, diarrhea, and yellowing of skin and sclera.

Interventions

1. Prevent further hepatotoxicity by reporting elevations in liver function tests and signs of liver involvement to physician, as these are indications for changing medication regimen.
2. Assist with the treatment for hepatotoxicity by providing supportive nursing care to relieve symptoms, such as pain, fever, diarrhea, and jaundice.

NURSING CONSIDERATIONS FOR RENAL TOXICITY

Assessment

1. Obtain and assess the following renal function tests
   - BUN (normal values: 10–20 mg/dl)
   - Serum uric acid (normal values: 2.0–7.8 mg/dl)
   - Creatinine clearance (normal values: women, 0.8–1.7 g/24 hr; men, 1.0–1.9 g/24 hr)
   - Quantitative uric acid (normal values: 250–750 mg/day)
2. Observe and document any stomach pain, swelling of feet or lower legs, shakiness, unusual body movement, and stomatitis.

Interventions

1. Record intake and output.
2. Limit hyperuricemia by encouraging extra fluid intake to speed excretion of uric acid, and to decrease hazard of crystal and urate stone formation.
3. Test pH and assist with alkalinization of urine as ordered.

NURSING CONSIDERATIONS FOR IMMUNOSUPPRESSION

Assessment

1. Assess for the presence of fever, chills, or sore throat.
2. Note any changes in WBC count and differential.

Interventions

Assist with treatment of client with immunosuppression by
- preventing infection as noted above under bone marrow depression for leukopenia.
- advising delay of active immunization for several months after therapy is completed, as there may be either a hypo- or hyperactive response.

NURSING CONSIDERATIONS FOR GU ALTERATIONS

Assessment

1. Assess for altered GU function.
2. Determine client understanding that most symptoms, such as amenorrhea, cease after medication is discontinued.
3. Ascertain client's comprehension of risks before initiation of therapy, by asking whether physician has informed client that sterility may be a permanent result of therapy.

Intervention

Prevent teratogenesis by teaching client and partner of childbearing age to use contraceptive measures to avoid pregnancy, both during and for several months after therapy, as drug could have a teratogenic effect on the fetus if the woman were to conceive during this period.

NURSING CONSIDERATIONS FOR ALOPECIA

Assessment

Assess client understanding that body hair might fall out during therapy, but that it will grow back. Reinforce that hair may be of a different texture or color, but will start to grow in again about 8 weeks after therapy is completed.

Interventions

1. Minimize alopecia by
   - assisting with the application of scalp tourniquet 10–15 min before, during, and for 10–15 min after medication is administered.
   - applying ice packs to scalp 10–15 min before, during, and for 10–15 min after administration of medication.
2. Alternatives for managing alopecia include
   - encouraging client to shop for a wig before hair loss begins.
   - shaving head, if hair starts to fall out in large clumps, and using a wig or scarf until scalp hair has grown in again.
   - using a wig or scarf while hair is falling out and growing in again.
   - wearing a night cap at bedtime. This assures that hair that falls out during the night will be collected in one place and will not be all over the bed in the morning.
   - encouraging expression of feelings related to changes in self-image.

NURSING CONSIDERATIONS FOR ALTERATIONS IN SKIN

Assessment

1. Assess skin turgor and integrity. Document baseline data for comparison.
2. Anticipate and explain to family that some clients have slight changes in skin color during therapy.

Interventions

1. Maintain cleanliness of skin through bathing and frequent linen changes.
2. Prevent dryness and replenish moisture of skin with emollient lotions.
3. Prevent excessive exposure to sun or artificial ultraviolet light.
4. Use a special mattress or bed to redistribute weight on bony prominences and to minimize pressure and friction on pressure points.

ALKYLATING AGENTS

Action/Kinetics: Alkylating agents are highly reactive in that under physiologic conditions they donate an alkyl group (carbonium ion) to biologically important macromolecules, such as DNA. These reactions inactivate the molecule, bringing *cell division* to a halt. This cytotoxic activity is not limited to cancerous cells, but affects replication of the other cells of an organism, especially that of rapidly proliferating tissues, such as the bone marrow, intestinal epithelium, and hair follicles.

The toxic effects of the alkylating agents are usually cell-cycle nonspecific. The cytotoxic effect on cell division becomes apparent when the cell enters the S phase and cell division is blocked at the G_2 phase (premitotic phase), resulting in cells having a double complement of DNA.

Resistance of cancer cells to alkylating agents usually develops slowly and gradually. The resistance seems to be the sum total of several minor adaptations and not a reaction to a single one. Such mechanisms include decreased permeability of the cells, increased production of noncancer receptors (nucleophilic substances), and increased efficiency of the DNA repair system.

BUSULFAN   (byou-**SUL**-fan)
Myleran (Abbreviation: BUS) (Rx)

See also *Antineoplastic Agents,* p. 287, and *Alkylating Agents,* p. 313.

Classification: Antineoplastic, alkylating agent.

Action/Kinetics: Busulfan is cell cycle-phase nonspecific and is thought to act by alkylating cellular thiol groups. It is especially active against granulocytic cells. Busulfan may cause severe bone marrow depression. WBC count drops during the second or third week. Thus, close medical supervision, including weekly laboratory tests, is mandatory. Rapidly absorbed from the GI tract; appears in serum 0.5–2 hr after PO administration. **t½:** 2.5 hr. It is slowly excreted by the kidney.

Increased appetite and sense of well-being may occur a few days after therapy is started. Sometimes administered with allopurinol to prevent symptoms of clinical gout.

Uses: Acute and chronic myelocytic leukemia.

Contraindications: Use during lactation only if benefits outweigh risks.

Special Concerns: Pregnancy category: D.

Additional Side Effects: Pancytopenia (more severe than with other agents), bronchopulmonary dysplasia, pulmonary fibrosis, cataracts (after prolonged use), hyperpigmentation, adrenal insufficiency-like syndrome, gynecomastia, suppression of ovarian function, amenorrhea, cholestatic jaundice, myasthenia gravis.

Laboratory Test Interference: ↑ Uric acid in blood and urine.

Dosage: Tablets. Individualized according to WBC count. *Chronic myelocytic leukemia:* **Adults, induction, usual dose:** 4–8 mg daily until leukocyte count falls below 15,000/mm³; **maintenance:** 2 mg twice weekly to 4 mg daily. Discontinue therapy if there is a precipitous fall in WBC count. **Children, induction:** 0.06–0.12 mg/kg or 1.8–4.6 mg/m² daily; **maintenance:** dosage is titrated to maintain a leukocyte count of 20,000/mm³.

NURSING CONSIDERATIONS
See also *Nursing Considerations* for *Antineoplastic Agents,* p. 303.

Administration/Storage
1. Busulfan should be taken at the same time each day.
2. Extra fluid intake may be required during therapy.
3. Busulfan should not be administered without supervision and the availability of facilities for weekly complete blood counts.

CARBOPLATIN FOR INJECTION   (KAR-boh-plah-tin)

Paraplatin (Rx)

See also *Antineoplastic Agents,* p. 287, and *Alkylating Agents,* p. 313.

Classification: Antineoplastic, alkylating agent.

Action/Kinetics: Related to cisplatin. Carboplatin acts by producing interstrand DNA-cross links and is thus thought to be cell-cycle nonspecific. **t½, initial:** 1.1–2 hr; **post-distribution:** 2.6–5.9 hr. The drug is eliminated unchanged in the urine.

Uses: Palliative treatment of recurrent ovarian cancer either initially or previously treated with chemotherapy, including cisplatin. Also used to treat small cell and nonsmall cell lung carcinoma, tumors of the head and neck, seminoma, and nonseminomatous testicular cancer.

Additional Contraindications: History of severe allergy to mannitol or platinum compounds (including cisplatin). Severe bone marrow depression, significant bleeding, lactation.

Special Concerns: Pregnancy category: D.

Additional Side Effects: *Neurologic:* Central neurotoxicity, peripheral neuropathies, ototoxicity. *GU:* Nephrotoxicity (including increased BUN and serum creatinine). *Electrolytes:* Loss of calcium, magnesium, potassium, sodium. *Allergic:* Rash, urticaria, pruritus, erythema; bronchospasm and hypotension (rare). *Miscellaneous:* Pain, alopecia, asthenia. Cardiovascular, respiratory, mucosal side effects.

Drug Interactions: Carboplatin can react with aluminum (e.g., needles, IV administration sets) causing formation of a precipitate and loss of potency.

Laboratory Test Interference: ↑ Alkaline phosphatase, AST, total bilirubin.

Dosage: IV: *Ovarian cancer, as a single agent:* 360 mg/m² q 4 weeks on day 1. Lower doses are recommended in patients with low creatinine clearances.

NURSING CONSIDERATIONS

See also *Nursing Considerations* for *Antineoplastic Agents,* p. 303.

Administration/Storage

1. Single intermittent doses of carboplatin should not be repeated until the neutrophil count is at least 2,000/mm³ and the platelet count is 100,000/mm³.
2. The dose may be escalated by no more than 125% of the starting dose if platelet counts are greater than 100,000/mm³ and neutrophil counts are greater than 2,000/mm³. If platelet counts are less than 50,000/mm³ and neutrophil counts are less than 500/mm³, subsequent doses should be 75% of the prior dose.
3. The dose is administered by infusion lasting 15 min or longer.
4. For clients with impaired kidney function, the dose should be adjusted as follows: creatinine clearance of 41–59 mL/min, 250 mg/m² on Day 1; creatinine clearance of 16–40 mL/min, 200 mg/m². There is no recommended dose if the creatinine clearance is less than 15 mL/min.
5. Immediately before use, the drug should be reconstituted with either sterile water for injection, 5% dextrose in water, or sodium chloride injection to obtain a final concentration of 10 mg/mL. Carboplatin can be further diluted to concentrations as low as 0.5 mg/mL with 5% dextrose in water or sodium chloride injection.

6. Reconstituted solutions are stable for 8 hr at room temperature. Discard after this period of time as there is no antibacterial preservative in the formulation.
7. Unopened vials should be stored at room temperature protected from light.

Assessment

1. Note any evidence of kidney impairment.
2. Determine if client has a history of allergic responses to mannitol or platinum compounds.
3. Note any evidence of neurologic disorders as a means of determining if those that may occur at a later date are drug related or exacerbations of a prior condition.
4. Assess closely for drug-induced anemia, a frequent side effect of carboplatin therapy.

Interventions

1. Premedicate client with antiemetics as vomiting is a frequent side effect of drug therapy.
2. Anticipate reduced dose with impaired liver and/or renal function.
3. If the client has evidence of kidney impairment give 1–2 L of water before starting therapy. This may be given over a period of time. Have diuretics available should the client begin to show signs of overhydration.
4. Drug dose is based on CBC and creatinine clearance results; monitor carefully.
5. Ascertain that alkaline phosphatase, AST, and total bilirubin have been done. These results serve as baseline data against which to measure client reactions to the drug therapy.

Client/Family Teaching

1. Warn that client may experience nausea and vomiting.
2. Instruct clients to alert the physician if they notice a rash, pruritis, redness of the skin or bronchospasm.
3. Encourage clients to maintain adequate fluid intake. Favorite fluids may be given, especially those with potassium and calcium, since these electrolytes may be lost in excess as a result of therapy.

Evaluation

1. Note any evidence of the development of neurotoxicity, ototoxicity or nephrotoxicity and notify physician.
2. Assess client color and any complaints that may be indications of anemia.
3. Observe for myelosuppression which is usually most severe 21 days after the start of therapy, as symptoms occur rapidly.

CARMUSTINE   (kar-MUSS-teen)

BiCNU (Abbreviation: BCNU) (Rx)

See also *Antineoplastic Agents,* p. 287, and *Alkylating Agents,* p. 313.

Classification: Antineoplastic, alkylating agent.

Action/Kinetics: Carmustine acts by alkylating DNA and RNA as well as by inhibiting several enzymes. It is cell-cycle nonspecific. The drug is not cross-resistant with other alkylating agents. Drug rapidly cleared from plasma and metabolized. Crosses blood-brain barrier (concentration in CSF at least 50% greater than in plasma). $t^{1/2}$: 15–30 min. Thirty percent excreted in urine after 24 hr, 60–70% after 96 hr.

Uses: Alone or in combination with other antineoplastic agents for palliative treatment of primary and metastatic brain tumors, multiple myeloma (in combination with prednisone). Advanced Hodgkin's disease and non-Hodgkin's lymphomas (not the drug of choice). *Investigational:* GI cancer, malignant melanoma, mycosis fungoides.

Special Concerns: Pregnancy category: D. Not recommended for use during lactation.

Additional Side Effects: *GI:* Nausea and vomiting within 2 hr after administration, lasting 4–6 hr. *GU:* Renal failure, azotemia, decrease in kidney size. *Hepatic:* Reversible increases in alkaline phosphatase, bilirubin, and transaminase. *Other:* Rapid IV administration may produce transitory intense flushing of skin and conjunctiva (onset: after 2 hr; duration: 4 hr). Pulmonary fibrosis, ocular toxicity including retinal hemorrhage.

Drug Interaction: Additive bone marrow depression when used with cimetidine.

Dosage: IV: 150–200 mg/m² q 6–8 weeks as a single or divided dose (on consecutive days). Alternate dosing schedule: 75–100 mg/m² on 2 successive days q 6 weeks or 40 mg/m² on 5 successive days q 6 weeks. Subsequent dosage should be reduced if platelet levels are less than 100,000/mm³ and leukocyte levels are less than 4,000/mm³.

NURSING CONSIDERATIONS

See also *Nursing Considerations* for *Antineoplastic Agents,* p. 303.

Administration/Storage

1. Discard vials in which powder has become an oily liquid.
2. Store unopened vials at 2°–8°C and protect from light. Store diluted solutions at 4°C and protect from light.
3. Reconstitute powder with absolute ethyl alcohol (provided); then add sterile water. For injection, these dilutions are stable for 24 hr when stored as noted above.
4. Stock solutions diluted to 500 mL with 0.9% sodium chloride for injection or with 5% dextrose for injection are stable for 48 hr when stored as noted above.
5. Administer by IV over 1- to 2-hr period, as faster injection may produce intense pain and burning at site of injection.
6. Contact of reconstituted carmustine with skin may result in hyperpigmentation (transient). If contact occurs, the skin or mucosa should be washed thoroughly with soap and water.
7. *Do not use vial for multiple doses,* since there is no preservative in vial.

Interventions

1. Check for extravasation if client complains of burning or pain at site of injection. Discomfort may be due to alcohol diluent.
2. If there is no extravasation, reduce rate of flow if client complains of burning at site of injection.
3. Slow rate of IV infusion and notify physician if client demonstrates intense flushing of skin and/or redness of conjunctiva.

CHLORAMBUCIL   (klor-**AM**-byou-sil)

Leukeran (Abbreviation: CHL) (Rx)

See also *Antineoplastic Agents,* p. 287, and *Alkylating Agents,* p. 313.

Classification: Antineoplastic, alkylating agent.

Action/Kinetics: Chlorambucil is cell-cycle nonspecific although it is also cytotoxic to non-proliferating cells. The drug forms an unstable ethylenimmonium ion which binds (alkylates) with intracellular substances such as nucleic acids. The cytotoxic effect is due to cross-linking of strands of DNA and RNA and inhibition of protein synthesis. The drug also has immunosuppressant activity. Is rapidly absorbed from the GI tract. **Peak plasma levels:** 1 hr. Plasma $t^{1/2}$: about 90 min. Chlorambucil is 99% bound to plasma proteins, especially albumin. Is extensively metabolized by the liver and at least one metabolite is active. Sixty percent of the drug is excreted through the urine 24 hr after drug administration, and 40% is bound to tissues, including fat.

Uses: Chronic lymphocytic leukemia, malignant lymphomas (including lymphosarcoma), giant follicular lymphomas, and Hodgkin's disease. *Investigational:* Ovarian and testicular cancer, hairy cell leukemia, polycythemia vera, in combination with prednisone for nephrotic syndrome in adults and children unresponsive to other therapy.

Special Concerns: Pregnancy category: D. Use during lactation only if benefits outweigh risks. Safety and efficacy have not been established in children.

Additional Side Effects: *Note:* In humans, chlorambucil is carcinogenic, mutagenic, and teratogenic. It also affects human fertility.
   Hepatic: Hepatotoxicity with jaundice. *Pulmonary:* Pulmonary fibrosis, bronchopulmonary dysplasia. *CNS:* Children with nephrotic syndrome have an increased risk of seizures. *Miscellaneous:* Keratitis, drug fever, sterile cystitis, interstitial pneumonia, peripheral neuropathy.

Laboratory Test Interference: ↑ Uric acid levels in serum and urine.

Dosage: Tablets: *Leukemia, lymphomas: individualized* according to response of patient; **Adults, children, initial dose:** 0.1–0.2 mg/kg body weight (or 4–10 mg) daily in single or divided doses for 3–6 weeks; **maintenance:** 0.03–0.1 mg/kg daily. **Alternative for chronic lymphocytic leukemia: initial,** 0.4 mg/kg; **then,** repeat this dose every 2 weeks increasing by 0.1 mg/kg until either toxicity or control of condition is observed. *Nephrotic syndrome, immunosuppressant:* **Adults, children,** 0.1–0.2 mg/kg body weight daily for 8–12 weeks.

NURSING CONSIDERATIONS

See also *Nursing Considerations* for *Antineoplastic Agents,* p. 303.

Client/Family Teaching

1. The drug should be taken 1 hr before breakfast or 2 hr after the evening meal.
2. Instruct client/family how to monitor and record intake. From 80–96 oz of fluid should be consumed each day.
3. During drug therapy, advise clients that contraception should be practiced.

CYCLOPHOSPHAMIDE   (sye-kloh-**FOS**-fah-myd)

Cytoxan, Cytoxan Lyophilized, Neosar, Procytox❋ (Abbreviation: CYC) (Rx)

See also *Antineoplastic Agents,* p. 287, and *Alkylating Agents,* p. 313.

Classification: Antineoplastic, alkylating agent.

Action/Kinetics: Cyclophosphamide is metabolized in the liver to both active antineoplastic alkylating agents and inactive metabolites. The active metabolites alkylate nucleic acids, thus interfering with the growth of neoplastic and normal tissues. The cytotoxic action is due to cross-linking of strands of DNA and RNA and inhibition of protein synthesis. **$t^{1/2}$:** 3–12 hr, but remnants of drug and/or metabolites detectable in serum after 72 hr; in children, the **$t^{1/2}$** averages 4.1 hr. Metabolites are excreted through the urine with up to 20% of cyclophosphamide excreted unchanged. Cyclophosphamide is also excreted in milk.

Uses: Multiple myeloma. Malignant lymphomas: Hodgkin's disease, follicular lymphoma, lymphocytic lymphosarcoma, reticulum cell sarcoma, lymphoblastic lymphosarcoma, Burkitt's lymphoma. Mycosis fungoides. Leukemias: Chronic lymphocytic and granulocytic leukemia, acute myelogenous and monocytic leukemia, acute lymphoblastic leukemia in children. Neuroblastoma, adenocarcinoma of ovary, retinoblastoma. Carcinoma of breast. *Investigational:* Rheumatic diseases including rheumatoid arthritis and lupus erythematosus, multiple sclerosis, polyarteritis nodosa, Ewing's sarcoma, osteosarcoma, soft-tissue sarcomas, prophylaxis of rejection in organ transplants. Also, cancer of the cervix, lung, endometrium, bladder, prostate and testes; Wilms' tumor.

Contraindications: Lactation.

Special Concerns: Pregnancy category: D. Use with caution in patients with thrombocytopenia, leukopenia, previous radiation therapy, bone marrow infiltration of tumor cells, previous therapy causing cytotoxicity, and impaired liver and kidney function.

Additional Side Effects: Hemorrhagic cystitis. Bone marrow depression appears frequently during 9th to 14th day of therapy. Alopecia occurs more frequently than with other drugs. Secondary neoplasia (especially of urinary bladder), pulmonary fibrosis, cardiotoxicity, darkening of skin or fingernails.

Drug Interactions	
Allopurinol	↑ Chance of bone marrow toxicity
Chloramphenicol	↓ Metabolism of cyclophosphamide to active metabolites → ↓ pharmacologic effect
Insulin	↑ Hypoglycemia
Phenobarbital	↑ Rate of metabolism of cyclophosphamide in liver
Succinylcholine	↑ Succinylcholine-induced apnea due to ↓ breakdown in plasma
Thiazide diuretics	↑ Chance of bone marrow toxicity

Laboratory Test Interference: ↑ Uric acid in blood and urine; false + Pap test; ↓ serum pseudocholinesterase. Suppression of certain skin tests.

Dosage: IV. Adults, loading dose: 40–50 mg/kg in divided doses over 2–5 days. Alternative therapy: 10–15 mg/kg q 7–10 days, 3–5 mg/kg twice weekly, or 1.5–3 mg/kg daily. **Children, induction:** 2–8 mg/kg (or 60–250 mg/m^2 daily in divided doses for 6 or more days); **maintenance:** 10–15 mg/kg q 7–10 days or 30 mg/kg q 3–4 weeks (or when bone marrow recovery occurs).

Oral Solution, Tablets: Adults: 1–5 mg/kg depending on patient tolerance. **Maintenance** (various schedules): **PO:** 1–5 mg/kg/day. **Children, induction:** 2–8 mg/kg (or 60–250 mg/m^2 in divided doses for 6 or more days); **maintenance:** 2–5 mg/kg (or 50–150 mg/m^2) twice a week.

Attempt to maintain leukocyte count at 3,000–4,000/mm³. Dosage should be adjusted for kidney or liver disease.

NURSING CONSIDERATIONS

See also *Nursing Considerations* for *Antineoplastic Agents,* p. 303.

Administration/Storage

1. IV/IM: Dissolve 100 mg cyclophosphamide in 5 mL sterile water for injection or bacteriostatic water.
2. The reconstituted solution may be stored at room temperature for 24 hr and for 6 days if refrigerated at 2°–8°C (36°–46°F).
3. An oral solution may be prepared by dissolving injectable cyclophosphamide in aromatic elixir.
4. PO: Administer preferably on empty stomach. Give with meals in case of GI disturbance.
5. Fluid intake should be increased before, during, and for 24 hr after cyclophosphamide administration.
6. The initial loading dose may need to be reduced by 1/3– 1/2 in clients who have previously received cytotoxic drugs or radiation therapy.

Assessment

Note any client history of prior radiation therapy and/or chemotherapy as this is an indication for dose reduction of cyclophosphamide.

Interventions

1. Keep client well hydrated to help prevent hemorrhagic cystitis due to excessive concentration of drug in urine.
2. Administer the drug in the morning so that kidneys can eliminate the drug before bedtime. Encourage frequent voiding.
3. Observe for any evidence of dysuria and hematuria.
4. Monitor for cardiotoxicity: client complaints of shortness of breath, presence of pulmonary crackles, or tachycardia.
5. Observe for increased coughing, or shortness of breath. Obtain periodic chest x-rays and pulmonary function tests.
6. See *Nursing Considerations* for *Neuromuscular Blocking Agents,* p. 959, if client is also receiving succinylcholine, as apnea may be induced.

Client/Family Teaching

1. Take medication on an empty stomach unless otherwise ordered.
2. Increase consumption of fluids during and for 24 hr after cyclophosphamide therapy.
3. Reassure client with alopecia that hair should grow back when drug is stopped or when a maintenance dosage is given.
4. Advise women that drug may cause a false + Pap test.
5. Contraception should be practiced by both men and women during therapy.
6. Advise diabetic client that signs and symptoms of hypoglycemia may be precipitated by drug interactions with insulin. Instruct to monitor sugars closely and to consult with physician for possible insulin dosage adjustment.

DACARBAZINE   (dah-**KAR**-bah-zeen)

DTIC✲, DTIC-Dome, Imidazole Carboxamide (Abbreviation: DTIC) (Rx)

See also *Antineoplastic Agents,* p. 287, and *Alkylating Agents,* p. 313.

Classification: Antineoplastic, alkylating agent.

Action/Kinetics: The drug is thought to act by three mechanisms including: alkylation by an activated carbonium ion, antimetabolite to inhibit DNA synthesis, and by combining with protein sulfhydryl groups. The drug is cell-cycle nonspecific. **t½, biphasic: initial,** 19 min; **terminal,** 5 hr. Drug probably localizes in liver. Limited amounts (14% of plasma level) enter CSF. Approximately 40% of drug excreted in urine unchanged within 6 hr. Dacarbazine is secreted through the kidney tubules rather than filtered through the glomeruli.

Uses: Metastatic malignant melanoma. Hodgkin's disease (with other agents).

Contraindications: Use during lactation.

Special Concerns: Pregnancy category: C. Dosage has not been established in children.

Additional Side Effects: Especially serious (fatal) hematologic toxicity. More than 90% of patients develop nausea, vomiting, and anorexia 1 hr after initial administration, which persists for 12 to 48 hr. Rarely, diarrhea, stomatitis, and intractable nausea. Also, flu-like syndrome, severe pain along injected vein, facial flushing, alopecia, photosensitivity. Elevation of SGOT, SGPT and other enzymes, CNS symptoms.

Dosage: IV only. *Malignant melanoma:* 2–4.5 mg/kg daily for 10 days; may be repeated at 4-week intervals; or 250 mg/m²/day for 5 days; may be repeated at 3-week intervals. *Hodgkin's disease:* 150 mg/m²/day for 5 days; or 375 mg/m² on day 1, with other drugs repeated every 15 days.

NURSING CONSIDERATIONS

See also *Nursing Considerations* for *Antineoplastic Agents,* p. 303.

Administration/Storage

1. In order to minimize adverse GI effects, antiemetics, fasting and limited fluid intake (4–6 hr preceding treatment) have been suggested.
2. Extreme care should be taken to avoid extravasation.
3. Drug can be given by IV push over 1-min period or further diluted and administered by IV infusion (preferred) over 15- to 30-min period.
4. Protect dry vials from light and store at 2°–8°C.
5. Reconstituted solutions are stable for up to 72 hr at 4°C or for 8 hr at 20°C. More dilute solutions for IV infusions are stable for 24 hr when stored at 2°–8°C.

Interventions

1. Ascertain how physician wishes to handle fluid status (have client fast for 4–6 hr before treatment to reduce emesis, or allow client to have fluids up to 1 hr before administration to minimize dehydration following treatment).
2. Report nausea and vomiting, as these side effects may last for 12–48 hr after injection.
3. Have phenobarbital and/or prochlorperazine available for palliation of vomiting following administration of dacarbazine.
4. Clients may develop flu-like symptoms with fever, aches, fatigue, usually starting 7–10 days after dose of drug. Administer antipyretics and analgesics as needed.

Client/Family Teaching

1. Reassure client that after the first 1–2 days of dacarbazine therapy, vomiting ceases because tolerance develops to the drug.

2. Alert client to report to physician flu-like syndrome (fever, myalgia, and malaise) that may occur after treatment.

3. Advise client to avoid prolonged exposure to sun or ultraviolet light, as photosensitivity reaction may occur.

IFOSFAMIDE   (ih-**FOS**-fah-myd)

Ifex (Rx)

See also *Antineoplastic Agents,* p. 287, and *Alkylating Agents,* p. 313.

Classification: Antineoplastic, alkylating agent.

Action/Kinetics: Ifosfamide, a synthetic analog of cyclophosphamide, must be converted in the liver to active metabolites. The alkylated metabolites of ifosfamide then interact with DNA. **t½:** 7 hr.

Uses: As third line therapy, in combination with other antineoplastic drugs, for germ cell testicular cancer. Ifosfamide should always be given with mesna (see below) to prevent ifosfamide-induced hemorrhagic cystitis. *Investigational:* Cancer of the breast, lung, pancreas, ovary, and stomach. Also for sarcomas, acute leukemias (except AML), malignant lymphomas.

Special Concerns: Pregnancy category: D. Use with caution in patients with compromised bone marrow reserve, impaired renal function, and during lactation. Safety and efficacy have not been established in children.

Additional Side Effects: *GU:* Hemorrhagic cystitis, hematuria, dysuria, urinary frequency. *CNS:* Confusion, depressive psychosis, somnolence, hallucinations. Less frequently: dizziness, disorientation, cranial nerve dysfunction, seizures, coma. *GI:* Salivation, stomatitis. *Miscellaneous:* Alopecia, infection, liver dysfunction, phlebitis, fever of unknown origin, dermatitis, fatigue, hypertension, hypotension, polyneuropathy, pulmonary symptoms, cardiotoxicity, interference with normal wound healing.

Laboratory Test Interferences: ↑ Liver enzymes, bilirubin.

Dosage: IV: 1.2 g/m²/day for 5 consecutive days. Treatment may be repeated q 3 wks or if platelet counts are at least 100,000/μL and white blood cells are at least 4,000/μL.

NURSING CONSIDERATIONS

See also *Nursing Considerations* for *Antineoplastic Agents,* p. 303.

Administration/Storage

1. To prevent bladder toxicity, ifosfamide should be given with at least 2 L of oral or IV fluid per day as well as with mesna.

2. Dosage should be administered slowly over 30 min.

3. The drug is reconstituted by adding either sterile water for injection or bacteriostatic water for injection for a final concentration of 50 mg/mL. Solutions may be further diluted to achieve concentrations from 0.6–20 mg/mL by adding 5% dextrose injection, 0.9% sodium chloride injection, sterile water for injection, or lactated Ringer's injection.

4. Reconstituted solutions (50 mg/mL) are stable for 1 week at 30°C or 3 weeks at 5°C.

Interventions

1. Anticipate concomitant administration with mesna to minimize occurrence of hemorrhagic cystitis.
2. Monitor input and output; promote high fluid intake during therapy.
3. Monitor CBC and platelets closely; obtain WBC and platelet parameters for drug administration.
4. Obtain and send urine for analysis prior to each dose of ifosfamide.
5. Note the presence of marked leukopenia and protect the client from possible infection. Immunosuppression may activate latent infections such as herpes.
6. Check client's mouth for furry patches on the tongue or oral membranes. Document and report to the physician.

Client/Family Teaching

1. Reinforce that hair loss, nausea, and vomiting are frequent side effects of drug therapy.
2. Stress that normal wound healing may be impaired during drug therapy.
3. Report any confusion, hallucinations, or marked drowsiness as these symptoms may necessitate discontinuation of drug therapy.
4. Warn clients that there may be hyperpigmentation.
5. Advise female clients to practice contraceptive measures during the treatment and for at least 4 months after treatments have ceased.
6. If the treatment is to last 6 months, the client should be told that infertility may result.
7. Report the presence of frothy dark urine, jaundice or light colored stools. These are signs of hepatotoxicity and adjustments may be needed in the dosage of drug or therapy may need to be changed.

Evaluation

1. Assess client response to therapy by reviewing blood studies before and during treatment.
2. Check for myelosuppression. This may indicate a need to adjust the drug to maintain the leukocyte count.
3. Client complaints of joint or flank pain may be caused by the increase in uric acid that results from the rapid cytolysis of tumor and red blood cells.
4. Note any evidence of neurotoxicity. Report these signs to the physician and document on client's record. During outpatient treatment it is particularly important to elicit the support of the family in making observations and evaluations, and to encourage them to keep a record of events and the times of their occurrence.

LOMUSTINE   (loh-MUS-teen)

CeeNu (Abbreviation: CCNU)(Rx)

See also *Antineoplastic Agents,* p. 287, and *Alkylating Agents,* p. 313.

Classification: Antineoplastic, alkylating agent.

Action/Kinetics: Lomustine is an alkylating agent with cross-reactivity to carmustine. The drug interferes with the function of DNA and RNA and is cell-cycle nonspecific. Lomustine also inhibits protein synthesis by inhibiting necessary enzyme reactions. Rapidly absorbed from the GI tract; crosses the blood-brain barrier resulting in concentrations higher than in plasma. **Peak plasma**

level: 1–6 hr; **t½:** biphasic; **initial,** 6 hr; **postdistribution:** 1–2 days. From 15% to 20% of drug remains in body after 5 days. Fifty percent of drug excreted within 12 hr through the kidney, 75% within 4 days. Small amounts are excreted through the lungs and feces. Metabolites present in milk.

Uses: Primary and metastatic brain tumors. Disseminated Hodgkin's disease (in combination with other antineoplastics). *Investigational:* Cancer of the lung, breast, kidney; multiple myeloma; malignant melanoma.

Contraindications: Use during lactation.

Special Concerns: Pregnancy category: D.

Additional Side Effects: High incidence of nausea and vomiting 3–6 hr after administration and lasting for 36 hr. Renal and pulmonary toxicity. Dysarthria. **Note:** Delayed bone marrow suppression may occur due to cumulative bone marrow toxicity.

Laboratory Test Interference: Elevated liver function tests (reversible).

Dosage: Capsules. Adults and children: initial, 100–130 mg/m² as a single dose q 6 weeks. If bone marrow function reduced, decrease dose to 100 mg/m² q 6 weeks. Subsequent dosage based on blood counts of patients (platelet count above 100,000/mm³ and leukocyte count above 4,000/mm³). Blood tests should be undertaken weekly.

NURSING CONSIDERATIONS

See also *Nursing Considerations* for *Antineoplastic Agents,* p. 287.

Administration/Storage

1. Store below 40°C.
2. Lomustine may be given alone or in combination with other drugs, surgery, or radiotherapy.

Client/Family Teaching

1. Client may have nausea and vomiting up to 36 hr after treatment; this period may be followed by 2–3 days of anorexia. Administer antiemetics as prescribed.
2. The client is often depressed by prolonged nausea and vomiting; ensure that psychological support is available as needed.
3. Explain to client that intervals of 6 weeks are necessary between doses for optimum effect with minimal toxicity.
4. GI distress may be reduced by the administration of antiemetics before drug is taken or by taking the drug after fasting.
5. Inform client that medication comes in capsules of 3 strengths and a combination of capsules will make up the correct dose; this combination should be taken at one time.

MECHLORETHAMINE HYDROCHLORIDE   (meh-klor-**ETH**-ah-meen)

Mustargen Hydrochloride, Nitrogen Mustard (Abbreviation: HN₂) (Rx)

See also *Antineoplastic Agents,* p. 287, and *Alkylating Agents,* p. 313.

Classification: Antineoplastic, alkylating agent.

Action/Kinetics: Mechlorethamine is cell-cycle nonspecific. It acts by forming an unstable ethylenimmonium ion which then alkylates or binds with various compounds, including nucleic acids. The cytotoxic activity is due to cross-linking of DNA and RNA strands and protein synthesis.

When used for intracavitary tumors, the drug exerts both an inflammatory reaction and sclerosis on serous membranes which causes adherence of the drug to serosal surfaces. It reacts rapidly with tissues and within minutes after administration the active drug is no longer present. Metabolites are excreted through the urine.

Uses: IV: Bronchogenic carcinoma; chronic lymphocytic and chronic myelocytic leukemia; Hodgkin's and non-Hodgkin's lymphomas; polycythemia vera, mycosis fungoides. **Intracavitary:** Intrapericardially, intraperitoneally, or intrapleurally for treatment of metastatic carcinoma resulting in effusion. *Topical:* Mycosis fungoides.

Contraindications: Use during lactation.

Special Concerns: Pregnancy category: D.

Additional Side Effects: High incidence of nausea and vomiting. Amyloidosis, hyperuricemia, petechiae, subcutaneous hemorrhages, tinnitus, deafness, herpes zoster, or temporary amenorrhea. Extravasation into subcutaneous tissue causes painful inflammation.

Drug Interaction: Amphotericin B: combination increases possibility of blood dyscrasias.

Dosage: IV, Adults, children, *total dose:* 0.4 mg/kg per course of therapy given as a single dose or in 2–4 divided doses over 2–4 days. Depending on blood cell count, a second course may be given after 3 weeks. **Intracavitary:** 0.4 mg/kg. **Intrapericardial:** 0.2 mg/kg. **Topical Ointment, Solution:** Apply to entire skin surface once daily until 6–12 months after a complete response is obtained; **then,** use once to several times a week for up to three years.

NURSING CONSIDERATIONS

See also *Nursing Considerations* for *Antineoplastic Agents,* p. 303.

Administration/Storage

1. Since drug is highly irritating, any contact with skin should be avoided; plastic or rubber gloves should be worn during preparation.
2. Drug is best administered through tubing of a rapidly flowing IV saline infusion.
3. Prepare solution immediately before administration.
4. Medication is available in a rubber-stoppered vial to which 10 mL of either sterile water for injection or sodium chloride injection should be added.
5. Insert the needle and keep it inserted until the medication is dissolved and the required dose withdrawn. Carefully discard the vial with the remaining solution so that no one will come in contact with it.
6. For intracavitary administration, turn client every 60 sec for 5 min to the following positions: prone, supine, right side, left side, and knee-chest. Lack of effect often results from failure to move the client often enough.

Interventions

1. Administer phenothiazine and/or a sedative as ordered, prior to medication and as needed, to control severe nausea and vomiting that usually occur 1–3 hr after administration of nitrogen mustard.
2. Administer in late afternoon, and follow with a sedative (sleeping pill) at an appropriate time to control untoward symptoms and induce sleep.
3. Monitor IV closely because extravasation causes swelling, erythema, induration, and sloughing.
4. In case of extravasation, remove IV, assist in infusion of area with isotonic sodium thiosulfate

(4.14% solution of USP salt), and apply cold compresses. If sodium thiosulfate is not available, use isotonic sodium chloride solution or 1% lidocaine. Apply ice for 6–12 hr.

5. Irrigate eye with copious amounts of saline solution and consult with an ophthalmologist if mechlorethamine comes in contact with eye.

6. Irrigate skin with water for 15 min and then with 2% solution of sodium thiosulfate in the event of accidental contact.

MELPHALAN   (MEL-fah-lan)

Alkeran, L-Pam, L-Phenylalanine Mustard (Abbreviation: MPL) (Rx)

See also *Antineoplastic Agents,* p. 287, and *Alkylating Agents,* p. 313.

Classification: Antineoplastic, alkylating agent.

Action/Kinetics: Melphalan is cell-cycle nonspecific. The drug forms an unstable ethylenimmonium ion which binds to or aklylates various intracellular substances including nucleic acids. It produces a cytotoxic effect by cross-linking of DNA and RNA strands as well as inhibition of protein synthesis. Absorption from GI tract is variable and incomplete. **t¹/₂:** 90 min. The drug is inactivated in tissues and body fluids although it will remain active in the blood for approximately 6 hr. Within 24 hr, 10% is excreted unchanged in the urine.

Uses: Multiple myeloma. Epithelial carcinoma of ovary (nonresectable). *Investigational:* Cancer of the breast and testes.

Contraindications: Use during lactation.

Special Concerns: Pregnancy category: D. Safety and efficacy have not been determined in children less than 12 years of age.

Additional Side Effects: Severe bone marrow depression, chromosomal aberrations, leukemia (acute, nonlymphatic) in patients with multiple myeloma. Also, pulmonary fibrosis, interstitial pneumonia, vasculitis, hemolytic anemia.

Laboratory Test Interferences: ↑ Uric acid and urinary 5-hydroxyindole acetic acid levels.

Dosage: Tablets. *Multiple myeloma:* (1) 0.15 mg/kg daily for 7 days followed by a rest period of at least three weeks. During the rest period, the leukocyte count will decrease; when white blood cell and platelet counts are increasing, a maintenance dose of 0.05 mg/kg daily may be given; or, (2) 0.1–0.15 mg/kg daily for 2–3 weeks (or 0.25 mg/kg daily for four days) followed by a rest period of 2–4 weeks. When leukocyte counts rise to 3,000–4,000/mm³ and platelet counts increase above 100,000/mm³ a maintenance dose of 2–4 mg daily may be given; or, (3) 7 mg/m² (or 0.25 mg/kg) daily for 5 days q 5–6 weeks (dose is adjusted to produce slight leukopenia and thrombocytopenia). *Ovarian cancer:* 0.2 mg/kg daily for five days repeated q 4–5 weeks (as long as blood counts return to normal).

NURSING CONSIDERATIONS

See also *Nursing Considerations* for *Antineoplastic Agents,* p. 303.

Interventions

1. Monitor hemoglobin and platelet levels and differential leukocyte count. Severe risk of infection exists if the absolute neutrophil count is less than 1,000/mm³, hemorrhage is possible if platelet

count drops below 50,000/mm³, and symptoms of anemia will develop if hemoglobin level falls below 9–10 g/d.

2. The client should be advised to use contraceptive measures during therapy.

MESNA   (MEZ-nah)

Mesnex (Rx)

Classification: Antidote for use with ifosfamide.

Action/Kinetics: Ifosfamide is metabolized to products that cause hemorrhagic cystitis. In the kidney, mesna reacts chemically with these ifosfamide metabolites to cause their detoxification. Following IV use, mesna is rapidly oxidized to mesna disulfide (dimesna) which is eliminated by the kidneys. **t¹/₂ in blood, mesna:** 0.36 hr; **dimesna:** 1.17 hr.

Uses: Prophylactically to reduce the incidence of hemorrhagic cystitis caused by ifosfamide. *Investigational:* Reduce incidence of hemorrhagic cystitis caused by cyclophosphamide.

Contraindications: Hypersensitivity to thiol compounds.

Special Concerns: Pregnancy category: B. Use with caution during lactation.

Side Effects: Since mesna is used with ifosfamide and other antineoplastic agents, it is difficult to identify those untoward reactions due to mesna. The following symptoms are believed possible. *GI:* Nausea, vomiting, diarrhea, bad taste in mouth.

Laboratory Test Interferences: False + test for urinary ketones.

Dosage: IV bolus: *prophylaxis of ifosfamide-induced hemorrhagic cystitis,* dosage of mesna equal to 20% of the ifosfamide dose given at the time of ifosfamide and at 4 and 8 hr after each dose of ifosfamide. Thus, the total daily dose of mesna is 60% of the ifosfamide dose (e.g., an ifosfamide dose of 1.2 g/m² would mean doses of mesna would be 240 mg/m² at the time the ifosfamide dose was given, 240 mg/m² after 4 hr, and 240 mg/m² after 8 hr). This dosage should be given on each day that ifosfamide is administered.

NURSING CONSIDERATIONS

Administration/Storage

1. If the dosage of ifosfamide is increased or decreased, the dosage of mesna should be adjusted accordingly.
2. The drug can be reconstituted to a final concentration of 20 mg mesna/mL fluid by adding either 5% dextrose injection, 5% dextrose and sodium chloride injection, 0.9% sodium chloride injection, or lactated Ringer's injection.
3. Diluted solutions are stable for 24 hr at 25°C. However, when mesna is exposed to oxygen, dimesna is formed; thus, a new ampule should be used for each administration.
4. Mesna is not compatible with cisplatin.

Interventions

1. Drug must be administered with each dose of ifosfamide to be effective against drug-induced hemorrhagic cystitis.
2. Obtain a morning urine specimen for analysis each day before ifosfamide therapy.

Client/Family Teaching

1. A bad taste may be experienced in the mouth of the client during drug therapy; use hard candy to mask taste.
2. Nausea, vomiting, and diarrhea are frequent side effects of drug therapy; report if persistent or bothersome.

PIPOBROMAN   (pip-oh-**BROH**-man)

Vercyte (Rx)

See also *Antineoplastic Agents,* p. 287, and *Alkylating Agents,* p. 313.

Classification: Antineoplastic, alkylating agent.

Action/Kinetics: The mechanism, metabolism, and excretion are not known. Well absorbed from the GI tract.

Uses: Polycythemia vera; chronic granulocytic leukemia (refractory to busulfan).

Additional Contraindication: Children under 15 years of age. Lactation.

Special Concerns: Pregnancy category: D.

Dosage: Tablets. *Polycythemia vera:* 1 mg/kg daily (up to 1.5–3 mg/kg daily may be required in patients refractory to other treatment). When hematocrit has been reduced to 50%–55%, **maintenance dosage** of 100–200 mcg/kg is instituted. *Chronic granulocytic leukemia:* **initial,** 1.5–2.5 mg/kg daily; **maintenance,** 7–175 mg daily, to be instituted when leukocyte count approaches 10,000/mm^3.

NURSING CONSIDERATIONS

See also *Nursing Considerations* for *Antineoplastic Agents,* p. 303.

Interventions

1. Administer drug in divided doses.
2. Be alert to persistent adverse reactions that may necessitate withdrawal of the drug.

STREPTOZOCIN   (strep-toe-**ZOH**-sin)

Zanosar (Rx)

See also *Antineoplastic Agents,* p. 287, and *Alkylating Agents,* p. 313.

Classification: Antineoplastic, alkylating agent.

Action/Kinetics: Streptozocin is cell-cycle nonspecific although it does inhibit progression out of the G$_2$ phase of cell division. The drug forms methylcarbonium ions which alkylate or bind with intracellular substances such as nucleic acids. It is also cytotoxic by virtue of cross-linking of DNA strands resulting in inhibition of DNA synthesis. It may also cause hyperglycemia. Streptozocin does not penetrate the blood-brain barrier well although within 2 hr after administration, metabolites do and produce levels similar to those in plasma. **t½, unchanged drug, initial,** 5–15 min. **t½, metabolites, initial:** 6 min; **intermediate:** 3.5 hr; **terminal:** 40 hr. Unchanged drug and metabolites excreted in urine.

Uses: Metastatic islet cell pancreatic carcinomas (functional and nonfunctional). *Investigational:* Malignant carcinoid tumors.

Contraindications: Use during lactation.

Special Concerns: Pregnancy category: C. Dosage has not been determined for children.

Additional Side Effects: Renal toxicity (up to two-thirds of patients) manifested by anuria, azotemia, glycosuria, hypophosphatemia, and renal tubular acidosis. Toxicity is dose-related and cumulative and may be fatal. Glucose intolerance (reversible) or insulin shock with hypoglycemia, depression.

Dosage: IV: *Daily schedule:* 500 mg/m^2 for 5 consecutive days every 6 weeks (until maximum benefit is achieved or toxicity occurs). Dose should not be increased. *Weekly schedule:* **Initial,** 1,000 mg/m^2 weekly for 2 weeks; **then,** if no response or no toxicity, dose can be increased, not to exceed a single dose of 1,500 mg/m^2. Response should be seen in 17–35 days.

NURSING CONSIDERATIONS

See also *Nursing Considerations* for *Antineoplastic Agents,* p. 303.

Administration/Storage

1. Drug should be reconstituted with dextrose injection or 0.9% sodium chloride injection.
2. No preservatives are found in the product; thus, total storage time for reconstituted drug is 12 hr. The ampule is not considered to be multiple dose.

Interventions

1. Measure fluid intake and urine output. If urine output decreases, report to physician, because streptozocin can cause anuria.
2. Perform finger sticks or test urine for glucose levels at least once a day and observe for symptoms of hypoglycemia.
3. Monitor blood sugar levels and renal function studies during therapy.

THIOTEPA   (thigh-oh-**TEE**-pah)

(Abbreviation: Thio) (Rx)

See also *Antineoplastic Agents,* p. 287, and *Alkylating Agents,* p. 313.

Classification: Antineoplastic, alkylating agent.

Action/Kinetics: Thiotepa is cell-cycle nonspecific; it is thought to act by causing the release of ethylenimmonium ions which bind or alkylate various intracellular substances such as nucleic acids. The drug is cytotoxic by virtue of cross-linking of DNA and RNA strands as well as by inhibition of protein synthesis. It is cleared rapidly from the plasma following IV use. Thiotepa may be significantly absorbed through the bladder mucosa. Approximately 85% is excreted through the urine, mainly as metabolites.

Uses: Adenocarcinoma of the breast or ovary. Control of serious effusions of pleural, pericardial, and peritoneal cavities. Superficial papillary carcinoma of the urinary bladder. Hodgkin's and non-Hodgkin's disease, lymphosarcoma, bronchogenic carcinoma. *Investigational:* Prevention of pterygium recurrences after surgery.

Contraindications: Use during lactation. Pregnancy. Renal, hepatic, or bone marrow damage. Acute leukemia.

Additional Side Effects: Anorexia or decreased spermatogenesis.

Drug Interaction: Thiotepa increases the pharmacologic and toxic effect of succinylcholine due to a decrease in breakdown by the liver.

Dosage: IV (may be rapid): 0.3–0.4 mg/kg at 1- to 4-week intervals or 0.2 mg/kg for 4–5 days q 2–4 weeks. **Intratumor or intracavitary administration:** 0.6–0.8 mg/kg q 1–4 weeks; **maintenance (intratumor):** 0.07–0.8 mg/kg at 1- to 4-week intervals, depending on condition of patient. *Carcinoma of bladder:* 30–60 mg in 30–60 mL distilled water instilled into the bladder and retained for 2 hr. Give once a week for 4 weeks. May be repeated monthly, if necessary.

NURSING CONSIDERATIONS

See also *Nursing Considerations* for *Antineoplastic Agents,* p. 303.

Administration/Storage

1. Minimize pain on injection and retard rate of absorption by simultaneous administration of local anesthetics. Drug may be mixed with procaine HCl 2% or epinephrine HCl 1:1,000, or both, upon order of the physician.
2. Store vials in the refrigerator. Reconstituted solutions may be stored for 5 days in the refrigerator without substantial loss of potency.
3. Since thiotepa is not a vesicant, it may be injected quickly and directly into the vein with the desired volume of sterile water. Usual amount of diluent is 1.5 mL.
4. Do not use normal saline as a diluent.
5. Discard solutions grossly opaque or with precipitate.
6. When used for bladder carcinoma, the client is dehydrated for 8–12 hr prior to each dose.

Interventions

1. Encourage clients who receive drug as bladder instillations to retain fluid for 2 hr.
2. Reposition client with a bladder instillation every 15 min to ensure maximum contact.

URACIL MUSTARD   (YOU-rah-sil)

(Rx)

See also *Antineoplastic Agents,* p. 287 and *Alkylating Agents,* p. 313.

Classification: Antineoplastic, alkylating agent.

Action/Kinetics: Uracil mustard is a bifunctional alkylating agent and is cell-cycle nonspecific. The drug forms unstable ethylenimmonium ions which bind or alkylate various intracellular substances. The drug cross-links with DNA and interferes with the function of DNA and RNA. The drug is excreted through the kidneys.

Uses: Chronic lymphocytic leukemia, non-Hodgkin's lymphomas (of the lymphocytic or histiocytic type), chronic myelogenous leukemia. Palliative therapy for polycythemia vera and mycosis fungoides.

Contraindications: Pregnancy and lactation. Leukopenia, thrombocytopenia, aplastic anemia.

Additional Side Effects: During therapy significant decreases in leukocyte and platelet counts occur. Also, hepatotoxicity, amenorrhea, azoospermia.

Laboratory Test Interference: ↑ Serum uric acid levels.

Dosage: Capsules. Adults: 0.15 mg/kg once weekly for 4 weeks. **Children:** 0.30 mg/kg once weekly for 4 weeks.

NURSING CONSIDERATIONS

See also *Nursing Considerations* for *Antineoplastic Agents,* p. 303.

Administration/Storage

1. Uracil mustard should not be administered until 2–3 weeks after the maximum effect of other cytotoxic drugs or x-ray therapy has been determined.
2. Complete blood counts should be done once or twice weekly during therapy and 1 month thereafter.
3. Effect of drug sometimes takes 3 months to become apparent, and drug should be given that long unless precluded by a toxicity reaction.
4. Capsules contain the dye tartrazine (FD & C yellow No. 5).

Client/Family Teaching

1. Encourage continuation with therapy, because beneficial effect may take as long as 3 months to appear.
2. Warn client not to have smallpox immunization during therapy with uracil mustard, since vaccinia may result as a complication of immunosuppression.
3. Encourage intake of large amounts of fluid during therapy to prevent hyperuricemia.

ANTIMETABOLITES

Action/Kinetics: Antimetabolites are able to disrupt DNA replication by interfering with an essential step in its synthesis and/or metabolism. Antimetabolites are thought to interfere with important enzymatic reactions in the synthesis of nucleic acids, purines, pyrimidines, and their precursors. Antimetabolites may also be incorporated into nucleic acids in place of corresponding nucleotides resulting in alterations in important cellular functions and inhibition of DNA synthesis. Antimetabolites are usually cell-cycle specific, being effective during the S and G_2 phases.

The antimetabolites fall into several categories: folic acid antagonists, pyrimidine antagonists, purine analogs, and miscellaneous agents.

CYTARABINE   (sye-**TAIR**-ah-been)

Ara-C, Cytosar✶, Cytosar-U, Cytosine Arabinoside (Rx)

See also *Antineoplastic Agents,* p. 287.

Classification: Antineoplastic, antimetabolite.

Action/Kinetics: Cytarabine is thought to act by inhibiting DNA polymerase as well as by being incorporated into both DNA and RNA. The drug is cell phase specific acting in the S phase and also blocking the progression of cells from the G_1 phase to the S phase. After oral administration, cytarabine is rapidly broken down by the GI mucosa and liver, resulting in systemic availability of less than 20%. **t½ after IV: distribution,** 10 min; **elimination,** 1–3 hr. The drug is metabolized in the liver to uracil arabinoside, which is excreted in the urine. Crosses blood-brain barrier. Eighty percent eliminated in urine in 24 hr.

Uses: Acute myelocytic leukemia in adults and children, acute lymphocytic leukemia, chronic myelocytic leukemia, erythroleukemia, and meningeal leukemia. In combination with other drugs for non-Hodgkin's lymphoma in children. *Investigational:* Hodgkin's lymphomas, myelodysplastic syndrome.

Contraindications: Use during lactation.

Special Concerns: Pregnancy category: D.

Additional Side Effects: "Cytarabine syndrome" (6–12 hr following drug administration) manifested by bone pain, fever, myalgia, maculopapular rash, conjunctivitis, chest pain, or malaise. Nephrotoxicity, neuritis, skin ulceration, sepsis, acute pancreatitis, pneumonia, hyperuricemia. Thrombophlebitis at injection site.

The incidence of side effects is higher in patients receiving rapid IV injection than in those receiving drug by IV infusion.

Dosage: Note: Cytarabine is frequently used in combination with other drugs; thus, dosage varies and must be carefully checked. *Acute myelocytic leukemia, acute lymphocytic leukemia:* **IV infusion:** 100–200 mg/m² as a continuous infusion over 24 hr or in divided doses (by rapid injection) for 5–10 days; repeat every 2 weeks. *Meningeal leukemia:* **intrathecal, usual:** 30 mg/m² every 4 days with hydrocortisone sodium succinate and methotrexate, each at a dose of 15 mg/m², until CSF findings are normal followed by one additional dose. *Refractory acute leukemia:* **IV:** 3 g/m² q 12 hr for 4–12 doses; repeat at 2–3 wk intervals.

The drug should be discontinued if platelet level falls to 50,000/mm³ or less or polymorphonuclear granulocyte level falls to 1,000/mm³ or less.

NURSING CONSIDERATIONS

See also *Nursing Considerations* for *Antineoplastic Agents,* p. 303.

Administration/Storage

1. Cytarabine may be given SC, IV infusion, or IV injection. It is ineffective orally.
2. The 100 mg vial of cytarabine should be reconstituted with 5 mL bacteriostatic water for injection with benzyl alcohol (0.9%) with the resultant solution containing 20 mg/mL. The 500 mg vial should be reconstituted with 10 mL of bacteriostatic water for injection with benzyl alcohol (0.9%) with the resultant solution containing 50 mg/mL cytarabine. Benzyl alcohol should not be used for reconstitution if the drug will be used intrathecally; rather, 0.9% saline or Elliott's B solution should be used.
3. Reconstituted solution should be stored at room temperature and used within 48 hr.
4. Discard hazy solution.
5. Systemic toxicity may result from intrathecal use of cytarabine.

FLOXURIDINE   (flox-YOU-rih-deen)

FUDR (Rx)

See also *Antineoplastic Agents,* p. 287.

Classification: Antineoplastic, antimetabolite.

Action/Kinetics: Floxuridine is cell-cycle specific for the S phase of cell division. The drug is rapidly metabolized to fluorouracil (see below). The drug inhibits DNA and RNA synthesis. Crosses blood-brain barrier. $t^{1/2}$: 5–20 min. From 60–80% of fluorouracil is excreted as respiratory CO_2 (8–12 hr); small amount (15%) excreted in urine (1–6 hr).

Uses: Intra-arterially as palliative treatment of GI adenocarcinoma metastatic to the liver (especially in patients incurable by surgery or other treatment). Used in patients with disease limited to an area capable of infusion by a single artery. *Investigational:* Cancer of the breast, ovaries, cervix, bladder, kidney, and prostate.

Contraindications: If patient is at poor risk, including depressed bone marrow function, nutritionally poor, or potentially serious infections. Lactation. Should not be used during pregnancy unless benefits clearly outweigh risks.

Additional Side Effects: Esophagopharyngitis, myocardial ischemia, angina, acute cerebellar syndrome, photophobia, lacrimation, decreased vision. Complications of intra-arterial administration are arterial aneurysm, arterial ischemia, arterial thrombosis, bleeding at catheter site, occluded, displaced, or leaking catheters, embolism, fibromyositis, infection at catheter site, thrombophlebitis.

Laboratory Test Interferences: ↑ Excretion of 5-hydroxyindoleacetic acid. ↑ Serum transaminase and bilirubin, lactic dehydrogenase, alkaline phosphatase. ↓ Plasma albumin.

Dosage: Intra-arterial infusion: 0.1–0.6 mg/kg/day by continuous infusion over 24 hr. Infusion is continued until a response or toxicity occurs (usually for 14–21 days with a rest period of 2 weeks between courses of therapy).

NURSING CONSIDERATIONS

See also *Nursing Considerations* for *Antineoplastic Agents,* p. 303.

Administration/Storage

1. Higher doses (0.4–0.6 mg) are best given by hepatic artery infusion because the liver metabolizes the drug, reducing the possibility of systemic toxicity.
2. The drug should be given until untoward effects are manifested. Resume therapy after untoward effects have subsided.
3. An infusion pump should be used to overcome pressure in the large arteries and to assure a uniform rate of infusion.
4. The drug should be reconstituted with 5 mL sterile water.

FLUOROURACIL (5-FLUOROURACIL, 5-FU) (floo-roh-**YOU**-rah-sil)

Adrucil, Efudex, Fluoroplex (Abbreviation: 5-FU) (Rx)

See also *Antineoplastic Agents,* p. 287.

Classification: Antineoplastic, antimetabolite.

Action/Kinetics: Pyrimidine antagonist inhibiting thymidylate desoxyuridylic acid, hence DNA, and to a lesser degree, RNA synthesis. The drug is cell-cycle specific for the S phase of cell division. $t^{1/2}$, **initial:** 5–20 min; **final:** 20 hr. From 60–80% eliminated as respiratory CO_2 (8–12 hr); small amount (15%) excreted unchanged in urine (1–6 hr).

Highly toxic; initiate use in hospital. Initially, topical creams cause ulcers, which might heal only 1–2 months after cessation of therapy.

Uses: Systemic: Palliative management of certain cancers of the rectum, stomach, colon, pancreas, and breast. Relieves pain and reduces size of tumor. **Topical (as solution or cream):** Actinic or solar keratosis, superficial basal cell carcinoma. *Investigational:* **Systemic:** Cancer of the bladder, ovaries, prostate, cervix, endometrium, lung, liver, head, and neck. Also, malignant pleural, peritoneal, and pericardial effusions. **Topical:** Actinic cheilitis, mucosal leukoplakia, Bowen's disease, radiodermatitis, erythroplasia of Queyrat.

Additional Contraindications: Systemic: Patients in poor nutritional state, with severe bone marrow depression, severe infection, or recent (4-week-old) surgical intervention. Lactation. To be used with caution in patients with hepatic or liver dysfunction.

Special Concerns: Use during pregnancy only if benefits clearly outweigh risks (pregnancy category: D).

Additional Side Effects: Esophagopharyngitis, myocardial ischemia, angina, acute cerebellar syndrome, photophobia, lacrimation, decreased vision. Also, arterial thrombosis, arterial ischemia, arterial aneurysm, bleeding or infection at site of catheter, thrombophlebitis, embolism, fibromyositis, abscesses.

Dosage: IV. Individualize dosage. Initial: 12 mg/kg/day for 4 days, not to exceed 800 mg/day. If no toxicity seen, administer 6 mg/kg on days 6, 8, 10, and 12. Discontinue therapy on day 12 even if there are no toxic symptoms. **Maintenance:** Repeat dose of first course every 30 days or when toxicity from initial course of therapy is gone; or, give 10–15 mg/kg/week as a single dose. Do not exceed 1 g/week. **If patient is debilitated or is a poor risk:** 6 mg/kg/day for 3 days; if no toxicity, give 3 mg/kg on days 5, 7, and 9 (daily dose should not exceed 400 mg). **Cream, Topical Solution:** *Actinic or solar keratoses:* Apply 1–5% cream or solution to cover lesion 1–2 times daily for 2–6 weeks. *Superficial basal cell carcinoma:* Apply 5% cream or solution to cover lesion b.i.d. for 3–6 weeks (up to 10–12 weeks may be required).

NURSING CONSIDERATIONS

See also *Nursing Considerations* for *Antineoplastic Agents,* p. 303.

Administration/Storage

IV

1. Store in a cool place (50°–80°F or 10°–27°C). Do not freeze. Excessively low temperature causes precipitation.
2. Do not expose the solution to light.
3. Solution may discolor slightly during storage, but potency and safety are not affected.
4. If precipitate forms, resolubilize by heating to 140°F with vigorous shaking. Allow to return to room temperature and allow air to settle out before withdrawing and administering medication.
5. Further dilution is not needed, and solution may be injected directly into the vein with a 25-gauge needle.
6. Drug can be administered by IV infusion for periods of 30 min–8 hr. This method has been reported to produce less systemic toxicity than rapid injection.
7. The drug should not be mixed with other drugs or IV additives.

Topical

1. Apply with fingertips, nonmetallic applicator, or rubber gloves. Wash hands immediately thereafter.

2. Avoid contact with eyes, nose, and mouth.

3. Limit occlusive dressings to lesions, since they are responsible for an increased incidence of inflammatory reactions in normal skin.

4. Complete healing of keratoses may require 2 months.

Assessment

1. Observe for intractable vomiting, stomatitis, and diarrhea, all of which are early signs of toxicity and thus indicate immediate discontinuation of drug.

2. The drug also should be discontinued if WBC and platelet counts are depressed below 3,500/mm³ and 100,000/mm³, respectively.

Interventions

1. Practice reverse isolation techniques when WBC count is below 2,000/mm³.

2. Prevent exposure to strong sunlight and other ultraviolet rays, because these rays intensify skin reaction to the drug.

HYDROXYUREA   (hy-DROX-ee-you-ree-ah)

Hydrea (Abbreviation: HYD)

See also *Antineoplastic Agents*, p. 287.

Classification: Antineoplastic, antimetabolite.

Action/Kinetics: Thought to be cell-cycle specific for the S phase of cell division. Believed to interfere with DNA but not synthesis of RNA or protein. Most active in inhibiting incorporation of thymidine into DNA. Rapidly absorbed from GI tract. **Peak serum concentration:** 2 hr. **t½:** 3–4 hr. The drug crosses the blood-brain barrier. Degraded in liver; 80% excreted through the urine with 50% unchanged; also excreted as respiratory CO_2.

Uses: Chronic, resistant, myelocytic leukemia. Carcinoma of the ovary (recurrent, inoperable, or metastatic). Melanoma. With irradiation to treat primary squamous cell carcinoma of the head and neck (but not the lip).

Contraindications: Leukocyte count less than 2,500/mm³ or thrombocyte count less than 100,000/mm³. Severe anemia.

Special Concerns: Use during pregnancy only if benefits clearly outweigh risks. Give with caution to patients with marked renal dysfunction. Dosage has not been established in children.

Additional Side Effects: Erythrocyte abnormalities including megaloblastic erythropoiesis. Constipation, redness of the face, maculopapular rash.

Laboratory Test Interference: ↑ Uric acid in serum; ↑ BUN and creatinine.

Dosage: Capsules. Dose individualized. *Solid tumors, intermittent therapy or when used together with irradiation:* 60–80 mg/kg as a single dose q third day; *solid tumors, continuous therapy:* 20–30 mg/kg daily as a single dose. Intermittent dosage offers advantage of reduced toxicity. If effective, maintain patient on drug indefinitely unless toxic effects preclude such a regimen. *Resistant chronic myelocytic leukemia:* 20–30 mg/kg/day in a single dose or two divided daily doses.

NURSING CONSIDERATIONS

See also *Nursing Considerations* for *Antineoplastic Agents,* p. 303.

Administration/Storage

1. Dosage should be calculated on the basis of actual or ideal weight (whichever is less).
2. Therapy should be continued for at least 6 weeks before efficacy is assessed.
3. If the client cannot swallow a capsule, contents may be given in glass of water that should be drunk immediately, even though some material may not dissolve and may float on top of glass.
4. Hydroxyurea should be started 7 days before irradiation.

Interventions

1. Observe for exacerbation of postirradiation erythema.
2. Monitor liver and renal function studies during therapy.

MERCAPTOPURINE   (mer-**KAP**-toe-**PYOU**-reen)

6-Mercaptopurine, 6-MP, Purinethol (Abbreviation: 6-MP) (Rx)

See also *Antineoplastic Agents,* p. 287.

Classification: Antimetabolite, purine analog.

Action/Kinetics: Mercaptopurine is cell-cycle specific for the S phase of cell division. The drug is converted to thioinosinic acid by the enzyme hypoxanthine-guanine phosphoribosyltransferase. Thioinosinic acid then inhibits reactions involving inosinic acid. Also, both thioinosinic acid and 6-methylthioinosinate (also formed from mercaptopurine) inhibit RNA synthesis. About 50% absorbed from GI tract. **Plasma t½:** 47 min in adults and 21 min in children. Metabolites are excreted in urine with up to 39% excreted unchanged. Cross-resistance with thioguanine has been observed.

Uses: Acute lymphocytic or myelocytic leukemia. Lymphoblastic leukemia, especially in children. Acute myelogenous and myelomonocytic leukemia. Effectiveness varies depending on use. The drug is not effective for leukemia of the CNS, solid tumors, lymphomas, or chronic lymphatic leukemia. *Investigational:* Inflammatory bowel disease, chronic myelocytic leukemia, polycythemia vera, non-Hodgkin's lymphoma, psoriatic arthritis.

Special Concerns: Pregnancy category: D. Use with caution in patients with impaired renal function. Use during lactation only if benefits clearly outweigh risks.

Additional Side Effects: Hepatotoxicity, oral lesions, hyperuricemia. Produces less GI toxicity than folic acid antagonists, and side effects are less frequent in children than in adults. Pancreatitis (when used for inflammatory bowel disease).

Drug Interaction: Allopurinol potentiates mercaptopurine by ↓ breakdown. Requires reduction of antineoplastic agent by 25%–33⅓%.

Dosage: Tablets. *Highly individualized:* 2.5 mg/kg/day. *Usual,* **adults:** 100–200 mg; **children:** 50 mg. Dosage may be increased to 5 mg/kg daily after 4 weeks if beneficial effects are not noted. Dosage is increased until symptoms of toxicity appear. **Maintenance after remission:** 1.5–2.5 mg/kg daily.

NURSING CONSIDERATIONS

See also *Nursing Considerations* for *Antineoplastic Agents,* p. 303.

Administration/Storage

1. Since the maximum effect of mercaptopurine on the blood count may be delayed and the blood count may drop for several days after drug has been discontinued, therapy should be discontinued at first sign of abnormally large drop in leukocyte count.
2. Administer drug in one dose daily at any convenient time.
3. Limit intake of alcoholic beverages.

METHOTREXATE   (meth-oh-**TREK**-sate)

Amethopterin, Folex (Abbreviation: MTX)(Rx)

METHOTREXATE SODIUM   (meth-oh-**TREK**-sate)

Folex PFS, Rheumatrex Dose Pack (Rx)

See also *Antineoplastic Agents,* p. 287.

Classification: Antimetabolite, folic acid analog.

Action/Kinetics: Methotrexate is cell-cycle specific for the S phase of cell division. The drug acts by inhibition of dihydrofolate reductase which prevents reduction of dihydrofolate to tetrahydrofolate; this results in decreased synthesis of purines and consequently DNA. The most sensitive cells are bone marrow, fetal cells, dermal epithelium, urinary bladder, buccal mucosa, intestinal mucosa, and malignant cells. The mechanism of action for use in rheumatoid arthritis is not known although the drug may affect immune function. Variable absorption from GI tract. **Peak serum levels, IM:** 30–60 min; **PO:** 1–2 hr. **t½:** initial, 1 hr; intermediate, 2–3 hr; final, 8–12 hr. Drug may accumulate in the body. Excreted by kidney (55–92% in 24 hr). Renal function tests are recommended before initiation of therapy; daily leukocyte counts should be taken during therapy.

Uses: Uterine choriocarcinoma (curative), hydatidiform mole, acute lymphocytic and lymphoblastic leukemia, lymphosarcoma, and other disseminated neoplasms in children; meningeal leukemia, some beneficial effect in regional chemotherapy of head and neck tumors, breast tumors, and lung cancer. Advanced mycosis fungoides. Severe, recalcitrant, disabling psoriasis. Rheumatoid arthritis (severe, active, classical or definite) in patients who have had inadequate response to NSAID's and at least one or more antirheumatic drugs (disease modifying). *Investigational:* Severe corticosteroid-dependent asthma to reduce corticosteroid dosage; adjunct to treat osteosarcoma.

Contraindications: Psoriasis patients with kidney or liver disease; blood dyscrasias as hypoplasia, thrombocytopenia, anemia, or leukopenia. Alcoholism, alcoholic liver disease or other chronic liver disease. Immunodeficiency syndromes. Pregnancy and lactation.

Special Concerns: Pregnancy category: X. Use with caution in impaired renal function and elderly patients. Safety and efficacy have not been established for juvenile rheumatoid arthritis.

Additional Side Effects: Severe bone marrow depression. Hepatotoxicity. Hemorrhagic enteritis, intestinal ulceration or perforation, acne, ecchymosis, hematemesis, melena, increased pigmentation, diabetes, chronic interstitial obstructive pulmonary disease. Intrathecal use may result in chemical arachnoiditis, transient paresis, or seizures. Concomitant exposure to sunlight may aggravate psoriasis.

Leucovorin, given as soon as possible, may decrease toxic effects. The dose used is 10 mg/m² PO or parenterally followed by 10 mg/m² PO q 6 hr for 72 hr.

Drug Interactions	
Alcohol, ethyl	Additive hepatotoxicity; combination can result in coma
Anticoagulants, oral	Additive hypoprothrombinemia
Chloramphenicol	↑ Effect of methotrexate by ↓ plasma protein binding
Folic acid-containing vitamin preparations	↓ Response to methotrexate
Ibuprofen	↑ Effect of methotrexate by ↓ renal secretion
Nonsteroidal anti-inflammatory drugs	Possible fatal interaction
PABA	↑ Effect of methotrexate by ↓ plasma protein binding
Phenylbutazone	↑ Effect of methotrexate by ↓ renal secretion
Phenytoin	↑ Effect of methotrexate by ↓ plasma protein binding
Probenecid	↑ Effect of methotrexate by ↓ renal clearance
Pyrimethamine	↑ Methotrexate toxicity
Salicylates (aspirin)	↑ Effect of methotrexate by ↓ plasma protein binding; also, salicylates ↓ renal excretion of methotrexate
Smallpox vaccination	Methotrexate impairs immunologic response to smallpox vaccine
Sulfonamides	↑ Effect of methotrexate by ↓ plasma protein binding
Tetracyclines	↑ Effect of methotrexate by ↓ plasma protein binding

Dosage: *Cancer chemotherapy. Methotrexate is administered* **PO (Tablets);** *methotrexate sodium is administered* **IM, IV, intra-arterially** *or* **intrathecally.** *Dose individualized. Choriocarcinoma,* **PO, IM:** 15–30 mg/day for 5 days. May be repeated 3–5 times with 1-week rest period between courses. *Leukemia,* **initial:** 3.3 mg/m² (with 60 mg/m² prednisone daily); **maintenance: PO, IM,** 30 mg/m² 2 times weekly or **IV,** 2.5 mg/kg q 14 days. *Meningeal leukemia,* **intrathecal:** 12 mg/m² q 2–5 days until cell count returns to normal. *Lymphomas,* **PO:** 10–25 mg/day for 4–8 days for several courses of treatment with 7- to 10-day rest periods between courses. *Mycosis fungoides:* **PO,** 2.5–10 mg/day for several weeks or months; **alternatively, IM,** 50 mg once weekly or 25 mg twice weekly. *Lymphosarcoma:* 0.625–2.5 mg/kg/day in combination with other drugs.

Psoriasis. **Individualized: usual (average adult): PO, IM, IV,** 10–25 mg weekly, continued until beneficial response observed. Weekly dose should not exceed 50 mg. **Alternate regimens: PO,** 2.5 mg q 12 hr for 3 doses or q 8 hr for 4 doses each week (not to exceed 30 mg weekly); **or** 2.5 mg **PO** daily for 5 days followed by 2 days of rest (dose should not exceed 6.25 mg daily). Once beneficial effects are noted, reduce dose to lowest possible level with longest rest periods between doses.

Rheumatoid arthritis: **initial,** single oral doses of 7.5 mg/week or divided PO doses of 2.5 mg at 12 hr intervals for 3 doses given once a week; **then,** adjust dosage to achieve optimum response, not to exceed a total weekly dose of 20 mg. Once response has been reached, the dose should be reduced to the lowest possible effective dose.

NURSING CONSIDERATIONS

See also *Nursing Considerations* for *Antineoplastic Agents,* p. 303.

Administration/Storage

1. Use only sterile, preservative-free sodium chloride injection to reconstitute powder for intrathecal administration.
2. Prevent inhalation of particles of medication and skin exposure.
3. When used for rheumatoid arthritis, improvement is thought to be maintained for up to 2 yr with continuous therapy. When the drug is discontinued, the arthritis usually worsens within 3–6 weeks.

Assessment

1. Determine if client is receiving other organic acids, such as aspirin, phenylbutazone, probenecid, and/or sulfa drugs, because these agents affect renal clearance of methotrexate and increase thrombocytopenic and GI side effects.
2. Assess for oral ulcerations, one of the first signs of toxicity.

Interventions

1. Monitor intake and output, and encourage fluid intake to facilitate excretion of drug.
2. Report oliguria, since this symptom may indicate need to discontinue drug.
3. Have calcium leucovorin—a potent antidote for folic acid antagonists—readily available in case of overdosage. Antidotes are ineffective if not administered within 4 hr of overdosage. Corticosteroids are sometimes given concomitantly with initial dose of methotrexate.
4. Advise client to avoid ingestion of alcohol when receiving methotrexate, as coma may result.
5. Do not vaccinate for smallpox when the client is receiving methotrexate, because the impaired immunologic response may result in vaccinia.
6. Anticipate reduction in anticoagulant dosage if administered concomitantly.

THIOGUANINE   (thigh-oh-**GWAH**-neen)

Lanvis ✹, TG, 6-Thioguanine (Abbreviation: 6-TG) (Rx)

See also *Antineoplastic Agents,* p. 287.

Classification: Antimetabolite, purine analog.

Action/Kinetics: Purine antagonist that is cell-cycle specific for the S phase of cell division. Thioguanine is converted to 6-thioguanylic acid which, in turn, interferes with the synthesis of guanine nucleotides and ultimately the synthesis of RNA and DNA. Partially absorbed (30%) from GI tract. **t½:** 80 min. Detoxified by liver and excreted in the urine. More effective in children than in adults. Cross-resistance with mercaptopurine. Perform platelet counts weekly; discontinue drug if abnormally large fall in blood count is noted, indicating severe bone marrow depression.

Uses: Acute lymphocytic and nonlymphocytic leukemias (usually in combination with other drugs). Chronic myelogenous leukemia.

Special Concerns: Pregnancy category: D. Use not recommended during lactation.

Additional Side Effects: Loss of vibration sense, unsteadiness of gait. Hepatotoxicity myelosuppression (common), hyperuricemia. Adults tend to show a more rapid fall in WBC count than children.

Laboratory Test Interference: ↑ Uric acid in blood and urine.

Dosage: Tablets: *Individualized* and determined by hematopoietic response; **adults and pediatric: initial:** 2 mg/kg daily (or 75–100 mg/m²). From 2 to 4 weeks may elapse before beneficial results become apparent. Compute dose to nearest multiple of 20 mg. If no response, dosage may be increased to 3 mg/kg daily. **Usual maintenance dose** (even during remissions): 2–3 mg/kg daily (or 100 mg/m²).

NURSING CONSIDERATIONS

See also *Nursing Considerations* for *Antineoplastic Agents,* p. 303.

Interventions

1. Provide assistance to ambulatory clients who may experience loss of vibration sense and thus have unsteady gait (these clients may be unable to rely on canes).
2. Encourage increased fluid intake to minimize hyperuricemia and hyperuricosuria.
3. Monitor liver function tests as a baseline before therapy is instituted and repeat monthly during course of therapy.

Client/Family Teaching

1. Withhold drug and report if jaundice occurs.
2. Emphasize to adult clients that contraceptive measures are advised with this drug.

ANTIBIOTICS

Action/Kinetics: A number of antineoplastic antibiotics are effective chemotherapeutic agents which are cell-cycle specific and interfere with the replication of DNA, RNA, and protein synthesis. Selected antineoplastic antibiotics are specific for certain tissues or organs, and many are part of combination therapy (See Table 7).

BLEOMYCIN SULFATE (blee-oh-**MY**-sin)

Blenoxane (Abbreviation: BLM) (Rx)

See also *Antineoplastic Agents,* p. 287.

Classification: Antineoplastic, antibiotic.

Action/Kinetics: Bleomycin is a glycopeptide antibiotic produced by *Streptomyces verticillus*. It is most effective in the G₂ and M phases of cell division although some activity is noted in noncycling cells. The action may be due to binding to DNA inducing lability of the DNA structure and decreasing synthesis of DNA and to a lesser extent RNA and protein. Drug currently used is mostly a mixture of bleomycin A₂ and B₂. Drug has relatively low bone marrow depressant activity, localizes in certain tissues, and is an important component of some combination regimens. **Peak plasma**

levels (after 4–5 days of therapy): 50 ng/mL. **t½, after rapid IV and intrapleural, adults:** 24 min and 4 hr; **children, less than 3 years of age:** 54 min and 3 hr. **t½, continuous IV, adults:** 79 min and 9 hr; **children, less than 3 years of age:** 2.3 hr (terminal phase). Two-thirds excreted in urine as active bleomycin.

Uses: Palliative treatment, either alone or in combination, for Hodgkin's and nonHodgkin's lymphomas (including lymphosarcoma and reticulum cell sarcoma), testicular carcinomas, and squamous cell carcinomas (especially of the head and neck, larynx, paralarynx, penis, cervix, vulva, and skin). *Investigational:* Soft-tissue sarcomas, osteosarcoma, malignant effusions (peritoneal, pleural), ovarian tumors. Also for severe, recalcitrant common warts (verruca vulgaris).

Additional Contraindications: Renal or pulmonary diseases. Pregnancy, lactation.

Additional Side Effects: Pulmonary fibrosis, especially in older patients. Mucocutaneous toxicity and hypersensitivity reactions. In approximately 1% of lymphoma patients, an idiosyncratic reaction manifested by hypotension, fever, chills, mental confusion, and wheezing has been reported.

Additional Drug Interaction: Bleomycin may ↓ plasma levels and renal excretion of digoxin.

Dosage: SC, IM, IV. *Hodgkin's disease, lymphosarcoma, reticulum cell sarcoma, testicular carcinoma, squamous cell carcinoma:* 0.25–0.5 units/kg (10–20 units/m²) once or twice weekly. **Maintenance, IM or IV,** *Hodgkin's disease:* 1 unit/day or 5 units/week. *Squamous cell carcinoma of head, neck, or cervix:* **Regional arterial infusion,** 30–60 units/day over a period of 1–24 hr. *Warts:* **intralesional,** 0.2–0.8 units (depending on the size) one or more times q 2–4 weeks (up to a maximum total dose of 2 units using a solution of 15 units of sterile bleomycin solution in 15 mL 0.9% saline or water for injection).

NURSING CONSIDERATIONS

See also *Nursing Considerations* for *Antineoplastic Agents,* p. 303.

Administration/Storage

1. For IM or SC use, the drug should be reconstituted with 1–5 mL sterile water for injection, 5% dextrose injection, sodium chloride for injection, or bacteriostatic water for injection.
2. Administer IV slowly over 10 min.
3. Hodgkin's disease and testicular tumors should respond within 2 weeks, while squamous cell cancers require at least 3 weeks.

Assessment

Assess client for basilar rales, cough, dyspnea on exertion, and tachypnea, all of which are dose-related symptoms of pulmonary toxicity.

Interventions

1. Clients receiving digoxin should be monitored closely and have digoxin levels monitored during therapy with bleomycin.
2. Teach client and/or family the idiosyncratic reaction (see additional side effects) that may occur in clients with lymphoma.

DACTINOMYCIN   (dack-tin-oh-**MY**-sin)

Actinomycin D, Cosmegen (Abbreviation: ACT) (Rx)

See also *Antineoplastic Agents,* p. 287.

Classification: Antineoplastic, antibiotic.

Action/Kinetics: Chromopeptide antibiotic produced by *Streptomyces parvullus*. Dactinomycin acts by intercalating into the purine—pyrimidine base pair, thereby inhibiting synthesis of messenger RNA. The activity is cell-cycle nonspecific; rapidly proliferating cells are more sensitive, however. The drug is concentrated in nucleated cells. **t½:** 36 hr. The drug does not cross the blood-brain barrier and is excreted mainly unchanged.

During therapy, leukocyte counts should be performed daily, and platelet counts q 3 days. Frequent liver and kidney function tests are recommended. Appearance of toxic manifestations may be delayed by several weeks. Irreversible bone marrow depression may occur in patients with preexisting renal, hepatic, or bone marrow impairment. The drug is corrosive to soft tissue.

Uses: In combination with vincristine, surgery and/or irradiation for treatment of Wilms' tumor (nephroblastoma) and its metastases. In combination with methotrexate to treat metastatic and nonmetastatic choriocarcinoma. In combination with cyclophosphamide, doxorubicin, and vincristine to treat rhabdomyosarcoma. Nonseminomatous testicular carcinoma. With cyclophosphamide and radiotherapy to treat Ewing's sarcoma. In combination with radiotherapy to treat sarcoma botryoides. Endometrial carcinoma. *Investigational:* Ovarian cancer, Kaposi's sarcoma, osteosarcoma, malignant melanoma.

Contraindications: Concurrent infection with chickenpox or herpes zoster (death may result). Lactation. Infants less than 6–12 months of age.

Special Concerns: Pregnancy category: C.

Additional Side Effects: Anaphylaxis. Due to corrosiveness, extravasation causes severe damage to soft tissues. Hypocalcemia. When combined with radiation, increased severity of skin reactions, GI toxicity, and bone marrow depression.

Dosage: IV, individualized. Adults, usual, 0.5 mg/m² once weekly for 3 weeks; or, 0.01–0.015 mg/kg daily for a maximum of 5 days q 4–6 weeks. **Pediatric:** 10–15 mcg/kg (0.45 mg/m²) daily for 5 days; **alternatively,** a total dose of 2.4 mg/m² over 1 week. Total daily dosage for both adults and children should not exceed 15 mcg/kg over a 5 day period. Course of treatment may be repeated after 3 weeks unless contraindicated due to toxicity. If no toxicity, second course can be given after 3 weeks. *Ewing's sarcoma/sarcoma botryoides,* **Isolation-perfusion:** 0.05 mg/kg for pelvis and lower extremities and 0.035 mg/kg for upper extremities.

NURSING CONSIDERATIONS

See also *Nursing Considerations* for *Antineoplastic Agents,* p. 303.

Administration/Storage

1. For IV use, dactinomycin is available in a lyophilized dactinomycin-mannitol mixture that turns a gold color upon reconstitution with sterile water. Use only sterile water without a preservative to reconstitute the drug for IV use, as it will precipitate. Solutions should not be exposed to direct sunlight.

2. *The drug is extremely corrosive.* It is most safely administered through the tubing of a running IV (e.g., 5% dextrose or sodium chloride). It may be given directly into the vein, but the needle used to draw up the solution should be discarded and another sterile needle attached, before injection, to prevent subcutaneous reaction and thrombophlebitis.

3. Extreme care should be exercised in reconstituting and administering dactinomycin so that the dust or vapors are not inhaled or come in contact with skin or mucous membranes. Special care should be exercised to prevent contact with the eyes.

4. Any portion of the solution not used for the injection should be discarded.

Assessment

Assess and report if client is pregnant, lactating, or infected with herpes, all of which are contraindications for dactinomycin therapy.

Interventions

1. Report erythema of the skin, which can lead to desquamation and sloughing, particularly in areas previously affected by radiation.
2. Warn client of the possibility of delayed toxic reactions and stress importance of returning for blood tests.
3. Anticipate that dactinomycin may be administered intermittently if nausea and vomiting persist even when an emetic is given.
4. Anticipate that penicillin will not be used if client contracts an infection, because dactinomycin inhibits the action of penicillin.

DAUNORUBICIN   (dawn-oh-ROOB-ih-sin)

Cerubidine (Abbreviation: DNR) (Rx)

See also *Antineoplastic Agents,* p. 287.

Classification: Antineoplastic, antibiotic.

Action/Kinetics: Anthracycline antibiotic produced by *Streptomyces peucetius.* Daunorubicin is most active in the S phase of cell division but is not cell-cycle specific. The drug inhibits synthesis of nucleic acid by inserting into the double helix of DNA. Daunorubicin also possesses immuno-suppressive, cytotoxic, and antimitotic activity. Rapidly cleared from the plasma. Metabolized to the active daunorubinicol. $t^{1}/_{2}$: daunorubicin, 18.5 hr; daunorubinicol, 27 hr. Drug rapidly taken up by heart, kidneys, lung, liver, and spleen. Chiefly excreted in bile (40%) and unchanged in urine (25%). Does not pass blood-brain barrier.

Uses: Acute nonlymphocytic leukemia in adults (myelogenous, erythroid, monocytic). When combined with cytarabine, effectiveness is increased. Acute lymphocytic leukemia in children (increased effectiveness when combined with vincristine and prednisone). *Investigational:* Ewing's sarcoma, chronic myeloctyic leukemia, neuroblastoma, non-Hodgkin's lymphomas, Wilms' tumor.

Special Concerns: Pregnancy category: D. Not recommended for use during lactation. Use with caution in preexisting heart disease or bone marrow depression, renal or hepatic failure.

Additional Side Effects: *Myocardial toxicity:* Potentially fatal congestive heart failure especially if total dosage exceeds 550 mg/m^2 for adults, 300 mg/m^2 for children more than 2 years of age, and 10 mg/kg for children less than 2 years of age. Mucositis (3–7 days after administration), red-colored urine, hyperuricemia. Severe tissue necrosis if extravasation occurs. Cross-resistance with doxorubicin (produced by similar microorganism) and vinca alkaloids.

Dosage: IV infusion (rapid). *Acute nonlymphocytic leukemia.* **Adults:** *daunorubicin,* 45 mg/m^2/day on days 1, 2, and 3 of first course and days 1 and 2 of additional courses; *cytosine arabinoside (Ara-c),* **IV infusion,** 100 mg/m^2/day for 7 days during first course and for 5 days during any additional courses of treatment. Some recommend reducing the dose of daunorubicin to 30 mg/m^2 in patients 60 years of age and older. Up to 3 courses may be required. *Acute lymphocytic leukemia:* **adults:** daunorubicin, 45 mg/m^2, **IV,** on days 1, 2, and 3; vincristine, **IV,** on days 1, 8, and 15; prednisone, **PO,** 40 mg/m^2 daily for days 1 to 22 and then taper between days 22 to 29; and, L-asparaginase, **IV,** 500 IU/kg/day on days 22 to 32.

Acute lymphocytic leukemia: **children:** daunorubicin, 25 mg/m², and vincristine, 1.5 mg/m² each **IV** on day 1 every week with prednisone, 40 mg/m² **PO** daily. Usually 4 courses will induce remission. (Note: Calculate the dose on the basis of mg/kg if the child is less than 2 years of age or the body surface is less than 0.5 m².)

Acute nonlymphocytic leukemia: **geriatric patients:** 30 mg/m² on days 1, 2, and 3 of the first course and days 1 and 2 of the second course in combination with cytarabine.

Dosage should be reduced in patients with renal or hepatic disease.

NURSING CONSIDERATIONS

See also *Nursing Considerations* for *Antineoplastic Agents,* p. 303.

Administration/Storage

1. Dilute in vial with 4 mL sterile water for injection USP. Agitate gently until dissolved (solution contains 5 mg daunorubicin/mL). Withdraw desired dose into syringe containing 10–15 mL isotonic saline; inject into tubing of rapidly flowing 5% glucose or normal saline IV. *Never administer daunorubicin IM or SC.*
2. Reconstituted solution stable for 24 hr at room temperature; for 48 hr when refrigerated.
3. Protect from sunlight.
4. Do not mix with other drugs or heparin.

Interventions

1. Assess client during and after termination of therapy for myocardial toxicity, manifested by changes in baseline ECG, edema, dyspnea, and cyanosis. Clients with a cardiac history who receive doses above 550 mg/m² are more susceptible to congestive heart failure.
2. Have digitalis preparations and diuretics readily available to treat congestive heart failure.

Client/Family Teaching

1. Review side effects and have client report any signs and symptoms of cardiac toxicity.
2. Urine may appear red for several days following therapy with daunorubicin.

DOXORUBICIN HYDROCHLORIDE   (dox-oh-**ROOB**-ih-sin)

Adriamycin PFS, Adriamycin RDF, Rubex (Abbreviation: ADR) (Rx)

See also *Antineoplastic Agents,* p. 287.

Classification: Antineoplastic, antibiotic.

Action/Kinetics: Anthracycline antibiotic produced by *Streptomyces peucetius.* Doxorubicin is cell-cycle specific for the S phase of cell division. Its antineoplastic activity may be due to binding to DNA by intercalating between base pairs resulting in inhibition of synthesis of DNA and RNA by template disordering and steric obstruction. The drug is metabolized in the liver to the active adriamycinol as well as inactive metabolites, which are excreted through the bile. **t½, doxorubicin:** biphasic: initial, 0.6 hr; **final,** 16.7 hr.

Uses: Acute lymphoblastic leukemia, acute myeloblastic leukemia, Wilms' tumor, soft tissue and osteogenic sarcomas, neuroblastoma, cancer of the breast, ovaries, lungs, bladder, and thyroid, lymphomas (Hodgkin's and non-Hodgkin's), bronchogenic carcinoma (especially small cell histologic type). *Investigational:* Cancer of the head and neck, cervix, liver, pancreas, prostate, testes, and endometrium.

Additional Contraindications: Lactation. Depressed bone marrow or cardiac disease. Use in pregnancy only if benefits outweigh risks. Use with caution in impaired hepatic function and necrotizing colitis.

Additional Side Effects: *Myocardial toxicity:* Potentially fatal congestive heart failure. Mucositis, lacrimation, conjunctivitis. Hyperpigmentation of nail beds. Facial flushing if injection is too rapid. Hyperuricemia, red-colored urine (initially). Extravasation may cause severe cellulitis and tissue necrosis. Drug may reactivate previous cardiac, skin, mucosal, and liver radiation damage. Cross-resistance with daunorubicin.

Drug Interactions

Cyclophosphamide	↑ Risk of hemorrhagic cystitis
Digoxin	↓ Digoxin plasma levels and renal excretion
6-Mercaptopurine	↑ Risk of hepatotoxicity

Dosage: IV only. *Adults, highly individualized:* 60–75 mg/m² q 21 days, or 25–30 mg/m² for 3 successive days q 3–4 weeks, or 20 mg/m² every week. Total dose should not exceed 550 mg/m² (440 mg/m² in patients with previous chest irradiation or medications increasing cardiotoxicity). **Pediatric:** 30 mg/m² on 3 successive days q 4 weeks. Use reduced dosage in patients with hepatic dysfunction, depending on serum bilirubin level. If bilirubin is 1.2–3 mg/100 mL, give 50% of usual dose; if it is greater than 3 mg/100 mL, give 25% of usual dose.

NURSING CONSIDERATIONS

See also *Nursing Considerations* for *Antineoplastic Agents,* p. 303.

Administration/Storage

1. Initiate therapy only in hospitalized patients.
2. The drug should be reconstituted with saline to give a final concentration of 2 mg/mL (e.g., dilute 10-mg vial with 5 mL). The reconstituted solution is stable for 24 hr at room temperature and 48 hr if stored at 2°–8° C (36°–46° F).
3. If the powder or solution comes in contact with the skin or mucous membranes, wash with soap and water thoroughly.
4. *Do not administer SC or IM, as severe necrosis of tissue may result.* In order to minimize danger of extravasation, inject slowly into tubing of free-flowing IV infusion of either 5% dextrose or sodium chloride injection.
5. Should not be mixed with heparin, dexamethasone sodium phosphate, or cephalothin since a precipitate may form. Mixing with aminophylline or 5-fluorouracil will result in a change from red to blue-purple indicating decomposition.

Interventions

1. Observe client for cardiac arrhythmias and/or respiratory difficulties that may be indicative of cardiac toxicity.
2. If medication reactivates previous radiotherapy damage, such as erythema, edema, and desquamation, reassure the client that these symptoms should disappear after 7 days.
3. Inform the client that urine will turn red for 1–2 days after initiation of therapy.
4. Advise the client that alopecia may occur but hair will grow back 2–3 months after discontinuation of therapy.

5. Monitor IV administration carefully. Stinging, burning, or edema at injection site is indicative of extravasation. Administration should be stopped, and injection site moved, to avoid tissue necrosis.

6. Be prepared with an injectable corticosteroid for local infiltration, and flood site with normal saline. Examine area frequently for ulceration that may necessitate early wide excision followed by plastic surgery.

MITOMYCIN   (my-toe-MY-sin)

Mutamycin (Abbreviation: MTC) (Rx)

See also *Antineoplastic Agents,* p. 287.

Classification: Antineoplastic, antibiotic.

Action/Kinetics: Antibiotic produced by *Streptomyces caespitosus,* which forms a mitomycin/DNA complex that inhibits RNA synthesis. Most active during late G_1 and early S stages. Not recommended as a single agent for primary treatment or in place of surgery and/or radiotherapy. **t½, initial:** 5–15 min; **final:** 50 min. Metabolized in liver, 10% excreted unchanged in urine, more when dose is increased.

Uses: Palliative treatment and adjunct to surgical or radiologic treatment of disseminated adenocarcinoma of the stomach and pancreas. Used in combination with other agents. *Investigational:* Superficial bladder cancer; cancer of the breast, head and neck, lung, cervix; colorectal cancer; biliary cancer; chronic myelocytic leukemia.

Contraindications: Pregnancy and lactation.

Special Concerns: Use with extreme caution in presence of impaired renal function.

Additional Side Effects: Severe bone marrow depression, especially leukopenia and thrombocytopenia. Pulmonary toxicity including dyspnea with nonproductive cough. Microangiopathic hemolytic anemia with renal failure and hypertension (hemolytic uremic syndrome), especially when used long-term in combination with fluorouracil. Cellulitis. Extravasation causes severe necrosis of surrounding tissue.

Drug Interaction: Severe bronchospasm and shortness of breath when used with vinca alkaloids.

Dosage: IV only: 10–20 mg/m² as a single dose via infusion q 6–8 wk. Subsequent courses of treatment are based on hematologic response and should not be repeated until leukocyte count is at least 3,000/mm³ and platelet count is at least 75,000/mm³.

NURSING CONSIDERATIONS

See also *Nursing Considerations* for *Antineoplastic Agents,* p. 303.

Administration/Storage

1. Drug is toxic, and extravasation is to be avoided.

2. Reconstitute 5- or 20-mg vial with 10–40 mL sterile water for injection, as indicated on label. Medication will dissolve if allowed to remain at room temperature.

3. Drug at concentration of 0.5 mg/mL is stable for 14 days under refrigeration or for 7 days at room temperature.

4. Diluted to a concentration of 20–40 mcg/mL, the drug is stable for 3 hr in D_5 W, for 12 hr in isotonic saline, and for 24 hr in sodium lactate injection.

5. Mitomycin (5–15 mg) and heparin (1,000–10,000 units) in 30 mL of isotonic saline is stable for 48 hr at room temperature.

MITOXANTRONE HYDROCHLORIDE (my-toe-**ZAN**-trohn)

Novantrone (Rx)

See also *Antineoplastic Agents,* p. 287.

Classification: Antineoplastic agent, antibiotic.

Action/Kinetics: Mitoxantrone is most active in the late S phase of cell division but is not cell-cycle specific. The drug appears to bind to DNA by intercalation between base pairs and a nonintercalative electrostatic interaction; this results in inhibition of DNA and RNA synthesis. Distribution to tissues such as the brain, spinal cord, spinal fluid, and eyes is low. **t½:** Approximately 6 days. Mitoxantrone is highly bound to plasma proteins. The drug is excreted through both the feces (via the bile) and the urine (up to 65% unchanged).

Uses: In combination with other drugs, for the initial treatment of acute nonlymphocytic leukemias, including monocytic, promyelocytic, myelocytic, and acute erythroid leukemias. *Investigational:* Breast and liver cancer; non-Hodgkin's lymphomas.

Contraindications: Preexisting myelosuppression (unless benefits outweigh risks). During lactation.

Special Concerns: Pregnancy category: D. Safety and efficacy have not been established in children.

Side Effects: *Hematologic:* Severe myelosuppression, ecchymosis, petechiae. *GI:* Nausea, vomiting, diarrhea, stomatitis, mucositis, abdominal pain, GI bleeding. *CNS:* Headache, seizures. *CV:* Congestive heart failure, decreases in left ventricular ejection fraction, arrhythmias, tachycardia, chest pain, hypotension. *Respiratory:* Cough, dyspnea. *Miscellaneous:* Conjunctivitis, urticaria, rashes, renal failure, hyperuricemia, alopecia, fever, phlebitis (at infusion site), tissue necrosis (as a result of extravasation), jaundice. In addition, there is an increased risk of pneumonia, urinary tract and fungal infections, and sepsis.

Dosage: IV infusion. *Initial therapy for acute nonlymphocytic leukemia, induction:* mitoxantrone, 12 mg/m²/day on days 1–3 combined with cytosine arabinoside, 100 mg/m² as a continuous 24-hr infusion on days 1–7. If the response is incomplete, a second induction course may be given using the same daily dosage, but giving mitoxantrone for 2 days and cytosine arabinoside for 5 days. *Consolidation therapy, approximately 6 weeks after final induction therapy:* mitoxantrone, 12 mg/m²/day on days 1 and 2 combined with cytosine arabinoside, 100 mg/m² as a continuous 24-hr infusion on days 1–5. A second consolidation course of therapy may be given 4 weeks after the first.

NURSING CONSIDERATIONS

See also *Administration* and *Nursing Considerations* for *Antineoplastic Agents,* p. 303.

Administration/Storage

1. The drug should not be frozen.

2. The client must be closely monitored for chemical, laboratory, and hematologic values.

3. Mitoxantrone should not be mixed in the same infusion with other drugs.

4. Mitoxantrone must be diluted prior to use with a minimum of 50 mL of either 5% dextrose injection or 0.9% sodium chloride injection.

5. The diluted solution is given into a freely running IV infusion of either 5% dextrose injection or 0.9% sodium chloride injection over a period of at least 3 minutes.

6. Care should be taken to avoid extravasation at the injection site. Also, the solution should not come in contact with the eyes, mucous membranes, or skin.

7. Hospital procedures for the handling and disposal of antineoplastic drugs should be followed closely.

Interventions

1. Obtain baseline hematologic and chemistry studies and monitor throughout therapy.
2. Maintain infusion on an electronic infusion device.
3. Monitor vital signs and closely observe client during therapy for any adverse side effects.
4. Initiate appropriate precautions for clients with severe myelosuppression.
5. Anticipate nausea, vomiting, mucositis, and stomatitis, and initiate appropriate protocol.

PLICAMYCIN (MITHRAMYCIN) (plye-kah-**MY**-sin, mith-rah-**MY**-sin)

Mithracin (Abbreviation: MTH) (Rx)

See also *Antineoplastic Agents,* p. 287.

Classification: Antineoplastic, antibiotic.

Action/Kinetics: Antibiotic produced by *Streptomyces plicatus, S. argillaceus,* and *S. tanashiensis.* Plicamycin complexes with DNA in the presence of magnesium (or other divalent cations), resulting in inhibition of cellular and enzymatic RNA synthesis. Drug affects calcium metabolism, leading to a decrease in blood calcium levels. Plicamycin is cleared rapidly from the blood and is concentrated in the Kupffer cells of the liver, renal tubular cells, and along formed bone surfaces. The drug crosses the blood-brain barrier. It is excreted through the urine.

Uses: Malignant testicular tumors usually associated with metastases. Hypercalcemia and hypercalciuria associated with advanced malignancy and not responsive to other therapy.

Additional Contraindications: Thrombocytopenia, coagulation disorders, and increased tendency to hemorrhage. Do not use for children under 15 years of age.

Special Concerns: Pregnancy category: X. Use with caution in impaired liver or kidney function.

Additional Side Effects: Severe thrombocytopenia, hemorrhagic tendencies. Facial flushing. Hepatic and renal toxicity. Extravasation may cause irritation or cellulitis.

Laboratory Test Interferences: ↓ Serum calcium, potassium, and phosphorus. ↑ Serum BUN, creatinine, SGOT, SGPT, alkaline phosphatase, bilirubin, isocitric dehydrogenase, ornithine carbamyltransferase, lactic dehydrogenase. ↑ BSP retention.

Dosage: IV only. *Individualized. Testicular tumor:* 25–30 (maximum) mcg/kg (given over a period of 4–6 hr) daily for 8–10 (maximum) days. A second approach is to use 25–50 mcg/kg on alternate days for an average of 8 doses. *Hypercalcemia, hypercalciuria:* 15–25 mcg/kg (given over a period of 4–6 hr) daily for 3–4 days. Additional courses of therapy may be warranted at weekly intervals if initial course is unsuccessful.

NURSING CONSIDERATIONS

See also *Nursing Considerations* for *Antineoplastic Agents*, p. 303.

Administration/Storage

1. *Store vials of medication in refrigerator at temperatures below 10°C (36°–46°F). Discard unused portion of drug.*
2. Reconstitute fresh for each day of therapy.
3. Drug is unstable in acid solution (pH 5 and below) and in reconstituted solutions (pH 7) and thus deteriorates rapidly.
4. Add sterile water to the vial as recommended on the package insert, and shake the vial to dissolve the drug.
5. Add the calculated dosage of the drug to the IV solution ordered (recommended 1 L of D_5W) and adjust the rate of flow as ordered (recommended time is 4–6 hr for 1 L).
6. Should be used only for hospitalized clients.

Assessment

Assess clients for evidence of hemorrhage, such as epistaxis, hemoptysis, hematemesis, purpura, or ecchymoses.

Interventions

1. Therapy should be interrupted if WBC count goes below $3,000/mm^3$ or if prothrombin time is more than 4 sec higher than that of the control. Daily platelet count should be performed on clients who have had x-ray films taken of abdomen and mediastinum.
2. If antiemetic drugs are ordered, administer before or during therapy with mithramycin.
3. Closely check peripheral IV for extravasation. Stop IV if extravasation occurs; apply moderate heat to disperse drug and to reduce pain and tissue damage. Restart IV at another site.
4. Prevent excessively rapid flow, because it precipitates more severe GI side effects.

NATURAL PRODUCTS AND MISCELLANEOUS AGENTS

ASPARAGINASE   (ah-SPAIR-ah-jin-ays)

Colaspase, Elspar, Kidrolase ✿ (Abbreviation: L-ASP) (Rx)

See also *Antineoplastic Agents*, p. 287.

Classification: Antineoplastic, miscellaneous.

Action/Kinetics: Drug isolated from *E. coli*. Cell cycle specific (G_1 phase). Neoplastic cells are unable to synthesize sufficient asparagine, an amino acid, to meet their metabolic needs. The supply of asparagine is further decreased by the enzyme asparaginase, which breaks down asparagine to aspartic acid and ammonia. Asparaginase interferes with synthesis of DNA, RNA, and protein and is cell-cycle specific for the G_1 phase of cell division. **Time to peak plasma levels, after IM:** 14–24 hr. **$t^{1/2}$, after IV:** 8 to 30 hr; **after IM:** 39–49 hr. The drug accumulates in plasma and tissue, and a small amount (1%) appears in CSF. Excretion is unknown. More toxic in adults than in children.

Use: Acute lymphocytic leukemia in children; mostly used in combination with other drugs. Not to be used for maintenance therapy. *Investigational:* Acute myelocytic and myelomonocytic leukemia, chronic lymphocytic leukemia, Hodgkin's and non-Hodgkin's lymphomas, melanosarcoma.

Contraindications: Anaphylactic reactions to asparaginase, acute hemorrhagic pancreatitis. Lactation. Institute retreatment with great care.

Special Concerns: Pregnancy category: C. Use with caution in presence of liver dysfunction.

Additional Side Effects: Hypersensitivity reaction including those with negative skin tests. Hyperglycemia, uricemia, azotemia, acute hemorrhagic pancreatitis, fatal hyperthermia. Hallucinations, Parkinson-like syndrome (rare).

Drug interactions	
Methotrexate	Asparaginase ↓ effect of methotrexate
Prednisone	Even though used with asparaginase, may cause ↑ toxicity
Vincristine	Even though used with asparaginase, may cause ↑ toxicity; ↑ hyperglycemic effect

Laboratory Test Interferences: ↑ Blood ammonia, BUN, glucose, uric acid, SGOT, SGPT, alkaline phosphatase, bilirubin (direct and indirect). ↓ Serum calcium albumin, cholesterol, plasma fibrinogen. Interference with interpretation of thyroid function tests.

Dosage: IV, IM, *individualized.* **When used as sole agent: Adults and children,** 200 IU/kg/day **IV** for 28 days. **In combination with prednisone and vincristine: asparaginase,** 1,000 IU/kg/day **IV** for 10 days beginning on day 22 of course of therapy; **vincristine:** 2 mg/m² **IV** once weekly on days 1, 8, and 15 of course of treatment (single dosage should not exceed 2 mg); **prednisone:** 40 mg/m²/day **PO** in 3 doses for 15 days; **then,** 20 mg/m² for 2 days, 10 mg/m² for 2 days, 5 mg/m² for 2 days, and 2.5 mg/m² for 2 days, followed by discontinuance of therapy.

   Alternative regimen: asparaginase, 6,000 IU/m² **IM** on days 4, 7, 10, 13, 16, 19, 22, 25, and 28 of course of treatment; **vincristine:** 1.5 mg/m² **IV** weekly on days 1, 8, 15, and 22 of course of treatment (maximum single dose should not exceed 2 mg); **prednisone:** 40 mg/m²/day **PO** in 3 divided doses for 28 days, followed by gradual discontinuation over a 2 week period.

NURSING CONSIDERATIONS

See also *Nursing Considerations* for *Antineoplastic Agents,* p. 303.

Administration/Storage

1. An intradermal skin test (0.1 mL of a 20-IU/mL solution) is to be done at least 1 hr before initial administration of drug and when 1 week or more has elapsed between treatments.
2. A desensitization procedure, with increasing amounts of asparaginase, is sometimes carried out in clients hypersensitive to the drug.
3. Treatment should be initiated only in hospitalized clients.
4. Asparaginase should not be used as the sole treatment agent unless a combined regimen is not possible due to toxicity or the client is refractory.
5. For IV use, reconstitute the 10,000-unit vial with either 5 mL sterile water for injection or sodium chloride injection. The solution may be given by direct IV administration or by infusion. When infused, give over at least 30 min in side of arm; use an infusion of either sodium chloride injection or dextrose injection (5%).

6. When used IM, no more than 2 mL should be given at a single injection site.

7. Reconstitute for IM use by adding 2 mL sodium chloride injection to the 10,000 unit vial. Do not use after 8 hr following reconstitution.

8. The drug should be handled with care as it is a contact irritant.

Interventions

1. Have emergency equipment readily available to counteract anaphylactic shock during each administration of asparaginase, since a severe reaction is more likely to occur with this drug.

2. Obtain baseline serum amylase levels and check periodically during therapy to detect pancreatitis.

3. Monitor client for hyperglycemia, glycosuria, and polyuria, all of which may be precipitated by asparaginase.

4. Have available IV fluids and regular insulin to treat hyperglycemia. Anticipate discontinuation of asparaginase.

5. Monitor intake and output; assess client for any evidence of renal failure.

6. Observe client for peripheral edema due to hypoalbuminemia triggered by asparaginase.

7. Assess for shakiness or unusual body movements. A Parkinson-like condition may be precipitated by asparaginase.

8. If ordered, administer vincristine and prednisone before asparaginase to reduce the toxic effect.

9. Administration of asparaginase 9–10 days before or within 24 hr after methotrexate may be ordered to reduce the GI and hematologic effects of methotrexate.

Client/Family Teaching

1. Advise client to promptly report any stomach pain, nausea, and vomiting, since these side effects may be symptoms of pancreatitis.

2. Alert client to report hyperthermia.

3. Caution that the drug may cause drowsiness, even several weeks after administration; therefore, the client should not drive a car or operate hazardous machinery.

CISPLATIN   (sis-PLAT-in)

Abiplatin✺, Platinol, Platinol-AQ (Abbreviation: CDDP) (Rx)

See also *Antineoplastic Agents,* p. 287.

Classification: Antineoplastic, miscellaneous.

Action/Kinetics: Cisplatin, a heavy metal inorganic coordination complex, acts similarly to alklyating agents in that it complexes with DNA and interferes with DNA function. The drug is cell-cycle nonspecific. $t^{1/2}$: initial, 25–49 min; **postdistribution,** 58–73 hr. Incomplete urinary excretion (only 27–43% after 5 days). Drug concentrates in liver, kidneys, large and small intestines, with low penetration of CNS. The drug is over 90% bound to plasma protein.

Uses: Treatment of metastatic testicular (in combination with bleomycin and vinblastine) and ovarian (in combination with doxorubicin) tumors in patients with prior radiotherapy or surgery. Advanced bladder cancer unresponsive to other treatment. *Investigational:* Cancer of the adrenal cortex, head and neck, breast, cervix, endometrium, stomach, lung, prostate. Neuroblastoma. Germ cell tumors of the ovary and in children. Osteosarcoma.

Additional Contraindications: Preexisting renal impairment, bone marrow suppression, hearing impairment, and allergic reactions to platinum. Lactation.

Special Concerns: Safe use during pregnancy has not been established.

Additional Side Effects: *Renal:* Severe cumulative renal toxicity including renal tubular damage and renal insufficiency. *Electrolytes:* Low levels of calcium, magnesium, potassium, phosphate, and sodium. *Neurological:* Seizures, taste loss, peripheral neuropathies. Neurotoxicity may occur 4–7 months after prolonged therapy. *Otic:* Ototoxicity characterized by tinnitus, especially in children. *Ophthalmologic:* Papilledema, cerebral blindness, optic neuritis. High doses have resulted in blurred vision and altered color perception. *Miscellaneous:* Anaphylactic reactions, hyperuricemia.

Additional Drug Interaction: When cisplatin is used with phenytoin, phenytoin plasma levels may be decreased.

Laboratory Test Interferences: ↑ Plasma iron levels. Nephrotoxicity results in ↑ serum uric acid, BUN, and creatinine and ↓ creatinine clearance.

Dosage: IV. *Metastatic testicular tumors:* **usual dosage,** cisplatin, 20 mg/m² daily for 5 days q 3 weeks for 3 courses; bleomycin sulfate, **IV (rapid infusion):** 30 units weekly (on day 2 of each week) for 12 consecutive weeks; vinblastine sulfate, **IV:** 0.15–0.2 mg/kg twice weekly (days 1 and 2) q 3 weeks for 4 courses (i.e., 8 doses total). *Metastatic ovarian tumor, as single agent:* 100 mg/m² once q 4 weeks. *In combination with doxorubicin hydrochloride,* cisplatin: 50 mg/m² once q 3 weeks (on day 1); doxorubicin hydrochloride: 50 mg/m² once q 3 weeks (on day 1). The drugs are given sequentially. *Advanced bladder cancer:* 50–70 mg/m² once q 3–4 weeks as a single agent. **Note:** Repeat courses should not be administered until (1) serum creatinine is below 1.5 mg/100 mL and/or the BUN is below 25 mg/100 mL; (2) platelets are equal to or greater than 100,000/mm³ and WBC count is equal to or greater than 4,000/mm³; and (3) auditory activity is within the normal range.

NURSING CONSIDERATIONS

See also *Nursing Considerations* for *Antineoplastic Agents,* p. 303.

Administration/Storage

1. Store unopened vials of dry powder in refrigerator at 2°–8°C to maintain stability for 2 years.
2. Reconstitute 10- and 50-mg vials with 10 or 50 mL of sterile water for injection as instructed on package insert.
3. Do not refrigerate reconstituted vials, as a precipitate will form. Reconstituted solution is stable at room temperature for 20 hr.
4. Use of a 0.45-μm filter is advised.
5. Before administration of cisplatin, hydrate client with 1–2 L of fluid by IV over a period of 8–12 hr.
6. Add dosage recommended from reconstituted vial to 2 L of 5% dextrose in one-half or one-third normal saline containing 37.5 g mannitol. Infuse over a period of 6–8 hr. Furosemide is ordered by some practitioners instead of mannitol.
7. Do not use any equipment with aluminum for preparing or administering, as a black precipitate will form and loss of potency will occur.

Interventions

1. Have emergency equipment readily available to treat any occurrence of an anaphylactic reaction to cisplatin.
2. *Assess*
   - for facial edema, bronchoconstriction, tachycardia, and shock.
   - for tremors that may progress to seizures due to hypomagnesemia.
   - for tetany, confusion, or signs of hypocalcemia associated with hypomagnesemia; monitor for appropriate levels.
3. Ascertain that baseline renal tests are performed before therapy is instituted, as cisplatin may cause severe cumulative renal toxicity.
4. Hydrate well and monitor for adequate hydration and output for 24 hr after treatment. Report oliguria.
5. Anticipate that additional doses of cisplatin will not be administered until the client's renal function has returned to baseline value.
6. Recommend client for audiometry before initiating therapy and before administering subsequent doses, to ascertain that client's hearing has not been affected.
7. Be alert to complaints of ringing in ears, difficulty in hearing, edema of lower extremities, and decreased urination and report.

ETOPOSIDE (VP-16–213) (eh-TOP-oh-syd)

VePesid (Rx)

See also *Antineoplastic Agents,* p. 287.

Classification: Antineoplastic, miscellaneous.

Action/Kinetics: Etoposide is a semisynthetic derivative of podophyllotoxin. Etoposide acts as a mitotic inhibitor at the A and G_2 portion of the cell cycle to inhibit DNA synthesis. At high doses, cells entering mitosis are lysed, whereas at low doses, cells will not enter prophase. **$t^{1/2}$:** biphasic, initial, 1.5 hr; final, 4–11 hr. **Effective plasma levels:** 0.3–10 mcg/mL. Poor penetration to the CNS. The drug is eliminated through both the urine and bile unchanged and as liver metabolites.

Uses: With combination therapy to treat refractory testicular tumors and small cell lung cancer. *Investigational:* Alone or in combination to treat acute monocytic leukemia, non-Hodgkin's lymphoma, Hodgkin's disease, AIDS-associated Kaposi's sarcoma, Ewing's sarcoma.

Contraindications: Lactation.

Special Concerns: Pregnancy category: D. Safety and efficacy in children have not been established.

Additional Side Effects: Anaphylactic-type reactions, hypotension, peripheral neuropathy, somnolence.

Dosage: IV. *Testicular carcinoma:* 50–100 mg/m²/day on days 1–5 or 100 mg/m²/day on days 1, 3, and 5 every 3–4 weeks (i.e., after recovery from toxic effects). Used in combination with other agents. *Small cell lung carcinoma:* 35 mg/m²/day for 4 days to 50 mg/m²/day for 5 days, repeated q 3–4 weeks. **Capsules.** *Small cell lung carcinoma:* 70 mg/m² (rounded to the nearest 50 mg) daily for 4 days to 100 mg/m² (rounded to the nearest 50 mg) daily for 5 days; repeat q 3–4 weeks.

NURSING CONSIDERATIONS

See also *Nursing Considerations* for *Antineoplastic Agents,* p. 303.

Administration/Storage

1. A slow IV infusion over 30–60 min will decrease the chance of hypotension. The drug should not be given by rapid IV push.
2. For IV use, the drug should be diluted with either 5% dextrose or 0.9% sodium chloride injection for a final concentration of 0.2 or 0.4 mg/mL.
3. Medical personnel should wear gloves when preparing this medication; if the drug comes in contact with the skin or mucosa, the area should be washed immediately and thoroughly with soap and water.
4. Diluted solutions to give a final concentration of 0.2 mg/mL are stable for 96 hr at room temperature, while final concentrations of 0.4 mg/mL are stable for 48 hr at room temperature.
5. Capsules must be stored at 2°–8°C (36°–46°F) but should not be frozen.

Interventions

1. Obtain baseline hemoglobin level and white blood cell count with differential before drug is administered.
2. Be prepared to treat anaphylactic reactions. Have available corticosteroids, pressor agents, antihistamines, and plasma expanders.
3. Monitor for signs of infection and bleeding, which are more likely to occur with this drug than with most antineoplastic agents.
4. Record BP at least twice a day and note any significant decreases.
5. Report any tingling sensations, numbness, and other signs of peripheral neuropathy.
6. Be aware that client may feel fatigued and be sleepy during and after drug administration. Schedule nursing activities accordingly.

INTERFERON ALFA-2A RECOMBINANT IFLrA, rIN-A   (in-ter-**FEER**-on **AL**-fa)

Roferon-A (Rx)

Classification: Antineoplastic, miscellaneous agent.

Action/Kinetics: Interferon alfa-2a is the product of recombinant DNA technology using strains of genetically engineered *Escherichia coli*. The activity of these drugs is expressed as International Units which are determined by comparing the antiviral activity of recombinant interferons with the activity of the international reference standard of human leukocyte interferon. Interferons bind to specific receptors on the cell surface, resulting in inhibition of virus replication in virus-infected cells, suppression of cell proliferation, increase in the phagocytic activity of macrophages, and enhancement of the toxic effects of leukocytes for target cells. **Peak serum levels:** 3.8–7.3 hr. **t½:** 3.7–8.5 hr. The drug is metabolized by the kidney.

Use: Hairy cell leukemia in patients older than 18 years of age. Can be used in splenectomized and nonsplenectomized patients. AIDS-related Kaposi's sarcoma in patients older than 18 years of age. *Investigational:* The drug has been used for a large number of other conditions. Significant activity has been noted against the following neoplastic diseases: locally for superficial bladder tumors, carcinoid tumor, chronic myelogenous leukemia, cutaneous T-cell lymphoma, essential thrombocythemia, low-grade non-Hodgkin's lymphoma. Interferon alfa-2a has also been used to treat the following viral infections: chronic non-A, non-B hepatitis, condylomata acuminata, cutaneous warts, cytomegaloviruses, herpes keratoconjunctivitis, herpes simplex, papillomaviruses, rhinoviruses, vaccinia virus, varicella zoster, and viral hepatitis B.

Contraindications: Lactation.

Special Concerns: Pregnancy category: C (use during pregnancy only if clearly required). Use with caution in patients with a history of unstable angina, uncontrolled congestive heart failure, chronic obstructive pulmonary disease, diabetes mellitus prone to ketoacidosis, thrombophlebitis, pulmonary embolism, seizure disorders, severe renal and hepatic disease, compromised CNS function, and severe myelosuppression. Safety and efficacy in individuals less than 18 years of age have not been established.

Side Effects: *Flu-like symptoms:* Fever, headache, fatigue, anorexia, myalgias, chills. *CV:* Hypotension, arrhythmias, syncope, hypertension, edema, chest pain, palpitations, transient ischemic attacks, pulmonary edema, myocardial infarction, congestive heart failure, stroke, hot flashes, Raynaud's phenomenon. *CNS:* Depression, confusion, dizziness, paresthesia, anxiety, nervousness, numbness, lethargy, sleep disturbances, visual disturbances, decreased mental status. *GI:* Anorexia, nausea, vomiting, diarrhea, hypermotility, abdominal fullness. *Hematologic:* Thrombocytopenia, neutropenia, leukopenia. *Musculoskeletal:* Myalgia, arthralgia, muscle contractions. *Dermatologic:* Rash, inflammation or dryness of the oropharynx, pruritus, dry skin, skin flushing, alopecia, urticaria. *Other:* Taste alteration, hepatitis, weight loss, diaphoresis, transient impotence, conjunctivitis, bronchospasm, night sweats, excessive salivation, tachypnea.

Laboratory Test Interferences: ↑ SGOT, SGPT, LDH, BUN, serum creatinine, alkaline phosphatase, bilirubin, uric acid, serum glucose, serum phosphorus. ↓ Hematocrit, hemoglobin. Hypocalcemia, proteinuria.

Dosage: IM, SC: *Hairy cell leukemia:* **induction,** 3 million IU/day for 16–24 weeks; **maintenance,** 3 million IU 3 times weekly. Doses higher than 3 million IU are not recommended. *AIDS-related Kaposi's sarcoma:* **IM, SC: induction,** 36 million IU/day for 10–12 weeks; or, 3 million IU/day on days 1–3; 9 million IU/day on days 4–6; and 18 million IU/day on days 7–9 followed by 36 million IU/day for the remainder of the 10–12 week induction period. **maintenance:** 36 million IU 3 times weekly. If severe untoward effects occur, the dose can be withheld or reduced by one-half.

NURSING CONSIDERATIONS

Administration/Storage

1. Treatment should be discontinued if the hairy cell leukemia does not respond within 6 months.
2. If severe reactions occur, the dose of the drug can be reduced by one-half or individual doses may be withheld. Also, assess the effect on bone marrow of previous x-ray therapy or chemotherapy.
3. Although the optimal duration of treatment has not been established, clients have been treated for up to 20 consecutive months.

Interventions

1. If the platelet count is less than 50,000/mm³ or if the client is at risk for bleeding, the drug should be given SC rather than IM.
2. Acetaminophen may be used to treat side effects of fever and headache.
3. Flu-like symptoms may be minimized by administering the drug at bedtime.
4. Clients should be well hydrated, especially when therapy is initiated.

Client/Family Teaching

1. The most common side effects are flu-like symptoms, such as fever, fatigue, headache, chills, nausea, and loss of appetite; these symptoms may be minimized by taking the drug at bedtime.
2. Flu-like symptoms usually diminish in severity as treatment continues.
3. Drink plenty of fluids during therapy.
4. Do not change brands of interferon without consulting physician, as changes in dosage may occur with a different brand.
5. Stress the importance of reporting for laboratory tests, including complete blood count, electrolyte levels, and liver function studies as scheduled.

INTERFERON ALFA-2B RECOMBINANT (IFN-alfa 2, rIFN-α2)
(in-ter-**FEER**-on **AL**-fa)

Intron A (Rx)

Classification: Antineoplastic, miscellaneous agent.

Action/Kinetics: Interferon alpha-2b is a product of recombinant DNA technology using strains of genetically engineered *Escherichia coli*. The activity is expressed as International Units which are determined by comparing the antiviral activity of the recombinant interferon with the activity of the international reference standard of human leukocyte interferon. Interferons bind to specific receptors on the cell surface, resulting in inhibition of virus replication in virus-infected cells, suppression of cell proliferation, increase in the phagocytic activity of macrophages, and enhancement of the toxic effects of leukocytes for target cells. **Peak serum levels after IM, SC:** up to 116 IU/mL after 3–12 hr. **t½, IM, SC:** 6–7 hr. **Peak serum levels after IV infusion:** up to 270 IU/mL at the end of the infusion. **t½, IV:** 2 hr. The main site of metabolism may be the kidney.

Use: Hairy cell leukemia in patients older than 18 years of age. Can be used in splenectomized and nonsplenectomized patients. Intralesional use for genital or venereal warts (*Condylomata acuminata*). AIDS-related Kaposi's sarcoma. *Investigational:* The drug has been used for a large number of conditions. Significant activity has been noted against the following neoplastic diseases: locally for superficial bladder tumors, carcinoid tumor, chronic myelogenous leukemia, cutaneous T-cell lymphoma, essential thrombocythemia, and low-grade non-Hodgkin's lymphoma. Interferon alfa-2b has also been used to treat the following viral infections: chronic non-A, non-B hepatitis, cutaneous warts, cytomegaloviruses, herpes keratoconjunctivitis, herpes simplex, papillomaviruses, rhinoviruses, vaccinia virus, varicella zoster, and viral hepatitis B.

Contraindications: Lactation.

Special Concerns: Pregnancy category: C (use only if clearly required). Use with caution in patients with a history of unstable angina, uncontrolled congestive heart failure, chronic obstructive pulmonary disease, diabetes mellitus prone to ketoacidosis, thrombophlebitis, pulmonary embolism, seizure disorders, severe renal and hepatic disease, compromised CNS function, and severe myelosuppression. Safety and efficacy in individuals less than 18 years of age have not been established.

Side Effects: *Flu-like symptoms:* Fever, headache, fatigue, anorexia, nausea, vomiting, chills. *CV:* Hypotension, arrhythmias, tachycardia, syncope, hypertension, coagulation disorders, chest pain. *CNS:* Depression, confusion, somnolence, dizziness, ataxia, headache, paresthesia, anxiety, nervousness, insomnia, emotional lability. *GI:* Nausea, vomiting, diarrhea, stomatitis, paralytic ileus, alteration of taste, weight loss, anorexia, dyspepsia, flatulence, dehydration, constipation. *Hematologic:* Thrombocytopenia, transient granulocytopenia. *Musculoskeletal:* Myalgia, arthralgia, leg cramps. *Other:* Pruritus, alopecia, skin rashes, urticaria, hot flashes, epistaxis, abnormal vision, pharyngitis, cold sores, purpura, sneezing, nasal congestion, increased salivation, hyperglycemia, oculomotor paralysis.

Laboratory Test Interferences: ↑ SGOT, SGPT, LDH, BUN, serum creatinine, alkaline phosphatase. ↓ Hematocrit, hemoglobin.

Dosage: IM, SC. *Hairy cell leukemia:* 2 million IU/m^2 3 times a week. Higher doses are not recommended. *AIDS-related Kaposi's sarcoma:* **IM, SC,** 30 million IU/m^2 3 times a week using only the 50 million IU vial. Using this dose, patients should tolerate an average dose of 110 million IU/week at the end of 12 weeks of therapy and 75 million IU/week at the end of 24 weeks of therapy.
    Intralesional. *Genital or venereal warts:* 1 million IU/lesion 3 times weekly for 3 weeks. For this purpose, use only the vial containing 10 million units and reconstitute using no more than 1 mL diluent.

NURSING CONSIDERATIONS

See also *Nursing Considerations* for *Interferon Alpha-2a Recombinant,* p. 355, and *Interferon Alpha-n3,* p. 358.

Administration/Storage

1. Prior to administration, the drug must be reconstituted with bacteriostatic water for injection, which is provided. After reconstitution, the solution is stable for 1 month at 2°–8°C.
2. Treatment for hairy cell leukemia should be discontinued if the client does not respond within 6 months.
3. When used for venereal or genital warts, maximum response usually occurs 4–8 weeks after therapy is initiated. If results are not satisfactory after 12–16 weeks, a second course of therapy may be undertaken.
4. Although the optimal duration of treatment has not been established, clients have been treated for up to 20 consecutive months.

Interventions

1. Prior to and periodically during therapy, the levels of hemoglobin, platelets, granulocytes and hairy cells, and bone marrow hairy cells should be determined.
2. If the platelet count is less than 50,000/mm^3, the drug should be given SC rather than IM.
3. Acetaminophen may be used to treat side effects of fever and headache.
4. Flu-like symptoms may be minimized by administering the drug at bedtime.
5. Clients should be well hydrated, especially when therapy is initiated.
6. If a response to the drug is manifested, treatment should be continued until no further beneficial effects are observed and laboratory values have been stable for 3 months.

INTERFERON ALFA-N3   (in-ter-FEER-on AL-fa)

Alferon N (Rx)

Classification: Antineoplastic.

Action/Kinetics: Interferon alfa-n3 is made from pooled human leukocytes induced by incomplete infection with Sendai (avian) virus. The product is a sterile, aqueous formulation of purified, natural, human interferon alpha proteins. The drug binds to receptors on cell surfaces leading to a sequence of events including inhibition of virus replication and suppression of cell proliferation. Also, interferon alfa-n3 causes immunomodulation characterized by enhanced phagocytosis by macrophages, augmentation of the cytotoxicity of lymphocytes, and enhancement of human leukocyte antigen expression. Intralesional use of interferon alfa-n3 does not result in detectable plasma levels of the drug.

Uses: Intralesional treatment of refractory or recurring external condylomata acuminata (genital or venereal warts) in patients 18 years of age or older. *Investigational:* Alpha interferons are being tested for use in a large number of neoplastic diseases and viral infections.

Contraindications: Hypersensitivity to human interferon alpha; patients who are allergic to mouse immunoglobulin (IgG), egg protein, or neomycin (the production process involves a nutrient medium containing neomycin although it has not been detected in the final product). Lactation.

Special Concerns: Pregnancy category: C (use only if clearly needed). Due to the manifestation of fever and flu-like symptoms with interferon alfa-n3 use, the drug should be used with caution in patients with debilitating diseases including unstable angina, uncontrolled congestive heart failure, chronic obstructive pulmonary disease, diabetes mellitus with ketoacidosis, thrombophlebitis, pulmonary embolism, hemophilia, severe myelosuppression, or seizure disorders. Safety and effectiveness have not been determined in children less than 18 years of age.

Side Effects: *Flu-like symptoms:* Commonly, fever, headache, myalgias which decrease with repeated doses. Also, chills, fatigue, malaise. *CNS:* Dizziness, lightheadedness, insomnia, depression, nervousness, decreased ability to concentrate. *GI:* Nausea, vomiting, heartburn, diarrhea, tongue hyperesthesia, thirst, altered taste, increased salivation. *Musculoskeletal/Skin:* Arthralgia, back pain, hot sensation at bottom of feet, tingling of legs/feet, muscle cramps. *Respiratory:* Nose or sinus drainage, nose bleed, throat tightness, pharyngitis. *Miscellaneous:* Pruritus, swollen lymph nodes, heat intolerance, visual disturbances, sensitivity to allergens, papular rash on neck, hot flashes, herpes labialis, dysuria, photosensitivity, decreased white blood count.

Note: When used for treatment of cancer, the incidence of many of the above untoward reactions was increased. Additional untoward reactions were noted including: *GI:* Constipation, anorexia, stomatitis, dry mouth, mucositis, sore mouth. *Laboratory Test Values:* Abnormal hemoglobin, white blood count, alkaline phosphatase, total bilirubin, platelet count, AST, and GGT. *Miscellaneous:* Insomnia, blurred vision, ocular rotation pain, sore injection site, chest pains, low blood pressure.

Dosage: Intralesional injection. *Condylomata acuminata:* 0.05 mL (250,000 IU) per wart twice a week for up to 8 weeks. The maximum recommended dose per treatment session is 0.5 mL (2.5 million IU). The safety and effectiveness of a second course of treatment have not been determined.

NURSING CONSIDERATIONS

See also *Nursing Considerations* for *Interferon Alfa-2a Recombinant,* p. 355.

Administration/Storage

1. The drug should be injected into the base of the wart using a 30-gauge needle.
2. For large warts, the drug can be injected at several points around the periphery of the wart using a total dose of 0.05 mL/wart.
3. The drug should be stored at 2°–8°C (36°–46°F). It should not be frozen or shaken.

Assessment

1. Take client history, especially noting any history of allergic reactions to egg protein or neomycin. These could indicate an increased sensitivity to interferon alfa-n3.
2. Note any client history of preexisting debilitating diseases.
3. For condylomata therapy, note the size of the wart. Measure it and document prior to initiating therapy.

Client/Family Teaching

1. Intralesional treatment should be continued for 8 weeks.
2. Genital warts may disappear both during treatment and after treatment has been discontinued. When this occurs, unless new warts appear or warts become enlarged, there should be a 3-month waiting period after the first 8 week course of therapy.
3. Do not change brands of interferon without consultation with the physician as the manufacturing process, strength, and type of interferon may vary.
4. Women should use contraceptive practices if fertile.
5. Review the early signs of hypersensitivity reactions (e.g., hives, chest tightness, generalized urticaria, hypotension, wheezing, anaphylaxis) and instruct client to contact their physician should these symptoms occur.

Evaluation

During therapy for condylomata, measure the size of the warts to determine the extent to which they are decreasing in size at each treatment session.

PROCARBAZINE HYDROCHLORIDE (pro-**KAR**-bah-zeen)

Matulane, MIH, N-Methylhydrazine, Natulan ✤ (Abbreviation: MIH) (Rx)

See also *Antineoplastic Agents*, p. 287.

Classification: Antineoplastic, miscellaneous.

Action/Kinetics: Procarbazine is both an alkylating agent and an inhibitor of monoamine oxidase. The drug is cell-cycle specific for the S phase of cell division. It inhibits synthesis of protein, RNA, and DNA, possibly because of autooxidation (production of hydrogen peroxide). Well absorbed from GI tract. Drug equilibrates between plasma and CSF (peak levels occur within 30–90 min). $t\frac{1}{2}$, **after IV:** 10 min. About 70% eliminated in urine, mostly as metabolites, after 24 hr. Procarbazine is mostly used in combination with other drugs (MOPP therapy).

Use: As an adjunct in the treatment of Hodgkin's disease (Stage III and Stage IV). *Investigational:* NonHodgkin's lymphomas, malignant melanoma, primary brain tumors, lung cancer, multiple myeloma, polycythemia vera.

Additional Contraindications: Hypersensitivity to drug. Depressed bone marrow. Low WBC and RBC or platelet counts. Lactation.

Special Concerns: Pregnancy category: D. Use with caution in impaired kidney or liver function.

Additional Side Effects: *GI:* Dysphagia, constipation or diarrhea. *CNS:* Psychosis, manic reactions, insomnia, nightmares, foot drop, decreased reflexes, tremors, coma, delirium, convulsions. *Dermatologic:* Hyperpigmentation, photosensitivity. *Miscellaneous:* Petechiae, purpura, arthralgia, hemolysis, acute myelocytic leukemia, malignant myelosclerosis, azoospermia. In geriatric patients, the MAO inhibitor effects may cause increased vascular accidents and increased sensitivity to hypotensive effects.

Drug Interactions

Alcohol	Antabuse-like reaction
Antihistamines	Additive CNS depression
Antihypertensive drugs	Additive CNS depression
Barbiturates	Additive CNS depression
Digoxin	↓ Digoxin plasma levels if combination therapy used
Guanethidine	Excitation and hypertension
Hypoglycemic agents, oral	↑ Hypoglycemic effect
Insulin	↑ Hypoglycemic effect
Levodopa	Flushing and hypertension
Methyldopa	Excitation and hypertension
Monoamine oxidase inhibitors	Possibility of hypertensive crisis
Narcotics	Additive CNS depression
Phenothiazines	Additive CNS depression; also, possibility of hypertensive crisis
Reserpine	Excitation and hypertension
Sympathomimetics	Possibility of hypertensive crisis
Tricyclic antidepressants	Possibility of hypertensive crisis
Tyramine-containing foods	Possibility of hypertensive crisis

Dosage: Capsules. Adults: 2–4 mg/kg daily for first week; **then,** 4–6 mg/kg/day until leukocyte count falls below 4,000/mm^3 or platelet count falls below 100,000/mm^3. If toxic symptoms appear, discontinue drug and resume treatment at rate of 1–2 mg/kg/day; **maintenance:** 1–2 mg/kg/day. **Children:** *highly individualized,* 50 mg/m^2/day for first week; then 100 mg/m^2 (to nearest 50 mg) until maximum response obtained.

NURSING CONSIDERATIONS

See also *Nursing Considerations* for *Antineoplastic Agents,* p. 303.

Client/Family Teaching

1. Unless approved by the physician, other prescription drugs should not be used.
2. Contraception should be practiced by both men and women.
3. Advise to observe and report untoward CNS reactions that may necessitate withdrawal of the drug, as noted in *Additional Side Effects*.
4. Do not drink alcohol, as a disulfiram-type reaction may occur.
5. Consult physician before taking any other medication, as procarbazine has monoamine oxidase inhibitory activity. The use of sympathomimetic drugs and foods that have a high tyramine content is contraindicated during therapy and for 2 weeks after discontinuing therapy.
6. For clients with diabetes, procarbazine increases effect of insulin and oral hypoglycemics. Hypoglycemic symptoms should be reported to physician, because adjustment of antidiabetic medication may be necessary.
7. Avoid exposure to sun or to ultraviolet rays, because a photosensitive skin reaction may occur.

VINBLASTINE SULFATE (vin-BLAS-teen)

Velban, Velbe ✿, Velsar (Abbreviation: VLB) (Rx)

See also *Antineoplastic Agents,* p. 287.

Classification: Antineoplastic, plant alkaloid.

Action/Kinetics: Alkaloid, isolated from the periwinkle plant, is believed to inhibit mitosis (metaphase in cell cycle). Rapidly cleared from plasma but poor penetration to the brain. About 75% bound to serum proteins. Almost completely metabolized in the liver after IV administration. **t½, triphasic:** initial, 3.7 min; intermediate 1.6 hr; final, approximately 25 hr. Metabolites are excreted in the bile with smaller amounts in the urine. No cross-resistance with vincristine.

Uses: Palliative treatment of Hodgkin's disease, lymphocytic leukemia, mycosis fungoides, advanced carcinoma of testis, histiocytic lymphoma, Kaposi's sarcoma, Letterer-Siwe disease, trophoblastic tumors, and breast cancer (especially cancer unresponsive to other drugs or surgery). Usually administered in combination with other drugs. *Investigational:* Cancer of the head and neck, bladder, lung, kidney, chronic myelocytic leukemia, and ovarian germ cell tumors.

Contraindications: Leukopenia, granulocytopenia. Bacterial infections. Lactation.

Special Concerns: Pregnancy category: D.

Additional Side Effects: Toxicity is dose-related and more pronounced in patients over age 65 or in those suffering from cachexia (profound general ill health) or skin ulceration. *GI:* Ileus, rectal bleeding, hemorrhagic enterocolitis, vesiculation of the mouth, bleeding from a former ulcer. *Dermatologic:* Total epilation, skin vesiculation. *Neurologic:* Paresthesias, neuritis, mental depression, loss of deep tendon reflexes, seizures. Extravasation may result in phlebitis and cellulitis with sloughing.

Drug Interactions	
Bleomycin sulfate	Combination of bleomycin and vinblastine may produce signs of Raynaud's disease in patients with testicular cancer
Glutamic acid	Inhibits effect of vinblastine
Mitomycin C	Severe bronchospasm with shortness of breath
Phenytoin	↓ Effect of phenytoin due to ↓ plasma levels
Tryptophan	Inhibits effect of vinblastine

Dosage: IV, *individualized, using WBC count as guide.* Vinblastine is administered once every 7 days. **Adults: initial,** 3.7 mg/m²; **then,** after 7 days, graded doses of 5.5, 7.4, 9.25, and 11.1 mg/m² at intervals of 7 days (maximum dose should not exceed 18.5 mg/m²). **Children: initial,** 2.5 mg/m²; **then,** after 7 days, graded doses of 3.75, 5.0, 6.25, and 7.5 mg/m² at intervals of 7 days (maximum dose should not exceed 12.5 mg/m²). **Maintenance** doses are calculated based on WBC count—at least 4,000/mm³.

NURSING CONSIDERATIONS

See also *Nursing Considerations* for *Antineoplastic Agents,* p. 303.

Administration/Storage

1. Dilute vinblastine with 10 mL of sodium chloride injection.
2. Inject into flowing infusion or directly into vein.

3. Remainder of solution may be stored in refrigerator for 30 days.
4. If the drug gets into the eye, wash eye thoroughly with water immediately to prevent irritation and ulceration.
5. To reconstitute, add 10 mL sodium chloride injection, which is preserved with either benzyl alcohol or phenol for a final concentration of 1 mg/mL.
6. The drug should not be reconstituted with solutions that raise or lower the pH from between 3.5 and 5.

Assessment

1. Take a thorough drug history.
2. Note any evidence of neuropathies prior to onset of therapy.
3. Obtain neutrophil and platelet count before starting therapy as a baseline against which to measure these counts once therapy has been initiated.

Interventions

1. Assess peripheral IV site for patency to prevent extravasation and local irritation and pain. If extravasation occurs, move infusion to other vein. Treat affected area with injection of hyaluronidase and application of moderate heat to decrease local reaction.
2. Observe client for cyanosis and pallor of extremities and for signs of Raynaud's disease if also receiving bleomycin.
3. Check clients for manifestations of neurotoxicity. Report these findings and document accordingly as the dosage of drug may need to be adjusted.
4. To prevent constipation, encourage client to eat a high-fiber diet, remain active and take stool softeners as prescribed.

Evaluation

1. Monitor neurologic toxicity by checking client reflexes and strength of hand grip.
2. Assess for jaw pain, numbness, tingling, and deep tendon loss as well as diminished reflexes in the lower extremities.

VINCRISTINE SULFATE   (vin-KRIS-teen)

Oncovin, Vincasar PFS, Vincrex (Abbreviation: VCR or LCR) (Rx)

See also *Antineoplastic Agents,* p. 287.

Classification: Antineoplastic, plant alkaloid.

Action/Kinetics: Vincristine is a vinca alkaloid. Vincristine inhibits mitosis at metaphase. The antineoplastic effect is due to interference with intracellular tubulin function. After IV use, drug is distributed within 15–30 min to tissues. Poorly penetrates blood-brain barrier. **t½, triphasic:** initial, 5 min; intermediate, 2.3 hr; final, 85 hr. Approximately 80% is excreted in the feces and up to 20% in the urine. No cross-resistance with vinblastine.

Uses: Frequently used in combination therapy. Acute lymphocytic leukemia in children. Hodgkin's and non-Hodgkin's lymphomas, Wilms' tumor, neuroblastoma, lymphosarcoma, rhabdomyosarcoma, reticulum cell sarcoma. *Investigational:* Idiopathic thrombocytopenic purpura; cancer of the breast, ovary, cervix, lung, colorectal area; malignant melanoma, osteosarcoma, multiple myeloma, ovarian germ cell tumors, mycosis fungoides, chronic lymphocytic leukemia, chronic myelocytic leukemia.

Contraindications: Patients with demyelinating Charcot-Marie-Tooth syndrome. Lactation. Use during radiation therapy.

Special Concerns: Pregnancy category: D. Geriatric patients are more susceptible to the neurotoxic effects.

Additional Side Effects: *Neurologic:* Paresthesias, depression of deep tendon reflexes, foot drop, seizures, difficulties in gait. *GI:* Intestinal necrosis or perforation. Constipation, paralytic ileus. *Renal:* Inappropriate antidiuretic hormone secretion (polyuria or dysuria). *Ophthalmic:* Blindness, ptosis, diplopia, photophobia. *Miscellaneous:* CNS leukemia, bronchospasm, shortness of breath. Less bone marrow depression than vinblastine.

Drug Interactions	
L-Asparaginase	Asparaginase ↓ liver clearance of vincristine
Calcium channel blocking drugs	↑ Accumulation of vincristine in cells
Digoxin	Vincristine ↓ effect of digoxin
Glutamic acid	Inhibits effect of vincristine
Methotrexate	Combination may cause hypotension
Mitomycin C	Severe bronchospasm and acute shortness of breath

Dosage: IV only (direct, infusion), *individualized with extreme care as overdose can be fatal.* **Adults: usual, initial,** 0.4–1.4 mg/m^2 (or 0.01–0.03 mg/kg) 1 time a week; **children:** 1.5–2 mg/m^2 1 time a week. **Children less than 10 kg or with body surface area less than 1 m^2,** 0.05 mg/kg 1 time a week. *For hepatic insufficiency:* if serum bilirubin is 1.5–3, administer 50% of the dose; if serum bilirubin is more than 3.1 or SGOT is more than 180, dose should be omitted.

NURSING CONSIDERATIONS

See also *Nursing Considerations* for *Antineoplastic Agents,* p. 303.

Administration/Storage

1. Dissolve powder in sterile water or isotonic saline injection to a concentration ranging from 0.01 to 1 mg/mL.
2. Medication is injected either directly into a vein or into the tubing of a flowing IV infusion over a period of 1 min.
3. Store in refrigerator. Dry powder is stable for 6 months. Solutions are stable for 2 weeks under refrigeration.
4. Protect drug from exposure to light.
5. Vincristine should not be mixed with any solution that alters the pH outside the range of 3.5–5.5.

Assessment

Assess for early signs and symptoms of neuromuscular side effects (e.g., sensory impairment and paresthesias) before neuritic pain and motor difficulties are apparent because neuromuscular manifestations are irreversible.

Interventions

1. Prevent constipation by encouraging increased intake of fluids and a high-fiber diet.
2. Assess for absence of bowel sounds indicative of paralytic ileus, which requires symptomatic care as well as temporary discontinuance of vincristine.

3. Be prepared with laxatives and high enemas to treat high colon impaction caused by vincristine.
4. If extravasation occurs, move infusion to another vein. Treat affected area with injection of hyaluronidase and application of moderate heat so as to decrease local reaction.

HORMONAL AND ANTIHORMONAL ANTINEOPLASTIC AGENTS

The growth of cancers affecting the male or female reproductive systems and the breasts is usually enhanced by the presence of the hormone normally controlling the function of these tissues. Administration of an antihormone or a different hormone, which alters the hormonal milieu by competing for hormone receptors, will often inhibit neoplastic growth.

NURSING CONSIDERATIONS
See also *Nursing Considerations* for *Antineoplastic Agents,* p. 303.

Assessment
1. Assess for insomnia, lethargy, anorexia, nausea, vomiting, coma, and vascular collapse—symptoms of hypercalcemia.
2. Ascertain that serum calcium concentrations are routinely done; assess results. (Normal: 4.5–5.5 mEq/L.) The effect of the steroid and osteolytic metastases may result in hypercalcemia.

Interventions
1. Withhold drug and report high serum calcium levels.
2. Encourage high fluid intake to minimize hypercalcemia.
3. Be prepared to assist with administration of IV fluids, diuretics, adrenocorticosteroids, and phosphate supplementation for severe hypercalcemia.
4. Closely monitor clients who resume therapy after drug-induced hypercalcemia is corrected.

DIETHYLSTILBESTROL   (dye-eth-ill-still-**BEST**-roll)
(Abbreviation: DES) (Rx)

DIETHYLSTILBESTROL DIPHOSPHATE   (dye-eth-ill-still-**BEST**-roll)
Honvol✹, Stilphostrol (Abbreviation: DES) (Rx)

See also *Estrogens,* p. 1181, and *Antineoplastic Agents,* p. 287.

Classification: Estrogen, synthetic, nonsteroidal.

Action/Kinetics: Synthetic estrogen, which competes with androgen receptors, thereby preventing androgen from inducing further growth of the neoplasm. Metabolized in the liver.

Uses: Postcoital contraceptive (emergency use only). Palliative treatment of prostatic cancer.

Contraindications: Known or suspected breast cancer, estrogen-dependent neoplasia, active thrombophlebitis, thromboembolic disease, markedly impaired liver function. **Not to be used during pregnancy because of the possibility of vaginal cancer in female offspring (pregnancy category: X).**

Special Concerns: Use with caution in presence of hypercalcemia, epilepsy, migraine, asthma, cardiac and renal disease. Use with caution in children in whom bone growth is incomplete.

Side Effects: *CV:* Thrombophlebitis, pulmonary embolism, cerebral thrombosis, neuro-ocular lesions. *GI:* Nausea, vomiting, anorexia. *CNS:* Headaches, malaise, irritability. *Skin:* Allergic rash, itching. *GU:* Gynecomastia, changes in libido. *Other:* Porphyria, backache, pain and sterile abscess at injection site, postinjection flare.

Dosage: *Diethylstilbestrol.* **Tablets.** *Menopausal symptoms, atrophic vaginitis, kraurosis vulvae:* 0.2–0.5 mg up to 2 mg daily, given cyclically. *Estrogen deficiency states:* 0.2–0.5 mg daily, given cyclically. *Breast cancer in males and females:* 15 mg daily. *Prostatic cancer:* **initial,** 1–3 mg; **then,** increase as needed but later reduce dose to 1 mg daily. *Postcoital contraceptive (emergency treatment only):* 25 mg b.i.d. for 5 consecutive days, beginning within 24 hr (and not later than 72 hr) after exposure.

Diethylstilbestrol diphosphate. Palliative treatment of prostatic carcinoma: **Tablets:** 50–166 mg t.i.d. up to 200 mg t.i.d., not to exceed 1 g daily. **IV:** 500 mg (in 250 mL 5% dextrose or saline) on day 1 followed by 1 g (in 250–500 mL 5% dextrose or saline) daily for 5 days. **Maintenance, IV:** 250–500 mg 1 to 2 times weekly. Maintenance dose may also be given orally.

NURSING CONSIDERATIONS

See also *Nursing Considerations* for *Antineoplastic Agents,* p. 303, and *Estrogens,* p. 1183.

Administration/Storage

1. Administer the diphosphate slowly by drip (20–30 drops/min for first 10–15 min); then adjust flow for a total administration period of 1 hr.
2. The diphosphate solution is stable for 5 days at room temperature if stored away from direct light. Do not use if solution appears cloudy or if a precipitate has formed.

Assessment

1. Assess client with poor cardiac function for edema.
2. The effect of the steroid and osteolytic metastases may result in hypercalcemia. Assess for symptoms of hypercalcemia: insomnia, lethargy, anorexia, nausea, vomiting, coma, and vascular collapse.

Interventions

1. Withhold drug and report high serum calcium levels.
2. Encourage high fluid intake to minimize hypercalcemia.
3. Be prepared to assist with administration of IV fluids, diuretics, adrenocorticosteroids, and phosphate supplements for severe hypercalcemia.
4. Closely monitor clients who resume therapy after drug-induced hypercalcemia is corrected.
5. Anticipate that gynecomastia in men may be prevented by low doses of radiation before therapy with diethylstilbestrol is initiated.

Client/Family Teaching

1. Report any nausea, vomiting, abdominal pain, and painful swelling of breasts to physician.
2. Instruct client that solid foods often relieve nausea.
3. Be alert for increased complications and/or edema in clients with poor cardiac function.

ESTRAMUSTINE PHOSPHATE SODIUM   (es-trah-MUS-teen)

Emcyt (Rx)

See also *Antineoplastic Agents,* p. 287.

Classification: Hormonal agent, alkylating agent.

Action/Kinetics: Estramustine is a water-soluble drug that combines estradiol and mechlorethamine (a nitrogen mustard). The estradiol facilitates uptake into cells containing the estrogen receptor while the nitrogen mustard acts as an alkylating agent. Chronic estramustine administration results in plasma levels and effects of estradiol similar to those of conventional estradiol therapy. It is well absorbed from the GI tract and dephosphorylated before reaching the general circulation. **t½:** 20 hr. Major route of excretion is in the feces.

Uses: Palliative treatment of metastatic and/or progressive prostatic carcinoma.

Contraindications: Active thrombophlebitis or thromboembolic disease unless the tumor mass is causing the thromboembolic disorder.

Special Concerns: Use with caution in presence of cerebrovascular disease, coronary artery disease, diabetes, hypertension, congestive heart failure, impaired liver or kidney function, and metabolic bone diseases associated with hypercalcemia.

Additional Side Effects: *CV:* Myocardial infarction, cardiovascular accident, thrombosis, congestive heart failure, increased blood pressure, thrombophlebitis, leg cramps, edema. *Respiratory:* Pulmonary embolism, dyspnea, upper respiratory discharge, hoarseness. *GI:* Flatulence, burning sensation of throat, thirst. *Dermatologic:* Easy bruising, flushing, peeling of skin or fingertips. *Miscellaneous:* Chest pain, tearing of eyes, breast tenderness or enlargement, decreased glucose tolerance.

Laboratory Test Interferences: ↑ Bilirubin, SGOT, LDH. ↓ Glucose tolerance.

Drug Interactions: Drugs or food containing calcium may ↓ absorption of estramustine phosphate sodium.

Dosage: Capsules: 14 mg/kg/day in 3–4 divided doses (range: 10–16 mg/kg/day) or 600 mg (base)/m² daily in 3 divided doses. Treat for 30–90 days before assessing beneficial effects; continue therapy as long as the drug is effective.

NURSING CONSIDERATIONS

See also *Nursing Considerations* for *Antineoplastic Agents,* p. 303.

Administration/Storage

1. Capsules should be stored in the refrigerator, although they may be kept at room temperature for 1–2 days without affecting potency.
2. Capsules should be taken with water 1 hr before or 2 hr after meals.

Assessment

1. Assess diabetic clients for hyperglycemia because glucose tolerance may be decreased. Ask clients about their tests at home and any difficulties or changes they may have noted in their condition such as increased fatigue, weakness, etc.
2. Assess for symptoms of hypercalcemia: insomnia, lethargy, anorexia, nausea, vomiting, coma, and vascular collapse.
3. Ascertain that serum calcium levels are routinely done; assess results (normal: 4.5–5.5 mEq/L). The effect of the steroid and osteolytic metastases may result in hypercalcemia.

Interventions

1. Take client blood pressure at each visit and teach the client and/or family member to take the blood pressure. BP elevation occurs in conjunction with this therapy.
2. Explain to male clients that impotence resulting from previous estrogen therapy may be reversed.
3. Estramustine phosphate sodium may cause genetic mutation. Therefore, contraceptive measures should be practiced to prevent teratogenesis.
4. Withhold drug and report high serum calcium levels. Encourage high fluid intake to minimize hypercalcemia.
5. For severe hypercalcemia, be prepared to assist with administration of IV fluids, diuretics, adrenocorticosteroids, and phosphate supplements.
6. Closely monitor clients who resume therapy after drug-induced hypercalcemia is corrected.

FLUTAMIDE (FLOO-tah-myd)

Eulexin (Rx)

See also *Antineoplastic Agents,* p. 287.

Classification: Antineoplastic, hormonal agent.

Action/Kinetics: Flutamide acts either to inhibit uptake of androgen or to inhibit nuclear binding of androgen in target tissues. Thus, the effect of androgen is decreased in androgen-sensitive tissues. Flutamide is rapidly metabolized to active (alpha-hydroxylated derivative) and inactive metabolites in the liver and mainly excreted in the urine. **$t^{1/2}$ of active metabolite:** 6 hr (8 hr in geriatric patients). 94%–96% is bound to plasma proteins.

Uses: In combination with leuprolide acetate (i.e., a LHRH-agonist) to treat stage D_2 metastatic prostatic carcinoma. Treatment must be initiated simultaneously with both drugs for maximum benefit.

Contraindications: Use during pregnancy (category: D).

Side Effects: Untoward reactions are listed for treatment of flutamide with LHRH-agonist. *GU:* Loss of libido, impotence. *CV:* Hot flashes, hypertension. *GI:* Nausea, vomiting, diarrhea, GI disturbances, anorexia. *CNS:* Confusion, depression, drowsiness, anxiety, nervousness. *Hepatic:* Elevated transaminases, bilirubin, or creatinine; hepatitis. *Dermatologic:* Rash, photosensitivity, irritation at injection site. *Miscellaneous:* Gynecomastia, edema, neuromuscular symptoms, pulmonary symptoms, hematopoietic symptoms.

Dosage: Capsules: 250 mg (2 capsules) t.i.d. q 8 hr for a total daily dose of 750 mg.

NURSING CONSIDERATIONS

See also *Nursing Considerations* for *Antineoplastic Agents,* p. 303.

Interventions

1. Anticipate concomitant administration with an LHRH-agonist (such as leuprolide acetate).
2. Periodic liver function tests should be performed in clients on long-term flutamide therapy.

Client/Family Teaching

1. Clients should be informed to take flutamide and the LHRH-agonist (leuprolide) at the same time.

2. Drug therapy should not be interrupted or discontinued without consulting the physician.

3. Hot flashes, impotence, and diarrhea are all potential side effects of drug therapy and should be reported if persistent or bothersome.

GOSERELIN ACETATE (GO-seh-rih-lin)
Zoladex (Rx)

Classification: Antineoplastic, hormonal agent.

Action/Kinetics: Goserelin acetate is a synthetic decapeptide analog of luteinizing hormone-releasing hormone (LHRH or GnRH). The drug is a potent inhibitor of gonadotropin secretion from the pituitary gland. Initially, there is actually an increase in serum luteinizing and follicle-stimulating hormones. This is followed by a long-term suppression of pituitary gonadotropins with serum levels of testosterone decreasing to those seen in surgically castrated males. **Peak serum levels after SC implantation:** 12–15 days. The drug is available as an implant in a preloaded syringe. For the first 8 days of the treatment cycle, the rate of absorption is slower than for the remainder of the period.

Uses: Palliative treatment of advanced prostatic carcinoma as an alternative to orchiectomy or estrogen administration when these are either unacceptable to the patient or not indicated.

Contraindications: Pregnancy (category: X). Lactation.

Special Concerns: Safety and effectiveness have not been determined in patients less than 18 years of age.

Side Effects: *GU:* Sexual dysfunction, decreased erections, lower urinary tract symptoms, renal insufficiency, urinary obstruction, urinary tract infection. *CNS:* Lethargy, dizziness, insomnia, anxiety, depression, headache. *GI:* Anorexia, nausea, constipation, diarrhea, vomiting, ulcer formation. *CV:* Edema, congestive heart failure, arrhythmias, cerebrovascular accident, myocardial infarction, peripheral vascular disorder, hypertension, chest pain. *Miscellaneous:* Hot flashes (common), upper respiratory tract infection, rash, sweating, chronic obstructive pulmonary disease, worsened pain for the first 30 days, breast swelling/tenderness, fever, chills, anemia, gout, hyperglycemia, weight increase.

Dosage: SC Implant: 3.6 mg every 28 days into the upper abdominal wall using sterile technique under the direction of a physician.

NURSING CONSIDERATIONS

See also *Nursing Considerations* for *Antineoplastic Agents,* p. 303.

Administration/Storage

1. The sterile syringe, in which the drug is contained, should not be removed until immediately before use. The syringe should be examined for damage and to ensure the drug is visible in the translucent chamber.

2. The area should be cleaned with an alcohol swab; a local anesthetic can be used prior to the injection.

3. To administer the drug, the client's skin should be stretched with one hand and the needle gripped with the fingers around the barrel of the syringe. The needle is inserted into the SC fat and should not be aspirated. If a large vessel is penetrated, blood will be seen immediately in the syringe; the needle should be withdrawn and the injection made elsewhere with a new syringe.

4. The direction of the needle is changed so it parallels the abdominal wall. The needle is then pushed in until the barrel hub touches the client's skin and then withdrawn approximately 1 cm to create a space to inject the drug. The plunger is depressed to deliver the drug.

5. The needle is then withdrawn and the area bandaged.

6. To confirm the drug has been delivered, ensure that the tip of the plunger is visible within the tip of the needle.

7. The drug should be stored at room temperature not exceeding 25°C (77°F).

8. There is no evidence the drug accumulates in clients with either hepatic and/or renal dysfunction.

Interventions

1. Goserelin should not be used in women who are likely to become pregnant or who are pregnant. Clients must be appraised of potential hazards to the fetus in the event of pregnancy.

2. Administration of the drug should be under the supervision of a physician.

3. The 28-day schedule should be adhered to as closely as possible.

4. If there is need to remove goserelin surgically, it can be located by ultrasound.

5. Be prepared to provide a lot of emotional support to clients and families.

Client/Family Teaching

Remind client that the most common adverse side effects (especially hot flashes, decreased erections, and sexual dysfunction) are due to decreased testosterone levels.

Evaluation

Be aware that there may be initial worsening of symptoms or the occurrence of new symptoms of prostatic cancer. This is the result of transient increases of testosterone. Clients may complain of an increase in bone pain and develop spinal cord compression or ureteral obstruction. Client and family should be reassured that these symptoms are usually only temporary.

LEUPROLIDE ACETATE   (loo-PROH-lyd)
Lupron, Lupron Depot (Rx)

See also *Antineoplastic Agents,* p. 287.

Classification: Antineoplastic agent, hormonal.

Action/Kinetics: Leuprolide inhibits secretion of gonadotropins by suppressing both ovarian and testicular steroidogenesis. The drug occupies gonadotropin-releasing hormone receptors, rendering them insensitive. Initially, however, there is an increase in LH and FSH levels leading to increases of sex hormones. However, decreases in these hormones will be observed within 2–4 weeks. **t½: 3 hr. Peak plasma level following depot injection:** 20 ng/mL after 4 hr and 0.36 ng/mL after 4 weeks.

Uses: Palliative treatment in advanced prostatic cancer. *Investigational:* Endometriosis, breast cancer, inducing fertility in hypogonadotropic hypogonadism.

Contraindications: Pregnancy category: X. Depot form is contraindicated during pregnancy and in women who may become pregnant while receiving the drug. Patients sensitive to benzyl alcohol (found in leuprolide injection).

Side Effects: Injection and Depot. *GI:* Nausea, vomiting, anorexia, diarrhea. *CNS:* Paresthesia, insomnia, pain. *CV:* Peripheral edema, angina, cardiac arrhythmias. *GU:* Hematuria, urinary frequency or urgency, dysuria, testicular pain. *Respiratory:* Dyspnea, hemoptysis. *Endocrine:* Gynecomastia, breast tenderness, impotency, hot flashes, sweating, decreased testicular size, decreased libido. *Other:* Myalgia, bone pain, dermatitis, asthenia, diabetes, fever, chills, increased calcium.

Injection. *CV:* ECG changes, hypertension, ischemia, heart murmur, congestive heart failure, thrombosis, phlebitis, myocardial infarction, hypotension, pulmonary emboli. *GI:* Constipation, GI bleeding, dysphagia, taste disorders, peptic ulcer, hepatic dysfunction, rectal polyps. *CNS:* Headache, dizziness, lightheadedness, lethargy, memory disorders, mood swings, anxiety, nervousness, syncope, blackouts, depression, fatigue. *Respiratory:* Sinus congestion, pneumonia, cough, pleural rub, pulmonary fibrosis or infiltrate. *Dermatologic:* Hair loss, skin pigmentation, skin lesions, carcinoma of ear or skin, dry skin, ecchymosis. *GU:* Urinary tract infection, bladder spasms, incontinence, penile swelling, prostate pain, increased libido, urinary obstruction. *Neuromuscular:* Joint pain, ankylosing spondylitis, pelvic fibrosis, peripheral neuropathy, numbness, spinal fracture, spinal paralysis. *Miscellaneous:* Blurred vision, hypoglycemia, ophthalmologic disorders, temporal bone swelling, enlarged thyroid, inflammation, infection, hypoproteinemia, decreased white blood cells.

Depot. *Miscellaneous:* Hair growth, weight gain, hard nodule in throat.

Laboratory Test Interferences: Injection: ↑ BUN, creatinine. **Depot:** ↑ LDH, alkaline phosphatase, AST, uric acid.

Dosage: SC: 1 mg daily, using the syringes provided. **Depot, IM:** 7.5 mg q 28–33 days.

NURSING CONSIDERATIONS

See also *Nursing Considerations* for *Antineoplastic Agents,* p. 303.

Administration/Storage

1. If unrefrigerated, injection should be stored below 30°C (86°F).
2. The injection should be administered using only the syringes provided.
3. Depot may be stored at room temperature.
4. The depot should be reconstituted only with the diluent provided; after reconstitution, the preparation is stable for 24 hours. However, since there is no preservative, it should be used immediately.
5. When injecting the depot form, needles smaller than 22 gauge should not be used.

Client/Family Teaching

Stress that hot flashes are a common side effect of drug therapy.

MEDROXYPROGESTERONE ACETATE (meh-drok-see-proh-**JESS**-ter-ohn)

Amen, Curretab, Cycrin, Depo-Provera, Provera (Rx)

See also *Progesterone/Progestins,* p. 1196, and *Antineoplastic Agents,* p. 287.

Classification: Progestational hormone, synthetic.

Action/Kinetics: Medroxyprogesterone acetate, a synthetic progestin, is devoid of estrogenic and androgenic activity. The drug prevents stimulation of endometrium by pituitary gonadotropins. Also available in depot form. Priming with estrogen is necessary before response is noted.

Additional Uses: Secondary amenorrhea, abnormal uterine bleeding due to hormonal imbalance (no organic pathology). Adjunct in palliative treatment of inoperable, recurrent, or metastatic endometrial or renal carcinoma. *Investigational:* Premenopausal and menopausal symptoms (injection). To stimulate respiration in obesity—hypoventilation syndrome (oral). The depot form has been used as a long-acting contraceptive and to treat advanced breast cancer.

Contraindications: Patients with or a history of thrombophlebitis, thromboembolic disease, cerebral apoplexy. Liver dysfunction. Known or suspected malignancy of the breasts or genital organs. Missed abortion; as a diagnostic for pregnancy. Undiagnosed vaginal bleeding.

Dosage: Tablets. *Secondary amenorrhea:* 5–10 mg/day for 5–10 days, with therapy beginning at any time. If endometrium has been estrogen primed: 10 mg medroxyprogesterone per day for 10–13 days (beginning on day 16–13, respectively). *Abnormal uterine bleeding with no pathology:* 5–10 mg/day for 5–10 days, with therapy beginning on day 16 or 21 of the menstrual cycle. If endometrium has been estrogen primed: 10 mg/day for 10 days, beginning on day 16 of the menstrual cycle. Bleeding usually begins within 3–7 days. **IM.** *Endometrial or renal carcinoma:* **initial,** 400–1,000 mg weekly; **then, if improvement noted,** 400 mg monthly. Medroxyprogesterone is not intended to be the primary therapy. *Long-acting contraceptive:* 150 mg of depot form q 3 months or 450 mg of depot form q 6 months.

NURSING CONSIDERATIONS

See *Nursing Considerations* for *Antineoplastic Agents,* p. 303, and *Progesterone and Progestins,* p. 1196.

Administration

Have IV fluids, diuretics, corticosteroids and phosphate supplements available in the event the client develops severe hypercalcemia.

Interventions

1. The combined effect of the drug and osteolytic metastases may result in hypercalcemia. Therefore, note especially client complaints of insomnia, lethargy, anorexia, nausea, and vomiting. Withhold the drug, obtain serum calcium levels and report if high to the physician.
2. Encourage a high fluid intake to minimize hypercalcemia.
3. Closely monitor the client who has resumed therapy after drug-induced hypercalcemia has been corrected.

MEGESTROL ACETATE   (meh-JESS-trohl)

Megace (Rx)

See also *Progesterone/Progestins,* p. 1196, and *Antineoplastic Agents,* p. 287.

Classification: Synthetic progestin.

Action/Kinetics: The antineoplastic activity is due to suppression of gonadotropins (antiluteinizing effect). Drug contains tartrazine, which can cause allergic-type reactions, including asthma, often occurring in patients sensitive to aspirin.

Uses: Palliative treatment of endometrial or breast cancer. Should not be used as sole treatment.

Additional Contraindications: Not to be used for diagnosis of pregnancy. Pregnancy.

Side Effects: *Few:* Abdominal pain, headache, nausea, vomiting, breast tenderness, carpal tunnel syndrome (soreness, weakness, and tenderness of muscles of thumbs), deep vein thrombosis, alopecia.

Dosage: Tablets. *Breast cancer:* 40 mg q.i.d. *Endometrial cancer:* 40–320 mg/day in divided doses. To determine efficacy, treatment should be continued for at least 2 months.

NURSING CONSIDERATIONS

See *Nursing Considerations* for *Antineoplastic Agents,* p. 303, *Progesterone and Progestins,* p. 1197, and *Medroxyprogesterone Acetate,* p. 1198.

MITOTANE (O,P'-DDD)   (MY-toe-tayn)

Lysodren (Rx)

See also *Antineoplastic Agents,* p. 287.

Classification: Antihormone.

Action/Kinetics: Mitotane directly suppresses activity of adrenal cortex. It also changes the peripheral metabolism of corticosteroids resulting in a decrease in 17-hydroxycorticosteroids. About 40% of drug absorbed from GI tract; detectable in serum for long periods of time (6–9 weeks after administration). Drug, however, mostly stored in adipose tissue. $t\frac{1}{2}$: After therapy terminated, 18–159 days. Unchanged drug and metabolites are excreted in the bile and eventually the feces.

Steroid replacement therapy may have to be instituted (i.e., increased) to correct adrenal insufficiency. Therapy is continued as long as drug seems effective. Beneficial results may not become apparent until after 3 months of therapy.

Use: Inoperable cancer of the adrenal cortex. *Investigational:* Cushing's syndrome.

Contraindications: Hypersensitivity to drug. Discontinue temporarily after shock or severe trauma.

Special Concerns: Pregnancy category: C. Use with caution in the presence of liver disease other than metastatic lesions. Long-term usage may cause brain damage and functional impairment. Use during lactation only if benefits outweigh risks.

Additional Side Effects: Adrenal insufficiency. *CNS:* Depression, sedation, vertigo, lethargy. *Ophthalmic:* Blurring, diplopia, retinopathy, opacity of lens. *Renal:* Hemorrhagic cystitis, hematuria, proteinuria. *Cardiovascular:* Flushing, orthostatic hypotension, hypertension. *Miscellaneous:* Hyperpyrexia, skin rashes, aching of body.

Drug Interactions: Mitotane may ↑ rate of metabolism of heparin requiring an increase of dosage.

Laboratory Test Interferences: ↓ PBI and urinary 17-hydroxycorticosteroids.

Dosage: Tablets: Adults, initial, 8–10 g/day in 3–4 equally divided doses (maximum tolerated dose may range from 2–16 g daily). Adjust dosage upward or downward according to severity of side effects or lack thereof. **Usual maintenance:** 8–10 g/day. **Children, initial:** 1–2 g/day in divided doses; **then,** dose can be increased gradually to 5–7 g daily. *Cushing's syndrome:* **initial,** 3–6 g daily in 3–4 divided doses; **then,** 0.5 mg two times a week to 2 g daily.

NURSING CONSIDERATIONS

See also *Nursing Considerations* for *Antineoplastic Agents,* p. 303.

Administration/Storage

1. Institute treatment in hospital until stable dosage schedule is achieved.
2. Treatment should be continued for 3 months to determine beneficial effects.

Assessment

1. Assess for symptoms of adrenal insufficiency, such as weakness, increased fatigue, lethargy, and GI effects (including weight loss and anorexia).
2. Assess for evidence of brain damage by performing behavioral and neurologic assessments of client.

Interventions

1. To counteract shock or trauma, be prepared to administer steroid medications in high doses, because depressed adrenals may not produce sufficient steroids.
2. Stress importance of wearing Medic Alert identification in case of trauma or shock.

POLYESTRADIOL PHOSPHATE   (pol-ee-es-trah-**DYE**-ol)
Estradurin (Rx)

See also *Estrogens,* p. 1181.

Classification: Estrogen, steroidal, synthetic.

Action/Kinetics: Estradiol is slowly split off from the parent compound, thus providing continuous levels for long periods of time. The estradiol combines with androgen receptors; 90% of the dose leaves the plasma in 24 hr and is stored in the reticuloendothelial system and slowly released.

Use: Palliation of cancer of the prostate.

Contraindications: Pregnancy (pregnancy category: X).

Dosage: Deep IM: 40–80 mg q 2–4 weeks. Response should be noted in approximately 3 months and drug continued until the disease begins progressing again.

NURSING CONSIDERATIONS

See also *Nursing Considerations* for *Estrogens,* p. 1183.

Administration/Storage

1. Add sterile diluent to the vial with a 20-gauge needle and 5-mL syringe. Swirl *gently* to dissolve.
2. Inject deeply. IM administration is painful, and may require concomitant administration of local anesthetic.
3. Stable at room temperature for 10 days. Shield from light.
4. Do not use solutions that have a deposit or are cloudy.

Assessment

1. Assess for symptoms of hypercalcemia: insomnia, lethargy, anorexia, nausea, vomiting, coma, and vascular collapse.
2. Steroids and osteolytic metastases may cause hypercalcemia. Thus, ascertain that serum calcium concentrations are routinely done; assess results (normal: 4.5–5.5 mEq/L).
3. Monitor serum acid phosphatase levels and the client's symptomatic improvement to determine dosage requirements.

Interventions

1. For severe hypercalcemia, be prepared to assist with administration of IV fluids, diuretics, adrenocorticosteroids, and phosphate supplements.

2. Encourage bedridden clients to do passive and active exercises to prevent calcium loss from the bone.

Client/Family Teaching

1. Review S&S of hypercalcemia.
2. Avoid eating foods high in calcium.
3. Increase fluid intake to dilute calcium and to prevent urinary calculi.
4. Advise to remain active and ambulatory as long as possible.

TAMOXIFEN   (tah-**MOX**-ih-fen)

Nolvadex, Nolvadex-D✹, Tamofen✹ (Rx)

See also *Antineoplastic Agents,* p. 287.

Classification: Antiestrogen.

Action/Kinetics: Antiestrogen is believed to occupy estrogen-binding sites in target tissue (breast). It also blocks uptake of estradiol. **Peak serum levels:** 0.06–0.14 mcg/mL attained after 7–14 hr. **t½, biphasic:** initial, 7–14 hr; distribution, 4 or more days. Metabolized to the equally active desmethyltamoxifen. Tamoxifen and metabolites are excreted mainly through the feces. Objective response may be delayed 4–10 weeks with bone metastases.

Uses: Palliative treatment of breast cancer in postmenopausal women, especially those with recent positive estrogen receptor tests. *Investigational:* Mastalgia, gynecomastia (to treat pain and size).

Contraindications: Lactation. Use with caution in patients with leukopenia or thrombocytopenia.

Special Concerns: Pregnancy category: D.

Side Effects: *GI:* Nausea, vomiting, distaste for food, anorexia. *CV:* Peripheral edema, pulmonary embolism, thromboembolic disorders (especially when tamoxifen is combined with other cytotoxic agents). *CNS:* Depression, dizziness, lightheadedness, headache. *GU:* Hot flashes, vaginal bleeding and discharge, menstrual irregularities, pruritus vulvae. *Other:* Skin rash, hypercalcemia, increased bone and tumor pain, mild to moderate thrombocytopenia and leukopenia, ophthalmologic effects.

Laboratory Test Interference: ↑ Serum calcium (transient).

Dosage: Tablets: 10–20 mg b.i.d. (morning and evening). **Enteric-coated Tablets:** 10–20 mg once daily.

NURSING CONSIDERATIONS

See also *Nursing Considerations* for *Antineoplastic Agents,* p. 303.

Assessment

The effect of the steroid and osteolytic metastases may result in hypercalcemia. Assess routinely for symptoms of hypercalcemia: insomnia, lethargy, anorexia, nausea, vomiting, coma, and vascular collapse.

Interventions

1. Be certain that client with increased pain has adequate orders for analgesics; provide analgesics as needed.

2. Monitor for and report high serum calcium levels.

3. Encourage high fluid intake to minimize hypercalcemia.

4. Closely monitor clients who resume therapy after drug-induced hypercalcemia is corrected.

Client/Family Teaching

1. Advise client to report side effects to the physician, because a reduction in dosage may be indicated.

2. Explain to client experiencing increased bone and lumbar pain or local disease flares that these symptoms may be associated with a positive response to medication.

3. Advise clients to have regular ophthalmologic examinations if doses of drug are much higher than those usually recommended for antihormonal antineoplastic agents.

TESTOLACTONE   (tes-toe-**LACK**-tohn)
Teslac (Rx)

See also *Antineoplastic Agents,* p. 287.

Classification: Antineoplastic, androgen.

Action/Kinetics: Synthetic steroid related to testosterone. The drug may act to reduce synthesis of estrone from adrenal androstenedione by inhibiting steroid aromatase activity. The drug is well absorbed from the GI tract. It is metabolized in the liver and unchanged drug and metabolites are excreted through the urine. Does not cause virilization.

Uses: Palliative treatment of advanced or disseminated mammary cancer in postmenopausal women or in premenopausal ovariectomized patients.

Additional Contraindications: Breast cancer in men; premenopausal women with intact ovaries.

Special Concerns: Pregnancy category: C. Safety and efficacy have not been determined in children.

Additional Side Effects: *GI:* Nausea, vomiting, glossitis, anorexia. *CNS:* Numbness or tingling of fingers, toes, face. *Miscellaneous:* Inflammation and irritation at injection site; increases BP during parenteral administration. Hypercalcemia. Maculopapular erythema, alopecia. See also *Testosterone,* p. 1230.

Drug Interactions: Testolactone may ↑ effect of oral anticoagulants.

Laboratory Test Interferences: ↑ Plasma calcium, urinary excretion of creatinine and 17-ketosteroids. ↓ Estradiol levels using radioimmunoassays.

Dosage: Tablets: 250 mg q.i.d. Therapy usually should be continued for 3 months.

NURSING CONSIDERATIONS

See also *Nursing Considerations* for *Antineoplastic Agents,* p. 303.

Interventions

1. Anticipate a reduction in dose of anticoagulants if client is on concomitant therapy.

2. The effect of the steroid and osteolytic metastases may result in hypercalcemia. Thus, assess routinely for symptoms of hypercalcemia: insomnia, lethargy, anorexia, nausea, vomiting, coma, and vascular collapse.

3. Withhold drug and report high serum calcium levels.
4. Encourage high fluid intake to minimize hypercalcemia.
5. Closely monitor clients who resume therapy after drug-induced hypercalcemia is corrected.

RADIOACTIVE ISOTOPES

CHROMIC PHOSPHATE P 32 (KROH-mick)

Phosphocol P 32 (Rx)

Classification: Antineoplastic, radioactive isotope.

Action/Kinetics: When introduced into a body cavity, the chromic phosphate P 32 is phagocytized by free macrophages and fixed to the lining of the cavity. This produces local irradiation to impede the growth of neoplastic cells. $t^{1/2}$: 14.3 days. Eliminated primarily through the urine.

Uses: Treatment of peritoneal or pleural effusions caused by metastatic disease (intracavitary) or localized disease (interstitial). Ovarian or prostatic carcinoma.

Additional Contraindications: Ulcerative tumors. Exposed cavities. Intravascular use. Lactation.

Special Concerns: Use during pregnancy only if the benefits clearly outweigh the risks. Safety and efficacy have not been determined in children.

Side Effects: Transitory radiation sickness, pleuritis, peritonitis, bone marrow depression, nausea and abdominal cramping. Radiation damage when injected accidentally interstitially or into a loculation (small space).

Dosage: For average (70 kg) patient: **Intraperitoneal instillation:** 10–20 mCi. **Intrapleural instillation:** 6–12 mCi. **Interstitial administration:** 0.1–0.5 mCi/g of estimated tumor weight.

NURSING CONSIDERATIONS

See also *Nursing Considerations* for *Antineoplastic Agents,* p. 303.

Administration/Storage

1. Administered by physician.
2. Measure client's dose using suitable radioactive calibration system immediately before administration.

Interventions

1. For radiation protection, follow specific and appropriate institutional guidelines.
2. Provide supportive nursing care to the client suffering from malaise and abdominal cramping caused by radiation.

SODIUM IODIDE I 131 (SO-dee-um EYE-oh-dyd)

Iodotope (Rx)

See *Thyroid and Antithyroid Drugs,* p. 1120.

SODIUM PHOSPHATE P 32   (SO-dee-um FOS-fayt)

(Rx)

Classification: Antineoplastic, radioactive isotope.

Action/Kinetics: The radioactive phosphorus of the drug concentrates in rapidly proliferating tissue. Upon decay, it emits beta particles. **t½:** 14.3 days. Initially the radioactivity decreases rapidly (25–50% in 4–6 days), then much more slowly (more than 1% a day). Remaining radioactivity concentrates in osseous tissue. Eliminated primarily through the urine with 5–10% within 24 hr and 20% within one week.

Uses: Polycythemia vera (with adjunctive phlebotomy), chronic myelocytic leukemia, chronic lymphocytic leukemia, or bone metastases.

Additional Contraindications: Lactation. Children younger than 18 years of age, or acute episodes of leukemia. Polycythemia vera in patients with leukocyte count of less than 5,000/mm³, platelet count of less than 150,000/mm³, or reticulocyte count of less than 0.2%. Chronic myelocytic leukemia with a leukocyte count of less than 20,000/mm³. Bone metastases with a leukocyte count of less than 5,000/mm³ or platelet count of less than 100,000/mm³. Sequential therapy with a chemotherapeutic agent.

Special Concerns: Pregnancy category: C. Geriatric patients may be more sensitive to the effects of radiation necessitating smaller doses and longer intervals between doses. Dosage has not been established in children.

Side Effects: Bone marrow depression. Radiation sickness (rare).

Dosage: IV only. *Polycythemia vera:* 3–5 mCi; dose may be repeated in 12 weeks if necessary. *Leukemias:* 1–3 mCi (with hormone manipulation).

NURSING CONSIDERATIONS

See also *Nursing Considerations* for *Antineoplastic Agents,* p. 303.

Administration/Storage

1. Store at room temperature in containers suitable for absorption of radiation.
2. Solution and container may darken, but this does not affect efficacy.
3. Note expiration date—should be 2 months after date of standardization.
4. Have client fast for 2 hr before and 6 hr after administration of drug to minimize the amount of unabsorbed radioactive material.
5. The dose should be measured by a radioactivity calibration system just before being administered.
6. Avoid using milk and milk products, iron, bismuth, and soft drinks for clients on sodium phosphate P 32.

Interventions

1. For radiation protection, follow specific and appropriate institutional guidelines for clients and staff.
2. Provide supportive nursing care for clients suffering from malaise and abdominal cramping caused by radiation.
3. Isotope (drug) should only be administered by trained personnel.
4. Initiate and follow appropriate dietary restrictions.

PART FOUR

Drugs Affecting Blood Formation and Coagulation

CHAPTER NINETEEN

Antianemic Drugs

General Statement: Anemia refers to the many clinical conditions in which there is a deficiency in the number of red blood cells (RBCs) or in the hemoglobin level within those cells. Hemoglobin is a complex substance consisting of a large protein (globin) and an iron-containing chemical referred to as heme. The hemoglobin is contained inside the RBCs. Its function is to combine with oxygen in the lungs and transport it to all tissues of the body, where it is exchanged for carbon dioxide (which is transported back to the lungs where it can be excreted). A lack of either RBCs or hemoglobin may result in an inadequate supply of oxygen to various tissues.

The average life span of a RBC is 120 days; thus, new ones have to be constantly formed. They are produced in the bone marrow, with both vitamin B_{12} and folic acid playing an important role in their formation. In addition, a sufficient amount of iron is necessary for the formation and maturation of RBCs. This iron is supplied in a normal diet and is also salvaged from old RBCs. There are many types of anemia. However, the two main categories are (1) iron-deficiency anemias, resulting from greater than normal loss or destruction of blood cells, and (2) megaloblastic anemias, resulting from deficient production of blood cells. Iron-deficiency anemia can result from hemorrhage or blood loss; the bone marrow is unable to replace the quantity of RBCs lost even when working at maximum capacity (due to iron-deficient diet or failure to absorb iron from the GI tract). The RBCs in iron-deficiency anemias (also called *microcytic* or *hypochromic anemias*) contain too little hemoglobin. When examined under the microscope, they are paler and sometimes smaller than normal. The cause of the iron deficiency must be determined before therapy is started.

Therapy consists of administering compounds containing iron so as to increase the body's supplies.

Megaloblastic anemias may result from insufficient supplies of the necessary vitamins and minerals needed by the bone marrow to manufacture blood cells. Pernicious anemia, for example, results from inadequate vitamin B_{12}. The RBCs characteristic of the megaloblastic anemias are enlarged and particularly rich in hemoglobin. However, the blood contains fewer mature RBCs than normal and usually contains a relatively higher number of immature RBCs (megaloblasts) that have been prematurely released from the bone marrow.

Iron Preparations

These agents are usually a complex of iron and another substance and are normally taken by mouth. The amount absorbed from the GI tract depends on the dose administered; therefore the largest dose that can be tolerated without causing side effects is given. Under certain conditions, iron compounds must be given parenterally, particularly (1) when there is some disorder limiting the amount of drug absorbed from the intestine or (2) when the patient is unable to tolerate oral iron.

Iron preparations are effective only in the treatment of anemias specifically resulting from iron deficiency. Blood loss is almost always the only cause of iron deficiency in adult males and postmenopausal females. The daily iron requirement is increased by growth and pregnancy, and iron deficiency is, therefore, particularly common in infants and young children on diets low in iron. Pregnant women and women with heavy menstrual blood loss may also be deficient in iron.

Iron is available for therapy in two forms: bivalent and trivalent. Bivalent (ferrous) iron salts are administered more often than trivalent (ferric) salts because they are less astringent and less irritating than ferric salts and are better absorbed.

Iron preparations are particularly suitable for the treatment of anemias in infants and children, in blood donors, during pregnancy, and in patients with chronic blood loss. Optimum therapeutic responses are usually noted within 2 to 4 weeks of treatment.

The RDA for iron is 90–300 mg daily.

Action/Kinetics: Iron is an essential mineral normally supplied in the diet. Iron salts and other preparations supply additional iron to meet the needs of the patient. Iron is absorbed from the GI tract through the mucosal cells where it combines with the protein transferrin. This complex is transported in the body to bone marrow where iron is incorporated into hemoglobin. Absorption kinetics depend on the iron salt ingested and on the degree of deficiency. Under normal circumstances, iron is well conserved by the body although small amounts are lost through shedding of skin, hair, and nails and in feces, perspiration, urine, breast milk, and during menstruation. Iron is highly bound to protein.

Uses: Prophylaxis and treatment of iron-deficiency anemia.

Contraindications: Patients with hemosiderosis, hemochromatosis, peptic ulcer, regional enteritis, and ulcerative colitis. Hemolytic anemia, pyridoxine-responsive anemia, and cirrhosis of the liver.

Drug Interactions	
Allopurinol	May ↑ hepatic iron levels
Antacids, oral	↓ Effect of iron preparations due to ↓ absorption from GI tract
Chloramphenicol	Chloramphenicol ↓ iron clearance from plasma and ↓ iron uptake into red blood cells
Cholestyramine	↓ Effect of iron preparations due to ↓ absorption from GI tract

Drug Interactions

Pancreatic extracts	↓ Effect of iron preparations due to ↓ absorption from GI tract
Penicillamine	↓ Effect of penicillamine due to ↓ absorption from GI tract
Tetracyclines	↓ Effect of tetracyclines due to ↓ absorption from GI tract
Vitamin E	Vitamin E ↓ response to iron therapy

Side Effects: *GI effects:* Constipation, gastric irritation, mild nausea, abdominal cramps, and diarrhea. These effects may be minimized by administering preparations as a coated tablet. Soluble iron preparations may stain the teeth.

Toxic reactions are more likely to occur after parenteral administration and include nausea and vomiting, fever, peripheral vascular collapse, and fatal anaphylactoid reactions. These symptoms may occur within 60 sec of a toxic dose. Symptoms may then disappear for 6 to 24 hr, followed by a second crisis. Symptoms including nausea and diarrhea or constipation may occur after use of oral preparations.

Treatment of Iron Toxicity

The treatment of iron intoxication is symptomatic. It concentrates on removing iron from the body and combating shock and acidosis. Vomiting should be induced immediately, followed by the administration of eggs and milk. Other measures include gastric lavage with aqueous solutions of sodium bicarbonate or sodium phosphate, followed by oral bismuth subcarbonate as a protectant and IV dextrose and sodium chloride injection to correct dehydration. Plasma, whole blood, calcium disodium edetate, deferoxamine, methionine, oxygen, and antibiotics may be ordered.

Some patients may report late manifestations 1 to 2 months after toxic overdosage. These late manifestations include GI distress caused by necrotic alterations of the gastric or intestinal mucosa. Residual effects may also include pyloric stenosis, fibrosis of the liver, and dilatation of the right side of the heart with pulmonary congestion and hemorrhage.

Laboratory Test Interference: Iron-containing drugs may affect electrolyte balance determinations.

Dosage: See individual drugs. Most replacement iron is given orally in daily doses of 90–300 mg elemental iron. Duration of therapy: 2–4 months longer than the time needed to reverse anemia, usually 6 or more months.

NURSING CONSIDERATIONS

Administration/Storage

For infants and young children, administer liquid preparation with a dropper. Deposit liquid well back against the cheek.

Assessment

1. Prior to administering medication, assess client and take a complete drug history, including:
   - client use of antacids and any other drugs that may interact with these preparations.
   - any over the counter drugs such as iron compounds or vitamin E that are in use.
2. Ask client about any evidence of GI bleeding such as tarry stools or bright red blood.
3. Note any complaints of fatigue, pallor, poor skin turgor, or change in mental status, especially among the elderly.

4. Assess diet through questioning as well as observation of intake if possible.

5. Pregnancy has generally been considered an indication for prescribing iron prophylactically.

Interventions

1. Establish goals for therapy with client and other members of the health care team.

2. Check for occult blood if GI bleeding is suspected, as drugs alter stool color.

3. Encourage persons with symptoms of anemia to seek medical assistance; discourage self-medication with iron based on symptoms only.

4. Coated tablets may be prescribed to diminish effects on the GI tract such as nausea, constipation or diarrhea, gastric irritation, and abdominal cramps.

5. Be prepared to assist with treatment of clients who may develop symptoms of iron intoxication, (most likely to occur after parenteral administration). If a client has iron poisoning, stop iron administration, notify physician, and monitor vital signs for 48 hours since a second crisis is likely to occur within 12–48 hrs. of the first one. Follow guidelines for *Treatment of Iron Toxicity*.

6. Anticipate that the medication will be discontinued if 500 mg of iron daily does not cause a rise of at least 2 mg/100 mL of hemoglobin in 3 weeks.

7. Iron will reduce the absorption of tetracycline. If a client is to receive tetracyclines as well as iron products, establish a schedule that allows at least two hours to elapse between administering the iron product and the tetracycline.

Client/Family Teaching

1. Many clients will be taking their medications at home and without constant supervision. Therefore, it is important to teach them to adhere to the prescribed regimen and report any problems with medication therapy immediately.

2. Advise clients to take iron preparations with meals to reduce gastric irritation.

3. Taking iron preparations with citrus juices enhances the absorption of iron.

4. Unless taking ferrous lactate, advise the client *NOT* to take iron compounds with milk products or antacids as these will interfere with absorption.

5. Discuss with the client the possibility of indigestion, change in stool color (black and tarry or dark green), and constipation.

6. Explain the possible untoward effects that may occur (gastric irritation, constipation or diarrhea, abdominal cramps) and encourage immediate reporting of these symptoms as they may be relieved by changing the medication, dosage, or time of administration.

7. Encourage clients to eat a well balanced diet, stressing the intake of foods high in iron. When working with poor families, explore the kinds of foods they can afford to assure that the diet prescribed is one they have access to (ex. raisins, green vegetables and liver may be more affordable than apricots or prunes).

8. Iron preparations are extremely dangerous for children. An overdosage can be fatal so keep iron preparations out of the reach of children.

9. When administering liquid iron medications to young children dilute well with water or fruit juice and use a straw to minimize the possibility of staining the teeth.

10. When working with pregnant women review their need for an iron rich diet. Also, The American Academy of Pediatrics recommends an iron supplement for infants during their first year of life.

11. Follow administration guidelines for each product to minimize side effects.

Evaluation

1. Evaluate client changes in exercise tolerance.
2. Check client compliance with the drug regimen.
3. Compare client condition against the baseline data prior to drug administration (skin pallor, color of nail beds, prior blood studies, changes in stool color, etc.).
4. Assess blood pressure, pulse rate, respirations, and any skin lesions for evidence of appropriate drug response.

FERROUS FUMARATE   (FEHR-rus)

Femiron, Feostat, Feostat Drops, Fumasorb, Fumerin, Hemocyte, Ircon, NeoFer✱, Novofumar✱, Palafer✱, Palafer Pediatric Drops✱, Palmiron, Span-FF (OTC)

See also *Antianemic Drugs,* p. 379.

Classification: Antianemic, iron.

Action/Kinetics: Better tolerated than ferrous gluconate or ferrous sulfate. Contains 33% elemental iron.

Dosage: Extended-release Capsules: Adults: 325 mg daily (for prophylaxis) or 325 mg b.i.d. (to treat anemia). Capsules are not recommended for use in children. **Oral Solution, Oral Suspension, Tablets, Chewable Tablets: Adults:** 200 mg daily (for prophylaxis) or 200 mg t.i.d.–q.i.d. (to treat anemia). **Children:** 3 mg/kg daily (prophylaxis) or 3 mg/kg t.i.d., up to 6 mg/kg daily, if needed (to treat anemia).

NURSING CONSIDERATIONS

See *Nursing Considerations* for *Antianemic Drugs,* p. 381.

FERROUS GLUCONATE   (FEHR-rus)

Apo-Ferrous Gluconate✱, Fergon, Ferralet, Fertinic✱, Novoferrogluc✱, Simron (OTC)

See also *Antianemic Drugs,* p. 379.

Classification: Antianemic, iron.

Use: Particularly indicated for patients who cannot tolerate ferrous sulfate because of gastric irritation.

Dosage: Preparation contains 11.6% elemental iron. **Capsules, Tablets. Adults:** 325 mg daily (prophylaxis) or 325 mg q.i.d. (for anemia). Can be increased to 650 mg q.i.d. if needed and tolerated. **Children, 2 years and older:** 8 mg/kg daily (prophylaxis) or 16 mg/kg t.i.d. (for anemia). **Elixir, Syrup. Adults:** 300 mg daily (prophylaxis) or 300 mg q.i.d. (for anemia). Can be increased to 600 mg q.i.d. as needed and tolerated. **Children, 2 years and older:** 8 mg/kg daily (prophylaxis) or 16 mg/kg t.i.d. (for anemia).
The physician must determine dosage for children less than 2 years of age.

NURSING CONSIDERATIONS

See *Nursing Considerations* for *Antianemic Drugs,* p. 381.

FERROUS SULFATE   (FEHR-rus)

Apo-Ferrous Sulfate✣, Feosol, Fer-In-Sol, Fer-Iron, Fero-Grad✣, Ferogradumet, Ferospace, Ferra-TD, Ferralyn Lanacaps, Mol-Iron, Novoferrosulfa✣, PMS Ferrous Sulfate✣ (OTC)

FERROUS SULFATE, DRIED   (FEHR-rus)

Feosol, Fer-in-Sol, Slow-Fe (OTC)

See also *Antianemic Drugs,* p. 379.

Classification: Antianemic, iron.

Action/Kinetics: Least expensive, most effective iron salt for oral therapy. Ferrous sulfate products contain 20% elemental iron, while ferrous sulfate dried products contain 30% elemental iron. The exsiccated form is more stable in air.

Dosage: *Ferrous Sulfate.* **Extended-release Capsules. Adults:** 150–250 mg 1–2 times daily. This dosage form is not recommended for children. **Elixir, Oral Solution, Tablets, Enteric-Coated Tablets. Adults:** 300 mg daily (prophylaxis) or 300 mg b.i.d. increased to 300 mg q.i.d. as needed and tolerated (for anemia). **Children:** 5 mg/kg daily (prophylaxis) or 10 mg/kg t.i.d. (for anemia). The enteric-coated tablets are not recommended for use in children. **Extended-Release Tablets. Adults:** 525 mg 1–2 times daily. This dosage form is not recommended for use in children.
Ferrous Sulfate, Dried. **Capsules. Adults:** 300 mg daily (prophylaxis) or 300 mg b.i.d. up to 300 mg q.i.d. as needed and tolerated (for anemia). **Children:** 5 mg/kg daily (prophylaxis) or 10 mg/kg t.i.d. (for anemia). **Tablets. Adults:** 200 mg daily (prophylaxis) or 200 mg t.i.d. up to 200 mg q.i.d. as needed and tolerated (for anemia). **Children:** Same dosage as ferrous sulfate, dried capsules. **Extended-release Tablets. Adults:** 160 mg 1–2 times daily. This dosage form is not recommended for use in children.

NURSING CONSIDERATIONS

See *Nursing Considerations* for *Antianemic Drugs,* p. 381.

IRON DEXTRAN INJECTION   (DEX-tran)

Dex Iron, Feostat, Imferon, Irodex, Norefmi, Nor-Feran, Proferdex, Z-Tex (Rx)

Classification: Iron preparation, parenteral.

Action/Kinetics: Iron dextran injection is a complex containing ferric oxyhydroxide and low molecular weight dextran. Following absorption from IM sites, the complex is split in the reticuloendothelial system to dextran and iron. The iron is then used by the body to replenish hemoglobin. The amount of available elemental iron varies. Most of an IM injection is absorbed within 72 hr with the remaining iron absorbed over 3–4 weeks. Although not recommended, the drug may be administered IV. **t½, after IV:** 5–20 hr (does not represent clearance of iron from the body).

Uses: IM or IV for iron deficiency anemias only when oral administration of iron is not possible.

Contraindications: Pernicious anemia, acute leukemia in the absence of iron depletion by blood loss, anemia associated with chronic leukemia or bone marrow depression, and other anemias not resulting from iron deficiency. Hypersensitivity to drug. Siderosis, hemochromatosis, or severe renal or hepatic failure. Infants less than 4 months of age. Use with oral iron preparations.

Special Concerns: Pregnancy category: C. Use with caution during lactation and in individuals with a history of asthma or allergies.

Side Effects: *Allergic:* Anaphylaxis, rashes, itching, myalgia, arthralgia, fever, allergic purpura, dyspnea, urticaria. *GI:* Nausea, vomiting, diarrhea, abdominal pain. *CV:* Hypotension, tachycardia, shock, chest pain (all due to rapid IV injection). *Hematologic:* Leukocytosis, lymphadenopathy. *CNS:* Headache, weakness, syncope, seizures. *Miscellaneous:* Reactivation of arthritis, paresthesia, chills, hematuria, bronchospasm, sweating.

Due to IM administration: Abscess formation, atrophy, fibrosis, necrosis, cellulitis, swelling, tissue discoloration (brown skin), soreness or pain at injection site. *Due to IV administration:* Phlebitis at site.

Laboratory Test Interferences: Falsely elevated serum bilirubin, prolongation of partial thromboplastin time, falsely decreased serum calcium, interference with bone scans involving Tc-99m diphosphonate.

Dosage: Test dose prior to therapeutic regimen: IM, IV: 25 mg (0.5 mL); observe patient for at least 1 hr. *Iron-deficiency anemia:* **IM:** Use dosage formula. **Maximum daily doses of iron: Adults over 50 kg:** 250 mg; **adults and children 9–50 kg:** 100 mg; **infants 3.5–9 kg:** 50 mg; **infants under 3.5 kg:** 25 mg. **IV:** Calculate dosage according to formula and dilute needed dose in 200–250 mL saline. If no reaction to test dose, give needed dose over 1–2 hrs.

NURSING CONSIDERATIONS

See also *Nursing Considerations* for *Antianemic Drugs,* p. 381.

Administration/Storage

1. No more than 2 mL/day should be given as an IV injection.
2. Although not a labeled indication, some physicians recommend giving the entire dose of iron dextran by a single IV infusion. If this approach is used, the amount of iron needed should be diluted with normal saline to 200–250 mL.
3. A test dose of 25 mg should be given over 5 min and, if no untoward reactions occur, the rest given over 1–2 hr.
4. Iron dextran should never be mixed with other medications or added to parenteral nutrition solutions for IV infusion.

Assessment

1. Take a complete drug history, noting any evidence of prior untoward reactions to drugs in this category.
2. Prior to initiating therapy check that a small test dose has been ordered and administered without any adverse effects.
3. Ascertain that appropriate blood studies have been done.
4. Assure that the client is properly hydrated before therapy begins. Otherwise, dextran may attract water to the extravascular spaces and result in further dehydration of the client.

Interventions

1. Obtain blood pressure and pulse. Check specific gravity of urine and other evidence of renal function to serve as baseline data against which to determine client response to therapy.
2. For Intramuscular Injection:
   - If the client is standing to receive the injection instruct him/her to bear weight on the leg

opposite from the injection site. Clients in bed should be positioned laterally, with the injection site uppermost.
- Check prior injection site and alternate. Chart the site of injection and discuss the importance of the alternate site with the client to facilitate accurate transfer of information.
- Prevent staining of skin by using a separate needle to withdraw medication from the container and by using the Z-track method of injection.
- Using a 2-inch needle, 19–20 gauge, insert the solution deeply into the upper outer quadrant of the gluteus muscle. Do not inject more than 5 mL IM/day. *Never* inject into the arm or other exposed areas.
- Before injecting the medication, withdraw the plunger of the syringe to check that the needle is not in a blood vessel.

3. Iron dextran can alter certain tests for blood glucose, urinary protein, and bilirubin. Therefore, alert the laboratory if any of these tests are ordered for clients receiving iron dextran.
4. Iron dextran can interfere with blood typing and cross-matching. If these procedures are to be done, be sure they are performed before administering iron dextran.
5. Monitor pulse, blood pressure and urine output every 5–15 minutes for the first hour after dextran has been administered. The drug should be discontinued if there is any evidence of renal dysfunction.

Evaluation

1. Note changes in the client's overall condition.
2. Assess for evidence of allergic responses that may occur (i.e. rashes, itching, fever, dyspnea).
3. Note any evidence of abscess formation, necrosis, swelling, tissue discoloration or soreness at the injection site.
4. Assess pretreatment and posttreatment lab studies. Check for prolonged bleeding and clotting times, decreased hematocrit or decreased plasma levels that may result from excessive dilution of blood constituents.
5. Check for any evidence of renal dysfunction.

IRON POLYSACCHARIDE   (EYE-urn pol-ee-SACK-ah-ryd)

Hytinic, Niferex, Niferex-150, Nu-Iron, Nu-Iron 150 (OTC)

Classification: Antianemic, iron-polysaccharide complex.

Action/Kinetics: Easily absorbable complex with relatively little GI upset and low toxicity. This product is the ferric form with the percentage elemental iron variable. Tablets contain 50 mg iron, the elixir contains 100 mg iron/5 mL, and the capsules contain 150 mg iron. This product does not stain teeth.

Dosage: Capsules, Tablets. Adults: 150 mg (elemental ferric iron) daily (prophylaxis) or 150 mg (elemental ferric iron) b.i.d. increased to q.i.d. as needed and tolerated (for anemia). **Children:** 1.5 mg (elemental ferric iron)/kg daily. **Elixir. Adults:** 100 mg (elemental ferric iron) daily (prophylaxis) or 100 mg (elemental ferric iron) b.i.d. up to q.i.d. as needed and tolerated (for anemia). **Children:** 1.5 mg (elemental ferric iron)/kg daily.

NURSING CONSIDERATIONS
See *Nursing Considerations* for *Antianemic Drugs,* p. 381.

CHAPTER TWENTY

Anticoagulants And Hemostatics

20

General Statement: Blood coagulation is a precise mechanism that can be defined as follows:

1. The process of coagulation is initiated when an inactive precursor escapes from the damaged platelets and activates *thromboplastin.*
2. The activated thromboplastin helps convert the protein *prothrombin* into *thrombin.*
3. *Thrombin* mediates the formation of the threadlike *fibrin*—an insoluble protein—from the soluble *fibrinogen.* The latter forms a clot, trapping blood cells and platelets. Vitamin K, calcium, and various accessory factors manufactured in the liver are essential for blood coagulation.

Once formed, the blood clot is dissolved by another enzymatic chain reaction involving a substance called fibrinolysin.

Blood coagulation can be affected by a number of diseases. An excessive tendency to form blood clots is one of the main factors involved in cardiovascular disorders, and a defect in the clotting mechanism is the cause of hemophilia and related diseases.

Since several of the factors that participate in blood clotting are manufactured by the liver, severe liver disease can also affect blood clotting, as does vitamin K deficiency.

Drugs that influence blood coagulation can be divided into three classes: (1) *anticoagulants,* or drugs that prevent or slow blood coagulation; (2) *thrombolytic agents,* which increase the rate at which an existing blood clot dissolves; and (3) *hemostatics,* which prevent or stop internal bleeding. Protamine sulfate, whose sole use is to correct heparin overdosage, is listed at the end of the anticoagulant section.

The dosage of all agents discussed in this chapter must be carefully adjusted since overdosage can have serious consequences.

ANTICOAGULANTS

General Statement: There are three major types of anticoagulants: (1) dicumarol and warfarin, (2) anisindione (indanedione-type) and (3) heparin. The following considerations are pertinent to each type.

Anticoagulant drugs are used mainly in the management of patients with thromboembolic disease; they do not dissolve previously formed clots, but they do forestall their enlargement and prevent new clots from forming.

Uses: Venous thrombosis, pulmonary embolism, acute coronary occlusions with myocardial infarctions, and strokes caused by emboli or cerebral thrombi.

Prophylactically for rheumatic heart disease, atrial fibrillation, traumatic injuries of blood vessels, vascular surgery, major abdominal, thoracic, and pelvic surgery, prevention of strokes in patients with transient attacks of cerebral ischemia, or other signs of impending stroke.

Contraindications: Patients with possible defects in the clotting mechanism (hemophilia) or with frail or weakened blood vessels, peptic ulcer, chronic ulcerations of the GI tract, hepatic and renal dysfunction, subacute bacterial endocarditis, or severe hypertension. Also after neurosurgery or recent surgery of the eye, spinal cord, or brain, or in the presence of drainage tubes in any orifice. Alcoholism.

NURSING CONSIDERATIONS

Assessment

1. Obtain a thorough nursing history and complete drug profile prior to initiating therapy. Note any potential drug interactions.
2. Through the health history profile identify client complaints that may indicate defects in the clotting mechanism.
3. Observe for any evidence of weakened blood vessel walls (capillary fragility).
4. Review past health problems (peptic ulcer, evidence of chronic ulcerations of the GI tract, renal or liver dysfunction, infections of the endocardium, hypertension) as evidence for contraindications to this therapy.
5. Note any evidence of alcoholism as anticoagulants are contraindicated. This is particularly important when working with clients who are homeless. Also, such evidence suggests the client may have problems with drug compliance.
6. Determine that appropriate blood tests have been conducted to serve as a baseline against which to measure response of the client to treatment.

Warfarin and Indanedione-type Anticoagulants

Action/Kinetics: These drugs act only in vivo by preventing the formation of factors II, VII, IX, and X in the liver due to inhibition of vitamin K-mediated gamma-carboxylation of precursor proteins. There is a delay in reaching full beneficial effects since circulating coagulating factors must first be removed by normal catabolism. Highly bound to albumin (99%). The drugs are metabolized by the liver and excreted through the urine.

Uses: Prophylaxis and treatment of deep venous thrombosis, pulmonary thromboembolism, thrombophlebitis. Prophylaxis of thromboembolism due to chronic atrial fibrillation or myocardial infarction. *Investigational:* Reduce risk of postconversion emboli; prophylaxis of recurrent, cerebral thromboembolism; prophylaxis of myocardial reinfarction; treatment of transient ischemic attacks in men and women; reduce the risk of thromboembolic complications in patients with certain types of prosthetic heart valves; reduced risk of thrombosis and/or occlusion following coronary bypass surgery.

Heparin is often used concurrently during the therapeutic initiation period.

Contraindications: Hemorrhagic tendencies, blood dyscrasias, ulcerative lesions of the GI tract, diverticulitis, colitis, subacute bacterial endocarditis, threatened abortion, recent operations on the eye, brain, or spinal cord, regional anesthesia and lumbar block, vitamin K deficiency, leukemia with bleeding tendencies, thrombocytopenic purpura, open wounds or ulcerations, acute nephritis, impaired hepatic or renal function, or severe hypertension.

Special Concerns: The drugs should be used with caution in menstruating women, in pregnant women (because they may cause hypoprothrombinemia in the infant), during lactation, during the postpartum period, and following cerebrovascular accidents. Geriatric patients may be more susceptible to the effects of anticoagulants.

Side Effects: *CV:* Hemorrhagic accidents are the chief danger of anticoagulant therapy. Frequent prothrombin time determinations should be performed for patients on long-term therapy to ascertain that values remain within safe levels. *GI:* Nausea, vomiting, diarrhea, abdominal cramps, anorexia. *Dermatologic:* Necrosis or gangrene of the skin and other tissues, alopecia, dermatitis, urticaria. *Hematologic:* Agranulocytosis, eosinophilia, leukopenia. *Other:* Fever, delayed hypersensitivity reactions, priapism, urine that becomes red-orange in color, mouth ulcers, nephropathy, hepatotoxicity, jaundice.

Blood in urine may be a first warning of impending hemorrhage.

Antidotes

Coumarin-type drugs can be counteracted by oral (100–200 mg) or IV (50–100 mg) administration of vitamin K (phytonadione).

Fresh whole blood or plasma transfusions may be required in emergencies.

Drug Interactions: These drugs are responsible for more adverse drug interactions than any other group. Patients on anticoagulant therapy must be monitored carefully each time a drug is added or withdrawn.

Monitoring usually involves determination of prothrombin time. In general, a lengthened prothrombin time means potentiation of the anticoagulant. Since potentiation may mean hemorrhages, a lengthened prothrombin time warrants **reduction of the dosage of the anticoagulant.** However, the anticoagulant dosage must again be increased when the second drug is discontinued.

A shortened prothrombin time means inhibition of the anticoagulant and may require an increase in dosage.

Drug Interactions

Acetaminophen	Slight ↑ in hypoprothrombinemia
Alcohol, ethyl	↑ or ↓ Effect of oral anticoagulants
Allopurinol	↑ Effect of anticoagulants due to ↓ breakdown by liver
Aminoglycoside antibiotics	Potentiate pharmacologic effect of anticoagulants
Anabolic steroids	Potentiate pharmacologic effect of anticoagulants
Antacids, oral	↓ Effect of anticoagulants due to ↓ absorption from GI tract
Antidepressants, tricyclic	↑ Effect of anticoagulants due to ↓ breakdown by liver
Barbiturates	↓ Effect of anticoagulants due to ↑ breakdown by liver
Carbamazepine	↓ Effect of anticoagulants due to ↑ breakdown by liver
Cephalosporins	↑ Effect of anticoagulants due to ↑ prothrombin time
Chloral hydrate	↑ Effect of anticoagulants by ↓ plasma protein binding
Chloramphenicol	↑ Effect of anticoagulant due to ↓ breakdown by liver
Cholestyramine	↓ Anticoagulant effect due to binding in and ↓ absorption from GI tract
Cimetidine	↑ Anticoagulant effect due to ↓ breakdown by liver
Clofibrate	↑ Anticoagulant effect by ↓ plasma protein binding
Colestipol	↓ Effect of anticoagulants due to ↓ absorption from GI tract
Contraceptives, oral	↓ Anticoagulant effect by ↑ activity of certain clotting factors (VII and X)
Contrast media containing iodine	↑ Effect of anticoagulants by ↑ prothrombin time
Corticosteroids, corticosterone	↓ Effect of anticoagulants by ↓ hypoprothrombinemia; also ↑ risk of GI bleeding due to ulcerogenic effect of steroids
Danazol	↑ Effect of anticoagulants
Dextrothyroxine	↑ Effect of anticoagulants
Disulfiram	↑ Effect of anticoagulants by ↓ breakdown by liver
Estrogens	↓ Anticoagulant response by ↑ activity of certain clotting factors
Ethchlorvynol	↓ Effect of anticoagulants due to ↑ breakdown by liver
Glucagon	↑ Effect of anticoagulants by ↑ hypoprothrombinemia

Drug Interactions

Glutethimide	↓ Effect of anticoagulants due to ↑ breakdown by liver
Griseofulvin	↓ Effect of anticoagulants due to ↑ breakdown by liver
Haloperidol	↓ Effect of anticoagulants due to ↑ breakdown by liver
Heparin	↑ Effect by ↑ prothrombin time
Hypoglycemics, oral	↑ Effect of anticoagulants due to ↓ plasma protein binding; also, ↑ effect of sulfonylureas
Indomethacin	↑ Effect of anticoagulants by ↓ plasma protein binding; also, indomethacin is ulcerogenic and may inhibit platelet function, leading to hemorrhage
Methotrexate	Additive hypoprothrombinemia
Methylthiouracil	Additive hypoprothrombinemia
Metronidazole	↑ Effect of anticoagulants due to ↓ breakdown by liver
Mineral oil	↑ Hypoprothrombinemia by ↓ absorption of vitamin K from GI tract; also mineral oil may ↓ absorption of anticoagulants from GI tract
Penicillin	Penicillin may potentiate the pharmacologic effect of anticoagulants
Phenylbutazone	↑ Effect of anticoagulants by ↓ plasma protein binding and ↓ breakdown by liver; phenylbutazone may also produce GI ulceration and therefore ↑ chance of bleeding
Phenytoin	↑ Effect of phenytoin due to ↓ in breakdown by liver; also possible ↑ in anticoagulant effect by ↓ plasma protein binding
Propylthiouracil	Additive hypoprothrombinemia
Quinidine, quinine	Additive hypoprothrombinemia
Rifampin	↓ Anticoagulant effect due to ↑ breakdown by liver
Salicylates	↑ Effect of anticoagulants by ↓ plasma protein binding, ↓ plasma prothrombin, and ↓ platelet aggregation; also, ↑ risk of GI bleeding due to ulcerogenic effect of salicylates
Sulfinpyrazone	↑ Anticoagulant effect due to ↓ breakdown by liver and inhibition of platelet aggregation
Sulfonamides	↑ Effect of sulfonamides by ↑ blood levels; also ↑ anticoagulant effect due to ↓ plasma protein binding and ↓ breakdown by liver
Sulfonylureas	↑ Effect of anticoagulant due to ↓ plasma protein binding; also, ↑ effect of sulfonylureas

Drug Interactions

Sulindac	↑ Effect of anticoagulants
Tetracyclines	IV tetracyclines ↑ hypoprothrombinemia
Thyroid hormones	↑ Anticoagulant effect due to ↑ breakdown of clotting factors
Triclofos	↑ Effect of anticoagulants due to ↓ plasma protein binding
Xanthines	↓ Effect of anticoagulants by ↑ plasma prothrombin and factor V

Laboratory Test Interferences: False ↓ levels of serum theophylline determined by Schack and Waxler UV method (warfarin and dicumarol). Metabolites of indanedione derivatives may color alkaline urine red; color disappears upon acidification.

Dosage: See individual drugs, below.

NURSING CONSIDERATIONS

See also *Nursing Considerations* for *Anticoagulants,* p. 388.

Administration/Storage

1. Patients on anticoagulant therapy should not ingest alcohol or salicylates.
2. Patients should be informed that their urine may become red-orange in color.
3. Strict adherence to the dosage regimen is required.

Assessment

1. Take a complete drug history prior to initiating therapy.
2. Determine that prothrombin levels have been obtained prior to beginning therapy. This should serve as a baseline against which to evaluate the effectiveness of the therapy.
3. Discuss with the client any of the possible health problems that may indicate that coumarin or other anticoagulants may be contraindicated.
4. Review with the client any prior problems he/she may have had with bleeding tendencies, ulcerative lesions of the GI tract, colitis, or history of leukemia.
5. Note if the client is a woman in the childbearing years and if she is sexually active. Include in the history if the woman is postpartum or is nursing a baby. In these instances, anticoagulant therapy must be used with caution.

Interventions

1. Assist the health team in evaluating the client's ability to take medication without supervision.
2. Monitor prothrombin levels closely; anticipate dose adjustment of the anticoagulant if the client is also receiving one of the many drugs known to interact with anticoagulants.
3. Question client for evidence of bleeding (bleeding gums, hematuria, tarry stools, hematemesis, ecchymosis and/or petechiae) during initial therapy and also during therapy with a medication that increases the anticoagulant effect.
4. Report the sudden appearance of lumbar pain in clients receiving anticoagulant therapy, since this symptom may indicate retroperitoneal hemorrhage.
5. Report symptoms of GI dysfunction in a client on anticoagulant therapy, since these symptoms may indicate intestinal hemorrhage. Anticipate that a client who has a history of ulcers or who

has recently undergone surgery should have frequent laboratory tests for blood in the urine and feces, as well as measurement of hemoglobin and hematocrit to assess for GI bleeding.

6. Have vitamin K available for parenteral emergency use.

Client/Family Teaching

1. Establish a routine that allows the medication to be taken at the same time every day or as otherwise prescribed.

2. Discuss the possibility of bleeding and symptoms of impending hemorrhage. Clients should be encouraged to report immediately dizziness, headaches, bleeding gums or wounds, or vomiting of coffee ground material. This is particularly important when working with an elderly client.

3. Bleeding or the presence of black and blue areas on the skin, or blood in the urine, is an indication that the medication should be stopped and the physician notified for further instructions.

4. Indanedione-type anticoagulants turn alkaline urine a red-orange color. Discoloration that results from the drug can be differentiated from hematuria by acidifying urine and reevaluating its color.

5. Clients receiving coumarin-type therapy should carry a card with the name of the drug therapy, the dosage, the client's name, and the name of the physician who is providing care so that appropriate persons may be contacted by paramedical personnel if excessive bleeding occurs or if emergency surgery is required.

6. Clients and families need to be aware of the necessity of remaining under medical supervision for blood tests and adjustment of drug dosages. If necessary, ask a reliable relative or friend of the client to report any untoward effects and to make sure that the client takes medication and comes in for blood tests as ordered.

7. Other medications and changes in diet or physical state may affect the action of the anticoagulant. Illness should be promptly reported to the physician.

8. Check with the prescribing physician prior to taking any nonprescription drugs such as aspirin, vitamin preparations with high levels of vitamin K, mineral preparations from health food stores, or alcohol. If the physician is not available, the client should discuss this with the pharmacist from whom he/she receives the prescription drugs.

9. Carry vitamin K capsules at all times.

10. To prevent cuts, clients should use an electric razor for shaving instead of a razor blade.

11. To reduce the potential of bleeding gums, use a soft bristle toothbrush.

12. Arrange furniture in the home to allow open space for ambulation. This diminishes the chance of bumping into objects that may cause bruising and bleeding.

13. When the client has severe problems with sight, teach family members that it is important that furniture not be moved from usual places. This creates confusion for someone without full vision and can cause accidents resulting in bleeding and/or bruising.

14. The client should always wear a Medic-Alert bracelet.

15. Clients should be warned against ingesting alcohol in any form.

Evaluation

1. If clients have discolored urine, determine cause. Check to see if discoloration is from drug therapy or if it is hematuria.

2. Check prothrombin times for cumulative effects of the drug and to determine if the effects of the drug therapy are consistent.

3. Observe closely for any evidence of bleeding (bleeding gums, petechiae, hematuria, and/or occult blood in stools. Assess hemoglobin and hemastocrit).

Special Concerns

1. Elderly people are more prone to developing bleeding complications than are other groups. Therefore, special attention must be given to this problem.
2. Unusual hair loss and itching are common problems with the elderly during drug therapy and should be reported immediately.
3. Since many elderly people use many different pharmacies to fill prescriptions, make sure that they have a printed form with the name and dosage of all drugs they are currently taking.

ANISINDIONE   (an-iss-in-**DYE**-ohn)
Miradon (Rx)

See also *Anticoagulants,* p. 387

Classification: Anticoagulant, indandione-type.

Action/Kinetics: Well absorbed from the GI tract. Anisindione is a long-acting anticoagulant. **Time to peak effect, as determined by prothrombin time:** 2–3 days. **Duration:** 1–3 days. **t½:** 3–5 days.

Side Effects: Dermatitis, fever, diarrhea, urticaria, jaundice, nephropathy, agranulocytosis.

Dosage: Tablets. Adults: 25–250 mg daily as determined by prothrombin times. Dosage has not been determined for children.

> **NURSING CONSIDERATIONS**
> See *Nursing Considerations* for *Anticoagulants,* p. 388, and *Warfarin and Indanedione-type Anticoagulants,* p. 395.

DICUMAROL (BISHYDROXYCOUMARIN, DICOUMAROL)   (dye-**KOO**-mah-rol)
(Rx)

See also *Anticoagulants,* p. 387.

Classification: Anticoagulant.

Action/Kinetics: Slowly and incompletely absorbed from the GI tract. **Onset:** 1–5 days. **Duration of action:** 2–10 days. **t½:** 1–4 days.

Dosage: Tablets. Adults: 25–200 mg daily as determined by prothrombin times. Dosage has not been determined for children.

> **NURSING CONSIDERATIONS**
> See also *Nursing Considerations* for *Anticoagulants,* p. 388, and *Warfarin and Indanedione-type Anticoagulants,* p. 395.
>
> **Client/Family Teaching**
> Explain to client and stress the importance for prothrombin times to be monitored as ordered. The effect of the drug is cumulative and persistent.

WARFARIN SODIUM   (WAR-fah-rin)

Carfin, Coumadin, Panwarfin, Sofarin, Warfilone✱ (Rx)

See also *Anticoagulants,* p. 387.

Classification: Anticoagulant.

Action/Kinetics: Well absorbed from the GI tract although food affects the rate (but not the extent) of absorption. Suitable for parenteral administration. **Onset:** 0.5–3 days; **duration:** 2–5 days. **t½:** 1.5–2.5 days. Response to drug more uniform than with other anticoagulants.

Additional Contraindications: Liver or kidney disease.

Dosage: Tablets, IM, IV. Adults: Doses are identical regardless of route. 10–15 mg/day for 2–4 days; **then,** 2–10 mg daily, depending on prothrombin times. Dosage has not been established for children.

NURSING CONSIDERATIONS

See also *Nursing Considerations* for *Anticoagulants,* p. 388.

Administration/Storage

1. Daily monitoring of prothrombin time is recommended during the first week of therapy and weekly thereafter.
2. After reconstitution, sodium warfarin injection may be stored for several days at 4°C. Discard solution if precipitate becomes noticeable. Store in light-resistant containers.
3. Client should not change brands of warfarin sodium. There may be differences in bioavailability.
4. If client is receiving anticoagulants, intramuscular injections should be avoided.

Assessment

1. Determine if client may be taking any of the drugs with which warfarin may unfavorably interact.
2. Note any history of bleeding tendencies.
3. When working with sexually active females check for pregnancy. Fetal malformations have been documented. In addition, there is danger of hemorrhage.

Interventions

1. Obtain baseline liver and renal function studies prior to initiating therapy.
2. Monitor prothrombin times and check the most recent laboratory findings prior to administering warfarin.
3. Query physician and determine the accepted therapeutic range for client prothrombin time.

Client/Family Teaching

1. Stress the importance of reporting as scheduled for lab studies to evaluate the effectiveness of therapy as dosage may need to be adjusted.
2. Instruct client to take oral warfarin before meals.
3. Do not change brands of drug unless approved by physician as dosage may be altered.
4. Advise women who are sexually active to use birth control measures (or abstinence) as there is an added risk involved when pregnant women are taking anticoagulant drugs.
5. Remind clients to wear an identification band that states that they are on anticoagulant therapy.

6. Advise client to avoid activities that may cause injury or cuts and bruises.
7. Advise clients to carry vitamin K with them. The usual dosage is 5–20 mg, to be used in the event of excessive bleeding.
8. Provide clients with a list of foods high in vitamin K that should be avoided.
9. Clients should be made aware that they may develop skin eruptions as an allergic reaction and to notify physician in this event.

Evaluation

1. Therapeutic range obtained for prothrombin time.
2. Freedom from complications of therapy, such as bleeding or allergic reactions.
3. Assess client/family knowledge and understanding of illness, response to therapy and to teaching.

HEPARIN AND PROTAMINE SULFATE

HEPARIN CALCIUM   (HEH-pah-rin)
Calcilean✽, Calciparine (Rx)

HEPARIN SODIUM INJECTION   (HEH-pah-rin)
Hepalean✽, Heparin Leo✽, Liquaemin Sodium, Liquaemin Sodium Preservative Free (Rx)

HEPARIN SODIUM IN DEXTROSE INJECTION   (HEH-pah-rin)
(Rx)

HEPARIN SODIUM IN SODIUM CHLORIDE INJECTION   (HEH-pah-rin)
(Rx)

See also *Anticoagulants,* p. 387.

Classification: Anticoagulant.

General Statement: Heparin is a naturally occurring substance isolated from porcine intestinal mucosa or bovine lung tissue. Must be given parenterally. Heparin does not interfere with wound healing. Leukocyte counts should be performed in heparinized blood within 2 hr after adding heparin. Heparinized blood should not be used for complement, isoagglutin, erythrocyte fragility test, or platelet counts.

Action/Kinetics: Heparin potentiates the inhibitory action of antithrombin III on various coagulation factors including factor IIa, IXa, Xa, XIa, and XIIa. This occurs due to the formation of a complex with and causing a conformational change in the antithrombin III molecule. Inhibition of factor Xa results in interference with thrombin generation; thus, the action of thrombin in coagulation is inhibited. Heparin also increases the rate of formation of antithrombin III-thrombin complex causing inactivation of thrombin and preventing the conversion of fibrinogen to fibrin. By inhibiting the activation of fibrin stabilizing factor by thrombin, heparin also prevents formation of a stable fibrin clot. Therapeutic doses of heparin prolong thrombin time, whole blood clotting time, activated clotting time, and partial thromboplastin time. Heparin also decreases the levels of triglycerides by releasing lipoprotein lipase from tissues; the resultant hydrolysis of triglycerides causes increased blood levels of free fatty acids. **Onset: IV,** immediate; **deep SC:** 20–60 min. **t$\frac{1}{2}$:** 60–90 min in healthy persons. **t$\frac{1}{2}$** increases with dose, severe renal disease, cirrhosis, and in anephric patients and decreases with pulmonary embolism and liver impairment other than cirrhosis. *Metabolism:* probably by reticuloendothelial system. Clotting time returns to normal within 2–6 hr.

Uses: As an anticoagulant, heparin is used to prevent the extension of clots or to prevent thrombi and emboli from recurring. It is also used prophylactically in the management of thromboembolic disease and to prevent complications after many kinds of surgery including cardiac and vascular surgery. To treat hyperlipemia and to prevent clotting in renal dialysis and blood transfusions. Diagnosis and treatment of disseminated intravascular coagulation (DIC). Prophylaxis of cerebral thrombosis in stroke. Coronary occlusion following myocardial infarction. Atrial fibrillation with embolization.

Contraindications: Active bleeding, blood dyscrasias (or other disorders characterized by bleeding tendencies such as hemophilia), purpura, thrombocytopenia, liver disease with hypoprothrombinemia, suspected intracranial hemorrhage, suppurative thrombophlebitis, inaccessible ulcerative lesions (especially of the GI tract), open wounds, extensive denudation of the skin, and increased capillary permeability (as in ascorbic acid deficiency).

The drug should not be administered during surgery of the eye, brain, or spinal cord or during continuous tube drainage of the stomach or small intestine. Use is also contraindicated in subacute endocarditis, shock, advanced kidney disease, threatened abortion, severe hypertension, or hypersensitivity to drug.

Use with caution during menstruation and in the postpartum period, as well as in patients with a history of asthma, allergies, mild liver or kidney disease, or in alcoholics. Should not be used in premature neonates due to the possibility of a fatal "gasping syndrome."

Special Concerns: Pregnancy category: C. Women over aged 60 may be more susceptible to hemorrhage during heparin therapy.

Side Effects: Hemorrhage ranging from minor local ecchymoses to major hemorrhagic complications. Such reactions are more likely to occur in prophylactic administration during surgery than in the treatment of thromboembolic disease. Thrombocytopenia.

Rare allergic reactions characterized by chills, fever, pruritus, urticaria, burning feet, rhinitis, conjunctivitis, lacrimation, asthma-like reactions, hyperemia, arthralgia, and anaphylactoid reactions have been noted. Use a test dose of 1,000 units in patients with a history of asthma or allergic disease. Long-term therapy may cause osteoporosis and/or spontaneous fractures and hypoaldosteronism.

Discontinuance of heparin has resulted in rebound hyperlipemia, priapism, transient alopecia, and decreased aldosterone synthesis. Heparin resistance has been observed in some elderly patients. In these cases, large doses may be required.

IM injections of heparin may produce local irritation, hematoma, and tissue sloughing.

Overdosage

Symptoms: nosebleeds, hematuria, tarry stools, petechiae, and easy bruising may be the first signs.

Treatment: Drug withdrawal is usually sufficient to correct heparin overdosage. In some cases, blood transfusion or the administration of a heparin antagonist (protamine sulfate) may be necessary.

Drug Interactions

ACTH	Heparin antagonizes effect of ACTH
Alteplase, recombinant	↑ Risk of bleeding, especially at arterial puncture sites
Anticoagulants, oral	Additive ↑ prothrombin time
Antihistamines	↓ Effect of heparin
Aspirin	Additive ↑ prothrombin time
Corticosteroids	Heparin antagonizes effect of corticosteroids
Dextran	Additive ↑ prothrombin time
Diazepam	Heparin ↑ plasma levels of diazepam
Digitalis	↓ Effect of heparin
Dipyridamole	Additive ↑ prothrombin time
Hydroxychloroquine	Additive ↑ prothrombin time
Ibuprofen	Additive ↑ prothrombin time
Indomethacin	Additive ↑ prothrombin time
Insulin	Heparin antagonizes effect of insulin
Phenylbutazone	Additive ↑ prothrombin time
Quinine	Additive ↑ prothrombin time
Tetracyclines	↓ Effect of heparin

Laboratory Test Interferences: ↑ SGOT and SGPT.

Dosage: Adjusted for each patient on the basis of laboratory tests. **Deep SC: initial loading dose,** 10,000–20,000 units (preceded by 5,000 units IV); **maintenance:** 8,000–10,000 units q 8 hr or 15,000–20,000 units q 12 hr. *Use concentrated solution.* **Intermittent IV: initially,** 10,000 units undiluted or in 50–100 mL saline; **then,** 5,000–10,000 units q 4–6 hr undiluted or in 50–100 mL saline. **Continuous IV infusion:** 20,000–40,000 units/day in 1,000 mL saline (preceded initially by 5,000 units IV).

Prophylaxis of postoperative thromboembolism: **Deep SC:** 5,000 units of concentrated solution 2 hr before surgery and 5,000 units q 8–12 hr thereafter for 7 days or until patient is ambulatory. *Surgery of heart and blood vessels:* **initial,** 150–400 units/kg (dose depends on estimated length of surgery); to prevent clotting in the tube system, add heparin to fluids in pump oxygenator. *Extracorporeal renal dialysis:* See instructions on equipment. *Blood transfusion:* 400–600 units/100 mL whole blood. *Laboratory samples:* 70–150 units/10- to 20-ml sample to prevent coagulation.

NURSING CONSIDERATIONS

See also *Nursing Considerations* for *Anticoagulants,* p. 388.

Administration/Storage

1. Client should be hospitalized for IV heparin therapy.
2. Protect solutions from freezing.
3. Heparin should not be administered IM.
4. Administer by deep SC injection to minimize local irritation, hematoma, and tissue sloughing and to prolong action of drug.
   - Z-track method: Use any fat roll, but abdominal fat rolls are preferred. Use a ½-inch or ⅝-inch needle. Grasp the skin layer of the fat roll and lift it up. Insert the needle at about a 45-degree angle to the skin surface and then administer the medication. With this medication, it is not necessary to check whether or not the needle is in a blood vessel. Rapidly withdraw the needle while releasing the skin.

- "Bunch technique" method: Grasp the tissue around the injection site, creating a tissue roll of about ½ inch in diameter. Insert the needle into the tissue roll at a 90-degree angle to the skin surface and inject the medication. It is not necessary to check whether or not the needle is in a blood vessel. Withdraw the needle rapidly when the skin is released.
- Do not administer within 2 inches of the umbilicus because of increased vascularity of area.

5. Do not massage before or after injection.
6. Change sites of administration.
7. Caution should be used to prevent negative pressure (with a roller pump), which would increase the rate at which heparin is injected into the system. Administer with a constant rate infusion pump.

Assessment

1. Inquire about any bleeding incidents a client may have had, i.e., bleeding tendencies, family history of bleeding tendencies, or any incidents of active bleeding.
2. Inquire about any history of peptic ulcer. This may be an indication for a potential site of bleeding.
3. Note any evidence of possible intracranial hemorrhage.

Interventions

1. Assure that all appropriate blood work has been completed prior to initiating therapy (Lee-White whole blood clotting time tests and activated partial thromboplastin times- APTT) and that the results are reported promptly to the physician.
2. With full-dose heparin administered by continuous IV, the APTT should be done before onset of therapy, q 4 hr during the early stages, and then daily.
3. During full-dose therapy, the accepted therapeutic range for the APTT is 1.5–2.5 times the control value in seconds. The activated coagulation time (ACT) may also be used.
   - ACT can be done at the bedside, (although it is time consuming), thus it is convenient for monitoring the degree of anticoagulation in clients with extracorporeal circulation.
   - The accepted therapeutic range for the ACT is two to three times the control value.
4. With full-dose intermittent IV heparin therapy, the APTT should be done before the start of therapy. In the early stages it may be repeated before each dose of drug, and then daily.
5. Anticipate that heparin therapy will be ordered on an individual basis after the coagulation time has been evaluated by the physician. Exceptions are when small doses are administered for prophylaxis.
6. If the client is receiving one of the many drugs that interact with anticoagulants anticipate an adjustment in the dosage of heparin.
7. Have protamine sulfate, a heparin antagonist, available should the client develop excessive bleeding and anticoagulant effects.
8. IV infusions should be administered utilizing an electronic infusion device (infusion pump).

Client/Family Teaching

1. Instruct and stress the importance of reporting any signs of active bleeding.
2. That in women of childbearing age, any excessive menstrual flow should be reported, since increased flow may be caused by the drug, necessitating a reduction in dosage.
3. Alopecia, if it occurs, is generally only temporary.
4. Alterations in GU function and any injury should be immediately reported to the physician prescribing heparin.

5. Use an electric razor for shaving.

6. Use a soft-bristle toothbrush to decrease gum irritation.

7. Arrange furniture in the home to allow open space for unimpeded ambulation and to diminish chances of bumping into objects that may cause bruising and bleeding.

8. Use a night light to provide illumination during trips to the bathroom at night.

9. Encourage clients to eat potassium-rich foods (e.g. baked potato, orange juice, bananas, beef, flounder, haddock, sweet potato, turkey, raw tomato).

10. Advise clients against eating large amounts of vitamin K foods. These are mostly yellow and dark green vegetables.

Evaluation

1. Monitor client for bruising, bleeding of nose, mouth, gums, tarry stools or GI upset.

2. Note any increase in hair loss or presence of skin rash.

3. If client has been using alcohol, monitor for increased anticoagulant response.

4. Monitor range of prothrombin time and/or partial thromboplastin time.

HEPARIN LOCK FLUSH SOLUTION   (HEH-pah-rin)

Hepalean-Lok✿. Hep-Lock (Rx)

See also *Anticoagulants,* p. 387.

Classification: Anticoagulant flushing agent.

Use: Dilute solutions of heparin sodium (100 USP units/mL) are used to maintain patency of indwelling catheters used for IV therapy or blood sampling. Not to be used therapeutically. See *Heparin* for all other information.

NURSING CONSIDERATIONS

See also *Nursing Considerations* for *Anticoagulants,* p. 388.

Interventions

1. Aspirate lock to determine patency. Maintain patency by injecting 1 mL of heparin lock flush solution into the diaphragm of the device after each use. This dose should maintain patency for up to 8 hr for a converted (capped) catheter.

2. When a drug incompatible with heparin is to be administered, flush the device with 0.9% sodium chloride injection or sterile water for injection before and immediately after the incompatible drug is administered. After the final flush, inject another dose of heparin lock flush solution.

3. When repeated blood samples are drawn from the venipuncture device, the presence of heparin or normal saline may cause interference with laboratory tests.

   • Clear the heparin lock flush solution by aspirating and discarding 1 mL of fluid from the device before withdrawing the blood sample.

   • Inject another 1 mL of heparin lock flush solution into the device after blood samples are drawn.

   • Because this is not the most reliable method of acquiring serum levels, if there are any excessively abnormal results, obtain a repeat sample from another site before treatment.

Evaluation

1. Note any allergic reactions to heparin due to various biological sources of the product.
2. Clients with underlying coagulation disorders may be at a risk for bleeding, observe coagulation times carefully.
3. Assess for evidence of thrombocytopenia, a possible side effect of heparin therapy.
4. Recent studies have shown that 0.9% NaCl is effective in maintaining patency of peripheral (noncentral) intermittent infusion devices. The following procedure has been recommended:
   - Determine patency by aspirating lock.
   - Flush with 2 cc NSS.
   - Administer medication therapy. (Flush between drugs.)
   - Flush with 2 cc NSS.
   - This does *NOT* apply to central venous access devices.

PROTAMINE SULFATE (PROH-tah-meen)

(Rx)

Classification: Heparin antagonist.

Action/Kinetics: Protamine sulfate is a strongly basic polypeptide that complexes with strongly acidic heparin to form an inactive stable salt. The complex has no anticoagulant activity. **Onset:** 30–60 sec. **Duration:** 2 hr (but is dependent on body temperature). Upon metabolism, the complex may liberate heparin (heparin rebound).

Use: Only for treatment of heparin overdose resulting in hemorrhage. Administration of whole blood or fresh frozen plasma may also be needed if hemorrhage is severe.

Contraindications: Previous intolerance to protamine. Not suitable for treating spontaneous hemorrhage, postpartum hemorrhage, menorrhagia, or uterine bleeding.

Special Concerns: Pregnancy category: C. Use with caution during lactation. Safety and efficacy have not been determined in children.

Side Effects: *CV:* Sudden fall in blood pressure, bradycardia, transitory flushing, warm feeling. *GI:* Nausea, vomiting. *CNS:* Lassitude. *Other:* Anaphylaxis, dyspnea.

Dosage: Slow IV. No more than 50 mg of protamine sulfate should be given in any 10-min period. One mg protamine sulfate can neutralize about 90 USP units of heparin derived from lung tissue or about 115 USP units of heparin derived from intestinal mucosa. **Note:** The dose of protamine sulfate is dependent on the amount of time that has elapsed since IV heparin administration. For example, if 30 min has elapsed, one-half the usual dose of protamine sulfate may be sufficient since heparin is cleared rapidly from the circulation.

NURSING CONSIDERATIONS

Administration/Storage

1. Protamine sulfate is incompatible with several penicillins and with cephalosporins.
2. If dilution of the product is required, use either dextrose 5% or normal saline. After reconstitution, the solution may be stored in the refrigerator for 24 hr.

Assessment

Note any history of previous intolerance to protamine.

Interventions

1. To minimize side effects, give protamine sulfate slowly over 1–3 min.
2. When administering heparin infusions, anticipate potential for heparin overdose and have protamine sulfate readily available.
3. Observe client closely in a monitored environment.
4. Coagulation studies should be performed 5–15 min after protamine sulfate has been administered to evaluate its effectiveness.
5. Observe client closely for increased bleeding, lowered BP, and/or shock. These are signs of heparin rebound and should be reported immediately as repeated doses of protamine sulfate may be indicated.

Evaluation

1. Note any sudden fall in BP, bradycardia, dyspnea, transitory flushing, or client complaint of a sensation of warmth.
2. Record vital signs and intake and output, assess closely for alterations.

HEMOSTATICS

General Statement: These drugs are used to control excessive bleeding in persons who have an inborn clotting defect, who suffer from a disease that affects the clotting mechanism, or who exhibit continuous leakage from a capillary that cannot be controlled by other (physical, surgical) means.
Hemostatic agents are divided into (1) topically active agents and (2) systemic agents.

Topical Agents

CELLULOSE, OXIDIZED   (SELL-you-lows)

Oxycel, Surgicel (Rx)

Classification: Hemostatic, topical.

Action/Kinetics: Upon contact with blood, oxidized cellulose (cellulosic acid) forms a tenacious, almost black mass that adheres to bleeding surfaces. This mass becomes gelatinous after 1–2 days and can then be removed without causing more bleeding. If left in place, it will be absorbed at a rate depending on the amount used, the location, and the amount of blood.

Oxidized cellulose also possesses antibacterial activity against a number of gram-positive and gram-negative organisms.

Uses: Surgery, to control moderate bleeding when suturing or ligation is impractical (such as biliary tract surgery), partial hepatectomy, resections or injuries of the pancreas, spleen, or kidneys, and bowel resections. Dental and oral surgery.

Contraindications: The material should not be used on open, external wounds because it interferes with new skin formation. It also should not be used for permanent packing because it interferes with bone regeneration. To control hemorrhage from large arteries or oozing surfaces (does not react with other body fluids). Vascular surgery; around optic nerve and chiasm.

Side Effects: *Following internal use:* Retention of fluid, infection, foreign body reaction, urinary difficulty or urethral obstruction after prostatectomy, prolonged drainage after cholecystectomies, intestinal obstruction following gallbladder surgery. *Following topical use:* Burning, stinging. *When used in the nose:* Burning, headache, sneezing, stinging, necrosis or perforation if material packed too tightly.

Dosage: Minimum amount necessary. Pledgets are especially indicated in dentistry.

NURSING CONSIDERATIONS

Administration/Storage

1. Use sterile technique in removing from containers.
2. Apply minimal amount necessary to control hemorrhage.
3. Apply in dry form.
4. Oxidized cellulose cannot be resterilized; thus unused material should be discarded.
5. Never pull oxidized cellulose from wound without irrigating material. Otherwise, fresh bleeding may be initiated.
6. Artificial scab can be removed after it becomes gelatinous.

Assessment

Assess client and note any history that may indicate that these agents should not be used. (ex. They should not be used on open, external wounds as they interfere with new skin formation.)

Evaluation

1. Following internal use, note any evidence of untoward responses such as client complaints of difficulty urinating, or retention of fluid.
2. Note incidence of infection (fever, leukopenia, etc.)
3. Following use during prostatectomy, observe for evidence of urethral obstruction.
4. When the agent has been used during gallbladder surgery, assess for evidence of intestinal obstruction.
5. Note any client complaints of stinging or burning sensation following topical administration.
6. Evaluate for the efficacy of treatment.

GELATIN FILM, ABSORBABLE STERILE   (JEH-lah-tin)

Gelfilm, Gelfilm Ophthalmic (Rx)

Classification: Hemostatic, topical.

Action/Kinetics: This is a thin, absorbable gelatin film that takes up to 50 times its weight of blood and water. Like absorbable gelatin sponge (see below), it can be left in place and is absorbed within 8 days to 6 months.

Uses: Neurosurgery, thoracic surgery, and ocular surgery.

Contraindications: Use in infected or contaminated surgical wounds.

Dosage: Topical: As required; after soaking, cut to desired size and shape.

NURSING CONSIDERATIONS

Administration/Storage

1. Moisten gelatin with sterile isotonic saline solution before applying it to bleeding surface.
2. Use immediately upon withdrawal from package to ensure sterility.

GELATIN SPONGE, ABSORBABLE   (JEH-lah-tin)
Gelfoam (Rx)

Classification: Hemostatic, topical.

Action/Kinetics: Specially prepared gelatin that absorbs approximately 50% of its weight in blood or other fluid. **Onset:** instantaneous. Absorbed systemically within 4–6 weeks. When applied to bleeding surfaces or mucosal membranes (nasal, rectal, or vaginal), liquefies within 2–5 days.

Uses: During surgery to control capillary bleeding including dental, oral, and prostatic surgery.

Contraindications: Frank infection, sole agent in presence of blood dyscrasias or abnormal bleeding, postpartum bleeding, menorrhagia. To close skin incisions.

Side Effects: *CNS:* Giant cell granuloma in the brain, compression of brain and spinal cord due to fluid accumulation. *Miscellaneous:* Infection, abscess formation.

Dosage: Enough of the sponge, pack, or dental pack used dry or saturated with sterile isotonic saline to cover bleeding surface. Prostatectomy cones are also available for use with the Foley bag catheter.

NURSING CONSIDERATIONS

Administration/Storage

1. Moisten material with sterile isotonic sodium chloride before applying to bleeding surface. Squeeze to remove air bubbles and replace in the solution so material can swell to original size prior to application.
2. Whether applied wet or dry, the material should be held with moderate pressure for 10–15 sec.
3. When used in dentistry, the material should be compressed to the diameter of the cavity to be filled. After insertion, light pressure should be applied for 1–2 min.
4. Resterilization by heating changes the absorption time.

MICROFIBRILLAR COLLAGEN HEMOSTAT   (my-kroh-FIB-rihl-lahr COLL-ah-jen HEE-moh-stat)
Avitene (Rx)

Classification: Hemostatic, topical.

Action/Kinetics: This product is purified bovine corium collagen prepared as the partial hydrochloric acid salt. Attracts platelets, which then release clotting factors that initiate formation of a fibrinous mass. Absorbable, water insoluble.

Uses: During surgery to control capillary bleeding and as an adjunct to hemostasis when conventional procedures are ineffectual or insufficient. It is ineffective in controlling systemic coagulation disorders.

Contraindications: Closure of skin incisions, because preparation may interfere with healing. On bone surfaces to which prosthetic materials will be attached. Intraocular use or for injection.

Special Concerns: Use during pregnancy only when benefits clearly outweigh risks.

Side Effects: Potentiation of infections, abscess formation, hematomas, wound dehiscence, mediastinitis. Formation of adhesions, foreign body or allergic reactions. *Following dental use:* Alveolalgia. *Following tonsillectomy:* Laryngospasm due to inhalation of dry material.

Dosage: *Individualized,* depending on severity of bleeding. *Usual for capillary bleeding:* 1 gm for 50 cm². More for heavier flow.

NURSING CONSIDERATIONS

Administration/Storage

1. Before applying dry product, compress surface to be treated with dry sponge. Use dry smooth forceps to handle.
2. Apply hemostat directly to source of bleeding.
3. After hemostat is in place, apply pressure with a dry sponge (not a gloved hand) for up to five minutes, depending on severity of bleeding.
4. When controlling oozing from porous (cancellous) bone, pack hemostat tightly into affected area. Tease off excess material after 5–10 min. Apply more hemostat in case of breakthrough bleeding.
5. Avoid spillage on nonbleeding surfaces, especially in the abdomen or thorax.
6. Remove excess material after a few minutes.
7. Do not reautoclave. Discard unused portion.
8. Avoid contacting nonbleeding surfaces with microfibrillar collagen hemostat.
9. Dry forceps should be used to handle hemostat as it will adhere to wet gloves or instruments.

Intervention

Monitor BP and pulse, and assess for shock because hemostat may mask a deeper hemorrhage by sealing off its exit site.

THROMBIN, TOPICAL   (THROM-bihn)

Thrombinar, Thrombostat (Rx)

Classification: Hemostatic, topical.

Action/Kinetics: Derived from bovine sources. Thrombin catalyzes conversion of fibrinogen to fibrin. It is most effective when thrombin can mix with blood as soon as it reaches the surface. **Onset:** 5 mL of saline containing 5,000 NIH units will clot an equal volume of blood in approximately 1 sec.

Use: During surgery, to control capillary bleeding. May be used with absorbable gelatin sponges.

Contraindications: Thrombin should never be injected, particularly IV. IV injections may be fatal.

Special Concerns: Pregnancy category: C. Safety and effectiveness in children have not been determined.

Side Effects: Fever, allergy when used to control nose bleeds.

Dosage: Topical: usual, 100 units/mL solution; if bleeding profuse, 1,000–2,000 units/mL may be needed. Also, may be applied dry to oozing surfaces.

NURSING CONSIDERATIONS

Administration/Storage

1. Dry powder may be stored indefinitely.
2. The powder should be reconstituted with sterile distilled water or isotonic saline.
3. Thrombin solution may be applied by a spray or with a sterile syringe and needle.
4. If used with absorbable gelatin sponge, the sponge strips should be soaked in the thrombin solution, then compressed to remove air bubbles, and then saturated with the solution. When applied to the area, the sponge should be held in place 10–15 seconds.
5. Thrombin solutions should be used immediately after reconstitution. However, solutions may be refrigerated for up to 3 hr.

Systemic Agents

AMINOCAPROIC ACID   (ah-me-noh-kah-**PROH**-ick **AH**-sid)

Amicar (Rx)

Classification: Hemostatic, systemic.

Action/Kinetics: Inhibits action of plasminogen (clotting factor), thereby preventing fibrinolysis (clot dissolution). Rapidly absorbed from the GI tract. **Peak plasma levels:** 2 hr. **Effective plasma levels:** 0.13 mg/mL. **Duration (after IV):** 3 hr or less. Rapidly excreted through the kidney, mostly unchanged.

Uses: Excessive bleeding associated with systemic hyperfibrinolysis and urinary fibrinolysis. Surgical complications following heart surgery and portacaval shunt in cancer of the lung, prostate, cervix, stomach, and other types of surgery associated with heavy postoperative bleeding. Aplastic anemia. *Investigational:* Prevention of recurrence of subarachnoid hemorrhage, megakaryocytic thrombocytopenia, prophylaxis and treatment of hereditary angioneurotic edema, acute promyelocytic leukemia with accompanying coagulopathy.

Contraindications: Patients with active, intravascular clotting possibly associated with fibrinolysis and bleeding.

Special Concerns: Use with caution, or not at all, in patients with uremia or cardiac, renal, or hepatic disease. Use during pregnancy only if benefits clearly outweigh risks.

Side Effects: *GI:* Nausea, cramping, diarrhea. *CNS:* Dizziness, malaise, headache, delirium; auditory, visual, and kinesthetic hallucinations. *CV:* Hypotension, thrombophlebitis. *Other:* Tinnitus, conjunctival suffusion, myopathies, nasal stuffiness, skin rash, prolongation of menses, reversible acute renal failure.

Drug Interactions

Anticoagulants, oral	↓ Anticoagulant effects
Contraceptives, oral (Estrogen)	Combination with aminocaproic acid may lead to hypercoagulable condition

Laboratory Test Interferences: ↑ Serum aldolase, SGOT, creatinine phosphokinase, and potassium.

Dosage: Syrup, Tablets. *Acute bleeding:* **Initial priming dose,** 5 g during first hour; **then,** 1–1.25 g q hr for 8 hr or until bleeding is controlled. **Maximum daily dose:** 30 g. *After prostatic surgery:* 6 g over the first 24 hr may be sufficient. *Prevention of hemorrhage after dental surgery:* 6 g immediately after surgery followed by 6 g q 6 hr for 9–19 days.

    IV infusion. *Acute bleeding:* **Initial priming dose:** 4–5 g during first hour; **then,** 1 g q hr for 8 hr (or until desired response is obtained). *Subarachnoid hemorrhage, recurrent:* 36 g daily (18 g in 400 mL 5% dextrose solution infused over 12 hr) for 10 days. Switch to oral therapy after this time.

NURSING CONSIDERATIONS

Administration/Storage

1. For IV use, may be mixed with saline, 5% dextrose, sterile water, or Ringer's solution. It should *never* be injected undiluted.
2. For IV, priming dose is dissolved in 250 mL of solution; continuous infusion is at the rate of 1—1.25 g/hr for 8 hr in 50 mL of diluent.

Assessment

1. Obtain complete blood count, platelet count, bleeding parameters, liver and renal function studies prior to instituting therapy.
2. Determine baseline BP and pulse before starting IV therapy.
3. Note any history of prior incidence of uremia, cardiac, renal or hepatic disease.
4. Determine if client is taking any oral contraceptives (estrogen). Interaction with aminocaproic acid can lead to hypercoagulable condition.
5. Note presence of menses.

Interventions

1. Infusions should be administered utilizing an electronic infusion device.
2. Assess client frequently for hypotension, bradycardia, and arrhythmias, symptoms that may indicate that the rate of IV administration is too fast. Slow rate of IV infusion and report if such symptoms occur.
3. With all systemic hemostatics, observe carefully for signs and symptoms of thrombosis, such as leg pain, chest pain, or respiratory distress.
4. Have available vitamin K or protamine sulfate for emergency use.
5. Keep tablets and raspberry-flavored syrup out of the reach of children.

Evaluation

1. Assess appropriate lab data to determine response to therapy.
2. Note presence of untoward effects such as nausea, cramping or diarrhea.
3. If client is experiencing menses, observe for excessive bleeding.

ANTIHEMOPHILIC FACTOR (AHF, FACTOR VIII) (an-tie-hee-moh-**FILL**-ick)
Hemofil M, Koate-HS, Koate-HT, Monoclate (Rx)

Classification: Hemostatic, systemic.

Action/Kinetics: Antihemophilic factor (AHF) is either isolated from pooled normal human blood or is derived from monoclonal antibodies. AHF is essential for blood coagulation. The potency and purity of preparation vary but each lot is standardized. Details on the package should be noted. Plasma protein (factor VIII) accelerates abnormally slow transformation of prothrombin to thrombin. **t½:** 9–15 hr. One AHF unit is the activity found in 1 mL of normal pooled human plasma.

Use: Control of bleeding in patients suffering from hemophilia A (factor VIII deficiency and acquired factor VIII inhibitors).

Contraindications: Use of monoclonal antibody-derived AHF in patients hypersensitive to mouse protein.

Special Concerns: Pregnancy category: C.

Side Effects: *Allergic:* Nausea, fever, hives, chills, urticaria, wheezing, hypotension, chest tightness, stinging at infusion site, anaphylaxis. Antibodies may form to the mouse protein found in AHF derived from monoclonal antibodies.

Antihemophilic factor contains traces of blood group A and B isohemagglutins. These may cause intravascular hemolysis in patients with types A, B, or AB blood.

Both hepatitis and AIDS may be transmitted from AHF prepared from human plasma.

Dosage: IV only. Individualized, depending on severity of bleeding, degree of deficiency, body weight, and presence of inhibitors of factor VIII. **Note:** AHF levels may rise 2% for every unit of AHF/kg administered. Dosages given are only guidelines. *Mild hemorrhage:* Single infusion to achieve AHF levels of at least 30%. Dosage should not be repeated. *Minor surgery, moderate hemorrhage:* AHF levels should be raised to 30–50% of normal. **Initial:** 15–25 IU/kg; **maintenance:** 10–15 IU/kg q 8–12 hr. *Severe hemorrhage:* Increase AHF levels to 80%–100% of normal. **Initial:** 40–50 IU/kg; **maintenance:** 20–25 IU/kg q 8–12 hr. *Major surgery:* Raise AHF levels to 80–100% of normal. Administer 1 hr before surgery; one-half the priming dose may be given 5 hr after the first dose. AHF levels should be maintained at 30% of normal for at least 10–14 days.

NURSING CONSIDERATIONS

Administration/Storage

1. Antihemophilic factor is labile and is inactivated rapidly: within 10 min at 56° C and within 3 hr at 49° C. Store vials at 2°–8° C. Check expiration date. **Do not freeze.**
2. Warm the concentrate and diluent to room temperature before reconstitution.
3. Place one needle in the concentrate to act as an airway and then aseptically with a syringe and needle add the diluent to the concentrate.
4. Gently agitate or roll the vial containing diluent and concentrate to dissolve the drug. **Do not shake vigorously.**
5. Administer drug within 3 hr of reconstitution, to avoid incubation if contamination occurred during mixing.
6. Do not refrigerate drug after reconstitution, because the active ingredient may precipitate out.
7. Keep reconstituted drug at room temperature during infusion because, at a lower temperature, precipitation of active ingredients may occur.
8. Administer IV only using a plastic syringe (solutions stick to glass syringes). Medication should be administered at a rate of 2 mL/min although rates up to 10 mL/min can be used if necessary.

Assessment

Take client's pulse and blood pressure prior to starting IV. In utilizing this information for baseline data it is well to realize that several readings at spaced intervals may be necessary to assure that the readings are typical for that particular client.

Interventions

1. Obtain and monitor hemoglobin and hematocrit and perform Coombs' test during therapy.
2. Monitor pulse and blood pressure during administration. If tachycardia and hypotension occur, slow IV and report incident to the physician.
3. If the client complains of headaches, flushing, numbness, back pain, visual disturbances, or chest constriction or if you notice the client flushing, slow the IV and report. Be certain to note the incident on the client record.

Client/Family Teaching

1. Review the appropriate method for storing and administering antihemophilic factor at home.
2. Explain that the product is prepared from human plasma and outline the associated potential risks, such as hepatitis, and HIV.
3. Stress that local support groups may assist them to understand and cope with their illness.

Evaluation

1. Assess client/family knowledge and understanding of illness, response to therapy and to teaching.
2. Check appropriate lab data.
3. Observe for freedom from complications of drug therapy.

ANTI-INHIBITOR COAGULANT COMPLEX

Autoplex T, Feiba VH Immuno (Rx)

Classification: Antihemophilic.

Action/Kinetics: This product is obtained from pooled human plasma; it contains both precursor and activated clotting factors. Autoplex T consists of dried anti-inhibitor coagulant complex as well as 2 units of heparin and 2 mg polyethylene glycol per mL of reconstituted product. Feiba VH Immuno is a heparin free, freeze-dried anti-inhibitor coagulant complex product. One unit of Factor VIII correctional activity is defined as the quantity of activated prothrombin complex which, when added to an equal volume of Factor VIII deficient or inhibitor plasma, will correct the clotting time to normal (i.e., 35 seconds).

Uses: The drug is most useful for patients with Factor VIII inhibitors. Patients who manifest Factor VIII inhibitor levels greater than 10 Bethesda units and whose inhibitor levels will rise to more than 10 Bethesda units after treatment with antihemophilic factor, should be treated with anti-inhibitor coagulant complex. Patients who manifest Factor VIII inhibitor levels between 2 and 10 Bethesda units, and whose inhibitor levels remain between 2 and 10 Bethesda units following treatment with antihemophilic factor, may be treated with either antihemophilic factor or anti-inhibitor coagulant complex. The drug may also be used in patients manifesting minor bleeding episodes, in order to maintain the inhibitor at low levels; this regimen allows use of other approaches should an acute emergency arise.

Contraindications: Disseminated intravascular coagulation, fibrinolysis, patients with normal coagulation times. Feiba VH Immuno should not be used in newborns but Autoplex T may be used with caution in this group. Concomitant use of epsilon-aminocaproic acid or tranexamic acid.

Special Concerns: Pregnancy category: C. Use Autoplex T with caution in patients with impaired liver function.

Side Effects: *Hematologic:* Disseminated intravascular coagulation including symptoms of respiratory distress, changes in pulse rate and blood pressure, cough, prolonged thrombin time, and prothrombin time, decreased fibrinogen levels, and decreased platelet count. *Hypersensitivity:* Fever, chills, allergic symptoms including urticaria and anaphylaxis. *Miscellaneous:* Headache, changes in blood pressure and pulse rate, and flushing all due to a rapid rate of infusion.

Laboratory Test Interference: Activated partial thromboplastin time may not correlate with the clinical response of this drug.

Dosage: IV Injection or Drip Only. *Hemorrhage of soft tissue:* 100 U/kg q 12 hr, not to exceed 200 U/kg daily. *Hemorrhage of joints:* 50–100 U/kg q 12 hr. Treatment should be continued until there is reduced swelling, pain relief, or improved mobility. *Bleeding of mucous membranes:* 50 U/kg q 6 hr with constant monitoring of hematocrit; dosage may be increased to 100 U/kg, if necessary, but should not exceed 200 U/kg daily. *CNS hemorrhage:* 100 U/kg q 12 hr (may be administered q 6 hr if necessary).

NURSING CONSIDERATIONS

Administration/Storage

1. The drug may be infused at rates up to 10 mL/min as long as symptoms such as headache, flushing, or changes in blood pressure or pulse rate do not occur. If these symptoms occur, the infusion should be stopped and restarted at a rate of 2 mL/min.
2. The drug should not be refrigerated after reconstitution. Autoplex T should be administered within 1 hr and Feiba VH Immuno within 3 hr after being reconstituted.
3. The unreconstituted drug should be stored between 2°–8° C (35°–46° F).
4. If these drugs are required for children, fibrinogen levels should be determined prior to therapy and monitored during treatment.

Assessment

1. Obtain baseline hematological studies and bleeding time.
2. Obtain documented Factor VIII inhibitor levels and assure that these have been recorded on the client's record.
3. Note any propensity clients may have for headaches or vacillating blood pressure readings or pulse rates. This information could be important when confronted with a client who exhibits these tendencies under "normal" conditions.

Interventions

1. Monitor vital signs throughout infusion.
2. Observe client for allergic reactions and have emergency equipment readily available.
3. The drug is for IV use only. Therefore, use the recommended precautions for IV administration.

Client/Family Teaching

1. Explain that product is prepared from human plasma and outline the associated potential risks.
2. Stress that local support groups may assist them to understand and cope with chronic disorders.

Evaluation

1. Observe client for symptoms of respiratory distress, changes in pulse rate or blood pressure.
2. Note any client complaint of headache or chest pain and notify the physician immediately.
3. Monitor client for tachycardia. This and the above symptoms may require terminating the infusion or decreasing the rate of infusion until the client can be reevaluated by the physician.
4. Using baseline data obtained prior to beginning therapy evaluate and record observations. This includes evaluation of blood studies and calling to the attention of other health team members any evidence of improvement or untoward reactions.
5. Note client complaints of chills, fever or urticaria. These are often allergic responses and need to be reported immediately to the physician for further evaluation of client response and possible treatment.

FACTOR IX COMPLEX (HUMAN)   (FAK-tor 9)

Konyne-HT, Profilnine Heat-Treated, Proplex SX-T, Proplex T (Rx)

Classification: Hemostatic, systemic.

Action/Kinetics: This product provides factors II, VII, IX, and X; thus, homeostasis can be restored. $t^{1}/_2$: 24 hr. A unit is the activity present (as factor IX) in 1 mL of normal plasma less than 1 hr old.

Uses: For patients with factor IX deficiency, especially hemophilia B and Christmas disease. Patients with inhibitors to factor VIII. To reverse hemorrhage induced by coumarin. To control or prevent bleeding in patients with factor VII deficiency (Proplex T only).

Contraindications: Factor VII deficiency, except for Proplex T. Liver disease with suspected intravascular coagulation or fibrinolysis.

Special Concerns: Pregnancy category: C. Assess benefit versus risk prior to use in liver disease or elective surgery.

Side Effects: *CV:* Disseminated intravascular coagulation, thrombosis. High doses may cause myocardial infarction, venous or pulmonary thrombosis. *Miscellaneous:* Chills, fever. *Symptoms due to rapid infusion:* Nausea, vomiting, headache, fever, chills, tingling, flushing, urticaria, and changes in blood pressure.

Most of these side effects disappear when rate of administration is slowed.

The preparation also contains trace amounts of blood groups A and B and isohemagglutins, which may cause intravascular hemolysis when administered in large amounts to patients with blood groups A, B, and AB.

Both hepatitis and AIDS may be transmitted using factor IX Complex since it is derived from pooled human plasma.

Drug Interaction: ↑ Risk of thrombosis if administered with aminocaproic acid.

Dosage: IV. Individualized, depending on severity of bleeding, degree of deficiency, body weight, and level of factor required. Minimum factor IX level required in surgery or following trauma is 25% of normal, which is maintained for 1 week after surgery. As a guide in determining the units required to raise blood level percentages of factor IX, use the following formula:

1 unit/kg x body weight (kg) x desired increase (% of normal).

For factor VII deficiency, use 0.5 unit/kg x body weight (kg) x desired increase (% of normal). The dose may be repeated q 4–6 hr.

The package insert should be checked carefully as a guideline for doses for various factor deficiencies.

Bleeding in Hemophilia A patients with factor VIII inhibitors: 75 IU/kg followed in 12 hr by a second dose. *Prophylaxis of bleeding in Hemophilia B patients:* 10–20 IU/kg once or twice a week.

NURSING CONSIDERATIONS

Administration/Storage

1. The rate of administration varies with the product. As a general guideline, infuse about 100 IU/min at a rate of 2–3 mL/min, not to exceed 3 mL/min.
2. Store at 2°–8° C.
3. Avoid freezing the diluent provided with drug.
4. Discard 2 years after date of manufacture.
5. Before reconstitution, warm diluent to room temperature but not above 40° C.
6. Agitate the solution gently until the powder is dissolved.
7. Administer drug within 3 hr of reconstitution to avoid incubation in case contamination occurred during preparation.
8. Do not refrigerate after reconstitution, because the active ingredient may precipitate out.

Asessment

1. Assess baseline BP and pulse and record before starting IV.
2. Obtain client's weight and height and record.
3. Note client complaints that may seem to suggest presence of liver disease (urticaria, fever, pruritus, anorexia, nausea, vomiting).

Interventions

1. If client complains of a tingling sensation, headache, chills or has a fever, reduce the rate of flow of IV, document and report to the physician.
2. Avoid aminocaproic acid administration. It may precipitate the development of thrombosis.
3. Monitor client closely for disseminated intravascular coagulation if Factor IX level is increased above 50% of normal.

Client/Family Teaching

1. Explain that product is prepared from human plasma and outline the associated potential risks.
2. Stress that local support groups may assist them to understand and cope with their disease.

Evaluation

1. Review appropriate lab data; assess response to therapy.
2. Observe for further evidence of side effects once IV rate of flow has been decreased.

TRANEXAMIC ACID (tran-ex-**AM**-ick **AH**-sid)

Cyklokapron (Rx)

Classification: Hemostatic, systemic.

Action/Kinetics: Tranexamic acid acts by competitively inhibiting activation of plasminogen thus decreasing the conversion of plasminogen to plasmin (the enzyme that breaks down fibrin clots). Up to 50% of an oral dose is absorbed from the GI tract; absorption is not affected by food. **Peak plasma levels:** 8 mg/L 3 hr after 1 g and 15 mg/L 3 hr after 2 g. **Effective tissue levels:**

Maintained for 17 hr. **Effective serum levels:** Maintained for 7–8 hr. **t½:** 2 hr (after IV use of 1 g). Over 95% of the drug is excreted via the kidney unchanged.

Uses: Short-term (2–8 days) in hemophiliacs to reduce or prevent hemorrhage (and to decrease need for replacement therapy) during and following tooth extraction. *Investigational:* Postsurgical hemorrhage, hyperfibrinolysis-induced hemorrhage, hereditary angioedema.

Contraindications: Subarachnoid hemorrhage, acquired defective color vision.

Special Concerns: Pregnancy category: B (use during pregnancy only if necessary). Use with caution during lactation.

Side Effects: *GI:* Nausea, vomiting, diarrhea. *Ophthalmologic:* Visual abnormalities. *Other:* Hypotension following rapid IV injection, giddiness.

Dosage: *Hemophiliacs requiring tooth extraction:* **IV, immediately before surgery,** 10 mg/kg; **then, after surgery, tablets,** 25 mg/kg t.i.d.–q.i.d. for 2–8 days. **Alternative regimen: PO,** 25 mg/kg t.i.d.–q.i.d. one day prior to surgery. If patient unable to take PO medication, give **IV,** 10 mg/kg t.i.d.–q.i.d.

The dosage should be reduced in patients with moderately to severely impaired renal function according to information provided by the manufacturer.

NURSING CONSIDERATIONS

Administration/Storage

1. Tranexamic acid may be mixed with any of the following solutions for IV infusion: carbohydrate, amino acid, electrolyte, dextran.
2. The drug should *not* be mixed with either blood or penicillin.
3. The mixture should be prepared on the day of use.
4. Heparin may be added to the solution for injection.
5. To minimize hypotension, IV administration should not exceed 1 mL/min.

Assessment

1. Take client's blood pressure and pulse before starting IV infusion of drug to establish a baseline against which to measure findings during and after drug therapy.
2. Note client history for evidence of defective color vision.
3. Assess for any evidence of nausea, vomiting or diarrhea.
4. When working with female clients check for potential pregnancy. With pregnancy, this drug should only be used if absolutely necessary.

Interventions

1. Monitor client frequently for hypotension during IV infusion, which indicates that the rate of infusion is too fast. Slow the rate of infusion and report to the physician.
2. Observe and report for signs and symptoms of thrombosis, such as leg pain, respiratory distress, or chest pain.
3. Anticipate reduced dosage in clients with impaired renal function.
4. Stress to client the importance of reporting for ophthalmologic examinations at regular intervals during drug therapy.

Evaluation

1. Assess response to therapy; review appropriate lab data.
2. Observe for freedom from complication of therapy.

CHAPTER TWENTY-ONE
Blood, Blood Components, and Blood Substitutes

General Statement: Blood, blood fractions, and blood extenders are not drugs in the ordinary sense. However, since they are often administered and monitored by nurses, they are discussed here briefly.

Blood falls into certain well-defined groups that can be exchanged relatively freely between members of the same group. Nevertheless, the transfusion of whole blood is associated with certain risks such as hypersensitivity and transmission of diseases (hepatitis, AIDS). The advent of blood components represents a major advance in therapy because the patient can now receive only the components necessary for treatment. The type of blood or blood substitute to be administered is determined by the need of the patient and the availability of the most suitable preparation.

Uses: Replacement of blood loss resulting from trauma, surgery, or disease. Plasma volume expansion, severe clotting defects, hemostasis (disease or drug-induced), and agranulocytosis. Burns, hypoproteinemia.

Side Effects: These depend on the blood or blood fraction being administered. *Viral Hepatitis* (onset 4 weeks to 6 months after transfusion): Characterized by anorexia, nausea, fever, malaise, tenderness and enlargement of liver, jaundice, and GI and skin reactions. *Hypersensitivity reactions:* Mild: urticaria, pruritus. Severe: bronchospasms. *Febrile reactions:* Characterized by fever (103°–104° F, or 39.4°–40.0° C), tremors, chills, and headaches. Onset: during initial 15 min of transfusion. *Hemolysis:* Potentially fatal complication caused by mismatching or mislabeling of blood or other human errors. Characterized by flushing, tachycardia, restlessness, dyspnea, chills, fever, headache, sharp pain in lumbar region, pressure feeling in chest, feeling of head fullness, nausea, and vomiting. Also hemoglobinuria and hemoglobinemia, and oliguria and acute renal failure. Usual onset: after administration of 100–200 mL incompatible blood. Shock and/or death occasionally occurs within min after initiation of transfusion. *Jaundice:* Caused by larger than normal number of hemolyzed RBCs that may be present in blood approaching its expiration date. Occurs more frequently in patients with inadequate liver function. *Hypervolemia (overexpanded blood volume):* Characterized by labored breathing, cough, dyspnea, cyanosis, and pulmonary edema. Occurs more frequently in the young, in the elderly, or in patients with cardiac or pulmonary disease. *Pyrogenic febrile reaction from contaminated products (especially bacteria:)* Characterized by chills, fever, profound shock, coma, convulsions, and often death. Onset: after transfusion of 50–100 mL.

NURSING CONSIDERATIONS FOR BLOOD, BLOOD EXPANDERS, FRACTIONS, AND SUBSTITUTES

Administration

1. Use normal saline as part of the Y setup (parallel setup) for blood transfusions.
2. Do not use dextrose injection. This will cause clumping of RBCs.
3. **Never use distilled water as this will cause hemolysis.**
4. Never add medication to blood or plasma.
5. Whenever possible, use plastic bags for transfusion to reduce the danger of air embolism.

Assessment

1. Review client history, asking client or family about any prior experience with blood transfusion.
2. Check chart to be certain that the proper blood work has been completed (type and cross match).
3. Prior to administration, check client name and blood type. Have two professionals verify client and check blood, following guidelines established by the institution.

Interventions

1. Prior to starting the transfusion, have available epinephrine, antihistamines, corticosteroids and resuscitative equipment.
2. Regulate IV to 20 drops/min and remain with the client to assess for any untoward reactions.
3. **Stop the infusion immediately and notify the physician if any of the following untoward reactions occur:**
   - *Anaphylactic reaction:* Client may complain of tightness of the chest; develops urticaria, wheezing, hypotension, nausea, and vomiting. Utilize emergency drugs and/or equipment as indicated.
   - *Circulatory embarrassment:* Client may first develop a persistent cough, often an early warning sign. Client then develops dyspnea, becomes cyanotic, and experiences frothy sputum (late sign). If this develops, position the client upright with lower extremities dependent. Utilize emergency drugs and equipment as necessary.
   - *Febrile (pyrogenic) reaction:* Client complains of sudden chills, headache—often suggesting that he/she must be catching a cold. Fever, nausea, and vomiting may also occur. Take temperature every 30 min after chills. Repeat until temperature is within normal range.
   - *Bacterial contamination:* Client develops severe chills, high fever, hypotension, and shock-like state. Take temperature every 30 min after chills. Repeat until temperature is within normal range.
   - *Hemolytic reaction:* Client develops chills and complains of a fullness in the head. Client complains of feeling pressure in the chest, and sharp pain in the lumbar region. The face is flushed, there is distention of neck veins, and hypotension, and circulatory collapse soon follow.
     - Have emergency drugs and equipment readily available.
     - Encourage client to ingest oral fluids for next few hours.
     - Measure and save all urine voided.
     - Monitor and record intake and output.
     - Have citrated blood tube available for blood to be drawn to check for free hemoglobin in plasma.
4. Check blood pressure, temperature and pulse according to institutional procedures (usually at the beginning of the infusion, 15 min after the infusion has started, and when the infusion is completed).

21

5. Report lack of response to therapy or any significant deviations from client's baseline values whether elevated or depressed.

6. Increase to rate of flow ordered if there are no reactions evident after the first 15 min. of therapy.

7. Unless otherwise indicated, anticipate that the rate of flow will be slower for the elderly and for clients with cardiac problems.

8. Document any untoward reaction and follow institutional guidelines for a transfusion reaction.

9. If an untoward reaction occurs, send the remainder of the material and the equipment used for the infusion to the laboratory for analysis.

ALBUMIN, NORMAL HUMAN SERUM, 5%   (al-BYOU-mihn)

Albuminar-5, Albutein 5%, Buminate 5%, Normal Serum Albumin (Human) 5% Solution, Plasbumin-5 (Rx)

ALBUMIN, NORMAL HUMAN SERUM, 25%   (al-BYOU-mihn)

Albuminar-25, Albutein 25%, Buminate 25%, Normal Serum Albumin (Human) 25% Solution, Plasbumin-25 (Rx)

Classification: Blood volume expander.

Action/Kinetics: Prepared from whole blood, serum, plasma, or placentas from healthy human donors. It is supplied as a 5% (isotonic and isosmotic with normal human plasma) and 25% (salt-poor solution of which each 50 mL is osmotically equivalent to 250 mL of citrated plasma) strength. It contains sodium, 130–160 mEq/liter.

Uses: Blood volume expander in shock, following surgery, hemorrhage, burns, or other trauma. Hypoproteinemia due to toxemia of pregnancy, anuria, acute hepatic cirrhosis or coma, acute nephrotic syndrome, tuberculosis, and premature infants. As an adjunct to exchange transfusions in hyperbilirubinemia and erythroblastosis fetalis. Adult respiratory distress syndrome, cardiopulmonary bypass (presurgically to dilute blood), acute liver failure (with or without coma), renal dialysis, acute nephrosis. Sequestration of protein-rich fluids as in extensive cellulitis, mediastinitis, pancreatitis, and acute peritonitis. To avoid excessive hypoproteinemia in exchange transfusions or where large volumes of washed or previously frozen red blood cells have been used.

Contraindications: Severe anemia, cardiac failure, allergy to albumin, renal insufficiency, presence of increased intravascular volume, chronic nephrosis, patients on cardiopulmonary bypass.

Special Concerns: Pregnancy category: C. This product is not a substitute for whole blood.

Side Effects: *Allergic:* Chills, fever, headache, rash, nausea, vomiting, flushing, urticaria, tachycardia, hypotension, respiratory and blood pressure changes, increased salivation. *CV:* Hypotension in patients on cardiopulmonary bypass. Rapid administration may cause pulmonary edema, dyspnea, and vascular overload.

Laboratory Test Interference: ↑ Serum alkaline phosphatase.

Dosage: 5%, IV infusion, individualized. *Hypoproteinemia:* rate not to exceed 5–10 mL/min. *Burns:* Sufficient solution to establish and maintain a plasma albumin level of 2–3 gm/100 mL (total serum protein of approximately 5.2 g/100 mL). *Shock:* **adults and children, initial,** 500 mL as rapidly as tolerated; repeat after 30 min if response inadequate. **Infants and neonates:** 10–20 mL/kg.

   25%, *Hypoproteinemia with or without edema:* **Adults,** 50–75 g/day; **pediatric:** 25 g/day. Rate should not exceed 2 mL/min. *Nephrosis:* 100 mL daily for 7–10 days, given with a loop diuretic. *Burns:* determined by extent; dose must be sufficient to maintain plasma albumin levels of 2–3 g/100 mL with a plasma oncotic pressure of 20 mm Hg. *Shock:* dose determined by condition of patient. For significantly reduced blood volume, give as rapidly as desired; for normal or slightly low blood volume, give 1 mL/min. *Hyperbilirubinemia and erythroblastosis fetalis:* 4 mL/kg (1 g/kg) 1–2 hr before transfusion of blood. *Erythrocyte resuspension:* Usually, 25 g/L of erythrocytes. *Renal dialysis:* 100 mL (avoid fluid overload).

NURSING CONSIDERATIONS

See also Nursing Considerations for *Blood, Blood Expanders, Fractions,* and *Substitutes,* p. 415.

Administration/Storage

1. Do not use turbid or sedimented solution.
2. Preparation does not contain preservatives. Use each opened bottle at once.
3. May be given as rapidly as needed initially. However, as plasma volume approaches normal, the 5% solution should not be given faster than 2–4 mL/min and the 25% solution should not be given faster than 1 mL/min.
4. In hypoproteinemia, the 5% solution should not be given faster than 5–10 mL/min and the 25% solution should not be given faster than 2–3 mL/min in order to minimize the possibility of circulatory overload and pulmonary edema.
5. Albumin should not be considered as a nutrient.
6. These products should be stored at room temperature, not to exceed 30°C (86°F).

Assessment

1. Note laboratory reports that may indicate the presence of any contraindications to therapy (e.g. anemia, renal insufficiency).
2. Obtain client blood pressure, pulse and respirations and record to use as a baseline against which to measure subsequent readings.
3. Weigh client if possible, before the start of therapy.

Interventions

1. Note symptoms of pulmonary edema, demonstrated by cough, dyspnea, rales and cyanosis. **Stop** the administration of albumin and notify the physician immediately if any of these symptoms occur. Obtain CXR.
2. Record intake and output and client weight.
3. Observe client for diuresis and reduction of edema if present.
4. Check client for evidence of dehydration such as dry, cracked lips, flushed, dry skin, reduced urinary output, dark colored urine, or loss of skin turgor. This necessitates further administration of IV fluids.
5. Take blood pressure and pulse frequently (usually every 15 min).
6. Note evidence of hemorrhage or shock that may occur following surgery or trauma. A rapid increase in blood pressure causes bleeding in severed blood vessels that had not been noted previously.
7. When administering commercial vials of blood volume expanders, use the accompanying vented IV administration sets.

BLOOD, WHOLE

Classification: Blood replacement.

Note: Because of the danger of hepatitis, mismatching errors, and allergic reactions, whole blood is only given when absolutely necessary. Individuals have also been infected with the AIDS virus in blood improperly screened although this problem has been greatly reduced by improved screening procedures.

Uses: Anemia, severe blood loss, and hypovolemia.

Side Effects: Serum hepatitis and hemolytic (chills, fever, flushing, restlessness, headache, nausea, vomiting) and allergic (bronchospasms) reactions.

Dosage: IV: 500 mL; repeat as necessary.

ADDITIONAL NURSING CONSIDERATIONS

See also *Nursing Considerations* for *Blood, Blood Expanders, Fractions, and Substitutes,* p. 415.

Administration/Storage

1. Obtain one unit of blood from blood bank just before transfusion unless there is an emergency situation.
2. Blood should be stored at 1°–10° C. Do not store blood in the ward or floor refrigerator. Temperature fluctuations make storage unsuitable in these areas.
3. Do not add any medication to blood bag or blood line.

Assessment

Assess baseline vital signs before transfusion is started and record.

Interventions

1. Review agency policy for administration of blood.
2. Explain to client the primary potential risks related to blood transfusions e.g., hepatitis, CMV, AIDS, syphilis, etc. Obtain appropriate consent.
3. Check client's name band and compare with blood identification slip to verify name and hospital number.
4. Check blood type on blood bag with the lab report on the client's chart. They must be ABO identical. Check for blood expiration dates (21 days for citrated blood and 4 days for heparinized blood).
5. Do not infuse cold blood. Warm blood at room temperature for 20–30 min before infusion.
6. Gently invert blood bag to remix plasma and RBCs before starting transfusion.
7. Use an in-line micron filter or filtered blood infusion sets to prevent microembolization, particularly pulmonary and cerebral embolization, from microaggregates present in stored blood.
8. Take vital signs at least hourly during the transfusion and then after the completion of the transfusion.
9. Allow a maximum of 4 hr for infusion of a unit of whole blood. Adjust flow according to client's age and condition. Consult the physician regarding the speed of transfusion.

DEXTRAN 1   (DEX-tran)

Promit (Rx)

Classification: Dextran adjunct.

Action/Kinetics: Dextrans 40, 70, and 75 are not antigenic; however, they are polysaccharides. Polysaccharide-reacting antibodies, due to antigenic polysaccharides, may react with dextran causing an anaphylactic reaction. Dextran 1, given prior to the administration of a clinical dextran solution, will prevent the formation of immune complexes with the polyvalent clinical dextrans, thus preventing anaphylaxis. Dextran 1 (molecular weight 1,000) is rapidly and completely excreted through the kidney. **t½:** 41 min.

Uses: Prevention of anaphylactic reactions due to IV infusion of dextrans 40, 70, or 75.

Contraindications: Same as those for the dextrans.

Special Concerns: Pregnancy category: B.

Side Effects: *CV:* Severe hypotension, bradycardia. *Miscellaneous:* Skin reactions, nausea, shivering, pallor.

Dosage: IV only. Adults: 20 mL (of the 150 mg/mL solution) rapidly 1–2 min before IV infusion of dextran solutions. **Pediatric:** 0.3 mL (of the 150 mg/mL solution) given the same way as the adult dose.

ADDITIONAL NURSING CONSIDERATIONS

See also *Nursing Considerations for Dextran 75,* p. 420.

Administration/Storage

1. The injection should not be diluted or mixed with clinical dextran.
2. No more than 15 min should elapse between the administration of dextran 1 and clinical dextran solutions. Should this period be exceeded, administer another dose of dextran 1.
3. If more than 48 hr has elapsed between infusions of clinical dextran, the dose of dextran 1 should be repeated.
4. Dextran 1 may be administered through a Y injection site or through a heparin lock but should not be given through an IV set used to infuse clinical dextran.
5. Dextran 1 should not be frozen and should be stored at a temperature not exceeding 25° C (77°F).

Assessment

Take client blood pressure prior to administering drug therapy.

Interventions

1. Monitor blood pressure and pulse closely during therapy.
2. Follow specific administration guidelines.

DEXTRAN, LOW MOLECULAR WEIGHT (DEXTRAN 40)   (DEX-tran)

10% LMD, Gentran 40, Rheomacrodex (Rx)

DEXTRAN, HIGH MOLECULAR WEIGHT (DEXTRAN 70)   (DEX-tran)

Gentran 70, Hyskon✿, Macrodex (Rx)

DEXTRAN 75   (DEX-tran)

Gentran 75 (Rx)

Classification: Blood volume expander.

Action/Kinetics: Dextrans are water-soluble, synthetic polysaccharides, which are available in various molecular weights; dextran 40, 70, and 75 have average molecular weights of 40,000, 70,000, and 75,000, respectively. The lower molecular weight products cause fewer allergic reactions. The preparation is a blood volume expander but is not a substitute for whole blood or its fractions. About one-half the dose of dextran 40 is excreted by the kidneys within 3 hr; the remaining dextran 40 is partly hydrolyzed and excreted in the urine or is taken back into the system where it is slowly metabolized by dextranase to glucose.

Uses: *Dextran 40:* Fluid replacement, treatment of shock due to surgery, hemorrhage, burns, or other trauma. As a priming fluid, alone or with other agents, in pump oxygenators for perfusing during extracorporeal circulation. Prophylaxis of acute thrombosis and pulmonary embolism in high risk surgical patients (i.e., hip surgery).

Dextran 70/75: Treatment of shock (or impending shock) due to surgery, hemorrhage, burns, or other trauma. It is not a substitute for whole blood.

Contraindications: Renal failure, severe bleeding disorders, marked cardiac decompensation, thrombocytopenia, hypofibrinogenemia, hypervolemic conditions, and known hypersensitivity. Products containing sodium chloride in patients with congestive heart failure, severe renal insufficiency, in edema, and in patients on corticosteroids.

Special Concerns: Pregnancy category: C. Use with caution in presence of renal, hepatic, or myocardial disease and during lactation.

Side Effects: *Allergic:* Nausea, vomiting, fever, urticaria, hypotension, headache, dyspnea, bronchospasm, tightness in chest, wheezing, anaphylaxis (rare). *Due to infusion technique:* Infection at injection site, phlebitis, venous thrombosis, hypervolemia. *Miscellaneous:* Hypernatremia, exacerbation of congestive heart failure. Dextran 70/75 may also cause nausea, vomiting, fever, marked hypotension, and joint pain.

Laboratory Test Interference: Falsely ↑ glucose, interference with bilirubin assays using alcohol, interference with total protein assays. Unreliable results in blood typing and cross matching procedures using enzyme techniques.

Dosage: Dextran 40. IV only. *Shock therapy:* **Adults and children, IV: first day,** 20 mL/kg with the first 10 mL/kg infused rapidly; **then,** daily dose should not exceed 10 mL/kg for more than 5 days. *Prophylaxis of venous thrombosis, pulmonary embolism:* On day of surgery, 10 mL/kg (500–1,000 mL); **then,** 500 mL daily for 2–3 days followed by 500 mL q 2–3 days up to 14 days. *Hemodiluent in extracorporeal circulation:* **Usual,** 10–20 mL/kg added to the perfusion circuit, not to exceed 20 mL/kg.

Dextran 70 and Dextran 75, IV only. Individualized, adults, usual: 500–1,000 mL. Total dose for first 24 hr should not exceed 20 mL/kg. Beyond 24 hr, dosage should not exceed 0.6 gm/kg (10 mL/kg). **Pediatric:** Dosage calculated on basis of body weight or surface area but total dose should not exceed 20 mL/kg.

ADDITIONAL NURSING CONSIDERATIONS

See also *Nursing Considerations* for *Blood, Blood Expanders, Fractions, and Substitutes,* p. 415.

Administration/Storage

1. Do not administer unless solution is clear.
2. Dissolve flakes in solution by heating the solution in water bath at 100° C for 15 min or by autoclaving at 110° C for 15 min.
3. Store unopened solution bottles at constant temperature, preferably 25° C (77° F), to prevent flake formation.
4. Discard partially used bottles, since they do not contain preservatives.

5. In emergencies, Dextran 70 or 75 may be administered to adults at a rate of 20–40 mL/min. In clients with normal or nearly normal plasma volume, the rate of infusion should not exceed 4 mL/min.

Assessment

1. Obtain a complete blood count, liver and renal function studies before administering dextran. These values may serve as a baseline against which to measure future values since they are all affected by the drug.
2. Note any signs of dehydration prior to onset of therapy.
3. Determine the presence of any bleeding disorders or any prior evidence of hypersensitivity to the drug.
4. Assess for the presence of edema.
5. Note if client is taking corticosteroids since Dextran is contraindicated in this instance.
6. Assess for the presence or any evidence of renal, hepatic, or cardiovascular disease. These conditions require particular caution and close monitoring during drug therapy.
7. Inquire if client follows a sodium restricted diet.

Interventions

1. If Dextran 70 or 75 is to be administered, perform all blood typing and cross match testing prior to starting therapy. Monitor laboratory values and report any changes to the physician.
2. Use finger sticks to determine blood sugar levels before and during therapy.
3. Have epinephrine and antihistamines readily available to counteract anaphylactic reactions that may occur.
4. Note any evidence of dehydration. Additional fluids may be necessary if dehydration develops.
5. Determine specific gravity of urine and record (normal: 1.005–1.025). Low values may indicate that dextran is not being eliminated and may mandate discontinuation of drug.
6. Measure output and assess for evidence of oliguria or anuria, which also may necessitate withdrawal of the drug.
7. Observe for sudden increases in central venous pressure, and/or pulmonary capillary wedge pressures, which may indicate circulatory overload. If this occurs, slow rate of IV infusion, document and report to the physician.
8. Observe client for elevated BP, cough, moist rales and cyanosis, especially if client has been on a sodium restricted diet. Dextran solutions contain sodium, which may precipitate pulmonary edema.
9. Note client complaints of nausea, vomiting or the presence of fever and arthralgia.
10. If the client is anesthetized and receiving Dextran 70 or 75, be alert for vomiting or for involuntary defecation.
11. Observe client for signs of bleeding (especially 3–9 hr after administration) from orifices and from the site of trauma.

Evaluation

1. Note any evidence of purpura, record and report to the physician.
2. Check hematocrit after administration of Dextran is completed.
3. Check client skin for signs of infection, venous thrombosis or phlebitis at the site of injection.
4. Note any client complaints of nausea, urticaria, headache or wheezing. These symptoms may appear mild but could result in severe allergic reaction.

HETASTARCH (HES) (HEH-tah-starch)

Hespan (Abbreviation: HES) (Rx)

Classification: Plasma expander.

Action/Kinetics: Hetastarch is a mixture of synthetic, water-soluble ethoxylated amylopectin molecules with molecular weights ranging from 10,000 to 1,000,000. The colloidal properties of 6% hetastarch are similar to albumin. Its action is similar to dextran, but it produces fewer allergic reactions and does not interfere with blood cross matching. Hetastarch is not a substitute for whole blood or its fractions. Molecules with a molecular weight less than 50,000 are eliminated quickly by the kidney whereas larger molecules are broken down to smaller ones. **t½:** 17 days for 90% of the dose and 48 days for 10% of the dose.

Use: Shock (burns, hemorrhages, sepsis, and surgery). Fluid replacement, plasma volume expansion. Adjunct in removal of WBCs (leukopheresis).

Contraindications: Severe bleeding disorders, severe CHF, or renal failure with oliguria or anuria.

Special Concerns: Use during pregnancy, especially in early pregnancy, only if benefits outweigh risks to the fetus.

Side Effects: *Hematologic:* Prolonged prothrombin, partial thromboplastin, and clotting times; decreased hematocrit. *GI:* Vomiting, enlargement of submaxillary and parotid glands. *Miscellaneous:* Chills, fever, itching, influenza-like syndrome, muscle pain, edema of the lower extremities, anaphylaxis, circulatory overload, dilution of plasma proteins.

Dosage: IV infusion only. Individualized, usual, *plasma expansion:* 500–1,000 mL of 6% solution up to maximum of 1,500 mL (20 mL/kg/day). *For acute hemorrhage:* rapid rate up to 20 mL/kg/hr. Use slower rates for burns and septic shock. *Leukopheresis:* 250–700 mL infused at a constant ratio, usually 1:8 to venous whole blood.

NURSING CONSIDERATIONS

Administration/Storage

1. The solution should not be used if it is turbid deep brown or if a crystalline precipitate forms.
2. The solution should not be frozen; store at room temperature not exceeding 40° C (104° F).
3. Discard partially used bottles.

Assessment

1. Determine hematocrit and record prior to administration of drug.
2. Inquire if client follows a sodium restricted diet.
3. Note any history of severe bleeding disorders, severe CHF, and/or renal dysfunction.
4. Assess women of childbearing age for pregnancy.

Interventions

1. Monitor output and assess for the presence of oliguria or anuria. If these occur, withdraw hetastarch and notify physician.
2. Check specific gravity of urine (normal: 1.005–1.025). Low values indicate that hetastarch is not being excreted and may require discontinuing administration of plasma expanders.
3. After administration of 500 mL of hetastarch, obtain a hematocrit. Hematocrit values lower than 30% by volume should be avoided.

4. Note any sudden increase in central venous pressure and/or pulmonary capillary wedge pressure. This may indicate a circulatory overload and congestive heart failure.

5. If client has been following a salt-restricted diet, watch closely for evidence of edema (elevated BP, cough, moist rales, cyanosis). Sodium in hetastarch may precipitate pulmonary edema in clients with cardiac disease or kidney dysfunction.

6. Observe client for purpura or other signs of bleeding from orifices or wounds, especially 3–9 hr after drug administration has been completed. Hetastarch may temporarily cause prolonged bleeding times.

Evaluation

1. Note any evidence of purpura, record and report to the physician.
2. Check hematocrit after administration of Hetastarch is completed.
3. Evaluate response to therapy and assess for complications of drug therapy.

PLASMA, PROTEIN FRACTION (PLAHZ-mah)
Plasmanate, Plasma-Plex, Plasmatein, Protenate (Rx)

Classification: Blood volume expander.

Action/Kinetics: The cell-free portion of the blood, or a 5% solution of human plasma proteins in sodium chloride injection, is used when whole blood is unnecessary or unavailable. Preparations contain albumin, globulins, and electrolytes. Contains sodium 130–160 mEq/liter.

Uses: Hypovolemic shock, hypoproteinemia.

Contraindications: Cardiopulmonary bypass surgery, severe anemia, renal insufficiency, cardiac failure, in normal or increased intravascular volume.

Special Concerns: Pregnancy category: C. Use with caution in renal or hepatic failure.

Side Effects: *CV:* Hypotension, vascular overload, pulmonary edema, dyspnea due to rapid infusion or intra-arterial use in patients on cardiopulmonary bypass. *Allergic:* Fever, chills, headache, rash, nausea, vomiting, flushing, urticaria, back pain, tachycardia, increased salivation, changes in respiration, pulse, and blood pressure.

Dosage: IV infusion, individualized. *Hypovolemic shock:* **initial,** 250–500 mL at a rate not to exceed 10 mL/min; **pediatric, infants and young children: initial,** 20–30 mL/kg at a rate not to exceed 10 mL/min. Subsequent dosage depends on response. *Hypoproteinemia:* 1,000–1,500 mL (50–75 gm protein) at a rate not to exceed 5–8 mL/min.

NURSING CONSIDERATIONS

Administration/Storage

1. The products are ready to use without further preparation.
2. Plasma protein fraction can be given without regard to the blood group or type of the client.
3. The solution should not be used if it is turbid, has been frozen, if there is a sediment in the bottle, or if more than 4 hr have elapsed after the vial has been entered.
4. Since there are no preservatives in these products, vials should be used only on one occasion. Unused portions should be discarded.
5. Plasma protein fraction should not be administered through the same IV set as amino acid solutions, protein hydrolysates, or alcohol since the proteins may precipitate.

6. Check administration rate with physician. Usual rate of administration: adult and infants, 5–10 mL/min. As plasma volume approaches normal, rate should not exceed 5–8 mL/min.

7. Not to be given near any site of infection or trauma.

8. If more than 250 g is required over 48 hr, consideration should be given to administering whole blood or plasma, rather than additional albumin.

Assessment

1. Obtain complete blood count and record, to serve as baseline data.
2. Determine that renal and liver function studies have been completed.
3. Document blood pressure and pulse prior to beginning therapy.

Interventions

1. Monitor BP and pulse closely. Document and report any evidence of hypotension to the physician.
2. Observe central venous pressure and/or pulmonary capillary wedge pressure for any sudden increases. Slow the rate of the infusion, document and report immediately to the physician.
3. Record and report any client complaints such as fever, chills, headache, rash or flushing. These side effects may indicate an allergic response to drug therapy.

RED CELLS, PACKED

Classification: Blood replacement.

Action/Kinetics: Packed red blood cells or concentrates are prepared by removing plasma from whole blood. The preparation sometimes goes through a freeze-thaw process that yields a purer product. Administration of packed red cells reduces the risk of circulatory overload and the amount of transfused blood antibodies and electrolytes (sodium, potassium, citrate). Other dangers associated with blood transfusions (hepatitis, allergic reactions, mismatching) are not reduced.

Uses: Aplastic anemia, hemorrhages, and when it is desirable to replace red cells without expanding blood volume. Especially suitable for the elderly, infants, and patients with cardiopulmonary or renal disease.

Side Effects: See *Blood, Whole.*

Dosage: Equivalent of indicated amount of whole blood.

ADDITIONAL NURSING CONSIDERATIONS

See also *Nursing Considerations* for *Blood, Blood Expanders, Fractions, and Substitutes,* p. 415 and *Blood, Whole,* p. 418.

Administration/Storage

1. Store between 1°–6° C.
2. Check label for expiration date and to ascertain correct typing and cross matching blood and client.
3. Allow 45–90 minutes for administration of packed cells.
4. *Must* be ABO compatible.

CHAPTER TWENTY-TWO

Thrombolytic Agents

General Statement: Alteplase, a product of recombinant DNA technology, has markedly changed the manner by which acute myocardial infarction is treated. Thrombolytic agents are used to promote the dissolution (lysis) of the insoluble fibrin trapped in intravascular emboli and thrombi. By activating the patient's own fibrinolytic system, the thrombolytic enzymes increase the degradation of the fibrin clots in the blood vessels. In thrombolytic therapy the enzymes interfere with the clotting mechanism of the body, the most serious complication of which is hemorrhage. Heparin therapy usually follows treatment with these agents.

ALTEPLASE, RECOMBINANT (AL-teh-playz)

Activase, Activase rt-PA✸ (Rx)

Classification: Thrombolytic agent (tissue plasminogen activator).

Action/Kinetics: Alteplase, a tissue plasminogen activator, is synthesized by a human melanoma cell line using recombinant DNA technology. This enzyme binds to fibrin in a thrombus, causing a conversion of plasminogen to plasmin. This conversion results in local fibrinolysis and a decrease in circulating fibrinogen. Within 10 min following termination of an infusion, 80% of the alteplase has been cleared from the plasma by the liver. The enzyme activity of alteplase is 580,000 IU/mg. $t^{1}/_{2}$, **initial:** 4 min; **final:** 35 min (elimination phase).

Uses: Lysis of coronary thrombi following acute myocardial infarction. The drug thus reduces the incidence of congestive heart failure and improves ventricular function. Acute pulmonary thromboembolism. *Investigational:* Unstable angina pectoris.

Contraindications: Severe (uncontrolled) hypertension. Patients with a risk of internal bleeding and history of cerebrovascular accident, intracranial or intraspinal surgery or trauma (within 2 months), aneurysm, bleeding diathesis, intracranial neoplasm, arteriovenous malformation or aneurysm, severe uncontrolled hypertension, and active internal bleeding.

Special Concerns: Use with caution in the presence of recent GI or GU bleeding (within 10 days), subacute bacterial endocarditis, acute pericarditis, significant liver dysfunction, concomitant use of oral anticoagulants, diabetic hemorrhagic retinopathy, septic thrombophlebitis or occluded AV cannula (at infected site), pregnancy (category: C) and lactation, mitral stenosis with atrial fibrillation. Use with caution within 10 days of major surgery (e.g., obstetrics, coronary artery bypass) and in patients over 75 years of age. Safety and efficacy have not been established in children.
  Note: Doses greater than 150 mg have been associated with an increase in intracranial bleeding.

Side Effects: *Bleeding tendencies:* Internal bleeding (including the GI and GU tracts and

22

intracranial or retroperitoneal sites). Superficial bleeding (e.g., sites of recent surgery, venous cutdowns, arterial punctures). *GI:* Nausea, vomiting. *Miscellaneous:* Fever, urticaria, hypotension.

Drug Interactions

Acetylsalicylic acid	↑ Risk of bleeding
Dipyridamole	↑ Risk of bleeding
Heparin	↑ Risk of bleeding, especially at arterial puncture sites

---

Dosage: IV infusion only. 100 mg total dose subdivided as follows: 60 mg (34.8 million IU) the first hour with 6–10 mg given in a bolus over the first 1–2 min and the remaining 50–54 mg given over the hour; 20 mg (11.6 million IU) over the 2nd hr and 20 mg given over the 3rd hr. **Patients less than 65 kg:** 1.25 mg/kg given over 3 hr, with 60% given the first hour with 6–10% given by direct IV injection within the first 1–2 min; 20% is given the 2nd hr and 20% during the 3rd hr. Doses of 150 mg have caused an increase in intracranial bleeding.

NURSING CONSIDERATIONS

Administration/Storage

1. Alteplase therapy should be initiated as soon as possible after onset of symptoms.
2. Nearly 90% of clients also receive heparin concomitantly with alteplase and either aspirin or dipyridamole during or after heparin therapy.
3. The product must be reconstituted with only sterile water for injection without preservatives immediately prior to use. The reconstituted preparation contains 1 mg/mL and is a colorless to pale yellow transparent solution.
4. Using an 18-gauge needle, the stream of sterile water for injection should be directed into the lyophilized cake. The product should be left undisturbed for several minutes to allow dissipation of any large bubbles.
5. If necessary, the reconstituted solution may be further diluted immediately prior to use in an equal volume of 0.9% sodium chloride injection or 5% dextrose injection to yield a concentration of 0.5 mg/mL. Dilution should be accomplished by gentle swirling or slow inversion.
6. Either glass bottles or polyvinyl chloride bags may be used for administration.
7. Alteplase is stable for up to 8 hr following reconstitution or dilution. Stability will not be affected by light.
8. Other medications should not be added to the infusion solution.
9. Lyophilized alteplase should be stored at room temperatures not to exceed 30° C or under refrigeration between 2°–8° C.

Assessment

1. Assure that bleeding times have been completed before initiating therapy. These serve as baseline data against which to determine client response to therapy and any associated changes that may need to occur.
2. Note any client history of hypertension or internal bleeding.
3. Record client age and determine whether or not client has had recent surgery.
4. Assess client's overall physical condition and document.
5. Obtain a drug history and determine if client is currently taking any oral anticoagulant drugs.

Interventions

1. Carefully review and follow instructions for drug reconstitution.
2. Review the contraindications carefully before initiating therapy.
3. Anticipate concurrent heparin administration by infusion.
4. Have available emergency drugs and resuscitative equipment.
5. Clients receiving therapy should be observed in a closely monitored environment.
6. Anticipate and assess for reperfusion reactions such as:
   - reperfusion arrhythmias usually of short duration. These may include accelerated idioventricular rhythm and sinus bradycardia.
   - a reduction of chest pain.
   - a return of the elevated ST segment to near baseline levels.
7. Check all access sites for any evidence of bleeding.
8. During IV therapy, arterial sticks require 30 min of manual pressure followed by application of a pressure dressing.
9. Use an electronic infusion device for medication administration. Do not add any other medications to the line.
10. In the event of any uncontrolled bleeding, terminate the alteplase and heparin infusions and notify the physician immediately.

Client/Family Teaching

1. Review the inherent risks of drug therapy with the client and family.
2. Stress that to be effective, the therapy should be instituted within 4–6 hours of onset of symptoms of acute myocardial infarction.

Evaluation

1. Note response to therapy, such as improved circulation or improved left ventricular function.
2. Evaluate for evidence of side effects such as rust colored urine, GI bleeding, or signs of intracranial bleeding (increased ICP).
3. Assess for any evidence of bleeding. Attempt to control bleed, document site and note extent of bleeding.

ANISTREPLASE   (an-ih-**STREP**-layz)

Eminase (Rx)

Classification: Thrombolytic enzyme.

Action/Kinetics: Anistreplase is prepared by acylating human plasma derived from lys-plasminogen and purified streptokinase derived from group C beta-hemolytic streptococci. When prepared, anistreplase is an inactive derivative of a fibrinolytic enzyme although the compound can still bind to fibrin. Anistreplase is activated by deacylation and subsequent release of the anisoyl group in the blood stream. The production of plasmin from plasminogen occurs in both the blood stream and the thrombus leading to thrombolysis. The drug will lyse thrombi obstructing coronary arteries and reduce the size of infarcts. **t½:** 70–120 min.

Uses: Management of acute myocardial infarction in adults resulting in improvement of ventricular function and reduction of mortality. Treatment should be initiated as soon as possible after the onset of symptoms of acute myocardial infarction.

Contraindications: Use in active internal bleeding; within 2 months of intracranial or intraspinal surgery or trauma; history of cerebrovascular accident; intracranial neoplasm, arteriovenous malformation, or aneurysm; known bleeding diathesis; severe, uncontrolled hypertension; severe allergic reactions to streptokinase.

Special Concerns: Pregnancy category: C. Use with caution in nursing mothers. Safety and effectiveness have not been determined in children.

Note: The risks of anistreplase therapy may be increased in the following conditions; thus, benefit versus risk must be assessed prior to use: within 10 days of major surgery (e.g., coronary artery bypass graft, obstetrical delivery, organ biopsy, previous puncture of noncompressible vessels); cerebrovascular disease; within 10 days of GI or GU bleeding; within 10 days of trauma including cardiopulmonary resuscitation; systolic blood pressure greater than 180 mm Hg or diastolic blood pressure greater than 110 mm Hg; likelihood of left heart thrombus (e.g., mitral stenosis with atrial fibrillation); subacute bacterial endocarditis; acute pericarditis; hemostatic defects including those secondary to severe hepatic or renal disease; pregnancy; patients older than 75 years of age; diabetic hemorrhagic retinopathy or other hemorrhagic ophthalmic conditions; septic thrombophlebitis or occluded AV cannula at seriously infected site; patients on oral anticoagulant therapy; any condition in which bleeding constitutes a significant hazard or would be difficult to manage due to its location.

Side Effects: *Bleeding:* Including at the puncture site (most common), nonpuncture site hematoma, hematuria, hemoptysis, GI hemorrhage, intracranial bleeding, gum/mouth hemorrhage, epistaxis, anemia, eye hemorrhage. *CV:* Arrhythmias, conduction disorders, hypotension; cardiac rupture, chest pain, emboli (causal relationship to use of anistreplase unknown). *Allergic:* Anaphylaxis, bronchospasm, angioedema, urticaria, itching, flushing, rashes, eosinophilia, delayed purpuric rash which may be associated with arthralgia, ankle edema, mild hematuria, GI symptoms, and proteinuria. *GI:* Nausea, vomiting. *Hematologic:* Thrombocytopenia. *CNS:* Agitation, dizziness, paresthesia, tremor, vertigo. *Respiratory:* Dyspnea, lung edema. *Miscellaneous:* Chills, fever, headache, shock.

Drug Interactions: Increased risk of bleeding or hemorrhage if used with heparin, oral anticoagulants, vitamin K antagonists, aspirin, or dipyridamole.

Laboratory Test Interferences: ↑ Transaminase levels, thrombin time, activated partial thromboplastin time, and prothrombin time. ↓ Plasminogen and fibrinogen.

Dosage: IV only: 30 units over 2–5 min into an IV line or vein as soon as possible after onset of symptoms.

NURSING CONSIDERATIONS

See also *Nursing Considerations* for *Alteplase, Recombinant*, p. 426.

Administration/Storage

1. The drug is to be reconstituted by slowly adding 5 mL of sterile water for injection. To minimize foaming, gently roll the vial after directing the stream of sterile water against the side of the vial. The vial should not be shaken.
2. The reconstituted solution should be colorless to pale yellow without any particulate matter or discoloration.
3. The reconstituted solution should not be further diluted before administration.
4. The reconstituted solution should not be added to any infusion fluids and no other medications should be added to the vial or syringe containing anistreplase.
5. The solution should be discarded if not administered within 30 min of reconstitution.

Assessment

1. Note any history and any evidence of bleeding.
2. Obtain client blood pressure and pulse readings as baseline data, before initiating therapy.
3. Take a full drug history. Note especially if client has been taking aspirin, anticoagulants or vitamin K antagonists.
4. Determine that appropriate laboratory studies have been completed prior to starting drug therapy.

Interventions

1. Invasive procedures should be avoided in order to minimize bleeding tendencies.
2. If an arterial puncture is necessary following use of anistreplase, an upper-extremity vessel that is accessible to manual compression should be used. Apply 30 min. of manual pressure followed by application of a pressure dressing. Puncture site should be checked frequently for any evidence of bleeding.

Evaluation

1. Resistance to the effects of anistreplase may be observed if the drug is given more than 5 days after a previous dose, after streptokinase therapy, or after a streptococcal infection.
2. Increased antistreptokinase antibody levels between 5 days and 6 months after anistreplase or streptokinase administration may increase the risk of allergic reactions.

STREPTOKINASE   (strehp-toe-**KYE**-nayz)

Kabikinase, Streptase (Rx)

Classification: Thrombolytic agent.

Action/Kinetics: Most patients have a natural resistance to streptokinase that must be overcome with the loading dose before the drug becomes effective. Thrombin time and streptokinase resistance should be determined before initiation of the therapy. Streptokinase acts with plasminogen to produce an "activator complex," which enhances the conversion of plasminogen to plasmin. Plasmin then breaks down fibrinogen, fibrin clots, and other plasma proteins. Thus, the drug promotes the dissolution (lysis) of the insoluble fibrin trapped in intravascular emboli and thrombi. Also, inhibitors of streptokinase, such as alpha-2-macroglobulin, are rapidly inactivated by streptokinase. **Onset:** rapid; **duration:** 12 hr. **t½, activator complex:** 23 min.

Uses: Deep vein thrombosis; arterial thrombosis and embolism; acute evolving transmural myocardial infarction. Also, clearing of occluded arteriovenous and IV cannulae.

Contraindications: Any condition presenting a risk of hemorrhage, such as recent surgery or biopsies, delivery within 10 days, ulcerative disease. Arterial emboli originating from the left side of the heart. Also, hepatic or renal insufficiency, TB, recent cerebral embolism, thrombosis, hemorrhage, subacute bacterial endocarditis, rheumatic valvular disease, thrombocytopenia. Streptokinase resistance in excess of 1 million IU.

Special Concerns: Pregnancy category: C. The use of streptokinase in septic thrombophlebitis may be hazardous. History of significant allergic response. Safety in children has not been established.

Side Effects: *CV:* Superficial bleeding, severe internal bleeding. *Allergic:* Nausea, headache, breathing difficulties, bronchospasm, angioneurotic edema, urticaria, flushing, musculoskeletal pain, vasculitis, interstitial nephritis, periorbital swelling. *Other:* Fever, possible development of Guillain-Barre Syndrome, development of antistreptokinase antibody (i.e., streptokinase may be ineffective if administered between 5 days and 6 months following prior use of streptokinase or following streptococcal infections).

Drug Interactions: The following drugs ↑ the chance of bleeding when given concomitantly with streptokinase: Anticoagulants, aspirin, heparin, indomethacin, and phenylbutazone.

Laboratory Test Interferences: ↓ Fibrinogen, plasminogen. ↑ Thrombin time, prothrombin time, and activated partial thromboplastin time.

Dosage: *Venous or arterial thrombosis, arterial or pulmonary embolism.* **IV infusion, initial,** 250,000 IU over 30 min (use the 1,500,000 IU vial diluted to 90 mL); **maintenance:** 100,000 IU/hr for 24–72 hr for arterial thrombosis or embolism, 72 hr for deep vein thrombosis, and 24 hr for pulmonary embolism. **Intracoronary infusion:** Same dose as IV infusion; however, the 1,500,000 IU vial should be diluted to 45 mL with a rate of infusion of 15 mL/hr for the loading dose and 3 mL/hr for maintenance doses. May be followed by continuous IV heparin infusion to prevent recurrent thrombosis (start only after thrombin time has decreased to less than twice the normal control value, usually 3–4 hr).

Acute evolving transmural myocardial infarction. **IV infusion:** 1,500,000 IU within 60 min (use the 1,500,000 IU vial diluted to a total of 45 mL). **Intracoronary infusion,** 20,000 IU by bolus; **then,** 2,000 IU/min for 60 min (total dose of 140,000 IU). Use the 250,000 IU vial diluted to 125 mL. *Arteriovenous cannula occlusion:* 250,000 IU in 2-mL IV solution into each occluded limb of cannula; **then,** after 2 hr aspirate cannula limbs, flush with saline, and reconnect cannula.

NURSING CONSIDERATIONS

See also *Nursing Considerations* for *Alteplase Recombinant,* p. 426.

Administration/Storage

1. Sodium chloride injection USP or 5% dextrose injection is the preferred diluent for IV use.
2. For AV cannulae, dilute 250,000 units with 2 mL of sodium chloride injection or 5% dextrose injection.
3. Reconstitute gently, as directed by manufacturer, without shaking vial.
4. Use within 24 hr after reconstitution.
5. Use an electronic infusion device to administer streptokinase and do not add any other medications to the line.

Assessment

1. Ensure that baseline bleeding studies have been completed prior to initiation of therapy.
2. Identify other drugs the client may be taking such as aspirin or similar products that could increase bleeding times.
3. During the nursing history, note any history of prior conditions that might contraindicate the use of streptokinase. (e.g. TB, SBE, ulcerative disease, recent surgery).
4. Determine from client or family any history or evidence of bleeding tendencies.
5. Note any evidence of heart disease and/or allergic reaction to any drugs.

Interventions

1. Assure that the client understands the purpose of the therapy.
2. Check that the client has had blood typed and cross matched before initiating thrombolytic therapy.

3. Review all contraindications before initiating therapy.

4. Have emergency drugs and equipment available. Have corticosteroids and aminocaproic acid available in the event there is excessive bleeding.

5. Clients receiving therapy should be observed in a closely monitored environment.

6. When administering thrombolytic agents, monitor plasma thrombin time q 4–12 hr. Thrombin time values should be 2–5 times higher than the normal control values.

7. Check access sites for evidence of bleeding. Check stools for evidence of occult blood.

8. During IV therapy, arterial sticks require 30 min of manual pressure followed by application of a pressure dressing.

9. To prevent bruising, avoid unnecessary handling of client.

10. If an IM injection is necessary, apply pressure after withdrawing the needle to prevent a hematoma and bleeding from the puncture site.

11. If excessive bleeding develops from an invasive procedure, discontinue therapy and call for packed RBCs and plasma expanders *other than dextran*.

12. To prevent new thrombus formation, anticipate the use of IV heparin and oral anticoagulants when the thrombolytic therapy is concluded.

13. Geriatric clients have an increased risk of bleeding during therapy.

14. Monitor BP and pulse. Have atropine available for hypotension and bradycardia.

15. Observe injection sites and postoperative wounds for bleeding during thrombolytic therapy. Document and report.

16. Note evidence of allergic reactions, ranging from anaphylaxis to moderate and mild reactions. These usually can be controlled with antihistamines and corticosteroids.

17. Note any redness and/or pain at the site of infusion. It may be necessary to further dilute the solution to prevent phlebitis.

18. Anticipate concomitant administration with aspirin.

19. Provide symptomatic treatment for fever reaction.

20. Following recanalization of an occluded coronary artery, clients may develop reperfusion reactions, these may include:
    - reperfusion arrhythmias, usually of short duration. These may include accelerated idioventricular rhythm and sinus bradycardia.
    - a reduction of chest pain.
    - a return of the elevated ST segment to near baseline levels.

Client/Family Teaching

1. Review the inherent risks of drug therapy with the client and family.

2. Stress that to be effective, the therapy should be instituted within 4–6 hours of onset of symptoms of acute myocardial infarction.

3. Explain the importance of reporting any symptoms or side effects to the nurse immediately.

Evaluation

1. Evaluate response to therapy utilizing pretreatment parameters for comparison.

2. Note any evidence of superficial or severe uncontrolled bleeding. In this event, stop therapy, attempt to control bleeding and notify physician immediately.

UROKINASE   (you-roh-**KYE**-nayz)

Abbokinase, Abbokinase Open-Cath (Rx)

Classification: Thrombolytic agent.

Action/Kinetics: Urokinase converts plasminogen to plasmin; plasmin then breaks down fibrin clots and fibrinogen. **Onset:** rapid; **duration:** 12 hr. **t½:** Less than 20 min, although effect on coagulation disappears after a few hours.

Uses: Acute pulmonary thromboembolism. To clear IV catheters that are blocked by fibrin or clotted blood. *Investigational:* Acute arterial thromboembolism, acute arterial thrombosis, acute arterial coronary thrombosis, to clear arteriovenous cannula.

Contraindications: Any condition presenting a risk of hemorrhage, such as recent surgery or biopsies, delivery within 10 days, pregnancy, ulcerative disease. Also hepatic or renal insufficiency, TB, recent cerebral embolism, thrombosis, hemorrhage, subacute bacterial endocarditis, rheumatic valvular disease, thrombocytopenia.

Special Concerns: Pregnancy category: B. The use of the drugs in septic thrombophlebitis may be hazardous. Use with caution during lactation. Safe use in children has not been established.

Side Effects: *CV:* Superficial bleeding, severe internal bleeding. *Allergic:* Rarely, skin rashes, bronchospasm. *Other:* Fever.

Drug Interactions: The following drugs ↑ the chance of bleeding when given concomitantly with urokinase: Anticoagulants, aspirin, heparin, indomethacin, and phenylbutazone.

Dosage: IV infusion only. *Acute pulmonary embolism:* **loading dose,** 4,400 IU/kg administered over 10 min at a rate of 90 mL/hr; **maintenance, IV:** 4,400 IU/kg administered continuously at a rate of 15 mL/hr for 12 hr. May be followed by continuous IV heparin infusion to prevent recurrent thrombosis (start only after thrombin time has decreased to less than twice the normal control value). *Coronary artery thrombi:* **Initial,** heparin, as a bolus of 2,500–10,000 units **IV; then,** begin infusion of urokinase at a rate of 6,000 IU/min (4 mL/min) for up to 2 hr (average total dose of urokinase may be 500,000 IU). Urokinase should be administered until the artery is opened maximally (15–30 min after initial opening although it has been given for up to 2 hr). *Clear IV catheter:* instill into the catheter 1–1.8 mL of a solution containing 5,000 IU/mL.

NURSING CONSIDERATIONS

See also *Nursing Considerations* for *Streptokinase,* p. 429, and *Alteplase, Recombinant,* p. 426.

Administration/Storage

1. Reconstitute only with sterile water for injection without preservatives. Do not use bacteriostatic water.
2. The vial should be rolled and tilted, but not shaken, during reconstitution.
3. Reconstitute immediately before using.
4. Discard any unused portion.
5. Dilute reconstituted urokinase before IV administration in 0.9% normal saline or 5% dextrose injection.

Part Five

Cardiovascular Drugs

5

CHAPTER TWENTY-THREE

Cardiac Glycosides

23

General Statement: Cardiac glycosides, such as digitoxin, are plant alkaloids. They are probably the oldest, yet still the most effective, drugs for treating congestive heart failure (CHF). By improving myocardial contraction, they improve blood supply to all organs, including the kidney, thereby improving function. This action results in diuresis, thereby correcting the edema often associated with cardiac insufficiency. Digitalis glycosides are also used for the treatment of cardiac arrhythmias, since they decrease pulse rate as well.

The cardiac glycosides are cumulative in action. This effect is partially responsible for the difficulties associated with their use.

Action/Kinetics: Cardiac glycosides increase the force of myocardial contraction (positive inotropic effect). This effect is due to inhibition of movement of sodium and potassium ions across myocardial cell membranes due to complexing with adenosine triphosphatase. This results in an increase of calcium influx and an increased release of free calcium ions within the myocardial cells which then potentiate the contractility of cardiac muscle fibers. The digitalis glycosides also decrease the rate of conduction and increase the refractory period of the AV node. This effect is due to an increase in parasympathetic tone and a decrease in sympathetic tone. The cardiac glycosides are absorbed from the GI tract. Absorption varies from 40 to 90%, depending on the preparation and brand. With most preparations, peak plasma concentrations are reached within 2–3 hr. Half-life ranges from 1.7 days for digoxin to 7 days for digitoxin. The drugs are primarily excreted through the kidneys, either unchanged (digoxin) or metabolized (digitoxin). The initial dose of digitalis glycosides is larger (loading dose) and is traditionally referred to as the *digitalizing dose (DD)*; subsequent doses are referred to as *maintenance doses (MD)*.

Uses: Congestive heart failure, especially secondary to hypertension, coronary artery or atherosclerotic heart disease, valvular heart disease. Control of rapid ventricular contraction rate in patients with atrial fibrillation or flutter. Slow heart rate in sinus tachycardia due to congestive heart failure. Supraventricular tachycardia. Prophylaxis and treatment of recurrent paroxysmal atrial tachycardia with paroxysmal AV junctional rhythm. In conjunction with propranolol for angina. Cardiogenic shock (value not established).

Contraindications: Coronary occlusion or angina pectoris in the absence of CHF or hypersensitivity to cardiogenic glycosides.

Special Concerns: Use with caution in patients with ischemic heart disease, acute myocarditis, ventricular tachycardia, hypertrophic subaortic stenosis, hypoxic or myxedemic states, Adams-Stokes or carotid sinus syndromes, cardiac amyloidosis, or cyanotic heart and lung disease, including emphysema and partial heart block. Electric pacemakers may sensitize the myocardium to cardiac glycosides.

The cardiac glycosides should also be given cautiously and at reduced dosage to elderly, debilitated patients, pregnant women and nursing mothers, and to newborn, term, or premature infants who have immature renal and hepatic function. Similar precautions also should be observed for patients with reduced renal and/or hepatic function, since such impairment retards excretion of cardiac glycosides.

Side Effects: Cardiac glycosides are extremely toxic and have caused death even in patients who have received the drugs for long periods of time. There is a narrow margin of safety between an effective therapeutic dose and a toxic dose. Overdosage caused by the cumulative effects of the drug is a constant danger in therapy with cardiac glycosides. Digitalis toxicity is characterized by a wide variety of symptoms, which are hard to differentiate from those of the cardiac disease itself.

CV: Changes in the rate, rhythm, and irritability of the heart and the mechanism of the heartbeat. Extrasystoles, bigeminal pulse, coupled rhythm, ectopic beat, and other forms of arrhythmias have been noted. Death most often results from ventricular fibrillation. Cardiac glycosides should be discontinued in adults when pulse rate falls below 60 beats/minute. All cardiac changes are best detected by the electrocardiogram (ECG), which is also most useful in patients suffering from intoxication. Acute hemorrhage.

GI: Anorexia, nausea, vomiting, excessive salivation, epigastric distress, abdominal pain, diarrhea, bowel necrosis. Patients on digitalis therapy may experience two vomiting stages. The first is an early sign of toxicity and is a direct effect of digitalis on the GI tract. Late vomiting indicates stimulation of the vomiting center of the brain, which occurs after the heart muscle has been saturated with digitalis.

CNS: Headaches, fatigue, lassitude, irritability, malaise, muscle weakness, insomnia, stupor. Psychotomimetic effects (especially in elderly or arteriosclerotic patients or neonates) including disorientation, confusion, depression, aphasia, delirium, hallucinations, and, rarely, convulsions. *Neuromuscular:* Neurologic pain involving the lower third of the face and lumbar areas, paresthesia. *Visual disturbances:* Blurred vision, flickering dots, white halos, borders around dark objects, diplopia, amblyopia, color perception changes. *Hypersensitivity (5–7 days after starting therapy):* Skin reactions (urticaria, fever, pruritus, facial and angioneurotic edema). *Other:* Chest pain, coldness of extremities.

Children: Atrial arrhythmias and atrial tachycardia with AV block are the most common signs of toxicity; in neonates excessive slowing of sinus rate, sinoatrial (SA) arrest, and prolongation of PR interval occur.

Patients suffering from digitalis intoxication should be admitted to the intensive care area for continuous monitoring of ECG. Administration of digitalis should be halted. If serum potassium is below normal, potassium salts should be administered. Antiarrhythmic drugs, such as phenytoin or lidocaine, can be given if ordered by the physician.

Drug Interactions: One of the most serious side effects of digitalis-type drugs is hypokalemia (lowering of serum potassium levels). This may lead to cardiac arrhythmias, muscle weakness, hypotension, and respiratory distress. Other agents causing hypokalemia reinforce this effect and increase the chance of digitalis toxicity. Such reactions may occur in patients who have been on digitalis maintenance for a long time.

Drug Interactions	
Aminoglycosides	↓ Effect of digitalis glycosides due to ↓ absorption from GI tract
Aminosalicylic acid	↓ Effect of digitalis glycosides due to ↓ absorption from GI tract
Amphotericin B	↑ K depletion caused by digitalis; ↑ incidence of digitalis toxicity
Antacids	↓ Effect of digitalis glycosides due to ↓ absorption from GI tract
Calcium preparations	Cardiac arrhythmias if parenteral calcium given with digitalis
Chlorthalidone	↑ K and Mg loss with ↑ chance of digitalis toxicity
Cholestyramine	Cholestyramine binds digitoxin in the intestine and ↓ its absorption
Colestipol	Colestipol binds digitoxin in the intestine and ↓ its absorption
Ephedrine	↑ Chance of cardiac arrhythmias
Epinephrine	↑ Chance of cardiac arrhythmias
Ethacrynic acid	↑ K and Mg loss with ↑ chance of digitalis toxicity
Furosemide	↑ K and Mg loss with ↑ chance of digitalis toxicity
Glucose infusions	Large infusions of glucose may cause ↓ in serum K and ↑ chance of digitalis toxicity
Hypoglycemic drugs	↓ Effect of digitalis glycosides due to ↑ breakdown by liver
Methimazole	↑ Chance of toxic effects of digitalis
Metoclopramide	↓ Effect of digitalis glycosides by ↓ absorption from GI tract
Muscle relaxants, nondepolarizing	↑ Risk of cardiac arrhythmias
Propranolol	Propranolol potentiates digitalis-induced bradycardia
Reserpine	↑ Chance of cardiac arrhythmias
Spironolactone	Either ↑ or ↓ toxic effects of digitalis glycosides
Succinylcholine	↑ Chance of cardiac arrhythmias

Drug Interactions

Sulfasalazine	↓ Effect of digitalis glycosides by ↓ absorption from GI tract
Sympathomimetics	↑ Chance of cardiac arrhythmias
Thiazides	↑ K and Mg loss with ↑ chance of digitalis toxicity
Thyroid hormones	↑ Effectiveness of digitalis glycosides

Laboratory Test Interferences: May ↓ prothrombin time. Alters tests for 17-ketosteroids and 17-hydroxycorticosteroids.

Dosage: PO, IM, or IV. *Highly individualized.* See individual drugs: digitoxin, digoxin.

Initially, the drugs are usually given at higher ("digitalizing" or loading) doses. These are reduced as soon as the desired therapeutic effect is achieved or undesirable toxic reactions develop. The response of the patient to cardiac glycosides is gauged by clinical and ECG observations.

There are considerable differences in the rates at which patients become digitalized. Patients with mild signs of congestion can often be digitalized gradually over a period of several days. Patients suffering from more serious congestion, for example, those showing signs of acute left ventricular failure, dyspnea, or lung edema, can be digitalized more rapidly by parenteral administration of a fast-acting cardiac glycoside.

Once digitalization has been attained (pulse 68–80 beats/min) and symptoms of CHF have subsided, the patient is put on maintenance dosage. Depending on the drug and the age of the patient, the daily maintenance dose is often approximately 10% of the digitalizing dose.

NURSING CONSIDERATIONS

Administration/Storage

1. Many cardiac glycosides have similar names. However, their dosage and duration of their effect differ markedly. Therefore, check the doctor's order, the medication record and the bottle label of the medication to be administered. If a client questions the drug (size, color, etc.) recheck the drug order, bottle label and the name of the client to whom the drug is to be given.
2. Measure all PO liquid cardiac medications precisely, using a calibrated dropper or a syringe.
3. The half-life of cardiac glycosides is prolonged in the elderly. When working with elderly clients, anticipate the doses of drug will be smaller than for those in other age groups.
4. Obtain written physician's orders indicating the pulse rates, both high and low, at which cardiac glycosides are to be withheld. Any change in rate or rhythm may indicate digitalis toxicity.

For Clients Starting on a Digitalizing Dose

Assessment

1. Note any drugs the client may be taking that would adversely interact with digitalis glycosides.
2. Obtain and review the following laboratory tests before administering medication: hemoglobin, hematocrit, serum electrolytes, calcium, magnesium, and liver and renal function tests.
3. Ascertain that an ECG has been completed and reviewed before administration.

For Clients Being Digitalized and for Clients on a Maintenance Dose of a Cardiac Glycoside

Interventions

1. Observe cardiac monitor for evidence of bradycardia and/or arrhythmias, or count the apical pulse rate for at least 1 min before administering the drug.

- If the adult pulse rate is below 60 beats/min or if an arrhythmia not previously noted occurs, withhold the drug, notify the physician and document.
- If a child's pulse rate is 90–110 beats per minute, or if there is an arrhythmia, withhold the drug and notify the physician.

2. With another nurse simultaneously take the client's apical/radial pulse for 1 minute. If there is a pulse deficit, withhold the drug, and report to the physician. A pulse deficit may indicate that the client is having an adverse reaction to the drug.
3. Weigh the client prior to initiating therapy and daily after beginning therapy. Weight gain may indicate the presence of edema.
4. Place the client on intake and output. Assure the client is adequately hydrated and that elimination is in line with the intake. Adequate intake will help prevent cumulative toxic effects of the drug.
5. Provide the client with foods such as orange juice and bananas which are high in potassium.
6. Anticipate that clients taking nonpotassium-sparing diuretics as well as a cardiac glycoside will require potassium supplements.
7. If a potassium supplement is needed, ask the pharmacist to provide the client with the most palatable preparation available. (Potassium preparations are usually bitter.)
8. If the client complains of gastric distress an antacid preparation may be ordered. Antacids containing aluminum or magnesium and kaolin/pectin mixtures should be given 6 hr before or 6 hr after dose of cardiac glycoside to prevent a decreased therapeutic effect of the glycoside.
9. When the drug is given to newborns, use a cardiac monitor to identify early evidence of toxicity. Any excessive slowing of sinus rate, sinoatrial arrest, or prolonged P-R interval should be reported immediately and the drug withheld.
10. Be especially alert to cardiac arrhythmias in children. This sign of toxicity occurs more frequently in children than in adults.
11. Monitor serum digoxin levels (therapeutic range 0.5–2.0 ng/mL) and become familiar with medications that enhance the effects of digoxin.
12. Elderly clients must be observed for early signs and symptoms of toxicity, because their rate of drug elimination is slower than with other clients. Nausea, vomiting, anorexia and/or confusion may be signs of toxicity and should be immediately reported.
13. During digitalization the client should be in a closely monitored environment where emergency equipment is readily available.
14. Have digoxin antidote available [Digoxin Immune FAB-(Ovine)].

Client/Family Teaching

1. Stress the need for close medical and nursing supervision and the importance of reporting any signs of change however minor they may seem.
2. How to count the pulse accurately before taking the medication.
3. To maintain a written record of pulse rates and medication administration for review by health care provider.
4. Emphasize guidelines for withholding medication and reporting abnormal pulse rate to physician.
5. To use the same brand of cardiac glycoside that was administered in the hospital. Different preparations have varying degrees of potency and pharmacokinetics and should not be used unless designated by the physician.

6. Follow directions carefully for taking medication.

7. If one dose of drug is accidentally missed do not double up on the next dose. Call the physician and report the incident.

8. Assist the client to develop a checklist that can be marked after taking medications. This is particularly important when working with elderly clients who may tend to have memory loss.

9. Administer medication after meals to lessen gastric irritation.

10. To avoid taking medications by mistake, discard any previously prescribed cardiac glycoside.

11. Review the toxic symptoms of prescribed drugs. Provide a printed list of the toxic symptoms, stressing early recognition and prompt reporting to the physician. Anorexia is often the earliest symptom.

12. Weight should be taken every morning at the same time before breakfast, and in similar clothing. Report any rapid weight gain and bring written record of weight to physician at time of appointment.

13. How to maintain a sodium restricted diet. Provide with a list of foods low in sodium.

14. To follow a potassium rich diet and provide with a list of potassium rich foods. This is particularly important when working with clients on a limited income as it enables them to make choices they can afford.

15. Review and explain any dietary and activity restrictions.

16. Consult with the physician before taking any other medications, whether prescribed or OTC, because drug interactions occur frequently with cardiac glycosides.

17. Instruct to report any persistent cough, difficulty breathing, or edema, to the physician. These are all signs of congestive heart failure and demand immediate medical attention.

18. Review all written instructions with the client and family at least several times in the days prior to discharge.

19. Assist clients to contact community health agencies designed to assist them in maintaining health.

Evaluation

1. Assess for evidence of dyspnea, rales and persistent cough, indicating congestive heart failure.

2. Evaluate for positive response to digitalization, as evidenced by improvement in rate and rhythm of heartbeat, improvement in breathing, reduction in weight, and diuresis.

3. Observe for symptoms of toxicity noted under *Side Effects* and monitor serum levels of drug.

DESLANOSIDE (dez-LAN-oh-syd)

Cedilanid ✤, Cedilanid-D (Rx)

See also *Cardiac Glycosides,* p. 433.

Action/Kinetics: Onset, IV: 10–30 min. **Peak effect:** 1–3 hr. **t½:** About 36 hr. **Duration:** 2–5 days. Low protein binding (25%). Is excreted mainly unchanged by the kidneys.

Uses: Rapid digitaliziation in emergency situations or when cardiac glycosides cannot be taken orally.

Dosage: IV. Adults, *digitalization:* 1.6 mg as a single dose or 0.8 mg initially and repeated after 4 hr. **IM. Adults,** *digitalization:* 0.8 mg given at each of two injection sites.

  IV, IM. Pediatric, 3 years or older: *digitalization,* 0.0225 mg/kg divided into 2–3 equal doses and given at 3–4 hr intervals (may be given as a single dose in emergencies). **Children, 2 weeks–3 years:** 0.025 mg/kg divided into 2–3 equal doses and given at 3–4 hr intervals (may be given as a single dose in emergencies). **Premature, full-term neonates, patients with reduced renal function or myocarditis:** 0.022 mg/kg divided into 2–3 equal doses and given at 3–4 hr intervals (may be given as a single dose in emergencies).

NURSING CONSIDERATIONS

See *Nursing Considerations* for *Cardiac Glycosides,* p. 436.

Administration/Storage

1. The injection vehicle contains ethyl alcohol and glycerin.
2. The product should be protected from light.

DIGITOXIN   (dih-jih-**TOX**-in)

Crystodigin (Rx)

See also *Cardiac Glycosides,* p. 433.

Classification: Cardiac glycoside.

Action/Kinetics: Most potent of the digitalis glycosides. Its slow onset of action makes it unsuitable for emergency use. Almost completely absorbed from GI tract. **Onset: PO,** 1–4 hr; maximum effect: 8–12 hr. **t¹/₂:** 5–9 days. **Duration:** 2 weeks. Significant protein binding (over 90%). Metabolized by the liver and excreted as inactive metabolites through the urine. **Therapeutic serum levels:** 14–26 ng/mL. Withhold drug and check with physician if serum level exceeds 35 ng/mL, indicating toxicity.

Use: Drug of choice for maintenance in congestive heart failure.

Special Concerns: Pregnancy category: C. Digitalis tablets may not be suitable for small children; thus, other digitalis products should be considered.

Additional Drug Interactions	
Aminoglutethimide	↓ Effect of digitoxin due to ↑ breakdown by liver
Barbiturates	↓ Effect of digitoxin due to ↑ breakdown by liver
Diltiazem	May ↑ serum levels of digitoxin
Phenylbutazone	↓ Effect of digitoxin due to ↑ breakdown by liver
Phenytoin	↓ Effect of digitoxin due to ↑ breakdown by liver
Quinidine	May ↑ serum levels of digitoxin
Rifampin	↓ Effect of digitoxin due to ↑ breakdown by liver
Verapamil	May ↑ serum levels of digitoxin

Dosage: Tablets. Adults. Digitalizing dose: Rapid, 0.6 mg followed by 0.4 mg in 4–6 hr; **then,** 0.2 mg q 4–6 hr until therapeutic effect achieved. **Digitalizing dose: Slow,** 0.2 mg b.i.d. for 4 days. **Maintenance dose: PO,** 0.05–0.3 mg/day (**usual:** 0.15 mg/day).

NURSING CONSIDERATIONS

See *Nursing Considerations* for *Cardiac Glycosides,* p. 436.

Administration/Storage

1. Incompatible with acids and alkali.
2. Protect from light.

DIGOXIN   (dih-**JOX**-in)

Lanoxicaps, Lanoxin, Novodigoxin ✽ (Rx)

See also *Cardiac Glycosides,* p. 433.

Classification: Cardiac glycoside.

Action/Kinetics: Action prompter and shorter than that of digitoxin. **Onset: PO,** 0.5–2 hr; **time to peak effect:** 2–6 hr. **Duration:** 6 days. **Onset, IV:** 5–30 min; **time to peak effect:** 1–4 hr. **Duration:** 6 days. **t½:** 35 hr. **Therapeutic serum level:** 0.5–2.0 ng/mL. Serum levels above 2.5 ng/mL indicate toxicity. 50–70% is excreted unchanged by the kidneys. Bioavailability depends on the dosage form: tablets (60–80%), capsules (90–100%), and elixir (70–85%). Thus, changing dosage forms may require dosage adjustments.

Uses: May be drug of choice for congestive heart failure because of rapid onset, relatively short duration, and ability to be administered PO or IV.

Special Concerns: Pregnancy category: A.

Additional Drug Interactions:

1. The following drugs increase serum digoxin levels, leading to possible toxicity: Aminoglycosides, amiodarone, anticholinergics, benzodiazepines, captopril, diltiazem, erythromycin, esmolol, flecainide, hydroxychloroquine, ibuprofen, indomethacin, nifedipine, quinidine, quinine, tetracyclines, tolbutamide, verapamil.
2. Disopyramide may alter the pharmacologic effect of digoxin.
3. Penicillamine decreases serum digoxin levels.

Dosage: Capsules. Adults, Digitalization: Rapid, 0.4–0.6 mg initially followed by 0.1–0.3 mg q 6–8 hr until desired effect achieved. **Digitalization: Slow,** a total of 0.05–0.35 mg daily divided in two doses for a period of 7–22 days in order to reach steady-state serum levels. **Maintenance:** 0.05–0.35 mg once or twice daily. **Pediatric. Digitalizing dosage is divided into 3 or more doses with the initial dose being about one-half the total dose; doses are given q 4–8 hr. Children, 10 years and older:** 0.008–0.012 mg/kg. **5–10 years of age:** 0.015–0.03 mg/kg. **2–5 years of age:** 0.025–0.035 mg/kg. **1 month–2 years of age:** 0.03–0.05 mg/kg. **Neonates, full-term:** 0.02–0.03 mg/kg. **Neonates, premature:** 0.015–0.025 mg/kg. **Maintenance, premature neonates:** 20–30% of total digitalizing dose divided and given in 2–3 daily doses. **Maintenance, neonates to 10 years of age:** 25–35% of the total digitalizing dose divided and given in 2–3 daily doses.

   Elixir, Tablets. Adults, Digitalization: Rapid, a total of 0.75–1.25 mg divided into 2 or more doses each given at 6–8 hr intervals. **Digitalization: Slow,** 0.125–0.5 mg once daily for 7 days. **Maintenance:** 0.125–0.5 mg daily. **Pediatric. Digitalizing dose is divided into 2 or more doses and given at 6–8 hr intervals. Children, 10 years and older, rapid or slow:** Same as adult dose. **5–10 years of age:** 0.02–0.035 mg/kg. **2–5 years of age:** 0.03–0.05 mg/kg. **1**

month–2 years of age: 0.035–0.06 mg/kg. **Premature and newborn infants to 1 month of age:** 0.02–0.035 mg/kg. **Maintenance:** one-fifth to one-third the total digitalizing dose daily. **Note:** An alternate regimen (referred to as the "small-dose" method) is 0.017 mg/kg daily. This dose causes less toxicity.

IV. Adults, digitalization: Same as Capsules. **Maintenance:** 0.125–0.5 mg daily in divided doses or as a single dose. **Pediatric: Same as Capsules.**

NURSING CONSIDERATIONS

See *Nursing Considerations* for *Cardiac Glycosides,* p. 436.

Administration/Storage

1. IV injections should be given over 5 min (or longer) either undiluted or diluted fourfold or greater with sterile water for injection, 0.9% sodium chloride injection, lactated Ringer's injection, or 5% dextrose injection.
2. Lanoxicaps gelatin capsules are more bioavailable than tablets. Thus, the 0.05 mg capsule is equivalent to the 0.0625 mg tablet; the 0.1 mg capsule is equivalent to the 0.125 mg tablet, and the 0.2 mg capsule is equivalent to the 0.25 mg tablet.
3. Differences in bioavailability have been noted between products; thus, clients should be monitored when changing from one product to another.
4. Protect from light.

DIGOXIN IMMUNE FAB (OVINE) (dih-**JOX**-in)

Digibind (Rx)

Classification: Digoxin antidote.

Action/Kinetics: Digoxin immune Fab are antibodies that bind to digoxin. The antibody is produced in sheep by immunization with digoxin bound to human albumin. In cases of digoxin toxicity, the antibodies can bind to digoxin and the complex is excreted through the kidneys. As serum levels of digoxin decrease, digoxin bound to tissue is released into the serum to maintain equilibrium and this is then bound and excreted. The net result is a decrease in both tissue and serum digoxin. **Onset:** Less than 1 min. **t½:** 15–20 hr (after IV administration). Each vial contains 40 mg of pure digoxin immune Fab, which will bind approximately 0.6 mg digoxin or digitoxin.

Uses: Life-threatening digoxin or digitoxin toxicity or overdosage. Symptoms of toxicity include severe sinus bradycardia, second- or third-degree heart block which does not respond to atropine, ventricular tachycardia, ventricular fibrillation.

Note: Cardiac arrest can be expected if a healthy adult ingests more than 10 mg digoxin or a healthy child ingests more than 4 mg. Also, steady-state serum concentrations of digoxin greater than 10 ng/mL or potassium concentrations greater than 5 mEq/L as a result of digoxin therapy require use of digoxin immune Fab.

Special Concerns: Use with caution during pregnancy (category: C) and lactation. Use in infants only if benefits outweigh risks. Patients sensitive to products of sheep origin may also be sensitive to digoxin immune Fab.

Side Effects: *CV:* Worsening of congestive heart failure or low cardiac output, atrial fibrillation (all due to withdrawal of the effects of digoxin). *Other:* Hypokalemia.

Dosage: IV. Dosage depends on the serum digoxin concentration. A large dose has a faster onset but there is an increased risk of allergic or febrile reactions. The package insert should be carefully consulted.

NURSING CONSIDERATIONS

Administration/Storage

1. The lyophilized material should be reconstituted with 4 mL of sterile water for injection to give a concentration of 10 mg/mL. If small doses are required (e.g., in infants), reconstituted antibody can be further diluted with 36 mL sterile isotonic saline to obtain a concentration of 1 mg/mL.
2. The reconstituted antibody should be used immediately. However, it may be stored for up to 4 hr at 2°–8°C (36°–46°F).
3. The dose should be administered over a 30-min period through a 0.22 μm membrane filter. A bolus injection may be used if there is immediate danger of cardiac arrest.
4. The total number of vials of antibody needed can be determined by dividing the total body load (in mg) by the amount of digoxin bound by each vial (0.6 mg).
5. If acute digoxin ingestion results in severe symptoms and a serum concentration is not known, 800 mg (20 vials) of digoxin immune Fab may be given. However, volume overload must be monitored in small children.
6. The dosage in infants should be administered with a tuberculin syringe.

Assessment

1. Evaluate laboratory data for electrolyte imbalance.
2. Note the presence of hypokalemia or evidence of increased congestive heart failure and document.

Interventions

1. In the event of a hypersensitivity reaction, have epinephrine (1:1,000) immediately available.
2. Monitor vital signs and cardiac rhythm in a monitored environment. Have emergency drugs and equipment readily available.
3. Clients with known allergy to sheep proteins should be appropriately identified and this information should be documented in their records. Do not administer digoxin immune Fab to these persons.

Evaluation

1. Observe for return to baseline cardiac rhythm.
2. Review serum digoxin level to evaluate response to therapy.

INOTROPIC AGENT

AMRINONE LACTATE   (AM-rih-nohn)

Inocor (Rx)

Classification: Cardiac inotropic agent.

Action/Kinetics: Amrinone causes an increase in cardiac output by increasing the force of contraction of the heart, probably by inhibition of phosphodiesterase. It reduces afterload and preload by directly relaxing vascular smooth muscle. **Time to peak effect:** 10 min. **t½, after rapid IV:** 3.6 hr; **after IV infusion:** 5.8 hr. **Plasma levels:** 3.0 mcg/mL. **Duration:** 30 min–2 hr, depending on the dose. The drug is excreted primarily in the urine both unchanged and as metabolites.

Uses: Congestive heart failure (short-term therapy in patients unresponsive to digitalis, diuretics, and/or vasodilators). Can be used in digitalized patients.

Contraindications: Hypersensitivity to bisulfites. Severe aortic or pulmonary valvular disease in lieu of surgery. Acute myocardial infarction.

Special Concerns: Safety and efficacy in pregnancy (category: C), lactation, and in children not established.

Side Effects: *GI:* Nausea, vomiting, abdominal pain, anorexia. *CV:* Hypotension, arrhythmias. *Allergic:* Pericarditis, pleuritis, ascites. *Other:* Thrombocytopenia, hepatotoxicity, fever, chest pain, burning at site of injection.

Drug Interactions: Excessive hypotension when used with disopyramide.

Dosage: IV. Initial: 0.75 mg/kg as bolus slowly over 2–3 min; may be repeated after 30 min if necessary. **Maintenance, IV infusion:** 5–10 mcg/kg/min. Daily dose should not exceed 10 mg/kg although up to 18 mg/kg/day has been used in some patients for short periods.

NURSING CONSIDERATIONS

Administration/Storage

1. Amrinone may be administered undiluted or diluted in 0.9% or 0.45% saline to a concentration of 1–3 mg/mL. Diluted solutions should be used within 24 hr.
2. Amrinone should not be diluted with solutions containing dextrose (glucose) prior to injection. However, the drug may be injected into running dextrose (glucose) infusions through a Y-connector or directly into the tubing.
3. Amrinone should not be administered in an IV line containing furosemide since a precipitate will form.
4. Protect from light and store at room temperature.

Assessment

1. Determine that a baseline ECG has been performed.
2. Clients should be on a cardiac monitor while receiving amrinone lactate.
3. Obtain baseline electrolytes, complete blood count and platelet count.
4. Note and record baseline blood pressure readings.

Interventions

1. Monitor serum potassium levels, complete blood count, and platelets; report any bruises or bleeding.
2. Monitor BP frequently, note any drop in blood pressure because drug can cause hypotension.
3. Administer solution with an electronic infusion device.

Evaluation

1. Evaluate for unusual hypersensitivity reactions, including pericarditis, pleuritis, and ascites.
2. Assess for a positive response to therapy such as improvement in cardiac output, decrease in preload and afterload, improvement in congestive heart failure, etc.

CHAPTER TWENTY-FOUR

Coronary Vasodilators (Antianginal Drugs)

General Statement: Angina pectoris may occur as a result of coronary atherosclerotic disease where there is an imbalance between the demand for oxygen by the myocardium and the oxygen supply (called secondary angina). The oxygen supply is compromised due to the inability of coronary blood flow to increase proportionally to increases in myocardial oxygen requirements. Angina pectoris may also result from vasospasm of large, surface coronary vessels or one of their major branches (called primary angina). In some patients, angina is due to a combination of constriction of coronary vessels and an insufficient oxygen supply.

There are three groups of drugs which are currently used for the treatment of angina. These agents include the nitrates/nitrites, beta-adrenergic blocking agents, and calcium channel blocking drugs. These drugs reduce the frequency and/or severity of angina by either increasing myocardial oxygen supply and/or decreasing the oxygen demand of the myocardium.

Drugs specifically used for the treatment of peripheral vascular disease are discussed under *Peripheral Vasodilators*, p. 468.

NITRATES / NITRITES

Action/Kinetics: Systemically, the primary effect of the coronary vasodilators is to reduce the oxygen requirements of the myocardium. This is accomplished by a reduction in left ventricular preload and afterload due to venous (predominately) and arterial dilation which causes more efficient redistribution of blood flow in myocardial tissue. For nitrates, there are several dosage forms available including sublingual, topical, transdermal, parenteral, oral, and buccal. The onset and duration is dependent on the product and route of administration.

Uses: Treatment and prophylaxis of acute angina pectoris, treatment of chronic angina pectoris. IV nitroglycerin is used to decrease blood pressure in surgical procedures, resulting in hypertension as well as an adjunct in treating hypertension or congestive heart failure associated with myocardial infarction. Nitroglycerin ointment has been used as an adjunct in treating Raynaud's disease.

Contraindications: Sensitivity to nitrites, which may result in severe hypotensive reactions, MI, or tolerance to nitrites. Severe anemia, cerebral hemorrhage, recent head trauma, glaucoma, impaired hepatic function, hypertrophic cardiomyopathy, hypotension, recent myocardial infarction. Oral dosage forms should not be used in patients with GI hypermotility or with malabsorption syndrome. The injection should not be used in patients with hypovolemia or with normal or low pulmonary capillary wedge pressure.

Special Concerns: Safety and efficacy have not been determined during lactation and in children.

Side Effects: Severe toxicity is rarely encountered with therapeutic use. *CNS:* Headaches (most common), syncope, dizziness, weakness, apprehension, vertigo. *CV:* Postural hypotension (common) with or without paradoxical tachycardia, palpitations, transient flushing, cardiovascular collapse. *GI:* Nausea, vomiting, dry mouth. *Miscellaneous:* Rash, exfoliative dermatitis, skin pallor, sweating, muscle twitching, methemoglobinemia, cold sweating, involuntary urination and/or defecation, blurred vision. **Topical use:** Peripheral edema, contact dermatitis.

Tolerance can occur following chronic use. Nitrites convert hemoglobin to methemoglobin, which impairs the oxygen-carrying capacity of the blood, resulting in anemic hypoxia. This interaction is dangerous in patients with preexisting anemia.

24

Drug Interactions	
Acetylcholine	Effects ↓ when used with nitrates
Alcohol, ethyl	Hypotension and cardiovascular collapse due to vasodilator effect of both agents
Antihypertensive drugs	Additive hypotension
Beta-adrenergic blocking drugs	Additive hypotension
Calcium channel blocking drugs	Additive hypotension
Dihydroergotamine	↑ Effect of dihydroergotamine due to increased bioavailability
Narcotics	Additive hypotensive effect
Phenothiazines	Additive hypotension
Sympathomimetics	↓ Effect of nitrates; also, nitrates may ↓ effect of sympathomimetics resulting in hypotension

Laboratory Test Interference: ↑ Urinary catecholamines. False-negative decrease in serum cholesterol.

NURSING CONSIDERATIONS

Administration/Storage

1. Nitrites and nitrates are available in a variety of dosage forms including sublingual, chewable, topical, transdermal, oral, inhalation, and parenteral. It is important to understand the appropriate use of each of these dosage forms.
2. Tablets and capsules should be stored tightly closed in their original container. Avoid exposure to air, heat, and moisture.
3. Inhalation products should be used either lying or sitting down.
4. Inhalation products are flammable and should not be used under situations where they might ignite.

Assessment

1. Note any history of sensitivity to nitrites.
2. If client has a history of anemia or glaucoma document and administer this category of drugs with extreme caution.
3. Determine client experience with self-administered medications and if physician has ordered sublingual tablets at the bedside.

Interventions

1. If hospitalized clients are instructed to keep sublingual tablets at the bedside, instruct them so that accurate records of attacks and the extent of medication relief are noted.
2. While caring for the client in the hospital, mutually record how much drug the client requires to keep angina under control. Record:
   - How frequently the drug is given.
   - The duration of the attacks.
   - Whether the relief is partial or complete.
   - How long it takes for relief to occur.
   - Whether or not there are any side effects.
3. Clients should be advised to wear a medic alert bracelet.

Client/Family Teaching

1. These medications should be taken on an empty stomach.
2. To carry sublingual tablets for use in aborting an attack, to observe the expiration date on the bottle, and to obtain a fresh bottle when needed.
3. The presence of a burning sensation under the tongue attests to the potency of the drug. If there is no burning sensation, the potency may have diminished and a fresh supply should be obtained.
4. Carry sublingual tablets in a *glass* bottle, tightly capped. Do not use plastic containers because drug will deteriorate in plastic; also, do not use bottles with child-proof caps since client must get to the tablets quickly.
5. That if anginal pain is not relieved in 5 min by first sublingual tablet, to take up to 2 more tablets at 5-min intervals. If pain has not subsided 5 min after third tablet, client should be taken to emergency room by a family member or by ambulance. Client should **not** drive himself.

6. Take sublingual tablets 5–15 min prior to any situation likely to cause anginal pain (e.g., climbing stairs, sexual intercourse, exposure to cold weather).

7. Take sublingual tablet while sitting or lying down to prevent postural hypotension.

8. Elderly clients should be encouraged to sit or lie down when taking nitroglycerine. Elderly clients are more prone to hypotensive side effects and may become dizzy and fall.

9. Do not drink alcohol. Nitrite syncope, a severe shock-like state, may occur.

10. Instruct specifically on how to apply topical nitroglycerin.

11. Prescriptions should generally be renewed/replaced every 6 months.

Evaluation

1. Be alert for signs of tolerance which may begin several days after treatment is started. This is manifested by absence of response to the usual dose. (Nitrites may be discontinued temporarily until such tolerance is lost, and then reinstituted. During the interim, other vasodilators may be ordered).

2. Observe clients for nausea, vomiting, client complaint of drowsiness, headache or visual disturbances during long-term prophylaxis. These are prolonged effects and may require a change in medication.

3. For symptoms of sensitivity to the hypotensive effects of nitrites. These may include the presence of nausea, vomiting, pallor, restlessness, and cardiovascular collapse.

4. Evaluate clients for presence of hypotension when they are receiving additional drugs that may cause hypotension. Drug dosage adjustment may be necessary.

5. Note change in client activity and response to the drug therapy.

6. Determine if client experiences less discomfort when performing regular activity.

AMYL NITRITE (AY-mil)

Amyl Nitrite Aspirols, Amyl Nitrite Vaporole (Rx)

See also *Nitrates/Nitrites,* p. 445.

Classification: Coronary vasodilator, antidote for cyanide poisoning.

Action/Kinetics: Amyl nitrite is believed to act by reducing systemic and pulmonary arterial pressure (afterload) and by decreasing cardiac output due to peripheral vasodilation as opposed to causing coronary artery dilation. As an antidote to cyanide poisoning, amyl nitrite promotes formation of methemoglobin which combines with cyanide to form the nontoxic cyanmethemoglobin. **Onset (inhalation):** 30 sec. **Duration:** 3–5 min. About 33% is excreted through the kidneys.

Uses: Acute attacks of angina pectoris, acute cyanide poisoning. *Investigational:* Diagnostic aid to assess reserve cardiac function.

Special Concerns: Pregnancy category: X. Use of amyl nitrite in children has not been studied. Hypotensive effects are more likely to occur in geriatric patients.

Dosage: Inhalation. *Angina pectoris:* 0.18–0.3 mL (1 container crushed). Usually, 1–6 inhalations from one container produces relief. Dosage may be repeated after 3–5 min. *Antidote for cyanide poisoning:* Administer for 30–60 sec q 5 min until patient is conscious; is then repeated at longer intervals for up to 24 hr.

NURSING CONSIDERATIONS

See also *Nursing Considerations* for *Nitrates/Nitrites,* p. 446.

Administration/Storage

1. Administer only by inhalation.
2. Containers should be protected from light and stored at a temperature of 46°F–59°F (8°C–15°C).
3. *Amyl nitrite vapors are highly flammable. Do not use near flame or intense heat.*

Assessment

1. Take a history of common precipitating incidents that immediately precede the onset of chest pain.
2. Note the presence of risk factors.
3. Determine and document the degree, location, type and duration of chest pain, and the direction in which it radiates.

Client/Family Teaching

1. Discuss and mutually set the goals of therapy with client and family.
2. Assist client to identify changes in lifestyle that may reduce the need for amyl nitrite.
3. To enclose fabric-covered ampule in a handkerchief or piece of cloth and to crush by hand.
4. To sit down during inhalation to avoid hypotension.
5. That drug has a pungent odor, but several deep breaths must nevertheless be taken in order to attain drug effects.
6. Always to store medication out of reach of children.
7. The medication has the potential for abuse and should be stored appropriately.

ERYTHRITYL TETRANITRATE   (eh-**RITH**-rih-til)

Cardilate (Rx)

See also *Nitrates/Nitrites,* p. 445.

Classification: Coronary vasodilator.

Action/Kinetics: Sublingual: Onset, 5 min; maximum effect: 30–45 min. **Duration:** 2–3 hr. **PO: Onset,** 15–30 min; maximum effect: 1–1.5 hr. **Duration:** 4–6 hr. Tolerance may develop.

Uses: Prophylaxis and chronic treatment of angina. Diffuse esophageal spasm. May improve exercise tolerance. As a vasodilator in congestive heart failure.

Additional Contraindication: To treat acute attacks of angina pectoris.

Special Concerns: Pregnancy category: C. Dosage has not been established for children.

Dosage: Sublingual, Oral, Buccal: 5–10 mg t.i.d.–q.i.d. Dose may be increased to 100 mg daily if necessary (chance of side effects increases).

NURSING CONSIDERATIONS

See also *Nursing Considerations* for *Nitrates/Nitrites,* p. 446.

Interventions

1. Report symptoms of headaches and/or GI upset. These symptoms call for a reduction in dosage early in therapy.
2. Anticipate that analgesics will be ordered for headaches.

Client/Family Teaching

1. Explain that all restrictions on activity cannot be removed, even though drug may permit more normal activity.
2. Sublingual tingling sensations may be relieved by placing tablet in buccal pouch.

ISOSORBIDE DINITRATE CAPSULES (eye-so-**SOR**-byd)

(Rx)

ISOSORBIDE DINITRATE CHEWABLE (eye-so-**SOR**-byd)

Sorbitrate (Rx)

ISOSORBIDE DINITRATE EXTENDED-RELEASE TABLETS (eye-so-**SOR**-byd)

Cedocard-SR

ISOSORBIDE DINITRATE SUBLINGUAL (eye-so-**SOR**-byd)

Apo-ISDN✿, Coronex✿, Isonate, Isorbid, Isordil, Sorbitrate (Rx)

ISOSORBIDE DINITRATE TABLETS (eye-so-**SOR**-byd)

Apo-ISDN✿, Coronex✿, Isonate, Isorbid, Isordil, Novosorbide✿, Sorbitrate (Rx)

See also *Nitrates/Nitrites,* p. 445.

Classification: Coronary vasodilator.

Action/Kinetics: Sublingual, chewable. Onset: 2–5 min; **duration:** 1–2 hr. **Oral Capsules/ Tablets. Onset:** 15–40 min; **duration:** 4–6 hr. **Extended-release. Onset:** up to 30 min; **duration:** 12 hr.

Additional Uses: Diffuse esophageal spasm. Oral tablets are only for prophylaxis while sublingual and chewable forms may be used to terminate acute attacks of angina.

Special Concerns: Pregnancy category: C. Dosage has not been established in children.

Additional Side Effects: Vascular headaches occur especially frequently.

Additional Drug Interactions	
Acetylcholine	Isosorbide antagonizes the effect of acetylcholine
Norepinephrine	Isosorbide antagonizes the effect of norepinephrine

Dosage: Sublingual/Buccal: *Acute attack:* 2.5–5 mg q 2–3 hr as required. *Prophylaxis:* 5–10 mg q 2–3 hr. **Chewable tablets:** *Acute attack:* **initial,** 5 mg q 2–3 hr. *Prophylaxis:* 5–10 mg q 2–3 hr. **Oral capsules/tablets:** 5–20 mg q 6 hr as needed (range: 5–40 mg q.i.d.). **Extended-release tablets:** 20–80 mg q 8–12 hr.

NURSING CONSIDERATIONS

See also *Nursing Considerations* for *Nitrates/Nitrites,* p. 446.

Client/Family Teaching

1. Administer with meals to eliminate or reduce headaches; otherwise, take on an empty stomach.
2. None of the products should be crushed or chewed, unless specifically ordered by the physician.
3. Review appropriate method for administration. Remind client not to chew sublingual tablets.
4. Stress that chewable tablets should be held in the mouth for 1–2 min to allow for absorption through the buccal membranes.

NITROGLYCERIN IV   (nye-troh-**GLIH**-sih-rin)

Nitro-Bid IV, Nitrol, Nitrostat IV, Tridil (Rx)

See also *Nitrates/Nitrites,* p. 445

Classification: Coronary vasodilator.

Action/Kinetics: Onset: immediate; **duration:** 3–5 min (dose-dependent).

Additional Uses: Hypertension associated with surgery and congestive heart failure associated with acute myocardial infarction. Angina unresponsive to usual doses of organic nitrate or beta-adrenergic blocking agents. Cardiac-load reducing agent.

Special Concerns: Pregnancy category: C. Dosage has not been established in children.

Dosage: IV infusion only. Initial: 5 mcg/min delivered by precise infusion pump. May be increased by 5 mcg/min q 3–5 min until response seen. If no response seen at 20 mcg/min, dose can be increased by 10–20 mcg/min until response noted. Monitor continuously to titrate each patient to desired level of response.

NURSING CONSIDERATIONS

See also *Nursing Considerations* for *Nitrates/Nitrites,* p. 446.

Administration/Storage

1. Dilute with 5% dextrose USP, or 0.9% sodium chloride injection. Nitroglycerin injection is not for direct IV use; it must first be diluted.
2. Use only a glass IV bottle and administration set provided by the manufacturer because nitroglycerin is readily adsorbed onto many plastics. Avoid adding unnecessary plastic to IV system.
3. Aspirate medication into a syringe and then inject immediately into a glass bottle (or polyolefin bottle) to minimize contact with plastic.
4. Administer with a volumetric infusion pump rather than a peristaltic pump to regulate flow more accurately.
5. Do not administer with any other medications in the IV system.
6. Do not interrupt IV nitroglycerin for administration of a bolus of any other medication.

7. To provide correct dosage, remove 15 mL of solution from the IV tubing if concentration of solution is changed.

Interventions

1. Obtain written parameters for BP and pulse and monitor closely throughout drug therapy.

2. Be prepared to monitor central venous pressure and/or pulmonary artery pressures as ordered.

3. Have emergency drugs readily available.

4. Administer IV solution with an electronic infusion device and in a closely monitored environment.

5. Monitor VS. Note any evidence of hypotension, client complaint of nausea, sweating and/or vomiting. Document presence of tachycardia or bradycardia. These symptoms may indicate that the dosage of drug is more than the client can tolerate.
   - Elevate the legs to restore blood pressure.
   - Be prepared to reduce the rate of flow of the solution or to administer additional IV fluids.

6. Assess for thrombophlebitis at the IV site. Remove the IV from the reddened area and assist with reinsertion.

7. Anticipate that after the initial positive response to therapy the dosage increments will be smaller. Adjustments in dosage will also be made at longer intervals.

8. Sinus tachycardia may occur in a client with angina pectoris who is receiving a maintenance dose of nitroglycerin. Notify physician, because a heart rate of 80 beats/min or less reduces myocardial demand.

9. Check that topical, oral, or sublingual doses are adjusted if client is on concomitant therapy with IV nitroglycerin.

10. Anticipate that client will be weaned from IV nitroglycerin by gradually decreasing doses to avoid posttherapy or cardiovascular distress. Tapering off is usually initiated when the client is receiving the peak effect from oral or topical vasodilators. The IV flow is usually reduced, and the client is monitored for hypertension and angina which would require increased titration.

11. Obtain p.r.n. order for a nonnarcotic analgesic, as headache is a common side effect of drug therapy.

NITROGLYCERIN EXTENDED-RELEASE BUCCAL TABLETS (nye-troh-**GLIH**-sih-rin)

Nitrogard, Nitrogard-SR✴ (Rx)

See also *Nitrates/Nitrites,* p. 445.

Classification: Coronary vasodilator.

Action/Kinetics: Onset: 3 min; **duration:** 3–5 hr.

Uses: Treatment and prophylaxis of angina.

Special Concerns: Pregnancy category: C. Dosage has not been established in children.

Dosage: Initial: 1 mg q 3–5 hr during time patient is awake. Dose may be increased if necessary.

NURSING CONSIDERATIONS

See also *Nursing Considerations* for *Nitrates/Nitrites,* p. 446.

Administration/Storage

1. Tablet should be placed either between the lip and gum above the upper incisors or between the gum and cheek in the buccal area.

2. Allow tablet to dissolve in the mouth. The client should be warned not to swallow the tablet.

3. From 3 to 5 hours are required for tablet dissolution.

4. Store properly to maintain potency.
   * Do not expose to light, heat or air.
   * Keep in a tightly closed container below 30°C (86°F).
   * Do not keep cotton in the container once the bottle has been opened.

NITROGLYCERIN SUBLINGUAL   (nye-troh-**GLIH**-sih-rin)

Nitrostat (Rx)

NITROGLYCERIN SUSTAINED-RELEASE CAPSULES   (nye-troh-**GLIH**-sih-rin)

Nitro-Bid Plateau Caps, Nitrocap 6.5 and T.D., Nitrocine Timecaps, Nitroglyn, Nitrolin, Nitrospan (Rx)

NITROGLYCERIN SUSTAINED-RELEASE TABLETS   (nye-troh-**GLIH**-sih-rin)

Klavikordal, Niong, Nitronet, Nitrong, Nitrong SR✿ (Rx)

NITROGLYCERIN, TOPICAL OINTMENT   (nye-troh-**GLIH**-sih-rin)

Nitro-Bid, Nitrol, Nitrong, Nitrostat (Rx)

See also *Nitrates/Nitrites*, p. 445.

Classification: Coronary vasodilator.

Action/Kinetics: Sublingual. Onset: 1–3 min; **duration:** 30–60 min. **Sustained release: Onset:** 20–45 min; **duration:** 8–12 hr. **Topical ointment. Onset:** 30 min; **duration:** 4–8 hr.

Uses: Sublingual preparations are the agents of choice for prophylaxis and treatment of angina pectoris. Sustained release and ointment products are used to prevent anginal attacks.

Special Concerns: Pregnancy category: C. Dosage has not been established in children.

Dosage: Sublingual: 150–600 mcg under the tongue or in the buccal pouch at first sign of attack; may be repeated in 5 min if necessary (no more than 3 tablets should be taken within 15 min). For prophylaxis, tablets may be taken 5–10 min prior to activities that may precipitate an attack.

Sustained release capsules: *antianginal,* 2.5, 6.5, or 9 mg q 8–12 hr. **Sustained release tablets:** *antianginal,* 1.3, 2.6, or 6.5 mg q 8–12 hr. Sustained release tablets should not be chewed and are not intended for sublingual use. **Topical ointment (2%):** 1–2 inches (15–30 mg) q 8 hr [up to 5 (75 mg) inches q 4 hr may be necessary]. One inch equals approximately 15 mg nitroglycerin. Determine optimum dosage by starting with ½ inch q 8 hr and increasing by ½ inch with each successive dose until headache occurs; then, decrease to largest dose that does not cause headache. When ending treatment, reduce both the dose and frequency of administration over 4–6 weeks to prevent sudden withdrawal reactions.

NURSING CONSIDERATIONS

See also *Nursing Considerations* for *Nitrates/Nitrites*, p. 446.

Administration/Storage

1. Sublingual tablets should be placed under the tongue and allowed to dissolve; they should not be swallowed.

2. Sustained-release tablets should be swallowed whole and are not intended for sublingual use.

Administration

Nitroglycerin, Topical

1. Squeeze ointment carefully onto dose-measuring application papers, which are packaged with the medicine. Use applicator to spread ointment or fold paper in half and rub back and forth.

2. Use the paper to spread the ointment onto a nonhairy area of skin. Many clients find application to the chest psychologically helpful, but ointment may be applied to other nonhairy areas.

3. Rotate sites to prevent irritation. Keep a record of areas used to avoid unnecessary repetitive use of sites.

4. Apply ointment in a thin, even layer covering an area of skin 5–6 inches in diameter. Remember to remove last dose.

5. Tape the application paper over the area, or cover the area with a piece of plastic wrap-type material. A clear plastic cover causes less leakage of ointment, decreases skin irritation, increases the amount absorbed, and prevents clothing stains.

6. Once the dose is established, use the same type of covering to ensure that the same amount of drug is absorbed during each application.

7. Clean around tube opening and tightly cap tube after use.

8. To prevent systemic absorption into nurse's system, the nurse should protect her own skin from contact with the ointment. Wash hands thoroughly after application to prevent headache.

9. Remove at bedtime or as directed to prevent tolerance or loss of drug effect. Reapply upon arising.

NITROGLYCERIN TRANSDERMAL SYSTEM   (nye-troh-**GLIH**-sih-rin)

Deponit 5 mg/24 hr (16 mg) and 10 mg/24 hr (32 mg); Minitran 0.1 mg/hr, 0.2 mg/hr, 0.4 mg/hr, and 0.6 mg/hr; Nitrocine (62.5 mg, 125 mg, and 187.5 mg); Nitrodisc 5 mg/24 hr (16 mg), 7.5 mg/24 hr (24 mg), and 10 mg/24 hr (32 mg); Nitro-Dur 5 mg/24 hr (40 mg), 7.5 mg/24 hr (60 mg) and 10 mg/24 hr (80 mg); Nitro-Dur II 2.5 mg/24 hr (20 mg), 5 mg/24 hr (40 mg), 10 mg/24 hr (80 mg), and 15 mg/24 hr (120 mg)) ; NTS 5 mg/24 hr and 15 mg/24 hr; Transderm-Nitro 2.5 (12.5 mg), 5 (25 mg), 10 (50 mg), 15 (75 mg) (Rx)

See also *Nitrates/Nitrites,* p. 445.

Classification: Coronary vasodilator.

Action/Kinetics: Onset: 30–60 min; **duration:** 8–24 hr. The amount released each hour or each day is indicated by the name (e.g., Nitrodisc 5 mg releases 5 mg/day, Transderm-Nitro 2.5 releases 2.5 mg/day, etc.).

Uses: Prophylaxis of angina pectoris due to coronary artery disease.

Special Concerns: Pregnancy category: C. Dosage has not been established in children.

Dosage: Initial: 1 pad (initially the smallest available dose in the dosage series) applied each day to skin site free of hair and free of excessive movement (e.g., chest, upper arm). **Maintenance:** Additional systems or strengths may be added depending on the clinical response.

NURSING CONSIDERATIONS

See also *Nursing Considerations* for *Nitrates/Nitrites,* p. 446 and *Nitroglycerin, Topical,* p. 452.

Administration/Storage

1. Follow instructions for specific products on package insert.

2. To avoid skin irritation, the application site should be slightly different each day.

3. Do not apply to distal areas of extremities.

4. If the pad loosens, apply a new pad.

5. It is important to note that there is a wide variety between clients in the actual amount of nitroglycerin absorbed each day.

6. When terminating therapy, the dose and frequency of application should be gradually reduced over 4–6 weeks.

Client/Family Teaching

1. Apply only as directed.

2. Remember to remove old pad.

3. Rotate sites of application.

4. Date patch as a reminder that drug has been administered.

5. Once applied, do not disturb or open patch.

6. Remove at bedtime or as directed, to prevent a diminished response (tolerance) to the drug. Reapply upon awakening.

NITROGLYCERIN, TRANSLINGUAL AEROSOL   (nye-troh-**GLIH**-sih-rin)

Nitrolingual (Rx)

See also *Nitrates/Nitrites*, p. 445.

Classification: Coronary vasodilator.

Action/Kinetics: Onset: 2–4 min; **duration:** 30–60 min.

Uses: Coronary artery disease to relieve an acute attack or used prophylactically 10–15 min before beginning activities that can cause an acute anginal attack.

Special Concerns: Pregnancy category: C. Dosage has not been established in children.

Dosage: Spray. *Termination of acute attack:* 1–2 metered doses (400–800 mcg) on or under the tongue q 5 min as needed; no more than 3 metered doses should be administered within a 15-min period. *Prophylaxis:* 1–2 metered doses 5–10 min before beginning activities that might precipitate an acute attack.

NURSING CONSIDERATIONS

See also *Nursing Considerations* for *Nitrates/Nitrites*, p. 446.

Administration/Storage

1. The spray should *not* be inhaled.

2. Immediate medical attention should be sought if chest pain persists.

PENTAERYTHRITOL TETRANITRATE EXTENDED-RELEASE CAPSULES   (pen-tah-eh-**RITH**-rih-tol)

Duotrate, Pentritol (Rx)

PENTAERYTHRITOL TETRANITRATE EXTENDED-RELEASE TABLETS (pen-tah-eh-**RITH**-rih-tol)

Peritrate SA (Rx)

PENTAERYTHRITOL TETRANITRATE TABLETS (pen-tah-eh-**RITH**-rih-tol)

Naptrate, Pentylan, Peritrate, Peritrate Forte ✽ (Rx)

See also *Nitrates/Nitrites,* p. 445.

Classification: Coronary vasodilator.

Action/Kinetics: Onset, tablets: 30 min; **extended-release Capsules/tablets:** slow. **Duration, tablets:** 4–6 hr; **extended Release capsules/tablets:** 12 hr. Excreted in urine and feces.

Use: Prophylaxis of anginal attacks, but is not to be used to terminate acute attacks.

Special Concerns: Pregnancy category: C. Dosage has not been established in children.

Additional Side Effects: Severe rash, exfoliative dermatitis.

Additional Drug Interactions

Acetylcholine	Pentaerythritol antagonizes the effect of acetylcholine
Norepinephrine	Pentaerythritol antagonizes the effect of norepinephrine

Dosage: PO, Tablets. Initial, 10–20 mg q.i.d.; **then,** up to 40 mg q.i.d. **Extended-release:** 30–80 mg q 12 hr.

NURSING CONSIDERATIONS

See also *Nursing Considerations* for *Nitrates/Nitrites,* p. 446.

Client/Family Teaching

1. Drug is to be taken 30 min before or 1 hr after meals, as well as at bedtime.
2. Sustained-release tablets are to be taken on an empty stomach.
3. Sustained-release tablets are not to be chewed or crushed.
4. Remind client to take only as directed and to report any rash or bothersome side effects.

CALCIUM CHANNEL BLOCKING AGENTS

Action/Kinetics: Calcium ions are important for generation of action potentials and for excitation/contraction of muscles. For contraction of cardiac and smooth muscle to occur, extracellular calcium must move into the cell through openings called *calcium channels*. The calcium channel blocking agents (also called *slow channel blockers* or *calcium antagonists*) inhibit the influx of calcium through the cell membrane, resulting in a depression of automaticity and conduction velocity in both smooth and cardiac muscle. This leads to a depression of contraction in these tissues. Although all drugs in this class act similarly, they have different degrees of selectivity on vascular smooth muscle, myocardium, and conduction and pacemaker tissues.

In the myocardium, these drugs dilate coronary vessels and inhibit spasms of coronary arteries. They also decrease total peripheral resistance, thus reducing energy and oxygen requirements of the heart. These effects benefit various types of angina.

These agents also are effective against certain cardiac arrhythmias by slowing AV conduction and prolonging repolarization. In addition, they depress the amplitude, rate of depolarization, and conduction in atria.

Drug Interactions

Beta-adrenergic blocking agents	Beta-blockers may cause depression of myocardial contractility and AV conduction
Cimetidine	↑ Effect of calcium channel blockers due to ↓ first-pass metabolism

Treatment of Overdosage:

1. Hypotension: IV isoproterenol, metaraminol, norepinephrine, calcium, dopamine. Also, provide IV fluids. Place client in Trendelenburg position.
2. Ventricular tachycardia: IV procainamide or lidocaine; also, cardioversion may be necessary. Also, provide slow-drip IV fluids.
3. Bradycardia, asystole, AV block: IV atropine sulfate (0.6–1 mg), calcium gluconate (10%), isoproterenol, norepinephrine; also, cardiac pacing may be indicated. Provide slow-drip IV fluids.

NURSING CONSIDERATIONS

Assessment

Note if the client has had any experience with calcium channel blocking drugs in the past and, if so, the response of the client to the drugs.

Interventions

These drugs cause peripheral vasodilation. Therefore, clients should have their blood pressure and pulse monitored during the initial administration of the drug. Any excessive hypotensive response and increased heart rate may precipitate angina.

Client/Family Teaching

1. Discuss with the client and family the goals of therapy (ex. to decrease the diastolic BP by 10 mm Hg, to decrease the heart rate by 20 beats per minute etc.).
2. Teach the client and family how to take pulse and BP at home. This should be done at the same time of day and at least twice a week.
3. Assist clients to develop a method to maintain a written record of BP and pulse and to note any response after taking the drug. This record should be brought for the physician to review at each visit.
4. Instruct clients to report any untoward signs such as dizziness, vertigo, unusual flushing, facial warmth or headaches.
5. Review with the client benefits from the drug and any possible side effects. Encourage the client to report any new signs or symptoms to the health care provider.

6. If there is evidence of postural hypotension advise the client to change positions slowly, especially when standing up from a reclining position.

7. Advise client to sit down immediately if faintness occurs. Remind to move slowly from lying down to a sitting or standing position.

8. Explain that long periods of standing, excessive heat, hot showers or baths, and ingestion of alcohol may exacerbate postural hypotension.

9. Stress that if the client notices any swelling of the hands or feet, or if there is pronounced dizziness, the physician should be notified immediately.

10. Calcium channel blocking agents should be taken with meals to reduce GI irritation.

Evaluation

1. For a positive clinical response as demonstrated by decreased blood pressure and/or decreased pulse depending on the goals of therapy. Review the client's BP and pulse record with him/her and their progress in attaining a pain free state.

2. Evaluate client understanding and adherence to prescribed drug regimen. Correct any misunderstandings the client may have.

3. Note any symptoms or client complaints that could indicate negative side effects to the drug therapy.

DILTIAZEM HYDROCHLORIDE (dill-**TIE**-ah-zem)

Cardizem, Cardizem-SR (Rx)

See also *Calcium Channel Blocking Agents,* p. 455.

Classification: Calcium channel blocking agent (antianginal, antihypertensive).

Action/Kinetics: Decreases SA and AV conduction and prolongs AV node effective and functional refractory periods. **Tablets: Onset,** 30–60 min; **time to peak plasma levels:** 2–3 hr; **t½, first phase:** 20–30 min; **second phase:** about 3–4.5 hr (5–8 hr with high and repetitive doses); **duration:** 4–8 hr. **Extended-release capsules: Onset,** 2–3 hr; **time to peak plasma levels:** 6–11 hr; **t½:** 5–7 hr; **duration:** 12 hr. **Therapeutic serum levels:** 0.05–0.2 mcg/mL. Metabolized to desacetyldiltiazem, which manifests 25–50% of the activity of diltiazem. Excreted through both the bile and urine.

Uses: Vasospastic angina (Prinzmetal's variant); chronic stable angina (especially in patients who can not use beta-adrenergic blockers or nitrates or who remain symptomatic after clinical doses of these agents). *Sustained-release form:* Only used to treat essential hypertension. *Investigational:* Prophylaxis of reinfarction of non Q-wave myocardial infarction; tardive dyskinesia, Raynaud's syndrome.

Contraindications: Hypotension, second- or third-degree AV block, sick sinus syndrome. Acute myocardial infarction, pulmonary congestion.

Special Concerns: Use during pregnancy only if benefits outweigh risks (pregnancy category: C). Safety and effectiveness in children have not been determined. Excreted in breast milk. The half-life may be increased in geriatric patients. Use with caution in hepatic disease and in congestive heart failure.

Side Effects: *CV:* AV block, bradycardia, congestive heart failure, hypotension, syncope, palpitations, peripheral edema, arrhythmias, angina, tachycardia, abnormal ECG, ventricular extraystoles. *GI:*

Nausea, vomiting, diarrhea, constipation, anorexia, abdominal discomfort, cramps, dry mouth, dysgeusia. *CNS:* Fatigue, weakness, nervousness, dizziness, headache, depression, psychoses, hallucinations, disturbances in sleep, somnolence, insomnia, amnesia, abnormal dreams. *Dermatologic:* Rashes, dermatitis, pruritus, urticaria, erythema multiforme. *Other:* Photosensitivity, joint pain or stiffness, flushing, nasal or chest congestion, dyspnea, shortness of breath, nocturia/polyuria, sexual difficulties, weight gain, paresthesia, tinnitus, tremor, asthenia, gynecomastia, gingival hyperplasia, petechiae, leukopenia, double vision, epistaxis, eye irritation, thirst, alopecia, bundle branch block, abnormal gait, hyperglycemia.

Additional Drug Interactions	
Carabamazepine	↑ Effect of diltiazem due to ↓ breakdown by liver
Cyclosporine	↑ Effect of cyclosporine possibly leading to renal toxicity
Lithium	↑ Risk of neurotoxicity

Laboratory Test Interferences: ↑ Alkaline phosphatase, CPK, LDH, AST, ALT.

Dosage: Tablets, initial: 30 mg q.i.d. before meals and at bedtime; **then,** increase gradually to total daily dose of 180–360 mg given in 3–4 divided doses q 1–2 days. **Capsules, sustained-release, initial:** 60–120 mg b.i.d.; **then,** when maximum antihypertensive effect is reached (approximately 14 days), adjust dosage to a range of 240–360 mg daily.

NURSING CONSIDERATIONS

See also *Nursing Considerations* for *Calcium Channel Blocking Agents,* p. 456.

Administration/Storage

1. Sublingual nitroglycerin may be taken concomitantly for acute angina.
2. Diltiazem may be taken together with long-acting nitrates.

Assessment

1. Note any evidence of edema.
2. Review lab test results especially those that are indicative of hepatic and/or renal dysfunction and document.
3. Assess ECG for evidence of AV block.

Interventions

1. Anticipate reduced dosage of diltiazem in clients with impaired renal or hepatic function.
2. The plasma half-life of the drug may be prolonged in elderly clients. Therefore, monitor these clients closely.

Client/Family Teaching

1. That the drug may cause drowsiness or dizziness.
2. Review the symptoms of postural hypotension and what to do to minimize these effects.
3. The client may experience constipation, unusual tiredness or weakness. Report any persistent and bothersome side effects.
4. To continue carrying short-acting nitrites (nitroglycerin) at all times and to use as directed by the physician.

NICARDIPINE HYDROCHLORIDE   (nye-KAR-dih-peen)

Cardene (Rx)

See also *Calcium Channel Blocking Agents,* p. 455.

Classification: Calcium channel blocking agent (antianginal, antihypertensive).

Action/Kinetics: Onset of action: 20 min. **Maximum plasma levels:** 30–120 min. Significant first-pass metabolism by the liver. Steady-state plasma levels are reached after 2–3 days of therapy. **Therapeutic serum levels:** 0.028–0.050 mcg/mL. **$t^{1/2}$, at steady state:** 8.6 hr. **Duration:** 8 hr. The drug is highly bound to plasma protein (>95%) and is metabolized by the liver with excretion through both the urine and feces.

Uses: Chronic stable angina (effort-associated angina) alone or in combination with beta-adrenergic blocking agents. Hypertension alone or in combination with other antihypertensive drugs.

Contraindications: Patients with advanced aortic stenosis due to the effect on reducing afterload. During lactation.

Special Concerns: Use during pregnancy only if the potential benefits outweigh potential risks (pregnancy category: C). Safety and efficacy in children less than 18 years of age have not been established. Use with caution in patients with congestive heart failure, especially in combination with a beta-blocker. Use with caution in patients with impaired liver function, reduced hepatic blood flow, or impaired renal function.

Side Effects: *CV:* Pedal edema, flushing, increased angina, palpitations, tachycardia, other edema, abnormal ECG, hypotension, postural hypotension. *CNS:* Dizziness, headache, somnolence, syncope, malaise, nervousness, insomnia, abnormal dreams, vertigo, depression, confusion, anxiety. *GI:* Nausea, vomiting, dyspepsia, dry mouth, constipation, sore throat. *Neuromuscular:* Asthenia, myalgia, paresthesia, hyperkinesia, arthralgia. *Miscellaneous:* Rash, dyspnea, tremor, nocturia, allergic reactions, abnormal liver chemistries, hot flashes, impotence, rhinitis, sinusitis, tinnitus, abnormal or blurred vision, increased urinary frequency.

Drug Interactions	
Cyclosporine	↑ Plasma levels of cyclosporine possibly leading to renal toxicity
Digoxin	Nicardipine may ↑ blood levels of digoxin
Fentanyl	Possibility of severe hypotension, especially if both nicardipine and a beta-blocker are used

Dosage: Capsules, individualized. *Angina or hypertension:* **initial:** 20 mg t.i.d.; **maintenance:** ranges from 20–40 mg t.i.d. In renal impairment, the initial dose should be 20 mg t.i.d. In hepatic impairment, the initial dose should be 20 mg b.i.d.

NURSING CONSIDERATIONS

See also *Nursing Considerations* for *Calcium Channel Blocking Agents,* p. 456.

Administration/Storage

1. When used for treating clients with angina, nicardipine may be administered safely along with sublingual nitroglycerin, prophylactic nitrates, or beta-blockers.

2. When used to treat clients with hypertension, nicardipine may be administered safely along with diuretics or beta-blockers.
3. When used to treat clients with both angina and hypertension, at least three days should elapse before increasing the dose of nicardipine so that steady-state plasma levels can be attained.

Assessment

1. Note any history of congestive heart failure and if the client is taking beta-blockers. This indicates the drug should be used with caution and demands particularly close monitoring.
2. Determine other drugs the client may be taking that could cause unfavorable drug interactions.
3. Assure that renal and liver studies have been conducted prior to initiating therapy.
4. Take blood pressure reading prior to initiating therapy to obtain baseline data against which to measure results of therapy.

Interventions

1. When used for hypertension, the maximum lowering of blood pressure occurs 1–2 hr after dosing. Thus, during initiation of therapy blood pressure should be monitored at this interval. Also, blood pressure should be evaluated at the trough (8 hr after dosing).
2. Obtain lab studies to determine renal or hepatic dysfunction. Use cautiously and anticipate reduced dosage with these conditions.
3. Monitor serum drug levels (therapeutic level 0.028–0.050 µg/mL).

Client/Family Teaching

1. Remind client to take the medication at the same time each day.
2. Report any persistent and/or bothersome side effects such as dizziness, flushing, or increased incidents of angina.
3. Encourage client to maintain a proper intake of fluids to avoid constipation.
4. Advise male clients that they may experience impotence. If this occurs they should discuss with the physician.

Evaluation

1. Assess client for evidence of edema and report if evident.
2. Note any evidence of change in the client's psychological state—depression, anxiety, or decreased mental acuity. This may be particularly important when working with elderly clients since there may be a tendency to misdiagnose the problem as senility.
3. Discuss client sleep patterns to ascertain if there has been a change and if the change could be drug related.

NIFEDIPINE (nye-FEH-dih-peen)

Adalat, Adalat FT✹, Adalat P.A.✹, Apo-Nifed✹, Novo-Nifedin✹, Procardia, Procardia XL (Rx)

See also *Calcium Channel Blocking Agents,* p. 455.

Classification: Calcium channel blocking agent (antianginal, antihypertensive).

Action/Kinetics: Variable effects on AV node effective and functional refractory periods. **Onset:** 20 min. **Peak plasma levels:** 30 min (up to 4 hr for extended release). **t½:** 2–5 hr. **Therapeutic serum levels:** 0.025–0.1 mcg/mL. **Duration:** 4–8 hr (12 hr for extended release). Metabolized in the liver to inactive metabolites.

Uses: Angina due to coronary artery spasm, chronic stable angina including angina due to increased effort (especially in patients who can not take beta-blockers or nitrates or who remain symptomatic following clinical doses of these drugs). Essential hypertension. *Investigational:* Orally, sublingually, or chewed in hypertensive emergencies. Also prophylaxis of migraine headaches, hypertension, primary pulmonary hypertension, severe pregnancy-associated hypertension, esophageal diseases, Raynaud's phenomenon, congestive heart failure, asthma, premature labor, biliary and renal colic, and cardiomyopathy.

Contraindications: Hypersensitivity. Lactation. Use with caution in impaired hepatic or renal function and in elderly patients.

Special Concerns: Use during pregnancy only if benefits outweigh risks (pregnancy category: C).

Side Effects: *CV:* Peripheral and pulmonary edema, myocardial infarction, hypotension, palpitations, syncope, congestive heart failure, decreased platelet aggregation, arrhythmias. Increased frequency, length, and duration of angina when beginning nifedipine therapy. *GI:* Nausea, diarrhea, constipation, flatulence, abdominal cramps, dysgeusia. *CNS:* Dizziness, lightheadedness, giddiness, nervousness, sleep disturbances, headache, weakness, depression, psychoses, hallucinations, disturbances in equilibrium. *Dermatologic:* Rash, dermatitis, urticaria, pruritus, photosensitivity. *Respiratory:* Dyspnea, cough, wheezing, throat, nasal or chest congestion. *Musculoskeletal:* Muscle cramps or inflammation, joint pain or stiffness, myoclonic dystonia. *Hematologic:* Thrombocytopenia, leukopenia, purpura, anemia. *Other:* Fever, chills, sweating, blurred vision, sexual difficulties, flushing, transient blindness, hyperglycemia, hypokalemia, gingival hyperplasia, hepatitis, gynecomastia, polyuria, nocturia, dysomia, erythromelalgia.

Additional Drug Interactions

Anticoagulants, oral	Possibility of ↑ prothrombin time
Digoxin	↑ Effect of digoxin by ↓ excretion by kidney
Fentanyl	Severe hypotension or increased fluid volume requirements when used with a beta-blocker and nifedipine in coronary bypass surgery
Quinidine	Possible ↓ effect of quinidine
Theophylline	Possible ↓ effect of theophylline

Laboratory Test Interferences: ↑ Alkaline phosphatase, CPK, LDH, AST, ALT. Positive Coombs' test.

Dosage: Capsules/Tablets. Individualized. Initial: 10 mg t.i.d. (range: 10–20 mg t.i.d.); **maintenance:** 10–30 mg t.i.d.–q.i.d. Patients with coronary artery spasm may respond better to 20–30 mg t.i.d.–q.i.d. Doses greater than 180 mg daily are not recommended. **Extended release tablets, initial:** 20 mg b.i.d. Dosage can be increased as required and as tolerated. *Investigational, hypertensive emergencies:* 10–20 mg given orally, sublingually (by puncturing capsule and squeezing contents under the tongue), or chewed (capsule is punctured several times and then chewed).

NURSING CONSIDERATIONS

See also *Nursing Considerations* for *Calcium Channel Blocking Agents,* p. 456.

Administration/Storage

1. A single dose should not exceed 30 mg.
2. Before increasing the dose of drug, blood pressure should be carefully monitored.
3. Only the sustained-release tablets should be used to treat hypertension.
4. Sublingual nitroglycerin and long-acting nitrates may be used concomitantly with nifedipine.
5. Concomitant therapy with beta-adrenergic blocking agents may be used. In these cases, note any potential drug interactions.
6. Clients withdrawn from beta-blockers may manifest symptoms of increased angina which can not be prevented by nifedipine; in fact, nifedipine may increase the severity of angina in this situation.
7. Angina clients may be switched to the sustained-release product at the nearest equivalent total daily dose. However, doses greater than 90 mg daily should be used with caution.
8. Protect capsules from light and moisture and store at room temperature in the original container.

Assessment

1. Note any evidence of pulmonary edema, ECG abnormalities or client complaint of palpitations.
2. Record any history of hypersensitivity to other calcium channel blocking agents.
3. When working with women of childbearing age, determine if pregnant since drug is contraindicated.

Interventions

1. During the titration period, note evidence of hypotensive response and increased heart rate that results from peripheral vasodilation. These untoward effects may precipitate angina.
2. Although beta-blocking drugs may be used concomitantly in clients with chronic stable angina, the combined effects of the drugs can not be predicted (especially in clients with compromised left ventricular function or cardiac conduction abnormalities). Thus, blood pressure should be monitored closely since severe hypotension may occur.
3. If therapy with a beta-blocker is to be discontinued, gradually decrease dosage to prevent withdrawal syndrome.

Client/Family Teaching

1. Sustained-release tablets should not be chewed or divided.
2. There is no cause for concern if an empty tablet appears in the stool.
3. Instruct clients to maintain a fluid intake of 2,000–3,000 mL/day to avoid constipation, unless contraindicated.
4. Caution not to use OTC drugs unless first discussed with the physician.

Evaluation

1. If the client is also receiving beta-adrenergic blocking agents note the development of severe hypotension, exacerbation of angina or evidence of heart failure.
2. Note any client complaint of dizziness or lightheadedness.

3. Once beta-blocking agents have been discontinued note any client complaint of increased anginal pain. This is a common withdrawal symptom and should be reported to the physician.

4. Evaluate the client for peripheral edema that may result from arterial vasodilatation that is precipitated by nifedipine or that may indicate increasing ventricular dysfunction.

NIMODIPINE (nye-**MOH**-dih-peen)

Nimotop (Rx)

See also *Calcium Channel Blocking Agents,* p. 455.

Classification: Calcium channel blocking agent.

Action/Kinetics: Nimodipine acts similarly to other calcium channel blocking agents although it has a greater effect on cerebral arteries than arteries elsewhere in the body (probably due to its highly lipophilic properties). Its mechanism, however, is not known when used to reduce neurological deficits following subarachnoid hemorrhage. **Peak plasma levels:** 1 hr. **t½:** 1–2 hr. Significantly bound (over 95%) to plasma protein. Undergoes first-pass metabolism in the liver; metabolites are excreted through the urine.

Uses: Improvement of neurological deficits due to spasm following subarachnoid hemorrhage from ruptured congenital intracranial aneurysms; patients should have Hunt and Hess Grades of I–III.

Contraindications: Lactation.

Special Concerns: Use during pregnancy only if the potential benefits outweigh potential risks (pregnancy category: C). Safety and efficacy have not been established in children. Use with caution in patients with impaired hepatic function. The half-life may be increased in geriatric patients.

Side Effects: *CV:* Hypotension, peripheral edema, congestive heart failure, ECG abnormalities, tachycardia, bradycardia, palpitations, rebound vasospasm, hypertension, hematoma, disseminated intravascular coagulation, deep vein thrombosis. *GI:* Nausea, dyspepsia, diarrhea, abdominal discomfort, cramps, GI hemorrhage, vomiting. *CNS:* Headache, depression, lightheadedness, dizziness. *Hepatic:* Abnormal liver function test, hepatitis, jaundice. *Hematologic:* Thrombocytopenia, anemia, purpura, ecchymosis. *Dermatologic:* Rash, dermatitis, pruritus, urticaria. *Miscellaneous:* Dyspnea, muscle pain or cramps, acne, itching, flushing, diaphoresis, wheezing, hyponatremia.

Laboratory Test Interference: ↑ Non-fasting serum glucose, LDH, alkaline phosphatase, ALT. ↓ Platelet count.

Dosage: Capsules, Adults: 60 mg q 4 hr beginning within 96 hr after subarachnoid hemorrhage and continuing for 21 consecutive days. The dosage should be reduced to 30 mg q 4 hr in patients with hepatic impairment.

NURSING CONSIDERATIONS

See also *Nursing Considerations* for *Calcium Channel Blocking Agents,* p. 456.

Administration/Storage

1. If the client can not swallow the capsule (e.g., unconscious or at time of surgery), a hole should be made in both ends of the capsule (soft gelatin) with an 18 gauge needle and the contents withdrawn into a syringe. The medication can then be administered into the nasogastric tube of the client and washed down the tube with 30 mL of normal saline.

2. Adult clients should be given 60 mg q 4 hr for 21 consecutive days after subarachnoid hemorrhage. The drug dosage should be reduced to 30 mg q 4 hr if the client has hepatic failure.

Assessment

1. Determine that laboratory studies for hepatic dysfunction have been performed.
2. If the client is of childbearing age ascertain if pregnant.

Interventions

1. Anticipate initiation of nimodipine therapy within 96 hours of subarachnoid hemorrhage.
2. Perform baseline neuro scores and thoroughly document deficits.
3. Monitor I & O, BP and pulse throughout therapy.
4. Anticipate reduction of dosage in clients with impaired liver function.
5. Inform the client that it is important to give the drug on time. Therefore, sleep must be interrupted to give the medication every 4 hours around the clock (RTC) for 21 days.

Client/Family Teaching

1. Discuss with the client and family and stress the importance of maintaining around-the-clock therapy.
2. Explain the importance of reporting any untoward side effects of the drug therapy, such as nausea, lightheadedness, dizziness, muscle cramps or muscle pain.

Evaluation

1. Note any client complaint of shortness of breath, the need to take deep breaths on occasion, wheezing or any other evidence of untoward reactions. These should be immediately reported.
2. Assess for evidence of improvement of client symptoms such as improved neuro scores and reduction of neurological deficits.

VERAPAMIL   (veh-RAP-ah-mil)

Calan, Calan SR, Isoptin, Isoptin SR, Novo-Veramil✿, Verelan (Rx)

See also *Calcium Channel Blocking Agents,* p. 455.

Classification: Calcium channel blocking agent (antianginal, antiarrhythmic).

Action/Kinetics: Slows AV conduction and prolongs effective refractory period. **Onset: PO,** 1–2 hr; **IV,** 3–5 min. **Time to peak plasma levels (PO):** 1–2 hr (5–7 hr for extended release). **$t^{1/2}$, PO:** 4.5–12 hr with repetitive dosing; **IV, initial:** 4 min; **final:** 2–5 hr. **Therapeutic serum levels:** 0.08–0.3 mcg/mL. **Duration, PO:** 8–10 hr (24 hr for extended release); **IV,** 10–20 min for hemodynamic effect and 2 hr for antiarrhythmic effect. Verapamil is metabolized to norverapamil, which possesses 20% of the activity of verapamil.

Uses: PO: Angina pectoris due to coronary artery spasm (Prinzmetal's variant), chronic stable angina including angina due to increased effort, unstable angina (preinfarction, crescendo); with digitalis to control rapid ventricular rate in chronic atrial flutter or atrial fibrillation; essential hypertension. Sustained-release tablets are used to treat essential hypertension (Step I therapy). **IV:** Supraventricular tachyarrhythmias. *Investigational:* Orally for prophylaxis of migraine, manic depression (alternate therapy), exercise-induced asthma, recumbent nocturnal leg cramps, treatment of PSVT.

Contraindications: Severe hypotension, second- or third-degree AV block, cardiogenic shock, severe congestive heart failure, sick sinus syndrome (unless patient has artificial pacemaker), severe left ventricular dysfunction. Cardiogenic shock and severe congestive heart failure unless secondary to supraventricular tachycardia which can be treated with verapamil. Lactation.

Special Concerns: Use during pregnancy only if benefits outweigh risks (pregnancy category: C). Infants less than 6 months of age may not respond to verapamil. Use with caution in hypertrophic cardiomyopathy, impaired hepatic and renal function, and in the elderly.

Side Effects: *CV:* Congestive heart failure, AV block, bradycardia, asystole, premature ventricular contractions and tachycardia (after IV use), peripheral and pulmonary edema, hypotension, syncope, palpitations, myocardial infarction. *GI:* Nausea, constipation, abdominal discomfort or cramps, dyspepsia, diarrhea, dry mouth. *CNS:* Dizziness, headache, fatigue, sleep disturbances, depression, amnesia, paranoia, psychoses, hallucinations, jitteriness, confusion, drowsiness, vertigo. *Dermatologic:* Rash, dermatitis, alopecia, urticaria, pruritus. *Respiratory:* Nasal or chest congestion, dyspnea, shortness of breath, wheezing. *Musculoskeletal:* Paresthesia, asthenia, muscle cramps or inflammation. *Other:* Blurred vision, sexual difficulties, spotty menstruation, sweating, rotary nystagmus, flushing, gingival hyperplasia, polyuria, nocturia, gynecomastia, claudication, hyperkeratosis, purpura, petechiae, bruising, hematomas.

Additional Drug Interactions

Antihypertensive agents	Additive hypotensive effects
Calcium salts	↓ Effect of verapamil
Carbamazepine	↑ Effect of carbamazepine due to ↓ breakdown by liver
Cyclosporine	↑ Plasma levels of cyclosporine possibly leading to renal toxicity
Digoxin	↑ Risk of digoxin toxicity due to ↑ plasma levels
Disopyramide	Additive depressant effects on myocardial contractility and AV conduction
Lithium	↓ Lithium plasma levels
Muscle relaxants, nondepolarizing	↑ Neuromuscular blockade due to effect of verapamil on calcium channels
Prazosin	Acute hypotensive effect
Quinidine	Effect of quinidine altered by verapamil
Rifampin	↓ Effect of verapamil
Theophyllines	↑ Effect of theophyllines
Vitamin D	↓ Effect of verapamil
Warfarin	Possible ↑ effect of either drug due to ↓ plasma protein binding

---

Note: Since verapamil is significantly bound to plasma proteins, interaction with other drugs bound to plasma protein may occur.

Laboratory Test Interferences: ↑ Alkaline phosphatase, transaminase.

Dosage: Tablets. *Angina.* **Individualized. Adults: initial,** 80–120 mg t.i.d. (40 mg t.i.d. if patient is sensitive to verapamil); **then,** increase dose to total of 240–480 mg/day. *Arrhythmias.* Dosage range in digitalized patients with chronic atrial fibrillation: 240–320 mg daily. For prophylaxis of nondigitalized patients: 240–480 mg daily in divided doses t.i.d.–q.i.d. *Essential hypertension.* **Initial, when used alone:** 80 mg t.i.d. In the elderly or in people with small stature, initial dose should be 40 mg t.i.d. *Essential hypertension.* **Extended-release tablets:** 180–240 mg daily (120 mg daily in the elderly or people of small stature). If response is inadequate, 240 mg may be given b.i.d. **IV, slow.** *Supraventricular tachyarrhythmias:* **Adults: initial,** 5–10 mg over 2 min (over 3 min in older patients); **then,** 10 mg 30 min later if response is not adequate. **Infants, up to 1 year:** 0.1–0.2 mg/kg over 2 min; **1–15 years:** 0.1–0.3 mg/kg (not to exceed 5 mg total dose) over 2 min. If response to initial dose is inadequate, it may be repeated after 30 min.

NURSING CONSIDERATIONS

See also *Nursing Considerations* for *Calcium Channel Blocking Agents,* p. 456.

Administration/Storage

1. Before administration, ampules should be inspected for particulate matter or discoloration.
2. IV dosage should be administered under continuous ECG monitoring with resuscitation equipment readily available.
3. Give as a slow IV bolus over 2 min (3 min to elderly clients) to minimize toxic effects.
4. Ampules should be stored at 15°–30°C and protected from light.
5. Do not give verapamil in an infusion line containing 0.45% sodium chloride with sodium bicarbonate because a crystalline precipitate will form.
6. Do not give verapamil by IV push in the same line used for nafcillin infusion since a milky white precipitate will form.
7. Verapamil should not be mixed with albumin, amphotericin B, hydralazine, trimethoprim/sulfamethoxazole, or diluted with sodium lactate in polyvinyl chloride bags.
8. Verapamil will precipitate in any solution with a pH greater than 6.
9. Dosage of verapamil in the elderly should always be individualized.
10. In the elderly, the pharmacological effects are more pronounced and more prolonged.
11. Verapamil interacts with and raises digoxin blood levels in the elderly.

Assessment

Note presence of hypotension. Verapamil may lower blood pressure to dangerously low levels if the client already has a low blood pressure.

Interventions

1. If the drug is to be administered IV, have continuous ECG monitoring and emergency drugs and resuscitative equipment readily available.
2. *Do not* administer concurrently with IV beta-adrenergic blocking agents.
3. If disopyramide is to be used, do not administer for at least 48 hr before verapamil to 24 hr after verapamil administration.
4. Unless treating verapamil overdosage, withhold any medication that elevates serum calcium levels and check with physician.
5. Anticipate reduced dosage for clients with hepatic or renal impairment.
6. Administer extended-release tablets with food to minimize fluctuations in serum levels.

Evaluation

1. Note return to normal sinus rhythm, usually attained 10 min after IV administration.
2. Assess for bradycardia and hypotension, symptoms that may indicate a need to treat overdosage.

OTHER VASODILATORS

DIPYRIDAMOLE   (dye-pih-**RID**-ah-mohl)

Apo-Dipyridamole✼, Dipimol, Dipridacot, Novodipiradol✼, Persantine, Pyridamole (Rx)

Classification: Adjunct to coumarin anticoagulants.

Action/Kinetics: Dipyridamole inhibits platelet adhesion by mechanisms that might include inhibition of uptake of adenosine, an inhibitor of platelet adhesion; inhibition of thromboxane A_2, a stimulator of platelet activity; or, inhibition of phosphodiesterase which increases cyclic-3',5'-AMP within platelets. **Peak plasma levels:** 75 min. **t½, initial:** 40 min; **terminal:** 10 hr. Highly protein bound. Dipyridamole is metabolized in the liver to inactive compounds which are excreted through the bile.

Uses: In combination with warfarin to prevent thromboembolism in patients with prosthetic heart valves. *Investigational:* In combination with aspirin to prevent myocardial infarction and coronary bypass graft occlusion. **Note:** Although used in the past to treat chronic angina, this combination is no longer recommended since it is no more effective than aspirin alone.

Contraindications: Sensitivity to dipyridamole.

Special Concerns: Pregnancy category: B. Use with caution in patients with hypotension and during lactation. Safety and efficacy have not been demonstrated in children less than 12 years of age.

Side Effects: *CNS:* Headaches, dizziness, weakness, or syncope. *GI:* Nausea, GI distress. *Other:* Flushing, skin rashes pruritus. Rarely, aggravation of angina pectoris.

Drug Interactions	
Alteplase	↑ Risk of bleeding
Aspirin	↑ Anticoagulant effect

Dosage: Tablets. *Adjunct to prevent thromboembolism after cardiac valve replacement:* 75–100 mg q.i.d. with warfarin. A dose of 100 mg daily when given with 1 g aspirin daily. **Note:** Differences in bioavailability between products may occur. **IV infusion.** *Platelet aggregation inhibitor:* 250 mg daily at a rate of 10 mg/hr.

NURSING CONSIDERATIONS

Assessment

Determine if client is taking or receiving any drugs such as aspirin or alteplase that may interact with dipyridamole.

Client/Family Teaching

1. Do not take any unprescribed drugs, such as aspirin, without first consulting the physician.
2. Do not switch brands without physician approval since there may be differences in drug bioavailability.
3. Report any symptoms such as weakness, dizziness, or faintness. These may have been potentiated by the medication and may indicate a need to change the drug regimen.

4. Clinical responses to drug therapy may be delayed from 1–3 months. Therefore, clients need to be encouraged to continue to comply with the drug regimen even if discouraged by the delay in clinical response.

Evaluation

1. Assess for a positive clinical response as demonstrated by increased exercise tolerance, reduced nitroglycerin requirements, and a reduction or elimination of anginal attacks.
2. For aggravation of angina pectoris, which necessitates discontinuation of therapy.
3. Note any untoward reactions, such as client complaint of headaches, dizziness, weakness, nausea, flushing or skin rash as dosage adjustment may be necessary.

NADOLOL   (NAY-doh-lol)
Corgard (Rx)

See Chapter 26, p. 491.

PROPRANOLOL HYDROCHLORIDE   (proh-PRAN-oh-lol)
Inderal (Rx)

See Chapter 26, p. 493.

CHAPTER TWENTY-FIVE
Peripheral Vasodilators

General Statement: Many conditions, including arteriosclerosis, reduce blood flow to the limbs. The resulting peripheral vascular disease may have serious consequences, such as tissue hypoxia and gangrene. Treatment usually involves relaxation of the muscles surrounding the small arteries and capillaries. Many of the drugs that act on various components of the autonomic nervous system (see Part 6,) p. 581 are used for the treatment of peripheral vascular disease. The drugs that specifically act on the peripheral blood vessels are discussed here.

CYCLANDELATE   (sigh-**KLAN**-deh-layt)
Cyclospasmol (Rx)

Classification: Peripheral vasodilator.

Action/Kinetics: Cyclandelate directly dilates peripheral smooth muscle of blood vessels. The drug has little effect on blood pressure and heart rate. Beneficial effects become noticeable gradually. **Onset:** 15 min. **Peak effect:** 1–1½ hr. **Duration:** 3–4 hr. Metabolic rate uncertain.

Uses: Intermittent claudication, thrombophlebitis (to treat muscle ischemia and vasospasm), arteriosclerosis obliterans, nocturnal leg cramps, Raynaud's phenomenon, ischemic cerebral vascular disease (only selected cases). However, the FDA has classified this drug as being ineffective for the labeled indications. Not intended as a substitute for other therapy.

Contraindications: Should be used with extreme caution in patients with obliterative coronary artery or cerebrovascular disease.

Special Concerns: Safe use in pregnancy and during lactation has not been established. Administer with caution to patients with glaucoma.

Side Effects: *GI:* Heartburn, GI distress, eructation. *CNS:* Headaches, dizziness, weakness. *CV:* Flushing, tachycardia. *Miscellaneous:* Tingling of extremities, sweating.

Dosage: Capsules/Tablets. Initial, 1,200–1,600 mg daily in divided doses before meals and at bedtime; **then,** decrease dose by 200 mg decrements until maintenance dosage is reached. **Maintenance:** 100–200 mg q.i.d. **Note:** Beneficial effects may not be seen for several weeks.

NURSING CONSIDERATIONS

Assessment

1. Assess client for claudication, cold extremities or local cyanosis.
2. Note client's feet for lack of hair, ulcerated areas, or evidence of poor wound healing.
3. Discuss with client any signs of persistent infection.
4. Note any signs of client confusion.
5. Determine if client has glaucoma, as drug is contraindicated in this condition.
6. Discuss with sexually active clients the potential of pregnancy. Safe use during pregnancy has not yet been established.

Interventions

Monitor client for changes in circulatory problems and document.

Client/Family Teaching

1. Take the drug with meals or with an antacid if there is evidence of gastric distress.
2. Improvement of circulation occurs slowly with cyclandelate. Encourage client to continue therapy despite slow improvement.
3. Client may experience heartburn. This may be attributed to the peripheral vasodilation. The response should be reported, however, and the client monitored for more serious side effects.

25

4. Explain that flushing, headache, weakness, and tachycardia occur frequently during the first few weeks of therapy.

5. Discuss the importance of maintaining a low fat diet since fats seem to aggravate peripheral vascular disorders.

6. Review the importance of avoiding standing for prolonged periods of time and crossing the legs.

7. Encourage the client to exercise on a regular basis unless otherwise contraindicated.

Evaluation

1. Evaluate response to therapy and client compliance with the prescribed regimen.

2. Note decreased complaints of frequency of nocturnal leg cramps.

3. Assess peripheral pulses to determine the quality. Note any improvement in color or warmth of extremities.

ETHAVERINE HYDROCHLORIDE   (eth-ah-**VER**-een)

Ethaquin, Ethatab, Ethavex-100, Isovex (Rx)

Classification: Peripheral vasodilator.

Action/Kinetics: Closely resembles papaverine. Acts directly on heart muscle, depressing conduction and prolonging refractory period. Also acts as direct nonspecific relaxant on other smooth muscles.

Uses: Various circulatory disorders accompanied by spasms of the blood vessels resulting in circulatory insufficiency. Spastic conditions of the GU and GI tracts. Efficacy is uncertain.

Contraindications: Complete A-V block, serious arrhythmias, severe liver disease.

Special Concerns: Administer with extreme caution in presence of coronary insufficiency, pulmonary embolism, and glaucoma. Safe use during pregnancy and lactation not established.

Side Effects: *GI:* Nausea, anorexia, abdominal distress, dryness of throat. *CV:* Hypotension, cardiac depression, arrhythmias, flushing. *CNS:* Vertigo, headache, drowsiness, lassitude, dizziness, malaise. *Miscellaneous:* Skin rashes, sweating, respiratory depression.

Dosage: Capsules/Tablets: 100 mg t.i.d., up to 200 mg t.i.d.

NURSING CONSIDERATIONS

Assessment

1. Assure that liver function tests have been completed to determine the presence of liver disease.

2. Note any history of coronary heart disease and/or glaucoma.

Interventions

1. Encourage client to report any incidents of skin rashes, unusual sweating or respiratory difficulty. These may be indications of untoward drug reactions.

2. Report any untoward drug reactions to the physician as the dosage of drug may need to be reduced or the drug may need to be discontinued.

3. Be particularly cognizant of potential problems if the client has coronary insufficiency, pulmonary embolus, or glaucoma.

- Note presence of cough, fever, or client complaint of pain. These may be symptoms if pulmonary embolus.
- Any pain in the midchest radiating to the back should be reported to the physician.

Client/Family Teaching

1. Use caution when driving because the drug causes drowsiness and dizziness.
2. Review proper foot care and the inherent benefits.
3. Advise client to avoid going barefoot or in slippers. The client needs support for the feet and should adhere to safety practices.

Evaluation

1. Note evidence of CNS side effects from drug such as drowsiness or headache.
2. Assess for any incidence of increased blood pressure or peripheral vasodilation.
3. Observe extremities for improvement in color and increased warmth. These signs indicate there has been improvement in the client's circulation.

ISOXSUPRINE (eye-SOX-uh-preen)
Vasodilan, Vasoprine (Rx)

Classification: Peripheral vasodilator.

Action/Kinetics: Direct relaxation of vascular smooth muscle in skeletal muscle, increasing peripheral blood flow. The drug has alpha-adrenergic receptor blocking activity and beta-adrenergic receptor stimulant properties. Isoxsuprine also causes cardiac stimulation and uterine relaxation. Drug crosses placenta. In high doses it lowers blood viscosity and inhibits platelet aggregation. **Onset, PO:** 1 hr; **IV,** 10 min. **Peak serum levels:** 1 hr, persisting for approximately 3 hr. **t¹/₂:** 75 min. Mostly excreted in urine.

Uses: Symptomatic treatment of cerebrovascular insufficiency. Improves peripheral blood circulation in arteriosclerosis obliterans, Buerger's disease, and Raynaud's disease. *Investigational:* Dysmenorrhea, threatened premature labor.

Contraindications: Postpartum period, arterial bleeding.

Special Concerns: Use with caution parenterally in patients with hypotension and tachycardia. Safety for use during pregnancy has not been determined. Risk of drug-induced hypothermia may be increased in geriatric patients.

Side Effects: *CV:* Tachycardia, hypotension, chest pain. *GI:* Abdominal distress, nausea, vomiting. *CNS:* Lightheadedness, dizziness, nervousness, weakness. *Miscellaneous:* Severe rash.

Dosage: Tablets: 10–20 mg t.i.d.–q.i.d. **IM.** *Premature labor:* 5–10 mg b.i.d.–t.i.d. (Injection not available in the U.S.).

NURSING CONSIDERATIONS

Assessment

1. Note if the client is taking a beta blocking agent as this may diminish the response to isoxsuprine.
2. If administering the drug to a pregnant woman, determine if there is evidence of uterine relaxation.
3. Note any other drugs such as diuretics, or hypotensive agents that the client may be taking and document.

Interventions

1. If the client is postpartum, be aware that arterial bleeding may occur. Have emergency drugs available.
2. When the drug is used to control premature labor, monitor the intensity, frequency and duration of uterine contractions.
3. If the drug is used to counteract a threatened spontaneous abortion, monitor the fetal heart rate at regular intervals.

Client/Family Teaching

1. Review with the client the goals of therapy.
2. Discuss the potential of the drug to cause hypotension, lightheadedness and dizziness.
3. Instruct client to avoid the use of alcoholic beverages.

NYLIDRIN   (NYE-lih-drin)

Arlidin, Arlidin Forte ✳, PMS Nylidrin ✳ (Rx)

Classification: Peripheral vasodilator.

Action/Kinetics: Vasodilation, primarily of skeletal muscle, by beta-adrenergic receptor stimulation and by direct relaxation of vascular smooth muscle. The drug also increases cardiac output. **Onset:** 10 min; **time to peak effect:** 30 min. **Duration:** 2 hr. Excreted in urine.

Uses: "Possibly effective" in peripheral vascular disease, including Raynaud's disease, thromboangiitis obliterans, arteriosclerosis obliterans, diabetic vascular disease, frostbite, night leg cramps, ischemic ulcer, acrocyanosis, acroparesthesia, thrombophlebitis. Circulatory disturbances of inner ear. Not a drug of choice. *Investigational:* To treat cognitive, emotional, and physical impairment in elderly patients.

Contraindications: Acute myocardial infarctions, angina pectoris, paroxysmal tachycardia, thyrotoxicosis.

Special Concerns: Use with caution in all patients with cardiac disease. Safety for use during pregnancy has not been determined. Risk of drug-induced hypothermia may be increased in geriatric patients. Patients intolerant to lactose, milk, or milk products may also be intolerant to nylidrin tablets as they contain lactose.

Side Effects: *CV:* Palpitations, orthostatic hypotension. *CNS:* Tremors, weakness, dizziness, nervousness. *GI:* Nausea, vomiting.

Dosage: Tablets: *Peripheral vascular disease, circulatory disturbances of the inner ear:* 3–12 mg t.i.d.–q.i.d. *Elderly patients to treat cognitive, emotional, and physical impairment:* 6–24 mg daily.

NURSING CONSIDERATIONS

Assessment

1. Note any history of heart disease. This drug must be used cautiously with clients who have cardiac dysfunction.
2. Assess BP and determine any evidence of pulse/pressure deficit.
3. Determine extent of client discomfort with alteration of vascularity.
4. Note any evidence of edema, numbness, and assess skin color.

Client/Family Teaching

1. Review mutually set goals of therapy with client.
2. Advise to avoid wearing restrictive garments.
3. Palpitations may occur but they should subside as therapy continues.
4. Improvement may not be apparent for several weeks, but advise client to continue to take medication as prescribed.
5. Report any symptoms that persist to the physician.
6. Warn clients of possible circulatory disorders that could cause them to have ringing in the ears or feelings of dizziness.
7. Caution clients to sit up slowly and to sit a few minutes on the side of the bed before standing up.
8. Advise client to take nylidrin with meals or with an antacid to avoid gastric distress.

Evaluation

1. Assess extremities for improvement in color or increased warmth.
2. Note quality of pedal pulses and determine if any evidence of improvement since therapy was initiated. Validate findings with client.
3. Assess for complaints of palpitations or persistent weakness or tremors. Report to the physician.

PAPAVERINE   (pah-**PAV**-eh-reen)

Cerespan, Genabid, Pavabid HP Capsulet, Pavabid Plateau Caps, Pavacap, Pavacen, Pavagen, Pavarine Spancaps, Pavased, Pavatine, Pavatym, Paverolan Lanacaps (Rx)

Classification: Peripheral vasodilator.

Action/Kinetics: Direct spasmolytic effect on smooth muscle, possibly by inhibiting cyclic nucleotide phosphodiesterase, thus increasing levels of cyclic AMP. This effect is seen in the vascular system, bronchial muscle, and in the GI, biliary, and urinary tracts. Large doses produce CNS sedation and sleepiness as well as depressing AV nodal and intraventricular conduction. The drug may also directly relax cerebral vessels as it increases cerebral blood flow and decreases cerebral vascular resistance. Absorbed fairly rapidly. Localized in fat tissues and liver. Steady plasma concentration maintained when drug is given q 6 hr. **Peak plasma levels:** 1–2 hr. **t½:** 30–120 min. Sustained-release products may be poorly and erratically absorbed. Metabolized in the liver and inactive metabolites excreted in the urine.

Uses: PO. Cerebral and peripheral ischemia due to arterial spasm and myocardial ischemia complicated by arrhythmias. Smooth muscle relaxant. **Parenteral.** Various conditions in which muscle spasm is observed including acute myocardial infarction, angina pectoris, peripheral vascular disease (with a vasospastic element), peripheral and pulmonary embolism, certain cerebral angiospastic states; ureteral, biliary, and GI colic. *Investigational:* Alone or with phentolamine as an intracavernous injection for impotence.

Contraindications: Complete AV block; administer with extreme caution in presence of coronary insufficiency and glaucoma.

Special Concerns: Safe use during pregnancy (pregnancy category: C) and lactation or for children not established.

Side Effects: *CV:* Flushing of face, hypertension, increase in heart rate. *GI:* Nausea, anorexia, abdominal distress, constipation or diarrhea, dry mouth and throat. *CNS:* Headache, drowsiness, sedation, vertigo. *Miscellaneous:* Sweating, malaise, pruritus, skin rashes, increase in depth of respiration, hepatitis, jaundice, eosinophilia, altered liver function tests.

Note: Both acute and chronic poisoning may result from use of papaverine. Symptoms are extensions of untoward effects. Also, acute poisoning symptoms include nystagmus, diplopia, coma, cyanosis, respiratory depression. Additional chronic poisoning symptoms include ataxia, blurred vision, erythematous macular eruptions, blood dyscrasias.

Drug Interactions	
Diazoxide IV	Additive hypotensive effect
Levodopa	Papaverine ↓ effect of levodopa by blocking dopamine receptors.

Laboratory Test Interferences: ↑ SGOT, SGPT, and bilirubin.

Dosage: Tablets: 100–300 mg 3–5 times/day; **Capsules, extended-release:** 150 mg q 12 hr up to 150 mg q 8 hr or 300 mg q 12 hr for severe cases. **IM, IV:** 30–120 mg given slowly (over 1–2 min, if IV) q 3 hr. *Cardiac extrasystoles:* Two doses 10 min apart either IM or IV (given slowly over 2 min). **Pediatric:** 6 mg/kg. **Intra-arterial:** 40 mg given slowly over 1–2 min. **Intracavernosal:** *impotence therapy:* 30 mg (of the injectable) mixed with 0.5–1 mg phentolamine mesylate for injection.

NURSING CONSIDERATIONS

Administration/Storage

1. IV injections must be given by the physician or under his/her immediate supervision.
2. Do not mix with Ringer's lactate solution because a precipitate will form.
3. Have available emergency drugs and equipment.

Assessment

Note in the client drug history if he/she is taking any drugs that would interact with papaverine therapy.

Interventions

1. Closely monitor pulse, respirations, and BP for at least 30 min after IV injection of papaverine.
2. Report any symptoms of autonomic nervous system distress such as nystagmus, diplopia or blurred vision to the physician.
3. Assess for GI reactions such as nausea or anorexia that should be reported to the physician. These may be symptoms of acute poisoning which require the immediate withdrawal of the drug and institution of emergency measures.

PHENOXYBENZAMINE HYDROCHLORIDE   (fen-ox-ee-**BENS**-ah-meen)

Dibenzyline (Rx)

See *Adrenergic Blocking Drugs, (Sympatholytic),* Chapter 45, p. 912.

TOLAZOLINE HYDROCHLORIDE   (toe-**LAZ**-oh-leen)

Priscoline HCl, Vasodil (Rx)

See *Adrenergic Blocking Drugs, (Sympatholytic),* Chapter 45, p. 912.

CHAPTER TWENTY-SIX
Antihypertensive Agents

26

Combination Drugs Commonly Used to Treat Hypertension

General Statement: Hypertension is a condition in which the mean arterial blood pressure is elevated. It is one of the most widespread chronic conditions for which medication is prescribed and taken on a regular basis. Most cases of hypertension are of unknown etiology and result from a generalized increase in resistance to flow in the peripheral vessels (arterioles). Such cases are known as primary or essential hypertension. Treatment of essential hypertension is aimed at reducing blood pressure to normal or near-normal levels, because this is believed to prevent or halt the slow, albeit permanent, damage caused by constant excess pressure.

Essential hypertension is commonly classified according to its severity as mild, moderate, or severe. Most early cases of hypertension are mild. Moderate or severe (malignant) hypertension can result in degenerative changes in the brain, heart, and kidneys and can be fatal.

Other types of hypertension (secondary hypertension) have a known etiology and can result from a complication of pregnancy (toxemic hypertension) or certain other diseases that cause impairment of kidney function. It can also be caused by a tumor of the adrenal gland (pheochromocytoma) or by blockage of certain arteries leading into the kidney (renal hypertension). The latter two cases can be corrected by surgery.

Most pharmacologic agents used to treat hypertension lower blood pressure by relaxing the constricted arterioles leading to a decrease in the resistance to peripheral blood flow. These drugs exert this effect by decreasing the influence of the sympathetic nervous system on smooth muscle of arterioles, by directly relaxing arteriolar smooth muscle, or by acting on the centers in the brain that control blood pressure.

Antihypertensive drug therapy is usually initiated when the diastolic blood pressure is greater than 90 mm Hg. Initial approaches of antihypertensive treatment include weight reduction, sodium restriction, alcohol restriction, stopping smoking, exercise, and behavior modification. Antihypertensive drug therapy is undertaken in a stepped care fashion. A single drug from one of the following classes should be considered as initial therapy: diuretic, beta-adrenergic blocking agent, calcium channel blocker, or an angiotensin converting enzyme (ACE) inhibitor. This therapy should be continued for one to three months. If the response to the drug is inadequate, the patient is adhering to the dosage regimen, and the patient is not experiencing significant side effects, one of the following three options should be considered: (1) add a drug from a different drug class; (2) increase the dose of the first drug, provided it is less than the recommended maximum dose; or (3) discontinue the initial drug and begin therapy with a drug from another drug class. When additional drugs (up to three or four different drugs may be required to control blood pressure) are added to the regimen, they should act by different mechanisms than the drugs already being used. A diuretic should be considered as either the initial or the second drug for antihypertensive drug therapy. The goal of drug therapy is to control the hypertension with the fewest number of drugs at the lowest effective dose. Importantly, the physician should attempt to decrease the dosage or number of antihypertensive drugs at regular intervals along with insisting that the patient adhere to the regimen established (i.e., weight control, sodium restriction).

The following drugs are used for stepped care: thiazide diuretics, beta-adrenergic blocking agents, calcium channel blocking drugs, ACE inhibitors, centrally acting alpha-blockers (Step II), peripherally acting drugs (Step II), vasodilators (Step III), and miscellaneous agents. Certain drugs, such as guanethidine (Step IV) and captopril are reserved for later use due to their potential side effects.

Other drugs used to treat hypertension include: sedatives and antianxiety agents (See Chapter 31, p. 611), rauwolfia alkaloids, ganglionic blocking agents, and one of the monoamine oxidase inhibitors.

Each of the drugs mentioned is discussed in this chapter. Also presented are commonly used combination drugs for the treatment of hypertension.

NURSING CONSIDERATIONS

Assessment

1. Determine baseline blood pressure before starting any antihypertensive therapy. To assure accuracy of baseline readings, take blood pressure at least three times during one visit and record.
2. Evaluate the extent of client's understanding of the disease of hypertension and the therapy as prescribed.
3. Ascertain lifestyle changes clients may have to make to achieve the goal of lowered blood pressure.
4. Assess the probability of the client's willingness to adhere to prescribed therapy.
5. Determine client's ability to take his/her own blood pressure measurements.

Interventions

1. Periodically reassess blood pressure measurements as determined by the client's condition.
2. Record significant changes in blood pressure readings or lack of response to medication on the client's record and report to the physician.

Client/Family Teaching

1. Discuss goals of drug therapy in the management of hypertension.
2. Advise clients to adhere to a low sodium, low fat diet.
3. Explain the importance of adhering to the treatment plan prescribed by the physician. Review the importance of exercise, proper diet and rest, and of complying with the prescribed drug therapy.
4. Teach clients and a family member how to take blood pressure recordings. Explain the importance of keeping a written record to share with the health care provider so that prescribed therapy may be evaluated at each visit.
5. Discuss the expected drug responses and the toxic side effects of prescribed drugs. Advise clients to report these symptoms immediately to the physician.
6. Teach the client and family how to monitor accurately fluid intake and output and if indicated (ordered) the importance of keeping an I&O record for physician review.
7. Avoid the concomitant use of other medications that could lower blood pressure (e.g. alcohol, barbiturates, CNS depressants) or that could elevate blood pressure (e.g. over-the-counter cold remedies).
8. Advise clients that if they accidentally miss a dose of medication and if it is remembered at the time of the next dose of drug, the client should not double up or take two doses close together.

Evaluation

1. Assess client/family knowledge and understanding of illness, response to therapy and to teaching.

2. Review record of BP measurements performed by client and determine drug response.

3. Observe for freedom from complications/side effects of drug therapy.

Special Concerns

1. Remind clients to keep all medications out of the reach of children.

2. Monitor elderly clients closely. They tend to have greater sensitivity to drugs and may develop untoward side effects more quickly than younger clients.

AGENTS THAT DEPRESS THE ACTIVITY OF THE SYMPATHETIC NERVOUS SYSTEM

I. Angiotensin-Converting Enzyme Inhibitors

CAPTOPRIL   (KAP-toe-prihl)
Capoten (Rx)

Classification: Antihypertensive, inhibitor of angiotensin synthesis.

Action/Kinetics: Mechanism not fully understood, but drug seems to inhibit angiotensin I-converting enzyme which decreases the conversion of angiotensin I to angiotensin II, which increases BP. Captopril also reduces peripheral arterial resistance. The drug increases renin activity and decreases aldosterone secretion, leading to small increase in serum potassium. **Peak blood levels:** 1 hr; presence of food decreases absorption by 30–40%. **Plasma protein binding:** 25–30%. **Time to peak effect:** 60–90 min. **Duration:** 6–12 hr. **t½:** 2 hr; in 24 hr, 95% of absorbed dose excreted in urine (40–50% unchanged).

Uses: Antihypertensive, Step I therapy. Concomitant use with diuretic therapy may, however, cause precipitous hypotension.

In combination with diuretics and digitalis in treatment of congestive heart failure not responding to conventional therapy.

Investigational: Rheumatoid arthritis, hypertensive crisis.

Special Concerns: Use with caution in cases of impaired renal function. Use in pregnancy only if potential benefits outweigh risks (pregnancy category: C). Use in children only if other antihypertensive therapy has proven ineffective in controlling BP. Use with caution during lactation.

Side Effects: *Dermatologic:* Rash with pruritus, fever, eosinophilia. Angioedema of face, mucous membranes of mouth, or extremities. Flushing, pallor. *GI:* Gastric irritation, nausea, vomiting, anorexia, constipation or diarrhea, ulcers, dyspepsia, dry mouth. *CNS:* Headache, dizziness, insomnia, malaise, fatigue. *CV:* Hypotension, angina, congestive heart failure, myocardial infarction, Raynaud's phenomenon, chest pain, palpitations, tachycardia. *Renal:* Renal insufficiency or failure, proteinuria, urinary frequency, oliguria, polyuria. *Other:* Decrease or loss of taste perception with weight loss (reversible), neutropenia, paresthesias.

Drug Interactions

Antihypertensives, oral	↑ Effect of captopril if renin is released
Diuretics	Sudden ↓ BP within 3 hr
Potassium-sparing diuretics	↑ Serum potassium

Laboratory Test Interferences: False + urinary acetone. Transient ↑ BUN and creatinine. ↑ Serum potassium.

Dosage: Tablets. *Hypertension:* **Adults, initial:** 12.5 mg b.i.d.–t.i.d. If unsatisfactory response after 1–2 weeks, increase to 25 mg b.i.d.–t.i.d.; if still unsatisfactory after another 1–2 weeks, thiazide diuretic should be added (e.g., hydrochlorothiazide, 25 mg/day). Dosage may be increased to 100–150 mg b.i.d.–t.i.d., not to exceed 450 mg daily. *Heart failure:* **initial,** 12.5 mg b.i.d.–t.i.d.; **then,** if necessary, increase dose to 50 mg t.i.d. and evaluate response; **maintenance:** 50–100 mg t.i.d., not to exceed 450 mg daily. *For accelerated or malignant hypertension:* **initial,** 25 mg b.i.d.–t.i.d.; **then,** increase dose q 24 hr until satisfactory response obtained or maximum dose reached. For all uses, doses should be reduced in patients with renal impairment. **Note:** For adults, an initial dose of 6.25–12.5 mg (0.15 mg/kg t.i.d. in children) should be given b.i.d.–t.i.d. to patients who are sodium- and water-depleted due to diuretics, who will continue to be on diuretic therapy, and who have renal impairment.

   Children, initial: 0.3 mg/kg t.i.d.; **then,** increase dose, if needed, in increments of 0.3 mg/kg at intervals of 8–24 hr to reach the minimum effective dose. **Newborns, initial:** 0.01 mg/kg b.i.d.–t.i.d.; adjust dose as needed.

NURSING CONSIDERATIONS

See also *Nursing Considerations* for *Antihypertensive Agents,* p. 477.

Administration/Storage

1. In cases of overdosage, volume expansion with normal saline (IV) is the treatment of choice to restore BP.
2. Captopril should not be discontinued without the consent of a physician.

Assessment

1. Obtain baseline hematological studies and renal and liver function tests prior to beginning therapy.
2. Determine if the client is taking nitroglycerin or other antianginal nitrates. These may act in synergism with captopril and may cause a more pronounced response.
3. Determine the potential for the client to understand and comply with the prescribed therapy.

Interventions

1. Observe client closely for a precipitous drop in BP within 3 hr after initial dose of captopril if a client has been on diuretic therapy and a sodium-restricted diet.
2. If BP falls rapidly, place the client in a supine position and be prepared to assist with an IV infusion of saline.
3. Check for proteinuria monthly after the onset of treatment and for at least 9 months.
4. Withhold potassium-sparing diuretics and consult with physician if client is not hypokalemic, because hyperkalemia may result.
5. Be alert to hyperkalemia occurring several months after administration of spironolactone and captopril.

Client/Family Teaching

1. Take captopril 1 hr before meals, on an empty stomach. Food interferes with the absorption of the drug.

2. Report fever, skin rash, sore throat, mouth sores, fast or irregular heartbeat, or chest pain to the physician.

3. Advise that some people may develop dizziness, fainting or lightheadedness. These symptoms usually disappear once the body adjusts to the medication. Encourage client to avoid sudden changes in posture to prevent dizziness and fainting.

4. Explain to clients that they may experience a loss of taste for the first 2–3 months. If this persists and interferes with nutrition, the physician should be notified. This usually disappears in 2–3 months.

5. Carry identification and a list of medications currently prescribed. Always inform any physician they may visit that they are taking captopril.

6. Encourage clients to call the physician if they have any questions concerning symptoms or about the effects of drug therapy. Remind them not to stop taking the medication without physician consent.

ENALAPRIL MALEATE   (eh-NAL-ah-pril)

Vasotec, Vasotec I.V. (Rx)

See also *Captopril,* p. 478.

Classification: Antihypertensive, angiotensin-converting enzyme inhibitor.

Action/Kinetics: Enalapril is converted in the liver by hydrolysis to the active metabolite, enalaprilat. The parenteral product is enalaprilat injection. **Onset, PO:** 1 hr; **IV,** 15 min. **Time to peak action, PO:** 4–6 hr; **IV,** 1–4 hr. **Duration, PO:** 24 hr; **IV,** about 6 hr. Approximately 50–60% is protein bound. **t½, PO:** 1 hr; **IV,** 15 min. Enalapril is excreted unchanged through the kidneys.

Special Concerns: Pregnancy category: C. Use with caution during lactation.

Use: Alone or in combination with a thiazide diuretic for the treatment of hypertension (Step I therapy). As adjunct with digitalis and diuretic in acute and chronic congestive heart failure.

Side Effects: *CV:* Palpitations, hypotension, chest pain, syncope. *GI:* Nausea, vomiting, diarrhea, abdominal pain, alterations in taste. *CNS:* Insomnia, headache, fatigue, dizziness, paresthesias, nervousness, sleepiness. *Renal:* Transient increases in creatinine and BUN. *Hematologic:* Agranulocytosis, neutropenia, thrombocytopenia, hemolytic anemia, pancytopenia (may be fatal). *Other:* Rash, cough, angioedema, labored breathing, pruritus, muscle cramps, asthenia, impotence, elevated liver enzymes.

Dosage: Tablets. *In patients not taking diuretics:* **Initial:** 5 mg once daily; **then,** adjust dosage according to response (range: 10–40 mg daily in 1–2 doses). *In patients taking diuretics:* **Initial:** 2.5 mg. Since hypotension may occur following the initiation of enalapril, the diuretic should be discontinued, if possible, for 2–3 days before initiating enalapril. If blood pressure is not maintained with enalapril alone, diuretic therapy may be resumed. Dosage should be decreased in patients with a creatinine clearance less than 30 mL/min and a serum creatinine level greater than 3 mg/dl. *Heart failure:* **Initial:** 2.5 mg 1–2 times daily; **then,** depending on the response, 5–20 mg/day in two divided doses. Dose should not exceed 40 mg daily. Dosage must be adjusted in patients with renal impairment or hyponatremia.

IV. *Hypertension:* 1.25 mg over a 5-minute period; repeat q 6 hr. *In patients taking diuretics:* **Initial:** 0.625-mg over 5 min; if an adequate response is seen after 1 hr, administer another 0.625 mg dose. Thereafter, 1.25 mg q 6 hr.

NURSING CONSIDERATIONS

See also *Nursing Considerations* for *Antihypertensive Agents,* p. 477.

Administration/Storage

1. Following IV administration, the peak effect after the first dose may not be observed for 4 hr (whether or not the client is on a diuretic). For subsequent doses, the peak effect is usually within 15 min.
2. Enalapril should be given as a slow IV infusion (over 5 min) either alone or diluted up to 50 mL with an appropriate diluent. Any of the following can be used: 5% dextrose injection, 5% dextrose in lactated Ringer's injection, Isolyte E, 0.9% sodium chloride injection, or 0.9% sodium chloride injection in 5% dextrose.
3. To convert from IV to PO therapy in clients on a diuretic, begin with 2.5 mg once daily for clients responding to a 0.625-mg IV dose. Thereafter, 2.5 mg once daily may be given.
4. To convert from PO to IV enalapril therapy in clients not on a diuretic, use the recommended IV dose (i.e., 1.25 mg q 6 hr). To convert from IV to PO therapy, begin with 5 mg once daily.

Assessment

1. Obtain complete blood count, liver and renal function studies as baseline data.
2. Identify drugs the client may be taking that would interact with enalapril and record on the client's record.

Interventions

1. Anticipate lowered dosage for clients receiving diuretics.
2. Monitor CBC, serum electrolytes, liver and renal function studies throughout therapy.

Client/Family Teaching

1. Stress the importance of keeping scheduled laboratory and physician appointments.
2. If there is a conflict, clients should be advised to reschedule the appointment as soon as possible.
3. Report any weight loss that may result from the client's loss of taste.

LISINOPRIL   (lie-**SIN**-oh-pril)

Prinivil, Zestril (Rx)

Classification: Antihypertensive, angiotensin-converting enzyme inhibitor.

Action/Kinetics: By inhibiting angiotensin-converting enzyme, lisinopril prevents the conversion of angiotensin I to angiotensin II. Inhibiting angtiotensin I conversion results in decreased vasopressor activity, leading to decreased blood pressure and decreased secretion of aldosterone. Both supine and standing blood pressure are reduced, although the drug is less effective in blacks than in Caucasians. Although food does not alter the bioavailability of lisinopril, only 25% of an oral dose is absorbed. **Onset:** 1 hr. **Peak serum levels:** 7 hr. **Duration:** 24 hr. **t½:** 12 hr. 100% of the drug is excreted unchanged in the urine.

Uses: Alone or in combination with a diuretic to treat hypertension (Step I therapy). *Investigational:* In combination with digitalis and a diuretic for treating congestive heart failure not responding to other therapy.

Special Concerns: Pregnancy category: C. Use with caution during lactation. Safety and efficacy have not been established in children.

Side Effects: *CNS:* Dizziness, headache, fatigue, vertigo, insomnia, depression, sleepiness. *GI:* Diarrhea, nausea, vomiting, dyspepsia, anorexia, constipation, flatulence, abdominal pain. *Respiratory:* Upper respiratory symptoms, cough, dyspnea, bronchitis, sinusitis, pharyngeal pain. *CV:* Hypotension, orthostatic hypotension, angina, tachycardia, palpitations, rhythm disturbances. *Musculoskeletal:* Asthenia, muscle cramps, joint pain, shoulder pain. *Miscellaneous:* Angioedema (may be fatal if laryngeal edema occurs), hyperkalemia, neutropenia, agranulocytosis, paresthesia, back pain, nasal congestion, decreased libido, chest pain, fever, flushing, peripheral edema, oliguria, azotemia, acute renal failure, blurred vision, pruritus, urinary tract infection, vasculitis of the legs.

Drug Interactions

Diuretics	Excess ↓ blood pressure
Indomethacin	Possible ↓ effect of lisinopril
Potassium-sparing diuretics	Significant ↑ serum potassium

Laboratory Test Interferences: ↑ Serum potassium, BUN, serum creatinine. ↓ Hemoglobin, hematocrit.

Dosage: Tablets. *Essential hypertension, used alone:* 10 mg once daily. Adjust dosage depending on response (range: 20–40 mg daily). Doses greater than 80 mg daily do not give a greater effect. *Essential hypertension in combination with a diuretic:* **Initial,** 5 mg. The blood pressure-lowering effects of the combination are additive. Dosage should be reduced in patients with renal impairment. *Congestive heart failure:* **Initial,** 2.5–5 mg daily; **maintenance:** 10–40 mg daily.

NURSING CONSIDERATIONS

See also *Nursing Considerations* for *Antihypertensive Agents*, p. 477.

Administration/Storage

1. When considering use of lisinopril in a client taking diuretics, discontinue the diuretic, if possible, 2–3 days before beginning lisinopril therapy. If the diuretic can not be discontinued, the initial dose of lisinopril should be 5 mg and the client should be closely observed for at least 2 hr.
2. In some clients, maximum antihypertensive effects may not be observed for 2–4 weeks.
3. Clients whose blood pressure is controlled with lisinopril, 20 mg, plus hydrochlorothiazide, 25 mg, given separately should be given a trial of Prinzide 12.5 mg or Zestoretic 20–12.5 mg before Prinzide 25 mg or Zestoretic 20–25 mg is used (see p. 529).
4. The maximum recommended daily dose of lisinopril is 80 mg in a single daily dose. However, clients usually do not require hydrochlorothiazide in doses exceeding 50 mg daily, especially if combined with other antihypertensives.
5. Use of potassium supplements, potassium-sparing diuretics, or potassium salt substitutes with Prinzide or Zestoretic may lead to increases in serum potassium.
6. Prinzide or Zestoretic is recommended for those clients with a creatinine clearance greater than 30 mL/min.

Intervention

Anticipate reduced dosage if the client has renal insufficiency.

Client/Family Teaching

1. Advise client to take medication at bedtime to minimize potential side effects.
2. Explain how to avoid symptoms of orthostatic hypotension (i.e., rise slowly from sitting or lying position and wait until symptoms subside).
3. Avoid all potassium supplements as well as foods high in potassium.
4. Stress the importance of reporting for scheduled laboratory studies.

II. Beta-Adrenergic Blocking Agents

Action/Kinetics: Beta-adrenergic blocking agents combine reversibly with beta-adrenergic receptors to block the response to sympathetic nerve impulses, circulating catecholamines, or adrenergic drugs. Beta-adrenergic receptors have been classified as beta-1 (predominantly in the cardiac muscle) and beta-2 (mainly in the bronchi and vascular musculature). Blockade of beta-1 receptors decreases heart rate, myocardial contractility, and cardiac output; in addition, AV conduction is slowed. These effects lead to a decrease in blood pressure, as well as a reversal of cardiac arrhythmias. Blockade of beta-2 receptors increases airway resistance in the bronchioles and inhibits the vasodilating effects of catecholamines on peripheral blood vessels. The various beta-blocking agents differ in their ability to block beta-1 and beta-2 receptors (see individual drugs); also, certain of these agents have intrinsic sympathomimetic action.

Uses: Depending on the drug, these agents may be used to treat one or more of the following conditions: hypertension, angina pectoris, cardiac arrhythmias, myocardial infarction, prophylaxis of migraine, situational anxiety, and alcohol withdrawal syndrome. Propranolol is indicated for a number of other conditions (see information on propranolol).

Contraindications: Sinus bradycardia, greater than first degree heart block, cardiogenic shock, congestive heart failure unless secondary to tachyarrhythmia treatable with beta-blockers, overt cardiac failure. Most are contraindicated in chronic bronchitis, asthma, bronchospasm, emphysema.

Special Concerns: Use with caution in diabetes, thyrotoxicosis, and impaired hepatic and renal function. Safe use during pregnancy and lactation and in children has not been established. Also, see individual agents.

Side Effects: *CV:* Bradycardia, hypotension (especially following IV use), congestive heart failure, cold extremities, claudication, worsening of angina, strokes, edema, syncope, arrhythmias, chest pain, peripheral ischemia, flushing, shortness of breath, sinoatrial block, pulmonary edema, vasodilation, increased heart rate, palpitations, conduction disturbances, first and third degree heart block, worsening of AV block, thrombosis of renal or mesenteric arteries, precipitation or worsening of Raynaud's phenomenon. Sudden withdrawal of large doses may cause angina, ventricular tachycardia, fatal myocardial infarction, or sudden death. *GI:* Nausea, vomiting, diarrhea, flatulence, dry mouth, constipation, anorexia, cramps, bloating, gastric pain, dyspepsia, distortion of taste, weight gain or loss, retroperitoneal fibrosis, ischemic colitis. *Hepatic:* Hepatomegaly, acute pancreatitis, elevated liver enzymes. *Respiratory:* Asthma-like symptoms, bronchospasms, bronchial obstruction, wheeziness, laryngospasm with respiratory distress, worsening of chronic obstructive lung disease, dyspnea, cough, nasal stuffiness, rhinitis, pharyngitis, rales. *CNS:* Dizziness, fatigue, lethargy, vivid dreams, depression, hallucinations, delirium, psychoses, paresthesias, insomnia, nervousness, nightmares, headache, vertigo, disorientation of time and place, hypoesthesia or hyperesthesia, decreased concentration, short-term memory loss, change in behavior, emotional lability, slurred speech, lightheadedness. In the elderly, paranoia, disorientation, and combativeness have occurred. *Hematologic:* Agranulocytosis, thrombocytopenia. *Allergic:* Fever, sore throat, respiratory distress, rash, laryngospasm, pharyngitis, anaphylaxis. *Skin:* Pruritus, rashes, increased skin pigmentation, sweating, dry skin, alopecia, skin irritation, psoriasis (reversible). *Musculoskeletal:* Joint and muscle pain, arthritis, arthralgia, back pain, muscle cramps. *GU:* Impotence, decreased libido, dysuria, urinary tract infection, nocturia, urinary retention or frequency, pollakiuria. *Ophthalmic:* Visual disturbances, eye irritation, dry or burning eyes, blurred vision, conjunctivitis. *Other:* Hyperglycemia or hypoglycemia, lupus-like syndrome, Peyronie's disease, tinnitus, increased in symptoms of myasthenia gravis, facial swelling, decreased exercise tolerance, rigors, speech disorders.

Drug Interactions

Anesthetics, general	Additive depression of myocardium
Anticholinergic agents	Counteract bradycardia produced by beta-adrenergic blockers
Antihypertensives	Additive hypotensive effect
Chlorpromazine	Additive beta-adrenergic blocking action
Cimetidine	↑ Effect of beta blockers due to ↓ breakdown by liver
Clonidine	Paradoxical hypertension; also, ↑ severity of rebound hypertension
Disopyramide	↑ Effect of both drugs
Epinephrine	Beta blockers prevent beta-adrenergic action of epinephrine but not alpha-adrenergic action → ↑ systolic and diastolic blood pressure and ↓ heart rate
Furosemide	↑ Beta-adrenergic blockade
Hydralazine	↑ Beta-adrenergic blockade
Indomethacin	↓ Effect of beta blockers possibly due to inhibition of prostaglandin synthesis
Insulin	Beta blockers ↑ hypoglycemic effect of insulin
Lidocaine	↑ Effect of lidocaine due to ↓ breakdown by liver
Methyldopa	Possible ↑ blood pressure due to alpha-adrenergic effect
Nonsteroidal anti-inflammatory drugs	↓ Effect of beta blockers, possibly due to inhibition of prostaglandin synthesis
Oral contraceptives	↑ Effect of beta blockers due to ↓ breakdown by liver
Phenformin	↑ Hypoglycemia
Phenobarbital	Phenobarbital ↓ effect of beta blockers due to ↑ breakdown by liver
Phenothiazines	↑ Effect of both drugs
Phenytoin	Additive depression of myocardium; also phenytoin ↓ effect of beta blockers due to ↑ breakdown by liver
Prazosin	↑ First-dose effect of prazosin (acute postural hypotension)

Drug Interactions

Reserpine	Additive hypotensive effect
Rifampin	Rifampin ↓ effect of beta blockers due to ↑ breakdown by liver
Ritodrine	Beta blockers ↓ effect of ritodrine
Salicylates	↓ Effect of beta blockers, possibly due to inhibition of prostaglandin synthesis
Succinylcholine	Beta blockers ↑ effects of succinylcholine
Sympathomimetics	Reverse effects of beta-blockers
Theophylline	Beta blockers reverse the effect of theophylline; also, beta blockers ↓ renal clearance of theophylline
Tubocurarine	Beta blockers ↑ effects of tubocurarine
Verapamil	Possible untoward reactions since both drugs ↓ myocardial contractility or AV conduction.

Laboratory Test Interference: ↓ Serum glucose.

Dosage: See individual drugs.

Treatment of Overdosage: General supportive treatment such as inducing emesis or gastric lavage, artificial respiration, treatment of hypoglycemia or hypokalemia. *Excessive bradycardia:* atropine, 0.6 mg; if no response, give q 3 min for a total of 2–3 mg. Cautious administration of isoproterenol may be tried. Also, glucagon, 5–10 mg, may reverse bradycardia. *Cardiac failure:* Digitalis, diuretic, and oxygen; if failure is refractory, IV aminophylline or glucagon may be helpful. *Hypotension:* IV fluids; also vasopressors such as norepinephrine, dobutamine, dopamine. If refractory, glucagon may be helpful. *Premature ventricular contractions:* Lidocaine or phenytoin. *Bronchospasms:* Give a β_2-adrenergic agonist or theophylline. *Heart block:* Isoproterenol or transvenous cardiac pacing.

NURSING CONSIDERATIONS

Administration/Storage

Sudden cessation of beta-blockers may precipitate or worsen angina.

Assessment

1. Take the client's pulse and blood pressure prior to beginning therapy.
2. Obtain serum glucose level, liver and renal function studies as a baseline against which to measure results after medication regimen begins.
3. Note any history of diabetes or impaired renal function.

Interventions

1. Take pulse rate, as well as BP, at least once a day to assure that the client has not developed tachycardia or bradycardia.
2. When assessing the client's respirations note the rate and quality. Drugs in this category may cause dyspnea and bronchospasm.
3. Observe for increasing dyspnea, coughing, client complaint of difficulty breathing or fatigue or the presence of edema. These are symptoms of congestive heart failure and indicate that the client may require digitalization, diuretics, and/or discontinuation of drug therapy.

4. If working with a client with diabetes be especially cognizant of symptoms of hypoglycemia, such as hypotension or tachycardia. Most beta-adrenergic blocking agents mask these signs.

Client/Family Teaching

1. Instruct client and family in taking blood pressures and pulse rates.
2. Assist them to develop a method to maintain accurate written records of blood pressures and pulse rates. Instruct client to maintain a written record for review by the health care provider so that medication can be adjusted as needed.
3. Provide written instructions as to when to call the physician, for example if the pulse rate goes below 50 beats per minute or the blood pressure is less than 90 mm Hg systolic.
4. Once dose is established, take and record BP at least twice a week and take pulse rate immediately prior to first dose each day unless otherwise directed.
5. To consult a physician before interrupting therapy because abrupt withdrawal of most beta-adrenergic blocking agents may precipitate angina, myocardial infarction, or rebound hypertension.
6. Some drugs may cause blurred vision; do not engage in activities that require mental alertness until drug effects become apparent.
7. Dress warmly during cold weather because diminished blood supply to extremities may cause client to be more sensitive to the cold.
8. Consult with physician before taking any OTC preparations.
9. Diabetic clients should be attentive to symptoms of hypoglycemia and should perform finger sticks more often while on drug therapy.
10. Report any asthma-like symptoms, cough or nasal stuffiness to the physician as these may be early symptoms of congestive heart failure.
11. Report any bothersome side effects to the physician, especially new-onset depression.
12. Keep all medications out of the reach of children.

Evaluation

1. Assess client/family knowledge and understanding of illness, and level of compliance as based on response to therapy and teaching.
2. Evaluate any client complaints of having a cold, easy fatigue, or feeling of lightheadedness. These untoward side effects may indicate a need to have the medication changed.
3. Check extremities for warmth.
4. Note if the blood pressure is responding as would be anticipated for clients receiving these drugs. Review client's written records of daily BP measurements.
5. Review all laboratory data for any evidence of intolerance to therapy.

ACEBUTOLOL HYDROCHLORIDE   (ah-seh-BYOU-toe-lohl)

Monitan ♣, Sectral (Rx)

See also *Beta-Adrenergic Blocking Agents,* p. 483.

Classification: Beta-adrenergic blocking agent.

Action/Kinetics: Predominantly beta-1 blocking activity but will inhibit beta-2 receptors at higher doses. Acebutolol also has some intrinsic sympathomimetic activity. **t½:** 3–4 hr. Low lipid solubility. Metabolized in liver and excreted in urine and bile.

Uses: Hypertension (either alone or with other antihypertensive agents such as thiazide diuretics). Premature ventricular contractions.

Additional Contraindication: Severe, persistent bradycardia.

Special Concerns: Pregnancy category: B. Dosage has not been established in children.

Dosage: Capsules. *Hypertension:* **initial,** 400 mg once daily (although 200 mg b.i.d. may be needed for optimum control); **then,** 400–800 mg daily (range: 200–1,200 mg daily). *Premature ventricular contractions:* **initial,** 200 mg b.i.d.; **then,** increase dose gradually to reach 600–1,200 mg/day. Dosage should be decreased in geriatric patients (should not exceed 800 mg daily) and in those with impaired kidney or liver function (decrease dose by 50% when creatinine clearance is 50 mL/min/1.73 m² and by 75% when it is less than 25 mL/min/1.73 m²).

NURSING CONSIDERATIONS

See also *Nursing Considerations* for *Beta-Adrenergic Blocking Agents,* p. 485.

Administration/Storage

1. When treatment is discontinued, the drug should be withdrawn gradually over a two week period.
2. The bioavailability increases in elderly clients; thus, such clients may require lower maintenance doses (no more than 800 mg daily).
3. Acebutolol may be combined with another antihypertensive agent.

ATENOLOL   (ah-**TEN**-oh-lohl)

Tenormin (Rx)

See also *Beta-Adrenergic Blocking Agents,* p. 483.

Action/Kinetics: Predominantly beta-1 blocking activity. Has no membrane stabilizing activity or intrinsic sympathomimetic activity. Low lipid solubility. **Peak blood levels:** 2–4 hr. **t½:** 6–9 hr. 50% eliminated unchanged in the feces.

Uses: Hypertension (either alone or with other antihypertensives such as thiazide diuretics). Angina pectoris due to hypertension, coronary atherosclerosis, and acute myocardial infarction. *Investigational:* Prophylaxis of migraine, alcohol withdrawal syndrome, situational anxiety, ventricular arrhythmias, prophylactically to reduce incidence of supraventricular arrhythmias in coronary artery bypass surgery.

Special Concerns: Pregnancy category: C. Dosage has not been established in children.

Dosage: Tablets. *Hypertension:* **initial,** 50 mg once daily, either alone or with diuretics; if response is inadequate, 100 mg once daily. Doses higher than 100 mg daily will not produce further beneficial effects. Maximum effects will usually be seen within 1–2 weeks. *Angina:* **initial,** 50 mg once daily; if maximum response is not seen in 1 week, increase dose to 100 mg daily (some patients require 200 mg daily). *Alcohol withdrawal syndrome:* 100 mg daily. *Prophylaxis of migraine:* 50–100 mg daily. *Ventricular arrhythmias:* 50–100 mg daily. *Prior to coronary artery bypass surgery:* 50 mg daily started 72 hr prior to surgery. Adjust dosage in cases of renal failure to 50 mg daily if creatinine clearance is 15–35 mL/min/1.73 m² and to 50 mg every other day if creatinine clearance is less than 15 mL/min/1.73 m².

IV. *Acute myocardial infarction:* 5 mg over 5 min followed by a second 5 mg dose 10 min later. Treatment should begin as soon as possible after patient arrives at the hospital. In patients who tolerate the full 10 mg dose, a 50 mg tablet should be given 10 min after the last IV dose followed by another 50 mg dose 12 hr later. **Then,** 100 mg once a day or 50 mg b.i.d. for 6–9 days (or until discharge from the hospital).

NURSING CONSIDERATIONS

See also *Nursing Considerations* for *Beta-Adrenergic Blocking Agents,* p. 485.

Administration/Storage

1. For IV use, the drug may be diluted in sodium chloride injection, dextrose injection, or sodium chloride and dextrose injection.
2. For hemodialysis clients, 50 mg should be given in the hospital after each dialysis.

BETAXOLOL HYDROCHLORIDE   (beh-**TAX**-oh-lohl)
Kerlone (Rx)

See also *Beta-Adrenergic Blocking Agents,* p. 483.

Classification: Beta-adrenergic blocking agent.

Action/Kinetics: Inhibits beta-1 adrenergic receptors although beta-2 receptors will be inhibited at high doses. Has some membrane stabilizing activity but no intrinsic sympathomimetic activity. Low lipid solubility. **t½:** 14–22 hr. Metabolized in the liver with most excreted through the urine; about 15% is excreted unchanged.

Uses: Hypertension, alone or with other antihypertensive agents (especially diuretics).

Special Concerns: Pregnancy category: C. Use with caution during lactation. Safety and effectiveness have not been determined in children. Geriatric patients are at greater risk of developing bradycardia.

Dosage: Tablets. Initial: 10 mg once daily either alone or with a diuretic. If the desired effect is not reached, the dose can be increased to 20 mg although doses higher than 20 mg will not increase the therapeutic effect. In geriatric patients the initial dose should be 5 mg daily.

NURSING CONSIDERATIONS

See also *Nursing Considerations* for *Beta-Adrenergic Blocking Agents,* p. 485.

Administration/Storage

1. The full effect is usually observed within 7–14 days.
2. As the dose is increased, the heart rate decreases.
3. Drug therapy with betaxolol should be discontinued gradually over a 2 week period.

CARTEOLOL HYDROCHLORIDE   (**KAR**-tee-oh-lohl)
Cartrol

See also *Beta-Adrenergic Blocking Agents,* p. 483.

Action/Kinetics: Carteolol has both beta-1 and beta-2 receptor blocking activity. The drug has no membrane stabilizing activity but does have moderate intrinsic sympathomimetic effects. Low lipid solubility. **t½:** 6 hr. Approximately 50%–70% excreted unchanged in the urine.

Uses: Hypertension. *Investigational:* Reduce frequency of anginal attacks.

Special Concerns: Pregnancy category: C. Dosage has not been established in children.

Dosage: Tablets. *Hypertension:* **initial,** 2.5 mg once daily either alone or with a diuretic. In the event of an inadequate response, the dose may be increased gradually to 5 mg and then 10 mg daily as a single dose. **Maintenance:** 2.5–5 mg once daily. Doses greater than 10 mg daily are not likely to increase the beneficial effect and may decrease the response. The dosage interval should be increased in patients with renal impairment. *Reduce frequency of anginal attacks:* 10 mg daily.

NURSING CONSIDERATIONS

See also *Nursing Considerations* for *Beta-Adrenergic Blocking Agents,* p. 485.

Intervention

Anticipate reduced dose with impaired renal function.

Client/Family Teaching

Do not exceed prescribed dose because desired response may be altered.

ESMOLOL HYDROCHLORIDE   (ez-MOH-lohl)
Brevibloc (Rx)

See also *Beta-Adrenergic Blocking Agents,* p. 483.

Classification: Beta-adrenergic blocking agent.

Action/Kinetics: Esmolol preferentially inhibits beta-1 receptors. It has a rapid onset and a short duration of action. It has no membrane stabilizing or intrinsic sympathomimetic activity. Low lipid solubility. **t½:** 9 min. Is rapidly metabolized by esterases in red blood cells.

Uses: Supraventricular or noncompensatory tachycardia, sinus tachycardia.

Special Concerns: Pregnancy category: C. Dosage has not been established in children.

Additional Side Effects: *Dermatologic:* Inflammation at site of infusion, flushing, pallor, induration, erythema, burning, skin discoloration, edema. *Other:* Urinary retention, midscapular pain, asthenia, changes in taste.

Additional Drug Interactions	
Digoxin	Esmolol ↑ digoxin blood levels
Morphine	Morphine ↑ esmolol blood levels

Dosage: IV infusion. *Supraventricular tachycardia:* **Initial:** 500 mcg/kg/min for 1 min; **then,** 50 mcg/kg/min for 4 min. If after 5 min an adequate effect is not achieved, repeat the loading dose followed by a maintenance infusion of 100 mcg/kg/min for 4 min. This procedure may be repeated, increasing the maintenance infusion by 50 mcg/kg/min increments (for 4 min) until the desired heart rate or lowered blood pressure is approached. **Then,** omit the loading infusion and reduce incremental infusion rate from 50 to 25 mcg/kg/min or less. The interval between titrations may be increased from 5 to 10 min.

Once the heart rate has been controlled, the patient may be transferred to another antiarrhythmic agent. The infusion rate of esmolol should be reduced by 50% 30 min after the first dose of the alternative antiarrhythmic agent. If satisfactory control is observed for 1 hr after the second dose of the alternative agent, the esmolol infusion may be stopped.

NURSING CONSIDERATIONS

See also *Nursing Considerations* for *Beta-Adrenergic Blocking Agents,* p. 485.

Administration/Storage

1. Infusions of esmolol may be necessary for 24–48 hr.
2. Esmolol HCl is not intended for direct IV push administration.
3. The concentrate should not be diluted with sodium bicarbonate.
4. To minimize venous irritation and thrombophlebitis, infusion concentrations should not be greater than 10 mg/mL.
5. Diluted esmolol is compatible with 5% dextrose injection, 5% dextrose in Ringer's injection, 5% dextrose and 0.9% sodium chloride injection, 5% dextrose and 0.45% sodium chloride injection, 0.45% sodium chloride injection, or lactated Ringer's injection.

Interventions

1. Monitor client closely for evidence of hypotension and/or bradycardia. Interrupt infusion if values for blood pressure and heart rate fall below critical levels and notify physician immediately.
2. Infusions should be administered in a monitored environment and with an electronic infusion device.
3. Have emergency drugs and equipment readily available.

METOPROLOL   (meh-toe-**PROH**-lohl)

Apo-Metoprolol ✽, Apo-Metaprolol (Type L) ✽, Betaloc ✽, Lopressor, Novometoprolol (Rx)

See also *Beta-Adrenergic Blocking Agents,* p. 483.

Action/Kinetics: Exerts mainly beta-1 adrenergic blocking activity although beta-2 receptors are blocked at high doses. Has no membrane stabilizing or intrinsic sympathomimetic effects. Moderate lipid solubility. **Onset:** 15 min. **Peak plasma levels:** 90 min. **t½:** 3–7 hr. Effect of drug is cumulative. Food increases bioavailability. Exhibits significant first-pass effect. Metabolized in liver and excreted in urine.

Uses: Hypertension (either alone or with other antihypertensive agents, such as thiazide diuretics). Acute myocardial infarction in hemodynamically stable patients. Angina pectoris. *Investigational:* IV to suppress atrial ectopy in chronic obstructive pulmonary disease, aggressive behavior, prophylaxis of migraine, ventricular arrhythmias, enhancement of cognitive performance in geriatric patients, essential tremors.

Additional Contraindications: Myocardial infarction in patients with a heart rate of less than 45 beats/min, in second or third degree heart block, or if systolic blood pressure is less than 100 mm Hg. Cardiac failure.

Special Concerns: Pregnancy category: B. Dosage has not been established in children.

Additional Drug Interactions

Cimetidine	May ↑ plasma levels of metoprolol
Contraceptives, oral	May ↑ effects of metoprolol
Methimazole	May ↓ the effects of metoprolol
Phenobarbital	↓ Effect of metoprolol due to ↑ breakdown by liver
Propylthiouracil	May ↓ the effects of metoprolol
Quinidine	May ↑ effects of metoprolol
Rifampin	↓ Effect of metoprolol due to ↑ breakdown by liver

Laboratory Test Interferences: ↑ Serum transaminase, LDH, alkaline phosphatase.

Dosage: Tablets. *Hypertension:* **initial,** 100 mg daily in single or divided doses; **then,** dose may be increased weekly to maintenance level of 100–450 mg daily. A diuretic may also be used. *Prophylaxis of myocardial infarction:* **early treatment,** 50 mg q 6 hr beginning 15 min after the last IV dose (or as soon as patient's condition allows). This dose is continued for 48 hr followed by **late treatment: PO,** 100 mg b.i.d. as soon as feasible; continue for 1–3 months (although data suggest treatment should be continued for 1–3 years). *Aggressive behavior:* 200–300 mg daily. *Essential tremors:* 50–300 mg daily. *Prophylaxis of migraine:* 50–100 mg b.i.d. *Ventricular arrhythmias:* 200 mg daily. **IV.** *Myocardial infarction,* **early treatment:** 5 mg as an IV bolus q 2 min for a total of 3 doses (15 mg); **then,** if this dose is tolerated, give 50 mg PO q 6 hr for 48 hr, beginning 15 min after the last IV dose (see above). If patient cannot tolerate full IV dose, begin PO dose at 25 or 50 mg q 6 hr.

NURSING CONSIDERATIONS

See also *Nursing Considerations* for *Beta-Adrenergic Blocking Agents,* p. 485.

Client/Family Teaching

Doses of metoprolol should be taken at the same time each day.

NADOLOL   (NAY-doh-lohl)

Corgard (Rx)

See also *Beta-Adrenergic Blocking Agents,* p. 483.

Classification: Beta-adrenergic blocking agent.

Action/Kinetics: Manifests both beta-1 and beta-2 adrenergic blocking activity. Has no membrane stablizing or intrinsic sympathomimetic activity. Low lipid solubility. **Peak serum concentration:** 3–4 hr. **t½:** 20–24 hr (permits once-daily dosage). **Duration:** 17–24 hr. Absorption variable, averaging 30%; steady plasma level achieved after 6–9 days of administration. Excreted unchanged by the kidney.

Uses: Hypertension, either alone or with other drugs (e.g., thiazide diuretic). Angina pectoris. *Investigational:* Prophylaxis of migraine, ventricular arrhythmias, treatment of lithium-induced tremors, aggressive behavior, essential tremor, tremors associated with lithium or Parkinsonism, antipsychotic-induced akathisia, rebleeding of esophageal varices, situational anxiety, reduce intraocular pressure.

Special Concerns: Pregnancy category: C. Dosage has not been established in children.

Dosage: Tablets. *Hypertension:* **initial,** 40 mg once daily; **then,** may be increased in 40- to 80-mg intervals until optimum response obtained. **Maintenance:** 40–80 mg once daily although up to 320 mg once daily may be needed. *Angina:* **initial,** 40 mg once daily; **then,** increase dose in 40- to 80-mg increments q 3–7 days until optimum response obtained. **Maintenance:** 40–80 mg once daily, although up to 240 mg once daily may be needed. *Aggressive behavior:* 40–160 mg daily. *Antipsychotic-induced akathisia:* 40–80 mg daily. *Essential tremor:* 120–240 mg daily. *Lithium-induced tremors:* 20–40 mg daily. *Tremors associated with Parkinsonsim:* 80–320 mg daily. *Prophylaxis of migraine:* 40–80 mg daily. *Rebleeding from esophageal varices:* 40–160 mg daily. *Situational anxiety:* 20 mg. *Ventricular arrhythmias:* 10–640 mg daily. *Reduction of intraocular pressure:* 10–20 mg b.i.d. Dosage for all uses should be decreased in patients with renal failure.

NURSING CONSIDERATIONS

See *Nursing Considerations* for *Beta-Adrenergic Blocking Agents*, p. 485.

PENBUTOLOL SULFATE   (pen-**BYOU**-toe-lohl)

Levatol (Rx)

See also *Beta-Adrenergic Blocking Agents*, p. 483.

Action/Kinetics: Penbutolol has both beta-1 and beta-2 receptor blocking activity. It has no membrane-stabilizing activity but does possess minimal intrinsic sympathomimetic activity. High lipid solubility. **t½:** 5 hr. 80%–98% protein bound. Penbutolol is metabolized in the liver and excreted through the urine.

Uses: Mild to moderate arterial hypertension.

Special Concerns: Pregnancy category: C. Dosage has not been established in children. Geriatric patients may manifest increased or decreased sensitivity to the usual adult dose.

Dosage: Tablets. *Hypertension:* **initial,** 20 mg once daily either alone or with other antihypertensive agents. **Maintenance:** Same as initial dose. Doses greater than 40 mg daily do not result in a greater antihypertensive effect.

NURSING CONSIDERATIONS

See also *Nursing Considerations* for *Beta-Adrenergic Blocking Agents*, p. 485.

Administration/Storage

1. The full effect of a 20–40 mg dose may not be observed for 2 weeks.
2. Doses of 10 mg daily are effective but full effects are not seen for 4–6 weeks.

Client/Family Teaching

1. Review the signs and symptoms associated with postural hypotension and instruct client to rise slowly from a sitting or lying position.
2. Take medication only as prescribed since full effects may not be realized for a month or more.

PINDOLOL (PIN-doh-lohl)
Visken (Rx)

See also *Beta-Adrenergic Blocking Agents,* p. 483.

Action/Kinetics: Manifests both beta-1 and beta-2 adrenergic blocking activity. Pindolol also has significant intrinsic sympathomimetic effects and minimal membrane-stabilizing activity. Moderate lipid solubility. **t½:** 3–4 hr; however, geriatric patients have a variable half-life ranging from 7–15 hr, even with normal renal function. The drug is metabolized by the liver, and the metabolites and unchanged (35%–40%) drug are excreted through the kidneys.

Uses: Hypertension (alone or in combination with other antihypertensive agents as thiazide diuretics). *Investigational:* Ventricular arrhythmias and tachycardias, antipsychotic-induced akathisia, situational anxiety.

Special Concerns: Pregnancy category: B. Dosage has not been established in children.

Laboratory Test Interferences: ↑ SGOT and SGPT. Rarely, ↑ LDH, uric acid, alkaline phosphatase.

Dosage: Tablets. *Hypertension:* **Initial,** 5 mg b.i.d. (alone or with other antihypertensive drugs). If no response in 3–4 weeks, increase by 10 mg/day q 3–4 weeks to a maximum of 60 mg daily. *Antipsychotic-induced akathisia:* 5 mg daily.

NURSING CONSIDERATIONS
See also *Nursing Considerations* for *Beta-Adrenergic Blocking Agents,* p. 485.

Intervention
Anticipate reduced dosage in clients with liver dysfunction.

PROPRANOLOL HYDROCHLORIDE (proh-PRAN-oh-lohl)
Apo-Propranolol✿, Detensol✿, Inderal, Inderal 10, 20, 40, 60, 80, and 90, Inderal LA, Novopranol✿, PMS Propranolol✿, Propranolol Intensol (Rx)

See also *Beta-Adrenergic Blocking Agents,* p. 483.

Classification: Beta-adrenergic blocking agent; antiarrhythmic (Type II).

Action/Kinetics: Propranolol manifests both beta-1 and beta-2 adrenergic blocking activity. The antiarrhythmic action results from both beta-adrenergic receptor blockade and from a direct membrane-stabilizing action on the cardiac cell. Propranolol has no intrinsic sympathomimetic activity and has high lipid solubility. **PO: Onset,** 30 min. **Maximum effect:** 1–1.5 hr. **Duration:** 3–6 hr. **t½:** 3–5 hr (8–11 hr for long-acting). Onset after IV administration is almost immediate. Completely metabolized by liver and excreted in urine. Although food increases bioavailability of the drug, absorption may be decreased.

Uses: Hypertension (alone or in combination with other antihypertensive agents). Angina pectoris, hypertrophic subaortic stenosis, prophylaxis of myocardial infarction, pheochromocytoma, prophylaxis of migraine, essential tremor. Cardiac arrhythmias including ventricular tachycardias and arrhythmias, tachycardias due to digitalis intoxication, supraventricular arrhythmias, premature ventricular contractions (PVCs), resistant tachyarrhythmias due to anesthesia/catecholamines.

Investigational: Schizophrenia, tremors due to Parkinsonism, aggressive behavior, antipsychotic-induced akathisia, rebleeding due to esophageal varices, situational anxiety, acute panic attacks, gastric bleeding in portal hypertension, vaginal contraceptive, anxiety, alcohol withdrawal syndrome.

Special Concerns: Pregnancy category: C.

Additional Side Effects: Psoriasis-like eruptions, skin necrosis, systemic lupus erythematosus (rare).

Additional Drug Interactions

Haloperidol	Severe hypotension
Hydralazine	↑ Effect of both agents
Methimazole	May ↑ effects of propranolol
Phenobarbital	↓ Effect of propranolol due to ↑ breakdown by liver
Propylthiouracil	May ↑ the effects of propranolol
Rifampin	↓ Effect of propranolol due to ↑ breakdown by liver
Smoking	↓ Serum levels and ↑ clearance of propranolol

Laboratory Test Interferences: ↑ Blood urea, serum transaminase, alkaline phosphatase, LDH. Interference with glaucoma screening test.

Dosage: Tablets, Long-acting Capsules, Oral Solution. *Hypertension:* **initial,** 40 mg b.i.d. or 80 mg of sustained-release/day; **then,** increase dose to maintenance level of 120–240 mg daily given in 2–3 divided doses or 120–160 mg of sustained-release medication once daily. Maximum daily dose should not exceed 640 mg. *Angina, prophylaxis:* **initial,** 10–20 mg t.i.d.–q.i.d. or 80 mg of sustained-release once daily; **then,** increase dose gradually to maintenance level of 160 mg/day of sustained-release capsule. The maximum daily dose should not exceed 320 mg. *Arrhythmias:* 10–30 mg t.i.d.–q.i.d. given after meals and at bedtime. *Hypertrophic subaortic stenosis:* 20–40 mg t.i.d.–q.i.d. before meals and at bedtime or 80–160 mg of sustained-release medication given once daily. *Myocardial infarction prophylaxis:* 180–240 mg daily given in 2–3 divided doses. Total daily dose should not exceed 240 mg. *Pheochromocytoma, preoperatively:* 60 mg daily for 3 days before surgery, given concomitantly with an alpha-adrenergic blocking agent. *Inoperable tumors:* 30 mg/day in divided doses. *Migraine:* **initial,** 80 mg sustained-release medication given once daily; **then,** increase dose gradually to maintenance of 160–240 mg daily. If a satisfactory response has not been observed after 4–6 weeks, the drug should be discontinued and withdrawn gradually. *Essential tremor:* **initial,** 40 mg b.i.d.; **then,** 120 mg daily up to a maximum of 320 mg daily.

   IV. *Life-threatening arrhythmias:* 1–3 mg not to exceed 1 mg/min; a second dose may be given after 2 min, with subsequent doses q 4 hr. Patients should begin PO therapy as soon as possible.

   Pediatric. *Hypertension:* **PO, initial,** 1 mg/kg daily in divided doses (e.g., 0.5 mg/kg b.i.d.). May be increased at 3–5 day intervals to a maximum of 2 mg/kg daily. The dosage range should be calculated by weight and not by body surface area.

   Investigational uses. Aggressive behavior: 80–300 mg daily. *Antipsychotic-induced akathisia:* 20–80 mg daily. *Tremors associated with Parkinsonism:* 160 mg daily. *Rebleeding due to esophageal varices:* 20–180 mg daily. *Situational anxiety:* 40 mg. *Schizophrenia:* 300–5,000 mg daily. *Acute panic symptoms:* 40–320 mg daily. *Anxiety:* 80–320 mg daily. *Gastric bleeding in portal hypertension:* 24–480 mg daily.

NURSING CONSIDERATIONS
See also *Nursing Considerations* for *Beta-Adrenergic Blocking Agents,* p. 485.

Administration/Storage

1. Do not administer for a minimum of 2 weeks after client has received MAO inhibitor drugs.

2. If signs of serious myocardial depression occur following propranolol administration, iso-proterenol (Isuprel) should be slowly infused IV.

Interventions

1. Observe client for evidence of a rash, fever, and/or purpura. These may be symptoms of a hypersensitivity reaction.
2. Monitor intake and output. Observe for signs and symptoms of congestive heart failure, (e.g., shortness of breath, rales, edema and weight gain).
3. After IV administration, have available emergency drugs and equipment to combat hypotension or circulatory collapse.

Client/Family Teaching

Do not smoke. Smoking decreases serum levels of the drug and interferes with drug clearance.

TIMOLOL MALEATE   (TIH-moh-lohl)

Apo-Timol✿, Blocadren, Timoptic, Timoptic in Acudose (Rx)

See also *Beta-Adrenergic Blocking Agents,* p.483.

Classification: Ophthalmic agent, beta-adrenergic blocking agent.

Action/Kinetics: Timolol exerts both beta-1 and beta-2 adrenergic blocking activity. Timolol has minimal sympathomimetic effects, direct myocardial depressant effects, and local anesthetic action. It does not cause pupillary constriction or night blindness. The mechanism of the protective effect in myocardial infarction is not known. **Peak plasma levels:** 1–2 hr. **t½:** 4 hr. Metabolized in the liver. Metabolites and unchanged drug excreted through the kidney.

Timolol also reduces both elevated and normal intraocular pressure, whether or not glaucoma is present; it is thought to act by reducing aqueous humor formation and/or by slightly increasing outflow of aqueous humor. The drug does not affect pupil size or visual acuity. For use in eye: **Onset:** 30 min. **Maximum effect:** 1–2 hr. **Duration:** 24 hr.

Uses: Tablets: Hypertension (alone or in combination with other antihypertensives such as thiazide diuretics). Within 1–4 weeks of myocardial infarction to reduce risk of reinfarction. *Investigational:* Prophylaxis of migraine, ventricular arrhythmias and tachycardias, essential tremors.

   Ophthalmic solution: Chronic open-angle glaucoma, selected cases of secondary glaucoma, ocular hypertension, aphakic (no lens) patients with glaucoma.

Contraindications: Hypersensitivity to drug.

Special Concerns: Use ophthalmic preparation with caution in patients for whom systemic beta-adrenergic blocking agents are contraindicated. Safe use during pregnancy (pregnancy category: C) and in children not established.

Side Effects: *Systemic following use of tablets:* See *Beta-Adrenergic Blocking Agents,* p. 483.

   Following use of ophthalmic product: Few. Occasionally, ocular irritation, local hypersensitivity reactions, slight decrease in resting heart rate.

Drug Interactions: When used ophthalmically, possible potentiation with systemically administered beta-adrenergic blocking agents.

Laboratory Test Interferences: ↑ BUN, serum potassium, and uric acid. ↓ Hemoglobin and hematocrit.

Dosage: Tablets. *Hypertension, Angina:* **initial,** 10 mg b.i.d. alone or with a diuretic; **maintenance:** 20–40 mg/day (up to 80 mg/day in 2 doses may be required). If dosage increase is necessary, wait 7 days. *Myocardial infarction prophylaxis:* 10 mg b.i.d. *Glaucoma:* One drop of 0.25%–0.50% solution in each eye b.i.d.

NURSING CONSIDERATIONS

See also *Nursing Considerations* for *Beta-Adrenergic Blocking Agents,* p. 485.

Administration/Storage

1. When client is transferred from another antiglaucoma agent, continue old medication on day 1 of timolol therapy (one drop of 0.25% solution). Thereafter, discontinue former therapy. Initiate with 0.25% solution. Increase to 0.50% solution if response is insufficient. Further increases in dosage are ineffective.

2. When client is transferred from several antiglaucoma agents, the dose must be individualized. If one of the agents is a beta-adrenergic blocking agent, it should be discontinued before starting timolol. Dosage adjustments should involve one drug at a time at one week intervals. The antiglaucoma drugs should be continued with the addition of timolol, 1 gtt of 0.25% solution b.i.d. (if response is inadequate, 1 gtt of 0.5% solution may be used b.i.d.). The following day, one of the other antiglaucoma agents should be discontinued while the remaining agents should be continued or discontinued based on client response.

Client/Family Teaching

1. Review the appropriate procedure for administration. Have client or person administering therapy return demonstrate.

2. Instruct client to apply finger lightly to lacrimal sac for 1 minute following administration.

3. Stress the importance of continued regular intraocular measurements by an ophthalmologist, because ocular hypertension may recur and/or progress without overt signs or symptoms.

4. When timolol is used for long-term prophylaxis against myocardial infarction, do not interrupt therapy without consulting with the prescribing physician. Abrupt withdrawal may precipitate reinfarction.

III. Centrally Acting Agents

CLONIDINE HYDROCHLORIDE   (KLAH-nih-deen)

Catapres, Catapres-TTS-1, -2, and -3, Dixarit✳ (Rx)

Classification: Antihypertensive, centrally acting antiadrenergic.

Action/Kinetics: Stimulates alpha-adrenergic receptors of the CNS, which results in inhibition of the sympathetic vasomotor centers and decreased nerve impulses. Thus, bradycardia and a fall in both systolic and diastolic blood pressure occurs. Plasma renin levels are decreased, while peripheral venous pressure remains unchanged. The drug has few orthostatic effects. Although sodium chloride excretion is markedly decreased, potassium excretion remains unchanged. Tolerance to the drug may develop. **Onset, PO:** 30–60 min; **transdermal:** 2–3 days. **Peak plasma levels, PO:** 3–5 hr; **transdermal:** 2–3 days. **Maximum effect, PO:** 2–4 hr. **Duration, PO:** 12–24 hr; **transdermal:** 7 days (with system in place). **t½:** 12–16 hr. Approximately 50% excreted unchanged in the urine; 20% excreted through the feces.

The transdermal dosage form contains the following levels of drug: Catapres-TTS-1 contains 2.5 mg clonidine (surface area 3.5 cm²), with 0.1 mg released daily; Catapres-TTS-2 contains 5 mg clonidine (surface area 7 cm²), with 0.2 mg released daily; and Catapres-TTS-3 contains 7.5 mg clonidine (surface area 10.5 cm²), with 0.3 mg released daily.

Uses: Mild to moderate hypertension. A diuretic or other antihypertensive drugs, or both, are often used concomitantly. *Investigational:* Diabetic diarrhea, alcohol withdrawal, treatment of Gilles de la Tourette syndrome, detoxification of opiate dependence, constitutional growth delay in children, hypertensive urgency (diastolic > 120 mm Hg), menopausal flushing, diagnosis of pheochromocytoma, facilitate cessation of smoking, ulcerative colitis, postherpetic neuralgia, reduce allergen-induced inflammation in patients with extrinsic asthma.

Special Concerns: Pregnancy category: C. Use with caution in presence of severe coronary insufficiency, recent myocardial infarction, cerebrovascular disease, or chronic renal failure. Use with caution during lactation. Safe use in children not established. Geriatric patients may be more sensitive to the hypotensive effects; a decreased dosage may also be necessary in these patients due to age-related decreases in renal function.

Side Effects: *CNS:* Drowsiness (common), sedation, dizziness, headache, fatigue, malaise, nightmares, nervousness, restlessness, anxiety, mental depression, increased dreaming, insomnia, hallucinations, delirium, agitation. *GI:* Dry mouth (common), constipation, anorexia, nausea, vomiting, parotid pain, weight gain. *CV:* Congestive heart failure, Raynaud's phenomenon, abnormalities in ECG, palpitations, tachycardia and bradycardia, orthostatic symptoms, conduction disturbances, sinus bradycardia. *Dermatologic:* Urticaria, skin rashes, angioneurotic edema, pruritus, thinning of hair, alopecia. *GU:* Impotence, urinary retention, decreased sexual activity, loss of libido, nocturia, difficulty in urination. *Musculoskeletal:* Muscle or joint pain, leg cramps, weakness. *Other:* Gynecomastia, increase in blood glucose (transient), increased sensitivity to alcohol, dryness of mucous membranes of nose; itching, burning, dryness of eyes; skin pallor, fever.

Transdermal products: Localized skin reactions, pruritus, erythema, allergic contact sensitization and contact dermatitis, localized vesiculation, hyperpigmentation, edema, excoriation, burning, papules, throbbing, blanching, generalized macular rash.

Note: Rebound hypertension may be manifested if clonidine is abruptly withdrawn.

Drug Interactions	
Alcohol	↑ Depressant effects
Beta-adrenergic blocking agents	Paradoxical hypertension; also, ↑ severity of rebound hypertension following clonidine withdrawal
CNS depressants	↑ Depressant effect
Levodopa	↓ Effect of levodopa
Tolazoline	Blocks antihypertensive effect
Tricyclic antidepressants	Blocks antihypertensive effect

Laboratory Test Interferences: Transient ↑ of blood glucose and serum creatinine phosphokinase. Weakly + Coombs' test. Alteration of electrolyte balance.

Dosage: Tablets. *Hypertension:* **initial,** 0.1 mg b.i.d.; **then,** increase by 0.1–0.2 mg/day until desired response is attained; **maintenance:** 0.2–0.6 mg/day in divided doses (maximum: 2.4 mg/day). Tolerance necessitates increased dosage or concomitant administration of a diuretic.

Gradual increase of dosage after initiation minimizes side effects. **Note:** In hypertensive patients unable to take oral medication, clonidine may be administered sublingually at doses of 0.2–0.4 mg daily. **Pediatric:** 5–25 mcg/kg daily in divided doses q 6 hr; increase dose at 5–7 day intervals.

Transdermal, initial: Use 0.1 mg system; **then,** if after 1–2 weeks adequate control has not been achieved, can use another 0.1 mg system or a larger system. The antihypertensive effect may not be seen for 2–3 days.

Investigational uses. Gilles de la Tourette syndrome: 0.15–0.2 mg/day. *Withdrawal from opiate dependence:* 15–16 mcg/kg daily. *Alcohol withdrawal:* 0.3–0.6 mg q 6 hr. *Diabetic diarrhea:* 0.15–1.2 mg daily or 0.3 mg/24 hr patch. *Constitutional growth delay in children:* 0.0375–0.15 mg/m² daily. *Hypertensive urgency:* **initially,** 0.1–0.2 mg; **then,** 0.05–0.1 mg q hr to a maximum of 0.8 mg. *Menopausal flushing:* 0.1–0.4 mg daily or 0.1 mg/24 hr patch. *Diagnosis of pheochromocytoma:* 0.3 mg. *Postherpetic neuralgia:* 0.2 mg daily. *Reduce allergen-induced inflammation in extrinsic asthma:* 0.15 mg for 3 days. *Facilitate cessation of smoking:* 0.15–0.4 mg daily or 0.2 mg/24 hr patch. *Ulcerative colitis:* 0.3 mg t.i.d.

NURSING CONSIDERATIONS

Administration/Storage

1. If the transdermal system is used, apply the medication to a hairless area of skin, such as upper arm or torso once a week.
2. Use a different site with each application.
3. It may take 2–3 days to achieve effective blood levels using the transdermal system. Therefore, any prior drug dosage should be reduced gradually.
4. If the drug is to be taken orally, administer the last dose of the day at bedtime to ensure overnight control of blood pressure.
5. Clients with severe hypertension may require antihypertensive drug therapy in addition to transdermal clonidine.
6. If the drug is to be discontinued, it should be done gradually over a period of 2–4 days.
7. Have IV tolazoline readily available to treat acute toxicity caused by clonidine.

Assessment

Note the client's occupation. This drug may interfere with the client's ability to work and should be noted.

Interventions

1. Monitor BP closely during the initial therapy. A decrease in BP occurs within 30–60 min after administration of clonidine and may persist for 8 hr.
2. Weigh the client daily, in the morning, in clothing of the same weight, to determine if there is edema caused by sodium retention. Any fluid retention should disappear after 3–4 days.
3. Note any fluctuations in BP to determine whether it is preferable to use clonidine alone or concomitantly with a diuretic. A stable BP reduces orthostatic effects of postural changes.
4. Observe for a paradoxical hypertensive response if client is also receiving propranolol.
5. Note any evidence of depression that may be precipitated by the drug, especially in those clients with a history of mental depression.
6. If the client is concomitantly receiving tolazoline or a tricyclic antidepressant, be aware that these drugs may block the antihypertensive action of clonidine. An increased dosage of clonidine may be indicated.
7. Note any side effects clients experience. These can be minimized by starting with a low dose and increasing the dosage of clonidine gradually until the desired effects are obtained.

8. Drug dosage is based on the client's BP and tolerance to therapy. Therefore, side effects should be recorded and reported even if they may seem minor.

Client/Family Teaching

1. Do not engage in activities that require alertness, such as operating machinery or driving a car, because the drug may cause drowsiness.
2. Do not discontinue medication abruptly or without medical supervision. Also do not initiate any change in the medication regimen until this has been cleared by the physician.
3. If the drug is to be withdrawn, explain the need for gradual withdrawal to prevent rebound hypertension.
4. If the client has Parkinson's disease and is controlled with levodopa, advise to report any increase in signs and symptoms of the disease. Clonidine may reduce the effect of levodopa.

GUANABENZ ACETATE   (GWAHN-ah-benz)

Wytensin (Rx)

Classification: Antihypertensive, centrally acting antiadrenergic.

Action/Kinetics: Guanabenz stimulates alpha-adrenergic receptors in the CNS, resulting in a decrease in sympathetic impulses and in sympathetic tone. It also decreases the pulse rate, but postural hypotension has not been manifested. **Onset:** 60 min. **Peak effect:** 2–4 hr. **Peak plasma levels:** 2–5 hr. **t½:** 6 hr. **Duration:** 8–12 hr.

Uses: Hypertension, alone or as adjunct with thiazide diuretics.

Contraindications: Lactation, children under 12 years of age.

Special Concerns: Pregnancy category: C. Use with caution in severe coronary insufficiency, cerebrovascular disease, recent myocardial infarction, hepatic or renal disease. Geriatric patients may be more sensitive to the hypotensive and sedative effects of methyldopa; also, it may be necessary to decrease the dose in these patients due to age-related decreases in renal function.

Side Effects: *CNS:* Drowsiness and sedation (common), dizziness, weakness, headache, ataxia, depression, disturbances in sleep, excitement. *GI:* Dry mouth (common), nausea, vomiting, diarrhea, constipation, abdominal pain or discomfort. *CV:* Palpitations, chest pain, arrhythmias. *Miscellaneous:* Edema, blurred vision, muscle aches, dyspnea, rash, pruritus, nasal congestion, urinary frequency, gynecomastia, alterations in taste, disturbances of sexual function, taste disorders, aches in extremities.

Drug Interaction: Use with CNS depressants may result in significant sedation.

Dosage: Tablets. Adults: initial, 4 mg b.i.d. alone or with a diuretic; **then,** increase by 4–8 mg q 1–2 weeks until control achieved. Maximum recommended dose: 32 mg b.i.d.

NURSING CONSIDERATIONS

Administration/Storage

The drug should be kept tightly closed and protected from light.

Client/Family Teaching

1. How to take BP and pulse, and to maintain a written record for physician review.

2. Do not drive an automobile or operate machinery until the sedative effect of this drug has been assessed.

3. Be alert to disturbances in sleep that may indicate a depressive episode. Report these symptoms to the health care provider.

GUANFACINE HYDROCHLORIDE (GWAHN-fah-seen)

Tenex (Rx)

Classification: Antihypertensive, centrally acting.

Action/Kinetics: Guanfacine is thought to act by central stimulation of alpha$_2$ receptors resulting in a decrease in peripheral sympathetic output and heart rate resulting in a decrease in blood pressure. The drug may also manifest a direct peripheral alpha$_2$ receptor stimulant action. **Onset:** 2 hr. **Peak plasma levels:** 1–4 hr. **Peak effect:** 6–12 hr. **t½:** 12–23 hr. **Duration:** 24 hr. Approximately 50% is excreted through the kidneys unchanged.

Uses: Hypertension concomitantly with a thiazide diuretic. *Investigational:* Withdrawal from heroin use.

Contraindications: Hypersensitivity to guanfacine. Acute hypertension associated with toxemia. Children less than 12 years of age.

Special Concerns: Use with caution during pregnancy (category: B) and lactation. Use with caution in patients with recent myocardial infarction, cerebrovascular disease, chronic renal or hepatic failure, or severe coronary insufficiency. Geriatric patients may be more sensitive to the hypotensive and sedative effects.

Side Effects: *GI:* Dry mouth, constipation, nausea, abdominal pain, diarrhea, dyspepsia, dysphagia. *CNS:* Sedation, weakness, dizziness, headache, fatigue, insomnia, amnesia, confusion, depression. *CV:* Bradycardia, substernal pain, palpitations. *Ophthalmic:* Visual disturbances, conjunctivitis, iritis. *Dermatologic:* Pruritus, dermatitis, purpura, sweating. *Other:* Decreased libido, impotence, rhinitis, tinnitus, alterations in taste, leg cramps, dyspnea, urinary incontinence, paresthesia, paresis, asthenia, hypokinesia, malaise, testicular disorder.
Note: If therapy is abruptly discontinued, a rebound reaction may occur within 2–4 days, which is manifested by nervousness, anxiety, and increased blood pressure.

Drug Interactions: Additive sedative effects when used concomitantly with CNS depressants.

Dosage: Tablets. *Hypertension:* **initial:** 1 mg daily at bedtime; if satisfactory results are not obtained in 3–4 weeks, dosage may be increased by 1 mg at 1- to 2-week intervals up to a maximum of 3 mg daily in 1–2 divided doses. *Heroin withdrawal:* 0.03–1.5 mg daily.

NURSING CONSIDERATIONS

Administration/Storage

1. If a decrease in blood pressure is not maintained for over 24 hr, the daily dose may be more effective if divided, although the incidence of side effects increases.

2. Adverse effects increase significantly when the daily dose exceeds 3 mg.

3. Therapy should be initiated in clients already taking a thiazide diuretic.

Client/Family Teaching

1. Teach client how to take BP and assist to develop a method to maintain a written record for physician review.
2. Use caution in performing tasks that require mental alertness, such as driving or operating machinery because the drug may cause dizziness or drowsiness.
3. Stress the importance of not discontinuing the drug abruptly.
4. Avoid ingestion of alcohol and any other nonprescribed drugs.

METHYLDOPA   (meth-ill-**DOH**-pah)

Aldomet, Apo-Methyldopa ✤, Dopamet ✤, Novomedopa ✤ (Rx)

METHYLDOPATE HYDROCHLORIDE   (meth-ill-**DOH**-payt)

Aldomet Hydrochloride (Rx)

Classification: Antihypertensive, centrally acting antiadrenergic.

Action/Kinetics: Primary mechanism thought to be that the active metabolite, alpha-methyl-norepinephrine, lowers BP by stimulating central inhibitory alpha-adrenergic receptors, false neurotransmission, and/or reduction of plasma renin. It causes little change in cardiac output. **PO: Onset:** 7–12 hr. **Duration:** 12–24 hr. All effects terminated within 48 hr. Absorption is variable. **IV: Onset:** 4–6 hr. **Duration:** 10–16 hr. Seventy percent of drug excreted in urine. **Full therapeutic effect:** 1–4 days. $t^{1/2}$: 1.7 hr.
   Note: Methyldopa is a component of Aldoril.

Uses: Moderate to severe hypertension. Particularly useful for patients with impaired renal function, renal hypertension, resistant cases of hypertension complicated by stroke, coronary artery disease, or nitrogen retention, and for hypertensive crisis (parenterally).

Contraindications: Sensitivity to drug, labile and mild hypertension, pregnancy, active hepatic disease, or pheochromocytoma.

Special Concerns: Use with caution in patients with a history of liver or kidney disease. Use during pregnancy only if benefits clearly outweigh risks (pregnancy category: B). Geriatric patients may be more sensitive to the hypotensive and sedative effects of methyldopa; also, it may be necessary to decrease the dose in these patients due to age-related decreases in renal function.

Side Effects: *CNS:* Sedation (disappears with use), weakness, headache, asthenia, dizziness, paresthesias, Parkinson-like symptoms, psychic disturbances, choreoathetotic movements, Bell's palsy, decreased mental acuity, verbal memory impairment. *CV:* Bradycardia, orthostatic hypotension, hypersensitivity of carotid sinus, worsening of angina, hypertensive response (paradoxical), myocarditis. *GI:* Nausea, vomiting, abdominal distension, diarrhea or constipation, flatus, colitis, dry mouth, "black tongue," pancreatitis, sialoadenitis. *Hematologic:* Hemolytic anemia, leukopenia, granulocytopenia, thrombocytopenia, bone marrow depression. *Endocrine:* Gynecomastia, amenorrhea, galactorrhea, lactation, hyperprolactinemia. *Miscellaneous:* Edema, jaundice, hepatitis, liver disorders, abnormal liver function tests, rash (eczema, lichenoid eruption), toxic epidermal necrolysis, fever, lupus-like symptoms, impotence, failure to ejaculate, decreased libido, nasal stuffiness, joint pain, myalgia, septic shock-like syndrome.

Drug Interactions

Anesthetics, general	Additive hypotension
Antidepressants, tricyclic	Tricyclic antidepressants may block hypotensive effect of methyldopa
Ephedrine	Action of ephedrine ↓ in methyldopa-treated patients
Fenfluramine	↑ Effect of methyldopa
Haloperidol	Methyldopa ↑ toxic effects of haloperidol
Levodopa	↑ Effect of both drugs
Lithium	↑ Possibility of lithium toxicity
Methotrimeprazine	Additive hypotensive effect
Monoamine oxidase inhibitors	May reverse hypotensive effect of methyldopa and cause headache and hallucinations
Norepinephrine	↑ Pressor response to norepinephrine
Phenoxybenzamine	Urinary incontinence
Phenylpropanolamine	↑ Pressor response to phenylpropanolamine
Propranolol	Paradoxical hypertension
Sympathomimetics	Potentiation of hypertensive effect of sympathomimetics
Thiazide diuretics	Additive hypotensive effect
Thioxanthines	Additive hypotensive effect
Tolbutamide	↑ Hypoglycemia due to ↓ breakdown by liver
Tricyclic antidepressants	↓ Effect of methyldopa
Vasodilator drugs	Additive hypotensive effect
Verapamil	↑ Effect of methyldopa

Laboratory Test Interferences: False + or ↑ : Alkaline phosphatase, bilirubin, BUN, BSP, cephalin flocculation, creatinine, SGOT, SGPT, uric acid, Coombs' test, prothrombin time. Positive lupus erythematosus (LE) cell preparation and antinuclear antibodies.

Dosage: *Methyldopa:* **Oral Suspension, Tablets. Initial:** 250 mg b.i.d.–t.i.d. for 2 days. Adjust dose every 2 days. If increased, start with evening dose. **Usual maintenance:** 0.5–3.0 g daily in 2–4 divided doses; **maximum:** 3 g daily. Transfer to and from other antihypertensive agents should occur gradually, with initial dose of methyldopa not exceeding 500 mg. *Note:* Do not use combination medication to initiate therapy. **Pediatric: initial,** 10 mg/kg daily in 2–4 divided doses, adjusting maintenance to a maximum of 65 mg/kg/day (or 3 g daily, whichever is less).

    Methyldopate HCl: **IV infusion, adults:** 250–500 mg q 6 hr; **maximum:** 1 g q 6 hr for *hypertensive crisis.* Switch to oral methyldopa, at same dosage level, when blood pressure is brought under control. **Pediatric:** 20–40 mg/kg daily in divided doses q 6 hr; **maximum:** 65 mg/kg/day (or 3 g daily, whichever is less).

NURSING CONSIDERATIONS

Administration/Storage

1. If the drug is to be administered by IV, methyldopate HCl should be mixed with 100 mL of 5% dextrose or administered in 5% dextrose in water at a concentration of 10 mg/mL.
2. The IV should be administered over a 30- to 60-min period.
3. Tolerance may occur following 2–3 months of therapy.
4. Increasing the dose or adding a diuretic often restores effect on blood pressure.

Interventions

1. Ascertain that hematological studies, liver function tests, and a Coombs' test are done before and during drug therapy.
2. If the client requires a blood transfusion, ascertain that both direct and indirect Coombs' tests are done. If the indirect and direct Coombs' tests are positive, anticipate consultation with a hematologist.
3. Weigh client daily and observe for evidence of edema.
4. Place client on strict intake and output, observe for reduced urine volume.
5. Assess for signs of drug tolerance. These may occur during the second or third month of drug therapy.
6. Note any evidence of jaundice. The drug is contraindicated when the client has hepatic disease.

Client/Family Teaching

1. Advise client to rise from bed slowly and dangle legs over the edge of the bed to prevent dizziness and fainting.
2. Sedation may occur when therapy is first started, but it disappears once the maintenance dose is established.
3. In rare cases, methyldopa may darken urine or turn it blue, but this reaction is not harmful.
4. Instruct client to withhold drug and report to the physician any of the following symptoms: tiredness, fever, or yellowing of skin and whites of eyes.
5. Advise client to always carry a card detailing current medication regimen.

IV. Peripherally Acting Drugs

GUANADREL SULFATE   (GWAHN-ah-drel)

Hylorel (Rx)

Classification: Antihypertensive, peripherally acting antiadrenergic.

Action/Kinetics: Similar to that of guanethidine. Inhibits vasoconstriction by blocking efferent, peripheral sympathetic pathways by depleting norepinephrine reserves and inhibiting norepinephrine release. Causes increased sensitivity to norepinephrine. **Onset:** 2 hr. **Peak plasma levels:** 1.5–2 hr. **Peak effect:** 4–6 hr. **t½:** Approximately 10 hr. **Duration:** 4–14 hr. Excreted through the urine as unchanged drug (40%) and metabolites.

Uses: Hypertension (usually Step 2 therapy).

Contraindications: Pheochromocytoma, congestive heart failure, within 1 week of monoamine oxidase drug use, within 2–3 days of elective surgery.

Special Concerns: Use with caution in bronchial asthma and peptic ulcer. Safety not established during pregnancy (category: B), lactation and in children. Geriatric patients may be more sensitive to the hypotensive effects.

Side Effects: *CNS:* Fainting, fatigue, headache, drowsiness, paresthesias, confusion, depression, sleep disorders, visual disturbances. *CV:* Exertional or resting shortness of breath, chest pain, orthostatic hypotension, palpitations, peripheral edema. *GI:* Increase in number of bowel movements, constipation, anorexia, indigestion, flatus, glossitis, nausea and vomiting, dry mouth and throat. *GU:* Difficulty in ejaculation, impotence, nocturia, hematuria, urinary urgency or frequency. *Miscellaneous:* Cough, leg cramps, changes in weight (gain or loss), backache, neckache, joint pain.

Drug Interactions

Beta-adrenergic blocking agents	Excessive hypotension, bradycardia
Ephedrine	Reverses effect of guanadrel
Norepinephrine	Guanadrel ↑ effect of norepinephrine
Phenothiazines	Reverses effect of guanadrel
Phenylpropanolamine	↓ Effect of guanadrel
Reserpine	Excessive hypotension, bradycardia
Tricyclic antidepressants	Reverses effect of guanadrel
Vasodilators	↑ Risk of orthostatic hypotension

Dosage: Tablets. Individualized. Initial: 5 mg b.i.d.; **then,** increase dosage to maintenance level of 20–75 mg/day in 2–4 divided doses.

NURSING CONSIDERATIONS

Administration/Storage

1. Tolerance may occur with long-term therapy, necessitating a dosage increase.
2. While adjusting dosage, both supine and standing blood pressure should be monitored.

Client/Family Teaching

1. Instruct clients how and when to take BP. Assist them to develop a method to maintain a written record for physician review.
2. Explain that weakness, dizziness, and fainting may occur with rapid changes of position from supine to standing. The client should be instructed to rise from bed slowly and dangle legs from the edge of the bed before standing.
3. Stress that nonprescription drugs should not be taken without consultation with their physician. Sympathomimetic amines in products used to treat asthma, colds, and allergies are to be used with extreme caution.
4. Warn clients that they may develop a dry mouth and become drowsy. Therefore, care should be taken not to perform any tasks that require mental alertness, such as driving a car.
5. Clients may develop diarrhea. If this is persistent the condition should be called to the physician's attention. The client could develop a severe electrolyte imbalance. This is particularly true with elderly clients.

GUANETHIDINE SULFATE   (gwah-NEH-thih-deen)

Apo-Guanethidine ✤, Ismelin Sulfate (Rx)

Classification: Antihypertensive, peripherally acting antiadrenergic.

Action/Kinetics: Guanethidine produces selective adrenergic blockade of efferent, peripheral sympathetic pathways by depleting norepinephrine reserve and inhibiting norepinephrine release. It induces a gradual, prolonged drop in both systolic and diastolic blood pressure, usually associated with bradycardia, decreased pulse pressure, a decrease in peripheral resistance, and small changes in cardiac output. The drug is not a ganglionic blocking agent and does not produce central or parasympathetic blockade. In patients with depleted catecholamines, guanethidine can directly depress the myocardium and can cause an increase in the sensitivity of tissues to catecholamines.

Incompletely and variably absorbed from the GI tract (3–30%) but is relatively constant for any given patient. **Peak effect:** 6–8 hr. **Duration:** 24–48 hr. **Maximum effect:** 1–3 weeks. **Duration:** 7–10 days after discontinuation. **t½:** approximately 5 days. From 25–50% excreted through the kidneys unchanged.

Uses: Moderate to severe hypertension—used alone or in combination. Renal hypertension.

Contraindications: Mild, labile hypertension; pheochromocytoma, CHF not due to hypertension, use of MAO inhibitors.

Special Concerns: Use during pregnancy (category: C) only when benefits clearly outweigh risks. Administer with caution and at a reduced rate to patients with impaired renal function, coronary disease, cardiovascular disease, especially when associated with encephalopathy, or to those who have suffered a recent myocardial infarction. During prolonged therapy, cardiac, renal, and blood tests should be performed. Used with caution in peptic ulcer. Geriatric patients may be more sensitive to the hypotensive effects of guanethidine; also, it may be necessary to decrease the dose in these patients due to age-related decreases in renal function.

Side Effects: *CNS:* Dizziness, weakness, lassitude. Rarely, dyspnea, fatigue, psychic depression. *CV:* Syncope due to exertional or postural hypotension, bradycardia, fluid retention and edema with possible congestive heart failure. Less commonly, angina. *GI:* Persistent diarrhea, increased frequency of bowel movements. Nausea, vomiting, dry mouth, and parotid tenderness are less common. *Miscellaneous:* Inhibition of ejaculation. Less commonly, dyspnea, nocturia, urinary incontinence, dermatitis, alopecia, increased blood urea nitrogen, drooping of upper eyelid, blurred vision, myalgia, muscle tremors, chest paresthesia, nasal congestion, asthma in susceptible individuals, weight gain, blurred vision, ptosis of the lids. Rarely, impotence, anemia, thrombocytopenia, priapism, impotence.

Drug Interactions

Alcohol, ethyl	Additive orthostatic hypotension
Amphetamines	↓ Effect of guanethidine by ↓ uptake of the drug to its site of action
Anesthetics, general	Additive hypotension
Antidepressants, tricyclic	↓ Effect of guanethidine by ↓ uptake of the drug to its site of action
Antidiabetic drugs	Additive effect ↓ in blood glucose
Cocaine	↓ Effect of guanethidine by ↓ uptake of the drug at its site of action
Digitalis	Additive slowing of heart rate
Ephedrine	↓ Effect of guanethidine by ↓ uptake of the drug at its site of action
Epinephrine	Guanethidine ↑ effect of epinephrine
Haloperidol	↓ Effect of guanethidine by ↓ uptake of the drug at its site of action
Levarterenol	See norepinephrine
Metaraminol	Guanethidine ↑ effect of metaraminol

Drug Interactions

Methotrimeprazine	Additive hypotensive effect
Methoxamine	Guanethidine ↑ effect of methoxamine
Minoxidil	Profound drop in blood pressure
Monoamine oxidase inhibitors	Reverse effect of guanethidine
Norepinephrine	↑ Effect of norepinephrine probably due to ↑ sensitivity of norepinephrine receptor and ↓ uptake of norepinephrine by the neuron
Oral contraceptives	↓ Effect of guanethidine by ↓ uptake of the drug to its site of action
Phenothiazines	↓ Effect of guanethidine by ↓ uptake of the drug to its site of action
Phenylephrine	↑ Response to phenylephrine in guanethidine-treated patients
Phenylpropanolamine	↓ Effect of guanethidine by ↓ uptake of the drug to its site of action
Procainamide	Additive hypotensive effect
Procarbazine	Additive hypotensive effect
Propranolol	Additive hypotensive effect
Pseudoephedrine	↓ Effect of guanethidine by ↓ uptake of the drug at its site of action
Quinidine	Additive hypotensive effect
Reserpine	Excessive bradycardia, postural hypotension, and mental depression
Thiazide diuretics	Additive hypotensive effect
Thioxanthines	↓ Effect of guanethidine by ↓ uptake of the drug at its site of action
Vasodilator drugs, peripheral	Additive hypotensive effect
Vasopressor drugs	↑ Effect of vasopressor agents probably due to ↑ sensitivity of norepinephrine receptor and ↓ uptake of vasopressor agent by the neuron

Laboratory Test Interference: ↑ BUN, SGOT, and SGPT. ↓ Prothrombin time, serum glucose, and urine catecholamines. Alteration of electrolyte balance.

Dosage: Tablets. *Ambulatory patients:* **initial:** 10–12.5 mg once daily; increase in 10–12.5 mg increments q 5–7 days; **maintenance:** 25–50 mg once daily. *Hospitalized patients:* **initial:** 25–50 mg; increase by 25 or 50 mg daily or every other day; **maintenance:** estimated to be approximately one-seventh of loading dose. **Pediatric, initial:** 0.2 mg/kg/day (6 mg/m^2) given in one dose; **then,** dose may be increased by 0.2 mg/kg/day q 7–10 days to maximum of 3 mg/kg/day.

NURSING CONSIDERATIONS

Administration/Storage

1. The loading dose for severe hypertension is given t.i.d. at 6-hr intervals with no nighttime dose.
2. Drug should be given daily or every other day.
3. Often used concomitantly with thiazide diuretics to reduce severity of sodium and water

retention caused by guanethidine. When used together, the dose of guanethidine should be reduced.

4. When control is achieved, dosage should be reduced to the minimal dose required to maintain lowest possible BP.

5. Guanethidine sulfate should be discontinued or dosage decreased at least 2 weeks before surgery.

Interventions

1. Prior to starting therapy, take the client's BP with the client standing and then in a supine position, unless contraindicated by the condition.

2. Ascertain that hepatic and renal function studies are completed before therapy is initiated.

3. Note the presence of bradycardia and report to the physician. An anticholinergic drug, such as atropine, may be indicated for severe bradycardia.

4. Note client complaints of persistent diarrhea. Severe electrolyte imbalance could occur. Document and report such incidents to the physician.

5. Weigh the client daily and record. Note any sudden increases in weight as this could indicate the presence of edema.

6. Monitor intake and output; observe for any reduction in urine volume.

7. Assess client for any undue stress, which could precipitate cardiovascular collapse. Assist to reduce such stress whenever possible.

8. Observe client closely for drug interactions. Since guanethidine interacts with many drugs the dosage may need to be adjusted.

Client/Family Teaching

1. Instruct client how to take BP and pulse and assist to develop a method to maintain a written record for review by health care provider.

2. Limit alcohol intake; otherwise, orthostatic hypotension may be further precipitated.

3. Rise slowly from bed by sitting on the edge of the bed with legs dangling for a few minutes before standing. This is especially important in the morning when the client should be assisted after lying flat all night, since hypotension may be more severe.

4. Lie down or sit down with head bent low, if feeling weak or dizzy.

5. Avoid any sudden or prolonged standing or exercise.

6. Report any nausea, vomiting or diarrhea.

PHENOXYBENZAMINE HYDROCHLORIDE   (fen-ox-ee-**BEN**-zah-meen)

Dibenzyline (Rx)

Classification: Antihypertensive, Adrenergic Blocking Agent. (See Chapter 45.)

PHENTOLAMINE MESYLATE   (fen-**TOE**-lah-meen **MESS**-ill-ayt)

Regitine Mesylate (Rx)

Classification: Antihypertensive, Adrenergic Blocking Agent. (See Chapter 45.)

PRAZOSIN HYDROCHLORIDE   (PRAY-zoh-sin)

Minipress (Rx)

Classification: Antihypertensive, alpha$_1$ adrenergic blocking agent.

Action/Kinetics: Produces selective blockade of postsynaptic alpha$_1$ adrenergic receptors. Dilates arterioles and veins, thereby decreasing total peripheral resistance and decreasing diastolic blood pressure more than systolic blood pressure. Cardiac output, heart rate, and renal blood flow are not affected. Can be used to initiate antihypertensive therapy and is most effective when used with other agents (e.g., diuretics, beta-adrenergic blocking agents). **Onset:** 2 hr. **Maximum effect:** 2–3 hr; **duration:** 6–12 hr. **t½:** 2–4 hr. Full therapeutic effect: 4–6 weeks. Metabolized extensively; excreted primarily in feces.

Uses: Mild to moderate hypertension. *Investigational:* Congestive heart failure refractory to other treatment. Raynaud's disease, ergot alkaloid toxicity, pheochromocytoma.

Special Concerns: Safe use during pregnancy (pregnancy category: C) and childhood has not been established. Use with caution during lactation. Geriatric patients may be more sensitive to the hypotensive and hypothermic effects of prazosin; also, it may be necessary to decrease the dose in these patients due to age-related decreases in renal function.

Side Effects: First-dose effect: Marked hypotension and syncope 30–90 minutes after administration of initial dose (usually 2 or more mg), increase of dosage, or addition of other antihypertensive agent. *CNS:* Dizziness, drowsiness, headache, fatigue, paresthesias, depression, vertigo, nervousness, hallucinations. *CV:* Palpitations, syncope, tachycardia, orthostatic hypotension, aggravation of angina. *GI:* Nausea, vomiting, diarrhea or constipation, dry mouth, abdominal pain, pancreatitis. *GU:* Urinary frequency or incontinence, impotence, priapism. *Miscellaneous:* Asthenia, sweating, symptoms of lupus erythematosus, blurred vision, tinnitus, epistaxis, nasal congestion, reddening of sclera, rash, alopecia, pruritus, dyspnea, edema, fever.

Drug Interactions	
Antihypertensives (other)	↑ Antihypertensive effect
Diuretics	↑ Antihypertensive effect
Indomethacin	↓ Effect of prazosin
Nifedipine	↑ Hypotensive effect
Propranolol	Especially pronounced additive hypotensive effect
Verapamil	↑ Hypotensive effect

Laboratory Test Interferences: ↑ Urinary metabolites of norepinephrine, VMA.

Dosage: Capsules/Tablets: *individualized,* always initiate with 0.5–1 mg b.i.d.–t.i.d.; **maintenance:** if necessary, increase gradually to 6–15 mg daily in 2–3 divided doses. Daily dose should not exceed 20 mg. If used with diuretics or other antihypertensives, reduce dose to 1–2 mg t.i.d. **Pediatric, less than 7 years of age, initial:** 0.25 mg b.i.d.–t.i.d. adjusted according to response. **Pediatric, 7–12 years of age, initial:** 0.5 mg b.i.d.–t.i.d. adjusted according to response.

NURSING CONSIDERATIONS

Administration/Storage

1. The first dose should be taken at bedtime.
2. Due to the first-dose effect, clients should not drive or operate machinery for 24 hr after the first dose.

3. In the event of overdosage, treat for shock with plasma volume expanders and vasopressor drugs as necessary.

Client/Family Teaching

1. Instruct client how to take own BP and assist to develop a method to maintain a written record for review by the physician.
2. Food may delay absorption and minimize side effects of the drug.
3. Comply with drug regimen, since full effect of drug may not be evident for 4–6 weeks.
4. Report any bothersome side effects because reduction in dosage may be indicated.
5. Do not discontinue medication unless directed by medical supervision.
6. Avoid cold, cough, and allergy medications, unless physician approves. The sympathomimetic component of such medications will interfere with the action of prazosin.
7. Do not engage in activities requiring alertness such as operating machinery or driving a car, until drug effects are determined. The drug may cause dizziness and drowsiness.
8. Avoid rapid postural changes that may precipitate weakness, dizziness, and syncope.
9. Lie down or sit down and put head below knees to avoid fainting if a rapid heartbeat is felt.
10. Avoid dangerous situations that may lead to fainting.

TERAZOSIN   (teh-**RAY**-zoh-sin)

Hytrin (Rx)

Classification: Antihypertensive, alpha$_1$-adrenergic receptor blocking agent.

Action/Kinetics: Terazosin blocks postsynaptic alpha$_1$-adrenergic receptors, leading to a dilation of both arterioles and veins, and ultimately, a reduction in blood pressure. Both standing and supine blood pressure are lowered with no reflex tachycardia. Bioavailability is not affected by food. **Onset:** 15 min. **Peak plasma levels:** 1–2 hr. **t½:** 9–12 hr. **Duration:** 24 hr. Terazosin is excreted as unchanged drug and inactive metabolites in both the urine and feces.

Uses: Alone or in combination with diuretics or beta-adrenergic blocking agents to treat hypertension.

Special Concerns: Pregnancy category: C. Use with caution during lactation. Safety and efficacy have not been determined in children. Geriatric patients may be more sensitive to the hypotensive and hypothermic effects of terazosin.

Side Effects: *First-dose effect:* Marked postural hypotension and syncope. *CV:* Palpitations, tachycardia, postural hypotension, syncope, arrhythmias, vasodilation. *CNS:* Dizziness, headache, somnolence, nervousness, paresthesia, depression, anxiety, insomnia. *Respiratory:* Nasal congestion, dyspnea, sinusitis, epistaxis, bronchitis, cough, pharyngitis, rhinitis. *GI:* Nausea, constipation, diarrhea, dyspepsia, dry mouth, vomiting, flatulence. *Musculoskeletal:* Asthenia, arthritis, arthralgia, myalgia, joint disorders, back pain, pain in extremities, neck and shoulder pain. *Miscellaneous:* Peripheral edema, weight gain, blurred vision, impotence, chest pain, fever, gout, pruritus, rash, sweating, urinary frequency, tinnitus, conjunctivitis, abnormal vision.

Laboratory Test Interferences: ↓ Hematocrit, hemoglobin, white blood cells, albumin.

Dosage: Tablets. Individualized, initial: 1 mg at bedtime (this dose is not to be exceeded); **then,** increase dose slowly to obtain desired response. **Range:** 1–5 mg daily; doses as high as 20 mg may be required in some patients.

NURSING CONSIDERATIONS

Administration/Storage

1. The initial dosing regimen must be carefully observed to minimize severe hypotension.
2. Monitor blood pressure 2–3 hr after dosing as well as at the end of the dosing interval, to ensure blood pressure control has been maintained.
3. An increase in dose or b.i.d. dosing should be considered if blood pressure control is not maintained at 24 hr interval.
4. After the initial dose, the daily dose can be given in the morning.
5. If terazosin must be discontinued for more than a few days, the initial dosing regimen should be used if therapy is reinstituted.
6. Due to additive effects, caution must be exercised when terazosin is combined with other antihypertensive agents.

Client/Family Teaching

1. Instruct client how to take BP and pulse and assist to develop a method to maintain a written record for review by the health care provider.
2. Advise client to use caution when performing activities that require mental alertness until drug effects are realized.
3. Instruct not to drive or undertake hazardous tasks for 12 hr after the first dose, and after increasing the dose or reinstituting therapy following an interruption of dosage.
4. Advise to take medication at bedtime to minimize side effects.
5. Instruct how to avoid symptoms of orthostatic hypotension associated with medication, (i.e., rise slowly from sitting or lying position and wait until symptoms subside).
6. Do not interrupt therapy without physician approval.
7. Report any persistent side effects so dosage may be evaluated and adjusted accordingly.

V. Miscellaneous Agents

LABETALOL HYDROCHLORIDE   (lah-**BAY**-toe-lohl)

Normodyne, Trandate (Rx)

Classification: Alpha- and beta-adrenergic blocking agent.

Action/Kinetics: Labetalol decreases blood pressure by blocking both alpha- and beta-adrenergic receptors. Significant reflex tachycardia and bradycardia do not occur although AV conduction may be prolonged. **Onset: PO,** 2–4 hr; **IV,** 5 min. **Peak plasma levels, PO:** 1–2 hr. **Duration: PO,** 8–12 hr. $t\frac{1}{2}$: **PO,** 6–8 hr; **IV,** 5.5 hr. Significant first-pass effect; metabolized in liver. Food increases bioavailability of the drug.

Uses: PO: Alone or in combination with other drugs for hypertension. **IV:** Hypertensive emergencies. *Investigational:* Pheochromocytoma, clonidine withdrawal hypertension.

Contraindications: Cardiogenic shock, cardiac failure, bronchial asthma, bradycardia, greater than first degree heart block.

Special Concerns: Use with caution during pregnancy (pregnancy category: C) and lactation, in impaired renal and hepatic function, and diabetes (may prevent premonitory signs of acute hypoglycemia). Safety and efficacy in children have not been established.

Side Effects: *CV:* Postural hypotension, edema, flushing, ventricular arrhythmias, intensification of AV block. *GI:* Nausea, vomiting, diarrhea, altered taste, dyspepsia. *CNS:* Headache, drowsiness, fatigue, sleepiness, dizziness, vertigo, paresthesias, numbness. *GU:* Impotence, urinary bladder retention, difficulty in urination, failure to ejaculate, priapism, Peyronie's disease. *Dermatologic:* Rashes, facial erythema, alopecia, urticaria, pruritus, psoriasis-like syndrome, bullous lichen planus. *Respiratory:* Bronchospasm, dyspnea, wheezing. *Musculoskeletal:* Muscle cramps, asthenia, toxic myopathy. *Other:* Systemic lupus erythematosus, jaundice, cholestasis, difficulties with vision, dry eyes, nasal stuffiness, tingling of skin or scalp, sweating, fever.

There may be changes in laboratory values including increased serum transaminase, positive antinuclear factor, antimitochondrial antibodies, and increases in blood urea and creatinine.

Drug Interactions	
Beta-adrenergic bronchodilators	Labetalol ↓ bronchodilator effect of these drugs
Cimetidine	↑ Bioavailability of oral labetalol
Glutethimide	↓ Effects of labetalol due to ↑ breakdown by liver
Halothane	↑ Risk of severe myocardial depression → hypotension
Nitroglycerin	Additive hypotension
Tricyclic antidepressants	↑ Risk of tremors

Laboratory Test Interference: False + increase in urinary catecholamines.

Dosage: Tablets. Initial: 100 mg b.i.d. alone or with a diuretic; **maintenance:** 200–400 mg b.i.d. up to 1,200–2,400 mg daily for severe cases. **IV. Individualize. Initial:** 20 mg slowly over 2 min; **then,** 40–80 mg q 10 min until desired effect occurs or a total of 300 mg has been given. **IV infusion. Initial:** 2 mg/min; **then,** adjust rate according to response. **Usual dose range:** 50–300 mg. *Transfer from IV to PO therapy:* **initial,** 200 mg; **then,** 200–400 mg 6–12 hr later, depending on response. Thereafter, dosage based on response.

NURSING CONSIDERATIONS
See also *Nursing Considerations* for *Beta-Adrenergic Blocking Agents,* p. 485.

Administration/Storage
1. When transferring to PO labetalol from other antihypertensive therapy, slowly reduce dosage of current therapy.
2. To transfer from IV to PO therapy in hospitalized clients, begin when supine blood pressure begins to increase.
3. Labetalol is not compatible with 5% sodium bicarbonate injection.
4. The full antihypertensive effect of labetalol is usually seen within the first 1–3 hr after the initial dose or dose increment.

5. When given by IV infusion, labetalol should be administered using an infusion pump, a micro-drip regulator, or similar devices in order to allow precise control of flow rate.

Interventions

1. The effect of labetalol on standing blood pressure should be assessed before the client is discharged from the hospital. Perform measurements with the client standing at several different times during the day to determine full effects of the drug.

2. To reduce the chance of orthostatic hypotension, clients should remain supine for 3 hr after receiving parenteral labetalol.

METYROSINE   (meh-TIE-roh-seen)

Demser (Rx)

Classification: Tyrosine hydroxylase inhibitor.

Action/Kinetics: By inhibiting the enzyme tyrosine hydroxylase, which is the rate-limiting step in the biosynthesis of catecholamines, there is a decrease in both norepinephrine and epinephrine synthesis. **Peak effect:** over 6 hr. **Duration:** 2–3 days. Well absorbed from the GI tract. Approximately 70% is excreted in the urine as unchanged drug. **t½:** Approximately 3.5 hr.

Use: Pheochromocytoma (preoperatively or for chronic therapy). Not used in the treatment of essential hypertension.

Contraindications: Hypersensitivity to drug.

Special Concerns: Safe use during pregnancy (pregnancy category: C), lactation, and children under 12 years of age not established. A decrease in dose may be necessary in geriatric patients due to age-related decreases in renal function.

Side Effects: *CNS:* Sedation (100%), which decreases with usage; alteration in sleep patterns; insomnia and psychic stimulation upon drug removal; headache; extrapyramidal symptoms (drooling, speech difficulties, tremors); anxiety, depression, hallucinations, disorientation, confusion, headaches. *GI:* Diarrhea (10%), nausea, vomiting, abdominal pain, decreased salivation, dry mouth. *Other:* Galactorrhea, crystalluria, hematuria, transient dysuria, nasal stuffiness, impotence, swollen breasts. *Rarely:* Eosinophilia, peripheral edema, hypersensitivity reactions, thrombocytopenia, anemia, thrombocytosis. During anesthesia and surgery, life-threatening arrhythmias may result. These may be treated with lidocaine or a beta-adrenergic blocking agent.

Drug Interactions	
Alcohol	Additive CNS depression
Alpha-adrenergic blocking agents	Hypotension; ↓ perfusion of agents
CNS depressants	Additive CNS depression
Haloperidol	↑ Extrapyramidal side effects
Phenothiazines	↑ Extrapyramidal side effects

Laboratory Test Interferences: ↑ SGOT and urinary catecholamine levels.

Dosage: Capsules. Adults and children over 12 yr: Initial, 250 mg q.i.d.; **then,** increase by 250–500 mg every day to maximum of 4 g/day in divided doses. Usual optimum dosage: 2–3 g/day. Dose must be individually determined by BP response and control of clinical symptoms. Phenoxybenzamine may be added if adequate control not achieved.

NURSING CONSIDERATIONS

Client/Family Teaching

1. Stress that adequate fluid intake is essential to prevent low BP, crystalluria, and poor circulation to vital organs.
2. Do not drive a car or operate hazardous machinery, because drowsiness may occur within the first 24 hr of therapy. Explain to client that sedative effects usually stop after 1 week unless dosage is 2 g or more per day.
3. Avoid alcohol and any other unprescribed drugs during therapy.
4. Review symptoms noted under *Side Effects* and instruct client to report any evidence of these to the physician.
5. Stress the importance of reporting for follow-up visits and laboratory studies, as scheduled.

MINOXIDIL, ORAL (mih-NOX-ih-dil)

Loniten, Minodyl (Rx)

Classification: Antihypertensive, depresses sympathetic nervous system.

Action/Kinetics: Decreases elevated BP by decreasing peripheral resistance. Drug causes increase in renin secretion, increase in cardiac rate and output, and salt/water retention. It does not cause orthostatic hypotension. **Onset:** 30 min. **Peak plasma levels:** reached within 60 min; **plasma t½:** 4.2 hr. **Duration:** 24–48 hr. Ninety percent absorbed from GI tract; excretion: renal (90% metabolites). The time needed to reach the maximum effect is inversely related to the dose.

Minoxidil can produce severe side effects; it should be reserved for resistant cases of hypertension. Use generally requires concomitant administration of beta-adrenergic blocking agents and diuretics. Close medical supervision required, including possible hospitalization during initial administration.

Use: Hypertension not controllable by the use of a diuretic plus two other antihypertensive drugs. Usually taken with at least two other antihypertensive drugs (a diuretic and a drug to minimize tachycardia such as a beta-adrenergic blocking agent). Topically to promote hair growth in balding men (see p. 483).

Contraindications: Pheochromocytoma. Within 1 month after a myocardial infarction.

Special Concerns: Safe use during pregnancy (pregnancy category: C) and lactation not established. Use with caution and at reduced dosage in impaired renal function. Geriatric patients may be more sensitive to the hypotensive and hypothermic effects of minoxidil; also, it may be necessary to decrease the dose in these patients due to age-related decreases in renal function.

Side Effects: *CV:* Edema, pericardial effusion, tamponade (acute compression of heart caused by fluid or blood in pericardium), CHF, angina pectoris, increased heart rate. *GI:* Nausea, vomiting. *CNS:* Headache, fatigue. *Other:* Hypertrichosis (enhanced hair growth, pigmentation and thickening of fine body hair 3–6 weeks after initiation of therapy), skin rashes (hypersensitivity), breast tenderness.

Drug Interactions: Concomitant use with guanethidine may result in severe hypotension.

Laboratory Test Interferences: Nonspecific changes in ECG. ↓ Hematocrit, erythrocyte count, and hemoglobin. ↑ Alkaline phosphatase, serum creatinine, and BUN.

Dosage: Tablets. Adults and children over 12 years: Initial, 5 mg once daily. For optimum control, dose can be increased to 10, 20, and then 40 mg in single or divided doses/day. Daily dosage should not exceed 100 mg. **Children under 12 years: Initial,** 0.2 mg/kg once daily. Effective dose range: 0.25–1.0 mg/kg/day. Dosage must be titrated to individual response. Daily dosage should not exceed 50 mg.

NURSING CONSIDERATIONS

Administration/Storage

Can be taken with fluids and without regard to meals.

Interventions

1. Anticipate that minoxidil therapy will be initiated in the hospital. After medication administration, BP decreases within 30 min and the client reaches minimum BP within 2–3 hr.
2. Monitor vital signs and intake and output.
3. Weigh client daily and examine for evidence of edema.
4. Observe for and report tachycardia or evidence of respiratory dysfunction.
5. Anticipate that clients receiving guanethidine concomitantly may experience severe hypotensive effects that may be precipitated by drug interaction.

Client/Family Teaching

1. Review the technique for monitoring pulse and BP. Assist the client to develop and maintain a written record and instruct him to report any abnormal reading to the physician.
2. Record weight daily and report any weight gain of over 5 lb within 3 days, as well as edema of extremities, face, and abdomen.
3. Report any dyspnea that occurs when lying down.
4. Report angina, dizziness, or fainting.
5. Explain that the medication may cause elongation, thickening, and increased pigmentation of body hair, but that there is a return to pretreatment norm when drug is discontinued.
6. Use drug only in the dose and form prescribed.

AGENTS THAT ACT DIRECTLY ON VASCULAR SMOOTH MUSCLE

DIAZOXIDE   (dye-ah-**ZOX**-yd)

Hyperstat IV (Rx)

Classification: Antihypertensive, direct action on vascular smooth muscle.

Action/Kinetics: Diazoxide is thought to exert a direct action on vascular smooth muscle to cause arteriolar vasodilation and decreased peripheral resistance. **Onset:** 1–5 min. **Time to peak effect:** 2–5 min. **Duration** (variable): usual, 3–12 hr. Excreted through the kidney (50% unchanged).

Uses: May be the drug of choice for hypertensive crisis (malignant and nonmalignant hypertension). Often given concomitantly with a diuretic. Especially suitable for patients with impaired renal function, hypertensive encephalopathy, hypertension complicated by left ventricular failure, and eclampsia. Ineffective for hypertension due to pheochromocytoma.

Contraindications: Hypersensitivity to drug or thiazide diuretics.

Special Concerns: Pregnancy category: C. A decrease in dose may be necessary in geriatric patients due to age-related decreases in renal function.

Side Effects: *CV:* Hypotension (may be severe), sodium and water retention, arrhythmias, cerebral or myocardial ischemia, palpitations, bradycardia. *CNS:* Headache, dizziness, drowsiness, light-headedness. Confusion, seizures, paralysis, unconsciousness, numbness (all due to cerebral ischemia). *Respiratory:* Tightness in chest, cough, dyspnea, sensation of choking. *GI:* Nausea, vomiting, diarrhea, anorexia, parotid swelling, change in sense of taste, salivation, dry mouth, ileus, constipation. *Other:* Hyperglycemia (may be serious enough to require treatment), sweating, flushing, sensation of warmth, tinnitus, hearing loss, retention of nitrogenous wastes, acute pancreatitis. Pain, cellulitis, phlebitis at injection site.

Drug Interactions	
Anticoagulants, oral	↑ Effect of oral anticoagulants due to ↓ plasma protein binding
Nitrites	↑ Hypotensive effect
Phenytoin	Diazoxide ↓ anticonvulsant effect of phenytoin
Reserpine	↑ Hypotensive effect
Thiazide diuretics	↑ Hyperglycemic, hyperuricemic, and anti-hypertensive effect of diazoxide
Vasodilators, peripheral	↑ Hypotensive effect

Laboratory Test Interference: False + or ↑ uric acid.

Dosage: IV push (30 sec or less): **Adults:** 1–3 mg/kg up to a maximum of 150 mg; may be repeated at 5- to 15-min intervals until adequate blood pressure response obtained. Drug may then be repeated at 4- to 24-hr intervals for 4–5 days or until oral antihypertensive therapy can be initiated. **Pediatric:** 1–3 mg/kg (30–90 mg/m²) using the same dosing intervals as adults.

NURSING CONSIDERATIONS

Administration/Storage

1. Do not administer IM or SC. Medication is highly alkaline.
2. Inject rapidly (30 sec) undiluted into a peripheral vein to maximize response.
3. Protect from light, heat, and freezing.

Assessment

1. Note client history for hypersensitivity to thiazide diuretics or to diazoxide.
2. Particularly note if client has diabetes mellitus. Diazoxide can cause serious elevations in blood sugar levels.

Interventions

1. Inspect the IV line to ensure patency before administering the medication.
2. Have a sympathomimetic drug, such as norepinephrine, available to treat severe hypotension should it occur.

3. Explain to client the need to remain in a recumbent position during and for 30 min after injection.

4. Maintain the client in a recumbent position for 8 to 10 hr if furosemide is administered as part of the therapy.

5. Monitor BP after injection until it has stabilized and then every hour thereafter until hypertensive crisis is resolved.

6. Obtain final BP of client upon arising after injection.

7. Note client complaints of sweating, flushing, or evidence of hyperglycemia and be prepared to treat.

8. Assess the site of insertion for signs of irritation or extravasation. If extravasation should occur, apply ice packs.

Evaluation

1. Take BP after the final injection to determine effectiveness of therapy.

2. Note evidence of hyperuricemia and report to physician.

HYDRALAZINE HYDROCHLORIDE   (hy-DRAH-lah-zeen)

Apresoline, Novo-Hylazin✣ (Rx)

Classification: Antihypertensive, direct action on vascular smooth muscle.

Action/Kinetics: Exerts a direct vasodilating effect on vascular smooth muscle. It also increases blood flow to the kidneys and brain and increases cardiac output by a reflex action. To minimize the cardiac effects, hydralazine is often given with drugs which decrease activity of sympathetic nerves. For example, it is found in Apresazide and Ser-Ap-Es. Food increases bioavailability of the drug. **PO: Onset,** 45 min; **peak plasma level:** 2 hr; **duration:** 3–8 hr. **t½:** 3–7 hr. **IM: Onset,** 10–30 min; **peak plasma level:** 1 hr; **duration:** 2–6 hr. **IV: Onset,** 10–20 min; **maximum effect:** 10–80 min; **duration:** 2–6 hr. Metabolized in the liver and excreted through the kidney (2–5% unchanged after PO use and 11–14% unchanged after IV administration).

Uses: *PO:* In combination with other drugs for essential hypertension. *Parenteral:* Hypertensive emergencies. *Investigational:* To reduce afterload in congestive heart failure, severe aortic insufficiency after valve replacement.

Contraindications: Coronary artery disease, angina pectoris, advanced renal disease (as in chronic renal hypertension), rheumatic heart disease (e.g., mitral valvular) and chronic glomerulonephritis.

Special Concerns: Pregnancy category: C. Use with caution in stroke patients. Use with caution during lactation, in patients with advanced renal disease, and in patients with tartrazine sensitivity. Safety and efficacy have not been established in children. Geriatric patients may be more sensitive to the hypotensive and hypothermic effects of hydralazine; also, a decrease in dose may be necessary in these patients due to age-related decreases in renal function.

Side Effects: *CV:* Orthostatic hypotension, myocardial infarction, angina pectoris, palpitations, tachycardia. *CNS:* Headache, dizziness, psychoses, tremors, depression, anxiety, disorientation. *GI:* Nausea, vomiting, diarrhea, anorexia, constipation, paralytic ileus. *Allergic:* Rash, urticaria, fever, chills, arthralgia, pruritus, eosinophilia. Rarely, hepatitis, obstructive jaundice. *Hematologic:* Decrease in hemoglobin and red blood cells, purpura, agranulocytosis, leukopenia. *Other:* Peripheral neuritis, impotence, nasal congestion, edema, muscle cramps, lacrimation, conjunctivitis, difficulty in urination, lupus-like syndrome, lymphadenopathy, splenomegaly. Side effects are less severe when dosage is increased slowly.

Drug Interactions

Beta-Adrenergic blocking agents	↑ Effect of both drugs
Methotrimeprazine	Additive hypotensive effect
Procainamide	Additive hypotensive effect
Quinidine	Additive hypotensive effect
Sympathomimetics	↑ Risk of tachycardia and angina

Dosage: Tablets. Adult, initial: 10 mg q.i.d for 2–4 days; **then,** increase to 25 mg q.i.d. for rest of first week. For second and following weeks, increase to 50 mg q.i.d. **Maintenance:** individualized to lowest effective dose; maximum daily dose should not exceed 300 mg. **Pediatric, initial:** 0.75 mg/kg/day (25 mg/m²/day) in 2–4 divided doses; dosage may be increased gradually up to 7.5 mg/kg/day (or 300 mg daily). Food increases the bioavailability of the drug.

IV, IM. *Hypertensive crisis:* **adults, usual:** 20–40 mg, repeated as necessary. Blood pressure may fall within 5–10 min, with maximum response in 10–80 min. Usually switch to PO medication in 1–2 days. Dosage should be decreased in patients with renal damage. **Pediatric:** 1.7–3.5 mg/kg/day (50–100 mg/m²/day) divided into 4–6 divided doses.

NURSING CONSIDERATIONS

Administration/Storage

1. Parenteral injections should be made as quickly as possible after being drawn into the syringe.
2. To enhance bioavailability, the tablets should be taken with food.
3. The presence of a metal filter will cause a change in color of hydralazine.

Assessment

1. Note any drug history of hypersensitivity to the drug.
2. Document other drugs the client may be taking that would interact with hydralazine.

Interventions

1. Weigh the client before initiating the drug therapy and daily thereafter. Record the weights and compare them, observe for any evidence of edema.
2. Place the client on intake and output. Note especially any reduction in urine output.
3. If the client is to receive the drug by parenteral injection, take the BP within 5 min and p.r.n. following the injection.
4. Monitor serum electrolytes.
5. The BP should be taken several times a day under standardized conditions, either sitting or standing, as ordered by the physician.
6. Anticipate that client's cardiac condition may require monitoring during drug therapy.

Client/Family Teaching

1. Instruct client how to take BP and assist to develop a method to maintain a written record for physician review.
2. Take oral prescribed drugs with meals to avoid gastric irritation.
3. Explain the possible side effects of the drug which the client may experience after taking the first dose. These may include headaches, palpitations, and possibly mild postural hypotension which may persist for 7–10 days with continued treatment.

4. If the client feels weak or dizzy, lie down or sit down with the head lowered.

5. Remind to change slowly from a supine to a sitting position.

6. Take weight daily and record. Also note if there is evidence of edema such as increased tightness of rings or clothing. These signs should be reported to the physician.

7. Advise clients to report tingling sensations or discomfort in the hands or feet. These generally are signs of peripheral neuropathies and need to be reported. The problem may be reversed with the use of other drugs, usually pyridoxine.

8. Avoid the use of alcohol or other drugs that could also lower blood pressure.

9. Do not take any OTC drugs without first discussing with the physician.

Evaluation

1. Assess client/family knowledge and understanding of illness, response to therapy and to teaching.

2. Note the development of arthralgia, dermatoses, fever, anemia or splenomegaly. These may require discontinuation of drug therapy.

3. Evaluate for the development of a rheumatoid-like or influenza-like syndrome which would necessitate discontinuing hydralazine therapy.

NITROPRUSSIDE SODIUM   (nye-troh-**PRUS**-zyd)

Nipride, Nitropress (Rx)

Classification: Antihypertensive, direct action on vascular smooth muscle.

Action/Kinetics: Direct action on vascular smooth muscle, leading to peripheral vasodilation. The drug acts on excitation-contraction coupling of vascular smooth muscle by interfering with both influx and intracellular activation of calcium. Nitroprusside has no effect on smooth muscle of the duodenum or uterus. The drug may also improve congestive heart failure by decreasing systemic resistance, preload and afterload reduction, and improved cardiac output. **Onset** (drug must be given by IV infusion): 0.5–1 min; **peak effect:** 1–2 min; **duration:** Up to 10 min after infusion stopped. Nitroprusside is converted to thiocyanate in the liver and is slowly excreted over several days.

Uses: Hypertensive crisis to reduce BP immediately. To produce controlled hypotension during anesthesia to reduce bleeding. *Investigational:* Severe refractory congestive heart failure (may be combined with dopamine); in combination with dopamine for acute myocardial infarction; adjunct in treatment of valvular regurgitation; peripheral vasospasm due to ergot alkaloid overdosage.

Contraindications: Compensatory hypertension. Use to produce controlled hypotension during surgery in patients with known inadequate cerebral circulation.

Special Concerns: Use with caution in hypothyroidism, liver or kidney impairment, during pregnancy (pregnancy category: C) and lactation. Geriatric patients may be more sensitive to the hypotensive effects of nitroprusside; also, a decrease in dose may be necessary in these patients due to age-related decreases in renal function.

Side Effects: Large doses may lead to cyanide toxicity. *Following rapid injection:* Dizziness, nausea, restlessness, headache, sweating, muscle twitching, palpitations, abdominal pain, apprehension, retching, retrosternal discomfort. *Other symptoms:* Bradycardia, tachycardia, increased intracranial pressure, ECG changes, venous streaking, rash, methemoglobinemia, decreased platelet count, flushing. *Symptoms of thiocyanate toxicity:* Blurred vision, tinnitus, confusion, hyperreflexia, seizures. *CNS symptoms (transitory):* restlessness, agitation, and muscle twitching. Vomiting or skin rash.

Drug Interaction: Concomitant use of other antihypertensives, volatile liquid anesthetics, or certain depressants ↑ response to nitroprusside.

Dosage: IV infusion only. Adults: average, 3 mcg/kg/min. **Range:** 0.5–10 mcg/kg/min. Smaller dose is required for patients receiving other antihypertensives. **Pediatric:** 1.4 mcg/kg/min adjusted slowly depending on the response.

Monitor BP and use as guide to regulate rate of administration so as to maintain desired antihypertensive effect. Rate of administration should not exceed 10 mcg/kg/min.

NURSING CONSIDERATIONS

Administration/Storage

1. Protect drug from heat, light, and moisture.
2. Protect dilute solutions during administration by wrapping flask with opaque material, such as aluminum foil.
3. The contents of the vial (50 mg) should be dissolved in 2–3 mL of 5% dextrose in water. This stock solution is then diluted in 250–1,000 mL 5% dextrose in water.
4. If properly protected from light, the reconstituted solution is stable for 24 hr.
5. Discard solutions that are any color but light brown.
6. Do not add any other drug or preservative to solution.

Interventions

1. Administer IV solution with an electronic infusion device in a monitored environment.
2. Obtain written parameters for BP and monitor closely throughout drug therapy. Titrate infusion accordingly.
3. Observe for symptoms of thiocyanate toxicity listed under side effects. Evaluate laboratory values for thiocyanate levels generally every other day during therapy.
4. Cover IV bag and tubing with aluminum foil or foil-lined bags and change setup every 24 hours, unless otherwise indicated. Explain to client that covering the IV bag protects the medication from light and maintains drug stability.

GANGLIONIC BLOCKING AGENTS

Action/Kinetics: These drugs block transmission of nerve impulses at the ganglia of the autonomic nervous system. This action results in inhibition of nerve impulses, including those that constrict the vascular walls, thereby causing a reduction in blood pressure. Baroreceptor reflexes are also blocked, thus preventing an increase in heart rate due to the decreased blood pressure.

These drugs are of limited value in long-term management of chronic hypertension due to side effects including orthostatic hypotension, adynamic ileus, and urinary retention.

Side Effects: Most untoward reactions are related to the blocking of parasympathetic and sympathetic nervous systems because the drugs block ganglia to all organs of the body—not just to the blood vessels. As with other powerful drugs that cause a major alteration of physiologic processes, it is often difficult to decide when an untoward reaction becomes excessive.

CV: Postural hypotension, interstitial pulmonary edema, and fibrosis. *GI:* Anorexia, diarrhea followed by constipation, paralytic ileus, dry mouth, nausea, vomiting, glossitis. *CNS:* Weakness, fatigue, dizziness, syncope, sedation. Rarely, seizures, chorieform movements, tremors, and mental disturbances especially with high doses. *GU:* Urinary retention, impotence, decreased libido. *Other:* Paresthesias.

Patients on low-sodium diets or those who have had sympathectomy and hypertensive encephalopathy are particularly sensitive to the ganglionic blocking agents.

Drug Interactions	
Alcohol	↑ Hypotensive effect
Antihypertensive drugs	Additive hypotensive effects
General anesthetics	Additive hypotensive effects
Thiazide diuretics	Additive hypotensive effects; concomitant use permits reduction of dosage of ganglionic blocking agents to about one-half

Dosage: Highly individualized. (See individual drug entries.) The required amount of drug depends on the time of day (higher doses are generally required at night), on the season (lower doses are required in warm weather), and on the position of the patient (higher doses are required for an ambulatory patient than for one confined to bed).

It is important always to measure blood pressure in patients taking ganglionic blocking agents in the standing position or as the physician orders.

NURSING CONSIDERATIONS

Interventions

1. Take BP and pulse at the specific times ordered.
2. Make sure that the client is in positions ordered for all readings, whether sitting or standing. If this is not possible, alterations in time and position should be indicated on the client's record.
3. Weigh the client daily and check for edema to determine if any weight gain is the result of retained fluid or due to increased appetite.
4. Measure intake and output to detect evidence of oliguria, a result of excessive hypotension.
5. Note client complaint of constipation. Check with the physician regarding orders for laxatives, which can be administered if the client fails to have regular bowel movements. If constipation persists, the drug must be discontinued, bulk-producing cathartics are ineffective.
6. Note evidence of additive hypotensive effects if any other hypotensive agents or diuretics are concomitantly administered. Adjustment in the dosage of drug may be required.

Client/Family Teaching

1. Instruct client how to take BP and pulse and assist to develop a method to maintain a written record for review by health care provider.
2. Advise the client that orthostatic hypotension may occur. This is manifested by weakness,

dizziness, and fainting. Since these symptoms occur when arising rapidly from a supine position, advise clients to rise slowly. First to a sitting position, dangling the legs for a few minutes, then when feeling stable, stand up. If this is a persistent problem have a family member present to assist.

3. Allow more time to prepare for the day's activities than usual to permit the body time to adjust to changes of position.

4. If weak, dizzy, or faint after standing or exercising for a long time, lie down if possible or otherwise sit down and lower head between knees.

5. Encourage the client to eat a diet high in fiber and provide a list of food and fluids that will help to avoid constipation.

MECAMYLAMINE HYDROCHLORIDE (meh-kah-**MILL**-ah-meen)

Inversine (Rx)

Classification: Ganglionic blocking agent, antihypertensive.

Action/Kinetics: The drug is less apt than other ganglionic blocking agents to induce tolerance. Withdraw or substitute mecamylamine slowly since sudden withdrawal or switching to other antihypertensive agents may result in severe hypertensive rebound. Since mecamylamine reduces peristalsis, it is a useful addition to a thiazide-guanethidine regimen in patients who experience persistent diarrhea with guanethidine.

Onset (gradual): 1/2–2 hr. **Duration:** 6–12 hr. May take 2–3 days to achieve full therapeutic potential. Mecamylamine is excreted unchanged by the kidneys. The rate of excretion is influenced by urinary pH in that alkalinization of the urine decreases (and acidification increases), renal excretion.

Uses: Moderate to severe hypertension including uncomplicated malignant hypertension.

Contraindications: Mild, moderate, labile hypertension; coronary insufficiency, patients with recent myocardial infarction, uremia, patients being treated with antibiotics and sulfonamides, glaucoma, pyloric stenosis, uncooperative patients.

Special Concerns: Pregnancy category: C. Safe use during lactation has not been established. Dosage has not been established in children. Geriatric patients may be more sensitive to the hypotensive effects of mecamylamine; also, a decrease in dose may be required in these patients due to age-related decreases in renal function. Use with caution in marked cerebral and coronary arteriosclerosis, after recent cerebral vascular accident, prostatic hypertrophy, urethral stricture, bladder neck obstruction. Abdominal distention, decreased bowel signs, and other symptoms of adynamic ileus are reasons for discontinuing the drug.

Dosage: Tablets. Adults: **initial,** 2.5 mg b.i.d. Increase by increments of 2.5 mg every 2 or more days; **maintenance:** 25 mg daily in 3 divided doses.

NURSING CONSIDERATIONS

See *Nursing Considerations* for *Antihypertensive Agents*, p. 477.

Administration

1. For better control of hypertension, administer after meals.

2. The morning dose may be small or omitted; larger doses are given at noon and in the evening.

Interventions

1. Take BP and pulse at the specific times ordered.
2. Make sure that the client is in positions ordered for all readings, whether sitting or standing. If this is not possible, alterations in time and position should be indicated on the client's record.
3. Weigh the client daily and check for edema to determine if any weight gain is the result of retained fluid or due to increased appetite.
4. Measure intake and output to detect evidence of oliguria, a result of excessive hypotension.
5. Note client complaint of constipation. Check with the physician regarding orders for laxatives, which can be administered if the client fails to have regular bowel movements. If constipation persists, the drug must be discontinued; bulk-producing cathartics are ineffective.
6. Note evidence of additive hypotensive effects if any other hypotensive agents or diuretics are concomitantly administered. Adjustment in the dosage of drug may be required.

Client/Family Teaching

1. Instruct client how to take BP and pulse and assist to develop a method to maintain a written record for review by health care provider.
2. Advise the client that orthostatic hypotension may occur. This is manifested by weakness, dizziness, and fainting. Since these symptoms occur when arising rapidly from a supine position, advise clients to rise slowly. First to a sitting position, dangling the legs for a few minutes, then when feeling stable, stand up. If this is a persistent problem have a family member present to assist.
3. Allow more time to prepare for the day's activities than usual to permit the body time to adjust to changes of position.
4. If weak, dizzy, or faint after standing or exercising for a long time, lie down if possible or otherwise sit down and lower head between knees.
5. Encourage the client to eat a diet high in fiber and provide a list of food and fluids that will help to avoid constipation.

TRIMETHAPHAN CAMSYLATE (try-METH-ah-fan)

Arfonad (Rx)

Classification: Ganglionic blocking agent, antihypertensive.

Action/Kinetics: In addition to acting as a ganglionic blocking agent, this drug directly dilates blood vessels as well as releases histamine. The antihypertensive effect is due to a reduction in sympathetic tone and vasodilation. **Onset:** immediate. **Duration:** extremely short (10–15 min). BP increases 10 min after discontinuance of IV infusion. Eliminated mostly unchanged through the kidney.

Uses: During surgery when controlled hypotension is desirable, as in the case of brain tumors, cerebral aneurysms, AV fistula repair, aortic grafts and transplants, coarctation, anastomosis, and fenestration operations. Trimethaphan is also indicated in hypertensive crisis and in pulmonary edema resulting from hypertension.

Contraindications: Pregnancy, anemia, shock, asphyxia, respiratory insufficiency, hypovolemia.

Special Concerns: Use with caution in arteriosclerosis, cardiac, hepatic, or renal disease, Addison's disease, diabetes, degenerative CNS disease, patients taking steroids. The drug should also be used with caution in debilitated patients or in children. Geriatric patients may be more sensitive to the hypotensive effects of mecamylamine; also, a decrease in dose may be required in these patients due to age-related decreases in renal function.

Drug Interactions

Anesthetics, general	Additive hypotension
Antihypertensive drugs	Additive hypotension
Diuretics	↑ Effect of trimethaphan
Muscle relaxants, nondepolarizing	Additive muscle relaxation
Succinylcholine	↑ Muscle relaxation

Dosage: IV infusion. *Controlled hypotension during surgery:* **Adults, initial,** 3–4 mg/min; **then,** 0.2–6 mg per min. *Hypertensive emergency:* **Adults, initial,** 0.5–1 mg/min adjusted according to response; **then,** 1–15 mg/min. **Pediatric:** 0.1 mg/kg/min adjusted according to the response. Check BP frequently.

NURSING CONSIDERATIONS

See also *Nursing Considerations* for *Ganglionic Blocking Agents,* p. 520.

Administration/Storage

1. Trimethaphan must always be diluted before being administered and should always be given by IV infusion.
2. Trimethaphan should be diluted with dextrose 5% to a concentration of 1 mg/mL.
3. Trimethaphan is an extremely potent hypotensive agent. Thus, its use should be limited to physicians with appropriate training.
4. Administration should be stopped before wound closure to allow blood pressure to return to normal (usually within 10 min).
5. Client should be positioned to avoid cerebral anoxia.

Assessment

1. If the client is within the childbearing age, determine if she is pregnant as the drug is contraindicated in this condition.
2. Note the age of the client. The drug should be used cautiously since the elderly tend to develop side effects more frequently than other age groups.

Interventions

1. Monitor BP closely. Systolic BP should be maintained above 60 mm Hg or at two-thirds the usual value in clients with hypertension.
2. Note excessive hypotension, rapid pulse, cold clammy skin, and cyanosis. These are evidence of peripheral vascular collapse and require drugs to be administered to counteract these reactions.
3. Levarterenol, ephedrine, methoxamine, and phenylephrine should be available to correct undesirably low BP.

Client/Family Teaching

If the client has a history of angina, the client needs to be taught the importance of reporting any further anginal attacks, or change in severity. The medication may precipitate such attacks.

MONOAMINE OXIDASE (MAO) INHIBITOR

PARGYLINE HYDROCHLORIDE (PAR-jih-leen)
Eutonyl (Rx)

Classification: Antihypertensive, monoamine oxidase (MAO) inhibitor.

Action/Kinetics: Mechanism of antihypertensive effect not known. Hypotensive effect is primarily orthostatic (similar to ganglionic blocking agents); thus, the drug may act by interfering with sympathetic vasoconstriction. **Discontinue at least 2 weeks before elective surgery. Onset:** Slow. Full therapeutic effect may take up to 3 weeks. **Duration:** Residual effects persist 3 weeks after drug discontinued. Pargyline is extensively metabolized by the liver and excreted by the kidneys.

For *Side Effects, Drug Interactions, Laboratory Test Interferences,* See Part 6, Chapter 33, *Antidepressants,* p. 656.

Uses: Moderate to severe essential or secondary hypertension. Used in conjunction with thiazides or with other antihypertensive drugs, or both.

Contraindications: Labile and mild hypertension; malignant hypertension, advanced renal failure, pheochromocytoma, paranoid schizophrenia, or hyperthyroidism. Children under 12 years.

Special Concerns: Pregnancy category: C. In geriatric patients there is an increased risk of vascular accidents and increased sensitivity to the hypotensive effects; also, a decrease in dose may be required in these patients due to age-related decreases in renal function.

Dosage: Tablets. Adult, initial: 25 mg once daily for 1 week; increase at weekly intervals by 10 mg until desired therapeutic effect is attained (total daily dose should not exceed 200 mg). **Maintenance, usual:** 25–50 mg once daily. **Initial dose** *for elderly or sympathectomized patients:* 10–25 mg. *When added to an established antihypertensive regiment:* **initial,** no more than 25 mg.

NURSING CONSIDERATIONS

Client/Family Teaching

1. Instruct client how to take BP and assist to develop a method to maintain a written record for review by the health care provider.
2. Avoid any other medication (particularly decongestants) unless physician is consulted first.
3. Avoid aged or natural cheese (e.g. Cheddar, Camembert, and Stilton), as well as other foods that require the actions of molds or bacteria for their preparation, such as pickled herring. Alcoholic beverages in any form should not be ingested. Concomitant use of pargyline with such foods may lead to hypertensive crisis.
4. Explain that the client may feel dizzy or faint, particularly when changing position from supine to standing. Client should rise slowly from bed. If he/she feels dizzy or faint, lie down or sit down with the head lowered.
5. Report headache or other unusual symptoms.
6. Avoid increase in physical activity while on medication, even though he/she may feel better. (This is particularly important for clients suffering from angina or coronary heart disease.)

7. Instruct client to weigh himself daily, to check for edema, and to report any significant changes.
8. How to monitor intake and output and maintain a record if ordered by the physician.
9. Report constipation to the physician to determine whether a laxative is needed.
10. Encourage to practice good mouth care to counteract nausea and dry mouth.

RAUWOLFIA ALKALOIDS

Action/Kinetics: Reserpine is believed to exert its action by depleting nerve terminals of norepinephrine, epinephrine, and serotonin. Thus less neurotransmitter is available to interact with receptors following nerve stimulation, resulting in a decreased heart rate and a lowering of blood pressure. Postural hypotension is not usually seen with reserpine. Reserpine also acts directly to depress myocardial function, to increase gastric acid secretion, and to produce a variety of endocrine changes. It also produces antipsychotic effects. **PO, Onset:** Several days to three weeks with multiple doses. **PO, Time to peak effect:** 3–6 weeks with multiple doses. **PO, Duration:** 1–6 weeks. **t½, initial:** 4.5 hr; **terminal:** 45–168 hr. Excreted mainly in the feces (60% unchanged) with less than 10% through the urine.

Uses: Mild essential hypertension. Adjunct with other drugs for severe hypertension. Psychoses, although such use is less common due to use of other more effective and safer drugs. See individual agents in Table 8.

Contraindications: Pheochromocytoma, history of mental depression, electroconvulsive therapy, colitis, or peptic ulcer.

Special Concerns: Use with caution in the presence of cardiac arrhythmias, impaired renal function, or asthma. The drugs pass the placental barrier and may cause the following reactions in the neonate: nasal congestion, increased respiratory secretions, hypothermia, lethargy, anorexia, cyanosis, and retractions. Through breast milk, they may cause nasal congestion, cyanosis, anorexia, and increased respiratory secretions in the infant. Thus, use during pregnancy (pregnancy category: C) and lactation should not be undertaken. Safety and efficacy have not been determined in children. Geriatric patients may be more sensitive to the hypotensive and CNS depressant effects of rauwolfia alkaloids; also, a decrease in dose may be required in these patients due to age-related decreases in renal function.

Side Effects: *CNS:* Drowsiness, depression (may be severe and lead to suicide attempts). Headache, dizziness, nightmares, increased dreaming, nervousness, paradoxical anxiety, extrapyramidal symptoms, deafness, dull sensorium. *CV:* Bradycardia, severe hypotension, angina-like symptoms, arrhythmias. *GI:* Nausea, vomiting, diarrhea, anorexia, cramps, increased gastric acid secretion (may aggravate peptic ulcer), dry mouth, GI bleeding. *Allergy:* Pruritus, rash, asthma symptoms in asthmatics. *Endocrine:* Impotence, decreased libido, breast engorgement, gynecomastia, pseudo-lactation. *Ophthalmic:* Glaucoma, conjunctival injection, uveitis, optic atrophy. *Other:* Nasal congestion (common), flushing, thrombocytopenic purpura, epistaxis, increased bleeding time, muscle aches, blurred vision, ptosis, dysuria, dyspnea, weight gain.

Overdosage is characterized by: CNS depression, hypotension, miosis, hypothermia, bradycardia, diarrhea, impaired consciousness, flushing of skin, conjunctival injection.

Table 8   Rauwolfia alkaloids

Drug	Dosage	Remarks
Alseroxylon (Rauwiloid) (Rx)	**Tablets: initial,** 2–4 mg daily in single or divided doses; **maintenance:** 2 mg daily.	1 mg equals approximately 0.1 mg reserpine. Pregnancy category: D. *Additional Drug Interactions:* 1. Ethanol ↑ CNS depressant and hypotensive effects of alseroxylon. 2. Levodopa and methyldopa ↑ hypotensive effects of alseroxylon.
Deserpidine (Harmonyl) (Rx)	**Tablets:** *Hypertension:* **initial,** 0.25–0.5 mg 1–2 times daily. **maintenance:** 0.25 mg daily.	Used for mild, essential hypertension and as an adjunct with other drugs to treat more severe hypertension. *Special Concerns:* Pregnancy category: C. Geriatric patients may be more sensitive to the usual adult dose.
Rauwolfia, whole root (Raudixin, Rauval, Rauverid, Wolfina) (Rx)	**Tablets: initial,** 50–200 mg daily in single or divided doses.	A dose of 200–300 mg of this preparation is equivalent to 0.5 mg of reserpine. *Uses:* See *Deserpidine*, above. *Special Concerns:* Pregnancy category: C. Geriatric patients may be more sensitive to the usual adult dose.
Reserpine (Novoreserpine♣, Reserfia♣, Reserpine, Serpalan) (Rx)	**Tablets.** 0.1–0.25 mg daily. **Pediatric:** 0.005–0.02 mg/kg (0.15–0.6 mg/m²) daily in 1–2 divided doses, although not usually recommended for children.	*Uses:* Hypertension. Raynaud's disease. Causes less bradycardia than does deserpine. Reserpine preferred for institutionalized patients. Drug of choice for institutionalized patients. May cause postural hypotension and respiratory depression. Determine BP before each administration. 10 mg or more may cause delayed hypotensive reaction. Geriatric patients may be more sensitive to the usual adult dose. When used alone, may not provide reliable control of hypertension. Most often used with thiazide diuretics or combined with hydralazine (e.g., Diupres, Hydropres, Regroton, Salutensin, Ser-Ap- Es).

Drug Interactions

Anticholinergics	Rauwolfia alkaloids ↓ effect of anticholinergics due to ↑ gastric acid secretion
Anticonvulsant drugs	Reserpine ↓ convulsive threshold and shortens seizure latency. Anticonvulsant drug dose may have to be adjusted.
Antidepressants, tricyclic	↑ Stimulating effect in depressed patients
Beta-adrenergic blocking agents	Additive hypotension and bradycardia
Diazoxide	Additive hypotensive effects
Digitalis glycosides	↑ Possibility of cardiac arrhythmias
Ephedrine	↓ Pressor response of ephedrine
General anesthetics	Hypotension, bradycardia
Guanadrel	Additive hypotensive effects
Guanethidine	Additive hypotensive effects
Hydralazine	Additive hypotensive effects
Levodopa	↑ Symptoms of Parkinsonism
Mephentermine	↓ Pressor response of mephentermine
Methotrimeprazine	Additive hypotensive effects
Methyldopa	Additive hypotensive effects
Monoamine oxidase inhibitors	Reserpine-induced release of accumulated norepinephrine caused by monoamine oxidase inhibitors results in excitation and hypertension
Phenothiazines	Additive hypotensive effects
Procarbazine	Additive hypotensive effects
Quinidine	Additive hypotensive effect and ↑ chance of cardiac arrhythmias
Sympathomimetics, directly-acting	Rauwolfia alkaloids may prolong sympathomimetic effects
Sympathomimetics, indirectly-acting	Rauwolfia alkaloids may inhibit sympathomimetic effects
Theophylline	↑ Chance of tachycardia
Thiazide diuretics	Additive hypotensive effect
Thioxanthines	Additive hypotensive effect
Tricyclic antidepressants	Symptoms of hypotension, flushing, diarrhea, and manic reactions
Vasodilator drugs, peripheral	Additive hypotensive effect

Laboratory Test Interference: ↑ Serum glucose, urine glucose, serum prolactin.   ↓ Urine catecholamines, 17-hydroxycorticosteroids, 17-ketosteroids, and vanillylmandelic acid.

Dosage: Given PO. See individual drugs, Table 8. Often combined with other antihypertensive drugs to decrease the incidence of side effects due to reserpine and to increase efficacy.

NURSING CONSIDERATIONS

Administration/Storage

Rauwolfia alkaloids must be discontinued 1 week before electroshock therapy.

Assessment

1. Obtain a thorough drug and nursing history. Note other drugs the client may be taking that could precipitate an unfavorable interaction.
2. Assess women of childbearing age for pregnancy as the drug is contraindicated in this circumstance.

Interactions

1. Observe client for personality changes, nightmares, or changes in sleep patterns. These are early symptoms of depression that may lead to suicide attempts.
2. Monitor BP under standard conditions and compare with baseline and other previous BP readings. Report any significant changes and obtain specific guidelines for each client from physician.
3. Weigh the client at least twice weekly under standard conditions (e.g. before breakfast and with similar weight clothing).
4. Monitor for fluid retention and evaluate severity and document.
5. Anticipate concomitant use with a diuretic.
6. Have a sympathomimetic agent such as ephedrine, available to treat overdose.

Client/Family Teaching

1. Instruct client how to take BP and pulse and assist to develop a method to maintain a written record for review by health care provider.
2. Review signs that may precede depression, such as changes in sleep patterns, nightmares or personality changes. Stress the importance of medical supervision should these occur.
3. Discuss possible side effects of rauwolfia alkaloid therapy. Advise clients to report any untoward side effects.
4. Instruct clients to weigh themselves twice a week and record. Any excess weight gain as well as evidence of edema should be reported.
5. Take with food or milk if GI upset occurs.

Evaluation

1. Assess client/family knowledge and understanding of illness, response to therapy and to teaching.
2. Review record of BP, pulse and weight to determine response to medication therapy as well as client compliance.
3. Observe for freedom from complications of drug therapy.

NURSING CONSIDERATIONS FOR PARENTERAL RAUWOLFIA

Interventions

1. Assess the client for respiratory depression.
2. Observe for evidence of postural hypotension.
3. Caution the client not to get out of bed without assistance.
4. Monitor BP before each parenteral dose of reserpine.

COMBINATION DRUGS COMMONLY USED TO TREAT HYPERTENSION

AMILORIDE AND HYDROCHLOROTHIAZIDE
(ah-**MILL**-oh-ryd, hy-droh-kloh-roh-**THIGH**-ah-zyd)

Moduretic, Moduret✿ (Rx)

See also *Amiloride*, p. 1269, and *Hydrochlorothiazide*, p. 1282.

Classification/Content: *Diuretic, potassium-sparing:* Amiloride HCl, 5 mg. *Antihypertensive/diuretic:* Hydrochlorothiazide, 50 mg.

Uses: Hypertension or congestive heart failure, especially when hypokalemia occurs.

Special Concerns: Pregnancy category: C. Use with caution during lactation. Geriatric patients may be more sensitive to the hypotensive and electrolyte effects of this combination; also, age-related decreases in renal function may require a decrease in dosage.

Dosage: Tablets. Initial: 1 tablet daily; **then,** dosage may be increased to 2 tablets daily.

NURSING CONSIDERATIONS

Administration/Storage

1. This drug should be taken with food.
2. The daily dose may be given as a single dose or in divided doses.
3. More than two tablets daily are not usually necessary.

LISINOPRIL AND HYDROCHLOROTHIAZIDE   (lie-**SIN**-oh-pril, hy-droh-kloh-roh-**THIGH**-ah-zyd)

Prinzide, Zestoretic (Rx)

See also *Lisinopril*, p. 481, and *Hydrochlorothiazide*, p. 1282.

Classification/Contents: Lisinopril is an angiotensin-converting enzyme inhibitor and hydrochlorothiazide is a diuretic. Prinzide 12.5 and Zestoretic 20–12.5: Lisinopril, 20 mg and hydrochlorothiazide, 12.5 mg. Prinzide 25 and Zestoretic 20–25: Lisinopril, 20 mg and hydrochlorothiazide, 25 mg.

Uses: Hypertension in patients in whom combination therapy is appropriate. Not for initial therapy.

Special Concerns: Pregnancy category: C.

Dosage: Individualized. PO, usual: 1 or 2 tablets once daily of Prinzide 12.5, Prinzide 25, Zestoretic 20–12.5, or Zestoretic 20–25.

NURSING CONSIDERATIONS

See also *Nursing Considerations* for *Lisinopril*, p. 482, and *Thiazide Diuretics*, p. 1276.

Administration

1. Clients whose blood pressure is controlled with lisinopril, 20 mg plus hydrochlorothiazide, 25 mg given separately should be given a trial of Prinzide 12.5 or Zestoretic 20–12.5 before Prinzide 25 or Zestoretic 20–25 mg is used.
2. The maximum recommended daily dose of lisinopril is 80 mg in a single daily dose. However,

clients usually do not require hydrochlorothiazide in doses exceeding 50 mg daily, especially if combined with other antihypertensives.

3. Use of potassium supplements, potassium-sparing diuretics, or potassium salt substitutes with Prinzide or Zestoretic may lead to increases in serum potassium.

4. Prinzide or Zestoretic is recommended for those clients with a creatinine clearance greater than 30 mL/min.

Client/Family Teaching

1. Stress the importance of reporting for scheduled laboratory studies.
2. Avoid all potassium supplements as well as foods high in potassium.
3. Instruct how to take blood pressure and maintain written record for physician review.

METHYLDOPA AND HYDROCHLOROTHIAZIDE (meth-ill-**DOH**-pah, hy-droh-kloh-roh-**THIGH**-ah-zyd)

Aldoril, Novodoparil✽, PMS Dopazide✽ (Rx)

See also *Methyldopa,* p. 501, and *Hydrochlorothiazide,* p. 1282.

Content/Classification: *Antihypertensive:* Methyldopa, 250–500 mg. *Diuretic/antihypertensive:* Hydrochlorothiazide, 15–50 mg.

Uses: Hypertension (not for initial treatment).

Special Concerns: Use in pregnancy only if benefits outweigh risks.

Dosage: Tablets. Adults: one tablet b.i.d.–t.i.d. for first 48 hr; **then,** increase or decrease dose, depending on response, in intervals of not less than two days. Maximum daily dosage: methyldopa, 3.0 g; hydrochlorothiazide, 100–200 mg.

NURSING CONSIDERATIONS

See also *Nursing Considerations* for *Methyldopa,* p. 502, and *Thiazides and Related Diuretics,* p. 1276.

Administration/Storage

1. If Aldoril is given together with antihypertensives other than thiazides, the initial dose of methyldopa should not be more than 500 mg daily in divided doses.
2. Additional methyldopa may be given separately if Aldoril alone does not control blood pressure adequately.
3. If tolerance is observed after 2–3 months of therapy, the dose of either methyldopa and/or hydrochlorothiazide may be increased to restore control.

PROPRANOLOL AND HYDROCHLOROTHIAZIDE (proh-**PRAN**-oh-lohl, hy-droh-kloh-roh-**THIGH**-ah-zyd)

Inderide, Inderide LA (Rx)

See also *Propranolol,* p. 493, and *Hydrochlorothiazide,* p. 1282.

Classification/Content: *Antihypertensive/diuretic:* Hydrochlorothiazide, 25 mg (Inderide) or 50 mg (Inderide LA).

Beta-adrenergic blocking agent: Propranolol HCl, 40 or 80 mg (Inderide) or 80, 120, or 160 mg (Inderide LA).

Uses: Hypertension (not indicated for initial therapy).

Special Concerns: Pregnancy category: C. Dosage has not been established in children. The risk of hypothermia is increased in geriatric patients.

Dosage: PO. Individualized. *Inderide:* 1–2 tablets b.i.d. up to 320 mg propranolol HCl daily. *Inderide LA:* 1 capsule once daily.

NURSING CONSIDERATIONS

See also *Propranolol, p. 494,* and *Hydrochlorothiazide,* p. 1283.

Administration/Storage

1. Because of side effects from hydrochlorothiazide, Inderide should not be used if propranolol must be given in excess of 320 mg daily.
2. If another antihypertensive agent is required, initial dosage should be one-half the usual recommended dose in order to prevent an excessive drop in blood pressure.
3. Inderide LA should not be considered a milligram-to-milligram substitute for Inderide as the LA produces lower blood levels.

RESERPINE AND CHLOROTHIAZIDE   (**REH**-sir-peen, kloh-roh-**THIGH**-ah-zyd)
Diupres, Diurigen with Reserpine (Rx)

See also *Chlorothiazide,* p. 1280, *Rauwolfia Alkaloids,* p. 525

Classification/Content: *Antihypertensive:* Reserpine, 0.125 mg. *Antihypertensive/diuretic:* Chlorothiazide, 250 or 500 mg.

Uses: Hypertension—not to be used for initial treatment.

Special Concerns: Use during pregnancy only if benefits outweigh risks. Geriatric patients may be more sensitive to the usual adult dose.

Dosage: PO: 1–2 tablets 1–2 times daily.

NURSING CONSIDERATIONS

See also *Nursing considerations* for *Duiretics,* p. 1250, *Thiazide Duiretics,* p. 1276, and *Rauwolfia Alkaloids,* p. 527.

Administration/Storage

Monitor blood pressure carefully if Diupres is used with other antihypertensive agents.

RESERPINE, HYDRALAZINE, AND HYDROCHLOROTHIAZIDE
(**REH**-sir-peen, hy-**DRAL**-ah-zeen, hy-droh-kloh-roh-**THIGH**-ah-zyd)

Cam-Ap-Es, Cherapas, Ser-A-Gen, Seralazide, Ser-Ap-Es, Serpazide, Tri-Hydroserpine, Unipres (Rx)

See also *Hydralazine,* p. 516, and *Hydrochlorothiazide,* p. 1282, and *Rauwolfia alkaloids,* p. 525.

Classification/Content: *Antihypertensive:* Hydralazine, 25 mg. *Antihypertensive:* Reserpine, 0.1 mg. *Antihypertensive/diuretic:* Hydrochlorothiazide, 15 mg.

Uses: Treatment of hypertension (not to be used for initial therapy).

Special Concerns: Pregnancy category: C. Geriatric patients may be more sensitive to the adult dose.

Dosage: PO. Individualized. Usual: 1–2 tablets t.i.d.

NURSING CONSIDERATIONS

See also *Nursing Considerations* for *Hydralazine*, p. 517, and *Hydrochlorothiazide*, p. 1283, and Rauwolfia Alkaloids, p. 527

Administration/Storage

1. It may take up to 2 weeks to manifest the maximum effect on blood pressure reduction.
2. Clients should be maintained on the lowest dose possible (requires titration).
3. If additional antihypertensive medication is necessary, initial doses should be 50% of the usual recommended dose.

TRIAMTERENE AND HYDROCHLOROTHIAZIDE CAPSULES (try-**AM**-teh-reen, hy-droh-kloh-roh-**THIGH**-ah-zyd)

Dyazide (Rx)

TRIAMTERENE AND HYDROCHLOROTHIAZIDE TABLETS (try-**AM**-teh-reen, hy-droh-kloh-roh-**THIGH**-ah-zyd)

Apo-Triazide ✤, Dyazide ✤, Maxzide, Novo-Triamzide ✤ (Rx)

See also *Triamterene*, p. 1272, and *Hydrochlorothiazide*, p. 1282.

Classification/Content: Capsules. *Diuretic:* Hydrochlorothiazide, 25 or 50 mg. *Diuretic:* Triamterene, 50 or 100 mg.

Tablets. *Diuretic:* Hydrochlorothiazide, 25 or 50 mg. *Diuretic:* Triamterene, 37.5 or 75 mg. (In Canada the tablets contain 25 mg of hydrochlorothiazide and 50 mg triamterene.)

Uses: To treat hypertension or edema in patients who manifest hypokalemia on hydrochlorothiazide alone. In patients requiring a diuretic and in whom hypokalemia cannot be risked (i.e., patients with cardiac arrhythmias, or those taking digitalis). Usually not the first line of therapy, except for patients in whom hypokalemia should be avoided.

Special Concerns: Pregnancy category: C. Use with caution during lactation. Geriatric patients may be more sensitive to the hypotensive and electrolyte effects of this combination; also, age-related decreases in renal function may require a decrease in dosage.

Dosage: Capsules. Adults: 1–2 capsules b.i.d. determined by individual titration with the components. Some patients may be controlled using 1 capsule every day or every other day. No more than 4 capsules should be taken daily.

Tablets. Adults: 1 tablet daily determined by individual titration with the components. In Canada, 1–2 tablets may be taken daily.

NURSING CONSIDERATIONS

See also *Nursing Considerations* for *Hydrochlorothiazide*, p. 1283, and *Triampterene*, p. 1272.

Administration

Clients who are transferred from less bioavailable formulations of triamterene and hydrochlorothiazide should be monitored for serum potassium levels following the transfer.

General Statement: The orderly sequence of contraction of the heart chambers, at an efficient rate, is necessary so that the heart can pump enough blood to the body organs. Normally the atria contract first, then the ventricles.

Altered patterns of contraction, or marked increases or decreases in the rate of the heart, reduce the ability of the heart to pump blood. Such altered patterns are called *cardiac arrhythmias*. Some examples of cardiac arrhythmias are:

1. *Premature ventricular beats* or beats that occasionally originate in the ventricles instead of in the sinus node region of the atrium. This causes the ventricles to contract before the atria and ultimately results in a decrease in the volume of blood pumped into the aorta.

2. *Ventricular tachycardia*. A rapid heartbeat with a succession of beats originating in the ventricles.

3. *Atrial flutter*. Rapid contraction of the atria at a rate too fast to enable it to force blood into the ventricles efficiently.

4. *Atrial fibrillation*. The rate of atrial contraction is even faster than that noted during atrial flutter and more disorganized.

5. *Ventricular fibrillation*. Rapid, irregular, and uncoordinated ventricular contractions that are unable to pump any blood to the body. This condition will cause death if not corrected immediately.

6. *Atrioventricular heart block*. Slowing or failure of the transmission of the cardiac impulse from atria to ventricles, in the atrioventricular junction. This can result in atrial contraction *not* followed by ventricular contraction.

The effective treatment of arrhythmias is dependent on accurate diagnosis, changing the causative factors, and, if appropriate, selection of an antiarrhythmic drug. The various antiarrhythmic drugs are classified according to both their mechanism of action and their effects on the action potential of

27

cardiac cells. Importantly, one drug in a particular class may be more effective and safer in an individual patient. The antiarrhythmic drugs are classified as follows:

1. Type I. These drugs decrease the rate of entry of sodium during cardiac membrane depolarization, decrease the rate of rise of phase O of the cardiac membrane action potential, prolong the effective refractory period of fast-response fibers, and require that a more negative membrane potential be reached before the membrane becomes excitable (and thus can propagate to other membranes). Drugs classified as Type I are further listed in subgroups as follows:

   • Type IA: Depress phase O and prolong the duration of the action potential. The drugs are disopyramide, procainamide, quinidine.
   • Type IB: Slightly depress phase O and are thought to shorten the action potential. The drugs include lidocaine, mexiletine, phenytoin, tocainide.
   • Type IC: Slight effect on repolarization but marked depression of phase O of the action potential. Significant slowing of conduction. The drugs in this group are encainide, flecainide, and indecainide.

2. Type II. The drugs of this type competitively block beta adrenergic receptors. These drugs may also cause a membrane-stabilizing effect. Acebutolol, esmolol, and propranolol and type II antiarrhythmics.

3. Type III. The drugs in this group prolong the duration of the membrane action potential without changing the phase of depolarization or the resting membrane potential. Drugs in this group include amiodarone and bretylium.

4. Type IV. The drug in this group (verapamil) slows conduction velocity and increases the refractoriness of the A-V node.

It is important to monitor serum levels of antiarrhythmic drugs since some drugs can cause toxic side effects which can be confused with the purpose for which the drug is used. For example, toxicity from quinidine can result in cardiac arrhythmias.

NURSING CONSIDERATIONS

Assessment

1. Assess the extent of the client's palpitations, fluttering sensations or missed beats prior to initiating the therapy.
2. Obtain pretreatment ECG and evaluate.
3. Note client complaints of chest pains or fainting episodes.
4. Obtain client blood pressure, pulse, and listen to heart sounds and record findings. These should serve as baseline data against which to measure the outcome of the prescribed therapy.
5. Assure that laboratory tests for liver and renal function and electrolytes and blood glucose levels have been completed.

Interventions

1. Attach client to a cardiac monitor if administering antiarrhythmic drugs by IV route.
2. Establish specific written guidelines with the physician concerning what to do should the client develop unusual changes in heart rate or rhythm.
3. If the client is to receive continuous drip infusion, microdrip tubing and an infusion control device or electronic infusion pump should be used.
4. Monitor blood pressure and pulse. A heart rate of less than 60 beats per minute or greater than 120 should generally be avoided, depending on the client's baseline.

5. Persistent bradycardia of new onset may indicate approaching cardiac collapse.

6. Have emergency drugs and equipment available in the event of an adverse reaction to therapy. Be prepared to help withdraw the medication, administer emergency drugs, and use resuscitative techniques.

7. Monitor for changes in cardiac rhythm. Document with rhythm strips and report to the physician as the drug administration may need to be altered.

8. Note any depression of cardiac activity, such as the prolongation of the P-R interval, widening of the QRS complex, increased A-V block, or aggravation of the arrhythmia and report.

9. Monitor serum concentrations of the antiarrhythmic agent throughout initial therapy.

Client/Family Teaching

1. Explain the desired effects of the drug therapy to the client.

2. Review the signs and symptoms of adverse reactions that should be reported.

3. Stress the importance of taking the drugs as ordered. If a dose of medication is missed the client should not double up on the next dose unless this is specifically ordered by the physician.

4. Assist the client to establish a time and a method of recording that would enable them to remember to take the medications as ordered.

5. Do not drink alcohol, as this may alter drug absorption.

6. Stress the importance of returning for follow-up visits as scheduled.

7. Remind clients to inform all health care providers that they are taking antiarrhythmic agents. An ID bracelet may be helpful.

Evaluation

1. Assess client/family knowledge and understanding of illness, response to teaching and level of compliance.

2. Obtain ECG to compare to pretreatment ECG to determine response to therapy.

3. Review serum drug concentrations to determine if levels are therapeutic.

4. Observe for any side effects that may be drug related.

5. Evaluate the client's electrolyte levels, diet and drug regimens to determine if the serum potassium levels are sufficient to enhance drug effectiveness.

ADENOSINE   (ah-DEN-oh-seen)

Adenocard (Rx)

Classification: Antiarrhythmic.

Action/Kinetics: Adenosine is found naturally in all cells of the body. The substance has been found to slow conduction time through the AV node, interrupt the reentry pathways through the AV node, and can restore normal sinus rhythm in paroxysmal supraventricular tachycardia (including those patients with Wolff-Parkinson-White Syndrome). **t½:** Less than 10 seconds (taken up by erythrocytes and vascular endothelial cells). Exogenous adenosine becomes part of the body pool and is metabolized mainly to inosine and adenosine monophosphate (AMP).

Uses: Conversion of sinus rhythm of paroxysmal supraventricular tachycardia. Symptomatic relief of varicose vein complications with stasis dermatitis.

Contraindications: Second- or third-degree AV block or sick sinus syndrome (except in patients with a functioning artificial pacemaker). Also, atrial flutter, atrial fibrillation, ventricular tachycardia.

Special Concerns: Use during pregnancy only when clearly needed (pregnancy category: C). Use with caution in patients with asthma.

Side Effects: *CV:* Facial flushing (common), headache, chest pain, sweating, palpitations, hypotension. *CNS:* Lightheadedness, dizziness, numbness, tingling in arms, heaviness in arms, blurred vision, apprehension. *GI:* Nausea, metallic taste, tightness in throat. *Respiratory:* Shortness of breath or dyspnea (common), chest pressure, hyperventilation. *Miscellaneous:* Pressure in head, burning sensation, neck and back pain, pressure in groin.

Drug Interactions

Caffeine	Competitively antagonizes effect of adenosine
Carbamazepine	↑ Degree of heart block
Dipyridamole	↑ Effect of adenosine
Theophylline	Competitively antagonizes effect of adenosine

Dosage: Rapid IV bolus only, initial: 6 mg over 1–2 sec. If the first dose does not reverse the supraventricular tachycardia within 1–2 min, 12 mg should be given as a rapid IV bolus. The 12 mg dose may be repeated a second time, if necessary. Doses greater than 12 mg are not recommended.

NURSING CONSIDERATIONS

See also *Nursing Considerations* for *Antiarrhythmic Drugs,* p. 534.

Administration/Storage

1. Store the drug at room temperature. Do not refrigerate as crystallization may occur.
2. The solution should be clear at the time of use.
3. Discard any unused portion as the product contains no preservatives.
4. The drug should be administered directly into a vein. If it is to be given into an IV line, introduce the drug in the most proximal line and follow with a rapid saline flush.

Interventions

1. Document client complaints of chest pressure, shortness of breath, heaviness of the arms, palpitations, or dyspnea.
2. Note any facial flushing and reassure the client. This is a common side effect of therapy and should be shared with the physician.
3. If client complains of numbness, tingling in the arms, blurred vision or appears apprehensive, check BP and pulse. Then notify the physician as this may be an indication to discontinue the drug therapy.

AMIODARONE HYDROCHLORIDE   (am-ee-**OH**-dah-rohn)

Cordarone (Rx)

See also *Antiarrhythmic Drugs,* p. 533.

Classification: Antiarrhythmic, type III.

Action/Kinetics: The antiarrhythmic activity is due to an increase in the duration of the myocardial cell action potential as well as alpha- and beta-adrenergic blockade. **Onset:** Several days up to 1–3 weeks. Drug may accumulate in the liver, lung, spleen, and adipose tissue. **Therapeutic serum levels:** 0.5–2.5 mcg/mL. **t½:** Biphasic: initial t½: 2.5–10 days; final t½: 40–55 days (usual). Effects may persist for several weeks or months after therapy is terminated. Effective plasma concentrations are difficult to predict although concentrations below 1 mg/L are usually ineffective while those above 2.5 mg/L are not necessary. Neither amiodarone nor its metabolite, desethylamiodarone, is dialyzable.

Uses: This drug should be reserved for life-threatening ventricular arrhythmias which do not respond to other therapy. Amiodarone has been used for recurrent ventricular fibrillation and recurrent, hemodynamically unstable ventricular tachycardia.

Contraindications: Marked sinus bradycardia due to severe sinus node dysfunction, second- or third-degree AV block, syncope caused by bradycardia (except when used with a pacemaker). Lactation.

Special Concerns: Should be used in pregnancy only when benefits outweigh the potential risks (pregnancy category: C). Safety and efficacy in children have not been determined. The drug may be more sensitive in geriatric patients, especially on thyroid function.

Side Effects: Adverse reactions, some potentially fatal, are common with doses greater than 400 mg/day. *Pulmonary:* Interstitial pneumonitis, alveolitis, pulmonary inflammation or fibrosis. *CV:* Worsening of arrhythmias, symptomatic bradycardia, sinus arrest, SA node dysfunction, congestive heart failure, edema, hypotension, cardiac conduction abnormalities, coagulation abnormalities. *Hepatic:* Increases in SGOT and SGPT, abnormal liver function tests. *CNS:* Malaise, tremor, lack of coordination, fatigue, ataxia, paresthesias, peripheral neuropathy, dizziness, insomnia, headache, decreased libido. *Ophthalmologic:* Corneal microdeposits (asymptomatic) in patients on therapy for 6 months or more, photophobia, dry eyes, blurred vision, halos. *GI:* Nausea, vomiting, constipation, anorexia, abdominal pain, abnormal smell and taste, abnormal salivation. *Dermatologic:* Photosensitivity, solar dermatitis, blue-gray pigmentation after prolonged exposure, rash, alopecia, spontaneous ecchymosis, flushing. *Miscellaneous:* Hypothyroidism or hyperthyroidism.

Drug Interactions	
Anticoagulants	↑ Effect → bleeding disorders
Beta-adrenergic blocking agents	↑ Chance of bradycardia, sinus arrest, or AV block
Digoxin, digitoxin	↑ Serum digoxin, digitoxin levels → toxicity
Phenytoin	↑ Serum phenytoin levels → toxicity
Procainamide	↑ Serum procainamide → toxicity
Quinidine	↑ Serum quinidine → toxicity

Dosage: Tablets. Due to the drug's side effects, unusual pharmacokinetic properties, and difficult dosing schedule, amiodarone should be administered in a hospital only by physicians trained in treating life-threatening arrhythmias. Loading doses are required to ensure a reasonable onset of action. *Life-threatening arrhythmias:* **PO, loading dose:** 800–1,600 mg/day for 1–3 weeks (or until initial response occurs); **then,** reduce dose to 600–800 mg/day for one month. **Maintenance dose:** 200–400 mg/day.

NURSING CONSIDERATIONS

See also *Nursing Considerations* for *Antiarrhythmic Drugs,* p. 534.

Administration/Storage

1. Daily doses of 1,000 mg or more should be administered in divided doses with meals.

2. To minimize side effects, the lowest effective dose should be determined. If side effects occur, the dose should be reduced.

3. If dosage adjustments are required, the client should be monitored for a prolonged period of time due to the long and variable half-life of the drug and the difficulty in predicting the time needed to achieve a new steady-state plasma drug level.

4. When initiating amiodarone therapy, other antiarrhythmic drugs should be gradually discontinued.

Assessment

1. Determine if the client is taking any other antiarrhythmic medications.
2. Note the client's baseline vital signs and skin color.
3. Assess quality of respirations and breath sounds.
4. Record client pulse rate several times in similar circumstances, where possible, to establish a baseline against which to measure responses after initiating therapy.
5. Obtain baseline data concerning the client's vision before starting therapy.

Interventions

1. When the client is hospitalized, observe ECG for increased arrhythmias and heart rates less than 60 bpm and report to the physician.
2. Monitor BP and assess for evidence of hypotension.
3. Note client complaints of shortness of breath, painful breathing or cough. Assess pulmonary status and document.
4. Observe for untoward CNS symptoms such as tremor, lack of coordination, paresthesias, and dizziness.
5. Anticipate reduced dosages of digoxin, warfarin, quinidine, procainamide, and phenytoin if administered concomitantly with amiodarone hydrochloride.
6. Monitor thyroid studies, as drug inhibits conversion of T_4 to T_3.
7. Note client complaints of headaches, depression or insomnia. Also observe for any change in client behavior such as decreased interest in personal appearance or apparent hallucinations. These findings may indicate a need for a change in drug therapy.
8. Clients should have periodic ophthalmic examinations since small corneal deposits may develop during prolonged therapy.

Client/Family Teaching

1. Some clients may develop crystals on the skin producing a bluish color. In this event, avoid exposure to the sun since the crystals create photosensitivity. Notify physician so that the dosage of drug can be adjusted.
2. Report any bleeding or bruising promptly, to enable the physician to avoid the development of coagulation disorders.
3. Report all side effects and avoid direct exposure to sunlight.
4. Wheezing, fever, coughing or dyspnea are all symptoms of pulmonary problems and require prompt attention.
5. Stress the importance of reporting for laboratory studies as scheduled.
6. Instruct the client to carry a medic alert card at all times.

BRETYLIUM TOSYLATE   (breh-**TIH**-lee-um **TOZ**-ill-ayt)

Bretylate Parenteral✳, Bretylol (Rx)

Classification: Antiarrhythmic, type III.

Action/Kinetics: Bretylium inhibits catecholamine release at nerve endings by decreasing excitability of the nerve terminal. The drug also increases the duration of the action potential and the effective refractory period, which may assist in reversing arrhythmias. **Peak plasma concentration and effect:** 1 hr after IM injection. Antifibrillatory effect within a few minutes after IV use. Suppression of ventricular tachycardia and ventricular arrhythmias takes 20–120 min while suppression of premature ventricular contractions does not occur for 6–9 hr. **Therapeutic serum levels:** 0.5–1.5 mcg/mL. **t½:** 5–10 hr. Up to 90% of drug is excreted unchanged in the urine after 24 hr.

Uses: Life-threatening ventricular arrhythmias that have failed to respond to other antiarrhythmics. Prophylaxis and treatment of ventricular fibrillation. For short-term use only.

Contraindications: Severe aortic stenosis, severe pulmonary hypertension.

Special Concerns: Safe use during pregnancy and in children has not been established.

Side Effects: *CV:* Hypotension (including postural hypotension), transient hypertension, increased frequency of premature ventricular contractions, bradycardia, precipitation of anginal attacks, initial increase in arrhythmias, sensation of substernal pressure. *GI:* Nausea, vomiting (especially after rapid IV administration), diarrhea, abdominal pain, hiccoughs. *CNS:* Vertigo, dizziness, lightheadedness, syncope, anxiety, paranoid psychosis, confusion, mood swings. *Miscellaneous:* Renal dysfunction, flushing, hyperthermia, shortness of breath, nasal stuffiness, diaphoresis, conjunctivitis, erythematous macular rash, lethargy.

Drug Interactions	
Digitoxin, Digoxin	Bretylium may aggravate digitalis toxicity due to initial release of norepinephrine
Procainamide, Quinidine	Concomitant use with bretylium ↓ inotropic effect of bretylium and ↑ hypotension

Dosage: IV. *Ventricular fibrillation:* 5 mg/kg of undiluted solution given rapidly. Can increase to 10 mg/kg and repeat as needed. **Maintenance, IV infusion:** 1–2 mg/min; or, 5–10 mg/kg q 6 hr of diluted drug infused over 10–30 min. *Other ventricular arrhythmias:* **IV infusion:** 5–10 mg/kg of diluted solution over 10–30 min, **Maintenance:** 5–10 mg/kg q 6 hr or 1–2 mg/min of continuous IV infusion.

IM. *Other ventricular arrhythmias:* 5–10 mg/kg of undiluted solution followed, if necessary, by the same dose at 1–2 hr intervals; **then,** give same dosage q 6–8 hr.

NURSING CONSIDERATIONS
See also *Nursing Considerations* for *Antiarrhythmic Drugs,* p. 534.

Administration/Storage
1. For IV infusion, dilute the 10 mL ampule up to a minimum of 50 mL with either 5% dextrose injection or sodium chloride injection.
2. For IM injection, use the drug undiluted.

3. Rotate the injection sites so that no more than 5 mL of drug is given at any site. This avoids localized atrophy, necrosis, fibrosis, vascular degeneration, or inflammation.

4. The client should be placed on an oral antiarrhythmic medication as soon as possible.

Assessment

Note if client is taking digitalis. Bretylium tosylate may aggravate digitalis toxicity.

Interventions

1. To reduce nausea and vomiting, administer the IV drug over an 8 min period.

2. IV solutions should be administered with the client lying down. BP should be monitored and documented every 15 min along with cardiac rhythm strips.

3. Bretylium often causes a fall in supine blood pressure within 1 hr of IV administration. If the pressure falls below 75 mm Hg, anticipate the need to use pressor agents.

4. Once the IV is finished, the client should continue to lie down until the blood pressure has stabilized.

5. Supervise the client once ambulation is permitted. Clients may develop lightheadedness and vertigo.

6. If clients develop side effects, stay with them, reorienting as needed.

7. Remember that the dose of bretylium to be administered is titrated based upon the client's response to therapy. Therefore careful recording of the drug effects is important as well as consultation with the physician.

DIGITALIS GLYCOSIDES   (dih-gih-**TAH**-lis **GLYE**-coh-syds)

See *Cardiac Glycosides,* Chapter 23, p. 433.

DILTIAZEM HYDROCHLORIDE   (dill-**TIE**-ah-zem)
Cardizem (Rx)

See *Calcium Channel Blocking Drugs,* Chapter 24, p. 455.

DISOPYRAMIDE   (dye-so-**PEER**-ah-myd)
Napamide, Norpace, Norpace CR, Rythmodan✿, Rythmodan-LA✿ (Rx)

Classification: Antiarrhythmic, type IA.

Action/Kinetics: Disopyramide reduces the excitability of cardiac muscle to electrical stimulation and prolongs the refractory period. It manifests anticholinergic effects, although it has fewer side effects than quinidine. The drug does not affect blood pressure significantly and it can be used in digitalized and nondigitalized patients. **Onset:** 30 min. **Peak plasma levels:** 2 hr. **Duration:** average of 6 hr (range 1.5–8 hr). **t½:** 5–8 hr. **Therapeutic serum levels:** 2–8 mcg/mL. Serum levels should not be used to adjust the dose because of variance in protein binding and potential toxicity of unbound drug. **Protein binding:** 40–60%. Both unchanged drug (50%) and metabolites (30%) are excreted through the urine. Approximately 15% is excreted through the bile.

Uses: Prevention, recurrence, and control of unifocal, multifocal, and paired premature ventricular contractions. Arrhythmias in coronary artery disease. *Investigational:* Ventricular arrhythmias in emergency conditions, paroxysmal supraventricular tachycardia.

Contraindications: Hypersensitivity to drug. Cardiogenic shock, heart failure, heart block, especially preexisting second- and third-degree AV block, glaucoma, urinary retention.

Special Concerns: Safe use during pregnancy (category: C), childhood, labor, and delivery has not been established. Geriatric patients may be more sensitive to the anticholinergic effects of this drug.

Side Effects: *CV:* Hypotension, congestive heart failure, edema, weight gain, cardiac conduction disturbances, hypotension, shortness of breath, syncope, chest pain. *Anticholinergic:* Dry mouth, urinary retention, constipation, blurred vision, dry nose, eyes, and throat. *GU:* Urinary frequency and urgency. *GI:* Nausea, pain, flatulence, anorexia, diarrhea, vomiting. *CNS:* Headache, nervousness, dizziness, fatigue, depression, insomnia, psychoses. *Dermatologic:* Rash/dermatoses. *Other:* Fever, respiratory problems, gynecomastia, anaphylaxis, malaise, muscle weakness, numbness, tingling, angle-closure glaucoma.

Drug Interaction: Phenytoin and rifampin ↓ effect due to ↑ breakdown by liver.

Dosage: Capsules. *Individualized.* **Initial loading dose:** 300 mg (200 mg if patient weighs less than 50 kg); **maintenance:** 400–800 mg/day in 4 divided doses (usual: 150 mg q 6 hr). *For patients less than 50 kg,* **maintenance:** 100 mg q 6 hr. If controlled release form used, administer q 12 hr. *Severe refractory tachycardia:* up to 400 mg q 6 hr may be required. *Cardiomyopathy:* do not administer a loading dose; give 100 mg q 6 hr. For all uses, dosage must be decreased in patients with renal or hepatic insufficiency. *Moderate renal failure or hepatic failure:* 100 mg q 6 hr (or 200 mg q 12 hr of sustained release form). *Severe renal failure:* 100 mg q 8–24 hr depending on severity.

    Capsules, extended-release. *Arrhythmias:* 300 mg q 12 hr (200 mg q 12 hr if patient weighs less than 110 lbs).

NURSING CONSIDERATIONS

See also *Nursing Considerations* for *Antiarrhythmic Agents,* p. 534.

Administration/Storage

1. Administer drug only after ECG assessment has been done.
2. Administer with caution to clients who are receiving or who have recently received other antiarrhythmic agents.
3. The extended-release capsule should not be used for initial dosage. These are intended for maintenance therapy.
4. When the client is being transferred from the regular oral capsule, the first extended-release capsule should be given 6 hr after the last regular dose.

Assessment

1. Determine if client has been taking other antiarrhythmic agents and the response to that therapy.
2. Check client history for any evidence of hypersensitivity to the drug.
3. Note any client complaint of dribbling, frequency of voiding, or sensation of bladder fullness. The condition may worsen once the client begins taking disopyramide.
4. Determine serum potassium levels and, if low, take corrective measures before initiating therapy.

Interventions

1. Clients who have been receiving other antiarrhythmic agents and who are now being placed on disopyramide therapy need to be monitored closely for anticholinergic effects.
2. Monitor BP frequently for hypotensive effect.
3. If the client is receiving the drug in the hospital, monitor ECG for QRS widening and QT prolongation. If this occurs, the drug should be discontinued.
4. Clients with poor left ventricular function are more likely to develop hypotension and require close monitoring.
5. Note symptoms of congestive heart failure, such as cough, dyspnea, moist rales, and cyanosis.
6. Monitor serum potassium levels to ensure effective response to disopyramide. Hyperkalemia increases drug toxicity.
7. Question clients about urinary hesitancy, difficulty voiding, or a sense of not completely emptying the bladder. This is particularly important in men with hypertrophy of the prostate and elderly clients who have had prior urinary tract problems. Palpate the bladder if hesitancy is severe and place client on I&O.
8. Weigh client daily and record.
9. Since the dose of medication is based on client's response and tolerance to the medication, report any untoward reactions.
10. If the ECG shows a new onset of first-degree heart block, do not administer the drug. Report the incident to the physician and anticipate the dosage of drug will be reduced.

Client/Family Teaching

1. Instruct clients how to take their own BP and assist to develop a method to maintain a written record for physician evaluation and review.
2. Increase intake of fruit juices and other bulk foods to prevent constipation.
3. For complaints of dry mouth suggest using frequent mouth rinses, chewing gum, or sucking on hard candy (use sugar-free varieties).
4. Avoid using alcohol.
5. Review the symptoms of congestive heart failure (edema, cough, sudden weight gain, dyspnea) and the importance of reporting these immediately to the physician.
6. Instruct clients to change positions slowly and to avoid hot showers, exposure to the sun, or prolonged standing.
7. Report any evidence of mental confusion.

ENCAINIDE HYDROCHLORIDE   (EN-kah-nyd)

Enkaid (Rx)

Classification: Antiarrhythmic, Class IC

Action/Kinetics: Encainide, and its active metabolites, slow conduction in the His—Purkinje system and the AV node, as well as increase the refractory period in AV pathways and in the AV node. These effects are due to a blockade of the sodium channel in the myocardium and Purkinje fibers. **Peak plasma levels:** 30–90 min. In 90% of patients, encainide is rapidly metabolized ($t^{1/2}$: 1–2 hr) to O-demethyl encainide (ODE) and 3-methoxy-O-demethyl encainide (MODE), both of which are more active than encainide. These metabolites are slowly excreted with a $t^{1/2}$ of 3–4 hr for ODE and

6–12 hr for MODE. **Time to peak plasma levels:** 30–90 min. **Time to steady-state plasma levels after multiple doses:** 3–5 days. **Therapeutic serum levels, ODE:** 0.1–0.3 mcg/mL. Ten percent of patients slowly metabolize encainide ($t\frac{1}{2}$: 6–11 hr) with few metabolites in plasma. In all patients, 3–5 days are required to achieve steady-state conditions.

Uses: Life-threatening arrhythmias such as sustained ventricular tachycardia.

Contraindications: Cardiogenic shock, preexisting second- or third-degree AV block, right bundle branch block when associated with bifascicular block (unless a pacemaker is present to sustain cardiac rhythm). Frequent premature ventricular complexes, symptomatic nonsustained ventricular arrhythmias.

Special Concerns: Use only if needed during pregnancy (category: B) and lactation. Use with caution in congestive heart failure, cardiomyopathy, sick sinus syndrome, with other drugs which affect cardiac conduction, in hepatic and renal impairment, and in electrolyte disturbances. Safety and efficacy in children under age 18 have not been determined. In geriatric patients, the dose may have to be reduced due to age-related impairment of renal function.

Side Effects: *CV:* New or worsened ventricular arrhythmias, second- or third-degree AV block, sinus bradycardia, sinus pause, sinus arrest, congestive heart failure, palpitations, premature ventricular contractions, ventricular tachycardia, syncope. *CNS:* Dizziness, headache, insomnia, nervousness, somnolence, tremor. *GI:* Nausea, vomiting, diarrhea, constipation, abdominal pain, anorexia, dyspepsia, dry mouth. *Respiratory:* Cough, dyspnea. *Other:* Asthenia, skin rash, blurred vision, abnormal vision, tinnitus, hepatitis, jaundice, increased blood glucose or increased insulin requirements in diabetic patients, paresthesia, chest pain, pain in upper and lower extremities, taste alterations.

Drug Interactions

Cardiovascular drugs	Additive effects on cardiac conduction
Cimetidine	↑ Plasma levels of encainide and active metabolites
Diuretics	Additive effects on cardiac conduction

Dosage: Capsules. Initial, adults: 25 mg q 8 hr. Increase to 35 mg t.i.d. after 3–5 days, if necessary. If desired response not achieved after an additional 3–5 days, increase dose to 50 mg t.i.d. *Patients with documented life-threatening arrhythmias:* 75 mg q.i.d. may be necessary. Maintenance doses should be lower.

NURSING CONSIDERATIONS
See also *Nursing Considerations* for *Antiarrhythmic Agents,* p. 534.

Administration/Storage
1. Clients at high risk for proarrhythmias should be hospitalized to initiate therapy. Clients should also be hospitalized if the daily dose is increased to 200 mg or greater.
2. Dosage adjustments may have to be made for clients with liver or renal impairment.
3. Three to five days should be allowed between dosage increments in order to allow for steady-state blood levels of encainide and its active metabolites to be attained.
4. The total daily dose may be given in two equally divided doses q 12 hr if the client is carefully monitored.
5. The maximum single dose should not exceed 75 mg.

6. Loading doses of encainide are not recommended.

7. Other antiarrhythmic therapy should be withdrawn for approximately two to four plasma half-lives before encainide is initiated.

Assessment

1. Determine if the client is taking other antiarrhythmic agents, ascertain last dose.

2. Check laboratory data prior to initiating therapy to detect any electrolyte imbalances or evidence of liver or renal dysfunction.

3. Note if the client has a history of fibrillation or ventricular tachycardia. Encainide may cause serious ventricular arrhythmias in these clients.

Interventions

1. If the drug is administered IV, monitor blood pressure and pulse every 5 min until stable. The client should be kept in a supine position until vital signs stabilize.

2. Some clients develop bradycardia and sinus pause. Therefore, monitor blood pressure and pulse frequently during therapy.

3. Note client complaints of dizziness, visual disturbances or headaches and report.

4. If the client has diabetes, note any increase in blood glucose levels. Anticipate the client will have increased insulin requirements.

5. If the client is also taking cimetidine, anticipate a reduced dosage of encainide will be ordered.

Client/Family Teaching

1. Review the desired effects of drug therapy with client and family.

2. Demonstrate how to take pulse and instruct to do so at least daily and record.

3. Report any side effects immediately.

4. Clients may develop an unpleasant metallic taste in their mouth. Explain that drug should not be discontinued without first reporting this side effect to the physician.

5. Stress the importance of reporting for laboratory tests and physician appointments as scheduled. If there needs to be a change, the lab and/or physician should be notified.

6. Emphasize the importance of maintaining a healthy diet, of limiting their intake of caffeine, and avoiding the use of alcoholic beverages.

FLECAINIDE ACETATE   (FLEH-kah-nyd AH-seh-tayt)

Tambocor (Rx)

See also *Antiarrhythmic Agents,* p. 533.

Classification: Antiarrhythmic, type IC.

Action/Kinetics: Flecainide produces its antiarrhythmic effect by a local anesthetic action, especially on the His—Purkinje system in the ventricle. The drug decreases single and multiple premature ventricular contractions and reduces the incidence of ventricular tachycardia. **Peak plasma levels:** 3 hr.; **steady state levels:** 3–5 days. **Effective plasma levels:** 0.2–1 mcg/mL. **t½:** 20 hr. Approximately 30% is excreted in urine unchanged. Impaired renal function decreases rate of elimination of unchanged drug. Food or antacids do not affect absorption.

Uses: Life-threatening arrhythmias manifested as sustained ventricular tachycardia.

Contraindications: Cardiogenic shock, preexisting second- or third-degree AV block, right bundle branch block when associated with bifascicular block (unless pacemaker is present to maintain cardiac rhythm). Frequent premature ventricular complexes and symptomatic nonsustained ventricular arrhythmias.

Special Concerns: Safe use has not been established in pregnancy (category: C) and lactation. Use with caution in sick sinus syndrome, congestive heart failure, myocardial infarction, in disturbances of potassium levels, in patients with permanent pacemakers or temporary pacing electrodes, renal and liver impairment. Safety and efficacy in children less than 18 years of age are not established. The incidence of proarrhythmic effects may be increased in geriatric patients.

Side Effects: *CV:* New or worsening ventricular arrhythmias, new or worsened congestive heart failure, palpitations, chest pain, sinus bradycardia, sinus pause, sinus arrest, ventricular fibrillation, ventricular tachycardia which cannot be resuscitated, second- or third-degree AV block, tachycardia, hypertension, hypotension, angina pectoris. *CNS:* Dizziness, faintness, syncope, lightheadedness, unsteadiness, headache, fatigue, paresthesia, paresis, insomnia, anxiety, malaise, vertigo, depression, seizures, euphoria, confusion, depersonalization, apathy, morbid dreams, speech disorders, stupor, amnesia, weakness. *GI:* Nausea, constipation, abdominal pain, vomiting, anorexia, dyspepsia, dry mouth, diarrhea, flatulence, change in taste. *Ophthalmic:* Blurred vision, difficulty in focusing, spots before eyes, diplopia, eye irritation, photophobia, eye pain, nystagmus, eye irritation, photophobia. *Hematologic:* Leukopenia, thrombocytopenia. *Genitourinary:* Decreased libido, impotence, urinary retention, polyuria. *Musculoskeletal:* Asthenia, tremor, ataxia, arthralgia, myalgia. *Other:* Edema, skin rashes, urticaria, exfoliative dermatitis, pruritus, dyspnea, fever, bronchospasm, flushing, sweating, swollen mouth, lips, and tongue.

Drug Interactions

Acidifying agents	↑ Renal excretion of flecainide
Alkalinizing agents	↓ Renal excretion of flecainide
Digitalis	↑ Digoxin plasma levels
Disopyramide	Additive negative inotropic effects
Propranolol	Additive negative inotropic effects; also, ↑ plasma levels of both drugs
Verapamil	Additive negative inotropic effects

Dosage: Tablets. *Sustained ventricular tachycardia:* **initial,** 100 mg q 12 hr; **then,** increase by 50 mg b.i.d. q 4 days until effective dose reached. **Usual effective dose:** 150 mg q 12 hr; dose should not exceed 400 mg daily.

NURSING CONSIDERATIONS

See also *Nursing Considerations* for *Antiarrhythmic Agents,* p. 534.

Administration/Storage

1. For most situations, therapy should be started in a hospital setting (especially in clients with symptomatic congestive heart failure, sustained ventricular arrhythmias, compensated clients with significant myocardial dysfunction, or sinus node dysfunction).

2. For clients with renal impairment, the dosage should be increased at intervals greater than 4 days. The client should be monitored carefully for adverse toxic effects.

3. The chance of toxic effects increases if the trough plasma levels exceed 1 mcg/mL.

4. If client is being transferred to flecainide from another antiarrhythmic, at least 2–4 plasma half-lives should elapse for the drug being discontinued before initiating flecainide therapy.

5. An occasional client may benefit from dosing at 8-hr intervals.

6. To minimize toxicity, the dose may be reduced once the arrhythmia is controlled.

Assessment

1. Obtain baseline ECG, electrolytes and renal function studies prior to initiating therapy.

2. Review client history for evidence of congestive heart failure, ventricular arrhythmias, sinus node dysfunction or abnormal ejection fractions.

Interventions

1. Monitor ECG for increased arrhythmias or AV block and report immediately to the physician.

2. Check serum potassium levels. Preexisting hypokalemia or hyperkalemia may alter the effects of the drug and should be corrected before starting therapy with flecainide.

3. Assess the client for labile blood pressure and document.

4. Note untoward CNS effects, such as client complaints of dizziness, visual disturbances, headaches, nausea, or depression.

5. Obtain urinary pH, to detect alkalinity or acidity. Alkalinity of the urine decreases renal excretion and acidity increases renal excretion. This in turn affects the rate of drug elimination.

6. Observe for any evidence of congestive heart failure.

7. Concomitant administration of flecainide with disopyramide, propranolol, or verapamil will promote additive negative inotropic effects.

Client/Family Teaching

1. Report any bruising or increased bleeding tendencies.

2. Observe for and report changes in elimination patterns.

3. Stress the importance of taking the medication in the dose and frequency prescribed.

INDECAINIDE HYDROCHLORIDE   (in-DEH-kah-nyd)

Decabid (Rx)

Classification: Antiarrhythmic drug, Class IC.

Action/Kinetics: Although the mechanism of action is not known with certainty, indecainide is thought to block sodium movement into Purkinje and myocardial cells resulting in stabilization of the cell membrane and a slowing of conduction of cardiac impulses. Both AV and intraventricular conduction velocities are slowed with an increase in the AV nodal effective refractory period. At doses of 200 mg daily, the drug significantly reduces left ventricular ejection fraction both at rest and during exercise. Food has no effect on absorption and there is no first-pass effect. **Peak serum levels:** 4 hr. **t½:** Approximately 8 hr in normal patients. Indecainide is metabolized in the liver to inactive and one active (desisopropylindecainide) metabolite. Approximately 80% excreted in the urine (65% unchanged) and 17% in the feces.

Uses: Treatment of life-threatening ventricular arrhythmias (such as sustained ventricular tachycardia). Use should be reserved for those patients in whom benefits outweigh the risks of using the drug.

Contraindications: Use for less severe ventricular arrhythmias. Pre-existing second- or third-degree AV block or right bundle branch block associated with a left hemiblock (unless patient has a pacemaker to sustain cardiac rhythm). Cardiogenic shock. Use during lactation.

Special Concerns: Pregnancy category: B. Safety and effectiveness have not been determined in children less than 18 years of age. Use with caution in patients with impaired renal function. Use with extreme caution in patients with sick sinus syndrome (drug may cause sinus bradycardia, sinus pause, or sinus arrest).

Side Effects: *CV:* Possibly increased mortality or nonfatal cardiac arrest in patients with asymptomatic non-life-threatening ventricular arrhythmias who experienced a myocardial infarction between 6 days and 2 years before use of the drug (this effect noted with use of encainide or flecainide). Proarrhythmic effects including new or worsening of arrhythmias; causing or worsening of congestive heart failure. Possibility of increased pacemaker thresholds. First- and third-degree AV block, syncope, sinus bradycardia, sinus pause, sinus arrest, angina pectoris, hypertension, hypotension, bundle branch block, palpitations. *GI:* Nausea, abdominal pain, constipation, diarrhea, dry mouth, dyspepsia, alteration in taste, vomiting. *CNS:* Dizziness, headache, circumoral paresthesia, insomnia, anxiety, emotional lability, vertigo, abnormal dreams, agitation, ataxia, confusion, nervousness, paresthesia, hypesthesia, seizures. *Respiratory:* Dyspnea, rhinitis, increased cough, chest pain. *Whole body:* Asthenia, back pain, general pain, fever, malaise. *Dermatologic:* Rash (including maculopapular or petechial), urticaria. *Hematologic:* Eosinophilia, anemia, leukopenia, thrombocytopenia. *Miscellaneous:* Hyperglycemia, tinnitus, diplopia, abnormal accommodation, arthralgia.

Drug Interactions

Antiarrhythmic drugs	Additive pharmacologic effects
Cimetidine	Significant ↑ in serum levels of indecainide

Laboratory Test Interfernces: ↑ BUN, creatinine clearance, AST, ALT.

Dosage: Extended-release tablets. Adults, initial: 50 mg b.i.d. at 12-hr intervals. After a minimum of 4 days, dose can be increased to 75 mg b.i.d. if necessary. If the desired effect is not observed after 4 more days, the dosage may be increased to 100 mg b.i.d. Some patients may require as much as 300 mg daily and should be hospitalized for initial dosing at this level. In patients with a creatinine clearance of 30 mL/min or less, therapy should be initiated with a single daily dose of 50 mg; the dose may be increased to 75 mg once daily after 7 days. Thereafter, increase dose slowly (no more frequently than q 7 days) up to a maximum of 150 mg daily if necessary.

NURSING CONSIDERATIONS
See also *Nursing Considerations* for *Antiarrhythmic Agents,* p. 534.

Administration/Storage
1. Therapy should be initiated in a hospital with facilities for monitoring cardiac rhythm as many of the serious proarrhythmic effects are observed within the first 1–2 weeks of therapy.
2. Extended-release tablets should be swallowed whole and not crushed or chewed.
3. Increments in dosage should not be undertaken more often than every 4 days.
4. When transferring clients from other antiarrhythmic drugs, the drug should be withdrawn for 2–5 plasma half-lives before beginning indecainide therapy. If withdrawal is potentially life-threatening, the client should be hospitalized and closely monitored.

Assessment
1. Obtain baseline ECG to determine if client has any evidence of advanced AV block, as drug is contraindicated under these circumstances.
2. Note any client history of congestive heart failure.

Interventions

1. Indecainide is only recommended for the treatment of life-threatening ventricular arrhythmias. Client should be in a closely monitored environment and have rhythm strips to document these arrhythmias before, during and throughout initial dosing adjustments.

2. Review serum electrolytes. Pre-existing hypokalemia or hyperkalemia should be corrected before administration of indecainide.

3. Note renal function studies to determine if there is any evidence of dysfunction. Anticipate reduced dose and dosing intervals of 7 days when adjusting the dosage for clients with renal dysfunction.

4. Clients treated successfully with indecainide usually manifested trough serum levels between 300–600 mcg/L. Thus, periodic monitoring of such levels may be useful in managing drug therapy.

5. Observe clients for complaints of dizziness, weakness, chest pain, or dyspnea as these are frequent side effects of drug therapy and should be documented and reported to the physician.

LIDOCAINE HYDROCHLORIDE   (LIE-doh-kayn)

IM: Lidopen Auto-Injector, Xylocaine HCl IM for Cardiac Arrhythmias (Rx). Direct IV or IV Admixtures: Lidocaine HCl without Preservatives, Xylocaine HCl IV for Cardiac Arrhythmias, Xylocard✳ (Rx). IV Infusion: Lidocaine HCl in 5% Dextrose (Rx)

See also *Antiarrhythmic Agents,* p. 533.

Classification: Antiarrhythmic, type IB.

Action/Kinetics: Lidocaine shortens the refractory period and suppresses the automaticity of ectopic foci without affecting conduction of impulses through cardiac tissue. It does not affect blood pressure, cardiac output, or myocardial contractility. **IV: Onset,** 45–90 sec; **duration:** 10–20 min. **IM, Onset,** 5–15 min; **duration,** 60–90 min. **t½:** 1–2 hr. **Therapeutic serum levels:** 1.5–6 mcg/mL. **Time to steady-state plasma levels:** 3–4 hr (8–10 hr in patients with acute myocardial infarction). **Protein-binding:** 40–80%. Since lidocaine has little effect on conduction at normal antiarrhythmic doses, it should be used in acute situations (instead of procainamide) in instances in which heart block might occur.

Uses: IV: Treatment of acute ventricular arrhythmias such as those following myocardial infarctions or occurring during surgery. The drug is ineffective against atrial arrhythmias. **IM:** Certain emergency situations (e.g., ECG equipment not available; mobile coronary care unit, under advice of a physician).

Contraindications: Hypersensitivity to amide-type local anesthetics, Adams-Stokes syndrome, or total or partial heart block. Use with caution in the presence of liver or severe kidney disease, CHF, marked hypoxia, severe respiratory depression, or shock.

Special Concerns: Use with caution during pregnancy (pregnancy category: B), labor, and delivery and in children. In geriatric patients, the rate and dose for IV infusion should be decreased by one-half and slowly adjusted.

Side Effects: *CV:* Precipitation or aggravation of arrhythmias (following IV use), hypotension, bradycardia (with possible cardiac arrest), cardiovascular collapse. *CNS:* Dizziness, restlessness, apprehension, euphoria, stupor, convulsions, unconsciousness. *Respiratory:* Difficulties in breathing or swallowing, respiratory depression. *Allergic:* Rash, urticaria, edema, anaphylaxis. *Other:* Tinnitus, blurred vision, vomiting, numbness, sensation of heat or cold, twitching, tremors.

During anesthesia, cardiovascular depression may be the first sign of lidocaine toxicity. During other usage, convulsions are the first sign of lidocaine toxicity.

Drug Interactions

Aminoglycosides	↑ Neuromuscular blockade
Cimetidine	↑ Effects of lidocaine
Metoprolol	↓ Lidocaine clearance
Phenytoin	IV phenytoin → excessive cardiac depression
Procainamide	Additive neurologic side effects
Propranolol	↓ Lidocaine clearance
Succinylcholine	↑ Action of succinylcholine by ↓ plasma protein binding
Tubocurarine	↑ Neuromuscular blockade

Dosage: IV bolus: 50–100 mg at rate of 25–50 mg/min. Repeat if necessary after 5-min interval. Onset of action is 10 sec. **Maximum dose/hr:** 200–300 mg. **Infusion:** 20–50 mcg/kg at a rate of 1–4 mg/min. No more than 300 mg/hr should be given. **IM:** 4.5 mg/kg (approximately 300 mg for a 70-kg adult). Switch to IV lidocaine or PO antiarrhythmics as soon as possible.

Pediatric: initial IV bolus dose, *antiarrhythmic:* 1 mg/kg at a rate of 25–50 mg/min; the dose can be repeated after 5 min if needed but the total dose should not exceed 3 mg/kg. **Then,** infuse 30 mcg/kg/min (range: 20–50 mcg/min).

NURSING CONSIDERATIONS

See also *Nursing Considerations* for *Antiarrhythmic Agents,* p. 534.

Administration/Storage

1. *Do not add lidocaine to blood transfusion assembly.*
2. Lidocaine solutions that contain epinephrine should not be used to treat arrhythmias. Make certain that vial states, "For Cardiac Arrhythmias."
3. Use 5% dextrose in water to prepare solution; this is stable for 24 hr.
4. IV infusions should be administered with an electronic infusion device.
5. IV bolus dosage should be reduced in clients over 70 years of age, in those with CHF or liver disease, and in clients taking cimetidine or propranolol (i.e., where metabolism of lidocaine is reduced).

Assessment

1. Note the age of the client. Elderly clients who have hepatic or renal disease or who weigh less than 100 pounds will need to be watched especially closely for untoward effects.
2. Note any client history of hypersensitivity to amide-type local anesthetics. These clients can be expected to have untoward reactions to lidocaine.
3. Obtain blood pressure, pulse and respirations to use as baseline data against which to measure response to the drug therapy.

Interventions

1. All clients who receive lidocaine by the IV route should be in a monitored environment.

2. Check prefilled syringes closely to ensure the appropriate dose has been obtained. Lidocaine prefilled syringes come in both milligrams and grams.

3. Observe clients for myocardial depression, variations of rhythm or aggravation of the arrhythmia. Document and report these changes since drug administration may need to be altered.

4. Assess BP frequently during IV therapy. Antiarrhythmic clients are particularly susceptible to hypotension and cardiac collapse.

5. Monitor cardiac rate. Bradycardia may be a sign of impending cardiac collapse.

6. Note evidence of CNS effects such as twitching and tremors. These symptoms may precede convulsions.

7. Assess for respiratory depression, characterized by slow, shallow respirations.

8. Note any sudden changes in the client's mental status. Notify physician immediately, as the dose of drug may need to be decreased.

9. If an adverse reaction occurs, be prepared to discontinue the medication. Have emergency drugs and equipment readily available.

10. The administration of the drug should be titrated to the client's response and within the written guidelines the physician has established.

11. Anticipate reduced dosage in the elderly and clients with CHF, liver disease, and if concomitantly taking cimetidine or propranolol.

MEXILETINE HYDROCHLORIDE (mek-SIL-eh-teen)
Mexitil (Rx)

See also *Antiarrhythmic Agents,* p. 533.

Classification: Antiarrhythmic, type IB.

Action/Kinetics: Mexiletine is similar to lidocaine but is effective orally. The drug inhibits the flow of sodium into the cell, thereby reducing the rate of rise of the action potential. Blood pressure and pulse rate are not affected following use, but there may be a small decrease in cardiac output and an increase in peripheral vascular resistance. The drug also has both local anesthetic and anticonvulsant effects. **Onset:** 30–120 min. **Peak blood levels:** 2–3 hr. **Therapeutic plasma levels:** 0.5–2 mcg/mL. **Plasma t½:** 10–12 hr. Approximately 10% excreted unchanged in the urine; acidification of the urine enhances excretion, while alkalinization decreases excretion.

Uses: Frequent premature ventricular contractions, unifocal or multifocal, couplets and ventricular tachycardia.

Contraindications: Cardiogenic shock, preexisting second- or third-degree AV block (if no pacemaker is present). Lactation.

Special Concerns: Pregnancy category: C. Use with caution in hypotension and severe congestive heart failure. Dosage has not been established in children.

Side Effects: *CV:* Worsening of arrhythmias, palpitations, chest pain. *GI:* Nausea, vomiting, heartburn, diarrhea or constipation, changes in appetite. *CNS:* Lightheadedness, dizziness, tremor, coordination difficulties, changes in sleep habits, fatigue, weakness, tinnitus, paresthesias, depression, confusion, difficulty with speech, headache. *Miscellaneous:* Blurred vision, dyspnea, rash, edema, arthralgia, dry mouth, elevated liver SGOT.

Drug Interactions

Cimetidine	↑ Plasma levels of mexiletine
Phenobarbital	↓ Plasma levels of mexiletine
Phenytoin	↓ Plasma levels of mexiletine
Rifampin	↓ Plasma levels of mexiletine

Dosage: Capsules. Adults, individualized, initial: 200 mg q 8 hr if rapid control of arrhythmia not required; **then,** 300–400 mg q 8 hr, depending on response and tolerance of patient. If adequate response is achieved with 300 mg or less q 8 hr, the same total daily dose may be given in divided doses q 12 hr (i.e., 450 mg q 12 hr). *Rapid control of arrhythmias,* **initial loading dose:** 400 mg followed by a 200-mg dose in 8 hr.

If transferring to mexiletine from other Class I antiarrhythmics, mexiletine may be initiated at a dose of 200 mg and then titrated according to the response at the following times: 6–12 hr after the last dose of quinidine sulfate, 3–6 hr after the last dose of procainamide, 6–12 hr after the last dose of disopyramide, or 8–12 hr after the last dose of tocainide.

NURSING CONSIDERATIONS

See also *Nursing Considerations* for *Antiarrhythmic Agents,* p. 534.

Administration/Storage

1. Two to three days should elapse between dosage adjustments; the dose may be adjusted in 50- to 100-mg increments up or down.
2. When transferring to mexiletine, the client should be hospitalized if there is a chance that withdrawal of the previous antiarrhythmic may produce life-threatening arrhythmias.

Interventions

1. Review ECG for increased arrhythmias and report.
2. Observe for untoward CNS effects such as dizziness, tremor, impaired coordination, nausea, and vomiting.
3. Obtain urinary pH to determine alkalinity or acidity. Alkalinity decreases renal excretion and acidity increases renal excretion of the drug.

Client/Family Teaching

1. Take medication with food or an antacid.
2. Report any bruising, bleeding, fevers, or sore throat.
3. Note any increase in palpitations and report immediately.

PHENYTOIN (DIPHENYLHYDANTOIN) (FEN-ih-toyn, dye-FEN-ill-hy-DAN-toyn)
Dilantin Infatab, Dilantin-30 Pediatric, Dilantin-125 (Rx)

PHENYTOIN SODIUM, EXTENDED (FEN-ih-toyn)
Dilantin Kapseals (Rx)

PHENYTOIN SODIUM, PARENTERAL (FEN-ih-toyn)
Dilantin Sodium (Rx)

PHENYTOIN SODIUM PROMPT (DIPHENYLHYDANTOIN SODIUM) (FEN-ih-toyn)

Diphenylan Sodium (Rx)

See also *Anticonvulsants,* p. 719, and *Antiarrhythmics,* p. 533.

Classification: Anticonvulsant, hydantoin type; antiarrhythmic (Type I).

Action/Kinetics: Phenytoin acts in the motor cortex of the brain to reduce the spread of electrical discharges from the rapidly firing epileptic foci in this area. This is accomplished by stabilizing hyperexcitable cells possibly by affecting sodium efflux. Also, phenytoin decreases activity of centers in the brain stem responsible for the tonic phase of grand mal seizures. This drug has few sedative effects.

Serum levels must be monitored because the serum concentrations of phenytoin increase disproportionately as the dosage is increased. Phenytoin extended is designed for once-a-day dosage. It has a slow dissolution rate—no more than 35% in 30 min, 30%–70% in 60 min, and less than 85% in 120 min. Absorption is variable following oral dosage. **Peak serum levels: PO,** 4–8 hr. Since the rate and extent of absorption depend on the particular preparation, the same product should be used for a particular patient. **Peak serum levels (following IM):** 24 hr (wide variation). **Therapeutic serum levels:** 10–20 mcg/mL. **t½:** 8–60 hr (average: 20–30 hr). Steady state attained 7–10 days after initiation. Phenytoin is biotransformed in the liver. Both inactive metabolites and unchanged drug are excreted in the urine.

As an antiarrhythmic, phenytoin increases the electrical stimulation threshold of heart muscle, although it is less effective than quinidine, procainamide, or lidocaine. **Onset:** 30–60 min. **Duration:** 24 hr or more. **t½:** 22–36 hr. **Therapeutic serum level:** 10–20 mcg/mL.

Uses: Chronic epilepsy, especially of the tonic-clonic, psychomotor type. Not effective against absence seizures and may even increase the frequency of seizures in this disorder. Parenteral phenytoin is sometimes used to treat status epilepticus and to control seizures during neurosurgery.

Orally for certain premature ventricular contractions and IV for premature ventricular contractions and tachycardia. The drug is particularly useful for arrhythmias produced by digitalis overdosage.

Investigational: Paroxysmal choreoathetosis; to treat blistering and erosions in patients with recessive dystrophic epidermolysis bullosa; episodic dyscontrol; trigeminal neuralgia; as a muscle relaxant in neuromyotonia, myotonia congenita, or myotonic muscular dystrophy; to treat cardiac symptoms in overdosage of tricyclic antidepressants.

Contraindications: Hypersensitivity to hydantoins or exfoliative dermatitis. Administer with extreme caution to patients with a history of asthma or other allergies, impaired renal or hepatic function, and heart disease. Should not be administered to nursing mothers.

Special Concerns: Use with caution in porphyria.

Side Effects: *CNS:* Drowsiness, incoordination, ataxia, slurred speech, dizziness, extrapyramidal reactions, paradoxical increase in motor activity, psychotomimetic effects including hallucinations and delusions, fatigue, insomnia, and apathy. *GI:* Nausea, vomiting, either diarrhea or constipation. *Dermatologic:* Various dermatoses including a measles-like rash (common), scarlatiniform, maculopapular, and urticarial rashes. Rarely, drug-induced lupus erythematosus, Stevens-Johnson syndrome, exfoliative or purpuric dermatitis, and toxic epidermal necrolysis. Skin reactions may necessitate withdrawal of therapy. *Hematopoietic:* Megaloblastic anemia, lymph node hyperplasia, thrombocytopenia, leukopenia, agranulocytosis, pancytopenia, anemias including hemolytic and aplastic. *Hepatic:* Hepatitis, jaundice. *Miscellaneous:* Hyperglycemia, osteomalacia, gingival hyperplasia, hirsutism, pulmonary fibrosis, alopecia, edema, photophobia.

Rapid parenteral administration may cause serious cardiovascular effects, including hypotension, arrhythmias, cardiovascular collapse, and heart block, as well as CNS depression.

Overdosage is characterized by nystagmus, ataxia, dysarthria, coma, unresponsive pupils, and hypotension, as well as by some of the CNS effects described above.

Many patients have a partial deficiency in the ability of the liver to degrade phenytoin, and as a result, toxicity may develop after a small oral dose. Liver and kidney function tests and hematopoietic studies are indicated prior to and periodically during drug therapy.

Drug Interactions

Alcohol, ethyl	In alcoholics, ↓ effect of phenytoin due to ↑ breakdown by liver
Allopurinol	↑ Effect of phenytoin due to ↓ breakdown in liver
Antacids	↓ Effect of phenytoin due to ↓ GI absorption
Anticoagulants, oral	↑ Effect of phenytoin due to ↓ breakdown by liver. Also, possible ↑ in anticoagulant effect due to ↓ plasma protein binding
Antidepressants, tricyclic	May ↑ incidence of epileptic seizures or ↑ effect of phenytoin
Barbiturates	Effect of phenytoin may be ↑, ↓, or not changed; possible ↑ effect of barbiturates
Benzodiazepines	↑ Effect of phenytoin due to ↓ breakdown by liver
Carbamazepine	↓ Effect of phenytoin due to ↑ breakdown by liver
Chloral hydrate	↓ Effect of phenytoin due to ↑ breakdown by liver
Chloramphenicol	↑ Effect of phenytoin due to ↓ breakdown by liver
Cimetidine	↑ Effect of phenytoin due to ↓ breakdown by liver
Contraceptives, oral	Estrogen-induced fluid retention may precipitate seizures; also, ↓ effect of contraceptives due to ↑ breakdown by liver
Corticosteroids	Effect of corticosteroids ↓ due to ↑ breakdown by liver
Cyclosporine	↓ Effect of cyclosporine due to ↑ breakdown by liver
Diazoxide	↓ Effect of phenytoin due to ↑ breakdown by liver
Dicumarol	Phenytoin ↓ effect of dicumarol
Digitalis glycosides	↓ Effect of digitalis glycosides due to ↑ breakdown by liver
Disulfiram (Antabuse)	↑ Effect of phenytoin due to ↓ breakdown by liver
Dopamine	IV phenytoin results in hypotension and bradycardia
Doxycycline	↓ Effect of doxycycline due to ↑ breakdown by liver

Drug Interactions

Estrogens	See *Contraceptives, Oral*
Folic acid	↓ Phenytoin blood levels due to ↑ breakdown by liver
Furosemide	↓ Effect of furosemide due to ↓ absorption
Haloperidol	↓ Effect of haloperidol due to ↑ breakdown by liver
Isoniazid	↑ Effect of phenytoin due to ↓ breakdown by liver
Levodopa	Phenytoin ↓ effect of levodopa
Meperidine	↓ Effect of meperidine due to ↑ breakdown by liver
Methadone	↓ Effect of methadone due to ↑ breakdown by liver
Methotrexate	↓ Effect of phenytoin due to ↓ absorption from GI tract
Metyrapone	↓ Effect of metyrapone due to ↑ breakdown by liver
Phenacemide	↑ Effect of phenytoin due to ↓ breakdown by liver
Phenothiazines	↑ Effect of phenytoin due to ↓ breakdown by liver
Phenylbutazone	↑ Effect of phenytoin due to ↓ breakdown by liver and ↓ plasma protein binding
Primidone	Possible ↑ effect of primidone
Quinidine	↓ Effect of quinidine due to ↑ breakdown by liver
Salicylates	↑ Effect of phenytoin by ↓ plasma protein binding
Sulfonamides	↑ Effect of phenytoin due to ↓ breakdown in liver
Sulfonylureas	↓ Effect of sulfonylureas
Theophylline	↓ Effect of both drugs due to ↑ breakdown by liver
Trimethoprim	↑ Effect of phenytoin due to ↓ breakdown by liver
Valproic acid	↑ Chance of phenytoin toxicity
Vinblastine	↑ Effect of phenytoin due to ↓ breakdown by liver

Laboratory Test Interferences: Alters liver function tests, ↑ blood glucose values, and ↓ PBI values. ↑ Gamma globulins. Phenytoin ↓ immunoglobulins A and G. False + Coombs' test.

Dosage: Oral Suspension, Chewable Tablets. *Seizures.* **Adults:** 125 mg t.i.d. initially; adjust dosage at 7–10 day intervals until seizures are controlled; **usual, maintenance:** 300–400 mg/day, although 600 mg/day may be required in some. **Pediatric: initial,** 5 mg/kg/day in 2–3 divided doses; **maintenance,** 4–8 mg/kg (up to maximum of 300 mg/day). Children over 6 years may require up to 300 mg/day. **Geriatric:** 3 mg/kg initially in divided doses; **then,** adjust dosage according to serum levels and response. Once dosage level has been established, the extended capsules may be used for once-a-day dosage.

Capsules, Extended-release Capsules. *Seizures:* **Adults, initial** 100 mg t.i.d.; adjust dose at 7–10 day intervals until control is achieved. An initial loading dose of 12–15 mg/kg divided into 2–3 doses over 6 hr followed by 100 mg t.i.d. on subsequent days may be preferred if seizures are frequent. **Pediatric:** See dose for oral suspension and chewable tablets.

IV. *Status epilepticus:* 20 mg/kg at a rate not to exceed 50 mg/min; **then,** 100 mg q 6–8 hr at a rate not exceeding 50 mg/min. Oral administration at a dose of 5 mg/kg daily divided into 2–4 doses should begin 12–24 hr after a loading dose is given. **Pediatric:** 15–20 mg/kg given at a rate of 1 mg/kg, not to exceed 50 mg/min. **IM** dose should be 50% greater than the PO dose. *Neurosurgery:* 100–200 mg IM q 4 hr during and after surgery (during first 24 hr, no more than 1,000 mg should be administered; after first day, give maintenance dosage).

Arrhythmias: **PO:** 200–400 mg daily. **IV:** 100 mg q 5 min up to maximum of 1 g.

Full effectiveness of orally administered hydantoins is delayed and may take 6–9 days to be fully established. A similar period of time will elapse before effects disappear completely.

When hydantoins are substituted for or added to another anticonvulsant medication, their dosage is gradually increased, while dosage of the other drug is decreased proportionally.

NURSING CONSIDERATIONS

See also *Nursing Considerations* for *Anticonvulsants,* p. 720, and *Antiarrhythmics,* p. 534.

Administration/Storage

1. For parenteral preparations:
   - Only a clear solution of the drug may be used.
   - Dilute with special diluent supplied by manufacturer.
   - Shake the vials until the solution is clear. It may take about 10 min for the drug to dissolve.
   - To hasten the process, warm the vial in warm water after adding the diluent.
   - The drug is incompatible with acid solutions.
2. IV phenytoin may form a precipitate. Therefore flush tubing thoroughly with sodium chloride before and after IV administration. *Do not* use dextrose solutions. Use an in-line filter to collect microscopic particulate matter.
3. Following the IV administration of the drug, administer sodium chloride injection through the same needle or IV catheter to avoid local irritation of the vein. This is caused by alkalinity of the solution.
4. For treatment of status epilepticus, inject the IV slowly at a rate not to exceed 50 mg/min. If necessary, the dose may be repeated 30 min after the initial administration.
5. Avoid subcutaneous or perivascular injections. Pain, inflammation, and necrosis may be caused by the highly alkaline solutions.
6. *Do not* add phenytoin to an already running IV solution.
7. If the client is receiving tube feedings of Isocal or Osmolite there may be interference with the absorption of oral phenytoin. Therefore, do not administer them together.

Assessment

1. Note the history and nature of the client's epileptic seizures.
2. Determine if the client is hypersensitive to hydantoins or has exfoliative dermatitis.
3. If the client is female and pregnant note that she should not breast feed the baby following delivery.
4. Obtain liver and renal function studies as baseline data against which to measure alterations once therapy is initiated.

Interventions

1. Monitor serum drug levels on a routine basis. Check prefilled syringe for appropriate dose.
2. Seven to 10 days may be required to achieve recommended serum levels. The drug is metabolized much more slowly by elderly clients.
3. If the client is receiving drugs that interact with hydantoins or has impaired liver function, the serum phenytoin level should be done periodically. The clinically effective range is 10–20 μg/mL.
4. Monitor the complete blood cell count and white cell differential throughout drug therapy.
5. During the IV administration, monitor BP closely for hypotension.
6. If client complains of weakness, ease of fatigue, headaches, or feeling faint, assess for signs of folic acid deficiency. Document and report to the physician. Invite a dietitian to review food intake and diet with the client.
7. Note if the client is developing an overgrowth of hair, coarse hair or acne. Document and report these symptoms to the physician. Provide emotional support and discourage the client from discontinuing therapy because of these side effects. Consult a dermatologist as needed.
8. The drug may alter thyroid function results. If thyroid studies are conducted, for ensured accuracy, they should be repeated 10 days after therapy has been discontinued.

Client/Family Teaching

1. Review symptoms of overdose and instruct client to notify the physician should any of these occur.
2. Do not substitute phenytoin products or exchange brands, as bioavailability of phenytoin may vary. Seizure control may be lost, or toxic blood levels may develop if a substitution is made.
3. Prompt release forms of the medication cannot be substituted for another unless the dosage is also adjusted.
   - If the client is taking phenytoin extended, he should not substitute chewable tablets for capsules. The strengths of the medications are not equal.
   - Clients taking phenytoin extended should check the labels of the bottle carefully. Chewable tablets are never in the extended form.
   - Clients taking phenytoin extended should take only a single dose of medication a day. It should be taken as directed by the physician. Also, take only the brand prescribed by the physician.
4. If the client misses a dose of medication, take the dose as soon as it is remembered. Then resume the usual schedule. Do not, however, double up to make up for the missed dose of drug. If the doses of drug are scheduled throughout the day, and one of the doses is missed, take the drug as soon as it is realized that the dose has been missed unless it is within 4 hours of the next dose of drug. In that case, omit the missed dose unless otherwise instructed.
5. Take with food to minimize GI upset.
6. Avoid ingestion of alcohol.
7. Do not take any other medication without medical supervision. Hydantoins interact with many other medications, and the addition of other drugs may require adjustment of the anticonvulsant dose.
8. If the client has diabetes mellitus, blood glucose levels should be monitored frequently when initiating therapy, or if the client is having the dosage of phenytoin adjusted. It may be necessary to adjust insulin dosage and/or the client's diet.
9. Clients with diabetes should report any changes in glucose determinations with urine tests and/or finger sticks to the physician.

10. Warn that hydantoins may cause the urine to appear pink, red, or brown.

11. To minimize bleeding from the gums, practice good oral hygiene. Client should be encouraged to brush teeth with a soft toothbrush, massage the gums and floss every day.

12. Hydantoin has an androgenic effect on the hair follicle. Clients may develop acne. They should be encouraged to practice good skin care.

13. Report any excessive growth of hair on the face and trunk, and any discolorations or skin rash to the physician.

14. Stress the importance of reporting for laboratory studies as ordered including a complete blood count, drug levels, and renal and liver function studies on a regular basis.

15. Do not abruptly stop medications without physician consent.

16. Report all bothersome side effects as these effects may be dose-related.

17. Provide sexually active women of childbearing age with birth control information while receiving phenytoin therapy.

Evaluation

1. Assess client/family knowledge and understanding of illness, response to therapy and to teaching.

2. Observe for freedom from complications of drug therapy.

3. Note any evidence of noncompliance with the drug regimen and determine the cause.

4. Determine serum drug level.

PROCAINAMIDE HYDROCHLORIDE   (proh-**KAY**-nah-myd)

Procan SR, Promine, Pronestyl, Pronestyl-SR (Rx)

See also *Antiarrhythmic Agents,* p. 533.

Classification: Antiarrhythmic, type IA.

Action/Kinetics: Procainamide produces a direct cardiac effect to prolong the refractory period of the heart and depress the conduction of the cardiac impulse. Large doses may cause AV block. It has some anticholinergic and local anesthetic effects. **Onset: PO,** 30 min; **IV,** 1–5 min. **Time to peak effect, PO:** 60–90 min; **IM,** 15–60 min; **IV,** immediate. **Duration:** 3 hr. **t½:** 2.5–4.5 hr. **Therapeutic serum level:** 4–8 mcg/mL. **Protein binding:** 15%. From 50–60% excreted unchanged.

Uses: Ventricular tachycardia, atrial fibrillation, resistant paroxysmal atrial tachycardia. Emergency treatment of ventricular tachycardia, digitalis intoxication, prophylactic control of tachycardia for patients at risk during anesthesia or undergoing thoracic surgery.

Contraindications: Hypersensitivity to drug, complete AV heart block, second- or third-degree AV heart block, myasthenia gravis, or blood dyscrasias.

Special Concerns: Safe use during pregnancy (pregnancy category: C) and lactation has not been established. Use with extreme caution in patients for whom a sudden drop in BP could be detrimental, in patients with liver or kidney dysfunction, and in those with bronchial asthma or other respiratory disorders. Procainamide may cause more hypotension in geriatric patients; also, in this population, the dose may have to be decreased due to age-related decreases in renal function.

Side Effects: *CV:* Following IV use: Hypotension, ventricular asystole or fibrillation, partial or complete heart block. *GI:* Nausea, vomiting, diarrhea, anorexia, bitter taste, abdominal pain. *Hematologic:* Thrombocytopenia, agranulocytosis. *Allergic:* Urticaria, pruritus, angioneurotic edema, maculopapular rash. *CNS:* Depression, giddiness, psychoses, hallucinations. *Other:* Lupus erythematosus-like syndrome, especially in those on maintenance therapy. Also, granulomatous hepatitis, weakness, fever, chills.

Drug Interactions

Acetazolamide	↑ Effect of procainamide due to ↓ excretion by kidney
Anticholinergic agents, atropine	Additive anticholinergic effects
Antihypertensive agents	Additive hypotensive effect
Cholinergic agents	Anticholinergic activity of procainamide antagonizes effect of cholinergic drugs
Cimetidine	↑ Effect of procainamide due to ↓ excretion by kidney
Ethanol	↓ Effect of procainamide due to ↑ rate of breakdown by liver
Kanamycin	Procainamide ↑ muscle relaxation produced by kanamycin
Lidocaine	Additive neurologic side effects
Magnesium salts	Procainamide ↑ muscle relaxation produced by magnesium salts
Neomycin	Procainamide ↑ muscle relaxation produced by neomycin
Sodium bicarbonate	↑ Effect of procainamide due to ↓ excretion by the kidney
Succinylcholine	Procainamide ↑ muscle relaxation produced by succinylcholine

Laboratory Test Interferences: May affect liver function tests. False + ↑ serum alkaline phosphatase.

Dosage: Capsules/Tablets. Adults, initial: *Atrial arrhythmias:* **initial,** 1.25 g followed in 1 hr by 0.75 g; **then,** if no ECG changes, 0.5–1.0 g q 2 hr until arrhythmia stopped. **Maintenance:** 0.5–1.0 g q 4–6 hr. *Premature ventricular contractions:* 50 mg/kg daily in divided doses q 3 hr. *Ventricular tachycardia:* **initial,** 1.0 g; **then,** 6 mg/kg q 3 hr. **Pediatric,** *antiarrhythmic:* 12.5 mg/kg (375 mg/m²) q.i.d. **Sustained-release Tablets:** Not recommended for initial therapy. **Maintenance:** *Atrial arrhythmias,* 1 g/6 hr. **Maintenance:** *ventricular arrhythmias,* 50 mg/kg/day in divided doses q 6 hr.

IM: Adults, 0.5–1.0 g q 4–8 hr until PO therapy possible. *Arrhythmias associated with surgery or anesthesia:* 0.1–0.5 g IM.

Direct IV use: 100 mg q 5 min by slow IV injection at a rate not to exceed 25–50 mg/min; give until arrhythmia stops or until 0.5 g is administered; **maintenance:** IV infusion, 2–6 mg/min. **IV infusion: initial,** 500–600 mg over 25–30 min; **then,** 2–6 mg/min. Switch to PO therapy as soon as possible, but wait at least 3–4 hr after the last IV dose.

NURSING CONSIDERATIONS

See also *Nursing Considerations* for *Antiarrhythmic Agents,* p. 534.

Administration/Storage

1. IV use should be reserved for emergency situations.

2. For IV initial therapy, the drug should be diluted with 5% dextrose and administered slowly to minimize side effects.

3. For IV solutions, dose is usually 2–6 mg/min. Drug solutions should be administered with an electronic infusion device for safety and accuracy.

4. Discard solutions of drug that are darker than light amber or otherwise colored. Solutions that have turned slightly yellow on standing may be used. Consult with pharmacist for clarification.

5. Extended-release tablets are not recommended for use in children.

Interventions

1. Place client in a monitored environment during IV administration. Have emergency drugs and equipment readily available.

2. Place client in a supine position during IV infusion and monitor BP frequently. Be prepared to discontinue infusion if diastolic BP falls 15 mm Hg or more during administration, or if increased AV block is noted on ECG. Notify physician.

3. Assess clients on oral drug maintenance for symptoms of lupus erythematosus, as manifested by polyarthralgia, arthritis, pleuritic pain, fever, myalgia, and skin lesions.

4. Weigh clients and assess GI symptoms. If severe and persistent the physician may permit the client to take the medication with meals or with a snack to ensure compliance with therapy.

5. Monitor complete blood count, antinuclear antibody titers, and procainamide levels throughout therapy.

Client/Family Teaching

1. Review the anticipated results of therapy with the client and family.

2. Advise to take the medication with a full glass of water to lessen GI symptoms. The drug should be taken either 1 hour before or 2 hours after meals unless otherwise ordered by the physician.

3. Take medication only as directed. Set an alarm clock to awaken through the night to take the drug as ordered.

4. If prescribed sustained-release preparations, they should be swallowed whole. They should not be crushed, broken or chewed.

5. Report any sore throat, fever, rash, chills, bruising or diarrhea.

6. Stress the importance of reporting for scheduled laboratory studies.

PROPAFENONE HYDROCHLORIDE   (PROH-pah-feh-nohn)

Rythmol (Rx)

Classification: Antiarrhythmic, type IC.

Action/Kinetics: Propafenone manifests local anesthetic effects and a direct stabilizing action on the myocardium. The drug reduces upstroke velocity (Phase O) of the monophasic action potential, reduces the fast inward current carried by sodium ions in the Purkinje fibers, increases diastolic excitability threshold, and prolongs the effective refractory period. Also, spontaneous activity is decreased. The drug has slight beta-adrenergic blocking activity. **Peak plasma levels:** 3.5 hr. **Therapeutic plasma levels:** 0.5–3 mcg/mL. Significant first-pass effect. Most patients metabolize propafenone rapidly ($t^1/_2$: 2–10 hr) to two active metabolites: 5-hydroxypropafenone and N-depropylpropafenone. However, approximately 10% of patients (as well as those taking quinidine) metabolize the drug more slowly ($t^1/_2$: 10–32 hr). However, because the 5-hydroxy metabolite is not formed in slow metabolizers and because steady-state levels are reached after 4–5 days in all patients, the recommended dosing regimen is the same for all patients.

Uses: Sustained ventricular tachycardia that is life-threatening.

Contraindications: Uncontrolled congestive heart failure, cardiogenic shock, sick sinus node syndrome or atrioventricular block in the absence of an artificial pacemaker, bradycardia, marked hypotension, bronchospastic disorders, manifest electrolyte disorders, hypersensitivity to the drug. Myocardial infarction more than 6 days but less than 2 years previously.

Special Concerns: Use during pregnancy (pregnancy category: C) only if benefits clearly outweigh the risks. Use with caution during labor, delivery, and lactation. The safety and effectiveness have not been determined in children. Use with caution in patients with impaired hepatic or renal function.

Side Effects: *CV:* First-degree AV block, intraventricular conduction delay, palpitations, premature ventricular contractions, proarrhythmia, bradycardia, atrial fibrillation, angina, syncope, congestive heart failure, ventricular tachycardia, second-degree AV block, increased QRS duration, chest pain, hypotension, bundle branch block. Less commonly, atrial flutter, AV dissociation, flushing, hot flashes, sick sinus syndrome, sinus pause or arrest, supraventricular tachycardia, cardiac arrest. *CNS:* Dizziness, headache, anxiety, drowsiness, loss of balance, ataxia, insomnia. Less commonly, abnormal speech, abnormal dreams, abnormal vision, confusion, depression, memory loss, apnea, psychosis/mania, seizures, vertigo, coma. *GI:* Unusual taste, constipation, nausea and/or vomiting, dry mouth, anorexia, flatulence, abdominal pain, cramps, diarrhea, dyspepsia, liver abnormalities (cholestasis, hepatitis, elevated enzymes). *Hematologic:* Agranulocytosis, increased bleeding time, anemia, granulocytopenia, bruising, leukopenia, purpura, thrombocytopenia. *Miscellaneous:* Blurred vision, dyspnea, weakness, rash, edema, tremors, diaphoresis, joint pain, possible decrease in spermatogenesis. Less commonly, tinnitus, unusual smell sensation, apnea, alopecia, eye irritation, hyponatremia, impotence, increased glucose, kidney failure, lupus erythematosus, muscle cramps or weakness, nephrotic syndrome, pain, pruritus.

Drug Interactions	
Cimetidine	Cimetidine ↓ plasma levels of propafenone
Digoxin	Propafenone ↑ plasma levels of digoxin necessitating a ↓ in the dose of digoxin
Local anesthetics	May ↑ risk of CNS side effects
Metoprolol	Propafenone ↑ plasma levels of metoprolol due to inhibition of metabolism
Propranolol	Propafenone ↑ plasma levels of propranolol due to inhibition of metabolism
Warfarin	Propafenone may ↑ plasma levels of warfarin necessitating a ↓ in the dose of warfarin

Dosage: PO, initial: 150 mg q 8 hr; dose may be increased at a minimum of q 3–4 days to 225 mg q 8 hr and, if necessary, to 300 mg q 8 hr.

NURSING CONSIDERATIONS

See also *Nursing Considerations* for *Antiarrhythmic Agents,* p. 534.

Administration/Storage

1. Initiation of propafenone therapy should always be undertaken in a hospital setting.
2. The effectiveness and safety of doses exceeding 900 mg daily have not been determined.
3. There is no evidence that the use of propafenone will affect the survival or incidence of sudden death in clients with recent myocardial infarction or supraventricular tachycardia.

Assessment

1. Assess ECG and note any client history of cardiac problems.
2. Determine if there is any history of renal or hepatic disease. Propafenone must be used with caution in these clients.

Interventions

1. The dose of propafenone should be titrated in each client on the basis of response and tolerance.
2. Propafenone may induce new or worsened arrhythmias. Document with rhythm strips and monitor client closely.
3. Notify physician and anticipate reduction of dosage in clients that develop significant widening of the QRS complex or second- or third-degree AV block.
4. Anticipate that the dose of propafenone will be increased more gradually in elderly clients as well as in clients with previous myocardial damage.
5. Monitor liver and renal function studies. Anticipate reduced dosage in clients with impaired liver or kidney function.
6. Evaluate hematological studies during drug therapy to determine the presence of anemia, agranulocytosis, leukopenia, thrombocytopenia or altered prothrombin and coagulation times.
7. Weigh client and place on strict I&O.
8. Client may complain of an unusual taste in the mouth. This may interfere with eating and nutrition so observe closely.

Client/Family Teaching

1. Encourage to drink adequate quantities of fluid and to maintain adequate bulk in the diet to avoid constipation.
2. Report any incidence of increased or unusual bruising or bleeding.
3. Observe for indications of hepatic dysfunction such as yellow sclera, dark yellow urine or yellow pigmentation of the skin and report.
4. Report any evidence of urinary tract problems such as decreased urinary output.

PROPRANOLOL HYDROCHLORIDE   (proh-**PRAN**-ah-lol)

Apo-Propranolol✱, Detensol✱, Inderal, Inderal LA, Novopranol✱, PMS Propranolol✱ (Rx)

Classification: Antiarrhythmic (type II), beta-adrenergic blocking agent.
See *Antihypertensive Agents,* Chapter 26, p. 475, for all details on this drug.

QUINIDINE BISULFATE   (**KWIN**-ih-deen)

Bioquin Durules✱ (Rx)

QUINIDINE GLUCONATE   (**KWIN**-ih-deen **GLOO**-koh-nayt)

Duraquin, Quinaglute, Quinalan, Quinate✱ (Rx)

QUINIDINE POLYGALACTURONATE   (**KWIN**-ih-deen pah-lee-gah-**LACK**-tyou-**RAH**-nayt)

Cardioquin (Rx)

QUINIDINE SULFATE   (KWIN-ih-deen)

Apo-Quinidine ✿, Cin-Quin, Novoquinidin ✿, Quinidex, Quinora (Rx)

See also *Antiarrhythmic Agents,* p. 533.

Classification: Antiarrhythmic, type IA.

Action/Kinetics: Quinidine reduces the excitability of the heart and increases the refractory period by decreasing potassium efflux of cardiac fibers. It also decreases cardiac output and possesses anticholinergic, antimalarial, antipyretic, and oxytocic properties. **PO: Onset:** 0.5–3 hr. **Duration:** 6–8 hr for tablets/capsules and 12 hr for extended-release tablets. **t½:** 6–7 hr. **Time to peak levels, PO:** 3–4 hr for gluconate salt and 1–1.5 hr for sulfate salt; **IM:** 1 hr. **Therapeutic serum levels:** 2–6 mcg/mL. **Protein binding:** 60%–80%. **Duration:** 6–8 hr for tablets/capsules and 12 hr for extended-release tablets. Metabolized by liver. Rate of urinary excretion (10%–50% excreted unchanged) is affected by urinary pH.

Uses: Treatment and control of atrial flutter, established atrial fibrillation, paroxysmal atrial fibrillation and tachycardia, paroxysmal atrioventricular junctional rhythm, paroxysmal ventricular tachycardia not associated with complete heart block, premature atrial and ventricular contractions. Often the drug of choice for atrial fibrillation and atrial and ventricular arrhythmias. Not indicated for prophylaxis during surgery.

Contraindications: Hypersensitivity to drug or other cinchona drugs.

Special Concerns: Safety for use during pregnancy (pregnancy category: C) and lactation and in children has not been established. Quinidine should be used with extreme caution in patients in whom a sudden change in blood pressure might be detrimental or in those suffering from extensive myocardial damage, subacute endocarditis, bradycardia, coronary occlusion, disturbances in impulse conduction, chronic valvular disease, considerable cardiac enlargement, frank congestive heart failure, arrhythmias due to digitalis toxicity, renal disease. Cautious use is also recommended in patients with acute infections, hyperthyroidism, myasthenia gravis, muscular weakness, respiratory distress, and bronchial asthma. The dose in geriatric patients may have to be reduced due to age-related changes in renal function.

Side Effects: *CV:* Widening of QRS complex, hypotension, asystole, ectopic ventricular beats, ventricular tachycardia or fibrillation, arterial embolism, circulatory collapse, bradycardia, congestive heart failure, partial or total heart block. *GI:* Nausea, vomiting, abdominal pain, colic, anorexia, diarrhea, urge to defecate as well as urinate. *CNS:* Syncope, headache, confusion, excitement, vertigo, apprehension, tinnitus, decreased hearing acuity. *Dermatologic:* Skin eruptions, urticaria, exfoliative dermatitis, photosensitivity, flushing. *Allergic:* Acute asthma, angioneurotic edema, respiratory paralysis, dyspnea, fever, vascular collapse. *Hematologic:* Hypoprothrombinemia, acute hemolytic anemia, thrombocytopenic purpura, agranulocytosis. *Ophthalmologic:* Blurred vision, mydriasis, alterations in color perception, decreased field of vision, double vision, photophobia, optic neuritis, night blindness, scotomata. *Other:* Liver toxicity including hepatitis, lupus erythematosus (rare).

Drug Interactions

Acetazolamide, antacids	↑ Effect of quinidine due to ↓ renal excretion
Anticholinergic agents, atropine	Additive effect on blockade of vagus nerve action
Anticoagulants, oral	Additive hypoprothrombinemia
Barbiturates	↓ Effect of quinidine due to ↑ breakdown by liver

Drug Interactions

Cholinergic agents	Quinidine antagonizes effect of cholinergic drugs
Cimetidine	↑ Effect of quinidine due to ↓ breakdown by liver
Digoxin, digitoxin	↑ Symptoms of digoxin toxicity
Guanethidine	Additive hypotensive effect
Methyldopa	Additive hypotensive effect
Neuromuscular blocking agents	↑ Respiratory depression
Phenobarbital, phenytoin	↓ Effect of quinidine by ↑ rate of metabolism in liver
Phenothiazines	Additive cardiac depressant effect
Potassium	↑ Effect of quinidine
Propranolol	Both drugs produce a negative inotropic effect on the heart
Reserpine	Additive cardiac depressant effects
Rifampin	↓ Effect of quinidine due to ↑ breakdown by liver
Skeletal muscle relaxants	↑ Skeletal muscle relaxation
Sodium bicarbonate	↑ Effect of quinidine due to ↓ renal excretion
Thiazide diuretics	↑ Effect of quinidine due to ↓ renal excretion
Verapamil	Hypotension in patients with hypertrophic cardiomyopathy

Laboratory Test Interferences: False + or ↑ PSP, 17-ketosteroids, prothrombin time.

Dosage: Quinidine Gluconate Extended-Release Tablets. Adults, maintenance: 324–660 mg q 6–12 hr as needed. Use not recommended for children. **Quinidine Polygalacturonate Tablets. Adults, initial:** 275–825 mg q 3–4 hr for 3–4 doses; **then,** increase by 137.5–275 mg q third or fourth dose until rhythm is restored. **Maintenance:** 275 mg b.i.d.–t.i.d. as needed. **Pediatric:** 8.25 mg/kg (247.5 mg/m^2) 5 times a day.

    Quinidine Sulfate Capsules/Tablets. Adults, *premature atrial and ventricular contractions:* 200–300 mg t.i.d.–q.i.d. *Paroxysmal supraventricular tachycardias:* 400–600 mg q 2–3 hr until beneficial effect noted. *Conversion of atrial fibrillation:* 200 mg q 2–3 hr for 5–8 doses; dose may be increased daily as needed and tolerated. **Maintenance:** 200–300 mg t.i.d.–q.i.d. as needed. **Pediatric,** *antiarrhythmic:* 6 mg/kg (180 mg/m^2) five times daily. **Quinidine Sulfate Extended-release Tablets.** 300–600 mg q 8–12 hr as needed. Use not recommended in children.

    Quinidine Gluconate Injection. IM, initial: 600 mg; **then,** 400 mg repeated as frequently as q 2 hr if needed. **IV:** 800 mg in 40 mL of 5% dextrose injection at a rate of 1 mL/min.

    Quinidine Sulfate Injection. IV, 600 mg in 40 mL of 5% dextrose injection at a rate of 1 mL/min.

NURSING CONSIDERATIONS

See also *Nursing Considerations* for *Antiarrhythmic Agents,* p. 534.

Administration/Storage

1. A preliminary test dose may be given before instituting quinidine therapy. **Adults:** 200 mg quinidine sulfate or quinidine gluconate administered PO or IM. **Children:** Test dose of 2 mg of quinidine sulfate per kilogram of body weight.

2. IV solution can be prepared by diluting 10 mL of quinidine gluconate injection with 50 mL of 5% glucose; this should be given at a rate of 1 mL/min.

3. Use only colorless clear solution for injection, because light may cause quinidine to crystallize, which turns solution brownish.

Assessment

1. Note any history of allergic reactions to antiarrhythmic drugs or tartrazine which is found in some formulations.

2. Determine that pretreatment lab tests including blood glucose, CBC, liver and renal function studies have been performed.

3. Obtain client blood pressure, pulse and auscultate heart sounds to determine baseline information against which to measure postmedication responses.

Interventions

1. Evaluate ECG and report any evidence of increased AV block, cardiac irritability or suppression during IV administration.

2. Observe client for hypersensitivity reactions.

3. Monitor intake and output and vital signs; observe for evidence of hypotension.

4. Observe clients for neurological deficits or sensory impairment and report if evident.

5. Monitor serum electrolytes and CBC during prolonged therapy with quinidine.

6. Among the elderly, there is a higher risk of toxicity, reduced cardiac output and unpredictable effects from drug therapy.

7. Carefully monitor plasma concentrations of quinidine. The therapeutic range is 2–6 mcg/mL.

Client/Family Teaching

1. Administer with food to minimize GI effects.

2. Take only as directed and notify physician of any persistent bothersome side effects.

3. Palpitations or faintness may indicate quinidine-induced ventricular arrhythmias and should be reported immediately.

4. If any of the following symptoms occur, advise the client to call the physician:
   - severe skin rash, hives or itching
   - severe headache
   - unexplained fever
   - ringing in the ears, buzzing, or hearing loss
   - unusual bruising or bleeding
   - blurred vision
   - irregular heart beat
   - continued diarrhea

5. Stress the importance of reporting for laboratory studies and follow-up appointments as scheduled.

TOCAINIDE HYDROCHLORIDE   (TOE-kay-nyd)

Tonocard (Rx)

See also *Antiarrhythmic Agents*, p. 533.

Classification: Antiarrhythmic, type IB.

Action/Kinetics: Tocainide, which is similar to lidocaine, decreases the excitability of cells in the myocardium. Tocainide produces increases in pulmonary and aortic arterial pressure and slight increases in peripheral resistance. Is effective in both digitalized and nondigitalized patients. **Peak plasma levels:** 0.5–2 hr. **t½:** 15 hr. **Therapeutic serum levels:** 4–10 mcg/mL. **Duration:** 8 hr. Approximately 10% is bound to plasma protein. Forty percent is excreted unchanged in the urine.

Uses: Ventricular arrhythmias including premature ventricular contractions, unifocal or multifocal, couplets, and ventricular tachycardia.

Contraindications: Allergy to amide-type local anesthetics, second- or third-degree AV block in the absence of artificial ventricular pacemaker.

Special Concerns: Safety during pregnancy (pregnancy category: C) and lactation and in children has not been established. Geriatric patients may have an increased risk of dizziness and hypotension; the dose may have to be reduced in these patients due to age-related impaired renal function.

Side Effects: *CV:* Increased arrhythmias, increased ventricular rate, congestive heart failure, tachycardia, hypotension, conduction disturbances, bradycardia, chest pain, left ventricular failure. *CNS:* Lightheadedness, dizziness, vertigo, giddiness, headache, tremors, restlessness, confusion, disorientation, hallucinations, ataxia, paresthesias, numbness, nystagmus, drowsiness. *GI:* Nausea, vomiting, anorexia, diarrhea. *Hematologic:* Leukopenia, agranulocytosis, hypoplastic anemia, thrombocytopenia. *Other:* Pulmonary fibrosis, blurred vision, tinnitus, hearing loss, sweating, arthritis, myalgia, lupus-like syndrome.

Drug Interactions: Use with metaprolol may result in additive effects.

Dosage: Tablets. Adults, individualized, initial: 400 mg q 8 hr, up to a maximum of 2,400 mg/day; **maintenance:** 1,200–1,800 mg daily in divided doses. Total daily dose of 1,200 mg may be adequate in patients with liver or kidney disease.

NURSING CONSIDERATIONS

See also *Nursing Considerations* for *Antiarrhythmic Agents,* p. 534.

Client/Family Teaching

1. Report any evidence of bruising, bleeding, or signs of infection such as fever, sore throat, or chills. These symptoms may indicate a blood dyscrasia.
2. Stress the importance of reporting for scheduled laboratory tests and follow-up visits.
3. Pulmonary symptoms such as wheezing, coughing, or dyspnea, should be reported immediately. These may indicate pulmonary fibrosis and in this case the drug must be discontinued.

VERAPAMIL (veh-**RAP**-ah-mil)

Calan, Isoptin (Rx)

See *Calcium Channel Blocking agents,* Chapter 24, p. 455.

CHAPTER TWENTY-EIGHT

Antihyperlipidemic and Hypocholesterolemic Agents

General Statement: Atherosclerosis is characterized by a narrowing of the blood vessels by lipid deposits, as well as an increased incidence of stroke or myocardial infarction. The condition is associated with changes in the cholesterol, fat, and/or carbohydrate metabolism, although it is not known whether these changes are a cause or a consequence of the disease. Patients often manifest increased levels of plasma lipids, a complex mixture of triglycerides, phospholipids, free cholesterol, and cholesterol esters—all associated with protein. The lipoproteins are further subdivided into chylomicrons, low-density lipoproteins (VLDL or prebeta-lipoproteins), low-density lipoproteins (LDL or beta-lipoproteins), and high-density lipoproteins (HDL or alpha-lipoproteins). The latter are considered beneficial and protective. They occur in higher concentrations in women and are increased by exercise. On the basis of their lipoprotein patterns and other characteristics, patients can be separated into five types (see Table 9).

Guidelines have been established for the treatment of high blood cholesterol by the National Cholesterol Education Program of the National Heart, Lung and Blood Institute. Levels of total cholesterol less than 200 mg/dl are considered desirable while levels between 200 and 239 mg/dl are borderline-high and levels above 240 mg/dl are considered high.

A reduction of plasma lipids, especially cholesterol and LDL, to more normal levels is believed to be therapeutically useful in minimizing atherosclerosis and the closely related hyperlipoproteinemias (Table 9). Such a reduction is achieved primarily through diet (decreased intake of cholesterol, saturated fats, simple sugars, increased amounts of fiber), weight loss, exercise, and, depending on the total cholesterol and LDL-cholesterol levels, drug therapy. The drugs will not remove existing intrarterial lipid plaques (atheromas) but may reduce the rate at which new ones are formed. Along with dietary measures, drug therapy may be indicated in Type IIA, IIB, III, IV, and V hyperlipidemias.

NURSING CONSIDERATIONS

Assessment

1. Obtain a complete nursing history and conduct a baseline assessment before the start of drug therapy.
2. Determine that liver profiles including serum lipid and cholesterol levels have been obtained.
3. Ascertain that hematology, electrolytes, liver and kidney function studies have been completed prior to initiating therapy.

Table 9   Primary Hyperlipoproteinemias

Lipid Pattern	Characteristic Features	Treatment
Type I	High level of triglycerides and chylomicrons. No change or slight increase in cholesterol and VLDL. Decreases in LDL and HDL.	Low-fat diet. Treatment of underlying condition (diabetes, thyroid condition).
Type II a	High cholesterol and LDL levels. Normal levels of chylomicrons, HDL, triglycerides. Normal or decreased VLDL.	Diet. Drug therapy such as cholestyramine, colestipol, dextrothyroxine, lovastatin, nicotinc acid, probucol.
Type II b	Increased cholesterol, trigylcerides, LDL, VLDL. Normal chylomicrons and HDL.	Diet. Depending on lipid/lipoprotein profile: Cholestyramine, colestipol, clofibrate, gemfibrozil, lovastatin, nicotinic acid, probucol.
Type III	Increased LDL and ILDL (an abnormal lipoprotein). Normal to increased cholesterol, triglycerides, and VLDL. Normal chylomicrons and HDL.	Diet. Use of clofibrate or nicotinic acid.
Type IV	Increased triglycerides and VLDL. Normal (or slight increase) in cholesterol. Normal chylomicrons. Normal or slight decrease in LDL and HDL.	Diet. Use of clofibrate, gemfibrozil, or nicotinic acid.
Type V	Increased tryglycerides, chylomicrons, and VLDL. Normal or increased cholesterol. Decreased LDL and HDL.	Weight reduction. Use of clofibrate, gemfibrozil, or nicotinic acid.

28

3. Ascertain that hematology, electrolytes, liver and kidney function studies have been completed prior to initiating therapy.

Client/Family Teaching

1. Review drug side effects and the intended goals of therapy.
2. Instruct the client and family or (meal provider) concerning low cholesterol diets and if possible have a dietician assist the client with meal planning.
3. Provide a printed list of foods permitted on the diet in order to enable the client to follow a diet low in cholesterol. Include foods high in vitamins A and D. Absorption of fat soluble vitamins is seriously impaired when taking these drugs.
4. Report for all laboratory studies as scheduled in order to measure the effectiveness of prescribed therapy and to screen for any early adverse drug reactions.

the pharmacist should there need to be a change in pharmacies or a need to purchase over-the-counter drugs at a time when a physician is unavailable for guidance.

7. Wear a medical identification tag or bracelet and always carry a list of medications they are currently prescribed and taking.

Evaluation

1. Assess client/family knowledge and understanding of illness and response to teaching.
2. Evaluate lab studies to determine the effectiveness of the drug regimen.
3. Review family history of hyperlipidemia and client lifestyles. Offer encouragement to clients who have difficulty lowering their serum cholesterol as well as offer methods for achieving this goal.

CHOLESTYRAMINE RESIN (koh-leh-**STY**-rah-meen)
Cholybar, Questran, Questran Light (Rx)

Classification: Hypocholesterolemic agent, bile acid sequestrant.

Action/Kinetics: Cholestyramine binds sodium cholate (bile salts) in the intestine; thus, the principal precursor of cholesterol is not absorbed due to formation of an insoluble complex which is excreted in the feces. The drug decreases cholesterol and LDL and has either no effect or increases triglycerides, VLDL, and HDL. Also, there is relief of itching as a result of removing irritating bile salts. The antidiarrheal effect results from the binding and removal of bile acids. **Onset, to reduce plasma cholesterol:** within 24–48 hr but levels may continue to fall for 1 yr; **to relieve pruritus:** 1–3 weeks; **relief of diarrhea associated with bile acids:** 24 hr. Cholesterol levels return to pretreatment levels 2–4 wks after discontinuance.

Fat-soluble vitamins (A, D, K) and possibly folic acid may have to be administered IM during long-term therapy, since cholestyramine binds these vitamins in the intestine.

Uses: Pruritus associated with partial biliary obstruction. Hyperlipoproteinemia (type IIA). Diarrhea due to bile acids. *Investigational:* Treatment of poisoning by chlordecone (Kepone); antibiotic-induced *Pseudomonas* colitis; digitalis toxicity; postvagotomy diarrhea; and hyperoxaluria.

Contraindications: Complete obstruction or atresia of bile duct.

Special Concerns: Use during pregnancy only if benefits outweigh risks. Use with caution during lactation and in children. Geriatric patients may be more likely to manifest GI side effects as well as adverse nutritional effects.

Side Effects: *GI:* Constipation (may be severe), nausea, vomiting, diarrhea, heartburn, GI bleeding, anorexia, flatulence, belching, abdominal distention, aggravation of hemorrhoids. Fecal impaction in elderly patients. Large doses may cause steatorrhea. *Other:* Bleeding tendencies (due to hypoprothrombinemia). Osteoporosis, electrolyte imbalance, and CNS and musculoskeletal manifestations. Prolonged administration may interfere with absorption of fat-soluble vitamins. Irritation and rash of skin, tongue, and perianal area.

Drug Interactions	
Acetaminophen	↓ Effect of acetaminophen due to ↓ absorption from GI tract
Amiodarone	↓ Effect of amiodarone due to ↓ absorption from GI tract

Drug Interactions

Anticoagulants, oral	↓ Anticoagulant effect due to ↓ absorption from GI tract
Cephalexin	↓ Absorption of cephalexin from GI tract
Chenodiol	↓ Effect of chenodiol due to ↓ absorption from GI tract
Chlorothiazide	↓ Effect of chlorothiazide due to ↓ absorption from GI tract
Clindamycin	↓ Absorption of clindamycin from GI tract
Corticosteroids	↓ Effect of corticosteroids due to ↓ absorption from GI tract
Digitalis glycosides	Cholestyramine binds digitoxin in the intestine and ↓ its half-life
Iron preparations	↓ Effect of iron preparations due to ↓ absorption from GI tract
Lovastatin	Effects may be additive
Naproxen	↓ Effect of naproxen due to ↓ absorption from GI tract
Penicillin G	↓ Effect of penicillin G due to ↓ absorption from GI tract
Phenobarbital	↓ Absorption of phenobarbital from GI tract
Phenylbutazone	Absorption of phenylbutazone delayed by cholestyramine—may ↓ effect
Piroxicam	↓ Effect of piroxicam due to ↓ absorption from GI tract
Propranolol	↓ Effect of propranolol due to ↓ absorption from GI tract
Tetracyclines	↓ Effect of tetracyclines due to ↓ absorption from GI tract
Thiazide diuretics	↓ Effect of thiazides due to ↓ absorption from GI tract
Thyroid hormones	↓ Effect of thyroid hormones due to ↓ absorption from GI tract
Trimethoprim	↓ Effect of trimethoprim due to ↓ absorption from GI tract
Ursodiol	↓ Effect of ursodiol due to ↓ absorption from GI tract
Warfarin	↓ Effect of warfarin due to ↓ absorption from GI tract

Note: These drug interactions may also be observed with colestipol.

Dosage: Bar, Powder. Adults: 4 g 1–6 times daily of either the powder or the bar. After relief of pruritus, dosage may be reduced. Doses greater than 24 g daily result in an increased incidence of side effects. **Pediatric, 6–12 years of age:** 80 mg (anhydrous cholestyramine)/kg (2.35 g/m^2) t.i.d. The adult dose should be used in children older than 12 years. Not recommended for children less than 6 years of age.

NURSING CONSIDERATIONS

See also *Nursing considerations for Antihyperlipidemic Agents,* p. 566.

Administration/Storage

1. Always mix powder with 60–180 mL water or noncarbonated beverage before administering because resin may cause esophageal irritation or blockage. Highly liquid soups or pulpy fruits such as applesauce or crushed pineapple may also be used.
2. After placing contents of one packet of resin on the surface of 4–6 oz of fluid, allow it to stand without stirring for 2 min, occasionally twirling the glass, and then stir slowly (to prevent foaming) to form a suspension.
3. The bar should be chewed thoroughly and taken with plenty of fluids.

Assessment

Note color of client's skin and eyes for evidence of jaundice.

Interventions

1. Anticipate that vitamins A, D, K, and folic acid will be administered during long term therapy. These may be administered in a water-miscible form when the client is receiving medication.
2. Note client complaints of constipation, abdominal pain or abdominal bloating. Encourage a fluid intake of 2500–3000 mL/day, and encourage an increased intake of citrus fruits, fruit juices and high fiber foods as preventive measures. Also, a stool softener may be indicated.
3. Encourage clients to increase their daily exercise as a method to avoid constipation.
4. If symptoms are severe or if they persist, discuss a change in dosage of drug or change of medication with the physician.
5. If the client complains of diarrhea, monitor intake, output, electrolytes and weight. Note any evidence of dehydration and/or electrolyte imbalance.
6. Monitor the client's serum cholesterol and triglyceride levels. Clients should also have frequent serum transaminase and other liver function tests conducted routinely.
7. To assure that the clients are not developing anemia, leukopenia, eosinophilia, potential anticoagulant effects or renal dysfunction, blood counts and renal function tests should be done routinely.
8. If clients develop bleeding from any orifice or develop purpura, they should receive parenteral vitamin K.

Client/Family Teaching

1. Other prescribed medications should be taken at least 1 hr before or 4 hr after taking antihyperlipidemic medication. These drugs interfere with the absorption of other medications.
2. Discuss the constipating effects the drug may have and ways to control this problem. Encourage the client to drink extra fluids and to include extra roughage in the diet.
3. If the client has problems with persistent constipation despite efforts to avoid the problem, a stool softener may be required.
4. Instruct the client to report tarry stools or any abnormal bleeding. These symptoms may indicate a need for vitamin K supplement.
5. Pruritus may subside 1–3 weeks after taking the drug, but may return after the medication is discontinued. Corn starch or oatmeal baths may assist to alleviate this discomfort.

CLOFIBRATE   (kloh-**FYE**-brayt)

Atromid-S, Claripex✤, Novofibrate✤ (Rx)

Classification: Antihyperlipidemic agent.

Action/Kinetics: Clofibrate decreases triglycerides, VLDL, and cholesterol and either does not change or increases HDL and does not change or decreases LDL. The mechanism is not known with certainty but may be due to increased catabolism of VLDL to LDL and decreased synthesis of VLDL by the liver. The higher the cholesterol level, the more effective the drug. The drug may also increase the release of antidiuretic hormone from the posterior pituitary. **Peak plasma levels:** 2–6 hr. **t½:** 6–25 hr. **Therapeutic effect: Onset,** 2–5 days; **maximum effect:** 3 weeks. Triglycerides return to pretreatment levels 2–3 weeks after therapy is terminated. Clofibrate is hydrolyzed to the active p-chlorophenoxyisobutyric acid (CPIB) which is further metabolized and excreted in the urine. The drug may concentrate in fetal blood. Liver function tests should be performed during therapy.

Uses: As adjunct treatment for type III hyperlipidemia in patients with a significant risk of coronary heart disease who have not responded to diet or other measures. Limited use in type II hyperlipidemia. *Investigational:* Partial central diabetes insipidus in patients with some residual posterior pituitary function.

Contraindications: Impaired hepatic or renal function, primary biliary cirrhosis, pregnancy or expectation thereof, lactation, children.

Special Concerns: Use with caution in patients with gout and peptic ulcer. Reduced dosage may be required in geriatric patients due to age-related decreases in renal function. Dosage has not been established in children.

Side Effects: *GI:* Nausea, dyspepsia, weight gain, gastritis, vomiting, bloating, flatulence, abdominal distress, stomatitis, loose stools, hepatomegaly. *CNS:* Headaches, dizziness, fatigue, weakness, drowsiness. *CV:* Changes in blood-clotting time, arrhythmias, increased or decreased angina, thrombophlebitis, swelling and phlebitis at xanthoma site, pulmonary embolism. *Skeletal muscle:* Myositis, asthenia, myalgia, weakness, muscle aches, cramps. *GU:* Impotence, dysuria, hematuria, decreased urine output, decreased libido, proteinuria. *Hematologic:* Anemia, leukopenia, eosinophilia. *Dermatologic:* Urticaria, skin rash, dry skin, pruritus, dry brittle hair, alopecia. *Enzyme changes:* ↑ Creatine phosphokinase, increased serum transaminase (if levels continue to increase after maximum therapeutic response has been achieved, therapy should be discontinued). *Other:* Increased incidence of gallstones, dyspnea, polyphagia.

Drug Interactions	
Anticoagulants	Clofibrate ↑ anticoagulant effect by ↓ plasma protein binding
Antidiabetics (sulfonylureas)	Clofibrate ↑ effect of antidiabetics
Furosemide	Concurrent use may ↑ effects of both drugs
Insulin	Clofibrate ↑ effect of insulin
Probenecid	↑ Effect of clofibrate due to ↓ breakdown by liver and ↓ kidney excretion
Rifampin	↓ Effect of clofibrate due to ↑ breakdown by liver

Dosage: Capsules. Adults: *Antihyperlipidemic,* 500 mg q.i.d. Therapeutic response may take several weeks to become apparent. Drug must be administered on a continuous basis, since lowered levels of cholesterol and other lipids will return to elevated state within several weeks after administration is stopped. Discontinue after 3 months if response is poor.

NURSING CONSIDERATIONS

See also *Nursing Considerations for Antihyperlipidemic Agents,* p. 566.

Assessment

If client is of childbearing age, determine if pregnant.

Client/Family Teaching

1. Advise that nausea usually decreases with continued therapy or reduced dosage. Drug may be taken with food if GI upset occurs.
2. Observe for bleeding from any orifice or for purpura if client is also receiving anticoagulant therapy. A reduction in anticoagulant drug dosage is customary if clofibrate therapy is instituted.
3. Report symptoms of hypoglycemia because of possible drug interactions when taking oral antidiabetics.
4. Use contraception if appropriate because clofibrate may be teratogenic.
5. Do not discontinue contraception for several months after discontinuing drug therapy, if pregnancy is planned.
6. The drug must be taken as ordered to be effective.
7. Report any adverse side effects so that drug therapy can be evaluated.

COLESTIPOL HYDROCHLORIDE (koh-**LEH**-stih-pol)

Colestid (Rx)

Classification: Hypocholesterolemic, bile acid sequestrant.

Action/Kinetics: Colestipol, an anion exchange resin, binds bile acids in the intestine forming an insoluble complex which is excreted in the feces. The loss of bile acids results in increased oxidation of cholesterol to bile acids and a decrease in LDL and serum cholesterol. Colestipol does not affect (or may increase) triglycerides or HDL and may increase VLDL. The drug is not absorbed from the GI tract. **Onset:** 1–2 days; **maximum effect:** 1 month. Return to pretreatment cholesterol levels after discontinuance of therapy: 1 month.

Uses: Primary hypercholesterolemia (type IIa hyperlipidemia) with a significant risk of coronary artery disease in patients who have not responded to diet or other measures. *Investigational:* Digitalis toxicity, pruritus associated with partial biliary obstruction, diarrhea due to bile acids, hyperoxaluria.

Contraindications: Complete obstruction or atresia of bile duct.

Special Concerns: Use during pregnancy only if benefits outweigh risks. Use with caution during lactation and in children. Children may be more likely to develop hyperchloremic acidosis although dosage has not been established. Patients over 60 years of age may be at greater risk of GI side effects and adverse nutritional effects.

Side Effects: *GI:* Constipation (may be severe), nausea, vomiting, diarrhea, heartburn, GI bleeding, anorexia, flatulence, belching, abdominal distention, aggravation of hemorrhoids. Fecal impaction in elderly patients. Large doses may cause steatorrhea. *Other:* Bleeding tendencies (due to hypoprothrombinemia). Osteoporosis, electrolyte imbalance, and CNS and musculoskeletal manifestations. Prolonged administration may interfere with absorption of fat-soluble vitamins. Irritation and rash of skin, tongue, and perianal area.

Drug Interactions: See *Cholestyramine,* p. 568.

Dosage: Oral Suspension. Adults: *antihyperlipidemic:* 15–30 g daily before meals in 2 to 4 equally divided doses. *Digitalis toxicity:* 10 g followed by 5 g q 6–8 hr.

NURSING CONSIDERATIONS

See also *Nursing Considerations for Antihyperlipidemic Agents,* p. 566.

Administration/Storage

1. Always mix with fluid before administering, because resin may cause esophageal irritation or blockage.
2. Disguise unpalatable taste of drug by mixing it with fruit juice, soup, milk, water, applesauce, pureed fruit, or carbonated beverages.
3. Administer other drugs 1 hr before or 4 hr after colestipol to reduce interference with their absorption.

DEXTROTHYROXINE SODIUM   (dek-stroh-thigh-**ROX**-in)

Choloxin (Rx)

Classification: Antihyperlipidemic.

Action/Kinetics: Dextrothyroxine (the dextro isomer of thyroid hormone) increases the rate at which cholesterol is metabolized in the liver; excretion of cholesterol and metabolites is increased, leading to decreased serum levels of cholesterol and LDL; there is no change in levels of triglycerides or HDL. Dextrothyroxine has little effect on the basal metabolic rate (BMR) but is otherwise similar physiologically to levothyroxine. The effectiveness increases as cholesterol levels increase. Approximately 25% is absorbed from the GI tract, almost completely bound to plasma proteins. **t½:** 18 hr. **Duration:** Serum lipid levels return to pretreatment levels from 6–12 weeks after termination of drug therapy. Eliminated through both the kidneys and feces.

Uses: Only for patients with primary hypercholesterolemia (type IIa hyperlipidemia) who are at a significant risk for coronary artery disease and who have not responded to diet or other measures.

Contraindications: Euthyroid patients with hypertensive organic heart disease, including angina pectoris, history of myocardial infarction, cardiac arrhythmias or tachycardia, rheumatic disease, CHF, decompensated or borderline compensated cardiac status, hypertension (other than mild, labile, systolic). Pregnancy, lactation, advanced liver or kidney disease, or a history of hypersensitivity to iodine.

Special Concerns: Use with caution in impaired liver and kidney function. Patients intolerant to lactose, milk, or milk products may be intolerant to the tablet since it also contains lactose. Geriatric patients may be more sensitive to the effects of dextrothyroxine.

Side Effects: *CNS:* Insomnia, nervousness, fever, headache, decreased sensorium, paresthesia, dizziness, malaise, tiredness, psychic changes, tremors. *CV:* Angina pectoris, increase in heart size, ischemic myocardial changes (ECG changes), arrhythmias including ectopic beats, supraventricular tachycardia, extrasystoles, worsening of peripheral vascular disease, possibility of fatal or nonfatal myocardial infarction (relationship to drug uncertain). *GI:* Nausea, vomiting, diarrhea, constipation, anorexia, dyspepsia, weight loss, bitter taste, GI hemorrhages. *Other:* Drooping eyelids, changes in libido, sweating, hair loss, diuresis, menstrual irregularities, hoarseness, tinnitus, peripheral edema, visual disturbances, muscle pain, gallstones, increases in blood sugar of diabetic patients, skin rashes, itching, flushing.

Aggravation of existing cardiac disease is cause for discontinuation. Overdose is characterized by hyperthyroidism, diarrhea, cramps, vomiting, nervousness, twitching, tachycardia, and weight loss.

Drug Interactions

Anticoagulants, oral	↑ Effect of anticoagulants by ↑ hypoprothrombinemia
Antidiabetics, oral	↓ Diabetic control as dextrothyroxine ↑ blood glucose
Beta-adrenergic blocking agents	Dextrothyroxine ↓ effect of beta-blockers
Cholestyramine	↓ Effect of dextrothyroxine due to ↓ absorption from GI tract
Colestipol	↓ Effect of dextrothyroxine due to ↓ absorption from GI tract
Digitalis	Additive stimulation of myocardium
Epinephrine	In coronary artery disease, concomitant use → coronary insufficiency
Insulin	↓ Diabetic control as dextrothyroxine ↑ blood glucose
Thyroid drugs	↑ Sensitivity of hypothyroid patients to thyroid drugs
Tricyclic antidepressants	Use with dextrothyroxine → CNS stimulation, ↑ heart rate, cardiac arrhythmias, nervousness

Dosage: Tablets. Adults, initial: 1–2 mg daily. Daily dosage can be increased every 4 weeks by 1–2 mg; **maintenance:** 4–8 mg daily. **Maximum daily dosage:** 8 mg. It may take 2–4 weeks for the therapeutic response to become manifested. **Pediatric, initial:** 0.05 mg/kg (1.5 mg/m^2) daily. Increase by 0.05 mg/kg every month, up to maximum of 4 mg daily, until satisfactory control is established. **Maintenance:** 0.1 mg/kg (3 mg/m^2) daily. Withdraw drug 2 weeks before surgery.

NURSING CONSIDERATIONS

See also *Nursing Considerations for Antihyperlipidemic Agents,* p. 566.

Administration/Storage

Use should be discontinued if symptoms of cardiac disease develop.

Assessment

1. Obtain a baseline ECG prior to starting the client on therapy.
2. Determine if the client is taking cardiac glycosides. In this event, client may be more susceptible to cardiac side effects.

Interventions

1. Assess for and note client complaints of chest pain or any attacks of angina.
2. Monitor pulse and if it is greater than 120 beats per min, withhold the dosage (unless otherwise indicated) and report to the physician.
3. If the client complains of nausea or a decrease in appetite, taking the drug with meals may reduce the gastric irritation and assure better compliance with the drug regimen.
4. With diabetes, dextrothyroxine may increase blood glucose levels. Monitor serum glucose levels as the client may require an adjustment in oral hypoglycemic agents if on oral medication, or an adjustment in insulin dosage.
5. Check eyes routinely for exophthalmos.

Client/Family Teaching

Report any new signs or changes to the physician to assure that serious side effects are not developing.

GEMFIBROZIL   (jem-**FIB**-roh-zil)

Lopid (Rx)

Classification: Antihyperlipidemic.

Action/Kinetics: Gemfibrozil, which resembles clofibrate, decreases triglycerides, cholesterol, and VLDL and increases HDL; LDL levels either decrease or do not change. In addition, the drug decreases hepatic triglyceride production by inhibiting peripheral lipolysis and decreasing extraction of free fatty acids by the liver. Also, gemfibrozil decreases VLDL synthesis by inhibiting synthesis of VLDL carrier apolipoprotein B as well as inhibits peripheral lipolysis and decreases hepatic extraction of free fatty acids (thus decreasing hepatic triglyceride production). The drug may be beneficial in inhibiting development of atherosclerosis. **Onset:** 2–5 days. **Peak plasma levels:** 1–2 hr; **t½:** 1.5 hr. Nearly 70% is excreted unchanged.

Uses: Hypertriglyceridemia (type IV and type V hyperlipidemia) unresponsive to dietary control or in clients who are at risk of pancreatitis and abdominal pain. (Response variable; discontinue if significant improvement not observed within 3 months.) Reduce risk of coronary heart disease in patients with type IIb hyperlipidemia who have not responded to diet, weight loss, exercise, and other drug therapy.

Contraindications: Gallbladder disease, primary biliary cirrhosis, hepatic or renal dysfunction.

Special Concerns: Pregnancy category: B. Use with caution during lactation. Safety and efficacy have not been established in children. The dose may have to be reduced in geriatric patients due to age-related decreases in renal function.

Side Effects: Cholelithiasis; increased chance of viral and bacterial infections. *GI:* Abdominal or epigastric pain, nausea, vomiting, diarrhea, dyspepsia, constipation, acute appendicitis, colitis, pancreatitis, cholestatic jaundice, hepatoma. *CNS:* Dizziness, headache, fatigue, vertigo, somnolence, paresthesia, hypesthesia, depression, confusion, syncope, seizures. *CV:* Atrial fibrillation, extrasystole, peripheral vascular disease, intracerebral hemorrhage. *Hematopoietic:* Anemia, leukopenia, eosinophilia, thrombocytopenia, bone narrow hypoplasia. *Musculoskeletal:* Painful extremities; possibly arthralgia, muscle cramps, swollen joints, back pain, myalgia, myopathy, myasthenia, rhabdomyolysis. *Allergic:* Urticaria, lupus-like syndrome, angioedema, laryngeal edema, vasculitis, anaphylaxis. *Dermatologic:* Eczema, dermatitis, pruritus, skin rashes, exfoliative dermatitis, alopecia. *Miscellaneous:* Increased chance of viral and bacterial infections, taste perversion, impotence, decreased male fertility, weight loss.

Drug Interaction	
Anticoagulants, oral	Gemfibrozil may ↑ effect of anticoagulants; dosage adjustment necessary
Lovastatin	Rhabdomyolysis when combined with gemfibrozil

Laboratory Test Interference: ↑ AST, ALT, LDH, CPK, alkaline phosphatase, bilirubin. Hypokalemia. Positive antinuclear antibody. ↓ Hemoglobin, white blood cells, hematocrit.

Dosage: Capsules/Tablets. Adults: 600 mg 30 min before the morning and evening meal (range: 900–1,500 mg/day). Dosage has not been established in children.

NURSING CONSIDERATIONS

See *Nursing Considerations* for *Clofibrate,* p. 572, and *Antihyperlipidemic Agents,* p. 566.

Client/Family Teaching

1. Limit the intake of alcohol.
2. Observe for bruising or bleeding and report, especially if client is also on anticoagulant therapy. A reduction in anticoagulant drug dosage is indicated if gemfibrozil therapy is instituted.
3. Be alert for signs and symptoms associated with gallstones, such as abdominal pain and vomiting. Report any persistent GI symptoms to the physician.
4. The client should report any right upper quadrant abdominal pain or change in color and consistency of the stools.
5. Use caution when driving or performing other dangerous tasks, since drug may cause dizziness or blurred vision.

LOVASTATIN (MELVINOLIN)   (low-vah-**STAH**-tin, mel-**VIN**-oh-lin)

Mevacor (Rx)

Classification: Antihyperlipidemic.

Action/Kinetics: Lovastatin is a drug isolated from a strain of *Aspergillus terreus.* It specifically inhibits HMG-coenzyme A reductase, an enzyme that is necessary to convert HMG-coenzyme A to mevalonate (an early step in the biosynthesis of cholesterol). The levels of VLDL, LDL, cholesterol, and plasma triglycerides are reduced, while the plasma concentration of HDL cholesterol is increased. Since the enzyme is not completely inhibited, mevalonate is available in amounts necessary to maintain homeostasis. Absorption is decreased by about one-third if the drug is given on an empty stomach rather than with food. **Onset:** within 2 weeks using multiple doses. **Time to peak plasma levels:** 2–4 hr. **Time to peak effect:** 4–6 weeks using multiple doses. **Duration:** 4–6 weeks after termination of therapy. The drug is metabolized in the liver (its main site of action) to active metabolites. Over 80% of an oral dose is excreted in the feces, via the bile, and approximately 10% is excreted through the urine.

Uses: As an adjunct to diet in primary hypercholesterolemia (types IIa and IIb) in patients with a significant risk of coronary artery disease and who have not responded to diet or other measures. May also be useful in patients with combined hypercholesterolemia and hypertriglyceridemia.

Contraindications: During pregnancy and lactation, active liver disease, persistent elevations of serum transaminases.

Special Concerns: Pregnancy category: X. Use in children is not recommended. Use with caution in patients who have a history of liver disease or who are known heavy consumers of alcohol.

Side Effects: *GI:* Flatus (most common), abdominal pain, cramps, diarrhea, constipation, dyspepsia, nausea, heartburn. *CNS:* Headache, dizziness. *Musculoskeletal:* Myalgia, muscle cramps. *Miscellaneous:* Blurred vision, rash, pruritus, dysgeusia, lenticular opacities.

Drug Interactions

Cholestyramine	Additive effects with lovastatin
Colestipol	Additive effects with lovastatin
Warfarin	↑ Prothrombin time

Laboratory Test Interference: Lovastatin ↑ transaminase and creatine phosphokinase levels.

Dosage: Tablets. Adults/adolescents: initial, 20 mg once daily with the evening meal. If serum cholesterol levels are greater than 300 mg/dl, initial dose should be 40 mg daily. **Maintenance:** 20–80 mg daily, individualized and adjusted at intervals of every 4 weeks, if necessary.

NURSING CONSIDERATIONS

See also *Nursing Considerations for Antihyperlipidemic Agents,* p. 566.

Administration/Storage

1. Dosage modification is not necessary in clients with renal insufficiency.
2. The maximum dose for clients on immunosuppressive therapy is 20 mg/day.

Assessment

1. Note any evidence of hepatic disease and any heavy consumption of alcohol.
2. Determine if the client has had recent eye examinations and request a report to serve as a baseline against which to measure possible eye changes in the future. Slight changes have been noted in the lens of the eyes of some clients.
3. If woman of childbearing age, determine if pregnant.

Client/Family Teaching

1. Instruct client to take the medication with meals.
2. If of childbearing age, advise client to practice some form of birth control.
3. Report the development of malaise, muscle spasms or fever. These may be mistaken for the flu, but the symptoms could be serious side effects of drug therapy and should not be ignored.
4. Any right upper quadrant abdominal pain or change in color and consistency of the stool should be reported.
5. Stress the importance of periodic eye exams during therapy with lovastatin and to report any visual disturbances.

Evaluation

1. Assess liver function tests every 4–6 weeks for the first 15 months of therapy. A threefold increase in serum transaminase, or an indication of abnormal liver function is a sign the therapy should be discontinued.
2. Monitor cholesterol levels every 4 weeks and adjust drug dose according to levels.

NICOTINIC ACID (NIACIN)   (nih-koh-**TIN**-ick **AH**-sid, **NYE**-ah-sin)

Niac, Niacels, Nico-400, Nicobid, Nicolar, Nicotinex, Span-Niacin-150 (Both Rx and OTC)

Classification: Antihyperlipidemic.

Action/Kinetics: By altering fat metabolism in adipose cells (increasing lipolysis, stimulating lipoprotein lipase), nicotinic acid decreases serum cholesterol, triglycerides, VLDL, and LDL in types II, III, IV, and V hyperlipoproteinemia, while levels of HDL increase. It stimulates the release of histamine from mast cells and increases gastric secretion. **Onset:** 30 min. **Peak plasma concentration:** 45 min. **t½:** 45 min. **Therapeutic plasma concentration:** 0.5–1.0 mcg/mL. **Onset, decreased cholesterol levels:** several days. **Onset, decreased triglyceride levels:** several hours. Excreted by the kidneys.

Uses: Primary hyperlipidemia (types IIa, IIb, III, IV, or V hyperproteinemia) in patients with a significant risk of coronary artery disease and who have not responded to weight loss and diet.

Contraindications: Active peptic ulcer, hemorrhage, severe hypotension, hepatic dysfunction.

Special Concerns: Pregnancy category: C. Use with caution in gallbladder disease and in patients with a history of jaundice, liver disease, arterial bleeding, glaucoma, gout, or diabetes. Safety and efficacy have not been determined in children or geriatric patients.

Side Effects: *GI:* Nausea, vomiting, diarrhea, GI distress, activation of peptic ulcer, abdominal pain, hepatotoxicity. These reactions can be severe but usually respond to dosage reduction. Concomitant administration of antacids helps. *Ophthalmologic:* Blurred vision, amblyopia, ocular edema. *CNS:* Panic reactions, nervousness. *Dermatologic:* Flushing, pruritus, urticaria, dry skin, sensation of warmth, keratosis nigricans, skin rashes, itching and tingling of skin. *Alteration of glucose metabolism:* Hyperglycemia, glycosuria, precipitation of diabetes. *Other:* Hypotension, headache (transient).

Drug Interactions	
Adrenergic blocking agents	Additive vasodilating effect → hypotension
Anticoagulants	Aluminum nicotinate ↑ effect
Antidiabetic agents	Change in sugar metabolism caused by aluminum nicotinate may require change in dosage of antidiabetic drugs
Probenecid	Nicotinic acid ↓ uricosuric effect of probenecid
Sulfinpyrazone	Nicotinic acid ↓ uricosuric effect of sulfinpyrazone
Tetracyclines	Effect ↓ by aluminum nicotinate

Laboratory Test Interferences: ↓ Glucose tolerance. Hyperuricemia, abnormal liver function tests.

Dosage: Extended-release Capsules/Tablets, Oral Solution, Tablets. Adults/adolescents: *antihyperlipidemic:* 1 g t.i.d. with or following meals (to be taken with cold water). The dose can be increased in increments of 500 mg daily q 2–4 weeks as needed. **Maintenance:** 1–2 g t.i.d. (maximum dose: 6 g/day). **Pediatric:** Up to 300 mg daily using the oral solution or tablets.

NURSING CONSIDERATIONS

See also *Nursing Considerations for Antihyperlipidemic Agents,* p. 566.

Administration/Storage

If flushing is persistent or bothersome, one aspirin, given 30 min prior to each dose of nicotinic acid, may assist the client.

Client/Family Teaching

1. Limit alcohol intake.

2. Take drug in *divided* doses with cold water at mealtime. If GI side effects persist, report to physician, who may reduce dosage and/or order an antacid.

3. Avoid taking aluminum nicotinate on an empty stomach, because in addition to gastric side effects, the likelihood of flushing is increased.

4. Flushing, pruritus, and nausea may subside with continued therapy. Aspirin may assist to reduce discomfort from the flushing response.

5. Clients with diabetes should be alert to symptoms of hyperglycemia precipitated by nicotinic acid. Monitor finger sticks and report hyperglycemia to the physician as a change in antidiabetic agents may be indicated.

6. Clients on anticoagulant therapy need to observe for increased bruising or bleeding and to report this to the physician.

7. In clients where acanthosis nigricans develops as a side effect, instruct that growths generally disappear 2 months after discontinuing drug therapy.

PROBUCOL   (PROH-byou-kohl)
Lorelco (Rx)

Classification: Antihyperlipidemic.

Action/Kinetics: Mechanism for alteration of cholesterol metabolism unknown, although the drug increases excretion of fecal bile acids, inhibits early stages of cholesterol synthesis, and slightly inhibits absorption of cholesterol from the diet. Decreases LDL cholesterol, and HDL; produces no change in triglycerides and either does not change or increases VLDL levels. After prolonged administration, the drug becomes deposited in the adipose tissues, and after discontinuation persists in the body for up to 6 months. Absorption from the GI tract is variable (usually less than 10%). Food increases peak blood levels. **t½ (biphasic): initial** 24 hr; **final:** 20 days. **Therapeutic onset:** 2–4 weeks; maximum: 20–50 days. Excreted through the feces and the urine (mainly unchanged).

Uses: Primary hypercholesterolemia, especially of type IIa, not responding to diet or weight control and clients who have a significant risk of coronary artery disease.

Contraindications: Hypersensitivity. Serious ventricular arrhythmias, unexplained syncope or syncope of cardiovascular origin, recent or progressive myocardial damage. In situations where the QT interval at an observed heart rate is more than 15% above the upper limit of normal (see package insert). Should not be used in treatment of elevated blood lipids to prevent coronary heart disease.

Special Concerns: Safe use during pregnancy (pregnancy category: B) and lactation and in children has not been established.

Side Effects: *CV:* Prolongation of the QT interval on the ECG, syncope, ventricular arrhythmias; sudden death may occur. *GI:* Most common: diarrhea, anorexia, indigestion, flatulence, GI bleeding, abdominal pain, nausea, vomiting. *Ophthalmic:* Blurred vision, tearing, conjunctivitis. *CNS:* Headache, dizziness, insomnia, paresthesia. *Hematologic:* Thrombocytopenia, eosinophilia, low hemoglobin, low hematocrit. *Dermatologic:* Rash, pruritus, hyperhidrosis, fetid sweat, petechiae, ecchymosis. *Miscellaneous:* Angioneurotic edema, decreased taste and smell sensations, enlargement of multinodular goiter, tinnitus, peripheral neuritis.

During the beginning of therapy certain patients have manifested an idiosyncratic reaction including dizziness, syncope, nausea, vomiting, palpitations, and chest pain.

Laboratory Test Interferences: Transient ↑ AST, ALT, alkaline phosphatase, uric acid, bilirubin, creatine phosphatase, alkaline phosphatase, blood glucose, BUN.

Dosage: Tablets. Adults only: 500 mg b.i.d. with morning and evening meals. In some patients, 500 mg once daily may be as effective as giving the drug b.i.d.

NURSING CONSIDERATIONS

See also *Nursing Considerations for Antihyperlipidemic Agents,* p. 566.

Administration/Storage

1. To be taken with morning and evening meals since food seems to increase absorption from the GI tract.
2. Clofibrate and probucol should not be given together as the combination may cause a significant decrease of HDL.
3. Store in dry place, in light-resistant containers away from excessive heat.

Client/Family Teaching

1. Advise client to take with food, as directed, to enhance absorption.
2. If diarrhea occurs, it is usually transient. Roughage should be eliminated until diarrhea stops.
3. Report any GI symptoms to physician if bothersome or persistent.
4. Stress the importance of reporting any unexplained bruising or bleeding.
5. Clients may develop insomnia, dizziness and/or headaches. These should be reported and a record kept of the occurrences.
6. If blurred vision occurs, or if clientd develop dizziness, they should be advised to avoid driving or using heavy equipment. The effects of the medication need to be reevaluated.
7. Nocturia and impotence may occur. Discuss this with the client when therapy is initiated. Encourage the client to report these developments at once as another medication may be necessary. Offer emotional support.

PART SIX

Drugs Affecting the Central Nervous System

6

29

CHAPTER TWENTY-NINE

Barbiturates

General Statement: The barbiturates, especially their sodium salts, are readily absorbed after oral, rectal, or parenteral administration. They are distributed throughout all tissues, cross the placental barrier, and appear in breast milk. Toxic doses depress the activity of tissues in addition to the CNS, including the cardiovascular system. In some patients, barbiturates manifest an unusual action, including an excitatory response.

Action/Kinetics: Barbiturates produce all levels of CNS depression, ranging from mild depression (sedation) following low doses to hypnotic (sleep-inducing) effects, and even coma and death, as dosage is increased. Certain barbiturates are also effective anticonvulsants. The depressant and anticonvulsant effects may be related to their ability to increase and/or mimic the inhibitory activity of the neurotransmitter gamma-aminobutyric acid (GABA) on nerve synapses. For example, the sedative-hypnotic effects of barbiturates may be due to an effect in the thalamus to inhibit ascending conduction in the reticular activating system, thus interfering with the transmission of impulses to the cerebral cortex. The anticonvulsant effects are believed to result from depression of monosynaptic and polysynaptic impulses in the CNS; barbiturates may also increase the threshold for electrical stimulation in the motor cortex. Importantly, barbiturates are not analgesics and therefore should not be given to patients for the purpose of ameliorating pain.

The main difference between the various barbiturates is in the onset of action. *Ultrashort-acting:* **Onset: IV,** immediate; **duration:** up to 30 min. *Short-acting:* **Onset: PO,** 10–15 min; **peak effect:** 3–4 hr. *Intermediate-acting:* **Onset: PO,** 45–60 min; **peak effect:** 6–8 hr. *Long-acting:* **Onset: PO,** 60 or more minutes; **peak effect:** 10–12 hr. *Rectal administration:* Onset times are similar to PO. **Onset: IV,** from immediate for short-acting drugs up to 5 min for long-acting drugs. **Duration of sedation:** 3–6 hr after IV; 6–8 hr, for all other routes. *Note:* It is currently believed that there is little difference in the duration of hypnosis after the use of any barbiturate; however, there is a difference in the time of onset. Thus, although widely used, the classification by duration of action may be outdated. Barbiturates are metabolized almost completely in the liver (except for barbital and phenobarbital) and are excreted in the urine.

Uses: Preanesthetic medication, anesthesia (thiobarbiturates), sedation, hypnotic, and for the control of acute convulsive conditions (only phenobarbital, mephobarbital, metharbital), as in epilepsy, tetanus, and eclampsia. The benzodiazepines have replaced barbiturates for the treatment of many conditions. See also information on individual drugs.

Contraindications: Hypersensitivity to barbiturates, severe trauma, pulmonary disease, edema, uncontrolled diabetes, history of porphyria, and for patients in whom they produce an excitatory response.

Special Concerns: Barbiturates should be used with caution during pregnancy (pregnancy category: D) and lactation and in patients with CNS depression, hypotension, marked asthenia (characteristic of Addison's disease, hypoadrenalism, and severe myxedema), porphyria, fever, anemia, hemorrhagic shock, cardiac, hepatic or renal damage, history of alcoholism in suicidal patients. Geriatric patients usually manifest increased sensitivity to barbiturates manifested by confusion, excitement, mental depression, and hypothermia.

Side Effects: *CNS:* Depression of CNS (sleepiness, drowsiness), ataxia, vertigo, nightmares, lethargy, hangover, agitation, confusion, hyperkinesia, paradoxical excitement, nervousness, hallucinations, psychiatric disturbances, insomnia, dizziness, anxiety, delirium, stupor. *CV:* Bradycardia, hypotension, syncope, circulatory collapse. *Respiratory:* Respiratory depression, bronchospasm, hypoventilation, apnea, laryngospasm. *GI:* Nausea, vomiting, diarrhea, constipation, epigastric pain. *Allergic:* Skin rashes, angioneurotic edema, serum sickness, urticaria, morbilliform rash. Rarely, exfoliative dermatitis, Stevens-Johnson syndrome. *Miscellaneous:* Pain syndrome (myalgia, neuralgia, arthritic pain). *After SC use:* Tissue necrosis, pain, tenderness, redness, permanent neurological damage if injected near peripheral nerves. *After IV use:* Thrombophlebitis. *After IM use:* Pain at injection site.

Barbiturates can induce physical and psychological dependence if high doses are used regularly for long periods of time. Withdrawal symptoms usually begin after 12–16 hr of abstinence. Manifestations of withdrawal include anxiety, weakness, nausea, vomiting, muscle cramps, delirium, and even tonic-clonic seizures.

Drug Interactions:

General Considerations

1. Barbiturates stimulate the activity of enzymes responsible for the metabolism of a large number of other drugs by a process known as *enzyme induction*. As a result, when barbiturates are given to patients receiving such drugs, their therapeutic effectiveness is markedly reduced or even abolished.
2. The CNS depressant effect of the barbiturates is potentiated by many drugs. Concomitant administration may result in coma or fatal CNS depression. Barbiturate dosage should either be reduced or eliminated when other CNS drugs are given.
3. Barbiturates also potentiate the toxic effects of many other agents.

Drug Interactions	
Alcohol	Potentiation or addition of CNS depressant effects. Concomitant use may lead to drowsiness, lethargy, stupor, respiratory collapse, coma, or death
Anesthetics, general	See *Alcohol*
Anorexiants	↓ Effect of anorexiants due to opposite pharmacologic effects
Antianxiety drugs	See *Alcohol*
Anticoagulants, oral	↓ Effect of anticoagulants due to ↓ absorption from GI tract and ↑ breakdown by liver
Antidepressants, tricyclic	↓ Effect of antidepressants due to ↑ breakdown by liver
Antidiabetic agents	Prolong the effects of barbiturates
Antihistamines	See *Alcohol*
Beta-adrenergic agents	↓ Beta blockade due to ↑ breakdown by the liver
Chloramphenicol	↑ Effect of barbiturates by ↓ breakdown by the liver and ↓ effect of chloramphenicol by ↑ breakdown by liver
CNS depressants	See *Alcohol*
Corticosteroids	↓ Effect of corticosteroids due to ↑ breakdown by liver
Digitoxin	↓ Effect of digitoxin due to ↑ breakdown by liver
Doxorubicin	↓ Effect of doxorubicin
Doxycycline	↓ Effect of doxycycline due to ↑ breakdown by liver
Estrogens	↓ Effect of estrogen due to ↑ breakdown by liver
Furosemide	↑ Risk or intensity of orthostatic hypotension

Drug Interactions

Griseofulvin	↓ Effect of griseofulvin due to ↓ absorption from GI tract
Haloperidol	↓ Effect of haloperidol due to ↑ breakdown by liver
Methoxyflurane	↑ Kidney toxicity due to ↑ breakdown of methoxyflurane by liver to toxic metabolites
Monoamine oxidase inhibitors	↑ Effect of barbiturates due to ↓ breakdown by liver
Narcotic analgesics	See *Alcohol*
Oral contraceptives	↓ Effect of contraceptives due to ↑ breakdown by liver
Phenothiazines	↓ Effect of phenothiazines due to ↑ breakdown by liver; also see *Alcohol*
Phenytoin	↓ Effect variable; monitor carefully
Procarbazine	↑ Effect of barbiturates
Quinidine	↓ Effect of quinidine due to ↑ breakdown by liver
Rifampin	↓ Effect of barbiturates due to ↑ breakdown by liver
Sedative-hypnotics, nonbarbiturate	See *Alcohol*
Theophyllines	↓ Effect of theophyllines due to ↑ breakdown by liver
Valproic acid	↑ Effect of barbiturates due to ↓ breakdown by liver

Acute Toxicity

Characterized by cortical and respiratory depression; anoxia; peripheral vascular collapse; feeble, rapid pulse; pulmonary edema; decreased body temperature; clammy, cyanotic skin; depressed reflexes; stupor; and coma. After initial constriction the pupils become dilated. Death results from respiratory failure or arrest followed by cardiac arrest.

Chronic Toxicity

Prolonged use of barbiturates at high doses may lead to physical and psychological dependence, as well as tolerance. Doses of 600–800 mg daily for 8 weeks may lead to physical dependence. The addict usually ingests 1.5 g/day. Addicts prefer short-acting barbiturates. Symptoms of dependence are similar to those associated with chronic alcoholism, and withdrawal symptoms are equally severe. Withdrawal symptoms usually last for 5 to 10 days and are terminated by a long sleep.

Treatment consists of a cautious withdrawal of the hospitalized addict over a 2- to 4-week period. A stabilizing dose of 200–300 mg of a short-acting barbiturate is administered every 6 hr. The dose is then reduced by 100 mg daily until the stabilizing dose is reduced by one-half. The patient is then maintained on this dose for 2–3 days before further reduction. The same procedure is repeated when the initial stabilizing dose has been reduced by three-quarters. If a mixed spike and slow activity appear on the ECG, or if insomnia, anxiety, tremor, or weakness is observed, the dosage is maintained at a constant level or increased slightly until symptoms disappear.

Treatment of Acute Toxicity

This should consist of maintenance of an adequate airway, oxygen intake, and carbon dioxide removal. Absorption following SC or IM administration of the drug may be delayed by the use of ice packs or tourniquets. After oral ingestion, gastric lavage or gastric aspiration may delay absorption. Emesis should not be induced once the symptoms of overdosage are manifested, as the patient may aspirate the vomitus into the lungs. Also, if the dose of barbiturate is high enough, the vomiting center in the brain may be depressed. Maintenance of renal function and removal of the drug by peritoneal dialysis or an artificial kidney should be carried out. Supportive physiologic methods have proven superior to analeptic methods.

Laboratory Test Interferences:

1. **Interference with test method:** ↑ 17-Hydroxycorticosteroids.
2. **Caused by pharmacologic effects:** ↑ Creatinine phosphokinase, alkaline phosphatase, serum transaminase, serum testosterone (in certain women), urinary estriol, porphobilinogen, coproporphyrin, uroporphyrin. ↓ Prothrombin time in patients on coumarin. ↑ or ↓ Bilirubin. False + lupus erythematosus test.

Dosage: Aim for minimum effective dosage (see Table 10). As hypnotics, barbiturates should be administered intermittently because tolerance develops. Elderly patients should receive one-half of the adult dose, and children should receive one-quarter to one-half the adult dose.

NURSING CONSIDERATIONS

Administration/ Storage

1. When used as hypnotics, barbiturates should not be given for more than 14–28 days.
2. Aqueous solutions of sodium salts are unstable and must be used within 30 min after preparation.
3. Discard parenteral solutions that contain precipitate.
4. Maintain an accurate record of the barbiturates on hand and the amounts dispensed.

Assessment

1. Note any history of untoward side effects to any of the barbiturate family of drugs.
2. Discuss the client's sleeping pattern with the client and family. This information is important in the physician's decision concerning the type of barbiturate to prescribe.
3. Determine the client's usual bedtime and the usual wakening hours.
4. If the client is of childbearing age determine if there is a likelihood of pregnancy. Other measures should be found to encourage sleep if pregnancy is a probability.
5. Determine the cause of the client's inability to sleep. A person in pain who gains relief of the pain may not need sleeping medication. Note evidence of fear and anxiety that may interfere with sleep.
6. Assess the client's environmental preferences for sleep, such as room temperature, lights and sounds.
7. Note presence of sensory alterations that could cause sleeplessness or disruptions in sleep time.

Interventions

1. Prior to administering the drug, discuss the goals of the medication therapy with the client.
2. Review the treatment for chronic and acute toxicity associated with barbiturates.
3. Do not awaken a client to administer a sleeping medication.
4. Assist the client during ambulation and use side rails once the client is in bed. Clients who receive hypnotic medications may become confused and unsteady. This is a particular problem among the elderly.

5. Use supportive measures such as a back rub, warm drinks, a quiet atmosphere and a calm attitude to encourage relaxation.

6. When the drug is administered PO, remain with the client to determine that the drug has been swallowed. If the client is disoriented and/or wearing dentures, check the buccal cavity, under the tongue and under denture plates. Routinely check the bedside area to assure that the client is not hoarding medication.

7. Anticipate that some clients may experience a period of transitory elation, confusion, or euphoria before sedation, and provide appropriate nursing measures to calm the client and prevent injury.

8. If the client becomes confused after taking the barbiturate, do not apply cuffs or other restraints. Rather remain with the client, and try to soothe and orient him/her by turning on a light and talking quietly and calmly until he/she is relaxed.

9. If the client asks for a second sleeping medication during the night, try to determine the cause of the sleeplessness. Institute comfort measures. If the client has pain, relieve the pain first. Wait approximately 20–30 minutes and then give the second dose of sleeping medication if the client has not yet fallen asleep.

10. Keep a careful check of the length of time the client has been receiving barbiturates. Therapy that requires sedative doses of medication over an 8 week period of time will cause physical dependence. Remind the medical staff of the amount of time the client has been taking the medication.

11. Assess the client for evidence of physical and/or psychological dependence and tolerance. Note on the client's chart and report the evidence to the physician.

12. Be alert to signs and symptoms of porphyria, characterized by nausea, vomiting, abdominal pain, and muscle spasms. Document and report the incidence and anticipate that the drug will be discontinued.

13. If the client receiving barbiturates is a child, supervise the child's play activity, especially if he/she is riding a bicycle or engaging in other potentially dangerous forms of play.

14. If clients are receiving barbiturates on an outpatient basis, be alert to the number of times the client returns for prescription refills. Frequency of refills may indicate the client has developed a dependency or that the client may be selling the drug for profit.

15. Monitor the client's blood count, periodically ordering a CBC, differential and platelet count. Some clients may develop hematologic disorders such as agranulocytosis, megaloblastic anemia and/or thrombocytopenia.

16. If the barbiturate is administered IV to counteract acute convulsions or for anesthesia anticipate that the therapy will be of limited duration.
    - Closely monitor the IV administration for the correct rate of flow. A too rapid injection may produce respiratory depression, dyspnea, and shock.
    - Monitor the site of the IV injection closely for extravasation, which may cause pain, nerve damage, and necrosis.
    - Note any redness or swelling along the site of the vein. This is evidence of thrombophlebitis.

Client/Family Teaching

1. Avoid the use of alcoholic beverages. These potentiate the effects of barbiturates.
2. Do not drive a car or operate other hazardous machinery after taking the medication.
3. Take the medication only as prescribed.

4. Avoid the use of OTC drugs or other medications unless the physician has first been consulted.

5. If the client is taking barbiturates for insomnia, suggest that the drug be taken a half hour before bedtime.

6. To avoid an accidental overdose, keep the medication in a medicine closet or in a drawer away from the bedside.

7. Keep all medications out of the reach of children. Large doses may be fatal and the potential for abuse exists.

8. If a client has been taking a barbiturate for 8 or more weeks, he/she should not discontinue the drug suddenly. To do so may result in withdrawal symptoms such as weakness, anxiety, delirium, and tonic-clonic seizures.

9. Dosages of drug should not be reduced without first checking with the physician.

10. Report to the physician immediately any signs of hematologic toxicity such as signs of infection (sore throat or fever) or increased bleeding tendencies (nosebleeds or easy bruising).

11. Assist to identify alternative methods that may promote relaxation and sleep (such as progressive muscle relaxation, guided imagery or soft music); support the client in exploring these methods.

Evaluation

1. At each visit, review the goals of therapy with the client and the effectiveness of the medication regimen. Investigate any problems noted by the client.

2. Note any changes in the pulse rate, blood pressure or changes in temperature and condition of the client's skin.

3. If the client is not responding as anticipated, review the need to alter the dose and explore other related factors such as changing the environment, or the existence of psychological stress.

PENTOBARBITAL (pen-toe-**BAR**-bih-tal)
Nembutal (C-II, Rx)

PENTOBARBITAL SODIUM (pen-toe-**BAR**-bih-tal)
Nembutal Sodium, Novo Rectal✱ (C-II, Rx)

See also *Barbiturates,* p. 581.

Classification: Sedative-hypnotic, barbiturate type.

Action/Kinetics: Short-acting. **t½:** 19–34 hr. Is 60%–70% protein bound.

Uses: Short-term treatment of insomnia. Sedative. Anticonvulsant (parenteral use only). *Investigational:* Parenterally to induce coma to protect the brain from ischemia and increased intracranial pressure following stroke and head trauma.

Special Concerns: Pregnancy category: D.

Dosage: Elixir, Capsules. *Sedation:* **Adults,** 20 mg t.i.d.–q.i.d. **Pediatric:** 2–6 mg/kg daily (use elixir). *Preoperative sedation:* **Adults,** 100 mg. *Hypnotic:* **Adults,** 100 mg at bedtime. **Suppositories, rectal.** *Hypnotic:* **Adults,** 120–200 mg; **infants, 2–12 months:** 30 mg; **1–4 years:** 30–60 mg; **5–12 years:** 60 mg; **12–14 years:** 60–120 mg. **IV (slow). Adults (70 kg),** 100 mg. **IM. Adults,** *hypnotic/preoperative sedation:* 150–200 mg; **pediatric:** 2–6 mg/kg (not to exceed 100 mg).

IV. Adults, *sedative/hypnotic:* 100 mg followed in 1 min by additional small doses, if required, up to a total of 500 mg. *Anticonvulsant:* **Adults, initial,** 100 mg; **then,** after 1 min, additional small doses may be given, if needed, up to a total of 500 mg.

IM, IV. Pediatric, *Anticonvulsant:* **initially,** 50 mg; **then,** after 1 min, additional small doses may be given, if needed, until the desired effect is achieved.

NURSING CONSIDERATIONS

See also *Nursing Considerations* for *Barbiturates,* p. 585.

Administration/Storage

1. Since pentobarbital is a potent CNS depressant that may cause adverse respiratory and circulatory responses, the IV dose is given in fractions. Adults generally receive 100 mg initially; children and debilitated clients, 50 mg. Subsequent fractions are administered after 1-min observation periods. Overdose or too rapid administration may cause spasms of the larynx or pharynx, or both.
2. Pentobarbital solutions are highly alkaline.
3. The parenteral product is not for SC use.
4. Parental pentobarbital is incompatible with most other drugs; therefore, do not mix other drugs in the same syringe.
5. Administer no more than 5 mL at one site **IM** because of possible tissue irritation (pain, necrosis, gangrene).
6. Suppositories are not to be divided.

Interventions

1. Observe for signs of respiratory depression. This is usually the first sign of drug overdose.
2. If the medication is administered IV, assess for patency.
3. Note client complaint of pain at the site of injection or in the limb. Interrupt the injection, document and report to the physician.
4. Note any delay in the onset of hypnosis, pallor, cyanosis or patchy discoloration of the skin. These are all signs of intra-arterial injection and can cause gangrene. The IV injection should be halted immediately, the observations recorded on the client's chart and the incident reported to the physician.
5. Initiate appropriate safety measures once the medication has been administered. This is particularly important when working with confused or elderly clients.

PHENOBARBITAL   (fee-no-**BAR**-bih-tal)

Ancalixir✿, Barbita, Gardenal✿, Solfoton (C-IV, Rx)

PHENOBARBITAL SODIUM   (fee-no-**BAR**-bih-tal)

Luminal Sodium (C-IV, Rx)

See also *Barbiturates,* p. 581.

Classification: Sedative, anticonvulsant, barbiturate type.

Action/Kinetics: Long-acting. **t½:** 24–140 hr. **Anticonvulsant therapeutic serum levels:** 10–40 mcg/mL. **Time for peak effect, after IV:** up to 15 min. Distributed more slowly than other barbiturates due to lower lipid solubility. Is 50%–60% protein bound.

Uses: Sedative, preanesthetic, postoperative sedation, hypnotic, anticonvulsant (tonic-clonic or cortical focal seizures); emergency control of acute seizure disorders such as status epilepticus, meningitis, tetanus, eclampsia, toxicity of local anesthetics. Phenobarbital is considered a drug of choice for tonic-clonic seizures. *Investigational:* Prophylaxis and treatment of hyperbilirubinemia.

Special Concerns: Pregnancy category: D.

Additional Side Effects: Chronic use may result in headache, fever, and megaloblastic anemia.

Dosage: *Phenobarbital, Phenobarbitol Sodium.* **Capsules, Elixir, Tablets.** *Sedation:* **Adults,** 30–120 mg daily in 2–3 divided doses. **Pediatric,** 2 mg/kg (60 mg/m²) t.i.d. *Hypnotic:* **Adults,** 100–320 mg at bedtime. **Pediatric,** Dose should be determined by physician. *Preoperative sedation:* **Pediatric,** 1–3 mg/kg. *Anticonvulsant:* **Adults,** 60–250 mg daily in single or divided doses. **Pediatric,** 1–6 mg/kg daily in single or divided doses. *Antihyperbilirubinemic:* **Adults,** 30–60 mg t.i.d. **Pediatric, up to 12 years of age:** 1–4 mg/kg t.i.d. **Neonates,** 5–10 mg/kg for the first few days after birth.
   IM, IV. *Sedation:* **Adults,** 30–120 mg daily in 2–3 divided doses. *Preoperative sedation:* **Pediatric,** 1–3 mg/kg 60–90 min prior to surgery. *Hypnotic:* **Adults,** 100–325 mg. **Pediatric:** dose to be determined by physician.
   IV. *Anticonvulsant:* **Adults,** 100–320 mg, repeated, if necessary to a total daily dose of 600 mg. **Pediatric, initial loading dose,** 10–20 mg/kg; **then,** 1–6 mg/kg daily. *Status epilepticus:* **Adults,** 10–20 mg/kg (given slowly); may be repeated if needed. **Pediatric,** 15–20 mg/kg given over a 10–15 min period.
   IM only. *Preoperative sedation:* **Adults,** 130–200 mg 60–90 min before surgery. *Antihyperbilirubinemic:* **Pediatric,** 5–10 mg/kg daily for the first few days after birth.

NURSING CONSIDERATIONS
See also *Nursing Considerations* for *Barbiturates,* p. 585.

Administration/Storage
1. When used for seizures, give the major fraction of the dose according to when seizures are likely to occur (i.e., on arising for daytime seizures and at bedtime when seizures occur at night).
2. In most cases, when used for epilepsy, drug must be taken regularly to avoid seizures, even when no seizures are imminent.
3. The aqueous solution for injection must be freshly prepared.
4. Some ready-dissolved solutions for injection are available; the vehicle is propylene glycol, water, and alcohol.
5. For IV administration, inject slowly at a rate of 50 mg/min.

Interventions
1. Instruct client to report any bothersome side effects.
2. Monitor serum levels as indicated.
3. Be aware that phenobarbital may require an increase in vitamin D consumption.

SECOBARBITAL   (see-koh-**BAR**-bih-tal)

Seconal (C-II, Rx)

SECOBARBITAL SODIUM   (see-koh-**BAR**-bih-tal)

Seconal Sodium (C-II, Rx)

See also *Barbiturates,* p. 581.

Classification: Sedative-hypnotic, barbiturate type.

Action/Kinetics: Short-acting. Distributed quickly as it has the highest lipid solubility of the barbiturates. **t½:** 15–40 hr. Is 46%–70% protein bound.

Uses: Short-term treatment of insomnia. Sedative to relieve anxiety, tension, and apprehension. Preoperative sedative. May be used parenterally as an anticonvulsant in tetanus.

Special Concerns: Pregnancy category: D.

Dosage: Capsules. *Hypnotic:* **Adults:** 100 mg at bedtime. *Preoperative sedation:* **Adults:** 200–300 mg 1–2 hr before surgery; **pediatric:** 2–6 mg/kg (up to a maximum of 100 mg) 1–2 hr before surgery. *Daytime sedation:* **Adults:** 30–50 mg t.i.d.–q.i.d. **Pediatric:** 2 mg/kg (60 mg/m²) t.i.d.
 Rectal suppositories. *Hypnotic:* **Adults:** 200 mg. *Daytime sedation:* **Adults,** 200 mg daily in 3 divided doses. Suppositories are not for use in children.
 Rectal solution. *Hypnotic:* **Pediatric, up to 40 kg:** 5 mg/kg; **over 40 kg:** 4 mg/kg.
 IM, IV. *Anticonvulsant in tetanus:* **Adults:** 5.5 mg/kg q 3–4 hr as needed. **Pediatric:** 3–5 mg/kg (125 mg/m²) per dose. **IM.** *Hypnotic:* **Adults:** 100–200 mg. **Pediatric:** 3–5 mg/kg (125 mg/m²) up to a maximum of 100 mg per dose. *Preoperative sedative:* **Pediatric:** 4–5 mg/kg. *Sedative for dentistry:* **Adults,** 1.1–2.2 mg/kg 10–15 min prior to procedure. **IV.** *Nerve block for dentistry:* **Adults:** 100–150 mg.

NURSING CONSIDERATIONS

See also *Nursing Considerations* for *Barbiturates,* p. 585.

Administration/Storage

1. For adults, the aqueous parenteral solution is preferred to polyethylene glycol, which may be irritating to the kidneys, especially in clients with signs of renal insufficiency.
2. Aqueous solutions for injection should be freshly prepared from dry-packed ampules.

Interventions

1. Rapid IV administration may precipitate hypotension, respiratory depression, laryngospasm or apnea; do not exceed recommended rate (50 mg/15 sec).
2. Following prolonged use, taper dosage and withdraw drug slowly to prevent precipitating withdrawal symptoms.

Table 10 Barbiturates

Drug	Use	Dosage	Remarks
Amobarbital (Amytal) (C-II, Rx) Amobarbital sodium (Amytal) (C-II, Rx) Pregnancy category: D.	PO: Sedative, short-term, hypnotic. Parenteral: Preoperative medication; Parenteral: Seizures due to status epilepticus, meningitis, eclampsia, drugs Also, acute seizures due to tetanus. Narcoanalysis; diagnosis of schizophrenia; treat catatonic, negativisitc, and manic reactions. Has mostly been replaced by benzodiazepines.	Capsules, Tablets. *Sedation:* Adults, 50–300 mg daily in divided doses. Pediatric: 2 mg/kg t.i.d. for sedation 2–6 mg/kg, up to a maximum of 100 mg preoperatively. *Hypnotic:* 65–200 mg at bedtime. *During labor:* 200–400 mg q 1/2 hr up to a total of 1 g. IM, IV. *Sedative:* Adults, IM, IV, 30–50 mg b.i.d.–t.i.d. *Preoperative sedative:* Pediatric, IV 3–5 mg/kg. *Hypnotic:* Adults, IM, IV, 65–200 mg at bedtime. Pediatric, less than 6 years, IM: 2–3 mg/kg. Pediatric, over 6 years, IM: 2–3 mg/kg; IV, 65–200 mg/dose. *Anticonvulsant:* Pediatric, less than six years of age. IM, IV: 3–5 mg/kg; over 6 years of age, IV: 65–500 mg/dose.	Onset, PO. 45–60 min. Duration: 6–8 hr. t^1/2: 16–40 hr. Intermediate-acting. *Administration* 1. IM. Inject deeply, in large muscle, no more than 5 ml at one site. 2. For IM, 20% solution may be used to reduce the total volume required. 3. IV. Inject slowly at a rate not exceeding 1 mL/min. Faster rates may lead to severe respiratory depression. 4. Solutions that are not clear after 5 min should not be used. 5. No more than 30 min should elapse between opening of ampule and usage. 6. To reconstitute for parenteral use, add sterile water for injection; the vial should be rotated for mixing but not shaken.
Aprobarbital (Alurate) (C-II, Rx) Pregnancy category: D.	Daytime sedation, hypnotic.	Elixir. Adults: *Sedation:* 40 mg t.i.d. Hypnotic: 40–160 mg at bedtime, depending on severity of the insomnia.	Onset: 45–60 min. Duration: 6–8 hr. Intermediate-acting. t^1/2: 14–34 hr. One teaspoon (5 mL) contains 40 mg aprobarbital. Use not recommended in children. Geriatric patients may manifest confusion, excitement, or mental depression.
Butabarbital sodium (Barbased, Butalan, Buticaps, Butisol, Sarisol No. 2) (C-III, Rx) Pregnancy Category: D.	Sedative, preoperative medication.	Capsules, Elixir, Tablets. *Sedation:* Adults, 15–30 mg t.i.d.–q.i.d. for daytime sedation; 50/100 mg 60–90 min prior to surgery.	Onset: 45–60 min. Duration: 6–8 hr. Intermediate-acting. t^1/2: 66–140 hr. Also found in Fiorinal Plain and Fiorinal with Codeine.

Table 10 (Continued)

Drug	Use	Dosage	Remarks
		Pedriatic: 2 mg/kg t.i.d.; 2–6 mg/kg (up to 100 mg/dose) for preoperative sedation. *Hypnotic:* **Adults,** 50–100 mg before bedtime.	Physician must individualize hypnotic dose in children. **Geriatric patients:** *See Aprobarbital.*
Mephobarbital (Mebaral)(C-IV, Rx) Pregnancy category: D.	Recommended only as an anticonvulsant. Sometimes used as a sedative.	**Tablets.** *Anticonvulsant:* **Adults,** 200 mg at bedtime to 600 mg daily in divided doses. **Pediatric, age five years and older,** 32–64 mg t.i.d.–q.i.d. **Age five years and younger,** 16–32 mg t.i.d.–q.i.d. *Sedative:* **Adults,** 32–100 mg t.i.d.–q.i.d. **Pediatric:** 16–32 mg t.i.d.–q.i.d.	**Onset:** More than 1 hr. **Duration:** 10–12 hr. Long-acting. **t½:** 11–67 hr in liver to phenobarbital, which is the active form. Causes little drowsiness or lassitude. *Administration* 1. If mephobarbital is to replace another anticonvulsant drug, the dose of the other drug should be decreased slowly as the dose of mephobarbital is increased slowly. 2. May be used together with phenytoin; in such instances, the dose of phenytoin should be reduced but the full dose of mephobarbital should be used.
Metharbital (Gemonil) (C-III, Rx) Pregnancy category: D.	Indicated only to treat various types of seizures such as tonic–clonic, myoclonic, or mixed type.	**Tablets.** *Individualized,* **Adults,** usual, 100 mg 1–3 times daily, increased, if needed to 800 mg daily. **Pediatric:** 50 mg 1–3 times daily or 5–15 mg/kg daily.	**Onset:** More than 1 hr. **Duration:** 10–12 hr. Long-acting. May be more effective as an anticonvulsant if used with other drugs. When adding to or replacing other anticonvulsant therapy, the dose of the other medication should be reduced slowly while increasing the dose of metharbital. Metharbital is metabolized to barbital. Geriatric patients may manifest confusion, excitement, or depression.

Methohexital sodium
(Brevital sodium)
(C-IV, Rx)
Pregnancy category:
C.

General anesthetic for short
surgical procedures; induction
to anesthesia; to supplement
other anesthetics; to induce
hypnosis.

IV, Induction, Adults: 1–2 mg/kg;
maintenance, intermittent IV:
0.25–1 mg/kg as required. **IM,
Induction, pedriatic:** 5–10
mg/kg; **IV,** 1–2 mg/kg.

Onset: few seconds. **Duration:**
5–8 min. Ultra-short acting.
Administration
1. Use with extreme caution in
   patients with status asthmaticus.
2. Dilution may be made with
   sterile water for injection, 5%
   dextrose injection, or 0.9%
   sodium chloride injection.
   Bacteriostatic diluents and
   lactated Ringer's solution
   should not be used.
3. The 1% solution should not
   be used unless it is clear and
   colorless.
4. Methohexital is stable for 6
   weeks at room temperature
   when diluted with sterile water
   for injection but is stable for
   only 24 hr when diluted with
   either dextrose or sodium
   chloride.
5. Methohexital should not be
   mixed with solutions of
   atropine sulfate, metocurine
   iodide, or succinylcholine
   chloride.
6. Methohexital is incompatible
   with silicone, including syringes
   or rubber stoppers coated with
   silicone.
7. Contraindicated in porphyria.

Talbutal (Lotusate)
(C-III, Rx)
Pregnancy
category: D

Short-term hypnotic.

PO. *Hypnotic:* 120 mg 15–30 min
before bedtime. Dosage not
established for children less
than 15 years of age.

Onset: 45–60 min. **Duration:** 6–8
hr. Intermediate-acting. **t½:**
15 hr. Geriatric patients
may manifest confusion,
excitment, depression.

Table 10 *(Continued)*

Drug	**Use**	**Dosage**	**Remarks**
Thiamylal sodium (Surital) (C-III, Rx) Pregnancy category: C.	General anesthetic for short surgical procedures; induction of anesthesia; to supplement other anesthetics; to induce hypnosis. *Investigational:* Treatment of seizures caused by inhalation or local anesthetics.	**IV. Adults, induction:** 2–4 mL of a freshly prepared 2.5% solution; **maintenance, individualized, usual:** 2–4 mL of a 2.5% solution by intermittent IV. For children, dose should be individualized by the physician. *Treat seizures:* **Adults,** 2–5 mL of a 2.5% solution given as soon as possible after seizure begins.	**Onset:** Few seconds. **Duration:** 20–30 min. Ultra-short acting. *Administration* 1. Initially, a test dose of 2 mL of a 2.5% solution should be given to determine sensitivity. 2. For maintenance, a 0.3% solution can be used by continuous drip; the 2.5% solution should be used for induction and for maintenance by intermittent IV injection. 3. The preferred diluent is sterile water for injection. Bacteriostatic products or Ringer's solution should not be used. For continuous drip, dilute with 5% dextrose or 0.9% sodium chloride. 4. Use with extreme caution in patients with status asthmaticus. 5. Thiamylal should not be mixed with atropine sulfate, metocurine iodide, or succinylcholine chloride. 6. Refrigerated solutions are stable for 6 days whereas solutions kept at room temperature should be used within 24 hr. Only use solutions that are clear. 7. The rate of injection should be 1 mL q 5 sec for induction (2.5%). 8. Introduction of air into the solution may increase the risk of cloudiness. 9. Contraindicated in porphyria.

Thiopental Sodium (Pentothal) (C-III, Rx) Pregnancy category: C.

General anesthetic for short surgical procedures; induction of anesthesia; preanesthetic medication; to supplement other anesthetics; to induce hypnosis. Treat seizures cause by inhalation or local anesthetics. Treat cerebral hypertension due to Reye's syndrome, cerebral edema, or acute head injury. Narcoanalysis in psychiatry. Rectal suspension: preanesthetic sedation or basal narcosis.
Investigational: Treatment of cerebral hypoxia or ischemia.

IV. *Induction of anesthesia:* 50–100 mg (2–4 mL of a 2.5% solution) depending on response. *Maintenance of anesthesia:* 50–100 mg whenever patient moves. If used as the sole anesthetic, maintain by continuous IV drip of a 0.2% or 0.4% solution. *Seizures following anesthesia:* 50–125 mg (3–5 mL of 2.5% solution). Seizures due to a local anesthetic may require 125–250 mg over a 10 min period. *Cerebral hypertension:* **Adults,** 1.5–3.5 mg/kg repeated as needed to reduce intracranial pressure. *Narcoanalysis:* **Adults,** 2.5% IV at a rate of 100 mg/min with patient counting backward from one hundred. **Rectal Solution.** *Preanesthetic sedation:* **Adults,** 30 mg/kg. *Basal narcosis:* **Adults, children,** up to 9 mg/kg. Use a lower rectal dose in inactive or debilitated patients.

Onset: Few seconds. **Duration:** 20–30 min. Rectal solutions: **Onset,** 8–10 min. Ultra-short acting.

Contraindications: Porphyria, status asthmaticus. Use with caution during lactation as the drug appears in breast milk.

Administration

1. The drug may be diluted with sterile water for injection, sodium chloride injection, or 5% dextrose injection.
2. A concentration of 2% or 2.5% is most commonly used for intermittent injections.
3. Solutions less than 2% in sterile water for injection cause hemolysis.
4. Reconstituted solutions should be freshly prepared and used promptly. Any unused solution should be discarded after 24 hr.
5. Thiopental should not be mixed with atropine sulfate, succinylcholine, or tubocurarine.
6. Solutions with a visible precipitate should not be used.
7. A test dose of 25–75 mg should be given initially to determine sensitivity.
8. IV administration should be done cautiously to avoid serious respiratory depression.
9. Dosage should be individualized in children less than 15 years of age (usually IV, 3–5 mg/kg). *Drug Interaction:* Sulfisoxazole ↑ effects of thiopental by ↓ plasma protein binding.

CHAPTER THIRTY

Benzodiazepine and other Nonbarbiturate Sedative-Hypnotics

Action/Kinetics: The nonbarbiturate sedative-hypnotics act similarly to the barbiturates in that they are believed to increase and/or mimic the inhibitory activity of the neurotransmitter gamma-aminobutyric acid (GABA) on nerve synapses. This results in inhibition of ascending conduction in the reticular activating system, thus interfering with the transmission of impulses to the cerebral cortex. Many of the actions of the nonbarbiturate sedative-hypnotics are similar to those of barbiturates, including development of psychological dependence, physical dependence, and tolerance (See Chapter 29, p. 581).

Drug Interactions: Concomitant use of nonbarbiturate sedative-hypnotics with alcohol, anesthetics, antianxiety drugs, antihistamines, barbiturates, narcotics, or phenothiazines may result in addition or potentiation of CNS depressant effects. Symptoms manifested are drowsiness, lethargy, stupor, respiratory collapse, coma, and possible death.

NURSING CONSIDERATIONS

Assessment

1. Note any evidence of renal failure. Ensure that pre-treatment lab studies have been performed.
2. If the client is of childbearing age and likely to become pregnant, document and notify physician. Fetal damage has been reported with the use of some drugs in this category.
3. Determine the client's menstrual history where appropriate.
4. In taking the drug history, note if the client is taking any drugs such as cimetidine that could impede the metabolism of benzodiazepines.

Interventions

1. Be alert to client complaints of drowsiness, fatigue or dizziness. Also note any family complaint of the client appearing confused and report to the physician.
2. Supervise ambulation of clients, and when they are in bed, keep the side rails up, the bed in low position, and the call bell within easy reach.

3. Document any complaints of double or blurred vision and have the client's vision evaluated as necessary.

4. Observe for evidence of jaundice, client complaints of right upper quadrant pain or malaise. Document and report as these symptoms may indicate a need for a change in the prescribed therapy.

5. Weigh the client routinely to determine any significant changes such as excessive gains or losses. Any significant variations may indicate a need to change drug therapy.

6. If menstrual irregularities occur, or if they are severe or bothersome, document and report as a change in drug therapy may be indicated.

Client/Family Teaching

1. Avoid ingestion of alcohol with any of these drugs.

2. Use caution in driving or operating machinery until daytime sedative effects are evaluated.

3. Assess for tolerance and psychological and physical dependence and notify physician.

4. When suffering from simple insomnia, try warm baths, warm drinks, and other interventions to induce sleep rather than becoming dependent on drugs.

5. Discuss with the client/family the need to avoid prolonged exposure to the sun. Wear protective clothing and use a sun screen on the skin when outside for extended periods of time.

6. Stress the importance of reporting any unusual symptoms and persistent or bothersome side effects.

7. If the client smokes, strongly encourage him/her to stop. Refer for therapy and smoking cessation programs as needed.

Evaluation

1. Review the expected benefits anticipated with this drug therapy and if attained.

2. Evaluate for freedom from complications of drug therapy.

3. Determine response to therapy and if the client is adhering to the prescribed drug regimen.

30

ACETYLCARBROMAL   (ah-see-til-kar-**BROH**-mal)

Paxarel (Rx)

Classification: Nonbarbiturate, nonbenzodiazepine sedative-hypnotic.

Action/Kinetics: Liberates bromide, which causes sedation. Since the active principle of acetylcarbromal is bromide, intoxication (bromism) may result. If bromism develops, the drug should be discontinued and the excretion of bromide increased by administering sodium or ammonium chloride or a chloruretic diuretic. Hemodialysis is also effective. The drug is rarely used.

Uses: Anxiety, tension, insomnia. Premenstrual tension or menopausal syndrome. Preoperative, preprocedural, or postoperative sedative. Spastic colitis.

Contraindications: Sensitivity to bromides. Lactation.

Side Effects: Large doses: Bromide intoxication characterized by dizziness, impaired thoughts, irritability, motor incoordination, skin rash, vomiting, profound stupor, and bromide psychosis.

Dosage: Tablets. Adults: 250–500 mg b.i.d.–t.i.d. **Pediatric:** Dosage is less than adults and determined by age and weight.

See also *Nursing Considerations* for *Barbiturates,* p. 585, and *Benzodiazepine and Other Nonbarbiturate Sedative-Hypnotics,* p. 596.

Client/Family Teaching

Review the signs and symptoms of bromide intoxication listed under *Side Effects.* Instruct the client/family to discontinue taking the drug and report to the physician if symptoms of bromism are observed.

CHLORAL HYDRATE   (KLOH-ral)

Aquachloral Supprettes, Noctec, Novochlorhydrate ❀ (C-IV, Rx)

Classification: Nonbarbiturate, nonbenzodiazepine sedative-hypnotic.

Action/Kinetics: Chloral hydrate is metabolized to trichloroethanol, which is the active metabolite causing CNS depression. Chloral hydrate produces only slight hangover effects and is said not to affect REM sleep. High doses lead to severe CNS depression, as well as depression of respiratory and vasomotor centers (hypotension). Both psychological and physical dependence develop. **Onset:** within 30 min. **Duration:** 4–8 hr. **t½, trichloroethanol:** 7–10 hr. The drug is readily absorbed from the GI tract and is distributed to all tissues; it passes the placental barrier and appears in breast milk as well. Metabolites excreted by kidney.

Uses: Short-term hypnotic. Daytime sedative and sedation prior to EEG procedures. Preoperative sedative and postoperative as adjunct to analgesics. Prevent or reduce symptoms of alcohol withdrawal.

Contraindications: Marked hepatic or renal impairment, severe cardiac disease, lactation. Drugs should not be given orally to patients with esophagitis, gastritis, or gastric or duodenal ulcer.

Special Concerns: Pregnancy category: C. Use by nursing mothers may cause sedation in the infant. A decrease in dose may be necessary in geriatric patients due to age-related decrease in both hepatic and renal function.

Side Effects: *CNS:* Paradoxical paranoid reactions. Sudden withdrawal in dependent patients may result in "chloral delirium." Sudden intolerance to the drug following prolonged use may result in respiratory depression, hypotension, cardiac effects, and possibly death. *GI:* Nausea, vomiting, diarrhea, bad taste in mouth, gastritis, increased peristalsis. *GU:* Renal damage, decreased urine flow and uric acid excretion. *Miscellaneous:* Skin reactions, hepatic damage, allergic reactions, leukopenia, eosinophilia.

Chronic toxicity is treated by gradual withdrawal and rehabilitative measures such as those used in treatment of the chronic alcoholic. Poisoning by chloral hydrate resembles acute barbiturate intoxication; the same supportive treatment is indicated (see *Barbiturates,* p. 581).

Drug Interactions	
Anticoagulants, oral	↑ Effect of anticoagulants by ↓ plasma protein binding
CNS depressants	Additive CNS depression. Concomitant use may lead to drowsiness, lethargy, stupor, respiratory collapse, coma, or death
Furosemide (IV)	Concomitant use results in diaphoresis, tachycardia, hypertension, flushing

Laboratory Test Interferences: ↑ 17-Hydroxycorticosteroids. Interference with fluorescence tests for catecholamines and copper sulfate test for glucose.

Dosage: Capsules, Syrup. Adults: *Daytime sedative:* 250 mg t.i.d. after meals. *Preoperative sedative:* 0.5–1.0 g 30 min before surgery. *Hypnotic:* 0.5–1 g 15–30 min before bedtime. **Pediatric:** *Daytime sedative:* 8.3 mg/kg (250 mg/m²) up to a maximum of 500 mg t.i.d. after meals. *Hypnotic:* 50 mg/kg (1.5 g/m²) at bedtime (up to 1 g may be given as a single dose). *Premedication prior to EEG procedures:* 20–25 mg/kg.

Suppositories, rectal. Adults: *Daytime sedative:* 325 mg t.i.d. *Hypnotic:* 0.5–1 g at bedtime. **Pediatric:** *Daytime sedative:* 8.3 mg/kg (250 mg/m²) t.i.d. *Hypnotic:* 50 mg/kg (1.5 g/m²) at bedtime (up to 1 g as a single dose).

NURSING CONSIDERATIONS

See also *Nursing Considerations* for *Benzodiazepines and other Nonbarbiturate Sedative Hypnotics,* p. 596.

Administration/Storage

1. PO: give capsules after meals with a full glass of water. Give the syrup with half a glass of juice, water, ginger ale, or coke syrup.
2. Oral syrups have an unpleasant taste which can be reduced by chilling the syrup before administration.

Assessment

Assess client alertness and response to stimuli and document.

Interventions

1. Note the level of alertness of the client and compare with the premedication history.
2. Observe client respiratory and cardiac responses. Note any evidence of vasomotor depression and dilatation of cutaneous blood vessels.
3. Periodically perform liver and renal function studies to determine any evidence of impairment.
4. Observe client for psychological and physical dependence. Symptoms of dependence resemble those of acute alcoholism, but with more severe gastritis. These should be documented and reported.
5. Have emergency drugs and equipment available should the client require supportive, physiologic treatment of acute poisoning.

ETHCHLORVYNOL (eth-klor-**VYE**-nohl)

Placidyl (C-IV, Rx)

Classification: Nonbarbiturate, nonbenzodiazepine sedative-hypnotic.

Action/Kinetics: Manifests anticonvulsant and muscle relaxant properties, as well as sedative and hypnotic effects. Said to depress REM sleep. Chronic use produces psychological and physical dependence. Produces less respiratory depression than occurs with barbiturates. **Onset:** 15–60 min. **Peak blood levels:** 1–1.5 hr. **Duration:** 5 hr. **t½:** initial, 1–3 hr; final, 10–25 hr. Approximately 90% metabolized in liver and excreted in urine.

Uses: Short-term treatment of insomnia (treatment not to exceed 1 week). Has generally been replaced by other sedative-hypnotic drugs. *Investigational:* Sedation.

Contraindications: Porphyria, hypersensitivity.

Special Concerns: Pregnancy category: C. Use during the third trimester may result in CNS depression and withdrawal symptoms in the neonate. Geriatric patients may be more sensitive to the effects of this drug; also, a decrease in dose may be necessary in these patients due to age-related decreases in both hepatic and renal function.

Side Effects: *CNS:* Initial excitement, giddiness, vertigo, mental confusion, headache, blurred vision, hangover, fatigue, ataxia. *GI:* Bad aftertaste, nausea, vomiting, gastric upset. *CV:* Hypotension, fainting. *Miscellaneous:* Skin rash, thrombocytopenia, jaundice, pulmonary edema (following IV abuse). Overdose produces symptoms similar to those of barbiturate intoxication.

Drug Interactions

Anticoagulants, oral	↓ Effect of anticoagulants due to ↑ breakdown by liver
Antidepressants, tricyclic	Combination may result in transient delirium

---

Laboratory Test Interference: ↓ Prothrombin time (patients on coumarin).

Dosage: Capsules. Adult, usual: 500 mg at bedtime; up to 1,000 mg may be required if insomnia is severe. If patient awakens, a 100- to 200-mg supplemental dose can be given. Adjust dose carefully in geriatric or debilitated patients. *Sedation:* 100–200 mg b.i.d.–t.i.d.

NURSING CONSIDERATIONS

See also *Nursing Considerations* for *Benzodiazepine,* p. 596.

Interventions

1. Monitor liver and renal function studies and anticipate altered dose with organ dysfunction.
2. Advise client to use caution in driving or operating machinery until daytime sedative effects are evaluated. Milk or food taken with the medication may reduce these symptoms.
3. Assess closely for tolerance and for psychological and physical dependence.

ETHINAMATE   (eh-**THIN**-ah-mayt)

Valmid (C-IV, Rx)

Classification: Nonbarbiturate, nonbenzodiazepine sedative-hypnotic.

Action/Kinetics: Drug may have some weak anticonvulsant and weak local anesthetic effects. Therapeutic doses produce quiet sleep with little or no hangover. Larger doses produce euphoria. Ethinamate may cause psychological and physical dependence as well as tolerance. Withdrawal symptoms are similar to those of barbiturates. **Onset:** 20–30 min. **Peak plasma levels:** About 35 min. **Duration:** 3–5 hr. **t½, elimination:** 2.5 hr. A dose of 500 mg ethinamate is approximately equal to 100 mg secobarbital. Inactivated in liver and excreted in urine.

Uses: Short-term treatment of insomnia (use should not exceed 1 week). Has generally been replaced by other sedative-hypnotics.

Contraindications: Hypersensitivity to drug. Not useful in patients suffering pain. *Not recommended* for routine daytime sedation because prolonged use may lead to psychological and physical dependence.

Special Concerns: Safety in pregnancy (pregnancy category: C), during lactation, and in children less than 15 years of age has not been established. Geriatric patients may be more sensitive to this drug; also, a decrease in dose may be necessary in these patients due to age-related decreases in both hepatic and renal function.

Side Effects: Few. Thrombocytopenic purpura, fever, mild GI symptoms, skin rashes, and paradoxical excitement in children. Abrupt withdrawal of large doses may be dangerous.

Laboratory Test Interference: Interferes with test by ↑ 17-hydroxycorticosteroids and 17-ketosteroids.

Dosage: Capsules. Adults: 0.5–1 g 20 min before bedtime. Elderly or debilitated patients should receive no more than 0.5 g initially at bedtime.

NURSING CONSIDERATIONS

See also *Nursing Considerations* for *Barbiturates,* p. 585, and *Benzodiazepine and Other Nonbarbiturate Sedative-Hypnotics,* p. 596.

Administration/Storage

If insomnia persists after one week of therapy, a one week rest period should follow before a second course of therapy.

Interventions

1. Assess client receiving large dosages for symptoms of dependence.
2. See discussion of treatment for acute toxicity under *Barbiturates,* Chapter 29, p. 581.
3. Be prepared to assist with gastric lavage for acute poisoning. Lavage must be done immediately because the drug is rapidly absorbed from the GI tract.

Client/Family Teaching

1. Avoid driving or operating heavy equipment. The drug may cause drowsiness and dizziness.
2. Caution client not to abruptly discontinue the drug. Notify physician first since withdrawal symptoms may occur.

FLURAZEPAM HYDROCHLORIDE   (floo-**RAY**-zeh-pam)

Apo-Flurazepam ✤, Dalmane, Durapam, Novoflupam ✤, Somnol ✤, Som-Pam ✤ (C-IV, Rx)

See also *Benzodiazepines and other Nonbarbiturate Sedative Hypnotics,* p. 596.

Classification: Benzodiazepine sedative-hypnotic.

Action/Kinetics: Flurazepam acts at benzodiazepine receptors which are part of the benzodiazepine-GABA receptor-chloride ionophore complex. Interaction with the complex enhances the inhibitory action of GABA leading to interference of transmission of nerve impulses in the reticular activating system. **Onset:** 17 min. The major active metabolite, *N*-desalkyl-flurazepam, is active and has a $t^{1/2}$ of 47–100 hr. **Time to peak plasma levels, flurazepam:** 0.5–1 hr; **active metabolite:** 1–3 hr. **Duration:** 7–8 hr. **Maximum effectiveness:** 2–3 days (due to slow accumulation of active metabolite). Significantly bound to plasma protein. Elimination is slow as metabolites remain in the blood for several days. Exceeding the recommended dose may result in development of tolerance and dependence.

Use: Insomnia (all types). Flurazepam is increasingly effective on the second or third night of consecutive use and for 1 or 2 nights after the drug is discontinued.

Contraindications: Hypersensitivity. Pregnancy or in women wishing to become pregnant.

Depression, renal or hepatic disease, chronic pulmonary insufficiency, children under 15 years.

Special Concerns: Use during the last few weeks of pregnancy may result in CNS depression of the neonate. Use during lactation may cause sedation and feeding problems in the infant. Geriatric patients may be more sensitive to the effects of flurazepam.

Side Effects: *CNS:* Ataxia, dizziness, drowsiness/sedation, headache, disorientation. Symptoms of stimulation including nervousness, apprehension, irritability, and talkativeness. *GI:* Nausea, vomiting, diarrhea, gastric upset or pain, heartburn, constipation. *Miscellaneous:* Arthralgia, chest pains, or palpitations. Rarely, symptoms of allergy, shortness of breath, jaundice, anorexia, blurred vision.

Drug Interactions	
Cimetidine	↑ Effect of flurazepam due to ↓ breakdown by liver
CNS depressants	Addition or potentiation of CNS depressant effects—drowsiness, lethargy, stupor, respiratory depression or collapse, coma, and possible death.
Disulfiram	↑ Effect of flurazepam due to ↓ breakdown by liver
Ethanol	Additive depressant effects up to the day following flurazepam administration
Isoniazid	↑ Effect of flurazepam due to ↓ breakdown by liver
Oral contraceptives	Either ↑ or ↓ effect of benzodiazepines due to effect on breakdown by liver
Rifampin	↓ Effect of benzodiazepines due to ↑ breakdown by liver

Laboratory Test Interference: ↑ Alkaline phosphatase, bilirubin, serum transaminases.

Dosage: Capsules. Adults: 15–30 mg at bedtime; 15 mg for geriatric and/or debilitated patients.

NURSING CONSIDERATIONS

See also *Nursing Considerations* for *Benzodiazepines,* p. 596.

Client/Family Teaching

1. Avoid the ingestion of alcohol with flurazepam.
2. Advise client to use caution in driving or operating machinery until daytime sedative effects are evaluated.
3. Report tolerance and any symptoms of psychological and/or physical dependence.
4. Clients suffering from simple insomnia should be instructed to try warm baths, warm drinks, and other relaxation techniques to induce sleep.

GLUTETHIMIDE   (gloo-TETH-ih-myd)

Doriden, Doriglute (C-III, Rx)

Classification: Nonbarbiturate, nonbenzodiazepine sedative-hypnotic.

Action/Kinetics: Glutethimide produces CNS depressant effects comparable to barbiturates, including suppression of REM sleep and REM rebound. Other effects include anticholinergic with mydriasis, inhibition of salivary secretion, and decreased GI motility. At comparable doses, glutethimide produces less respiratory depression but greater hypotension than occurs with barbiturates. Psychological and physical dependence may develop. **Onset:** 30 min. **Peak plasma concentration:** 1–6 hr (erratically absorbed from GI tract). **t½:** 10–12 hr. **Duration:** 4–8 hr. About 50% is bound to plasma protein. Metabolized in liver and excreted in urine.

Uses: Short-term treatment of insomnia (use should not exceed 1 week). Has generally been replaced by other sedative-hypnotics.

Contraindications: Hypersensitivity to drug. Porphyria. Patients with a history of drug dependence, alcoholism, or emotional disorders. Use not recommended during pregnancy, during lactation, and in children. **Do not give to patient with glaucoma or to patients with a history of drug dependence, alcoholism, or emotional disorders.**

Special Concerns: Pregnancy category: C. Use during lactation may cause sedation in the infant. Dosage adjustment may be necessary in geriatric patients due to age-related prostatic hypertrophy and impairment of renal function.

Side Effects: *GI:* Nausea, vomiting, anorexia, xerostomia. *CNS:* Headache, hangover, dizziness, confusion, drowsiness. *Dermatologic:* Skin rash (cause for discontinuing drug), urticaria, purpura. *Miscellaneous:* Osteomalacia following long-term use. *Rarely:* Excitation, blurred vision, acute hypersensitivity, exfoliative dermatitis, intermittent porphyria, and blood dyscrasias including thrombocytopenia, aplastic anemia, and leukopenia. Abrupt withdrawal of large doses may be dangerous—withdrawal symptoms are similar to those of barbiturates. Occasionally, symptoms similar to withdrawal occur in patients who have been taking only moderate doses, even when there is no abstention (tremulousness, nausea, tachycardia, fever, tonic muscle spasms, generalized convulsions).

Chronic Toxicity

Characterized by psychosis, confusion, delirium, hallucinations, ataxia, tremor, hyporeflexia, slurred speech, memory loss, irritability, fever, weight loss, mydriasis, xerostomia, nystagmus, headache, and convulsions. Treatment consists of careful, cautious withdrawal of drug over a period of several days or weeks.

Acute Toxicity

Characterized by coma, hypotension, hypothermia, followed by fever, tachycardia, depression or absence of reflexes (including pupillary response), sudden apnea, cyanosis, tonic muscle spasms, convulsions, and hyperreflexia.

Treatment of acute toxicity is supportive, starting with gastric lavage, CNS stimulants (used with caution), vasopressors, and maintenance of pulmonary ventilation. Parenteral fluids are administered cautiously, and hemodialysis may be necessary. Endotracheal intubation or tracheotomy may be indicated.

Drug Interactions	
Anticoagulants, oral	↓ Effect of anticoagulants due to ↑ breakdown by liver
Antidepressants, tricyclic	Additive anticholinergic side effects
CNS depressants	Additive CNS depression

Laboratory Test Interference: ↑ or ↓ 17-ketogenic steroids, 17-hydroxycorticosteroids.

Dosage: Tablets. **Adults:** Individualize to minimize chance of overdosage. **Usual:** 500 mg at bedtime. Dose may be repeated but not less than 4 hr before patient arises. **Geriatric or debilitated patients:** Initial daily dose should not exceed 500 mg. **Not recommended for children.**

NURSING CONSIDERATIONS

Treatment of Overdosage

1. Be prepared to treat for overdosage.
   - Assist with gastric lavage for treatment of acute toxicity.
   - Monitor vital signs.
   - Have emergency drugs and equipment available.
   - Anticipate hemodialysis in severe cases.

Interventions

1. Incorporate safety measures such as side rails and assisted ambulation.
2. Provide special mouth care for clients to avoid or minimize xerostomia.
3. Check clients for bowel regularity. Provide extra fluids and increased dietary roughage. Consult with the physician regarding the need for a stool softener or laxative.
4. If the client seems to be depressed or have suicidal tendencies, withhold the drug, document and report to the physician.
5. Withdraw the drug gradually to minimize withdrawal symptoms.
6. The drug suppresses REM sleep. Therefore, try alternative methods to induce sleep, such as relaxation methods, having the client drink warm milk, or give client a backrub.

Client/Family Teaching

Warn clients receiving glutethimide not to drive a car or operate other machinery after taking medication because drug may cause drowsiness.

METHYPRYLON   (meth-ih-**PRYE**-lon)

Noludar (C-III, Rx)

Classification: Nonbarbiturate, nonbenzodiazepine sedative-hypnotic.

Action/Kinetics: The action of methyprylon is similar to that of the barbiturates in that it suppresses REM sleep and induces rebound when drug therapy is discontinued. **Onset:** 45 min. **Peak plasma level:** 1–2 hr; **duration:** 5–8 hr. **t½:** 3–6 hr. Inactive liver metabolites are excreted in the urine.

Uses: Hypnotic for no more than 7 days. Especially useful for patients allergic to barbiturates. The drug has generally been replaced by other sedative-hypnotics.

Contraindications: Hypersensitivity to drug. Children under 12 years.

Special Concerns: Administer with caution during pregnancy (pregnancy category: B), during lactation, in the presence of renal and hepatic disease, and in acute, intermittent porphyria. Geriatric patients may be more sensitive to the effects of methyprylon.

Side Effects: *CNS:* Morning drowsiness, dizziness, vertigo, headache, EEG changes, pyrexia, ataxia, seizures, hallucinations. Paradoxical excitation, anxiety, depression, nightmares; confusion and acute brain syndrome, especially in elderly patients. *GI:* Nausea, vomiting, diarrhea, constipation, esophagitis. *CV:* Syncope, hypotension. *Hematologic:* Neutropenia, aplastic anemia, thrombocytopenic purpura. *Miscellaneous:* Blurred vision, double vision, allergic reactions, rash, pruritus, hangover. Overdosage is characterized by somnolence, confusion, coma, constricted pupils, respiratory depression, hypotension, shock, edema, tachycardia, hepatic dysfunction.

Laboratory Test Interference: With test methods: ↑ 17-Hydroxycorticosteroids, 17-ketosteroids, 17-ketogenic steroids.

Dosage: Capsules, Tablets. Adults: 200–400 mg before bedtime. **Pediatric over 12 years:** (effectiveness extremely variable, dose must be individualized), **initial,** 50 mg. If ineffective, may be increased to 200 mg at bedtime.

NURSING CONSIDERATIONS

See also *Nursing Considerations* for *Benzodiazepine and Other Nonbarbiturate Sedative-Hypnotics,* p. 596.

Interventions

1. Have available equipment and drugs for treating toxicity.
   - Caffeine and sodium benzoate to stimulate respiration.
   - Norepinephrine or metaraminol for the management of hypotension.
2. Monitor clients closely for signs of toxicity.
3. In the event of toxicity, assist in lavaging the stomach.
4. Provide oxygen and assist with ventilation if necessary.
5. Monitoring IV fluids and electrolytes.
6. Monitor intake and output. Hemodialysis may be necessary if urinary output is too scant.
7. If the client is comatose, turn the client onto the side to prevent aspiration of vomitus.
8. Provide safety measures such as side rails.

Client/Family Teaching

1. Do not engage in hazardous activities such as driving because drowsiness may develop.
2. That when suffering from simple insomnia to try warm baths, warm milk, and relaxation techniques to induce sleep rather than becoming dependent on drugs.

PARALDEHYDE   (pah-**RAL**-deh-hyd)

Paral (C-IV) (Rx)

Classification: Nonbarbiturate sedative-hypnotic.

Action/Kinetics: Paraldehyde is bitter tasting (liquid) and has a strong, unpleasant odor. In usual doses, it has little effect on either respiration or blood pressure. In the presence of pain, paraldehyde may induce excitement or delirium; it is not analgesic. **Onset:** 10–15 min. **Duration:** 8–12 hr. **Peak serum levels:** After PO, 30–60 min; after rectal administration, 2.5 hr. Approximately 70%–90% is detoxified in the liver, with the remainder excreted unchanged by the lungs. **t½:** 3.4–9.8 hr.

Uses: Sedative and hypnotic, although such use has generally been replaced by other sedative-hypnotics. Delirium tremens and other excited states. Prior to EEG to induce artificial sleep. Emergency treatment of seizures, eclampsia, tetanus, status epilepticus, and overdose of stimulant or convulsant drugs.

Contraindications: Gastroenteritis, bronchopulmonary disease, hepatic insufficiency. Use with caution during labor and during lactation.

Special Concerns: Pregnancy category: C. Use during labor may lead to respiratory depression in the neonate.

Side Effects: *Dermatologic:* Skin rash, redness, swelling or pain at injection site; nerve damage (may be severe and permanent), especially of the sciatic nerve if drug injected too close to nerve. *Respiratory:* Rarely, difficulty in breathing, shortness of breath. *Miscellaneous:* Bradycardia, strong odor to breath up to 24 hr following use. *Following IV use:* Coughing; right heart edema, dilation and failure; massive pulmonary hemorrhage. *Following prolonged use:* Dependence, similar to alcoholism leading to withdrawal syndrome including hallucinations and delirium tremens. Also, prolonged use may result in hepatitis.

Drug Interactions	
Disulfiram	Combination may produce a Disulfiram–like-reaction
Sulfonamides	↑ Chance of sulfonamide crystalluria

Laboratory Test Interference: 17-hydroxycorticosteroids, 17-ketogenic steroids.

Dosage: Liquid, Oral or Rectal. *Hypnotic:* **Adults, PO,** 10–30 mL; **rectal,** 10–20 mL with 1–2 parts olive oil or isotonic sodium chloride. **Pediatric, PO, rectal:** 0.3 mL/kg. *Sedation:* **Adults, PO, rectal,** 5–10 mL. **Pediatric, PO, rectal,** 0.15 mL/kg. *Delirium tremens:* **Adults, PO,** 10–35 mL. *Anticonvulsant:* **Adults, PO,** Up to 12 mL via gastric tube q 4 hr, if needed; **rectal,** 10–20 mL. **Pediatric, PO, rectal,** 0.3 mL/kg.

 IM, IV. *Anticonvulsant:* **Adults, IM,** 5–10 mL; **IV infusion,** 5 mL diluted with at least 100 mL 0.9% sodium chloride given at a rate not to exceed 1 mL/min. **Pediatric, IM, IV,** 0.1–0.15 mL/kg.

NURSING CONSIDERATIONS

See also *Nursing Considerations* for *Chloral Hydrate,* p. 599.

Administration/Storage

1. *PO* Drug should be cold to minimize odor and taste as well as gastric irritation. Mask the taste and odor by mixing drug with syrup, milk, or fruit juice.
2. *Rectal* Mix with olive oil, cottonseed oil, or isotonic sodium chloride solution to minimize irritation—1 part medication to 2 parts diluent.
3. *IM* A pure sterile preparation should be used. Inject deeply into gluteus maximus and avoid extravasation into subcutaneous tissue as drug is irritating and may cause sterile abscesses and nerve injury and paralysis.
4. *IV* Only in an emergency, dilute with 20 volumes of 0.9% sodium chloride injection and inject at a rate not to exceed 1 mL/minute since circulatory collapse or pulmonary edema may occur. Use glass syringe and metal needles because the drug may react with the plastic used in disposable syringes and needles.
5. Store in a tight, light-resistant container, at temperatures not to exceed 25°C (77°F).
6. Should not be used if paraldehyde has a strong vinegar odor or is brownish in color.
7. Paraldehyde should not be used if the container has been opened for more than 24 hr.

Assessment

Obtain baseline liver and renal function studies against which to measure future organ function as the therapy progresses.

Interventions

1. Ensure that the room is well ventilated so as to remove exhaled paraldehyde.
2. Reassure the client disturbed by the odor of the drug.
3. Assess the client for evidence of dependency and toxicity. Do not withdraw the drug abruptly.
4. Report coughing during IV administration, as this symptom can indicate untoward effects on pulmonary capillaries.
5. Note evidence of pulmonary edema or respiratory depression, document and report to the physician immediately.
6. Assess the client for symptoms of overdosage as evidenced by labored breathing, a fast, feeble pulse, low blood pressure, and a characteristic odor of paraldehyde on the breath.

PROPIOMAZINE HYDROCHLORIDE (proh-pee-**OH**-may-zeen)

Largon (Rx)

Classification: Nonbarbiturate sedative, phenothiazine.

Action/Kinetics: At therapeutic dosages, this phenothiazine drug has sedative, antiemetic, antihistaminic, and anticholinergic effects. **Peak sedative effects: IV,** 15–30 min; **IM,** 40–60 min. **Time to peak serum levels:** 1–3 hr (following IM). **Duration** 3–6 hr. **t½, IV:** about 8 hr; **IM,** about 11 hr.

Uses: Preoperatively to reduce anxiety and during surgery to decrease emesis. Adjunct to narcotic analgesia during labor to relieve restlessness and apprehension.

Contraindications: Intra-arterial injection.

Special Concerns: Use with caution in pregnancy.

Side Effects: *GI:* Dry mouth, GI upset. *CNS:* Dizziness and confusion in the elderly. Transient restlessness. *CV:* Increase in blood pressure (may be desirable), hypotension, tachycardia. *Other:* Skin rashes, respiratory depression, altered respiratory pattern. Irritation and thrombophlebitis at injection site.

Dosage: IM and IV. Adults: *Preoperative sedation,* **usual,** 20 mg (up to 40 mg) with meperidine, 50 mg. *Obstetrics:* 20–40 mg in the early stages of labor; **then,** 20–40 mg given with meperidine, 25–75 mg. Doses may be repeated q 3 hr. *Sedation with local anesthesia:* 10–20 mg. **Pediatric.** *Pre- and postoperatively:* **children weighing less than 27 kg:** 0.55–1.1 mg/kg. *Alternative dosing:* **children, 2–4 years of age:** 10 mg; **4–6 years of age:** 15 mg; **6–12 years of age:** 25 mg.

NURSING CONSIDERATIONS

Administration/Storage

1. Inject into large, undamaged vein.
2. Avoid extravasation.
3. Never administer subcutaneously or intra-arterially.

4. Do not use solutions that are cloudy or contain precipitate.

5. Aqueous solutions are incompatible with barbiturate salts or alkaline solutions.

6. Store at 15°–30°C and protect from light.

7. If used with propiomazine, the dose of barbiturates should be reduced by at least ½; the dose of meperidine, morphine, or analgesic depressants should be reduced by ¼–½ if used with propiomazine.

Interventions

1. Anticipate reduction of dose by ¼ to ½ in strength of other sedatives administered concomitantly with propiomazine.

2. Anticipate that if vasopressor drugs are administered with propiomazine, norepinephrine should be used rather than epinephrine.

3. Provide mouth care to relieve xerostomia except for clients scheduled for surgery, for whom a dry mouth is desirable.

4. Monitor BP frequently after IM or IV administration because medication may have a hypotensive effect up to 5 hr.

5. Monitor and assess clients for any side effects (blood dyscrasias, hepatotoxicity, extrapyramidal symptoms, reactivation of psychotic processes, cardiac arrest, endocrine disturbances, dermatologic disorders, ocular changes, and hypersensitivity reactions) associated with long-term use of phenothiazines.

6. Provide a safe environment for elderly clients experiencing dizziness, confusion, or amnesia after administration of the drug.

7. The antiemetic effect of propiomazine may be masking other pathology, such as toxicity to other drugs, intestinal obstruction, or brain lesions, so assess the client carefully.

QUAZEPAM (KWAY-zeh-pam)

Doral (Rx, C-IV)

See also *Benzodiazpines,* p. 596.

Classification: Benzodiazepine, hypnotic.

Action/Kinetics: The drug will improve sleep induction time, duration of sleep, number of nocturnal awakenings, occurrence of early morning awakening, and sleep quality without producing an effect on REM sleep. Hangover effects are minimal. **Peak plasma levels:** 2 hr. Quazepam and two of its metabolites (2-oxoquazepam and N-desalkyl-2-oxoquazepam) are active on the CNS. **t½, quazepam and 2-oxoquazepam:** 39 hr; **t½, N-desalkyl-2-oxoquazepam:** 73 hr. Significantly (95%) bound to plasma protein.

Uses: Insomnia characterized by difficulty in falling asleep, frequent nocturnal awakenings, and/or early morning awakenings.

Contraindications: Patients with established sleep apnea. Pregnancy (pregnancy category: X), lactation.

Special Concerns: Use with caution in patients with impaired renal or hepatic function, in chronic pulmonary insufficiency, and in depression. Safety and effectiveness have not been established in children less than 18 years of age. Use during lactation may cause sedation and feeding problems in the infant. Geriatric and debilitated patients may be more sensitive to the effects of quazepam.

Side Effects: *CNS:* Daytime drowsiness (most common), headache, dizziness, fatigue, irritability, slurred speech, paradoxical stimulation, agitation, sleep disturbances, hallucinations. *GI:* Dry mouth, dyspepsia. *Miscellaneous:* Incontinence, urinary retention, jaundice, dysarthria, dystonia, changes in libido, menstrual irregularities. **Note:** Rapid withdrawal after continued use may cause signs and symptoms of withdrawal from CNS depressant drugs.

Drug Interactions: Additive CNS depressant effects when taken with antihistamines, ethanol, antipsychotics, anticonvulsants, and other drugs producing depression of the CNS.

Dosage: Tablets. Adults, initial: 15 mg until individual response has been determined. The dose may be reduced to 7.5 mg in some patients (especially in geriatric or debilitated patients).

NURSING CONSIDERATIONS

See also *Nursing Considerations* for *Benzodiazepine,* p. 596.

Client/Family Teaching

1. Do not use alcohol or any other drugs having CNS depressant effects while taking quazepam.
2. Do not drive a car or operate potentially dangerous machinery until the sedative effects of the drug are known.
3. The drug may produce daytime sedation even for several days after it has been discontinued.
4. Do not increase the dose of quazepam without first consulting with the physician.
5. Do not stop taking the drug abruptly following prolonged and regular use.

TEMAZEPAM (teh-**MAY**-zeh-pam)

Restoril (C-IV, Rx)

See also *Benzodiazepines,* p. 596.

Classification: Benzodiazepine hypnotic.

Action/Kinetics: Temazepam is a benzodiazepine derivative. Disturbed nocturnal sleep may occur the first one or two nights following discontinuance of the drug. Prolonged administration is not recommended, since physical dependence and tolerance may develop. See also *Flurazepam,* p. 601. **Peak blood levels:** 2–4 hr. **t½, initial:** 0.4–0.6 hr; **final:** 10 hr. **Steady-state plasma levels:** 382 ng/mL (2.5 hr after 30-mg dose). Accumulation of the drug is minimal following multiple dosage. Significantly bound (98%) to plasma protein. The drug is metabolized in the liver to inactive metabolites.

Uses: Insomnia in patients unable to fall asleep, with frequent awakenings during the night and/or early morning awakenings.

Contraindications: Pregnancy (pregnancy category: X).

Special Concerns: Use with caution in severely depressed patients. Use during lactation may cause sedation and feeding problems in the infant. Geriatric patients may be more sensitive to the effects of temazepam.

Side Effects: *CNS:* Drowsiness (after daytime use) and dizziness are common. Lethargy, confusion, euphoria, weakness, ataxia, lack of concentration, hallucinations. In some patients, paradoxical excitement (less than 0.5%), including stimulation and hyperactivity, occurs. *GI:* Anorexia, diarrhea. *Other:* Tremors, horizontal nystagmus, falling, palpitations. Rarely, blood dyscrasias.

Dosage: Capsules. Adults: usual, 15–30 mg at bedtime. **In elderly or debilitated patients: initial,** 15 mg; **then,** adjust dosage to response.

NURSING CONSIDERATIONS

See *Nursing Considerations* for *Benzodiazepines,* p. 596 and *Triazolam,* p. 610.

TRIAZOLAM   (try-**AY**-zoh-lam)

Halcion (C-IV, Rx)

See also *Benzodiazepines,* p. 596.

Classification: Benzodiazepine sedative-hypnotic.

Action/Kinetics: Triazolam decreases sleep latency, increases the duration of sleep, and decreases the number of awakenings. **Time to peak plasma levels:** 0.5–2 hr. **$t^{1/2}$:** 1.5–5.5 hr. Metabolized in liver and inactive metabolites excreted in the urine.

Uses: Insomnia (short-term management, not to exceed 1 month). May be beneficial in preventing or treating transient insomnia due to a sudden change in sleep schedule.

Contraindications: Pregnancy (pregnancy category: X).

Special Concerns: Safety and efficacy in children under 18 years of age not established. Use during lactation may cause sedation and feeding problems in the infant. Geriatric patients may be more sensitive to the effects of triazolam.

Side Effects: *CNS:* Rebound insomnia, anterograde amnesia, headache, ataxia, decreased coordination. Psychological and physical dependence. *GI:* Nausea, vomiting.

Dosage: Tablets. Adults: initial, 0.25–0.5 mg before bedtime. **Geriatric or debilitated patients, initial:** 0.125 mg; **then,** depending on response, 0.125–0.25 mg before bedtime.

NURSING CONSIDERATIONS

See also *Nursing Considerations* for *Benzodiazepines,* p. 596.

Interventions

1. Assess client for tolerance and for psychological and physical dependence.
2. When client suffers from simple insomnia, try warm baths, warm milk, and other interventions to induce sleep, such as soft music, guided imagery or progressive muscle relaxation.
3. Initiate safety precautions (i.e., side rails up, frequent observations) at bedtime, especially with elderly clients and confused clients.

Client/Family Teaching

1. Avoid the use of alcoholic beverages.
2. Use caution when driving or in operating machinery until daytime sedative effects have been evaluated.
3. Try warm baths, warm milk, and other methods to induce sleep, such as guided imagery or progressive muscle relaxation rather than become dependent on drugs for insomnia.
4. Report any unusual side effects including hallucinations or periods of confusion.

CHAPTER THIRTY-ONE

Antianxiety Agents

BENZODIAZEPINES

General Statement: The benzodiazepines exhibit a wide margin of safety between therapeutic and toxic doses. For example, ataxia and sedation are observed at doses higher than those required to achieve antianxiety effects. The major difference among benzodiazepines appears to be a function of duration of action and other pharmacokinetic properties.

All antianxiety agents have the ability to cause psychological and physical dependence. Withdrawal symptoms usually start within 12–48 hr after stopping the drug and last for 12–48 hr. When the patient has received large doses of these drugs for weeks or months, dosage should be reduced gradually over a period of 1–2 weeks. Alternatively, a short-acting barbiturate may be substituted and then withdrawn gradually. Abrupt withdrawal of high dosage of the drug may be accompanied by coma, convulsions, and even death.

Action/Kinetics: The major antianxiety agents include the benzodiazepines and meprobamate. The benzodiazepines are thought to affect the limbic system and reticular formation to reduce anxiety. This effect is believed to be mediated through the action of the benzodiazepines to increase or facilitate the inhibitory neurotransmitter activity of GABA which is one of the inhibitory CNS neurotransmitters. Meprobamate and the benzodiazepines also possess varying degrees of anticonvulsant activity, skeletal muscle relaxation, and the ability to alleviate tension. The rate of absorption from the GI tract will determine the onset and intensity of action of the various benzodiazepines. The benzodiazepines generally have long half-lives (1–8 days); thus cumulative effects can occur. Also, several of the benzodiazepines are metabolized to active metabolites in the liver, which prolongs their duration of action. Benzodiazepines are widely distributed throughout the body. Approximately 70–99% of an administered dose is bound to plasma protein. Metabolites of benzodiazepines are excreted through the kidneys.

Uses: Management of anxiety and tension occurring alone or as a side effect of other conditions, including menopausal syndrome, premenstrual tension, asthma, and angina pectoris. Neurologic conditions involving muscle spasm and tetanus. Adjunct in treatment of rheumatoid arthritis,

31

osteoarthritis, trauma, low back pain, torticollis, and selected convulsive disorders including status epilepticus. Premedication for surgery or electric cardioversion. Rehabilitation of chronic alcoholics, delirium tremens, nocturnal enuresis in childhood, and to induce sleep. *Investigational:* Irritable bowel syndrome.

Contraindications: Hypersensitivity, acute narrow-angle glaucoma, psychoses.

Special Concerns: Use with caution in impaired hepatic or renal function and in the geriatric or debilitated patient. Use during lactation may cause sedation, weight loss, and possibly feeding difficulties in the infant. Geriatric patients may be more sensitive to the effects of benzodiazepines.

Side Effects: *CNS:* Drowsiness, fatigue, confusion, ataxia, sedation, dizziness, vertigo, depression, apathy, lightheadedness, delirium, headache, lethargy, disorientation, hypoactivity, crying, antero-grade amnesia, slurred speech, stupor, coma, fainting, difficulty in concentration, euphoria, nervousness, irritability, akathisia, hypotenia, vivid dreams, "glassy-eyed", hysteria, suicidal attempt, psychosis. Paradoxical excitement manifested by anxiety, acute hyperexcitability, increased muscle spasticity, insomnia, hallucinations, sleep disturbances, rage, and stimulation. *GI:* Increased appetite, constipation, diarrhea, anorexia, nausea, vomiting, weight gain or loss, dry mouth, bitter or metallic taste, increased salivation, coated tongue, sore gums, difficulty in swallowing, gastritis, fecal incontinence. *Dermatologic:* Urticaria, rash, pruritus, alopecia, hirsutism, dermatitis, edema of ankles and face. *Endocrine:* Increased or decreased libido, gynecomastia, menstrual irregularities. *GU:* Difficulty in urination, urinary retention, incontinence, dysuria, enuresis. *CV:* Hypertension, hypotension, bradycardia, tachycardia, palpitations, edema, cardiovascular collapse. *Hematologic:* Anemia, agranulocytosis, leukopenia, eosinophilia, thrombocytopenia. *Ophthalmologic:* Diplopia, conjunctivitis, nystagmus, blurred vision. *Miscellaneous:* Joint pain, lymphadenopathy, muscle cramps, paresthesia, dehydration, lupus-like symptoms, sweating, shortness of breath, flushing, hiccoughs, fever, hepatic dysfunction.

Following IM use: Redness, pain, burning. *Following IV use:* Thrombosis and phlebitis at site.

Symptoms of Overdose

Severe drowsiness, confusion, tremors, slurred speech, staggering, coma, hypotension, shortness of breath, labored breathing, weakness, slow heart rate. *Note:* Geriatric patients, debilitated patients, young children, and patients with liver disease are more sensitive to the CNS effects of benzodiazepines.

Treatment of Overdose

Supportive therapy. Gastric lavage, provided that an endotracheal tube with an inflated cuff is used to prevent aspiration of vomitus. Emesis only if drug ingestion was recent and patient is fully conscious. Activated charcoal and saline cathartic may be given after emesis or lavage. Adequate respiratory function must be maintained. Hypotension may be reversed by IV fluids, norepineph-rine, or metaraminol. Infusion of physostigmine, 0.5–4 mg (1 mg/min) may reverse central anticholinergic symptoms such as confusion, hallucinations, delirium, visual disturbances, and disturbed memory.

Drug Interactions

Alcohol	Potentiation or addition of CNS depressant effects. Concomitant use may lead to drowsiness, lethargy, stupor, respiratory collapse, coma, or death
Anesthetics, general	See *Alcohol*
Antacids	↓ Rate of absorption of benzodiazepines

Drug Interactions

Antidepressants, tricyclic	Concomitant use with benzodiazepines may cause additive sedative effect and/or atropine-like side effects
Antihistamines	See *Alcohol*
Barbiturates	See *Alcohol*
Cimetidine	Cimetidine ↑ effect of benzodiazepines by ↓ breakdown in liver
CNS depressants	See *Alcohol*
Digoxin	Benzodiazepines ↑ effect of digoxin by ↑ serum levels
Disulfiram	Disulfiram ↑ effect of benzodiazepines by ↓ breakdown in liver
Erythromycin	Erythromycin ↑ effect of benzodiazepines by ↓ breakdown in liver
Fluoxetine	↑ Effect of benzodiazepines due to ↓ breakdown in liver
Isoniazid	↑ Effect of benzodiazepines due to ↓ breakdown in liver
Ketoconazole	↑ Effect of benzodiazepines due to ↓ breakdown in liver
Levodopa	Effect may be ↓ by benzodiazepines
Metoprolol	↑ Effect of benzodiazepines due to ↓ breakdown in liver
Narcotics	See *Alcohol*
Oral contraceptives	↑ Effect of benzodiazepines due to ↓ breakdown in liver; or, ↑ rate of clearance of benzodiazepines that undergo glucuronidation (e.g., lorazepam, oxazepam)
Phenothiazines	See *Alcohol*
Phenytoin	Concomitant use with benzodiazepines may cause ↑ effect of phenytoin due to ↓ breakdown by liver
Probenecid	↑ Effect of selected benzodiazepines due to ↓ breakdown by liver
Propoxyphene	↑ Effect of benzodiazepines due to ↓ breakdown by liver
Propranolol	↑ Effect of benzodiazepines due to ↓ breakdown by liver
Ranitidine	May ↓ absorption of benzodiazepines from the GI tract
Rifampin	↓ Effect of benzodiazepines due to ↑ breakdown by liver
Sedative-hypnotics, nonbarbiturate	See *Alcohol*
Theophyllines	↓ Sedative effect of benzodiazepines
Valproic acid	↑ Effect of benzodiazepines due to ↓ breakdown by liver

Laboratory Test Interference: ↑ SGPT, SGPT, LDH, alkaline phosphatase.

Dosage: See individual drugs.

NURSING CONSIDERATIONS

Administration/Storage

1. Persistent drowsiness, ataxia, or visual disturbances may require dosage adjustment.
2. Lower dosage is usually indicated for older clients.
3. GI effects are decreased when drugs are given with meals or shortly afterward.
4. Withdraw drugs gradually.
5. Review the list of drug interactions prior to taking the client's history and beginning drug therapy.

Assessment

1. Note any history of adverse reactions to this class of drugs.
2. Assess the client's life style and general level of health.
3. Note the manner in which the client responds to questions and discusses the problem.
4. Determine if the client has had any prior treatment for the same problems and the outcome.
5. Obtain baseline CBC, liver and renal function studies to determine potential problems or impaired function.
6. Review the client's physical history for any contraindications to drug therapy.

Interventions

1. In the event that treatment is required for overdosage, have emergency equipment and drugs available. Including
   - Equipment for gastric lavage.
   - Epinephrine, antihistamines, corticosteroids for hypersensitivity reactions.
   - Respiratory support equipment.
2. Determine the presence of any blood dyscrasias that could preclude administering the drug.
3. Monitor the blood pressure before and after the client receives an IV dose of antianxiety medication. Keep the client in a recumbent position for 2–3 hours after IV administration. Determine the presence and degree of hypotension and document.
4. Anticipate that the dosage of drug will be the lowest possible effective one, especially when administering the drug to the elderly or debilitated client.
5. When the drug is administered to a hospitalized client, remain with client until the drug is swallowed.
6. If the client exhibits ataxia, or complains of weakness or lack of coordination when ambulating, provide assistance. Use side rails once the client is back in bed.
7. Note any early symptoms of cholestatic jaundice, such as client complaint of nausea, diarrhea, upper abdominal pain, or the presence of high fever or rash. Check liver functions studies and report to the physician.
8. If there is any yellowing of the client's sclera, skin or mucous membranes, the client is exhibiting a late sign of cholestatic jaundice and biliary tract obstruction. Withhold the medication, document, and report to the physician.
9. If the client complains of a sore throat, fever or weakness, assess for blood dyscrasias. Obtain CBC with diff, notify the physician and anticipate that the drug may be withheld until appropriate data can be evaluated.

10. If the client appears overly sleepy, confused, or if the client becomes comatose, withhold the drug, document and report to the physician.

11. If the client has suicidal tendencies, anticipate that the drug will be prescribed in small doses. Be alert to signs of increased depression and report immediately.

12. If the prescription is for a client who has a history of alcoholism or of taking excessive quantities of drug, carefully supervise the amount of drug prescribed and dispensed.

13. Note any other evidences of client physical or psychological dependence.

14. Assess for manifestations of ataxia, slurred speech, and vertigo. Such symptoms are characteristic of chronic intoxication and are usually indications that the client is taking more than the recommended dose of drug.

15. For clients receiving the medication on an outpatient basis, determine the frequency of the requests for medication. Count the number of tablets or capsules left at the time of the request for refills or renewal of the prescription if the frequency seems out of the ordinary. The client may be taking larger doses than is recommended.

Client/Family Teaching

1. Stress that these drugs may reduce the client's ability to handle potentially dangerous equipment, such as automobiles and other machinery.

2. Avoid alcohol while taking antianxiety agents. Alcohol potentiates the depressant effects of both the alcohol and the medication.

3. Do not take any unprescribed or OTC medications without first consulting with the physician.

4. If feeling faint he/she should sit or lie down immediately and lower the head.

5. Arise slowly from a supine position and dangle the legs over the side of the bed for a few minutes before standing up.

6. Encourage working clients to allow extra time to prepare for their daily activities to enable them to take the necessary precautions before arising, thereby reducing one source of anxiety and stress.

7. Do not stop taking the drug suddenly. Any sudden withdrawal of the drug after a prolonged period of therapy or after excessive use may cause a recurrence of the preexisting symptoms of anxiety. It may also cause a withdrawal syndrome, manifested by increased anxiety, anorexia, insomnia, vomiting, ataxia, muscle twitching, confusion and hallucinations. Some clients may develop seizures and convulsions.

8. Instruct the client and family in several relaxation techniques that may assist in lowering their anxiety levels.

Evaluation

Assess for a positive clinical response. This may be evident when the client reports a reduction in the level of anxiety they are currently experiencing as well as the development of new coping strategies.

ALPRAZOLAM   (al-PRAYZ-oh-lam)

Xanax (C-IV, Rx)

See also *Benzodiazepines,* p. 611.

Classification: Antianxiety agent.

Action/Kinetics: Peak plasma levels: PO, 8–37 ng/mL after 1–2 hr. **t½:** 12–15 hr. 80% plasma protein bound. Metabolized to alpha-hydroxyalprazolam, an active metabolite. Excreted in urine.

Uses: Anxiety. Anxiety associated with depression. Antipanic drug. *Investigational:* Treatment of panic attacks.

Special Concerns: Pregnancy category: D.

Dosage: Tablets. Adults, initial, 0.25–0.5 mg t.i.d.; **then,** titrate to needs of patient, with total daily dosage not to exceed 4 mg. **In elderly or debilitated: initial,** 0.25 mg b.i.d.–t.i.d.; **then,** adjust dosage to needs of patient. *Antipanic agent:* 0.5 mg t.i.d.; increase dose as needed up to a maximum of 8 mg daily.

NURSING CONSIDERATIONS

See also *Nursing Considerations* for *Benzodiazepines,* p. 614.

Administration/Storage

The daily dose should not be decreased more than 0.5 mg every 3 days if therapy is terminated or the dose decreased.

Interventions

Use side rails and support devices as needed, especially at night because elderly clients tend to become somewhat confused.

CHLORDIAZEPOXIDE   (klor-dye-ay-zeh-**POX**-syd)

Apo-Chlordiazepoxide ✤, Libritabs, Librium, Lipoxide, Medilium ✤, Mitran, Novopoxide ✤, Reposans-10, Solium ✤ (C-IV, Rx)

See also *Benzodiazepines,* p. 611.

Classification: Antianxiety agent, benzodiazepine.

Action/Kinetics: Onset: PO, 30–60 min; **IM,** 15–30 min (absorption may be slow and erratic); **IV,** 3–30 min. **Peak plasma levels (PO):** 0.5–4 hr. **Duration: t½:** 5–30 hr. Is metabolized to four active metabolites: desmethylchlordiazepoxide, desmethyldiazepam, oxazepam, and demoxepam. Chlordiazepoxide has less anticonvulsant activity and is less potent than diazepam.

Special Concerns: Pregnancy category: D.

Uses: Anxiety, acute withdrawal symptoms in chronic alcoholics. Sedative-hypnotic. Preoperatively to reduce anxiety and tension. Tension headache. Antitremor agent (PO). Antipanic (parenteral).

Additional Side Effects: Jaundice, acute hepatic necrosis, hepatic dysfunction.

Laboratory Test Interferences

1. *Interference with test methods:* ↑ 17-Hydroxycorticosteroids, 17-ketosteroids.
2. *Caused by pharmacologic effects:* ↑ Alkaline phosphatase, bilirubin, serum transaminase, porphobilinogen. ↓ Prothrombin time (patients on coumarin).

Dosage: Capsules/Tablets. Adults: *Anxiety and tension,* 5–10 mg t.i.d.–q.i.d. (up to 20–25 mg t.i.d.–q.i.d. in severe cases). Reduce dose to 5 mg b.i.d.–q.i.d. in geriatric or debilitated patients.

Pediatric, over 6 years, initial, 5 mg b.i.d.–q.i.d. May be increased to 10 mg b.i.d.–q.i.d. *Preoperatively:* 5–10 mg t.i.d.–q.i.d. on day before surgery. *Alcohol withdrawal/Sedative-hypnotic:* 50–100 mg; may be increased to 300 mg/day; **then,** reduce to maintenance levels.

IM, IV (not recommended for children under 12 years): *Acute/severe agitation/anxiety:* **initial,** 50–100 mg; **then,** 25–50 mg t.i.d.–q.i.d. *Preoperatively:* **IM,** 50–100 mg 1 hr before surgery. *Alcohol withdrawal:* **IM, IV,** 50–100 mg; repeat in 2–4 hr if necessary. Dosage should not exceed 300 mg/day. *Antipanic:* **Adults, initial:** 50–100 mg; dose may be repeated in 4–6 hr if needed.

NURSING CONSIDERATIONS

See also *Nursing Considerations* for *Benzodiazepines,* p. 614.

Administration/Storage

1. **IM:** Prepare solution immediately before administration by adding diluent, which is provided, to ampule. Shake until dissolved. Discard any unused solution. Inject slowly into upper, outer quadrant of gluteal muscle.

2. **IV:** Prepare immediately before administration by diluting with 5 mL of sterile water for injection or sterile 0.9% sodium chloride solution. Inject directly into vein over 1-min period. Do not add to IV infusion because of instability of drug. Do not use IV solution for IM.

CLORAZEPATE DIPOTASSIUM   (kloh-**RAYZ**-eh-payt)

Gen-Xene, Novoclopate✳, Tranxene-SD, Tranxene-SD Half (C-IV, Rx)

See also *Benzodiazepines,* p. 611.

Classification: Antianxiety agent, benzodizepine type; anticonvulsant.

Action/Kinetics: Peak plasma levels: 1–2 hr. **t$\frac{1}{2}$:** 30–100 hr. Clorazepate is hydrolyzed in the stomach to desmethyldiazepam, the active metabolite. Oxazepam is also an active metabolite. **t$\frac{1}{2}$, desmethyldiazepam:** 30–100 hr; **t$\frac{1}{2}$, oxazepam:** 5–15 hr. **Time to peak plasma levels:** 0.5–2 hr. The drug is slowly excreted by the kidneys.

Uses: Anxiety, tension. Acute alcohol withdrawal, as adjunct in treatment of seizures. Adjunct for treating partial seizures.

Additional Contraindications: Depressive patients, nursing mothers. Give cautiously to patients with impaired renal or hepatic function.

Special Considerations: Pregnancy category: D.

Dosage: Capsules/Tablets. *Anxiety:* **initial,** 7.5–15 mg b.i.d.–q.i.d.; **maintenance:** 15–60 mg/day in divided doses. **Elderly or debilitated patients: initial,** 7.5–15 mg/day. **Alternative: Single daily dosage: Adult, initial,** 15 mg; **then,** 11.25–22.5 mg once daily. *Acute alcohol withdrawal: Day 1,* **initial,** 30 mg; **then,** 15 mg b.i.d.–q.i.d. the first day; *day 2,* 45–90 mg/day; *day 3,* 22.5–45 mg/day; *day 4,* 15–30 mg/day. Thereafter, reduce to 7.5–15 mg/day and discontinue as soon as possible. *Anticonvulsant, adjunct:* **Adults and children over 12 years: initial,** 7.5 mg t.i.d.; increase no more than 7.5 mg/week to maximum of 90 mg/day. **Children (9–12 years): initial,** 7.5 mg b.i.d.; increase no more than 7.5 mg/week to maximum of 60 mg/day. Not recommended for children under 9 years of age.

NURSING CONSIDERATIONS

See *Nursing Considerations* for *Benzodiazepines,* p. 614.

DIAZEPAM   (dye-AYZ-eh-pam)

Apo-Diazepam✢, Diazepam Intensol, E-Pam✢, Meval✢, Novodipam✢, Rival✢, Valrelease, Vivol✢, Zetran (C-IV, Rx)

See also *Benzodiazepines,* p. 611.

Action/Kinetics: Onset: PO, 30–60 min; **IM,** 15–30 min; **IV,** more rapid. **Peak plasma levels: PO,** 0.5–2 hr; **IM,** 0.5–1.5; **IV,** 0.25 hr. **Duration:** 3 hr. **t¹/₂:** 20–70 hr. Diazepam is broken down in the liver to the active metabolites desmethyldiazepam, oxazepam, and temazepam. Diazepam and metabolites are excreted through the urine.

Uses: Anxiety, tension (more effective than chlordiazepoxide), alcohol withdrawal, muscle relaxant, anticonvulsive agent, antipanic drug. Used prior to gastroscopy and esophagoscopy, preoperatively and prior to cardioversion. In dentistry to induce sedation. Treatment of status epilepticus. Adjunct in cerebral palsy, paraplegia, or tetanus. Relieve spasms of facial muscles in occlusion and temporomandibular joint disorders.

Additional Contraindications: Narrow-angle glaucoma, children under 6 months, and parenterally in children under 12 years. During lactation.

Special Concerns: Pregnancy category: D.

Additional Drug Interactions:

1. Diazepam potentiates antihypertensive effects of thiazides and other diuretics.
2. Diazepam potentiates muscle relaxant effects of *d*-tubocurarine and gallamine.
3. Ranitidine ↓ GI absorption of diazepam.
4. Isoniazid ↑ half-life of diazepam.
5. Fluoxetine ↑ half-life of diazepam.

Dosage: Tablets, Oral Solution. Adults: *Antianxiety, anticonvulsant, adjunct to skeletal muscle relaxants:* 2–10 mg b.i.d.–q.i.d. **Elderly, debilitated patients:** 2–2.5 mg 1–2 times daily. May be gradually increased to adult level. **Pediatric, over 6 months: initial,** 1–2.5 mg (0.04–0.2 mg/kg or 1.17–6 mg/m²) t.i.d.–b.i.d. *Alcohol withdrawal:* 10 mg t.i.d.–q.i.d. during the first 24 hr; **then,** decrease to 5 mg t.i.d.–q.i.d. as required.

Extended-release Capsules. Adults: *Antianxiety, skeletal muscle relaxant:* 15–30 mg once daily. To be used in children over 6 months of age only if the dose has been determined to be 5 mg t.i.d. (use one 15-mg capsule daily). **IM, IV. Adults: IM,** *Preoperative or diagnostic use:* 10 mg 5–30 min before procedure. *Adjunct to treat skeletal muscle spasm:* 5–10 mg initially; **then,** repeat in 3–4 hr if needed (larger doses may be required for tetanus). *Moderate anxiety:* 2–5 mg q 3–4 hr if necessary. *Severe anxiety, muscle spasm:* 5–10 mg q 3–4 hr, if necessary. *Acute alcohol withdrawal:* **initial,** 10 mg; **then,** 5–10 mg q 3–4 hr. *Preoperatively:* **IM,** 10 mg prior to surgery. *Endoscopy:* **IV,** 10 mg or less although doses up to 20 mg can be used; **IM,** 5–10 mg 30 min prior to procedure. *Cardioversion:* **IV,** 5–15 mg 5–10 min prior to procedure. *Tetanus in children,* **IM, IV, over 1 month:** 1–2 mg, repeated q 3–4 hr as necessary; **5 years and over:** 5–10 mg q 3–4 hr. **IV,** *Status epilepticus:* **Adults,** 5–10 mg initially; **then,** dose may be repeated at 10–15 min intervals up to a maximum dose of 30 mg. **Children, 1 month–5 years:** 0.2–0.5 mg q 2–5 min, up to a maximum of 5 mg. Can be repeated in 2–4 hr. **5 years and older:** 1 mg q 2–5 min up to a maximum of 10 mg; dose can be repeated in 2–4 hr, if needed.

Elderly or debilitated patients should not receive more than 5 mg parenterally at any one time.

NURSING CONSIDERATIONS

See also *Nursing Considerations* for *Benzodiazepines,* p. 614.

Administration/Storage

1. One 15-mg sustained-release diazepam capsule may be used if the daily dosage is 5 mg t.i.d.
2. The Intensol solution should be mixed with beverages such as water, soda, and juices, or soft foods such as applesauce or puddings. Only the calibrated dropper provided with the product should be used to withdraw the medication. Once the medication is withdrawn and mixed, it should be used immediately.
3. To reduce reactions at the site of IV administration, diazepam should be given slowly (5 mg/min). Also, small veins or intra-arterial administration should not be used.
4. When administering the drug IV, have emergency equipment and drugs available.
5. Due to the possibility of precipitation and instability, diazepam should not be infused.
6. Except for the deltoid muscle, absorption from IM sites is slow and erratic.
7. Review the drug interaction chart before administering the drug.

Assessment

1. Obtain a CBC, platelet count, liver and renal profiles as baseline data.
2. Note if the client has diabetes and the type of agent used for testing the urine as diazepam interferes with many of these agents. Have client convert to finger sticks for a more accurate blood glucose determination.

Interventions

1. Parenteral administration may cause bradycardia, respiratory or cardiac arrest. Monitor vital signs and client closely.
2. Elderly clients may experience adverse reactions more quickly than younger clients. Therefore, anticipate a lower dose of drug to be ordered in this group.

HALAZEPAM   (hal-AYZ-eh-pam)

Paxipam (C-IV, Rx)

See also *Benzodiazepines,* p. 611.

Classification: Antianxiety agent, benzodiazpine type.

Action/Kinetics: $t^{1/2}$: 14 hr. Metabolized in liver to *N*-desmethyldiazepam (active with a $t^{1/2}$ of 30–100 hr) and to inactive conjugates. **Maximum plasma levels of active metabolite:** 3–6 hr. Excreted through the kidneys.

Use: Short-term relief of anxiety.

Additional Contraindication: Acute narrow-angle glaucoma.

Special Concerns: Pregnancy category: D. Dose has not been established in children less than 18 years of age.

Dosage: Tablets. Adults: 20–40 mg t.i.d.–q.i.d. In elderly or debilitated patients: **initial,** 20 mg 1–2 times daily.

NURSING CONSIDERATIONS

See *Nursing Considerations* for *Benzodiazepines,* p. 614.

LORAZEPAM   (low-**RAYZ**-eh-pam)

Apo-Lorazepam ✿, Ativan, Novolorazepam ✿ (C-IV, Rx)

See also *Benzodiazepines,* p. 611.

Classification: Antianxiety agent, benzodiazepine.

Action/Kinetics: Absorbed and eliminated faster than other benzodiazepines. **Peak plasma levels: PO,** 1–6 hr; **IM,** 1–1.5 hr. **t½:** 10–20 hr. Is metabolized to inactive compounds which are excreted through the kidneys.

Uses: PO: Anxiety, tension, anxiety with depression, insomnia, acute alcohol withdrawal symptoms. **Parenteral:** Amnesic agent, anticonvulsant, antitremor drug, adjunct to skeletal muscle relaxants, preanesthetic medication, adjunct prior to endoscopic procedures, treatment of status epilepticus, relief of acute alcohol withdrawal symptoms.

Additional Contraindications: Narrow-angle glaucoma. Use cautiously in presence of renal and hepatic disease. Parenterally in children less than 18 years.

Special Concerns: Pregnancy category: D. Oral dosage has not been established in children less than 12 years of age and IV dosage has not been established in children less than 18 years of age.

Additional Drug Interactions: With parenteral lorazepam, scopolamine → sedation, hallucinations, and behavioral abnormalities.

Dosage: Tablets. Adults: *Anxiety:* 1–3 mg b.i.d.–t.i.d. *Hypnotic:* 2–4 mg at bedtime. **Geriatric/debilitated patients: initial,** 0.5–2 mg/day in divided doses. Dose can be adjusted as required.
   IM. Adults: 0.05 mg/kg up to maximum of 4 mg 2 hr before surgery for maximum amnesic effect. **IV. Adults, initial:** 0.044 mg/kg or a total dose of 2 mg, whichever is less. *Amnesic effect:* 0.05 mg/kg up to a maximum of 4 mg administered 15–20 min prior to surgery.

NURSING CONSIDERATIONS

See also *Nursing Considerations* for *Benzodiazepines,* p. 614.

Administration/Storage

1. For IV use, dilute just before use with either sterile water for injection, sodium chloride injection, or 5% dextrose injection.
2. The IV rate of administration should not exceed 2 mg/min.
3. The solution should not be used if it is discolored or contains a precipitate.
4. If higher doses are required, the evening dose should be increased before the daytime doses.

OXAZEPAM   (ox-**AYZ**-eh-pam)

Apo-Oxazepam ✿, Novoxapam ✿, Ox-Pam ✿, PMS-Oxazepam ✿, Serax, Zapex ✿ (C-IV, Rx)

See also *Benzodiazepines,* p. 611.

Classification: Antianxiety agent, benzodiazepine.

Action/Kinetics: Absorbed more slowly than most benzodiazepines. **Peak plasma levels:** 2–4 hr. $t^{1/2}$: 5–20 hr. Broken down in the liver to inactive metabolites which are excreted through both the urine and feces. Drug is reputed to cause less drowsiness than chlordiazepoxide.

Uses: Anxiety, tension, anxiety with depression. Adjunct in acute alcohol withdrawal.

Special Concerns: Pregnancy category: D. Dosage has not been established in children less than 12 years of age; use is not recommended in children less than 6 years of age.

Additional Side Effects: Paradoxical reactions characterized by sleep disorders and hyperexcitability during first weeks of therapy. Hypotension has occurred with parenteral administration.

Dosage: Capsules, Tablets. Adults: *Anxiety, mild to moderate:* 10–30 mg t.i.d.–q.i.d. **Geriatric and debilitated patients,** *anxiety, tension, irritability, agitation:* 10 mg t.i.d.; can be increased to 15 mg t.i.d.–q.i.d. *Alcohol withdrawal:* 15–30 mg t.i.d.–q.i.d.

NURSING CONSIDERATIONS
See *Nursing Considerations* for *Benzodiazepines,* p. 614.

PRAZEPAM   (PRAYZ-eh-pam)
Centrax (C-IV, Rx)

See also *Benzodiazepines,* p. 611.

Classification: Antianxiety agent, benzodiazepine type.

Action/Kinetics: Significant first-pass effect results in biotransformation to the active metabolites desmethyldiazepam and oxazepam. **Peak plasma levels:** 2.5–6 hr for desmethyldiazepam. Slow onset. **$t^{1/2}$: desmethyldiazepam:** 30–100 hr; **oxazepam,** 5–15 hr.

Uses: Antianxiety agents. Psychoneurosis associated with various disease states.

Special Concerns: Pregnancy category: D. Dosage has not been established in children less than 18 years of age.

Dosage: Capsules, Tablets. Adults: 10 mg t.i.d. (range 20–60 mg daily); or may be administered in a single dose at night: 20–40 mg at bedtime. **Geriatric and debilitated patients: initial,** 10–15 mg daily in divided doses.

NURSING CONSIDERATIONS
See *Nursing Considerations* for *Benzodiazepines,* p. 614.

MEPROBAMATE AND OTHER AGENTS

BUSPIRONE HYDROCHLORIDE   (byou-SPYE-rohn)
BuSpar (Rx)

Classification: Antianxiety agent.

Action/Kinetics: The mechanism of action is unknown. Buspirone is not chemically related to the benzodiazepines; it does not manifest anticonvulsant or muscle relaxant properties. Significant sedation has not been observed. The drug binds to serotonin (5-HT$_{1A}$) and dopamine (D$_2$) receptors in the CNS; it is thus possible that dopamine-mediated neurological disorders may occur. These include dystonia, Parkinson-like symptoms, akathisia, and tardive dyskinesia. **Peak plasma levels:** 1–6 ng/mL 40–90 min after a single oral dose of 20 mg. **t½:** 2–3 hr. The drug undergoes extensive first-pass metabolism and active and inactive metabolites are excreted in the urine and through the feces.

Uses: Anxiety disorders, short-term use to relieve symptoms of anxiety due to motor tension, apprehension, autonomic hyperactivity, or hyperattentiveness. Not usually indicated for treatment of anxiety and tension due to stress of everyday living.

Contraindications: Psychoses, severe liver or kidney impairment, lactation.

Special Concerns: Use with caution in pregnancy (category: B). Safety and efficacy in children less than 18 years of age not established. A decrease in dose may be necessary in geriatric patients due to age-related impairment of renal function.

Side Effects: *CNS:* Dizziness, drowsiness, insomnia, fatigue, nervousness, excitement, dream disturbances, dysphoria, noise intolerance, euphoria, depersonalization, akathisia, hallucinations, suicidal ideation, seizures, decreased concentration, confusion, anger or hostility, depression. *CV:* Nonspecific chest pain, hypotension, palpitations, tachycardia, syncope, hypertension. *GI:* Nausea, vomiting, diarrhea, constipation, abdominal distress, dry mouth, altered taste, increased appetite, irritable colon. *Ophthalmologic:* Redness and itching of eyes, conjunctivitis, photophopia, eye pain. *Dermatologic:* Skin rash, pruritus, dry skin, edema of face, acne, easy bruising, flushing. *Neurological:* Paresthesia, tremor, numbness, incoordination. *GU:* Urinary hesitancy or frequency, enurersis, amenorrhea, pelvic inflammatory disease. *Miscellaneous:* Tinnitus, sore throat, nasal congestion, altered smell, muscle aches or pains, skin rash, headache, sweating, hyperventilation, shortness of breath, hair loss, galactorrhea, decreased or increased libido, delayed ejaculation.

Drug Interactions: Use of monoamine oxidase inhibitors may cause an increase in blood pressure.

Dosage: Tablets. Adults: 5 mg t.i.d. Dosage may be increased in increments of 5 mg/day every 2–3 days to achieve optimum effects; the total daily dose should not exceed 60 mg.

NURSING CONSIDERATIONS

See also *Nursing Considerations* for *Antianxiety Agents,* p. 614.

Administration/Storage

1. Buspirone does not manifest cross-tolerance with other sedative-hypnotic drugs, including benzodiazepines.
2. Buspirone will not block the withdrawal syndrome, which may occur following cessation of sedative-hypnotics. Thus, clients on chronic sedative-hypnotic therapy should be withdrawn gradually prior to beginning buspirone therapy.
3. To date, buspirone has not manifested potential for abuse, tolerance, or either physical or psychological dependence.
4. Up to 2 weeks may be required before beneficial anti-anxiety effects are manifested.

Interventions

1. Note any client complaints of weakness, restlessness, nervousness, headaches or feelings of depression. These should be reported to the prescribing physician.
2. Some clients may develop Parkinson-like symptoms or have suicide ideations. These should be reported immediately and anticipate that the physician will withdraw the drug.

3. Nausea is a common side effect that can be alleviated by advising the client to take the drug with a snack to lessen the effects. If the nausea persists or is severe, the physician should be notified.

Client/Family Teaching

1. Review with the client and family the goals of therapy. Review the possible side effects and advise the client to report any unexpected side effects.
2. The drug may cause drowsiness or dizziness. Use caution when operating a motor vehicle or performing tasks that require mental alertness.
3. Report any involuntary, repetitive movements of the face or neck muscles immediately.
4. Avoid the use of alcohol.
5. Discuss with the physician any decision to stop taking the drug. The client may experience withdrawal symptoms such as nausea, vomiting, dry mouth, nasal congestion, or sore throat. These syptoms may occur even with gradual withdrawal from the drug.
6. Caution the client to avoid using OTC preparations unless the physician has been consulted.

CHLORMEZANONE   (klor-MEZ-ah-nohn)

Trancopal (Rx)

Classification: Antianxiety agent, meprobamate-type.

Action/Kinetics: The mechanism of action is unknown but chlormezanone will relieve anxiety, usually without impairing consciousness. The drug does act on subcortical levels of the CNS. **Onset:** 15–30 min. **Duration:** 4–6 hr. **Peak plasma levels:** 1–2 hr. **t ½:** 24 hr. Metabolized in the liver to inactive metabolites which are excreted in both the feces and urine.

Uses: Anxiety, tension. The drug has generally been replaced by more effective antianxiety agents.

Special Concerns: Safety during pregnancy and lactation has not been established. Dosage has not been established in children less than 5 years of age. A decrease in dose may be required in geriatric patients due to age-related decreases in renal function.

Side Effects: *CNS:* Dizziness, drowsiness, depression, excitement, tremors, headache, confusion, weakness. *GI:* Nausea, dry mouth. *Miscellaneous:* Rash, edema, flushing, inability to void, cholestatic jaundice (rare).

Drug Interactions: Additive effects when used with other CNS depressants.

Dosage: Tablets. Adults: 100–200 mg t.i.d.–q.i.d.; **pediatric, 5–12 years:** 50–100 mg t.i.d.–q.i.d.

NURSING CONSIDERATIONS

See also *Nursing Considerations* for *Benzodiazepines,* p. 614.

Administration/Storage

1. Initial dosage should be the lowest possible, especially in children.
2. Can be taken on an empty stomach.
3. Clients should be warned about possible interference with driving or operating machinery.

Interventions

1. Clients may complain of drowsiness, headache, ataxia, and may develop slurred speech. These symptoms should be documented and reported to the physician.

2. Client's activities should be supervised when in the hospital. Family members need to be aware of the need for supervision when the client is at home.

3. Monitor the client's weight and observe for any excessive weight loss.

Client/Family Teaching

1. Review the benefits and the possible side effects associated with drug therapy.

2. Do not attempt to perform any tasks that require mental alertness.

3. Note and report any skin discolorations.

4. Caution the client about the importance of reporting any difficulty with voiding. Instruct the client to record intake and output and to share this with the physician.

5. Remind the client that the drug may be habit-forming. Note any frequent returns for prescription refills.

6. Excessive morning drowsiness should be reported to the physician. The dosage of drug may need to be reduced or the drug may need to be changed.

HYDROXYZINE HYDROCHLORIDE   (hy-DROX-ih-zeen))

Anxanil, Apo-Hydroxyzine✿, Atarax, Atozine, E-Vista, Hydroxacen, Hyzine-50, Multipax✿, Novohydroxyzin✿, Quiess, Vistaject-25 and -50, Vistaquel 50, Vistaril, Vistazine 50 (Rx)

HYDROXYZINE PAMOATE   (hy-DROX-ih-zeen)

Vamate, Vistaril (Rx)

Classification: Antianxiety agent, miscellaneous.

Action/Kinetics: The action of hydroxyzine may be due to a depression of activity in selected important regions of the subcortical areas of the CNS. Hydroxyzine manifests anticholinergic, antiemetic, antispasmodic, local anesthetic, antihistaminic, and skeletal relaxant effects. The drug also has mild antiarrhythmic activity and mild analgesic effects. **Onset:** 15–30 min. **t½:** 3 hr. **Duration:** 4–6 hr. Metabolized by the liver and excreted through the urine. The pamoate salt is believed to be converted to the hydrochloride in the stomach.

Uses: PO use: Psychoneurosis and tension states, anxiety and agitation. Anxiety observed in organic disease. Adjunct in the treatment of chronic urticaria. Control of nausea and vomiting accompanying various diseases. Preanesthetic medication. **IM use:** Acute hysteria or agitation, withdrawal symptoms (including delirium tremens) in the acute or chronic alcoholic, asthma, nausea and vomiting (except that due to pregnancy), pre- or postoperative and pre-or postpartum to allow decrease in dosage of narcotics.

Contraindications: Pregnancy (especially early) or lactation; not recommended for the treatment of morning sickness during pregnancy or as sole agent for treatment of psychoses or depression. Hypersensitivity to drug. Not to be used IV, SC, or intra-arterially.

Special Concerns: Geriatric patients may manifest increased anticholinergic and sedative effects.

Side Effects: Low incidence at recommended dosages. Drowsiness, dryness of mouth, involuntary motor activity, dizziness, urticaria, or skin reactions. Marked discomfort, induration, and even gangrene have been reported at site of IM injection.

Drug Interactions: Additive effects when used with other CNS depressants. See *Drug Interactions* for *Benzodiazepines,* p. 612.

Laboratory Test Interference: Hydroxycorticosteroids.

Dosage: Capsules, Oral Suspension, Syrup. Hydroxyzine hydrochloride and **hydroxyzine pamoate.** *Antianxiety:* **Adults,** 50–100 mg q.i.d.; **pediatric under 6 years:** 50 mg daily; **over 6 years:** 50–100 mg daily in divided doses. *Pruritus:* **Adults,** 25 mg t.i.d.–q.i.d.; **children under 6 years:** 50 mg daily in divided doses; **children over 6 years:** 50–100 mg/day in divided doses. *Preoperatively:* **Adults,** 50–100 mg; **children:** 0.6 mg/kg.

    IM. Hydroxyzine hydrochloride. *Acute anxiety, including alcohol withdrawal:* **Initial,** 50–100 mg repeated q 4–6 hr as needed. *Nausea, vomiting, pre- and postoperative, pre- and postpartum:* **Adults,** 25–100 mg; **pediatric,** 1.1 mg/kg. Switch to **PO** as soon as possible.

NURSING CONSIDERATIONS
See also *Nursing Considerations* for *Benzodiazepines,* p. 614.

Administration/Storage
Inject IM only. Injection should be made into the upper, outer quadrant of the buttocks or the midlateral muscles of the thigh.
    In children the drug should be injected into the midlateral muscles of the thigh.

Client/Family Teaching
1. Frequent rinsing of the mouth and increased fluid intake may relieve dryness of the mouth.
2. Wait and evaluate the sedative effects of hydroxyzine before performing any tasks that require mental alertness.
3. Avoid ingestion of alcohol.

MEPROBAMATE   (meh-proh-**BAM**-ayt)
Apo-Meprobamate✳, Equanil, Equanil Wyseals, Meditran✳, Meprospan 200 and 400; Miltown 200, 400, and 600; Neuramate, Novomepro✳, (C-IV) (Rx)

Classification: Antianxiety agent.

Action/Kinetics: Meprobamate is a carbamate derivative that also possesses muscle relaxant and anticonvulsant effects. It acts on the limbic system and the thalamus, as well as to inhibit polysynaptic spinal reflexes. **Onset:** 1 hr. **Blood levels, chronic therapy:** 5–20 mcg/mL. **t½:** 6–24 hr. Extensively metabolized in liver and inactive metabolites and some unchanged drug (8–19%) are excreted in the urine. Mebrobamate is also found in *Equagesic.*

Uses: Short-term treatment (no more than 4 months) of anxiety.

Contraindications: Hypersensitivity to meprobamate or carisoprodol. Porphyria. Children under 6 years of age. Children less than 6 years of age.

Special Concerns: Use with caution in pregnancy, lactation, epilepsy, liver and kidney disease. Geriatric patients may be more sensitive to the depressant effects of meprobamate; also, due to age-related impaired renal function, the dose of meprobamate may have to be reduced.

Side Effects: *CNS:* Ataxia, drowsiness, dizziness, weakness headache, paradoxical excitement, euphoria, slurred speech, vertigo. *GI:* Nausea, vomiting, diarrhea. *Miscellaneous:* Visual disturbances, allergic reactions including hematologic and dermatologic symptoms, paresthesias.

Drug Interactions: Additive depressant effects when used with CNS depressants, MAO inhibitors, and tricyclic antidepressants.

Laboratory Test Interferences: *With test methods:* ↑ 17-Hydroxycorticosteroids, 17-ketogenic steroids, and 17-ketosteroids. *Pharmacologic effects:* ↑ Alkaline phosphatase, bilirubin, serum transaminase, urinary estriol (colorimetric tests), porphobilinogen. ↓ Prothrombin time in patients on coumarin.

Dosage: Tablets. Adults, initial, 400 mg t.i.d.–q.i.d. (or 600 mg b.i.d.). May be increased, if necessary, up to maximum of 2.4 g daily. **Pediatric, 6–12 years of age:** 100–200 mg t.i.d.–t.i.d. (the 600-mg tablet is not recommended for use in children).

Extended-release Capsules: 400–800 mg in the morning and at bedtime. **Children 6–12 years:** 200 mg in the morning and at bedtime.

NURSING CONSIDERATIONS

See *Nursing Considerations* for *Benzodiazepines,* p. 614.

Administration/Storage

Tablets and sustained-release capsules should not be crushed or chewed.

CHAPTER THIRTY-TWO

Antipsychotic Agents

Phenothiazines

Thioxanthene Derivatives

Butyrophenone Derivatives

Miscellaneous Antipsychotic Agents

General Statement: The advent of antipsychotic drugs was responsible for a major change in the treatment of the mentally ill. Reserpine, an alkaloid derived from *Rauwolfia serpentina,* and chlorpromazine, both of which appeared during the early 1950s, almost singlehandedly revolutionized the care of the mentally ill, both inside and outside the hospital. Patients who had not been helped for decades with electroshock, insulin therapy, and/or other forms of treatment could now often be discharged from the hospital. Antipsychotic drugs do not cure mental illness, but they calm the intractable patient, relieve the despondency of the severely depressed, activate the immobile and withdrawn, and make some patients more accessible to psychotherapy.

PHENOTHIAZINES

General Statement: Most phenothiazines induce some sedation, especially during the initial phase of the treatment. Medicated patients can, however, be easily roused. In this manner, the phenothiazines differ markedly from the narcotic analgesics and sedative hypnotics. However, phenothiazines potentiate the analgesic properties of opiates and prolong the action of CNS depressant drugs.

The drugs also decrease spontaneous motor activity, as in parkinsonism, and many lower blood pressure.

According to their detailed chemical structure, the phenothiazines belong to three subgroups:

1. Dimethylaminopropyl compounds
2. Piperazine compounds
3. Piperidine compounds

Drugs belonging to the *dimethylaminopropyl subgroup,* which includes chlorpromazine, are often the first choice for patients in acute excitatory states. Drugs belonging to this subgroup cause more sedation than other phenothiazines and are especially indicated for patients exhausted by lack of sleep.

Members of the *piperazine subgroup* act most selectively on the subcortical sites. This accounts for the fact that they can be administered in relatively small doses. This, in turn, results in minimal drowsiness and undesirable motor effects. The piperazines also have the greatest antiemetic effects because they specifically depress the chemoreceptor trigger zone (CTZ) of the vomiting center. Members of the *piperidyl subgroup* are less toxic in terms of extrapyramidal effects. Mellaril, a member of this group, has little effectiveness as an antiemetic drug.

Action/Kinetics: It has been postulated that excess amounts of dopamine in certain areas of the CNS cause psychoses. Phenothiazines are thought to act by blocking postsynaptic mesolimbic dopamine receptors, leading to a reduction in psychotic symptoms. Phenothiazines block both D_1 and D_2 dopamine receptors. The antiemetic effects are thought to be due to inhibition or blockade of dopamine (D_2) receptors in the chemoreceptor trigger zone in the medulla as well as by peripheral blockade of the vagus nerve in the GI tract. Relief of anxiety is manifested as a result of an indirect decrease in arousal and increased filtering of internal stimuli to the brainstem reticular system. Alpha-blockade produces sedation. Phenothiazines also raise pain threshold and produce amnesia due to suppression of sensory impulses. In addition, these drugs produce anticholinergic and antihistaminic effects, and depress the release of hypothalamic and hypophyseal hormones. Peripheral effects include anticholinergic and alpha-adrenergic blocking properties. Kinetic information on the phenothiazines is scarce and often unreliable.

Generally, peak plasma levels occur 2–4 hr after oral administration. Phenothiazines are widely distributed throughout the body. They have an average half-life of 10–20 hr. Most are metabolized in the liver and excreted by the kidney. Studies have shown that both oral dosage forms and suppositories from different manufacturers differ in their bioavailability. It is therefore recommended that brands not be interchanged unless data indicating bioequivalance are available.

Uses: Psychoses, especially if excessive psychomotor activity manifested. Involutional, toxic, or senile psychoses. Used in combination with monoamine oxidase inhibitors in depressed patients manifesting anxiety, agitation, or panic (use with caution). With lithium in acute manic phase of manic-depressive illness. As an adjunct in alcohol withdrawal to reduce anxiety, tension, depression, nausea, and/or vomiting. For severe behavioral problems in children, manifested by hyperexcitable and/or combative behavior; also, for short-term use in hyperactive children who exhibit excess motor activity and conduct disorders.

Prophylaxis and control of severe nausea and vomiting due to cancer chemotherapy, radiation therapy, postoperatively. Intractable hiccoughs, intermittent porphyria, tetanus (as adjunct). As preoperative and/or postoperative medications. Some phenothiazines are antipruritics. See also individual drugs.

Contraindications: Severe CNS depression, coma, patients with subcortical brain damage, bone marrow depression, lactation. In patients with a history of seizures and in patients on anticonvulsant drugs. Geriatric or debilitated patients, hepatic or renal disease, cardiovascular disorders, glaucoma, prostatic hypertrophy. Contraindicated in children with chicken pox, CNS infections, measles, gastroenteritis, dehydration due to increased risk of extrapyramidal symptoms in these patients.

Special Concerns: Phenothiazines should be used with caution in patients exposed to extreme heat or cold and in those with asthma, emphysema, or acute respiratory tract infections. Safe use during pregnancy not established; thus use only when benefits outweigh risks. Children may be more sensitive to the neuromuscular or extrapyramidal effects (especially dystonias); those especially at risk include children with chicken pox, CNS infections, measles, dehydration, or gastroenteritis. Thus, generally, phenothiazines are not recommended for use in children less than 12 years of age. Geriatric patients often manifest higher plasma levels due to decreases in lean body mass, total body water and albumin, and an increase in total body fat. Also, geriatric patients may be more likely to manifest orthostatic hypotension, anticholinergic effects, sedative effects, and extrapyramidal side effects.

Side Effects: *CNS:* Depression, drowsiness, dizziness, lethargy, fatigue. Extrapyramidal effects, Parkinson-like symptoms including shuffling gait or tic-like movements of head and face, tardive dyskinesia (see below), akathisia, dystonia. Seizures, especially in patients with a history thereof. Neuroleptic malignant syndrome (rare). *CV:* Orthostatic hypotension, increase or decrease in blood pressure, tachycardia, fainting. *GI:* Dry mouth, anorexia, constipation, paralytic ileus, diarrhea. *Endocrine:* Breast engorgement, galactorrhea, gynecomastia, increased appetite, weight gain, hyper- or hypoglycemia, glycosuria. Delayed ejaculation, increased or decreased libido. *GU:* Menstrual irregularities, loss of bladder control, urinary difficulty. *Dermatologic:* Photosensitivity, pruritus, erythema, eczema, exfoliative dermatitis, pigment changes in skin (long-term use of high doses). *Hematologic:* Aplastic anemia, leukopenia, agranulocytosis, eosinophilia, thrombocytopenia. *Ophthalmologic:* Deposition of fine particulate matter in lens and cornea leading to blurred vision, changes in vision. *Respiratory:* Laryngospasm, bronchospasm, laryngeal edema, breathing difficulties. *Miscellaneous:* Fever, muscle stiffness, decreased sweating, muscle spasm of face, neck, or back, obstructive jaundice, nasal congestion, pale skin, mydriasis, systemic lupus-like syndrome.

Tardive dyskinesia has been observed with all classes of antipsychotic drugs, although the precise cause is not known. The syndrome is most commonly seen in older patients, especially women, and in individuals with organic brain syndrome. It is often aggravated or precipitated by the sudden discontinuance of antipsychotic drugs and may persist indefinitely after the drug is discontinued. Early signs of tardive dyskinesia include fine vermicular movements of the tongue and grimacing or tic-like movements of the head and neck. Although there is no known cure for the syndrome, it may not progress if the dosage of the drug is slowly reduced. Also, a few drug-free days may unmask the symptoms of tardive dyskinesia and help in early diagnosis.

Drug Interactions

Alcohol, ethyl	Potentiation or addition of CNS depressant effects. Concomitant use may lead to drowsiness, lethargy, stupor, respiratory collapse, coma, or death
Aluminum salts (antacids)	↓ Absorption from GI tract
Amphetamine	↓ Effect of amphetamine by ↓ uptake of drug to the site of action
Anesthetics, general	See *Alcohol*
Antacids, oral	↓ Effect of phenothiazines due to ↓ absorption from GI tract
Antianxiety drugs	See *Alcohol*
Anticholinergic drugs	Additive anticholinergic side effects and/or ↓ antipsychotic effect
Antidepressants, tricyclic	Additive anticholinergic side effects
Antidiabetic agents	↓ Effect of antidiabetic agents, since phenothiazines ↑ blood sugar
Bacitracin	Additive respiratory depression
Barbiturate anesthetics	↑ Chance of tremor, involuntary muscle activity, and hypotension
Barbiturates	See *Alcohol;* also, barbiturates may ↓ effect due to ↑ breakdown by liver
Bromocriptine	Phenothiazines ↓ effect
Capreomycin	Additive respiratory depression
Charcoal	↓ Effect of phenothiazines due to ↓ absorption from GI tract
CNS depressants	See *Alcohol;* also, ↓ effect of phenothiazines due to ↑ breakdown by liver
Colistimethate	Additive respiratory depression
Diazoxide, Epinephrine	Additive hyperglycemic effect
Guanethidine	↓ Effect of guanethidine by ↓ uptake of drug at the site of action
Hydantoins	↑ Risk of hydantoin toxicity
Lithium carbonate	↑ Risk of extrapyramidal symptoms, disorientation, or unconsciousness
Meperidine	↑ Risk of hypotension and sedation
Metoprolol	Additive hypotensive effects
Monoamine oxidase inhibitors	↑ Effect of phenothiazines due to ↓ breakdown by liver
Narcotics	See *Alcohol*

Drug Interactions

Phenytoin	↑ Effect of phenytoin due to ↓ breakdown by liver
Polymyxin B	Additive respiratory depression
Propranolol	Additive hypotensive effects
Quinidine	Additive cardiac depressant effect
Sedative-hypnotics, nonbarbiturate	See *Alcohol*
Succinylcholine	↑ Muscle relaxation
Tricyclic antidepressants	↑ Serum levels of tricyclic antidepressant

Laboratory Test Interference: False + : Bile (urine dipstick), ferric chloride, pregnancy tests, urinary porphobilinogen, urinary steroids, urobilinogen (urine dipstick). False − : Inorganic phosphorus, urinary steroids. *Caused by pharmacologic effects:* ↑ Alkaline phosphatase, bilirubin, serum transaminases, serum cholesterol, urinary catecholamines. ↓ Glucose tolerance, serum uric acid, 5-hydroxyindoleacetic acid (5-HIAA), FSH, growth hormone, luteinizing hormone, vanillylmandelic acid.

Dosage: See individual drugs. The phenothiazines are effective over a wide dosage range. Dosage is usually increased gradually to minimize side effects over a period of 7 days until the minimal effective dose is attained. Dosage is increased more gradually in elderly or debilitated patients, since they are more susceptible to the effects and side effects of drugs. After symptoms are controlled, dosage is gradually reduced to maintenance levels. It is usually desirable to keep chronically ill patients on maintenance levels indefinitely.

Medication, especially in patients on high dosages, should not be discontinued abruptly.

NURSING CONSIDERATIONS

Administration/Storage

1. Do not interchange brands of oral form of drug or suppositories. They may differ in bioavailability.
2. Do not use pink or markedly discolored solutions.
3. When preparing or administering parenteral solutions, both nurse and client should avoid contact of drug with skin, eyes, and clothing.
4. Do not mix antipsychotic drugs with other drugs in the same syringe.
5. A specific rate of flow of drug should be ordered when administering parenteral solutions.
6. To lessen the pain of the injection, dilute commercially available injectable solutions in saline or local anesthetic.
7. When administering the drug IM, inject the drug deeply into the muscle.
8. Massage the area of the injection site after IM administration to reduce the pain.
9. Prevent extravasation of the IV solution.
10. Store solutions in a cool dry place in amber-colored containers.

Note: These *Nursing Considerations* apply to all antipsychotic agents except lithium.

Assessment

1. Take a complete drug history noting any past incidence of drug hypersensitivity.

2. When performing the nursing history, determine if there is any history of seizures. The drugs in this class may lower the seizure threshold.

3. When working with elderly clients, note their baseline level of mental acuity and document.

4. If administering the drug to children, note the extent of the client's hyperexcitability.

5. If the client is a child, assess the possibility of the child having chicken pox or measles.

6. Note any history of asthma or emphysema.

7. Obtain baseline readings of blood pressure and pulse before administering any antipsychotic drug. Assess the client's blood pressure when the client is in a reclining position, standing position and sitting position.

8. Ensure that the client has a complete blood count with differential, liver function tests, urinalysis, an EEG, and ocular examination prior to initiating therapy.

9. Note all medications the client may be taking to determine if any may interact unfavorably with the antipsychotic agent being considered.

Interventions

1. If drug is administered IV, the rate of flow should be monitored carefully and the blood pressure taken at frequent intervals.

2. Note client complaints of undue distress when in a hot or cold room. The client's heat regulating mechanism may be affected by the drug.
   - If the client complains of feeling cold, provide extra blankets.
   - If the client complains of feeling too warm, suggest bathing in tepid water.
   - Clients should *NOT* use heating pads or hot water bottles if they feel cold.

3. If the client becomes excessively active or depressed, document and report to the physician. The medication may need to be changed.

4. Note the presence of spasms of the client's face, neck, back or tongue. The physician may determine that the condition can be treated with antihistamines, or the decision may be to discontinue the drug.

5. When working with elderly clients be particularly observant for symptoms of tardive dyskinesia. Clients may exhibit puffing of the cheeks or tongue, develop chewing movements, and involuntary movements of the extremities and trunk. Such symptoms should be reported immediately to the physician and the drug discontinued.

6. If the client develops a sore throat, persistent fever, malaise and weakness document and report. These may be signs associated with agranulocytosis. The drug should be withheld until the appropriate blood work has been performed and the tests are evaluated by the physician.

7. Measure intake and output and observe for abdominal distention. Report any urinary retention. The dosage of medication may need to be reduced, antispasmodics may be indicated, or the drug may need to be changed.

8. Question clients concerning constipation. Encourage them to maintain an adequate fluid intake and to eat a diet high in roughage. Laxatives may be required.

9. Conduct periodic ocular examinations to detect any early visual disturbances.

10. Note any changes in carbohydrate metabolism (e.g. glycosuria, weight loss, polyphagia, increased appetite, or excessive weight gain). These signs may require a change in diet or medication therapy. These symptoms can be particularly significant if the client has diabetes.

11. Premenopausal women need to know that the menstrual cycle may become irregular. They may develop engorged breasts and begin lactating. The client needs to be reassured that this condition may be altered by a change in the medication therapy.

12. Some clients may develop a hypersensitivity reaction such as fever, asthma, laryngeal edema, angioneurotic edema and anaphylactic reaction. Administer epinephrine, steroids, antihistamines and/or oxygen as needed.

13. Be aware that clients on long term therapy may develop a yellow-brown skin reaction that may turn grayish-purple.

14. Note evidence of early cholestatic jaundice, such as high fever, client complaint of upper abdominal pain, nausea, diarrhea and rash. Obtain liver function studies and compare with the baseline measurements.

15. If the client develops yellowing of the sclera, skin, or mucous membranes, withhold the drug. Record these observations and report to the physician as these signs may indicate that the client has a biliary obstruction.

16. The antiemetic effects of phenothiazines may mask other pathology such as toxicity to other drugs, intestinal obstruction or brain lesions. Careful client observations are essential.

17. If the client is receiving barbiturates to relieve anxiety during phenothiazine therapy, the dose of the barbiturate will be reduced.

18. If barbiturates are being administered as an anticonvulsant, the dosage of barbiturates will not be reduced.

19. If administering phenothiazines to a child, note neuromuscular reactions, especially if the child is dehydrated or has an acute infection. These children are more susceptible to adverse reactions.

20. If the medication is to be administered IV, keep the client recumbent for at least one hour after the IV is completed.
    - Monitor the blood pressure for hypotension, compare to the baseline measurements.
    - After one hour, slowly elevate the head of the bed, and observe for tachycardia, faintness, or complaint of dizziness.
    - Keep side rails up.

21. If the drug is to be discontinued, it should be done so gradually so as to minimize the possible onset of severe GI disturbances or symptoms of tardive dyskinesias.

22. If the client is in a hospital setting, remain with him/her to assure that the medication has been swallowed. It may be advisable to give a liquid preparation of the drug to permit better control over drug taking and improve compliance.

23. If the client develops respiratory symptoms, instruct him to take slow, deep breaths. The drug may depress the cough reflex.

24. When the client is being seen on an outpatient basis, check on the number of times they request prescription refills. The client may be hoarding medication, especially if depressed.

Client/Family Teaching

1. Advise young women that the drug may cause menstrual irregularity, and can cause false positive pregnancy tests. If the client suspects she may be pregnant, she should notify her physician.

2. Encourage female clients to keep an accurate record of their menstrual periods.

3. Male clients should be told they may experience decreased libido and develop breast enlargement. Reassure client and instruct him to report these symptoms to the physician so that the medication can be adjusted.

4. Many clients develop photosensitivity reactions. Advise them to wear protective clothing when in the sun and to avoid sunbathing. They should also use large quantities of sun screens.

5. Drug may turn the urine pink or reddish-brown.
6. To prevent a dry mouth, advise clients to rinse the mouth frequently, increase fluid intake, chew sugarless gum and/or to suck on hard candies.
7. Avoid drinking alcoholic beverages.
8. If the client develops blurred vision, avoid driving the car and notify physician.
9. Remind clients that long term therapy may affect their vision. Therefore they should schedule regular ophthalmic examinations.
10. Avoid driving a car or operating heavy machinery or engaging in any activities that require mental alertness for at least 2 weeks after the therapy has started. Consult with physician for evaluation of client's response to treatment before client resumes any of these activities.
11. Report any elevation of body temperature, feeling of weakness, or sore throat. These may be indications of blood dyscrasias and require immediate attention.
12. Advise clients not to stop taking the drug abruptly. An abrupt cessation of high doses of phenothiazines can cause nausea, vomiting, tremors, sensations of warmth and cold, sweating, tachycardia, headache and insomnia.
13. Remind the client and family that it may be weeks or months before the full effects of the medication will be noticed.
14. Stress the importance of taking the drug as prescribed after discharge.
15. Advise all health care providers of the medications currently prescribed.
16. Stress the importance of reporting for periodic laboratory studies and follow-up care for evaluation and adjustment of drug dosage.

Evaluation

1. Review goals of therapy with client and family and assess degree to which they have been attained.
2. Compare baseline evaluations of client behavior with present level.
3. Note client orientation as to time, place, and understanding of his/her illness.
4. Assess client for extrapyramidal effects of drug therapy.
5. Determine if the client is adhering to the prescribed drug regimen.

ACETOPHENAZINE MALEATE (ah-see-toe-**FEN**-ah-zeen)

Tindal (Rx)

See also *Phenothiazines,* p. 627.

Classification: Antipsychotic, piperazine-type phenothiazine.

Action/Kinetics: Acetophenazine manifests a low incidence of orthostatic hypotension, moderate sedation and anticholinergic effects but a high incidence of extrapyramidal effects.

Uses: Psychoses.

Special Concerns: Dosage has not been established in children less than 12 years of age.

Dosage: Tablets. Adults and children over 12 years, usual: 20 mg t.i.d. (range: 40–80 mg daily in divided doses); 80–120 mg daily in divided doses for hospitalized schizophrenic patients (doses as high as 400–600 mg/day may be needed in severe schizophrenia). Emaciated, geriatric, and debilitated patients require a lower initial dose.

NURSING CONSIDERATIONS

See also *Nursing Considerations* for *Phenothiazines,* p. 630.

Assessment

1. Note the age of the client since elderly clients usually require lower drug dosage.
2. Identify if the client is taking lithium. Acetophenazine potentiates CNS toxicity.

Client/Family Teaching

1. Administer 1 hr before bedtime if client has difficulty sleeping.
2. Provide clients with a list of potential drug reactions which they should report to the physician.
3. Remind client to call the physician if any adverse reactions occur and *not* to stop taking the medication abruptly.

CHLORPROMAZINE   (klor-**PROH**-mah-zeen)

Largactil✿, Thorazine (Rx)

CHLORPROMAZINE HYDROCHLORIDE   (klor-**PROH**-mah-zeen)

Chlorpromanyl-20 and -40✿, Largactil✿, Novo-Chlorpromazine✿, Ormazine, Thorazine, Thor-Prom (Rx)

See also *Phenothiazines,* p. 627.

Classification: Antipsychotic, dimethylamino-type phenothiazine.

Action/Kinetics: Chlorpromazine has significant antiemetic, hypotensive, and sedative effects; moderate to strong anticholinergic effects and weak to moderate extrapyramidal effects. **Peak plasma levels:** 2–3 hr after both PO and IM administration. **t½** (after IV, IM): **initial,** 4–5 hr; **final,** 3–40 hr. Chlorpromazine is extensively metabolized in the intestinal wall and liver; certain of the metabolites are active. **Steady-state plasma levels** (in psychotics): 10–1,300 ng/mL. After 2–3 weeks of therapy, plasma levels decline, possibly because of reduction in drug absorption and/or increase in drug metabolism.

Uses: Acute and chronic psychoses, including schizophrenia; manic phase of manic-depressive illness. Acute intermittent porphyria. Preanesthetic, adjunct to treat tetanus, intractable hiccoughs, severe behavioral problems in children, neuroses, nausea and vomiting. Treatment of choreiform movements in Huntington's disease.

Special Concerns: Use during pregnancy only if benefits outweigh risks. Oral dosage for psychoses and nausea/vomiting have not been established in children less than 6 months of age.

Additional Drug Interactions	
Epinephrine	Chlorpromazine ↓ peripheral vasoconstriction and may reverse action of epinephrine
Norepinephrine	Chlorpromazine ↓ pressor effect and eliminates bradycardia due to norepinephrine
Valproic acid	↑ Effect of valproic acid due to ↓ clearance

Dosage: Extended-release Capsules, Oral Concentrate, Syrup, Tablets. *Psychotic disorders:*

Adults and adolescents, 10–25 mg (of the base) b.i.d.–q.i.d.; dosage may be increased by 20–50 mg a day q 3–4 days as needed. Or, 30–300 mg (of the base) using the extended-release capsules 1–3 times daily (the 300 mg extended-release capsules are used only in severe neuropsychiatric situations). **Pediatric:** 0.55 mg/kg (15 mg/m^2) q 4–6 hr. *Nausea and vomiting:* **Adults and adolescents,** 10–25 mg (of the base) q 4 hr; dosage may be increased as needed. **Pediatric:** 0.55 mg/kg (15 mg/m^2) q 4–6 hr. *Preoperative sedation:* **Adults and adolescents,** 25–50 mg (of the base) 2–3 hr before surgery. **Pediatric:** 0.55 mg/kg (15 mg/m^2) 2–3 hr before surgery. *Hiccoughs or porphyria:* **Adults and adolescents,** 25–50 mg (of the base) t.i.d.–q.i.d.

IM. *Severe psychoses,* **Adults,** 25–50 mg (of the base) repeated in 1 hr if needed; **then,** repeat the dose q 3–4 hr as needed and tolerated (the dose may be increased gradually over several days). **Pediatric, over 6 months of age:** 0.55 mg/kg (15 mg/m^2) q 6–8 hr as needed. *Nausea and vomiting:* **Adults,** 25 mg (base) as a single dose; **then,** increase to 25–50 mg q 3–4 hr as needed until vomiting ceases. **Pediatric:** 0.55 mg/kg q 6–8 hr as needed. *Nausea and vomiting during surgery:* **Adults,** 12.5 mg (base) as a single dose; repeat in 30 min if needed. **Pediatric,** 0.275 mg/kg; repeat in 30 min if needed. *Preoperative sedative:* **Adults,** 12.5–25 mg (base) 1–2 hr before surgery. **Pediatric:** 0.55 mg/kg 1–2 hr before surgery. *Hiccoughs:* **Adults,** 25–50 mg (base) t.i.d.–q.i.d. *Porphyria:* **Adults,** 25 mg (base) q 6–8 hr until patient can take PO therapy. *Tetanus:* **Adults,** 25–50 mg (base) t.i.d.–q.i.d. (dose can be increased as needed and tolerated).

IV. *Nausea and vomiting during surgery:* **Adults,** 25 mg (base) diluted to 1 mg/mL with 0.9% sodium chloride injection given at a rate of no more than 2 mg q 2 min. **Pediatric:** 0.275 mg/kg diluted to 1 mg/mL with 0.9% sodium chloride injection given at a rate of no more than 1 mg q 2 min. *Tetanus:* **Adults,** 25–50 mg (base) diluted to 1 mg/mL with 0.9% sodium chloride injection and given at a rate of 1 mg/min. **Pediatric:** 0.55 mg/kg diluted to 1 mg/mL with 0.9% sodium chloride injection and given at a rate of 1 mg/2 min.

Suppositories. *Nausea and vomiting:* **Adults and adolescents,** 50–100 mg q 6–8 hr as needed up to a maximum of 400 mg daily. **Pediatric:** 1 mg/kg q 6–8 hr as needed (the 100 mg suppository should not be used in children).

NURSING CONSIDERATIONS

See also *Nursing Considerations* for *Phenothiazines,* p. 630.

Administration/Storage

1. Chlorpromazine should not be used to treat nausea and vomiting in children less than 6 months of age.
2. The maximum daily oral and parenteral dose for adults and adolescents should be 1 g of the base.
3. The maximum IM dose should be 40 mg daily for children up to 5 years of age and 75 mg daily for children 5–12 years of age.
4. Sustained-release capsules should be swallowed whole.
5. Solutions of chlorpromazine may cause contact dermatitis; thus, medical personnel should avoid getting solution on hands or clothing.
6. When used IV in children for tetanus, the preparation should be diluted to 1 mg/mL and given at a rate of 1 mg/2 min.
7. The concentrate (to be used in hospitals only) can be mixed with 60 mL or more of fruit or tomato juice, orange or simple syrup, milk, carbonated drinks, coffee, tea, water, or semisolid foods (e.g., soup, pudding).
8. Slight discoloration of injection or oral solutions will not affect the action of the drug.
9. Solutions with marked discoloration should be discarded. Consult with pharmacist if unsure of drug potency.

Assessment

1. Note any history of seizure disorders as the drug is contraindicated in these instances.
2. Conduct baseline studies of liver and kidney function.
3. Determine age of male clients and assess for prostatic hypertrophy.

Interventions

1. When administering the drug IM, select a large, well-developed muscle mass. Use the dorsogluteal site or rectus femoris in adults and the vastus lateralis in children.
2. Document and rotate injection sites.
3. Be alert for side effects and immediately report them.

FLUPHENAZINE DECANOATE   (flew-**FEN**-ah-zeen)

Modecate❋, Prolixin Decanoate (Rx)

FLUPHENAZINE ENANTHATE   (flew-**FEN**-ah-zeen)

Moditen Enanthate❋, Prolixin Enanthate (Rx)

FLUPHENAZINE HYDROCHLORIDE   (flew-**FEN**-ah-zeen)

Apo-Fluphenazine❋, Moditen HCl-H.P.❋, Permitil, Prolixin (Rx)

See also *Phenothiazines,* p. 627.

Classification: Antipsychotic, piperazine-type phenothiazine.

Action/Kinetics: Fluphenazine is accompanied by a high incidence of extrapyramidal symptoms and a low incidence of sedation, anticholinergic effects, antiemetic effects, and orthostatic hypotension. The enanthate and decanoate esters dramatically increase the duration of action. *Decanoate:* **Onset,** 24–72 hr; **peak plasma levels,** 24–48 hr; **t½** (approximate), 14 days; **duration:** up to 4 weeks. *Enanthate:* **Onset,** 24–72 hr; **peak plasma levels,** 48–72 hr; **t½** (approximate): 3.6 days; **duration:** 1–3 weeks.

Fluphenazine hydrochloride can be cautiously administered to patients with known hypersensitivity to other phenothiazines.

Fluphenazine enanthate may replace fluphenazine hydrochloride if desired response occurs with hypersensitivity reaction to fluphenazine.

Uses: Psychotic disorders. Adjunct to tricyclic antidepressants for chronic pain states (e.g., diabetic neuropathy, and patients trying to withdraw from narcotics).

Dosage: Fluphenazine hydrochloride is administered **PO and IM.** Fluphenazine enanthate and decanoate are administered **SC and IM.**

Elixir, Oral Solution, Tablets. *Psychotic disorders:* **Adults and adolescents, initial:** 2.5–10 mg/day in divided doses q 6–8 hr; **then,** reduce gradually to maintenance dose of 1–5 mg/day (usually given as a single dose, not to exceed 20 mg/day). *Geriatric, emaciated, debilitated patients:* **Initial:** 1–2.5 mg/day; **then,** dosage determined by response. **Pediatric:** 0.25–0.75 mg 1–4 times daily.

IM, Hydrochloride. Adults and adolescents: 1.25–2.5 mg q 6–8 hr as needed. Maximum daily dose: 10 mg. Elderly, debilitated, or emaciated patients should start with 1–2.5 mg daily.

IM, SC. Decanoate. *Psychotic disorders:* **Adults, initial,** 12.5–25 mg; **then,** the dose may be repeated or increased q 1–3 weeks. The usual maintenance dose is 50 mg q 1–4 weeks. Maximum adult dose: 100 mg/dose. **Pediatric, 12 years and older:** 6.25–18.75 mg weekly; the dose can be increased to 12.5–25 mg given q 1–3 weeks. **Pediatric, 5–12 years of age:** 3.125–12.5 mg with this dose being repeated q 1–3 weeks.

IM, SC. Enanthate. *Psychotic disorders:* **Adults and adolescents:** 25 mg; dose can be repeated or increased q 1–3 weeks. For doses greater than 50 mg, increases should be made in increments of 12.5 mg. Maximum adult dose: 100 mg/dose.

NURSING CONSIDERATIONS

See also *Nursing Considerations* for *Phenothiazines,* p. 630.

Administration/Storage

1. Protect all forms of medication from light.
2. Store at room temperature and avoid freezing.
3. Color of parenteral solution may vary from colorless to light amber. Do not use solutions that are darker than light amber.
4. The hydrochloride concentrate should not be mixed with any beverage containing caffeine, tannates (e.g., tea), or pectins (e.g., apple juice) due to a physical incompatibility.
5. Clients beginning therapy with phenothiazines should first receive a short-acting form of the drug; the decanoate and enanthate can be considered after the response to the drug has been evaluated.

Assessment

Note the age and condition of the client. Elderly and debilitated clients are particularly at risk for acute extrapyramidal symptoms.

MESORIDAZINE BESYLATE   (mez-oh-**RID**-ah-zeen)

Serentil (Rx)

See also *Phenothiazines,* p. 627.

Classification: Antipsychotic, piperidine-type phenothiazine.

Action/Kinetics: Mesoridazine has pronounced sedative and hypotensive effects, moderate anticholinergic effects, and a low incidence of extrapyramidal symptoms and antiemetic effects.

Uses: Schizophrenia, acute and chronic alcoholism, behavior problems in patients with mental deficiency and chronic brain syndrome, psychoneurosis.

Special Concerns: Use during pregnancy only if benefits clearly outweigh risks. Dosage has not been established in children less than 12 years of age. Geriatric, debilitated, and emaciated patients require a lower initial dose.

Dosage: Oral Solution, Tablets. *Psychotic disorders:* **Adults and adolescents,** 30–150 mg daily in 2–3 divided doses. *Alcoholism:* **initial,** 25 mg b.i.d.; **optimum total dose:** 50–200 mg/day.

IM. *Psychotic disorders:* **Adults and adolescents:** 25 mg (base); **then,** repeat the dose in 30–60 min as needed.

NURSING CONSIDERATIONS

See also *Nursing Considerations* for *Phenothiazines,* p. 630.

Administration/Storage

1. Maintain client supine for minimum of 30 minutes after parenteral administration to minimize orthostatic effect.

2. Acidified tap or distilled water, orange juice, or grape juice may be used to dilute the concentrate prior to use.
3. Bulk dilutions should not be prepared or stored.
4. For IM administration, give 25 mg initially, repeated at 30–60 minute intervals as needed.

PERPHENAZINE (per-**FEN**-ah-zeen)

Apo-Perphenazine ✱, Phenazine ✱, Trilafon (Rx)

See also *Phenothiazines,* p. 627.

Classification: Antipsychotic, antiemetic, piperazine-type phenothiazine.

Action/Kinetics: Resembles chlorpromazine. Use accompanied by a high incidence of extrapyramidal effects; strong antiemetic effects; moderate anticholinergic effects; and a low incidence of orthostatic hypotension and sedation. Perphenazine is also found in Triavil. **Onset, IM:** 10 min. **Maximum effect, IM:** 1–2 hr. **Duration, IM:** 6 hr (up to 24 hr).

Uses: Psychotic disorders. To treat severe nausea and vomiting.

Special Concerns: Use during pregnancy only if benefits clearly outweigh risks. Dosage has not been established in children less than 12 years of age. Geriatric, emaciated, or debilitated patients usually require a lower initial dose.

Dosage: Oral Solution, Syrup, Tablets. *Psychoses:* **Nonhospitalized patients:** 4–8 mg t.i.d. or 8–16 mg repeat-action tablets b.i.d. **Hospitalized patients:** 8–16 mg b.i.d.–q.i.d. or 8–32 mg repeat-action tablets b.i.d. Total daily dosage should not exceed 64 mg. *Severe nausea and vomiting:* 8–16 mg/day in divided doses (24 mg daily may be required in some patients).

IM. Adults and adolescents: *Psychotic disorders,* **Nonhospitalized patients:** 5 mg q 6 hr, not to exceed 15 mg daily. **Hospitalized patients: initial,** 5–10 mg; total daily dose should not exceed 30 mg. *Severe nausea and vomiting:* 5 mg (initially, 10 mg in severe cases) q 6 hr, not to exceed 15 mg in ambulatory patients or 30 mg in hospitalized patients.

IV. *Severe nausea and vomiting:* Up to 5 mg diluted to 0.5 mg/mL with 0.9% sodium chloride injection. Should be given in divided doses of not more than 1 mg q 1–3 hr. Can also be given as an infusion at a rate not to exceed 1 mg/min. Use should be restricted to hospitalized recumbent adults. Maximum single dose should not exceed 5 mg.

NURSING CONSIDERATIONS

See also *Nursing Considerations* for *Phenothiazines,* p. 630.

Administration/Storage

1. Each 5.0 mL of oral concentrate should be diluted with 60 mL of diluent, such as water, milk, carbonated beverage, or orange juice.
2. Do not mix with tea, coffee, cola, grape juice, or apple juice.
3. When rapid action is required, administer IM using 5 mg. Inject deep into the muscle, and repeat at 6-hour intervals as needed. The client should be in a recumbent position and remain in that position for at least 1 hour after IM administration.
4. Protect from light.
5. Store solutions in an amber-colored container.

Interventions

1. Monitor the client's blood pressure since the drug may cause hypotension.
2. Assess pulse rate for evidence of tachycardia and/or bradycardia.

PROCHLORPERAZINE   (proh-klor-**PER**-ah-zeen)

Compazine, Stemetil ❀ (Rx)

PROCHLORPERAZINE EDISYLATE   (proh-klor-**PER**-ah-zeen)

Compazine Edisylate (Rx)

PROCHLORPERAZINE MALEATE   (proh-klor-**PER**-ah-zeen)

Compazine Maleate, Stemetil ❀ (Rx)

See also *Phenothiazines,* p. 627.

Classification: Antipsychotic, antiemetic, piperazine-type phenothiazine.

Action/Kinetics: Prochlorperazine causes a high incidence of extrapyramidal and antiemetic effects; moderate sedative effects; and, a low incidence of anticholinergic effects and orthostatic hypotension. It also possesses significant antiemetic effects.

Uses: Psychoneuroses. Postoperative nausea and vomiting, radiation sickness, vomiting due to toxins. Generally not used for patients who weigh less than 9 kg or who are under 2 years of age. Severe nausea and vomiting.

Special Concerns: Safe use during pregnancy has not been established. Dosage has not been established in children less than 2 years of age or 9 kg body weight. Geriatric, emaciated, and debilitated patients usually require a lower initial dose.

Dosage: Edisylate Syrup, Maleate Extended-release Capsules, Tablets. *Psychotic disorders:* **Adults and adolescents,** 5–10 mg (base) t.i.d.–q.i.d. (dose can be increased gradually q 2–3 days as needed and tolerated). For extended-release capsules, up to 100–150 mg daily can be given. **Pediatric, 2–12 years:** 2.5 mg (base) b.i.d.–t.i.d. *Nausea and vomiting:* **Adults and adolescents,** 5–10 mg (base) t.i.d.–q.i.d. (up to 40 mg daily). For extended-release capsules, the dose is 15–30 mg once daily in the morning (or 10 mg q 12 hr, up to 40 mg daily). **Pediatric, 18–39 kg:** 2.5 mg (base) t.i.d. (or 5 mg b.i.d.), not to exceed 15 mg daily; **14–17 kg:** 2.5 mg (base) b.i.d.–t.i.d., not to exceed 10 mg daily; **9–13 kg:** 2.5 mg (base) 1–2 times daily, not to exceed 7.5 mg daily. The total daily dose for children should not exceed 10 mg the first day; on subsequent days, the total daily dose should not exceed 20 mg for children 2–5 years of age or 25 mg for children 6–12 years of age. *Anxiety:* **Adults and adolescents,** 5 mg (base) t.i.d.–q.i.d. up to 20 mg daily for no longer than 12 weeks.

   IM. Edisylate Injection. *Psychotic disorders, for immediate control of severely disturbed patients:* **Adults and adolescents:** 10–20 mg (base); dose can be repeated q 2–4 hr as needed (usually up to 3 or 4 doses). **Maintenance:** 10–20 mg (base) q 4–6 hr. **Pediatric:** 0.132 mg/kg. *Anxiety:* **Adults and adolescents,** 5–10 mg (base); dose can be repeated q 2–4 hr as needed. *Nausea and vomiting:* **Adults and adolescents,** 5–10 mg with the dose repeated q 3–4 hr as needed. **Pediatric, 2–12 years:** 0.132 mg/kg. *Nausea and vomiting during surgery:* **Adults and adolescents,** 5–10 mg (base) 1–2 hr before induction of anesthesia; to control symptoms during or after surgery, the dose can be repeated once after 30 min.

   IV. Edisylate Injection. *Nausea and vomiting:* **Adults and adolescents,** 2.5–10 mg as a slow injection or infusion (rate should not exceed 5 mg/min up to 40 mg daily). *Nausea and vomiting during surgery:* **Adults and adolescents,** 5–10 mg (base) given as a slow injection or infusion 15–30 min before induction of anesthesia; to control symptoms during or after surgery the dose can be repeated once. The rate of infusion should not exceed 5 mg/mL/min.

Rectal Suppositories. Pediatric, 2–12 years: 2.5 mg b.i.d.–t.i.d. with no more than 10 mg given on the first day. No more than 20 mg daily for children 2–5 years and 25 mg daily for children 6–12 years of age.

NURSING CONSIDERATIONS

See also *Nursing Considerations* for *Phenothiazines,* p. 630.

Administration/Storage

1. Store all forms of the drug in tight-closing amber-colored bottles; store the suppositories below 37°C.
2. Add the desired dosage of concentrate to 60 mL of beverage (e.g., tomato or fruit juice, milk, soup) or semisolid food just before administration to disguise the taste.
3. Drug should not be administered SC due to irritation.
4. Prochlorperazine should not be mixed with other agents in a syringe.
5. Prochlorperazine should not be diluted with any material containing the preservative parabens.
6. When given IM to children for nausea and vomiting, the duration of action may be 12 hr.
7. Parenteral prescribing limits are 20 mg daily for children 2–5 years of age and 25 mg daily for children 6–12 years of age.

Interventions

1. Have emergency equipment and drugs available when treating an overdose.
2. Monitor vital signs and incorporate safety precautions during the treatment of an overdose.
3. If the client was taking spansules, continue the treatment of overdosage until all signs of overdosage are no longer evident.
4. In treating clients for an overdosage of medication, anticipate that saline laxatives may be used to hasten the evacuation of pellets that have not yet released their medication.

Client/Family Teaching

1. Advise parents not to exceed the prescribed dose of drug.
2. If the child shows signs of restlessness and excitement, withhold the medication and notify the physician.

PROMAZINE HYDROCHLORIDE   (PROH-mah-zeen)

Prozine-50, Sparine (Rx)

See also *Phenothiazines,* p. 627.

Classification: Antipsychotic, dimethylaminopropyl-type phenothiazine.

Action/Kinetics: The use of promazine is accompanied by significant anticholinergic, sedative, and hypotensive effects; moderate antiemetic effect; and, weak extrapyramidal effects. This drug is ineffective in reducing destructive behavior in acutely agitated psychotic patients.

Uses: Psychotic disorders.

Special Concerns: Safe use during pregnancy has not been established. Dosage has not been established in children less than 12 years of age. Geriatric, emaciated and debilitated patients may require a lower initial dosage.

Dosage: Tablets. *Psychotic disorders:* **Adults:** 10–200 mg q 4–6 hr; adjust dose as needed and tolerated. Total daily dose should not exceed 1,000 mg. **Pediatric, 12 years and older:** 10–25 mg q 4–6 hr; adjust dose as needed and tolerated.

   IM. *Psychotic disorders, severe and moderate agitation:* **Adults, initial:** 50–150 mg; adjust dose if necessary after 30 min. **Maintenance:** 10–200 mg q 4–6 hr as needed and tolerated. Switch to PO therapy as soon as possible. **Children over 12 years:** 10–25 mg q 4–6 hr for chronic psychotic disorders (maximum dose: 1 g daily).

   The dose may be given IV.

NURSING CONSIDERATIONS

See also *Nursing Considerations* for *Phenothiazines,* p. 630.

Administration/Storage

1. Dilute concentrate as directed on bottle. Taste can be disguised when given with citrus fruit juice, milk, or flavored drinks.
2. IM injections should be given in the gluteal region.
3. IV doses should be diluted to 25 mg/mL with 0.9% sodium chloride injection and given slowly.

THIORIDAZINE HYDROCHLORIDE   (thigh-oh-**RID**-ah-zeen)

Apo-Thioridazine✽, Mellaril, Mellaril-S, Novoridazine✽, PMS Thioridazine✽, Thioridazine HCl Intensol Oral (Rx)

See also *Phenothiazines,* p. 627.

Classification: Antipsychotic, piperidine-type phenothiazine.

Action/Kinetics: The use of thioridazine is accompanied by a high incidence of hypotensive effects; a moderate incidence of sedative and anticholinergic effects and weak antiemetic and extrapyramidal effects. Thioridazine can often be used in patients intolerant of other phenothiazines. It has little or no antiemetic effects.

   Peak plasma levels (after PO administration): 1–4 hr. Thioridazine may impair its own absorption at higher doses due to the strong anticholinergic effects. **t½:** 10 hr. Metabolized in the liver to both active and inactive metabolites.

Uses: Acute and chronic schizophrenia; moderate to marked depression with anxiety; sleep disturbances. *In children:* treatment of hyperactivity in patients and those with retarded and behavior problems. Geriatric patients with organic brain syndrome. Alcohol withdrawal. Intractable pain.

Special Concerns: Safe use during pregnancy has not been established. Dosage has not been established in children less than 2 years of age. Geriatric, emaciated, or debilitated patients usually require a lower initial dose.

Additional Side Effects: More likely to cause pigmentary retinopathy than other phenothiazines.

Dosage: Oral Suspension, Oral Solution, Tablets. Highly individualized. *Neurosis, anxiety states, sleep disturbances, tension, alcohol withdrawal, senility,* **range:** 20–200 mg daily; **initial:** 25 mg t.i.d. **Maintenance,** mild cases: 10 mg b.i.d.–q.i.d.; severe cases: 50 mg t.i.d.–q.i.d. *Psychotic, severely disturbed hospitalized patients:* **initial,** 50–100 mg t.i.d. If necessary, increase to maximum of 200 mg q.i.d. When control is achieved, reduce gradually to minimum effective dosage. **Pediatric above 2 years:** 0.25–3.0 mg/kg daily. *Hospitalized psychotic children:* **initial,** 25 mg b.i.d.–t.i.d. *Moderate problems:* **initial,** 10 mg b.i.d.–t.i.d. Increase gradually if necessary. **Not recommended for children under 2 years of age.**

NURSING CONSIDERATIONS

See also *Nursing Considerations* for *Phenothiazines,* p. 630.

Administration/Storage

Dilute each dose just before administration with distilled water, acidified tap water, or suitable juices. Preparation and storage of bulk dilutions are not recommended.

TRIFLUOPERAZINE   (try-flew-oh-**PER**-ah-zeen)

Apo-Trifluoperazine ✤, Novo-Flurazine ✤, Solazine ✤, Stelazine, (Rx)

See also *Phenothiazines,* p. 627.

Classification: Antipsychotic, antiemetic, piperazine-type phenothiazine.

Action/Kinetics: Trifluoperazine is accompanied by a high incidence of extrapyramidal symptoms and antiemetic effects and a low incidence of sedation, orthostatic hypotension, and anticholinergic side effects. Recommended only for hospitalized or well-supervised patients. **Maximum therapeutic effect:** Usually 2–3 weeks after initiation of therapy.

Uses: Schizophrenia. Suitable for patients with apathy or withdrawal. Anxiety, tension, agitation in neuroses.

Special Concerns: Use during pregnancy only when benefits clearly outweigh risks. Dosage has not been established in children less than 6 years of age. Geriatric, emaciated, or debilitated patients usually require a lower initial dose.

Dosage: Oral Solution, Tablets. *Psychoses:* **Adults and adolescents, initial** 2–5 mg (base) b.i.d.; **maintenance:** 15–20 mg daily in 2 or 3 divided doses. **Pediatric, 6–12 years:** 1 mg (base) 1–2 times daily; adjust dose as required and tolerated. *Anxiety/tension:* **Adults and adolescents,** 1–2 mg daily up to 6 mg daily. Not to be given for this purpose longer than 12 weeks.

IM. *Pyschoses:* **Adults** 1–2 mg q 4–6 hr, not to exceed 10 mg daily. Switch to PO therapy as soon as possible. **Pediatric:** *Severe symptoms only:* 1 mg 1–2 times/day.

NURSING CONSIDERATIONS

See also *Nursing Considerations* for *Phenothiazines,* p. 630.

Administration/Storage

1. Dilute concentrate with 60 mL of juice (tomato or fruit), carbonated drinks, water, milk, orange or simple syrup, coffee, tea, or semisolid foods (e.g., applesauce, pudding, soup).
2. Dilute just before administration.
3. Protect liquid forms from light.

4. Discard strongly colored solutions.

5. Avoid skin contact with liquid form to prevent contact dermatitis.

6. To prevent cumulative effects, at least 4 hr should elapse between IM injections.

TRIFLUPROMAZINE HYDROCHLORIDE   (try-flew-**PROH**-mah-zeen)

Vesprin (Rx)

See also *Phenothiazines,* p. 627.

Classification: Antipsychotic, dimethylaminopropyl-type phenothiazine.

Action/Kinetics: This drug produces significant anticholinergic and antiemetic effects; moderate to strong extrapyramidal and sedative effects; and moderate hypotensive effects.

Uses: Severe nausea and vomiting. Psychotic disorders (should not be used for psychotic disorders with depression).

Special Concerns: Use during pregnancy only if benefits clearly outweigh risks. Dosage has not been established for children less than 30 months of age. IV use not recommended for children due to hypotension and rapid onset of extrapyramidal side effects. Geriatric, emaciated, or debilitated patients may require a lower initial dose.

Dosage: IM. *Psychoses.* **Adults and adolescents,** 60 mg up to maximum of 150 mg/day. **Pediatric,** 0.2–0.25 mg/kg to maximum of 10 mg/day. *Nausea and vomiting.* **Adults and adolescents,** 5–15 mg as single dose repeated q 4 hr up to maximum of 60 mg/day (for elderly or debilitated patients: 2.5 mg up to maximum of 15 mg/day). **Pediatric, over 2½ years:** 0.2–0.25 mg/kg up to maximum of 10 mg/day.

IV. *Psychoses.* **Adults and adolescents,** 1 mg as required, up to a maximum of 3 mg daily.

NURSING CONSIDERATIONS

See also *Nursing Considerations* for *Phenothiazines,* p. 630.

Administration/Storage

1. Avoid excessive heat and freezing.

2. Store in amber-colored containers.

3. Do not use discolored (darker than light amber) solutions.

4. Avoid skin contact with liquid form to prevent contact dermatitis.

5. When used in children for nausea and vomiting, the duration may be 12 hr.

THIOXANTHENE AND BUTYROPHENONE DERIVATIVES

General Statement: Drugs belonging to two other chemical families—the thioxanthene derivatives and the butyrophenone derivatives—are used as antipsychotic agents. The thioxanthene derivatives, chlorprothixene and thiothixene, are closely related to the phenothiazines from a chemical, pharmacologic, and clinical point of view.

Although the butyrophenone derivatives (haloperidol and droperidol) differ chemically from the phenothiazines, they are closely related in their pharmacologic actions.

For all general information pertaining to these agents, see *Phenothiazines*.

THIOXANTHENE DERIVATIVES

CHLORPROTHIXENE (klor-proh-**THIK**-seen)

Taractan (Rx)

Classification: Antipsychotic, thioxanthene derivative.

Action/Kinetics: The antipsychotic effect of chlorprothixene is thought to be manifested by blocking postsynaptic dopamine receptors in the brain. Chlorprothixene causes significant sedation and orthostatic hypotension and antiemetic effects with moderate anticholinergic and extrapyramidal effects. It is a more potent inhibitor of postural reflexes and motor coordination than is chlorpromazine, but has less pronounced antihistaminic effects. The drug also produces alpha-adrenergic blockade and depresses the release of most hypothalamic and hypophyseal hormones. **IM, Onset:** 30 min.; **duration:** up to 12 hr.

Uses: Neurosis, depression, schizophrenia, antiemesis, alcohol withdrawal. Adjunct in electroshock therapy. Drug may be effective in patients resistant to other psychotherapeutic drugs.

Special Concerns: Use during pregnancy only if benefits outweigh risks. Use with caution during lactation. Children are more prone to develop neuromuscular and extrapyramidal side effects (especially dystonias). Oral dosage has not been established in children less than 6 years of age and IM dosage has not been established in children less than 12 years of age. Adolescents may experience a higher incidence of hypotensive and extrapyramidal reactions than adults. Geriatric patients may be more prone to orthostatic hypotension and manifest an increased sensitivity to tardive dyskinesia and Parkinson-like symptoms. Geriatric or debilitated patients usually require a lower starting dose.

Side Effects: Drowsiness, lethargy, orthostatic hypotension, tachycardia, dizziness, and dry mouth occur especially frequently.

Drug Interactions: May cause additive hypotensive effects with methyldopa or reserpine.

Laboratory Test Interferences: False + immunologic urine pregnancy test.

Dosage: Oral Suspension, Tablets. *Antipsychotic:* **Adults and children over 12 years:** 25–50 mg t.i.d.–q.i.d. up to a maximum of 600 mg daily. **Pediatric, 6–12 years:** 10–25 mg t.i.d.–q.i.d.
    IM. *Antipsychotic:* **Adults and children over 12 years:** 25–50 mg t.i.d.–q.i.d. Doses exceeding 600 mg/day are rarely needed. Switch to oral dosage when feasible. **Geriatric or debilitated patients, initial:** 10–25 mg t.i.d.–q.i.d.

NURSING CONSIDERATIONS

See *Nursing Considerations* for *Phenothiazines*, p. 630.

Administration/Storage

1. Oral products should not be given to children less than 6 years of age, and parenteral products should not be given to children less than 12 years of age.

2. Inject deeply into large muscle mass.

3. Client should be supine during administration because of postural hypotension developing.

4. Protect from light.

5. The concentrate may be given undiluted or mixed with fruit juice, coffee, carbonated beverages, milk, or water.

THIOTHIXENE   (thigh-oh-**THIK**-seen)

Navane (Rx)

Classification: Antipsychotic, thioxanthine derivative.

Action/Kinetics: The antipsychotic action is due to blockade of postsynaptic dopamine receptors in the brain. Thiothixene causes significant extrapyramidal symptoms and antiemetic effects; minimal sedation, orthostatic hypotension, and anticholinergic effects. Its actions closely resemble those of chlorprothixene with respect to postural reflexes and motor coordination. The margin between a therapeutically effective dose and one that causes extrapyramidal symptoms is narrow. **Peak plasma levels, PO:** 1–3 hr. **t½:** 34 hr. **Therapeutic plasma levels** (during chronic treatment): 10–150 ng/mL.

Uses: Symptomatic treatment of acute and chronic schizophrenia, especially when condition is accompanied by florid symptoms.

Special Concerns: Safe use during pregnancy has not been established. Dosage has not been established for children under 12 years of age. Children are more prone to develop neuromuscular and extrapyramidal side effects (especially dystonias). Adolescents may experience a higher incidence of hypotensive and extrapyramidal reactions than adults. Geriatric patients may be more prone to orthostatic hypotension and manifest an increased sensitivity to tardive dyskinesia and Parkinson-like symptoms. Geriatric or debilitated patients usually require a lower starting dose.

Side Effects: See *Chlorprothixene,* p. 644.

Drug Interactions: See *Chlorprothixene,* p. 644.

Laboratory Test Interference: ↓ Serum uric acid.

Dosage: Capsules, Oral Solution. *Antipsychotic:* **Adults and adolescents, initial,** 2 mg t.i.d. for mild conditions and 5 mg b.i.d. for severe conditions; can be increased gradually to usual maintenance dose of 20–30 mg/day, although some patients require 60 mg/day.

   IM. *Antipsychotic:* **Adults and adolescents:** 4 mg b.i.d.–q.i.d.; **usual maintenance:** 16–20 mg/day, although up to 30 mg/day may be required in some cases. Switch to **PO** form as soon as possible. **Not recommended for children under 12 years of age.**

NURSING CONSIDERATIONS

See also *Nursing Considerations* for *Phenothiazines,* p. 630.

Administration/Storage

1. The powder for injection can be reconstituted by adding 2.2 mL of sterile water for injection.

2. Thiothixene is well absorbed.

Client/Family Teaching

Review with the client and family the purpose and goals of drug therapy. Discuss the responses they can anticipate, depending upon the method of administration.

Evaluation

1. Expect a therapeutic response in 1–6 hours after an IM injection.
2. Oral medications will require several days to observe therapeutic effects.

BUTYROPHENONE DERIVATIVES

DROPERIDOL   (droh-**PER**-ih-dol)

Inapsine (Rx)

Classification: Antipsychotic, butyrophenone; antianxiety agent.

Action/Kinetics: Droperidol causes sedation, alpha-adrenergic blockade, peripheral vascular dilation, and has antiemetic properties. For other details, see *Haloperidol,* p. 647, and *Phenothiazines,* p. 627.**Onset** (after IM, IV): 3–10 min. **Peak effect:** 30 min. **Duration:** 2–4 hr, although alteration of consciousness may last up to 12 hr. **t½:** 2.2 hr. Metabolized in the liver and excreted in both the feces and urine.

Uses: Preoperatively; induction and maintenance of anesthesia. To relieve nausea and vomiting and reduce anxiety in diagnostic procedures or surgery. Neuroleptanalgesia. Antiemetic in cancer chemotherapy (used IV).

Special Concerns: Pregnancy category: C. Use with caution during lactation; in the elderly, debilitated, or poor risk patient; and in renal or hepatic impairment. Safety for use during labor has not been established. Safety and efficacy have not been established in children less than 2 years of age.

Side Effects: *CNS:* Postoperative drowsiness (common), restlessness, hyperactivity, anxiety, dizziness, postoperative hallucinations; extrapyramidal symptoms (e.g., akathisia, dystonia, oculogyric crisis). *CV:* Hypotension and tachycardia (common), increase in blood pressure (when combined with fentanyl or other parenteral analgesics). *Respiratory:* Respiratory depression (when combined with fentanyl), laryngospasm, bronchospasm. *Miscellaneous:* Chills, shivering.

Drug Interactions	
Anesthetics, conduction (e.g., spinal)	Peripheral vasodilation and hypotension
CNS depressants	Additive or potentiating effects
Narcotic analgesics	↑ Respiratory depressant effects

Dosage: IM. *Preoperatively:* **Adults,** 2.5–10 mg 30–60 min before surgery (modify dosage in elderly, debilitated); **pediatric, 2–12 years,** 88–165 mcg/kg. *Diagnostic procedures:* **Adults,** 2.5–10 mg 30–60 min before procedure; **then,** if necessary, IV, 1.25–2.5 mg.
    IV. *Adjunct to general anesthesia:* **Adults,** 0.28 mg/kg with analgesic or anesthetic; **maintenance:** 1.25–2.5 mg (total dose). **IV (slow) or IM.** *Adjunct to regional anesthesia:* 2.5–5 mg.

NURSING CONSIDERATIONS

See also *Nursing Considerations* for *Phenothiazines,* p. 630.

Administration/Storage

1. At a concentration of 1 mg/50 mL, droperidol is stable for 7–10 days in glass bottles with 5% dextrose injection, lactated Ringer's injection, and 0.9% sodium chloride injection. Droperidol is stable for 7 days in polyvinyl chloride bags containing 5% dextrose injection or 0.9% sodium chloride injection.
2. If droperidol is used with Innovar injection (fentanyl plus droperidol), the dose of droperidol in the injection must be taken into consideration.
3. Droperidol is compatible at a concentration of 2.5 mg/mL for 15 min when combined in a syringe with the following: atropine sulfate, butorphanol tartrate, chlorpromazine hydrochloride, diphenhydramine hydrochloride, fentanyl citrate, glycopyrrolate, hydroxyzine hydrochloride, meperidine hydrochloride, morphine sulfate, perphenazine, promazine hydrochloride, promethazine hydrochloride, and scopolamine hydrobromide.
4. A precipitate will form if droperidol is mixed with barbiturates.

Intervention

Closely monitor BP and pulse during the immediate postoperative period until stabilized at satisfactory levels. Hypertension has been reported.

HALOPERIDOL   (HAH-low-PER-ih-dol)

Apo-Haloperidol✱, Haldol, Halperon, Novoperidol✱, Peridol✱ (Rx)

HALOPERIDOL DECANOATE   (HAH-low-PER-ih-dol)

Haldol Decanoate 50 and 100 (Rx)

HALOPERIDOL LACTATE   (HAH-low-PER-ih-dol)

Haldol Lactate (Rx)

Classification: Antipsychotic, butyrophenone.

Action/Kinetics: Although the precise mechanism is not known, haloperidol does competitively block dopamine receptors in the tuberoinfundibular system to cause sedation. The drug also causes alpha-adrenergic blockade, decreases release of growth hormone, and increases prolactin release by the pituitary. Haloperidol causes significant extrapyramidal effects, as well as a low incidence of sedation, anticholinergic effects, and orthostatic hypotension. The margin between the therapeutically effective dose and that causing extrapyramidal symptoms is narrow. The drug also has antiemetic effects. **Peak plasma levels: PO,** 2–6 hr; **IM,** 20 min; **IM, decanoate:** approximately 6 days. **Therapeutic serum levels:** 3–10 ng/mL. **t½, PO:** 12–38 hr; **IM:** 13–36 hr; **IM, decanoate:** 3 weeks; **IV:** approximately 14 hr. **Plasma protein binding:** 90%. Metabolized in liver, slowly excreted in urine and bile.

Uses: Psychotic disorders including manic states, drug-induced psychoses, and schizophrenia. Aggressive and agitated patients including chronic brain syndrome or mental retardation. Severe behavior problems in children. Short-term treatment of hyperactive children. Control of tics and vocal utterances associated with Gilles de la Tourette's syndrome.

Investigational: Antiemetic for cancer chemotherapy, infantile autism, Huntington's chorea.

Contraindications: Use with extreme caution, or not at all, in patients with parkinsonism. Lactation.

Special Concerns: Pregnancy category: C (decanoate form). Oral dosage has not been determined in children less than 3 years of age; IM dosage is not recommended in children. Geriatric patients are more likely to exhibit orthostatic hypotension, anticholinergic effects, sedation, and extrapyramidal side effects (such as parkinsonism and tardive dyskinesia).

Side Effects: Extrapyramidal symptoms, especially akathisia and dystonias, occur more frequently than with the phenothiazines. Overdosage is characterized by severe extrapyramidal reactions, hypotension, or sedation. The drug does not elicit photosensitivity reactions like those of the phenothiazines.

Drug Interactions	
Amphetamine	↓ Effect of amphetamine by ↓ uptake of drug at its site of action
Anticholinergics	↓ Effect of haloperidol
Antidepressants, tricyclic	↑ Effect of antidepressants due to ↓ breakdown by liver
Barbiturates	↓ Effect of haloperidol due to ↑ breakdown by liver
Guanethidine	↓ Effect of guanethidine by ↓ uptake of drug at site of action
Lithium	↑ Toxicity of haloperidol
Methyldopa	↑ Toxicity of haloperidol
Phenytoin	↓ Effect of haloperidol due to ↑ breakdown by liver

Laboratory Test Interferences: ↑ Alkaline phosphatase, bilirubin, serum transaminase; ↓ prothrombin time (patients on coumarin), serum cholesterol.

Dosage: Oral Solution, Tablets. Adults: 0.5–2 mg b.i.d.–t.i.d. up to 3–5 mg b.i.d.–t.i.d. for severe symptoms; **maintenance:** reduce dosage to lowest effective level. Up to 100 mg/day may be required in some. **Geriatric or debilitated patients:** 0.5–2 mg b.i.d.–t.i.d. **Pediatric, 3–12 years:** 0.05 mg/kg daily in 2–3 divided doses; if necessary the daily dose may be increased by 0.5-mg increments q 5–7 days for a total of 0.15 mg/kg daily for psychotic disorders and 0.075 mg/kg for nonpsychotic behavior disorders and Tourette's syndrome.

IM. *Acute psychoses:* **Adults and adolescents, initial:** 2–5 mg; may be repeated if necessary q 4–8 hr to a total of 100 mg daily. Switch to **PO** therapy as soon as possible. **IM, Decanoate:** *Chronic therapy,* **initial dose:** 10–15 times the daily oral dose; **then,** repeat q 4 weeks (decanoate is not to be given IV).

NURSING CONSIDERATIONS

See also *Nursing Considerations* for *Phenothiazines,* p. 630.

Interventions

1. Use with caution in the elderly as they tend to exhibit toxicity more frequently and may benefit from a drug "holiday" periodically.
2. Document any evidence of new onset of Parkinson's symptoms as drug has been reported to induce this disorder.

MISCELLANEOUS ANTIPSYCHOTIC AGENTS

CLOZAPINE   (KLOH-zah-peen)

Clozaril (Rx)

Classification: Antipsychotic.

Action/Kinetics: Clozapine interferes with the binding of dopamine to both D-1 and D-2 receptors; it is more active at limbic than at striatal dopamine receptors. Thus, it is relatively free from extrapyramidal side effects and it does not induce catalepsy. The drug also acts as an antagonist at adrenergic, cholinergic, histaminergic, and serotonergic receptors. Clozapine increases the amount of time spent in REM sleep. Food does not affect the bioavailability of clozapine. **Peak plasma levels:** 2.5 hr. **Average maximum concentration at steady state:** 122 ng/mL plasma after 100 mg b.i.d. Highly bound to plasma proteins. **t½:** 12 hr. Metabolized in the liver to inactive compounds and excreted through the urine (50%) and feces (30%).

Uses: Severely ill schizophrenic patients who do not respond adequately to conventional antipsychotic therapy, either because of ineffectiveness or intolerable adverse effects from other drugs.

Contraindications: Myeloproliferative disorders. Use in conjunction with other agents known to suppress bone marrow function. Severe CNS depression or coma due to any cause. Use with caution in patients with known cardiovascular disease, prostatic hypertrophy, narrow angle glaucoma, hepatic or renal disease.

Special Concerns: Pregnancy category: B.

Untoward Reactions: *Hematologic:* Agranulocytosis. *CNS:* Seizures (appear to be dose-dependent), drowsiness or sedation, dizziness, vertigo, headache, tremor. *GI:* Dry mouth, salivation, constipation, nausea. *CV:* Orthostatic hypotension (especially initially), tachycardia, syncope. *Neuroleptic malignant syndrome:* Hyperpyrexia, muscle rigidity, altered mental status, irregular pulse or blood pressure, tachycardia, diaphoresis, cardiac dysrhythmias. *Miscellaneous:* Sweating, visual disturbances, fever (transient).

Drug Interactions	
Anticholinergic drugs	Additive anticholinergic effects
Antihypertensive drugs	Additive hypotensive effects
Digoxin	↑ Effect of digoxin due to ↓ binding to plasma protein
Epinephrine	Clozapine may reverse effects if epinephrine is given for hypotension
Warfarin	↑ Effect of warfarin due to ↓ binding to plasma protein

Dosage: PO, initial: 25 mg 1–2 times daily; **then,** if drug is tolerated, the dose can be increased by 25–50 mg/day to a dose of 300–450 mg/day at the end of 2 weeks. Subsequent dosage increments should occur no more often than once or twice a week in increments not to exceed 100 mg. **Usual maintenance dose:** 300–600 mg/day (although doses up to 900 mg/day may be required in some patients). Total daily dose should not exceed 900 mg.

NURSING CONSIDERATIONS

Administration

1. Clozapine, marketed as Clozaril, is available only through the "Clozaril Patient Management System," which is a special program that combines client monitoring, white blood cell testing, pharmacy, and drug distribution services for the purposes of compliance with the required safety monitoring.
2. If the drug is effective, the lowest maintenance doses possible should be sought to maintain remission.
3. If termination of therapy is planned, there should be a gradual reduction of the dose over a 1–2 week period. If cessation of therapy is abrupt due to toxicity, the client should be observed carefully for recurrence of psychotic symptoms.
4. Clozapine therapy may be initiated immediately upon discontinuation of other antipsychotic medication; however, a 24 hr "washout period" is desirable.

Assessment

1. Observe and document client's behavior to determine baseline information against which to measure postmedication responses.
2. Obtain lab studies including CBC, prior to initiating therapy.
3. Note any history of seizure disorder.
4. Obtain baseline vital signs, including temperature and ECG.

Interventions

1. Periodically reassess the client to determine continued need for the drug.
2. If white blood counts fall below $2,000/mm^3$ or granulocyte counts fall below $1,000/mm^3$, the drug should be discontinued. Such clients should not be restarted on clozapine therapy.
3. Monitor vital signs and note any irregular pulse, tachycardia, hyperpyrexia, and hypotension and report to the physician.

Client/Family Teaching

1. Avoid driving or other potentially hazardous activity while taking clozapine due to the possibility of seizures.
2. Report immediately to the physician symptoms of lethargy, weakness, fever, sore throat, malaise, mucous membrane ulceration or other signs of infection.
3. There is a risk of orthostatic hypotension, especially during initial dosing. Use care when rising from a supine or sitting position.
4. Women of childbearing age should notify the physician if they become pregnant or intend to become pregnant during therapy.
5. Do not breast feed when taking clozaril.
6. Do not take any prescription or OTC drugs or alcohol without the permission of the physician.
7. Weekly blood tests are required to monitor for the occurrence of agranulocytosis. Clozaril is available only through a special program which ensures the required blood monitoring, so compliance is mandatory.

LITHIUM CARBONATE   (LIH-thee-um)

Carbolith✿, Cibalith-S, Duralith✿, Eskalith, Eskalith CR, Lithane, Lithizine✿, Lithobid, Lithonate, Lithotabs (Rx)

LITHIUM CITRATE   (LIH-thee-um)

Cibalith-S (Rx)

Classification: Antipsychotic agent, miscellaneous.

Action/Kinetics: Although the precise mechanism for the antimanic effect of lithium is not known, various hypotheses have been put forth. These include: (a) a decrease in catecholamine neurotransmitter levels caused by lithium's effect on Na + –K + ATPase to improve transneuronal membrane transport of sodium ion; (b) a decrease in cyclic AMP levels caused by lithium which decreases sensitivity of hormonal-sensitive adenyl cyclase receptors; or (c) interference by lithium with lipid inositol metabolism ultimately leading to insensitivity of cells in the CNS to stimulation by inositol.

Lithium also affects the distribution of calcium, magnesium, and sodium ions and affects glucose metabolism. **Peak serum levels** (regular release): 1–4 hr; (slow-release): 4–6 hr. **Onset:** 5–14 days. **Therapeutic serum levels:** 0.4–1.0 mEq/L (must be carefully monitored, as toxic effects may occur at these levels and significant toxic reactions occur at serum lithium levels of 2 mEq/L). $t^{1/2}$ (plasma): 24 hr (longer in presence of renal impairment and in the elderly). Lithium and sodium are excreted by the same mechanism in the proximal tubule. Thus, to reduce the danger of lithium intoxication, sodium intake must remain at normal levels.

Uses: Control of manic and hypomanic episodes in manic-depressive patients. Prophylaxis of bipolar depression. *Investigational:* To reverse neutropenia induced by cancer chemotherapy and in children with chronic neutropenia. Prophylaxis of cluster headaches and cyclic migraine headaches. Treatment of certain types of mental depression (e.g., schizoaffective disorder, augment the antidepressant effect of tricyclic or monoamine oxidase drugs in treating unipolar depression). Also for premenstrual tension, alcoholism accompanied by depression, tardive dyskinesia, bulimia, hyperthyroidism, excess ADH secretion. Lithium succinate, in a topical form, has been used for the treatment of genital herpes and seborrheic dermatitis.

Contraindications: Cardiovascular or renal disease. Brain damage. Dehydration, sodium depletion, patients receiving diuretics. Pregnancy (pregnancy category: D), lactation.

Special Concerns: Safety and efficacy have not been established for children less than 12 years of age. Use with caution in geriatric patients as lithium is more toxic to the CNS in these patients; also, geriatric patients are more likely to develop lithium-induced goiter and clinical hypothyroidism and are more likely to manifest excessive thirst and larger volumes of urine.

Side Effects: These are related to the blood lithium level. *CNS:* Fainting, drowsiness, slurred speech, confusion, dizziness, tiredness, lethargy, ataxia, dysarthria, aphasia, vertigo, stupor, restlessness, coma, seizures. Pseudotumor cerebri leading to papilledema and increased intracranial pressure. *GI:* Anorexia, nausea, vomiting, diarrhea, thirst, dry mouth, bloated stomach. *Muscular:* Tremors (especially of hand), muscle weakness, fasciculations and/or twitching, clonic movements of limbs, increased deep tendon reflexes, choreoathetoid movements, cogwheel rigidity. *Renal:* Nephrogenic diabetes insipidus (polyuria, polydypsia), oliguria, albuminuria. *Endocrine:* Hypothyroidism, goiter, hyperparathyroidism. *CV:* Changes in ECG, edema, hypotension, cardiovascular collapse, irregular pulse, tachycardia. *Ophthalmologic:* Blurred vision, downbeat nystagmus. *Dermatologic:* Acneform eruptions, pruritic-maculopapular rashes, drying and thinning of hair, alopecia, paresthesia, cutaneous ulcers, lupus-like symptoms. *Miscellaneous:* Hoarseness, swelling of feet, lower legs, or neck; cold sensitivity, leukemia, leukocytosis, dyspnea on exertion.

Drug Interactions

Acetazolamide	↓ Lithium effect by ↑ renal excretion
Aminophylline	↓ Lithium effect by ↑ renal excretion
Bumetanide	↑ Lithium toxicity due to ↓ renal clearance
Carbamazepine	↑ Risk of lithium toxicity
Diazepam	↑ Risk of hypothermia
Ethacrynic acid	↑ Lithium toxicity due to ↓ renal clearance
Fluoxetine	↑ Serum levels of lithium
Furosemide	↑ Lithium toxicity due to ↓ renal clearance
Haloperidol	↑ Risk of neurologic toxicity
Ibuprofen	↑ Chance of lithium toxicity due to ↓ renal clearance
Indomethacin	↑ Chance of lithium toxicity due to ↓ renal clearance
Iodide salts	Additive effect to cause hypothyroidism
Mannitol	↓ Lithium effect by ↑ renal excretion
Mazindol	↑ Chance of lithium toxicity due to ↑ serum levels
Methyldopa	↑ Chance of lithium toxicity due to ↑ serum levels
Naproxen	↑ Chance of lithium toxicity due to ↑ serum levels
Neuromuscular blocking agents	Lithium ↑ effect of these agents → respiratory depression and apnea
Phenothiazines	↓ Levels of phenothiazines and ↑ neurotoxicity
Phenylbutazone	↑ Chance of lithium toxicity due to ↓ renal clearance
Phenytoin	↑ Chance of lithium toxicity
Piroxicam	↑ Chance of lithium toxicity due to ↓ renal clearance
Probenecid	↑ Chance of lithium toxicity due to ↑ serum levels
Sodium bicarbonate	↓ Lithium effect by ↑ renal excretion
Sodium chloride	Excretion of lithium is proportional to amount of sodium chloride ingested; if patient is on salt-free diet, may develop lithium toxicity since less lithium excreted
Spironolactone	↑ Chance of lithium toxicity due to ↑ serum levels
Succinylcholine	↑ Muscle relaxation
Sympathomimetics	↓ Pressor effect of sympathomimetics
Tetracyclines	↑ Chance of lithium toxicity due to ↑ serum levels
Theophyllines	↓ Effect of lithium due to ↑ renal excretion
Thiazide diuretics, triamterene	↑ Chance of lithium toxicity due to ↓ renal clearance
Tricyclic antidepressants	↑ Effect of tricyclic antidepressants
Urea	↓ Lithium effect by ↑ renal excretion

Laboratory Test Interferences: False + urinary glucose test (Benedict's), ↑ serum glucose, creatinine kinase. False − or ↓ serum protein bound iodine (PBI), uric acid; ↑ thyroid-stimulating hormone; ↓ thyroxine.

Dosage: Capsules, Slow-release Capsules, Tablets, Extended-release Tablets, Syrup. *Acute mania:* Individualized and according to lithium serum level (not to exceed 1.4 mEq/L) and clinical response. **Usual initial:** 300–600 mg t.i.d. or 600–900 mg b.i.d. of slow-release form; **elderly and debilitated patients:** 0.6–1.2 g daily in 3 doses. **Maintenance:** 300 mg t.i.d.–q.i.d.

Administration of drug is discontinued when lithium serum level exceeds 1.2 mEq/L and resumed 24 hr after it has fallen below that level. *To reverse neutropenia:* 300–1,000 mg/day (to achieve serum levels of 0.5–1.0 mEq/liter) for 7–10 days. *Prophylaxis of cluster headaches:* 600–900 mg/day.

NURSING CONSIDERATIONS

Administration/Storage

1. To prevent toxic serum levels from occurring, blood levels should be determined 1 to 2 times per week during initiation of therapy, and monthly thereafter, on blood samples taken 8 to 12 hr after dosage. (Therapeutic level 0.4–1.0 mEq/L.)
2. Full beneficial effects of lithium therapy may not be noted for 6 to 10 days after initiation.

Assessment

1. Conduct a drug history and determine if the client is taking other medications that are likely to interact with lithium.
2. If the client has an arthritic condition, determine if he/she is taking any anti-inflammatory agents and document.
3. Obtain pretreatment thyroid function studies and monitor throughout therapy.

Intervention

Monitor cardiovascular function periodically during drug therapy as well as serum drug levels.

Client/Family Teaching

1. Review with the client and family the goals of medication therapy and the possible side effects associated with this drug.
2. Provide printed instructions regarding medication administration and possible side effects.
3. Caution the client and family to report any side effects that may occur. If diarrhea, vomiting, drowsiness, muscular weakness, and lack of coordination occur, lithium therapy must be discontinued immediately, and client must report for medical supervision.
4. The drug should be taken with food or immediately after meals. Report any episodes of persistent diarrhea as these symptoms may indicate a need for supplemental fluids or salt.
5. Avoid any caffeinated beverages/foods since these may aggravate mania.
6. Explain the relationship between lithium activity and dietary sodium. Instruct clients to maintain a constant level of sodium intake to avoid fluctuations in lithium action.
7. Advise client to drink 10–12 glasses of water each day and to avoid dehydration (e.g., sunbathing, sauna).
8. Tell client not to engage in physical activities that require alertness or physical coordination. Lithium therapy causes drowsiness and may impair these abilities.
9. Advise clients not to change brands of medication.

10. Reassure the client and family that it will take several weeks to realize a benefit from lithium therapy.
11. Provide the name and telephone number of persons to contact if the client has problems or if family members note behavioral changes or physical changes contrary to expectations.
12. Once lithium level is stabilized, blood tests to check serum levels (therapeutic serum concentration 0.4–1.0 mEq/L) should be completed monthly.
13. Establish a schedule of follow-up lab and medical appointments and stress the importance of adhering to this schedule.
14. Instruct clients to wear a medic alert tag or bracelet indicating the diagnosis and medication regimen.

Evaluation

1. Assess client knowledge and understanding of illness and response to teaching.
2. Monitor the stabilization of mood. Compare with pretreatment behavior.
3. Check neurological and psychiatric status. Assess neuromuscular, GI, cardiovascular, renal and thyroid function.
4. Evaluate client compliance with the therapeutic regimen.
5. Review serum drug levels to determine if dose is within therapeutic range.

LOXAPINE HYDROCHLORIDE   (LOX-ah-peen)
Loxitane C, Loxitane IM (Rx)

LOXAPINE SUCCINATE   (LOX-ah-peen)
Loxapac ✳, Loxitane (Rx)

See also *Phenothiazines,* p. 627.

Classification: Antipsychotic, miscellaneous.

Action/Kinetics: Loxapine belongs to a new subclass of tricyclic antipsychotic agents. The drug is thought to act by blocking dopamine at postsynaptic brain receptors. It causes significant extrapyramidal symptoms, moderate sedative effects, and a low incidence of anticholinergic effects, as well as orthostatic hypotension. **Onset:** 20–30 min. **Peak effects:** 1.5–3 hr. **Duration:** about 12 hr. **t½:** 3–4 hr. Partially metabolized in the liver; excreted in urine, and unchanged in feces.

Uses: Psychoses. *Investigational:* Anxiety neurosis with depression.

Additional Contraindications: History of convulsive disorders.

Special Concerns: Pregnancy category: C. Use with caution in patients with cardiovascular disease. Use during lactation only if benefits outweigh risks. Dosage has not been established in children less than 16 years of age. Geriatric patients may be more prone to developing orthostatic hypotension, anticholinergic, sedative, and extrapyramidal side effects.

Additional Side Effects: Tachycardia, hypertension, hypotension, lightheadedness, and syncope.

Dosage: Capsules, Oral Solution. Adults, initial, 10 mg (of the base) b.i.d. *Severe:* up to 50 mg daily. Increase dosage rapidly over 7–10 days until symptoms are controlled. **Range:** 60–100 mg up to 250 mg daily. **Maintenance:** If possible reduce dosage to 15–25 mg b.i.d.–q.i.d.
   IM: 12.5–50 mg (of the base) q 4–6 hr; once adequate control has been established, switch to PO medication after control achieved (usually within 5 days).

NURSING CONSIDERATIONS

See also *Nursing Considerations* for *Phenothiazines*, p. 630.

Administration/Storage

1. Measure the dosage of the concentrate *only* with the enclosed calibrated dropper.
2. Mix oral concentrate with orange or grapefruit juice immediately before administration to disguise unpleasant taste.

MOLINDONE   (moh-**LIN**-dohn)

Moban (Rx)

Classification: Antipsychotic, miscellaneous.

Action/Kinetics: This drug is related chemically to serotonin. Although the exact mechanism is not known, molindone may act by occupying D_2 receptors in the brain thus decreasing dopamine activity. It produces moderate sedation, extrapyramidal symptoms, and anticholinergic effects and a low incidence of orthostatic hypotension. **Peak blood levels:** 90 min. A single oral dose may exert effects for 24–36 hr. Drug extensively metabolized in liver and metabolites and small amount of unchanged drug eliminated through urine and feces.

Use: Psychoses (chronic, brief reactive, or schizophreniform).

Contraindications: Hypersensitivity to drug. Severe CNS depression caused by other agents. Used to manage behavior in mentally retarded patients.

Special Concerns: Use with caution during pregnancy and lactation. Dosage has not been established in children less than 12 years of age. Geriatric patients may be more prone to develop orthostatic hypotension, anticholinergic, sedative, and extrapyramidal effects.

Side Effects: *CNS:* Transient initial drowsiness, Parkinson-like reactions, akinesia, restlessness, insomnia, depression, hyperactivity, euphoria, headaches, increased libido. *GI:* Dry mouth, nausea, salivation, constipation. *CV:* Postural hypotension, tachycardia. *Miscellaneous:* Menstrual abnormalities, blurred vision.

Drug Interactions: Calcium sulfate is found in these tablets; may interfere with absorption of tetracyclines or phenytoin.

Dosage: Oral Solution, Tablets. Adults: Individualized and according to severity of symptoms. **Initial:** 50–75 mg/day in 3–4 divided doses, increased to 100 mg daily in 3–4 divided doses within 3–4 days. **Maintenance:** *Mild psychoses:* 5–15 mg t.i.d.–q.i.d.; *moderate psychoses:* 10–25 mg t.i.d.–q.i.d.; *severe psychoses:* 225 mg daily, up to maximum of 400 mg/day. Can be given once daily.

NURSING CONSIDERATIONS

See *Nursing Considerations* for *Phenothiazines*, p. 630.

Antidepressants

The diagnosis of depression is often difficult and is frequently based on the patient experiencing a persistent (nearly every day) mood of depression or dysphoria for at least 14 days which is interfering with daily function. If the patient has several of the following symptoms, a diagnosis of depression should be considered: insomnia or excessive sleep, significant weight loss or gain when not dieting, increase or decrease in appetite, depression of mood, decreased pleasure or interest in nearly all activities, loss of energy (fatigue), having feelings of being worthless or having excessive or inappropriate guilt, decreased ability to think or concentrate, psychomotor slowing or agitation, recurring thoughts of death, and suicide thoughts or attempts.

The treatment of depression has been revolutionized with the discovery of the tricyclic antidepressants as well as drugs such as bupropion, fluoxetine, maprotiline, and trazodone. Monoamine oxidase inhibitors have also been used to treat depression but are not as widely used due to an increased risk of side effects.

MONOAMINE OXIDASE (MAO) INHIBITORS

General Statement: Because of their relatively high toxicity, MAO inhibitors are prescribed only if tricyclic compounds are ineffective. MAO inhibitors may also interfere with detoxification mechanisms, and thus with biotransformation of certain drugs, which occurs in the liver. One MAO inhibitor—pargyline—is used as an antihypertensive (see Chapter 26, p. 524).

Action/Kinetics: Monoamine oxidase is one of the enzymes that breaks down biogenic amines (norepinephrine, epinephrine, serotonin) in the body. Drugs classified as MAO inhibitors prevent the enzyme from metabolizing biogenic amines; these amines therefore accumulate in the presynaptic granules, increasing the concentration of neurotransmitters released upon nerve stimulation. This increase is thought to be responsible for the antidepressant effects of the monoamine oxidase inhibitors. **Onset:** Few days to several months. Clinical effects of drug manifested for up to 2 weeks after termination of therapy.

Uses: See individual drugs. These drugs are rarely used as first drugs for therapy of depressive illness.

Contraindications: Hypersensitivity to MAO inhibitors. History of liver disease, abnormal liver function tests, pheochromocytoma (tumor of the adrenal medulla), impaired renal function, hyperthyroidism, paranoid schizophrenia, epilepsy, cerebrovascular disease, hypertension, cerebral or generalized arteriosclerosis, hypernatremia, atonic colitis, and cardiovascular disease. MAO inhibitors may aggravate glaucoma. They may also suppress anginal pain, which may serve as a warning sign for patients with angina pectoris.

Special Concerns: Use cautiously in elderly patients. Safety has not been determined for use during pregnancy and during lactation. Not to be used in children under 16 years of age.

Side Effects: *CNS:* Restlessness, headache, dizziness, drowsiness, insomnia, vertigo, hypomania, memory impairment, weakness, fatigue, euphoria, ataxia, confusion, impairment of memory, coma, akathisia, neuritis, chills. Symptoms of excitation including agitation, overactivity, jitteriness, restlessness, anxiety, mania. Rarely, convulsions, hallucinations, schizophrenic symptoms, toxic delirium. *CV:* Orthostatic hypotension, changes in cardiac rate and rhythm, tachycardia, palpitations. *GI:* Nausea, vomiting, abdominal pain, constipation or diarrhea, anorexia, dryness of mouth. *Neuromuscular:* Tremors, hyperreflexia, muscle twitching. *Genitourinary:* Urinary retention, dysuria, incontinence. Rarely, increased secretion of antidiuretic hormone. *Hepatic:* Rarely, hepatitis, reversible jaundice, fatal progressive necrotizing hepatocellular damage. *Miscellaneous:* Edema, blurred vision, sweating, skin rashes, glaucoma, nystagmus, photosensitivity, sexual disturbances, black tongue, hypernatremia, paresthesia. Rarely, leukopenia, tinnitus, edema of the glottis.

Drug Interactions: MAO inhibitors potentiate both the pharmacologic actions and the toxic effects of a wide variety of drugs. Because of the long duration of action of MAO inhibitors, adverse drug reactions may also occur if any of the drugs listed below are given to patients within 2–3 weeks after the administration of MAO inhibitors has been terminated.

Drug Interactions

Alcohol, ethyl	Tyramine-containing beverages (e.g., Chianti wine) may result in hypertensive crisis
Amphetamine	See *Sympathomimetic drugs*
Anesthetics, general	↑ Hypotensive effect; use together with caution
Anticholinergic agents, atropine	MAO inhibitors ↑ effects of anticholinergic drugs
Antidepressants, tricyclics	Concomitant use may result in excitation, sweating, tachycardia, tachypnea, hyperpyrexia, disseminated intravascular coagulation, delirium, tremors, and convulsions, and death. At least 7–10 days should elapse between discontinuing a monamine oxidase inhibitor and initiating a new drug. Such combinations have, however, been used successfully

33

Drug Interactions

Antidiabetic agents	MAO inhibitors ↑ and prolong hypoglycemic response to insulin and oral hypoglycemics
Antihypertensives	↑ Chance of hypotension
Barbiturates	↑ Effect of barbiturates due to ↓ breakdown by liver
Dopa	See *Levodopa*
Doxapram	MAO inhibitors ↑ adverse cardiovascular effects of doxapram (arrhythmias, increase in BP)
Ephedrine	See *Sympathomimetic drugs*
Fluoxetine	Possibility of severe side effects; five weeks should elapse between discontinuing fluoxetine and starting a monoamine oxidase inhibitor
Guanethidine	↓ Hypotensive effect of guanethidine
Levodopa	Concomitant administration may result in ↑ effects of levodopa resulting in hypertension, lightheadedness, and flushing
Meperidine	See *Narcotics*
Metaraminol	See *Sympathomimetic drugs*
Methyldopa	See *Sympathomimetic drugs*
Methylphenidate	See *Sympathomimetic drugs*
Narcotic analgesics	Possible potentiation of either MAO inhibitor (excitation, hypertension), or narcotic (hypotension, coma) effects—death has resulted
Phenothiazines	↑ Effect of phenothiazines due to ↓ breakdown by liver; also ↑ chance of severe extrapyramidal effects and hypertensive crisis
Phenylephrine	See *Sympathomimetic drugs*
Phenylpropanolamine	See *Sympathomimetic drugs*
Reserpine	Concomitant use may cause hypertensive crisis
Succinylcholine	↑ Effect of succinylcholine due to ↓ breakdown of drug in plasma by pseudocholinesterase
Sympathomimetic drugs—amphetamine, ephedrine, metaraminol, methylphenidate, phenylephrine, phenylpropanolamine. (Many OTC cold tablets and capsules, hay fever medications, and nasal decongestants contain one or more of these drugs)	All peripheral, metabolic, cardiac, and central effects are potentiated up to 2 weeks after termination of MAO inhibitor therapy (symptoms include acute hypertensive crisis with possible intracranial hemorrhage, hyperthermia, convulsions, coma—death may occur)
Tyramine-rich foods, such as beer, broad beans, cheeses (Brie, cheddar, Camembert, Stilton), Chianti wine, chicken livers, caffeine, cola beverages, figs, licorice, liver, pickled or kippered herring, tea, cream, yogurt, yeast extract, and chocolate	Severe headache, hypertension, intracranial hemorrhage, and even death have been reported if these foods are eaten by patient being treated with MAO inhibitor

Laboratory Test Interferences: ↑ Alkaline phosphatase, BUN, bilirubin, serum transaminase, urinary catecholamines, metanephrine, prothrombin time; ↓ urinary 5-HIAA.

Dosage: See individual drugs, Table 11. All agents are administered orally. The effectiveness of the MAO inhibitors is cumulative and it may take days or even months for the drugs to reach their full effectiveness. The effects of the drugs also take 2 to 3 weeks to wane. Therefore, if switching from one MAO inhibitor to another, the second drug should not be given for 2 weeks after the first drug has been discontinued. Also, all drug interactions between MAO inhibitors and other agents can occur up to 2 to 3 weeks after MAO inhibitor therapy has been discontinued. Rapid drug withdrawal in patients receiving high doses may cause a rebound effect characterized by headache, CNS excitability, and occasional hallucinations.

NURSING CONSIDERATIONS

Administration

1. All drugs are for oral administration.
2. The effectiveness of MAO inhibitors is cumulative. It may take days or months to become fully effective, and 2–3 weeks for the effects to wane. Therefore, if changing from one MAO drug to another, the second drug should not be started until 2 weeks after the first drug has been discontinued.
3. Drug dosages are titrated according to the level of improvement of the client's depression or the occurrence of adverse drug effects.

Assessment

1. Take a complete nursing history, noting any prior adverse effects to MAO inhibitors.
2. Note if the client is using antihistamines, sedatives, meperidine or alcohol. These drugs have a synergistic depressive effect when taken with MAO inhibitors.
3. Obtain baseline measurements of blood pressure, vital signs and ECG, especially in clients with a history of cardiovascular disease, before initiating therapy.
4. Note the client's age. If the client is female, sexually active, question about the possibility of pregnancy. MAO inhibitors cross the placental barrier and may be teratogenic.
5. Determine if the client is on any special diet and if foods on the diet affect MAO inhibitors.

Interventions

1. In the event of overdosage, have gastric lavage equipment available.
2. Have a rapid-acting alpha-adrenergic blocking agent such as phentolamine or a vasodilator-type drug available to counteract an excessive pressor response as in hypertensive crisis.
3. Phenothiazine tranquilizers, IM, should be on hand to treat excessive agitation.
4. Take the client's blood pressure every 4 to 8 hours when initiating therapy and at regular intervals thereafter to detect hypertension which may necessitate discontinuation of the drug.
5. Monitor the client's pulse rate as well as blood pressure to detect tachycardia and other potential arrhythmias.
6. Weigh the client prior to initiating therapy and bi-weekly thereafter. Some clients experience weight loss, nausea, anorexia and/or diarrhea.
7. Monitor clients closely during initiation of therapy for indications of suicidal ideations. Suicide attempts are more frequent during this period when the client emerges from the deepest phases of depression.
8. Observe for any early symptoms of congestive heart failure, such as the presence of peripheral edema.

Table 11 Antidepressants, MAO Inhibitor Type

Drug	Use	Dosage	Remarks
Isocarboxazid (Marplan) Rx	"Probably effective" for treating depression that is refractory to tricyclic antidepressants and in depressed patients in whom tricyclic drugs are contraindicated.	**Tablets. Initial,** 30 mg daily as a single dose or divided dose. Reduce when clinical improvement is noted. **Maintenance:** 10–20 mg daily.	Three to four weeks may be required for beneficial effects to be noticed. Use with caution during lactation. Use not recommended for children less than 16 years of age.
Phenelzine sulfate (Nardil) Rx	Major depression with or without melancholia or with atypical, nonendogenous depression or depressive neurosis; often manifest mixed anxiety and depression, phobic, or hypochondria. Panic disorders.	**Tablets. Initial,** 15 mg t.i.d.; increase dose gradually to 60 mg/day (some may require 90 mg/day). **Maintenance** (after maximum beneficial effects noted): 15 mg/day or every other day. **Geriatric, initial:** 0.8–1 mg/kg daily in divided doses; **then,** increase as needed to a maximum of 60 mg daily.	Beneficial effects may not be seen for 4 or more weeks. Use not recommended for children less than 16 years of age. During pregnancy and lactation, potential benefits versus risks should be assessed. Geriatric patients may manifest a greater risk of hypotension.
Tranylcypromine sulfate (Parnate) Rx	Major depressive episodes with or without melancholia. *Investigational:* Depressed phase of bipolar disorder and moderate to severe depressive neurosis.	**Tablets. Initial:** 10 mg in the morning and evening. If no response in 2–3 weeks, increase dose to 20 mg in the morning and 10 mg in the afternoon and re-evaluate after 1 week. **Usual maintenance:** 10–20 mg daily, not to exceed 60 mg daily. **Geriatric, initial:** 2.5–5 mg daily; **then,** increase gradually in increments of 2.5–5 mg q 3–4 days to a maximum of 45 mg daily.	This drug should be used only under close supervision and in patients who have not responded to drugs more commonly used for depression. Reduce dosage gradually when withdrawing this drug. Prior to use during pregnancy and lactation, assess benefits versus risks. Use not recommended in children less than 16 years of age.

9. Note any client complaint of red-green vision. This may be the first indication of ophthalmic damage.

10. Monitor liver and renal function studies periodically throughout therapy.

11. If anti-depressant drugs are employed, monitor for any evidence of drug interactions.

12. Report to the physician if the client appears agitated, anxious, manic, or has any marked changes in behavior.

13. MAO inhibitors potentiate the effect of insulin and sulfonylurea compounds. Therefore, clients with diabetes mellitus must be carefully assessed for hypoglycemia.

14. Because of the risk of insomnia, do not administer the drugs in the evening.

15. Urinary retention is common among elderly clients, males, and those who are immobilized. Monitor intake and output and note other evidence of urinary retention such as bladder distention, which may necessitate changes in drug therapy.

16. To avoid constipation provide clients with 2500–3000 mL of fluid per day and increase their intake of fruits, fruit juices and fiber.

17. If a client has been taking elevated doses of MAO inhibitors over a long period of time, any drug withdrawal should be accomplished by gradually reducing the dosage of drug to a maintenance level before discontinuing the drug entirely.

Client/Family Teaching

1. MAO drugs should be taken with meals to avoid GI irritation.

2. Provide a printed list of tyramine-containing foods to avoid. (ex. cheeses, alcoholic beverages, sour cream, yogurt, bananas, raisins, figs, dried fish, herring, salami, chicken or beef livers, tenderizers, game meats, avocados).

3. Instruct clients to avoid taking other medications while they are on MAO inhibitor therapy unless ordered by the physician. This includes any OTC preparations for coughs, colds, congestion or allergic reactions.

4. Avoid taking other medications for 2–3 weeks after therapy has been discontinued unless otherwise ordered by the physician.

5. Reassure the client that several weeks of therapy are required before they may see significant changes in their condition.

6. Remind them to continue taking the medication even if there appears to be improvement. Continued drug therapy is required to maintain proper blood levels of the drug as well as the feelings of improvement.

7. Advise to limit or eliminate the use of caffeinated coffee, tea and cola beverages. Excessive use of beverages with caffeine, accompanied by the use of MAO inhibitors, may cause a hypertensive crisis. Clients may experience a marked elevation of blood pressure, occipital headaches, palpitations, and constricting chest pain.

8. Caution clients with diabetes that the drug may interact with insulin or oral hypoglycemic agents. Advise them to monitor their blood glucose levels more often and report variations. The physician may need to alter their diet or the dose of prescribed hypoglycemic agents.

9. Caution clients to report immediately to the physician any visual changes, stiff neck, soreness, photophobia, sweating, or change in pupil size. These may be symptoms of hypertensive crisis and require immediate attention.

10. Advise women who think they may be pregnant to consult their physician. If the client is of childbearing age some form of birth control may be indicated.

11. Frequent mouth rinses, sugarless gum or hard candy, and increased fluid intake may diminish the drug effects of dry mouth.

12. Avoid all use of alcoholic beverages.

13. Lie down immediately if feeling faint. Rise slowly from a supine position and dangle legs before standing to minimize orthostatic hypotension.

14. Maintain activity in moderation. MAO inhibitors suppress anginal pain which is a warning sign of myocardial ischemia.

15. Advise clients to weigh themselves regularly. If weight gain becomes significant (ex. 3–5 pounds per week) the client may need to go on a calorie reducing diet, or a change in drug or drug dosage may be warranted. Clients should maintain a weight chart for physician review.

16. Stress the importance of keeping scheduled appointments, as dose will gradually be increased until desired response is obtained.

Evaluation

1. Note indications of positive clinical responses such as improvement in mood, energy and interest level, sleep patterns and level of activity.

2. Assess for a reduction in somatic complaints.

3. If there is no response observed by the third week of therapy, it is not likely that the client will respond to increased dosages of medication.

TRICYCLIC ANTIDEPRESSANTS

General Statement: The tricyclic antidepressants are chemically related to the phenothiazines and, as such, they exhibit many of the same pharmacologic effects (e.g., anticholinergic, antiserotonin, sedative, antihistaminic, and hypotensive). The tricyclic antidepressants are less effective for depressed patients in the presence of organic brain damage or schizophrenia. Also, they can induce mania; this possibility should be kept in mind when given to patients with manic-depressive psychoses.

Action/Kinetics: Tricyclic antidepressants prevent the reuptake of norepinephrine or serotonin, or both, into the storage granules of the presynaptic nerves. This results in increased concentrations of these neurotransmitters in the synapses, which alleviates depression. (*Note:* Endogenous depression is thought to be caused by low concentrations of norepinephrine and/or serotonin.) The tricyclic antidepressants are well absorbed from the GI tract. All these drugs have a long serum half-life. Up to 4 to 6 days may be required to reach steady plasma levels, and maximum therapeutic effects may not be noted for 2 to 4 weeks. Because of the long half-life, single daily dosage may suffice. The tricyclic antidepressants are more than 90% bound to plasma protein. They are partially metabolized in the liver and excreted primarily in the urine.

Uses: Endogenous and reactive depressions. Preferred over MAO inhibitors because they are less toxic. See individual drugs for special uses, such as use in depression associated with anxiety and disturbances in sleep.

Contraindications: Severely impaired liver function. Use during acute recovery phase from myocardial infarction. Concomitant use with MAO inhibitors.

Special Concerns: Use with caution in patients with epilepsy, cardiovascular diseases, glaucoma, benign prostatic hypertrophy, suicidal tendencies, a history of urinary retention, and the elderly. Concomitant use with MAO inhibitors should be undertaken with caution. Use during pregnancy only when benefits clearly outweigh risks. Use with caution during lactation. Generally not recommended for children less than 12 years of age. Geriatric patients may be more sensitive to the anticholinergic and sedative side effects.

Side Effects: Most frequent side effects are sedation and atropine-like reactions. *CNS:* Confusion, anxiety, restlessness, insomnia, nightmares, hallucinations, delusions, mania or hypomania, headache, dizziness, inability to concentrate, panic reaction, worsening of psychoses, fatigue, weakness. *Anticholinergic:* Dry mouth, blurred vision, mydriasis, constipation, paralytic ileus, urinary retention or difficulty in urination. *GI:* Nausea, vomiting, anorexia, gastric distress, unpleasant taste, stomatitis, glossitis, cramps, increased salivation, black tongue. *CV:* Fainting, tachycardia, hypo- or hypertension, arrhythmias, heart block, possibility of palpitations, myocardial infarction, stroke. *Neurologic:* Paresthesias, numbness, incoordination, neuropathies, extrapyramidal symptoms including tardive dyskinesia, dysarthria, seizures. *Dermatologic:* Skin rashes, urticaria, flushing, pruritus, petechiae, photosensitivity, edema. *Endocrine:* Testicular swelling and gynecomastia in males, increase or decrease in libido, impotence, menstrual irregularities and galactorrhea in females, hypo- or hyperglycemia, changes in secretion of antidiuretic hormone. *Miscellaneous:* Sweating, alopecia, nasal congestion, lacrimation, increase in body temperature, chills, urinary frequency including nocturia. Bone marrow depression including thrombocytopenia, leukopenia, agranulocytosis, eosinophilia.

High dosage increases the frequency of seizures in epileptic patients and may cause epileptiform attacks in normal subjects.

Drug Interactions	
Acetazolamide	↑ Effect of tricyclics by ↑ renal tubular reabsorption of the drug
Alcohol, ethyl	Concomitant use may lead to ↑ GI complications and ↓ performance on motor skill tests—death has been reported
Ammonium chloride	↓ Effect of tricyclics by ↓ renal tubular reabsorption of the drug
Anticholinergic drugs	Additive anticholinergic side effects
Anticoagulants, oral	↑ Hypoprothrombinemia due to ↓ breakdown by liver
Anticonvulsants	Tricyclics may ↑ incidence of epileptic seizures
Antihistamines	Additive anticholinergic side effects
Ascorbic acid	↓ Effect of tricyclics by ↓ renal tubular reabsorption of the drug
Barbiturates	Additive depressant effects; also, barbiturates may ↑ breakdown of antidepressants by liver
Benzodiazepines	Tricyclic antidepressants ↑ effect of benzodiazepines
Beta-adrenergic blocking agents	Tricyclic antidepressants ↓ effect of the blocking agents
Charcoal	↓ Absorption of tricyclic antidepressants → decreased effectiveness (or toxicity)
Chlordiazepoxide	Concomitant use may cause additive sedative effects and/or additive atropine-like side effects

Drug Interactions

Cimetidine	↑ Effect of tricyclics (especially serious anticholinergic symptoms) due to ↓ breakdown by liver
Clonidine	Dangerous ↑ in blood pressure and hypertensive crisis
Contraceptives, oral	Oral contraceptives may ↑ effect of tricyclic antidepressants
Diazepam	Concomitant use may cause additive sedative effects and/or additive atropine-like side effects
Dicumarol	Tricyclic antidepressants may ↑ the t½ of dicumarol → increased anticoagulation effects
Disulfiram	↑ Levels of tricyclic antidepressant; also, possibility of acute organic brain syndrome
Ephedrine	Tricyclics ↓ effects of ephedrine by preventing uptake at its site of action
Estrogens	Depending on the dose, estrogens may ↑ or ↓ the effects of tricyclics
Ethchlorvynol	Combination may result in transient delirium
Fluoxetine	Fluoxetine ↑ pharmacologic and toxic effects of tricyclic antidepressants (effect may persist for several weeks after fluoxetine is discontinued)
Furazolidone	Toxic psychoses possible
Glutethimide	Additive anticholinergic side effects
Guanethidine	Tricyclics ↓ the antihypertensive effect of guanethidine by preventing uptake at its site of action
Haloperidol	↑ Effect of tricyclics due to ↓ breakdown by liver
Levodopa	↓ Effect of levodopa due to ↓ absorption
Meperidine	Tricyclics enhance narcotic-induced respiratory depression; also, additive anticholinergic side effects
Methyldopa	Tricyclics may block hypotensive effects of methyldopa
Methylphenidate	↑ Effect of tricyclics due to ↓ breakdown by liver
Monoamine oxidase inhibitors	Concomitant use may result in excitation, increase in body temperature, delirium, tremors, and convulsions, although combinations have been used successfully
Narcotic analgesics	Tricyclics enhance narcotic-induced respiratory depression; also, additive anticholinergic effects
Oral contraceptives	↑ Plasma levels of tricyclic antidepressants due to ↓ breakdown by liver

Drug Interactions

Oxazepam	Concomitant use may cause additive sedative effects and/or atropine-like side effects
Phenothiazines	Additive anticholinergic side effects; also, phenothiazines ↑ effects of tricyclics due to ↓ breakdown by liver
Procainamide	Additive cardiac effects
Quinidine	Additive cardiac effects
Reserpine	Tricyclics ↓ hypotensive effect of reserpine
Sodium bicarbonate	↑ Effect of tricyclics by ↑ renal tubular reabsorption of the drug
Sympathomimetics	Potentiation of sympathomimetic effects → hypertension or cardiac arrhythmias
Tobacco (smoking)	↓ Serum levels of tricyclic antidepressants due to ↑ breakdown by liver
Thyroid preparations	Mutually potentiating effects observed
Vasodilators	Additive hypotensive effect

Laboratory Test Interferences: ↑ Alkaline phosphatase, bilirubin; ↑ or ↓ blood glucose. False + or ↑ urinary catecholamines.

Overdosage:

Symptoms

Drowsiness, ataxia, tachycardia, ECG abnormalities, congestive heart failure, convulsions, mydriasis, severe hypotension, stupor, coma, agitation, hyperactive reflexes, muscle rigidity, diaphoresis, respiratory depression, cyanosis, shock, vomiting, hyperpyrexia.

Treatment of Overdosage

1. Admit patient to hospital.
2. Empty stomach in alert patients by induced vomiting followed by gastric lavage and charcoal administration **after insertion of cuffed endotracheal tube.** Maintain respiration and avoid the use of respiratory stimulants.
3. Administer physostigmine salicylate to reverse CNS and cardiovascular effects. **Adults:** 1–3 mg; **pediatric:** 0.5 mg repeated q 5 min up to maximum of 2 mg, if necessary. For all patients, repeat, if needed, q 30–60 min.
4. Monitor ECG for at least 72 hr. Closely monitor cardiac function.
5. Control hyperpyrexia by external means (ice pack, cool baths, spongings).
6. To reduce possibility of convulsions, minimize external stimulation. If necessary, use diazepam, short-acting barbiturates, paraldehyde, or methocarbamol to control convulsions. Avoid barbiturates if MAO inhibitors have been used recently.
7. For life-threatening arrhythmias, lidocaine, propranolol, or phenytoin have been used. Monitor for myocardial depression caused by these agents.

Dosage: See individual drugs. Dosage levels vary greatly in effectiveness from one patient to another; therefore, dosage regimens must be carefully individualized.

NURSING CONSIDERATIONS

Administration/Storage

1. In adolescents and elderly clients, initial dosage should be lower than in adults; the dose may then be gradually increased as required.
2. The dosage of drug should be highly individualized according to the client's age, weight, physical and mental condition and response to the therapy.
3. For maintenance therapy, a single daily dose may suffice.
4. The dose is usually administered at bedtime, so that any anticholinergic and/or sedative effects will not be bothersome.
5. To reduce incidence of sedation and anticholinergic effects, small dosages of the drug should be used first and then gradually increased to the desired dosage levels.

Assessment

1. Obtain baseline complete blood counts and liver function studies before initiating therapy.
2. Record ECG, heart sounds, and evaluate neurological functioning as baseline data.
3. Note client report of sleep disturbances, lethargy, apathy, impaired thought processes or lack of responses.
4. Assess extent of dysphoric mood, appetite and any reports of weight changes.
5. Obtain baseline ophthalmic exam and note any reports of visual disturbances and the presence of glaucoma.
6. Note any evidence of urinary retention, especially among the elderly.

Interventions

1. Monitor clients for any changes in vision, such as client complaint of headaches, halos or eye pain.
2. Assess clients closely if they also develop dilated pupils or complain of nausea. These symptoms may be serious, especially if the client has angle-closure glaucoma and may require a change in medication.
3. Note any signs of an allergic response to the drug, such as skin rash, alopecia, and eosinophilia.
4. Note client complaints of constipation. Provide a diet high in fiber, an increased fluid intake, and a stool softener as needed.
5. Routinely check client's CBC for eosinophil count, thrombocytes, and leukocytes. Check for evidence of agranulocytosis, especially common among elderly women and during the second month of drug therapy. Document and report to the physician as the drug may need to be withheld.
6. Obtain ECG's periodically throughout drug therapy and compare to the baseline ECG. If the client has a history of cardiovascular disorders, assess the client for tachycardia and any increase in attacks of angina as these may lead to a myocardial infarction or stroke.
7. Note any client complaints of sore throat, fever, easy bruising, unusual bleeding, presence of petechiae or purpura. These are symptoms of blood dyscrasias. Withhold drug and notify the physician. Place client in protective isolation and practice universal precautions until the CBC with leukocyte counts has been evaluated.
8. Assess G.I. complaints of anorexia, nausea, vomiting, epigastric distress, diarrhea, a blackened tongue, and a peculiar taste in the mouth. Document and notify the physician as these symptoms require an adjustment of dosage. Administering the medication with or immediately following meals may reduce gastric irritation.

9. Query client concerning adverse endocrine disturbances such as increased or decreased libido, gynecomastia, testicular swelling and impotence. Discuss these with the client's physician and the client and mutually devise a plan to help deal with the problem.

10. Monitor clients with diabetes mellitus, especially when tricyclic therapy is initiated or discontinued. These drugs may alter blood sugar levels in either direction and require an adjustment in the dose of hypoglycemic agent.

11. In clients with a history of hyperthyroidism, be alert for cardiac arrhythmias that may be precipitated by tricyclic drugs.

12. Assess clients for changes in baseline behavior, indicating further psychological disturbances such as mood swings, increases in agitation and anxiety. Document and report as a change in medication may be indicated.

13. Monitor intake and output. Check for abdominal distention, urinary retention and for the absence of bowel sounds (as in paralytic ileus) as these conditions may require a reduction in drug dose.

14. Note symptoms of cholestatic jaundice and biliary tract obstruction such a high fevers, yellowing of the skin, mucous membranes and sclera, pruritus as well as upper abdominal pain. Document and report as a change in therapy may be indicated.

15. If the client has been receiving electroshock therapy, check with the physician before administering tricyclic drugs. The combination may be hazardous to the client.

16. Ascertain if the drug is to be discontinued several days prior to surgery. The tricyclic compounds may adversely affect blood pressure during surgery.

17. If withdrawal of the drug is required for any reason, expect the procedure to occur slowly in order to avoid any withdrawal symptoms.

18. MAO inhibitors are usually contraindicated with tricyclic antidepressants. If used in conjunction with tricyclic drugs, the dosages should be small and the client should be under close medical supervision.

Client/Family Teaching

1. Advise client not to ingest any other drugs while taking tricyclic antidepressants without the expressed consent of the physician. This rule should also be followed for 2 weeks after completing tricyclic drug therapy.

2. It may require 2 to 4 weeks for the client to realize a maximum clinical response. Apprise client of the delay in response and encourage him/her to stay on the treatment regimen.

3. Advise to rise gradually from a supine position and not to remain standing in one place for any length of time. If the client feels faint, lie down in order to minimize orthostatic hypotension. Review appropriate safety measures.

4. Provide nutritional guidance in order to avoid or counteract problems associated with drug therapy such as anorexia, nausea, or nervous eating. Take medication with meals to decrease G I upset.

5. Advise clients to increase oral hygiene and take frequent sips of water, suck on hard candy, or chew sugarless gum to maintain a moist mouth.

6. Instruct the family on methods to help clients alter their behavior.

7. Discuss changes in libido or reproductive function. Encourage involvement in marital and family therapy.

8. For diabetic clients to monitor blood glucose levels carefully because drug may affect carbohydrate metabolism, and adjustment of hypoglycemic drugs and diet may be indicated.

9. If the client becomes photosensitive, stay out of the sun.

10. Use caution when performing hazardous tasks requiring mental alertness or physical coordination, because the drug may cause drowsiness or ataxia.

11. Stress the importance of maintaining an environment conducive to regular sleep patterns during the initiation of tricyclic therapy.

12. Encourage client to report any alterations in perceptions, such as the development of hallucinations, blurred vision or excessive stimulations.

Evaluation

1. Review expected results of therapy and determine the client's need for continued drug therapy.

2. Ascertain if the client is hoarding drugs.

3. Evaluate for suicidal tendencies of clients recovering from depression.

4. Note if any epileptiform seizures are precipitated by the drug. Evaluate the client/family knowledge of seizure precautions.

AMITRIPTYLINE HYDROCHLORIDE   (ah-mih-**TRIP**-tih-leen)

Amitril, Apo-Amitriptyline ✺, Elavil, Endep, Enovil, Levate ✺, Novo-Triptyn ✺ (Rx)

See also *Tricyclic Antidepressants,* p. 662.

Classification: Tricyclic antidepressant.

Action/Kinetics: Amitriptyline is metabolized to an active metabolite, nortriptyline. Has significant anticholinergic and sedative effects with moderate activity to cause orthostatic hypotension. **Effective plasma levels of amitriptyline and nortriptyline:** Approximately 110–250 ng/mL. **t¹/₂:** 31–46 hr. Up to one month may be required for beneficial effects to be manifested.
Amitriptyline is also found in Limbritrol and Triavil.

Uses: Relief of symptoms of depression including depression accompanied by anxiety and insomnia. Chronic pain due to cancer or other pain syndromes. Prophylaxis of cluster and migraine headaches. *Investigational:* Pathologic laughing and crying secondary to forebrain disease, bulimia nervosa, antiulcer agent, enuresis.

Special Concerns: Pregnancy category: C.

Dosage: Syrup, Tablets. *Antidepressant:* **Adults (outpatients):** 75 mg/day in divided doses; may be increased to 150 mg/day. *Alternate dosage:* **initial,** 50–100 mg at bedtime; **then,** increase by 25–50 mg, if necessary, up to 150 mg daily. **Hospitalized patients: initial,** 100 mg/day; may be increased to 200–300 mg/day. **Maintenance: usual,** 40–100 mg/day (may be given as a single dose at bedtime). **Adolescent and geriatric:** 10 mg t.i.d. and 20 mg at bedtime up to a maximum of 100 mg daily. **Pediatric, 6–12 years of age:** 10–30 mg (1–5 mg/kg) daily in 2 divided doses. *Chronic pain:* 50–100 mg daily. *Enuresis:* **Pediatric, over 6 years:** 10 mg daily as a single dose at bedtime; dose may be increased up to a maximum of 25 mg. **Less than 6 years:** 10 mg daily as a single dose at bedtime.
IM only. *Antidepressant:* **Adults,** 20–30 mg q.i.d.; switch to **PO** therapy as soon as possible.

NURSING CONSIDERATIONS

See also *Nursing Considerations* for *Tricyclic Antidepressants,* p. 666.

Administration/Storage

1. Increases in dosage should be made in late afternoon or at bedtime.

2. Beneficial antidepressant effects may not be noted for 30 days.

3. Sedative effects may be manifested prior to antidepressant effects.

Client/Family Teaching

Warn clients not to drive a car or operate hazardous machinery, as drug causes a high degree of sedation.

AMITRIPTYLINE AND PERPHENAZINE   (ah-mih-**TRIP**-tih-leen, per-**FEN**-ah-zeen)

Triavil (Rx)

See also *Amitriptyline,* p. 668, and *Perphenazine,* p. 638.

Classification/Content: See also information on individual components.
Antidepressant: Amitriptyline HCl, 10–50 mg. *Antipsychotic:* Perphenazine, 2–4 mg.
There are five different strengths of Triavil: Triavil 2–10, Triavil 2–25, Triavil 4–10, Triavil 4–25, and Triavil 4–50. *Note:* the first number refers to the number of milligrams of perphenazine and the second number refers to the number of milligrams of amitriptyline.

Uses: Treatment of depressed patients who manifest anxiety and/or agitation, as well as depression and anxiety in patients with chronic physical disease. Also schizophrenic patients with symptoms of depression.

Contraindications: Use during pregnancy is not recommended.

Dosage: PO. Adults, initial: One tablet of Triavil 2–25 or 4–25 t.i.d.–q.i.d. or one tablet of Triavil 4–50 b.i.d. Schizophrenic patients should receive an initial dose of two tablets of Triavil 4–50 t.i.d., with a fourth dose at bedtime, if necessary. Initial dosage for geriatric or adolescent patients in whom anxiety dominates is Triavil 4–10 t.i.d.–q.i.d., with dosage adjusted as required. **Maintenance:** One tablet Triavil 2–25 or 4–25 b.i.d.–q.i.d. or one tablet Triavil 4–50 b.i.d.

NURSING CONSIDERATIONS

See *Nursing Considerations* for *Tricyclic Antidepressants,* p. 666.

Administration/Storage

1. Triavil is not recommended for children.

2. Total daily dosage of Triavil should not exceed four of the 4–50 tablets or eight tablets of all other dosage strengths.

3. The therapeutic effect may take up to several weeks to be manifested.

4. Once a satisfactory response has been observed, the dose should be reduced to the smallest amount required for relief of symptoms.

AMOXAPINE   (ah-**MOX**-ah-peen)

Asendin (Rx)

See also *Tricyclic Antidepressants,* p. 662.

Classification: Tricyclic antidepressant.

Action/Kinetics: In addition to its effect on monoamines, this drug also blocks dopamine receptors. Is metabolized to the active metabolites 7-hydroxy and 8-hydroxyamoxapine. **Peak blood levels:** 90 min. **Effective plasma levels:** 200–500 ng/mL. **t½:** 8 hr; t½ of major metabolite: 30 hr. Excreted in urine.

Uses: Endogenous and reactive depression. Antianxiety agent.

Contraindications: Avoid high dose levels in patients with a history of convulsive seizures. Not to be used during acute recovery period after myocardial infarction.

Special Concerns: Pregnancy category: C. Safe use in children under 16 years of age and during lactation not established.

Additional Side Effects: Tardive dyskinesia. Overdosage may cause seizures (common), neuroleptic malignant syndrome, testicular swelling, impairment of sexual function, and breast enlargement in males and females. Also, renal failure may be seen 2–5 days after overdosage.

Dosage: Tablets. Adults: *individualized,* **initial,** 50 mg t.i.d. Can be increased to 100 mg t.i.d. during first week. Doses greater than 300 mg daily should not be used unless this dose has been ineffective for at least 14 days. **Maintenance:** 300 mg as a single dose at bedtime. **Hospitalized patients:** Up to 150 mg q.i.d. **Geriatric, initial,** 25 mg b.i.d.–t.i.d. If necessary, increase to 50 mg b.i.d.–t.i.d. after first week. **Maintenance:** Up to 300 mg once daily at bedtime.

NURSING CONSIDERATIONS

See also *Nursing Considerations* for *Tricyclic Antidepressants,* p. 666.

Assessment

Observe client for early CNS manifestations of tardive dyskinesia.

CLOMIPRAMINE HYDROCHLORIDE (kloh-**MIP**-rah-meen)

Anafranil (Rx)

See also *Tricyclic Antidepressants,* p. 662.

Classification: Antidepressant, tricyclic.

Action/Kinetics: Clomipramine possesses a high degree of anticholinergic and sedative effects as well as moderate orthostatic hypotension. **t½:** 19–37 hr. **Effective plasma levels:** 80–100 ng/mL. The drug is metabolized to the active desmethylclomipramine.

Uses: Treatment of obsessive-compulsive disorder in which the obsessions or compulsions cause marked distress, significantly interfere with social or occupational activities, or are time-consuming. Also, to treat panic attacks and cataplexy associated with narcolepsy.

Contraindications: To relieve symptoms of depression.

Special Concerns: Safety has not been established for use during pregnancy and lactation. Safety has not been established in children less than 10 years of age.

Additional Side Effects: Hyperthermia, especially when used with other drugs. Increased risk of seizures. Aggressive reactions, asthenia, anemia, eructation, failure to ejaculate, laryngitis, vestibular disorders, muscle weakness.

Dosage: Capsules. Adult, initial: 25 mg daily; **then,** increase gradually to approximately 100 mg during the first 2 weeks (depending on patient tolerance). The dose may then be increased slowly to a maximum of 250 mg daily over the next several weeks. **Adolescents, children, initial:** 25 mg daily; **then,** increase gradually during the first 2 weeks to a maximum of 100 mg or 3 mg/kg, whichever is less. The dose may then be increased to a maximum daily dose of 3 mg/kg or 200 mg, whichever is less.

NURSING CONSIDERATIONS

See also *Nursing Considerations* for *Tricyclic Antidepressants,* p. 666.

Administration/Storage

1. Initially, the daily dosage should be divided and given with meals to reduce GI side effects.
2. After the optimum dose is determined, the total daily dose can be given at bedtime to minimize daytime sedation.
3. The dose for all ages should be adjusted to the lowest effective dose and be evaluated periodically to determine the continued need for treatment.
4. Although the efficacy of clomipramine has not been determined after 10 weeks of therapy, clients have successfully used the drug for up to 1 year without loss of beneficial effects.

DESIPRAMINE HYDROCHLORIDE   (deh-**ZIP**-rah-meen)

Norpramin, Pertofrane (Rx)

See also *Tricyclic Antidepressants,* p. 662.

Classification: Antidepressant, tricyclic.

Action/Kinetics: Has minimal anticholinergic and sedative effects and slight ability to cause orthostatic hypotension. **Effective plasma levels:** 125–300 ng/mL. **t½:** 12–24 hr. Patients who will respond to drug usually do so within the first week.

Uses: Symptoms of depression. Bulimia nervosa. To decrease craving and depression during cocaine withdrawal. To treat severe neurogenic pain. Cataplexy associated with narcolepsy. Attention deficit disorders with or without hyperactivity in children over 6 years of age.

Additional Side Effects: Bad taste in mouth, hypertension during surgery.

Dosage: Capsules, Tablets. *Antidepressant:* **initial,** 100–200 mg in single or divided doses. **Maximum daily dose:** 300 mg. **Maintenance:** 50–100 mg given once daily. **Geriatric patients:** 25–50 mg/day in divided doses up to a maximum of 150 mg daily. **Children, 6–12 years of age:** 10–30 mg daily (1–5 mg/kg) in divided doses. **Adolescents:** 25–50 mg daily in divided doses up to a maximum of 100 mg. *Cocaine withdrawal:* 50–200 mg daily.

NURSING CONSIDERATIONS

See also *Nursing Considerations* for *Tricyclic Antidepressants,* p. 666.

Administration/Storage

1. Clients requiring 300 mg daily should have treatment initiated in a hospital setting.
2. Maintenance doses should be given for at least 2 months following a satisfactory response.
3. Administration of a single daily dose, or any increases in the dosage should be administered at bedtime in order to reduce daytime sedation.

DOXEPIN HYDROCHLORIDE   (DOX-eh-peen)

Adapin, Sinequan, Triadapin ✻ (Rx)

See also *Tricyclic Antidepressants,* p. 662.

Classification: Antidepressant, tricyclic.

Action/Kinetics: Doxepin is metabolized to the active metabolite, desmethyldoxepin. It has moderate anticholinergic effects and ability to cause orthostatic hypotension and high sedative effects. **Minimum effective plasma level of both doxepin and desmethyldoxepin:** 100–200 ng/mL. **t½:** 8–24 hr.

Uses: Symptoms of depression. Antianxiety agent, depression accompanied by anxiety and insomnia, depression in patients with manic-depressive illness. Depression or anxiety due to organic disease or alcoholism. Chronic, severe neurogenic pain. Peptic ulcer disease. Dermatologic disorders including chronic urticaria, angioedema, and nocturnal pruritus due to atopic eczema.

Additional Contraindications: Glaucoma or a tendency for urinary retention.

Special Concerns: Safety has not been determined in pregnancy. Not recommended for use in children less than 12 years of age.

Additional Side Effects: Doxepin has a high incidence of side effects, including a high degree of sedation, decreased libido, extrapyramidal symptoms, dermatitis, pruritus, fatigue, weight gain, edema, paresthesia, breast engorgement, insomnia, tremor, chills, tinnitus, and photophobia.

Dosage: Capsules, Oral Solution. *Antidepressant, mild to moderate anxiety or depression:* **Adults:** 25 mg t.i.d. (or up to 150 mg can be given at bedtime); **then,** adjust dosage to individual response (usual optimum dosage: 75–150 mg/day). **Geriatric patients, initially:** 25–50 mg daily; dose can be increased as needed and tolerated. *Severe symptoms:* **Initial,** 50 mg t.i.d.; **then,** gradually increase to 300 mg/day. *Emotional symptoms with organic disease:* 25–50 mg daily. *Antipruritic:* 10–30 mg at bedtime.

NURSING CONSIDERATIONS

See also *Nursing Considerations* for *Tricyclic Antidepressants,* p. 666.

Administration/Storage

Oral concentrate is to be diluted with 4 oz water, fruit juice, or milk just before ingestion. The concentrate should not be mixed with carbonated beverages or grape juice.

IMIPRAMINE HYDROCHLORIDE   (ih-MIP-rah-meen)

Apo-Imipramine ✻, Impril ✻, Janimine, Novo-Pramine ✻, Tofranil (Rx)

IMIPRAMINE PAMOATE   (ih-MIP-rah-meen)

Tofranil-PM (Rx)

See also *Tricyclic Antidepressants,* p. 662.

Action/Kinetics: Imipramine is biotransformed into its active metabolite, desmethylimipramine (desipramine). **Effective plasma level of imipramine and desmethylimipramine:** 200–350 ng/mL. **t½:** 11–25 hr.

Uses: Symptoms of depression. Enuresis in children. Chronic, severe neurogenic pain. Bulimia nervosa.

Special Concerns: Pregnancy category: B.

Additional Side Effects: High therapeutic dosage may increase frequency of seizures in epileptic patients and cause seizures in nonepileptic patients. Elderly and adolescent patients may have low tolerance to the drug.

Laboratory Test Interferences: ↑ Metanephrine (Pisano test); ↓ Urinary 5-HIAA.

Dosage: Tablets, Capsules. *Depression:* **Hospitalized patients:** 50 mg b.i.d.–t.i.d. Can be increased by 25 mg every few days up to 200 mg daily. After 2 weeks, dosage may be increased gradually to maximum of 250–300 mg once daily at bedtime. **Outpatients:** 75–150 mg daily. Maximum dose for outpatients is 200 mg. Decrease when feasible to maintenance dosage: 50–150 mg once daily at bedtime. **Adolescent and geriatric patients:** 30–40 mg/day up to maximum of 100 mg/day. **Pediatric:** 1.5 mg/kg daily in 3 divided doses; can be increased 1–1.5 mg/kg daily q 3–5 days to a maximum of 5 mg/kg daily. *Childhood enuresis:* **age 6 years and over:** 25 mg/day 1 hr before bedtime. Dose can be increased to 50 mg/day up to 12 years of age and to 75 mg/day in children over 12 years of age.

IM. Adults: *Antidepressant:* up to 100 mg daily in divided doses. IM route not recommended for use in children less than 12 years of age.

NURSING CONSIDERATIONS

See also *Nursing Considerations* for *Tricyclic Antidepressants,* p. 666.

Administration/Storage

1. Crystals, which may be present in the injectable form, can be dissolved by immersing closed ampules into hot water for 1 min.
2. Total daily dose can be given once daily at bedtime.
3. Protect from direct sunlight and strong artificial light.
4. Parenteral therapy should be used only in clients unwilling or unable to take oral medication. Switch to oral medication as soon as possible.
5. Imipramine injection should not be given IV.
6. When used for the treatment of enuresis, the drug can be given in doses of 25 mg in midafternoon and 25 mg at bedtime (this regimen may increase effectiveness).
7. When used as an enuretic in children, the dose should not exceed 2.5 mg/kg daily.

Client/Family Teaching

Report increase in frequency of seizures in epileptics and any occurrence of seizures in nonepileptics.

MAPROTILINE HYDROCHLORIDE (mah-**PROH**-tih-leen)

Ludiomil (Rx)

See also *Tricyclic Antidepressants,* p. 662.

Classification: Antidepressant, tetracyclic.

Action/Kinetics: Maprotiline is actually a tetracyclic compound but has many similarities to the tricyclic drugs. It causes moderate anticholinergic, sedative, and orthostatic hypotensive effects.

Effective plasma levels: 200–300 ng/mL. **t½:** Approximately 21–25 hr. **Peak effect:** 12 hr. Beneficial effects may not be observed for 2–3 weeks.

Uses: Treat symptoms of depression. Depressive neuroses, depression in patients with manic-depressive illness, depression with anxiety.

Additional Contraindications: Known or suspected seizure disorders.

Special Concerns: Pregnancy category: B. Not recommended for patients under 18 years of age.

Additional Side Effects: Overdosage may cause increased incidence of seizures.

Dosage: Tablets. Adults, *mild to moderate depression,* **outpatients, initial:** 75 mg/day; can be increased to 150–225 mg/day if necessary. **Adult,** *severe depression,* **hospitalized, initial:** 100–150 mg/day; can be increased to 225 mg if necessary. Dosage should not exceed 225 mg/day. **Maintenance:** For all uses, 75–150 mg/day, adjusted depending on therapeutic response. **Geriatric patients:** 50–75 mg/day.

NURSING CONSIDERATIONS

See also *Nursing Considerations* for *Tricyclic Antidepressants,* p. 666.

Administration/Storage

1. May be given in single or divided doses.
2. Should be discontinued as long as possible before elective surgery.

NORTRIPTYLINE HYDROCHLORIDE   (nor-**TRIP**-tih-leen)

Aventyl, Pamelor (Rx)

See also *Tricyclic Antidepressants,* p. 662.

Classification: Antidepressant, tricyclic.

Action/Kinetics: Nortriptyline manifests moderate anticholinergic and sedative effects but slight orthostatic hypotensive effects. **Effective plasma levels:** 50–150 ng/mL. **t½:** 18–44 hr.

Uses: Treatment of symptoms of depression. Chronic, severe neurogenic pain. Dermatologic disorders including chronic urticaria, angioedema, and nocturnal pruritus in atopic eczema.

Special Concerns: Use with caution during pregnancy. Safety and efficacy have not been determined in children.

Laboratory Test Interference: ↓ Urinary 5-hydroxyindole acetic acid (5-HIAA).

Dosage: Capsules, Oral Solution. Adults: *Depression:* 25 mg t.i.d.–q.i.d. Dose individualized. **Doses above 150 mg daily are not recommended. Elderly patients:** 30–50 mg/day in divided doses. **Not recommended for children.** *Dermatologic disorders:* 75 mg daily.

NURSING CONSIDERATIONS

See also *Nursing Considerations* for *Tricyclic Antidepressants,* p. 666.

Administration/Storage

Give after meals and at bedtime.

PROTRIPTYLINE HYDROCHLORIDE   (proh-**TRIP**-tih-leen)

Triptil✿, Vivactil (Rx)

See also *Tricyclic Antidepressants,* p. 662.

Classification: Antidepressant, tricyclic.

Action/Kinetics: Significant anticholinergic effects but low sedative and orthostatic hypotensive effects. **Effective plasma levels:** 100–200 ng/mL. **t¹/₂:** Approximately 67–89 hr.

Uses: Symptoms of depression. Withdrawn and anergic patients. Obstructive sleep apnea. Has also been used with amphetamines to treat cataplexy associated with narcolepsy and to relieve symptoms of attention deficit disorders in some children over 6 years of age with or without hyperactivity.

Special Concerns: Use with caution during pregnancy. Administer with caution to patients with myocardial insufficiency and those in whom tachycardia or a drop in blood pressure might lead to serious complications. Safety and efficacy for treating depression have not been determined in children.

Dosage: Tablets. Adults: *Antidepressant,* **individualized,** 15–40 mg daily in 3–4 divided doses. Up to 60 mg daily (maximum) may be given. **Elderly patients, adolescents: initial,** 5 mg t.i.d.; increase dose slowly. Monitor cardiovascular system closely if dose exceeds 20 mg/day in the elderly. **Not recommended for children.** *Anticataleptic:* 15–20 mg daily at bedtime.

NURSING CONSIDERATIONS

See also *Nursing Considerations* for *Tricyclic Antidepressants,* p. 666.

Administration/Storage

If drug causes insomnia, give last dose no less than 8 hr before bedtime.

Interventions

Assess vital signs at least b.i.d. during initiation of therapy.

TRIMIPRAMINE MALEATE   (try-**MIP**-rah-meen)

Apo-Trimip✿, Surmontil (Rx)

See also *Tricyclic Antidepressants,* p. 662.

Classification: Antidepressant, tricyclic.

Action/Kinetics: Trimipramine causes moderate anticholinergic and orthostatic hypotensive effects and significant sedative effects. **Effective plasma levels:** 180 ng/mL. **t¹/₂:** 7–30 hr. Seems more effective in endogenous depression than in other types of depression.

Uses: Treatment of symptoms of depression. Peptic ulcer disease.

Special Concerns: Pregnancy category: C. Not recommended for use in children less than 12 years of age.

Dosage: Capsules. Adults, outpatients: initial, 75 mg/day in divided doses up to 150 mg/day. Daily dosage should not exceed 200 mg; **maintenance:** 50–150 mg/day. Total dose can be given at bedtime. **Adults, hospitalized: initial,** 100 mg/day in divided doses up to 200 mg/day. If no improvement in 2–3 weeks, increase to 250–300 mg/day. **Adolescent/geriatric patients: initial,** 50 mg/day up to 100 mg/day. Not recommended for children.

NURSING CONSIDERATIONS

See *Nursing Considerations* for *Tricyclic Antidepressants*. p. 666.

MISCELLANEOUS AGENTS

BUPROPION HYDROCHLORIDE   (byou-**PROH**-pee-on)

Wellbutrin (Rx)

Classification: Antidepressant, miscellaneous.

Action/Kinetics: Bupropion is an antidepressant whose mechanism of action is not known; the drug does not inhibit monoamine oxidase and it only weakly blocks neuronal uptake of epinephrine, serotonin, and dopamine. **Peak plasma levels:** 2 hr. **t½:** 8–24 hr. Metabolized to both active and inactive metabolites. Excreted through both the urine (87%) and the feces (10%).

Uses: Short-term (6 weeks or less) treatment of depression.

Contraindications: Seizure disorders; presence or history of bulimia or anorexia nervosa. Concomitant use of a monoamine oxidase inhibitor.

Special Concerns: Pregnancy category: B. Use with caution in patients with a history of seizures, cranial trauma, with drugs that lower the seizure threshold, and other situations that might cause seizures. Use with caution and in lower doses in patients with liver or kidney disease and in patients with a recent history of myocardial infarction or unstable heart disease. Assess benefits versus risks during lactation. Safety and efficacy have not been established in patients less than 18 years of age.

Side Effects: *CNS:* Dose-dependent risk of seizures; agitation, sedation, headache or migraine, insomnia, decreased concentration, euphoria, delusions, hallucinations, psychoses, confusion, paranoia, anxiety, manic episodes in bipolar manic depression, suicide. *GI:* Nausea, vomiting, constipation, anorexia, weight loss (up to 5 lb), diarrhea, dyspepsia, increased appetite, weight gain, dry mouth, increased salivation. *Neurologic:* Akinesia, bradykinesia, tremor, sensory disturbances, pseudoparkinsonism, akathisia, muscle spasms. *CV:* Dizziness, tachycardia, hypertension, hypotension, palpitations, cardiac arrhythmias, syncope. *GU:* Impotence, menstrual irregularities, urinary frequency or retention. *Miscellaneous:* Excessive sweating, blurred vision, auditory disturbances, alteration in taste, rash, pruritus, fever, chills, arthritis, fatigue, upper respiratory problems, temperature disturbances of the skin.

Drug Interactions	
Alcohol	Alcohol lowers seizure threshold; use with bupropion may precipitate seizures
Carbamazepine	Possible additive effect to ↑ drug metabolizing enzymes in the liver
Cimetidine	See *Carbamazepine*
Levodopa	↑ Risk of side effects
Monoamine oxidase inhibitors	Acute toxicity to bupropion may be increased especially if used with phenelzine

Drug Interactions	
Phenobarbital	See *Carbamazepine*
Phenytoin	See *Carbamazepine*

Dosage: Tablets. Adults, initial: 100 mg in the morning and evening for the first 3 days; **then,** 100 mg t.i.d., given in the morning, midday, and in the evening (6 hr should elapse between doses). If no response is observed after 4 weeks or longer, the dose may be increased to 450 mg daily with individual doses not to exceed 150 mg. Doses higher than 450 mg should not be administered. **Maintenance:** Lowest dose to control depression.

NURSING CONSIDERATIONS

Administration/Storage

1. To reduce the risk of seizures, the total daily dose should not exceed 450 mg, each single dose should not exceed 150 mg, and doses of drug should be increased gradually.
2. Several months of treatment may be necessary to control acute depression.
3. Review list of drugs with which this medication interacts.

Assessment

1. Obtain baseline weight, ECG, liver and renal function studies. Anticipate reduced dose with renal and/or liver dysfunction.
2. Determine if client has a history of seizures and/or recent myocardial infarction. Dose of bupropion may need to be reduced.
3. Note any client history of bulimia or anorexia nervosa.
4. Determine if the woman client is of childbearing age and lactating. Assess the benefits and risks and discuss with the physician. This information may serve as a guide when discussing the drug therapy with the client.

Client/Family Teaching

1. Discuss the side effects associated with drug therapy.
2. Explain the potential for a change in taste perceptions. The result could be loss of appetite and weight loss. These symptoms should be reported and an accurate accounting of weight loss should be recorded for the physician's review.
3. Young women should be informed about possible menstrual irregularities.
4. Men should be warned about possible symptoms of impotence. These symptoms should be reported.
5. The beneficial effects of the drug may not be noticed for 5–21 days. The client should continue taking the medication and not be discouraged by the delayed response.
6. Report any changes in urinary output. The client should be instructed how to record intake and output.
7. Dizziness may occur. Therefore, clients should not arise from a supine position suddenly. If dizziness occurs during the day, the client should sit down until the sensation subsides. If it persists, notify the physician.
8. Report any bothersome or persistent side effects, especially marked weight loss or diarrhea.
9. Stress the importance of reporting for follow-up lab studies and medical visits so that drug therapy and dosage may be evaluated and adjusted as needed.

FLUOXETINE HYDROCHLORIDE   (flew-**OX**-eh-teen)

Prozac (Rx)

Classification: Antidepressant, miscellaneous

Action/Kinetics: Fluoxetine is not related chemically to tricyclic, tetracyclic, or other antidepressants. The antidepressant effect is thought to be due to inhibition of uptake of serotonin into CNS neurons. The drug also binds to muscarinic, histaminergic, and alpha$_1$-adrenergic receptors, accounting for many of the side effects. Fluoxetine is metabolized in the liver to norfluoxetine, a metabolite with equal potency to fluoxetine. Norfluoxetine is further metabolized by the liver to inactive metabolites that are excreted by the kidneys. **t^1/$_2$, fluoxetine:** 2–3 days; **t^1/$_2$, norfluoxetine:** 7–9 days. Steady-state plasma levels are achieved after 4–5 weeks. Active drug will be maintained in the body for weeks after withdrawal.

Uses: Depression manifested by outpatients. Use in hospitalized patients or for longer than 5–6 weeks has not been studied adequately. *Investigational:* Treatment of obesity and bulimia nervosa, and obsessive-compulsive disorders.

Special Concerns: Use with caution during pregnancy (category: B) and lactation and in patients with impaired liver or kidney function. Safety and efficacy have not been determined in children.

Side Effects: A large number of untoward reactions have been reported for this drug. Listed are those untoward reactions with a reported frequency of greater than 1%. *CNS:* Headache (most common), activation of mania or hypomania, insomnia, anxiety, nervousness, dizziness, fatigue, sedation, decreased libido, drowsiness, lightheadedness, decreased ability to concentrate, tremor, disturbances in sensation, agitation, abnormal dreams. Although less frequent than 1%, some patients may experience seizures or attempt suicide. *GI:* Nausea (most common), diarrhea, vomiting, constipation, dry mouth, dyspepsia, anorexia, abdominal pain, flatulence, alteration in taste, gastroenteritis, increased appetite. *CV:* Hot flashes, palpitations. *GU:* Sexual dysfunction, frequent urination, infection of the urinary tract, dysmenorrhea. *Respiratory:* Upper respiratory tract infections, pharyngitis, cough, dyspnea, rhinitis, bronchitis, nasal congestion. *Skin:* Rash, pruritis, sweating. *Musculoskeletal:* Muscle, joint, or back pain. *Miscellaneous:* Flu-like symptoms, asthenia, fever, chest pain, allergy, visual disturbances, weight loss.

Drug Interactions	
Diazepam	Fluoxetine ↑ half-life of diazepam
Digitoxin	↑ Effect of fluoxetine due to ↓ plasma protein binding
Lithium	↑ Serum levels of lithium → possible neurotoxicity
MAO inhibitors	MAO inhibitors should be discontinued 14 days before initiation of fluoxetine therapy
Tricyclic antidepressants	↑ Pharmacologic and toxicologic effects of tricyclics
Tryptophan	Symptoms of agitation, GI distress, restlessness
Warfarin	↑ Effect of fluoxetine due to ↓ plasma protein binding

Dosage: Capsules. Adults, initial: 20 mg daily in the morning. If clinical improvement is not observed after several weeks, the dose may be increased to a maximum of 80 mg daily.

NURSING CONSIDERATIONS

Administration/Storage

1. Doses greater than 20 mg daily should be divided and given in the morning and at noon.
2. The maximum therapeutic effect may not be observed until 4 weeks after beginning therapy.
3. Elderly clients or clients taking multiple medications should take lower or less frequent doses.
4. Lower doses should be used in clients with liver or kidney dysfunction.

Assessment

1. Obtain baseline liver and renal function studies prior to initiating therapy. Anticipate reduced dose in clients with hepatic and/or renal insufficiency.
2. In women of childbearing age, determine if pregnant or lactating.

Client/Family Teaching

1. Use caution when driving or performing tasks that require mental alertness, as drug may cause drowsiness and/or dizziness.
2. Report any side effects, especially rashes, hives, increased anxiety, and loss of appetite.
3. Stress the importance of taking the medication at the specific times designated by the physician.
4. Remind client that it usually takes 1 month to note any significant benefits from therapy, and not to become discouraged and discontinue the medication before benefits are attained and evaluated.
5. Do not take any OTC medications without first consulting with physician.
6. Avoid ingestion of alcohol.
7. Stress the importance of reporting for all scheduled lab and medical visits.

TRAZODONE HYDROCHLORIDE   (TRAY-zoh-dohn)

Desyrel, Desyrel Dividose, Trazon, Trialodine (Rx)

Classification: Antidepressant, miscellaneous.

Action/Kinetics: Trazodone is a novel antidepressant that does not inhibit MAO and is also devoid of amphetamine-like effects. Response usually occurs after 2 weeks (75% of patients), with the remainder responding after 2–4 weeks. The drug may inhibit serotonin uptake by brain cells, therefore increasing serotonin concentrations in the synapse. It may also cause changes in binding of serotonin to receptors. The drug causes moderate sedative and orthostatic hypotensive effects and slight anticholinergic effects. **Peak plasma levels:** 1 hr (empty stomach). $t^{1/2}$: initial, 3–6 hr; final, 5–9 hr. **Effective plasma levels:** 800–1,600 ng/mL. Metabolized in liver and excreted through both the urine and feces.

Uses: Depression with or without accompanying anxiety. *Investigational:* In combination with tryptophan for treating aggressive behavior. Treatment of cocaine withdrawal. Chronic pain including diabetic neuropathy.

Contraindications: During the initial recovery period following myocardial infarction. Concurrently with electroshock therapy.

Special Concerns: Use with caution during pregnancy (pregnancy category: C) and lactation. Safety and efficacy in children less than 18 years of age have not been established. Geriatric patients are more prone to the sedative and hypotensive effects.

Side Effects: *General:* Dermatitis, edema, blurred vision, constipation, dry mouth, nasal congestion, skeletal muscle aches and pains. *CV:* Hypertension or hypotension, syncope, palpitations, tachycardia, shortness of breath, chest pain. *GI:* Diarrhea, nausea, vomiting, bad taste in mouth, flatulence. *GU:* Delayed urine flow, priapism, hematuria, increased urinary frequency. *CNS:* Nightmares, confusion, anger, excitement, decreased ability to concentrate, dizziness, disorientation, drowsiness, lightheadedness, fatigue, insomnia, nervousness, impaired memory. Rarely, hallucinations, impaired speech, hypomania. *Other:* Incoordination, tremors, paresthesias, decreased libido, appetite disturbances, red eyes, sweating or clamminess, tinnitus, weight gain or loss, anemia, hypersalivation. Rarely, akathisia, muscle twitching, increased libido, impotence, retrograde ejaculation, early menses, missed periods.

Drug Interactions	
Alcohol	↑ Depressant effects of alcohol
Antihypertensives	Additive hypotension
Barbiturates	↑ Depressant effects of barbiturates
Clonidine	Trazodone ↓ effect of clonidine
CNS depressants	↑ CNS depression
Digoxin	Trazodone may ↑ serum digoxin levels
MAO inhibitors	Initiate therapy cautiously if trazodone is to be used together with MAO inhibitors
Phenytoin	Trazodone may ↑ serum phenytoin levels

Dosage: Tablets. Adults and adolescents, initial, 150 mg/day; **then,** increase by 50 mg/day every 3–4 days to maximum of 400 mg/day in divided doses (outpatients). Inpatients may require up to, but not exceeding, 600 mg/day in divided doses. **Maintenance:** Use lowest effective dose. **Geriatric patients:** 75 mg daily in divided doses; dose can then be increased, as needed and tolerated, at 3–4 day intervals.

NURSING CONSIDERATIONS

Administration/Storage

1. Take with food to enhance absorption and minimize dizziness and/or lightheadedness.
2. To reduce side effects during the day, take major portion of dose at bedtime.
3. Dose should be initiated at the lowest possible level and increased gradually.
4. Beneficial effects may be observed within 1 wk with optimal effects in most clients seen within 2 weeks.

Assessment

1. Take a complete medication history, noting if the client is taking MAO inhibitors. Trazodone could cause an unfavorable interaction.
2. Determine if the client is taking drugs to treat hypertension, as trazodone may reduce the dosage required.
3. Note any history of recent myocardial infarction.

Intervention

1. Review potential side effects and if noted report to physician.
2. Observe closely for cues to suicide. Clients taking antidepressants and emerging from the deepest phases of depression are more prone to suicide.

Client/Family Teaching

1. Use caution when driving or when performing other hazardous tasks, since trazodone may cause drowsiness or dizziness.
2. Avoid alcohol and do not take any other depressant drugs during therapy with trazodone.
3. Encourage family to share responsibility for drug therapy in order to optimize treatment and to prevent overdosage.
4. Inform physician if elective surgery is planned so as to minimize interaction of trazodone with anesthetic agent.
5. Report any bothersome side effects.
6. Encourage client to take trazodone with food to enhance absorption and also to take the majority of the prescribed dose at bedtime in order to minimize adverse effects.

CHAPTER THIRTY-FOUR
Antiparkinson Agents

Antiparkinson Agents

Cholinergic Blocking Agents Used To Treat Parkinsonism

34

Parkinson's disease is a progressive disorder of the nervous system, affecting mostly people over the age of 50. The symptoms manifested include slowness of motor movements (bradykinesia and akinesia), stiffness or resistance to passive movements (rigidity), muscle weakness, tremors, speech impairment, sialorrhea (salivation), and postural instability.

Parkinsonism is a frequent side effect of certain antipsychotic drugs, including prochlorperazine, chlorpromazine, and reserpine. Drug-induced symptoms usually disappear when the responsible agent is discontinued. Extrapyramidal Parkinson-like symptoms can accompany brain injuries (strokes, tumors) or other diseases of the nervous system.

The cause of Parkinson's disease is unknown; however, it is associated with a depletion of the neurotransmitter dopamine in the nervous system. Administration of levodopa—the precursor of dopamine—relieves symptoms in 75–80% of the patients. Anticholinergic agents also have a beneficial effect by reducing tremors and rigidity and improving mobility, muscular coordination, and motor performance. They are often administered together with levodopa. Certain antihistamines, notably diphenhydramine (Benadryl), are also useful in the treatment of parkinsonism.

Patients suffering from Parkinson's disease need emotional support and encouragement because the debilitating nature of the disorder often causes depression. Comprehensive treatment also includes physical therapy.

ANTIPARKINSON AGENTS

AMANTADINE HYDROCHLORIDE   (ah-**MAN**-tah-deen)
Symadine, Symmetrel (Rx)

Classification: Antiviral and antiparkinson agent.

Action/Kinetics: As an antiviral agent, amantadine is believed to prevent penetration of the virus into cells, possibly by inhibiting uncoating of the RNA virus. Amantadine may also prevent the release of infectious viral nucleic acid into the host cell. The drug reduces symptoms of viral infections if given within 24–48 hr after onset of illness.

For the treatment of parkinsonism, either release of dopamine from synaptosomes or blockade of the reuptake of dopamine into presynaptic neurons. Either of these mechanisms results in an increase in the levels of dopamine in dopaminergic synapses in the corpus striatum. Well absorbed from GI tract. **Onset:** 48 hrs. **Peak serum concentration:** 0.2 mcg/mL after 1–4 hr. **t½:** range of 9–37 hr, longer in presence of renal impairment. Ninety percent excreted unchanged in urine.

Use: Influenza A viral infections of the respiratory tract (prophylaxis and treatment of high-risk patients with immunodeficiency, cardiovascular, metabolic, neuromuscular or pulmonary disease).

Symptomatic treatment of idiopathic parkinsonism and parkinsonism syndrome resulting from encephalitis, carbon monoxide intoxication, drugs, or cerebral arteriosclerosis. The drug decreases extrapyramidal symptoms, including akinesia, rigidity, tremors, excessive salivation, gait disturbances, and total functional disability. Favorable results have been obtained in about 50% of the patients. Improvements can last for up to 30 months, although some patients report that the effect of the drug wears off in 1 to 3 months. A rest period or an increased dosage may reestablish effectiveness. For parkinsonism, amantadine hydrochloride is usually used concomitantly with other agents, such as levodopa and anticholinergic agents.

Contraindications: Hypersensitivity to drug.

Special Concerns: Administer with caution to patients with liver and renal disease, history of epilepsy, CHF, peripheral edema, orthostatic hypotension, recurrent eczematoid dermatitis, or severe psychosis, to patients on CNS stimulant drugs, to those exposed to rubella, and to nursing mothers. Safe use for those who may become pregnant (category: C), for lactating mothers, and in children less than one year have not been established.

Side Effects: *GI:* Nausea, vomiting, constipation, anorexia, xerostomia. *CNS:* Depression, psychosis, convulsions, hallucinations, lightheadedness, confusion, ataxia, irritability, anxiety, headache, dizziness, fatigue, insomnia. *CV:* Congestive heart failure, orthostatic hypotension, peripheral edema. *Miscellaneous:* Urinary retention, leukopenia, neutropenia, mottling of skin of the extremities due to poor peripheral circulation (livedo reticularis), skin rashes, visual problems, slurred speech, oculogyric episodes, dyspnea, weakness, eczematoid dermatitis.

Drug Interactions	
Anticholinergics	Additive anticholinergic effects (including hallucinations, confusion), especially with trihexyphenidyl and benztropine
CNS stimulants	May ↑ CNS and psychic effects of amantadine; use cautiously together
Hydrochlorothiazide/triamterene combination	↓ Urinary excretion of amantadine → ↑ plasma levels
Levodopa	Potentiated by amantadine

Dosage: Capsules, Syrup. *Antiviral.* **Adults:** 200 mg daily as a single or divided dose. **Children, 1–9 years:** 4.4–8.8 mg/kg/day up to a maximum of 150 mg/day in 1 or 2 divided doses (use syrup); **9–12 years:** 100 mg b.i.d. *Prophylactic treatment:* institute before or immediately after exposure and continue for 10–21 days if used concurrently with vaccine or for 90 days without vaccine. *Symptomatic management:* initiate as soon as possible and continue for 24–48 hr after disappearance of symptoms. Dose should be decreased in renal impairment (see package insert). *Parkinsonism.* When used as sole agent, usual dose is 100 mg b.i.d.; may be necessary to increase up to 400 mg/day in divided doses. When used with other antiparkinson drugs: 100 mg 1–2 times/day. *Drug-induced extrapyramidal symptoms:* 100 mg b.i.d. (up to 300 mg/day may be required in some). Dosage should be reduced in patients with impaired renal function.

Treatment of Overdosage: Gastric lavage or induction of emesis followed by supportive measures. Ensure that patient is well hydrated; give IV fluids if necessary.

NURSING CONSIDERATIONS

See also *General Nursing Considerations For All Anti-Infectives* under *Penicillins,* p. 140.

Administration/Storage

Protect capsules from moisture.

Assessment

1. Obtain a thorough nursing history and note any history of seizures, CHF and renal insufficiency.
2. Anticipate that following loss of effectiveness of the drug, benefits may be regained by increasing the dosage or discontinuing the drug for several weeks and then reinstituting it.

Client/Family Teaching

1. Do not drive a car or work in a situation where alertness is important, because medication can affect vision, concentration, and coordination.
2. Rise slowly from a prone position, because orthostatic hypotension may occur.
3. Lie down if dizzy or weak, in order to relieve these symptoms of orthostatic hypotension.
4. Report patchy discoloration of the skin, but also that discoloration lessens when legs are elevated and usually fades completely within weeks after discontinuing drug.
5. Report any exposure to rubella, because drug may increase susceptibility to disease.

6. Susceptible individuals should avoid crowds during "flu" season.

7. Notify physician of any persistent or bothersome side effects.

8. Administer last daily dose several hours before retiring to prevent insomnia.

Evaluation

Assess

- clients with a history of epilepsy or other seizures for an increase in seizure activity and take appropriate precautions.
- clients with a history of CHF or peripheral edema for increased edema and/or respiratory distress and report promptly.
- clients with renal impairment for crystalluria, oliguria, and increased BUN or creatinine levels and report promptly.

BROMOCRIPTINE MESYLATE   (broh-moh-**KRIP**-teen)

Parlodel (Rx)

Classification: Prolactin secretion inhibitor; dopamine receptor agonist.

Action/Kinetics: Bromocriptine is a nonhormonal agent that inhibits the release of the hormone prolactin by the pituitary. The drug should be used only when prolactin production by pituitary tumors has been ruled out. Its effect in parkinsonism is due to a direct stimulating effect on dopamine type 2 receptors in the corpus striatum. Less than 30% of the drug is absorbed from the GI tract. **Onset, lower prolactin:** 2 hr; **antiparkinson:** 30–90 min; **decrease growth hormone:** 1–2 hr. **Peak plasma concentration:** 1–3 hr. $t^{1/2}$, **plasma:** 3 hr; **terminal:** 15 hr. **Duration, lower prolactin:** 24 hr (after a single dose); **decrease growth hormone:** 4–8 hr. Significant first-pass effect. Metabolized in liver, excreted mainly through bile and thus the feces.

Uses: Short-term treatment of amenorrhea/galactorrhea associated with hyperprolactinemia. Prevention of physiologic lactation. Acromegaly. Parkinsonism. Female infertility associated with hyperprolactinemia. *Investigational:* Hyperprolactinemia due to pituitary adenoma; male infertility.

Contraindications: Sensitivity to ergot alkaloids. Pregnancy, lactation, children under 15 years of age. Peripheral vascular disease, ischemic heart disease.

Special Concerns: Geriatric patients may manifest more CNS effects. Use with caution in liver or kidney disease.

Side Effects: The type and incidence of untoward reactions depends on the use of the drug. *When used for hyperprolactinemia. GI:* Nausea, vomiting, abdominal cramps, diarrhea, constipation. *CNS:* Headache, dizziness, fatigue, drowsiness, lightheadedness, psychoses. *Other:* Nasal congestion, mild hypotension.

When used to prevent physiological lactation. GI: Nausea, vomiting, cramps, diarrhea. *CNS:* Headaches, dizziness, fatigue, syncope. *CV:* Decreased blood pressure (transient).

When used for acromegaly. GI: Nausea, vomiting, anorexia, dry mouth, dyspepsia, indigestion, GI bleeding. *CNS:* Dizziness, syncope, drowsiness, tiredness, headache; rarely, lightheadedness, lassitude, vertigo, sluggishness, paranoia, insomnia, decreased sleep requirement, delusional psychosis, visual hallucinations. *CV:* Orthostatic hypotension, digital vasospasm, worsening of Raynaud's syndrome; rarely, arrhythmias, ventricular tachycardia, bradycardia, vasovagal attack; *Other:* Rarely, potentiation of effects of alcohol, hair loss, shortness of breath, paresthesia, tingling of ears, muscle cramps, facial pallor, reduced tolerance to cold.

When used for parkinsonism. GI: Nausea, vomiting, abdominal discomfort, constipation, anorexia, dry mouth, dysphagia. *CNS:* Confusion, hallucinations, fainting, drowsiness, dizziness, insomnia, depression, vertigo, anxiety, fatigue, headache, lethargy, nightmares. *GU:* Urinary incontinence, urinary retention, urinary frequency. *Other:* Abnormal involuntary movements, asthenia, visual disturbances, ataxia, hypotension, shortness of breath, edema of feet and ankles, blepharospasm, erythromelalgia, skin mottling, nasal stuffiness, paresthesia, skin rash, signs and symptoms of ergotism.

Drug Interactions

Alcohol	↑ Chance of GI toxicity; alcohol intolerance
Antihypertensives	Additive ↓ in blood pressure
Butyrophenones	↓ Effect of bromocriptine because butyrophenones are dopamine antagonists
Diuretics	Should be avoided during bromocriptine therapy
Phenothiazines	↓ Effect of bromocriptine because phenothiazines are dopamine antagonists

Laboratory Test Interference: ↑ BUN, SGOT, SGPT, GGPT, CPT, alkaline phosphatase, uric acid.

Dosage: Capsules, Tablets. *Amenorrhea/galactorrhea/female or male infertility due to hyperprolactinemia:* **Adults, initial,** 1.25–2.5 mg daily with meals; **then,** increase dose by 2.5 mg q 3–7 days until optimum response observed (usual: 5–7.5 mg daily; range: 2.5–15 mg daily). For amenorrhea/galactorrhea, do not use for more than 6 months. *Prevention of physiological lactation:* (begin no sooner than 4 hr after delivery): usual, 2.5 mg b.i.d. with meals; therapy should be continued for 14–21 days. *Parkinsonism:* **Initial,** 1.25 mg (one-half tablet) b.i.d. with meals while maintaining dose of levodopa, if possible. Dosage may be increased q 14–28 days by 2.5 mg/day with meals. Dose should not exceed 100 mg/day. *Acromegaly:* **initial,** 1.25–2.5 mg for 3 days with food and on retiring; **then,** increased by 1.25–2.5 mg q 3–7 days until optimum response observed. Usual optimum therapeutic range: 20–30 mg daily, not to exceed 100 mg daily. Patients should be reevaluated monthly and dosage adjusted accordingly.

NURSING CONSIDERATIONS

Administration/Storage

1. Before administering the first dose of drug, have the client lie down. This is due to the possibility of fainting or dizziness.
2. For doses less than 5 mg, tablets should be used.

Assessment

1. In taking a drug history, inquire about any sensitivity to ergot alkaloids.
2. Note the age of the client, if she is female and sexually active and likely to become pregnant.
3. If the client has any history of liver or kidney dysfunction, obtain baseline liver and renal function studies.
4. List other drugs the client is taking to determine the potential for drug interactions.

Interventions

Observe the client for complaints of fatigue, headache, nausea, drowsiness, cramps or diarrhea. Document and report these findings to the physician.

Client/Family Teaching

1. Advise client to take the drug with food to minimize GI upset.
2. Caution that drug may cause dizziness, drowsiness or syncope. If clients experience syncope or dizziness, instruct them to lie down. Advise clients to avoid activities that require mental alertness.
3. If the client is using oral contraceptives, advise her to use other contraceptive measures while taking bromocriptine.
4. When a menstrual period is missed, schedule the sexually active client for pregnancy tests every 4 weeks during the period of amenorrhea and after resumption of menses.
5. Discuss with the client the signs and symptoms of pregnancy. If there is a likelihood of pregnancy, advise withholding the drug and reporting to the physician. Explain that pregnancy tests may fail to diagnose early pregnancy and the medication may harm the fetus.

CARBIDOPA   (KAR-bih-doh-pah)
Lodosyn (Rx)

CARBIDOPA/LEVODOPA   (KAR-bih-doh-pah/LEE-voh-doh-pah)
Sinemet-10/100, -25/100, or -25/250 (Rx)

Classification: Antiparkinson agent.

Action/Kinetics: Carbidopa inhibits peripheral decarboxylation of levodopa but not central decarboxylation, since it does not cross the blood-brain barrier. Since peripheral decarboxylation is inhibited, this allows more levodopa to be available for transport to the brain, where it will be converted to dopamine, thus relieving the symptoms of parkinsonism. It is recommended that both carbidopa and levodopa be given together (e.g., Sinemet). However, *the dosage of levodopa must be reduced by up to 80% when combined with carbidopa.* This decreases the incidence of levodopa-induced side effects. *Note:* Pyridoxine will not reverse the action of carbidopa/levodopa. **$t\frac{1}{2}$, carbidopa:** 1–2 hr; when given with levodopa, the $t\frac{1}{2}$ of levodopa increases from 1 hr to 2 hr (may be as high as 15 hr in some patients). About 30% carbidopa is excreted unchanged in the urine.

Uses: All types of parkinsonism. *Investigational:* Postanoxic intention myoclonus. See *Levodopa,* p. 688.**Warning:** Levodopa must be discontinued at least 8 hr before carbidopa/levodopa therapy is initiated. Also, patients taking carbidopa/levodopa must not take levodopa concomitantly, because the former is a combination of carbidopa and levodopa.

Contraindications: See *Levodopa,* p. 688.History of melanoma. MAO inhibitors should be stopped 2 weeks before therapy. Lactation.

Special Concerns: Use during pregnancy only if benefits outweigh risks. Safety and efficacy in children less than 18 years of age have not been determined. Lower doses may be necessary in geriatric patients due to reduced tolerance for side effects.

Side Effects: See *Levodopa,* p. 688. Also, because more levodopa reaches the brain, dyskinesias may occur at lower doses with carbidopa/levodopa than with levodopa alone. Patients abruptly withdrawn from levodopa may experience neuroleptic malignant-like syndrome including symptoms of muscular rigidity, hyperthermia, increased serum phosphokinase, and changes in mental status.

Drug Interactions: Use with tricyclic antidepressants may cause hypertension and dyskinesia.

Dosage: Tablets. Individualized. *Patients not receiving levodopa:* **initial,** 1 tablet of 10 mg carbidopa/100 mg levodopa or 25 mg carbidopa/100 mg levodopa t.i.d.; **then,** increase by 1 tablet every 1–2 days until a total of 6 tablets/day is taken. If additional levodopa is required, substitute 1 tablet of 25 mg carbidopa/250 mg levodopa t.i.d.–q.i.d. *Patients receiving levodopa:* **initial,** carbidopa/levodopa dosage should be about 25% of prior levodopa dosage (levodopa dosage is discontinued 8 hr before carbidopa/levodopa is initiated); **then,** adjust dosage as required.

Carbidopa is available alone for patients requiring additional carbidopa, (i.e., inadequate reduction in nausea and vomiting); in such patients, carbidopa may be given at a dose of 25 mg with the first daily dose of carbidopa/levodopa. If necessary, additional carbidopa, at doses of 12.5 or 25 mg, may be given with each dose of carbidopa/levodopa.

NURSING CONSIDERATIONS

Administration

1. Note any potential drug interactions prior to starting drug therapy.
2. Do not administer with levodopa.

Assessment

1. Obtain baseline ECG, vital signs, respiratory assessment and determine level of bladder function.
2. Note any history of cardiovascular disease, cardiac arrhythmias, or chronic obstructive pulmonary disease.
3. Determine the client's usual sleep patterns as baseline data against which to measure possible adverse effects of drug therapy.
4. Assess and document motor function, reflexes, gait, strength of grip and amount of tremor.
5. Observe the extent of the tremors, muscle weakness, muscle rigidity, difficulty walking or changing directions.

Interventions

1. Monitor blood pressure with the client in supine and standing positions to facilitate the detection of postural hypotension.
2. Observe client closely during the dosage adjustment period. Note any involuntary movement that may require dosage reduction.
3. Assess for blepharospasm. This is an early sign of excessive dosage for some clients.
4. To facilitate the client's adjustment to changes in medication, administer the last dose of levodopa at bedtime and start carbidopa/levodopa when the client arises in the morning.

Client/Family Teaching

1. Review the side effects that may occur and advise the client to report these. The physician may reduce the dose of drug or temporarily discontinue the drug. They may also encourage the client to tolerate certain side effects because of the overall benefits gained with therapy.
2. Instruct that as clients improve with drug therapy, they may resume normal activity gradually. Also, remind clients that with increased activity, they must take other medical conditions into consideration.
3. Stress that antiparkinson drugs should not be withdrawn abruptly. When changing medication, one drug should be withdrawn slowly and the other started in small doses under medical supervision.

DIPHENHYDRAMINE HYDROCHLORIDE   (dye-fen-**HI**-drah-meen)

Allerdryl❋, AllerMax, Beldin Cough, Belix, Bena-D, Bena-D 50, Benadryl, Benadryl Complete Allergy, Benahist 10 and 50, Ben-Allergin-50, Benoject-10 and -50, Benylin Cough, Benaphen, Bydramine Cough, Diahist, Dihydrex, Diphenacen-10 and -50, Diphenadryl, Diphen Cough, Fenylhist, Fynex, Hydramine, Hydramine Cough, Hydril, Hyrexin-50, Noradryl, Nordryl, Nordryl Cough, Tusstat, Valdrene, Wehdryl (OTC and Rx).

Sleep-Aids: Compoz, Dormarex 2, Insomnal❋, Nervine Nighttime Sleep-Aid, Nytol with DPH, Sleep-Eze 3, Sominex 2, Twilite (OTC)

See also *Antihistamines,* p. 1003, *Antiemetics,* p. 1076, and *Antiparkinson Agents,* p. 681.

Classification: Antihistamine, antiemetic (ethanolamine type).

Additional Uses: Treatment of parkinsonism in geriatric patients unable to tolerate more potent drugs. Also for mild parkinsonism in other age groups. Drug-induced extrapyramidal symptoms. Motion sickness, antiemetic, as a sleep-aid. Coughs, including those due to allergy.

Special Concerns: Pregnancy category: B.

Dosage: Capsules, Elixir, Syrup, Tablets. *Antihistamine, antiemetic, antimotion sickness, parkinsonism:* **Adults,** 25–50 mg t.i.d.–q.i.d.; **pediatric, over 9 kg:** 12.5–25 mg t.i.d.–q.i.d. (or 5 mg/kg/day not to exceed 300 mg daily). *Sleep aid:* **Adults,** 50 mg at bedtime. *Antitussive:* **Adults,** 25 mg q 4 hr, not to exceed 150 mg daily; **pediatric, 6–12 years:** 12.5 mg q 4 hr, not to exceed 75 mg daily; **pediatric, 2–6 years:** 6.25 mg q 4 hr, not to exceed 25 mg daily.

IV, deep IM: Adults 10–50 mg up to 100 mg, not to exceed 400 mg daily; **pediatric:** 5 mg/kg/day, not to exceed 300 mg daily.

NURSING CONSIDERATIONS

See also *Nursing Considerations* for *Antihistamines,* p. 1007, *Antiemetics,* p. 1076, and *Antiparkinson Agents,* p. 681.

Administration/Storage

For motion sickness, the full prophylactic dose should be given 30 min prior to travel with similar doses administered with meals and at bedtime.

LEVODOPA   (**LEE**-voh-doh-pah)

Dopar, Larodopa, L-Dopa (Rx)

Classification: Antiparkinson agent.

Action/Kinetics: Levodopa, a dopamine precursor, is able to cross the blood-brain barrier to enter the CNS. It is decarboxylated to dopamine in the basal ganglia, thus replenishing depleted dopamine stores. **Peak plasma levels:** 1–2 hr (may be delayed if ingested with food). $t^{1/2}$: 1–3 hr. Onset occurs in 2–3 weeks although some patients may require up to 6 months. Levodopa is extensively metabolized both in the GI tract and the liver and metabolites are excreted in the urine.

Uses: Idiopathic, arteriosclerotic, or postencephalitic parkinsonism. Parkinsonism due to carbon monoxide or manganese intoxication. Levodopa only provides symptomatic relief and does not alter the course of the disease. When effective it relieves rigidity, bradykinesia, tremors, dysphagia, seborrhea, sialorrhea, and postural instability. Used in combination with carbidopa. *Investigational:* Pain from herpes zoster.

Contraindications: Concomitant use with monoamine oxidase inhibitors. History of melanoma or in patients with undiagnosed skin lesions. Lactation. Hypersensitivity to drug, narrow-angle glaucoma, blood dyscrasias, hypertension, coronary sclerosis.

Special Concerns: Use with extreme caution in patients with history of myocardial infarctions, convulsions, arrhythmias, bronchial asthma, emphysema, active peptic ulcer, psychosis or neurosis, wide-angle glaucoma. Use during pregnancy only if benefits clearly outweigh risks. Safety has not been established in children less than 12 years of age. Geriatric patients may require a lower dose as they have a reduced tolerance for the drug and its side effects (including cardiac effects). Patients may experience an "on-off" phenomenon in which patients experience an improved clinical status followed by loss of therapeutic effect.

Side Effects: The side effects of levodopa are numerous and usually dose-related. Some may abate with usage. *CNS:* Choreiform and/or dystonic movements, paranoid ideation, psychotic episodes, depression (with possibility of suicidal tendencies), dementia, seizures (rare), dizziness, headache, faintness, confusion, insomnia, nightmares, hallucinations, delusions, agitation, anxiety, malaise, fatigue, euphoria. *GI:* GI bleeding, development of duodenal ulcer, nausea, vomiting, anorexia, abdominal pain, dry mouth, sialorrhea, hiccups, diarrhea, constipation, burning sensation of tongue, bitter taste, flatulence, weight gain or loss. *CV:* Cardiac irregularities, palpitations, orthostatic hypotension, hypertension, phlebitis, hot flashes. *Ophthalmologic:* Diplopia, dilated pupils, blurred vision, development of Horner's syndrome, oculogyric crisis. *Hematologic:* Hemolytic anemia, agranulocytosis, leukopenia. *Musculoskeletal:* Muscle twitching, tonic contraction of the muscles of mastication, increased hand tremor, ataxia. *Miscellaneous:* Urinary retention, urinary incontinence, increased sweating, unusual breathing patterns, weakness, numbness, bruxism, blepharospasm, alopecia, priapism, hoarseness, edema, dark sweat and/or urine.

Levodopa interacts with many other drugs (see below) and must be administered cautiously.

Drug Interactions	
Amphetamines	Levodopa potentiates the effect of indirectly acting sympathomimetics
Antacids	↑ Effect of levodopa due to ↑ absorption from GI tract
Anticholinergic drugs	Possible ↓ effect of levodopa due to ↑ breakdown of levodopa in stomach (due to delayed gastric emptying time)
Antidepressants, tricyclic	↓ Effect of levodopa due to ↓ absorption from GI tract; also, ↑ risk of hypertension
Clonidine	↓ Effect of levodopa
Digoxin	↓ Effect of digoxin
Ephedrine	Levodopa potentiates the effect of indirectly acting sympathomimetics
Furazolidone	↑ Effect of levodopa due to ↓ breakdown by liver
Guanethidine	↑ Hypotensive effect of guanethidine
Hypoglycemic drugs	Levodopa upsets diabetic control with hypoglycemic agents
MAO inhibitors	Concomitant administration may result in hypertension, lightheadedness, and flushing due to ↓ breakdown of dopamine and norepinephrine formed from levodopa
Methyldopa	Additive effects including hypotension

Drug Interactions

Metoclopramide	↑ Bioavailability of levodopa
Papaverine	↓ Effect of levodopa
Phenothiazines	↓ Effect of levodopa due to ↓ uptake of dopamine into neurons
Phenytoin	Phenytoin antagonizes the effect of levodopa
Propranolol	Propranolol may antagonize the hypotensive and positive inotropic effect of levodopa
Pyridoxine	Pyridoxine reverses levodopa-induced improvement in Parkinson's disease
Reserpine	Reserpine inhibits response to levodopa by ↓ dopamine in the brain
Thioxanthines	↓ Effect of levodopa in Parkinson patients
Tricyclic antidepressants	↓ Absorption of levodopa → ↓ effect

Laboratory Test Interferences: ↑ BUN, SGOT, LDH, SGPT, bilirubin, alkaline phosphatase, protein-bound iodine. ↓ Hemoglobin, hematocrit, white blood cells. False + Coombs' test. Interference with tests for urinary glucose and ketones.

Dosage: Capsules, Tablets. Adults, initial: 250 mg b.i.d.–q.i.d. taken with food; **then,** increase total daily dose by 100–750 mg q 3–7 days until optimum dosage reached (should not exceed 8 g/day). Up to 6 months may be required to achieve a significant therapeutic effect.

NURSING CONSIDERATIONS

See also *Nursing Considerations* for *Cholinergic Blocking Agents* under *Antiparkinson Agents,* p. 693.

Administration/Storage

1. Administer to clients unable to swallow tablets or capsules by crushing tablets or emptying the capsule into a small amount of fruit juice at the time of administration.
2. Levodopa is often administered together with an anticholinergic agent.

Assessment

1. Obtain baseline ECG, complete blood count, liver and renal function studies and protein bound iodine tests prior to beginning therapy.
2. Review the client's medical history for contraindications to the drug therapy.

Interventions

1. Monitor vital signs, CBC, liver and renal function studies throughout drug therapy, especially during long-term therapy.
2. If the client is to have surgery, check with the physician to determine if the drug is to be stopped 24 hours before surgery. Also, determine when the drug is to be restarted following surgery.
3. Observe and document any signs of the client becoming depressed, psychotic or exhibiting any other unusual behavioral changes.
4. Offer emotional support and encouragement throughout the therapy.

Client/Family Teaching

1. Take levodopa with food.
2. Report the occurrence of headaches since these may indicate drug-induced glaucoma.

3. Stress that dosage of drug is not to exceed 8 g daily.

4. Advise clients to avoid taking multivitamin preparations containing 10–25 mg of vitamin B_6. This vitamin rapidly reverses the antiparkinson effect of levodopa.

5. Significant results may take up to 6 months to be realized. Therefore, instruct client to continue taking the drug even though immediate results are not evident.

6. Instruct the client and family how to take blood pressure and pulse readings and to monitor these during drug therapy. Provide parameters for which the physician should be notified.

7. Warn clients that their sweat and urine may appear dark. This is not harmful.

8. Male clients need to be warned that priapism may occur. This should be reported to the physician.

9. Stress the importance of reporting for all scheduled lab and medical visits so that the effectiveness of drug therapy can be evaluated and adjusted as needed.

PERGOLIDE MESYLATE   (PER-go-lyd)

Permax (Rx)

Classification: Antiparkinson agent.

Action/Kinetics: Pergolide is a potent dopamine receptor (both D_1 and D_2) agonist. The drug is believed to act by directly stimulating postsynaptic dopamine receptors in the nigrostriatal system, thus relieving symptoms of parkinsonism. The drug also inhibits prolactin secretion, causes a transient rise in serum levels of growth hormone, and a decrease in serum levels of luteinizing hormone. About 90% of the drug is bound to plasma proteins. The drug is metabolized in the liver and excreted through the urine.

Uses: Adjunctive treatment to levodopa/carbidopa in Parkinson's disease.

Special Concerns: Use during pregnancy only if clearly needed (pregnancy category: B). Benefit versus risk should be assessed when considered for use during lactation. Use with caution in patients prone to cardiac arrhythmias, in preexisting dyskinesia, and preexisting states of confusion or hallucinations. Safety and efficacy have not been determined in children.

Side Effects: The most common untoward reactions are listed.
   CV: Postural hypotension, palpitation, vasodilation, syncope, hypotension, hypertension, arrhythmias, myocardial infarction. *GI:* Nausea (common), vomiting, diarrhea, constipation, dyspepsia, anorexia, dry mouth. *CNS:* Dyskinesia (common), dizziness, dystonia, hallucinations, confusion, insomnia, somnolence, anxiety, tremor, depression, abnormal dreams, psychosis, personality disorder, extrapyramidal syndrome, akathisia, paresthesia, incoordination, akinesia, neuralgia, hypertonia, speech disorders. *Musculoskeletal:* Arthralgia, bursitis, twitching, myalgia. *Respiratory:* Rhinitis, dyspnea, hiccup, epistaxis. *Dermatologic:* Sweating, rash. *Ophthalmologic:* Abnormal vision, double vision, eye disorders. *GU:* Urinary tract infection, urinary frequency, hematuria. *Whole body:* Pain in chest, abdomen, neck, or back; headache, asthenia, flu syndrome, chills, facial edema, infection. *Miscellaneous:* Taste alteration, peripheral edema, anemia, weight gain.

Drug Interactions	
Butyrophenones	↓ Effect of pergolide due to dopamine antagonist effect
Metoclopramide	↓ Effect of pergolide due to dopamine antagonist effect

Drug Interactions

Phenothiazines	↓ Effect of pergolide due to dopamine antagonist effect
Thioxanthines	↓ Effect of pergolide due to dopamine antagonist effect

Dosage: Tablets. Adults, initial: 0.05 mg daily for the first two days; **then,** increase dose gradually by 0.1 or 0.15 mg/day every third day over the next 12 days. The dosage may then be increased by 0.25 mg/day every third day until the therapeutic dosage level is reached. The mean therapeutic daily dosage is 3 mg daily used concurrently with levodopa/carbidopa (expressed as levodopa) at a dose of 650 mg daily. The effectiveness of doses of pergolide greater than 5 mg daily has not been evaluated.

NURSING CONSIDERATIONS

Administration/Storage

1. Pergolide is usually given in divided doses 3 times daily.
2. When determining the therapeutic dose for pergolide, the dosage of concurrent levodopa/carbidopa may be decreased cautiously.

Client/Family Teaching

1. Pergolide is to be taken concurrently with a prescribed dose of levodopa/carbidopa.
2. Do not exceed prescribed daily dose.
3. Review the list of side effects associated with pergolide therapy and instruct the client and family to report any persistent and/or bothersome symptoms.
4. Remind client to rise slowly from a sitting or lying position to minimize hypotensive effects of drug therapy.
5. Stress the importance of reporting for all scheduled lab and medical appointments so that drug therapy may be evaluated and adjusted as needed.

SELEGILINE HYDROCHLORIDE   (seh-**LEH**-jih-leen)

Eldepryl (Rx)

Classification: Antiparkinson agent.

Action/Kinetics: Although the precise mechanism of action is not known, selegiline is known to inhibit monoamine oxidase, type B. Also, selegiline may act through other mechanisms to increase dopaminergic activity.

Uses: Adjunct in the treatment of Parkinson's disease in patients being treated with levodopa/carbidopa who have manifested a decreased response to this therapy. **Note:** There is no evidence that selegiline is effective in patients not taking levodopa.

Contraindications: Hypersensitivity to the drug. Doses greater than 10 mg daily.

Special Concerns: Pregnancy category: C. Use with caution during lactation. Safety and efficacy in children have not been established.

Side Effects: *CNS:* Dizziness, lightheadedness, fainting, confusion, hallucinations, vivid dreams/

nightmares, headache, anxiety, drowsiness, depression, mood changes, delusions, fatigue, disorientation, apathy, malaise, vertigo, overstimulation, sleep disturbance, transient irritability, weakness. *Skeletal muscle:* Tremor, chorea, loss of balance, blepharospasm, increased bradykinesia, facial grimace, dystonic symptoms, tardive dyskinesia, dyskinesia, involuntary movements, muscle cramps, heavy leg, falling down, stiff neck, freezing, festination, increased apraxia. *Altered sensations/pain:* Headache, tinnitus, migraine, back or leg pain, supraorbital pain, burning throat, chills, numbness of fingers/toes, taste disturbance, generalized aches. *CV:* Orthostatic hypotension, hypertension, arrhythmia, angina pectoris, palpitations, hypotension, tachycardia, syncope, peripheral edema, sinus bradycardia. *GI:* Nausea, vomiting, constipation, anorexia, weight loss, dry mouth, poor appetite, dysphagia, diarrhea, rectal bleeding, heartburn. *GU:* Nocturia, slow urination, urinary hesitancy or retention, prostatic hypertrophy, urinary frequency. *Miscellaneous:* Blurred vision, sexual dysfunction, increased sweating, diaphoresis, facial hair, hair loss, rash, photosensitivity, hematoma, asthma, diplopia, shortness of breath, speech affected.

Drug Interactions: Drugs inhibiting monoamine oxidase are often contraindicated for use with meperidine or other opioids.

Dosage: Tablets. Adults: 5 mg taken at breakfast and lunch, not to exceed 10 mg daily.

NURSING CONSIDERATIONS

Administration/Storage

1. No evidence exists that doses higher than 10 mg daily will result in additional beneficial effects.
2. Following 2 or 3 days of selegiline therapy, attempts may be made to decrease the dose of levodopa/carbidopa (10%–30%).

Client/Family Teaching

1. Selegiline is to be taken concurrently with prescribed dose of levodopa/carbidopa.
2. Do not exceed prescribed daily dose.
3. Review list of side effects associated with drug therapy and instruct client and family to report any bothersome and/or persistent symptoms.
4. Remind client to rise slowly from a sitting or lying position in order to minimize the hypotensive effects of drug therapy.

CHOLINERGIC BLOCKING AGENTS USED TO TREAT PARKINSONISM

Action/Kinetics: The cholinergic blocking agents prevent the neurotransmitter acetylcholine from combining with central cholinergic receptors located in the striatum. This results in a balance between cholinergic and dompaminergic activity in the basal ganglia. In therapeutic doses these drugs have little effect on transmission of nerve impulses across ganglia (nicotinic sites) or at the neuromuscular junction.

The main effects of cholinergic blocking agents are:

1. to reduce spasms of smooth muscles like those controlling the urinary bladder or spasms of bronchial and intestinal smooth muscle.
2. to block vagal impulses to the heart, resulting in an increase in the rate and speed of impulse conduction through the atrioventricular conducting system.

3. to suppress or decrease gastric secretions, perspiration, salivation, and secretion of bronchial mucus.
4. to relax the sphincter muscles of the iris and cause pupillary dilation (mydriasis) and loss of accommodation for near vision (cycloplegia).
5. to act in diverse ways on the CNS, producing such reactions as depression (scopolamine) or stimulation (toxic doses of atropine). Many of the anticholinergic drugs also have antiparkinsonism effects. They abolish or reduce the signs and symptoms of Parkinson's disease, such as tremors and rigidity, and result in some improvement in mobility, muscular coordination, and motor performance. These effects may be due to blockade of the effects of acetylcholine in the CNS. This section also discusses miscellaneous synthetic antispasmodics related to anticholinergic drugs.

The anticholinergics that are related to atropine are quickly absorbed following oral ingestion. These agents cross the blood-brain barrier and may exert significant CNS effects. Examples of these drugs are scopolamine, *l*-hyoscyamine, and belladonna alkaloids. The drugs classified as quaternary ammonium anticholinergic drugs are erratically absorbed from the GI tract and exert minimal CNS effects, since they do not cross the blood-brain barrier. Examples of these drugs are glycopyrrolate, methantheline, propantheline, tridihexethyl chloride, clidinium bromide, isopropamide, and others.

Uses: See individual drugs.

Contraindications: Glaucoma, tachycardia, partial obstruction of the GI and biliary tracts, prostatic hypertrophy, renal disease, myasthenia gravis, hepatic disease, paralytic ileus, intestinal atony, ulcerative colitis, obstructive uropathy. Cardiac patients, especially when there is danger of tachycardia; older persons suffering from atherosclerosis or mental impairment.

Special Concerns: Use with caution in pregnancy (pregnancy category: C) and lactation. Use with caution in hyperthyroidism, congestive heart failure, cardiac arrhythmias, hypertension, Down's syndrome, asthma, allergies, and chronic lung disease. Safety and efficacy have not been shown in children who may be more sensitive to the anticholinergic effects of these drugs. Geriatric patients (especially those with arteriosclerotic changes) may manifest impaired memory, mental confusion, agitation, disorientation, agitation, hallucinations, and psychoses.

Side Effects: These are desirable in some conditions and undesirable in others. Thus, the anticholinergics have an antisalivary effect that is useful in parkinsonism. This same effect is unpleasant when the drug is used for spastic conditions of the GI tract.

Most untoward reactions are dose-related and decrease when dosage decreases. Sometimes it helps to discontinue the medication for several days. With this in mind, anticholinergic drugs have the following untoward reactions. *GI:* Nausea, vomiting, dry mouth, dysphagia, constipation, heartburn, change in taste perception, paralytic ileus. *CNS:* Dizziness, drowsiness, nervousness, disorientation, headache, weakness, insomnia, fever. Large doses may produce CNS stimulation including tremor and restlessness. *GU:* Urinary retention or hesitancy, impotence. *Ophthalmologic:* Blurred vision, dilated pupils, photophobia, cycloplegia, precipitation of acute glaucoma. *Allergic:* Urticaria, skin rashes, anaphylaxis. *Other:* Flushing, decreased sweating, nasal congestion, suppression of glandular secretions including lactation.

Belladonna Poisoning: Infants and children are especially susceptible to the toxic effects of atropine and scopolamine. Poisoning (dose dependent) is characterized by the following symptoms: dry mouth, burning sensation of the mouth, difficulty in swallowing and speaking, blurred vision, photophobia, rash, tachycardia, increased respiration, increased body temperature (up to 109°F, 42.7°C), restlessness, irritability, confusion, muscle incoordination, dilated pupils, hot dry skin, respiratory depression and paralysis, tremors, seizures, hallucinations, and death.

Treatment of Belladonna Poisoning: *After PO intake:* gastric lavage or induction of vomiting followed by activated charcoal.

Systemic antidote: physostigmine (Eserine), 1–3 mg IV (effectiveness uncertain; thus use other agents if possible). Neostigmine methylsulfate, 0.5–2 mg IV, repeated as necessary. If there is excitation, diazepam or a short-acting barbiturate may be given. For fever, cool baths may be used. Keep patient in a darkened room if photophobia is manifested.

Drug Interactions

Amantadine	Additive anticholinergic side effects
Antacids	↓ Absorption of anticholinergics from GI tract
Antidepressants, tricyclic	Additive anticholinergic side effects
Antihistamines	Additive anticholinergic side effects
Benzodiazepines	Additive anticholinergic side effects
Corticosteroids	Additive increase in intraocular pressure
Cyclopropane	↑ Chance of ventricular arrhythmias
Digoxin	↑ Effect of digoxin due to ↑ absorption from GI tract
Disopyramide	Potentiation of anticholinergic side effects
Guanethidine	Reversal of inhibition of gastric acid secretion caused by anticholinergics
Haloperidol	Additive increase in intraocular pressure; also, ↑ in symptoms of schizophrenia
Histamine	Reversal of inhibition of gastric acid secretion caused by anticholinergics
Levodopa	Possible ↓ effect of levodopa due to ↑ breakdown of levodopa in stomach (due to delayed gastric emptying time)
Meperidine	Additive anticholinergic side effects
Methylphenidate	Potentiation of anticholinergic side effects
Metoclopramide	Anticholinergics block action of metoclopramide
Monoamine oxidase inhibitors	↑ Effects of anticholinergics due to ↓ breakdown by liver
Nitrates, nitrites	Potentiation of anticholinergic side effects
Nitrofurantoin	↑ Bioavailability of nitrofurantoin
Orphenadrine	Additive anticholinergic side effects
Phenothiazines	Additive anticholinergic side effects; also, ↓ effect of phenothiazines
Primidone	Potentiation of anticholinergic side effects
Procainamide	Additive anticholinergic side effects
Quinidine	Additive anticholinergic side effects
Reserpine	Reversal of inhibition of gastric acid secretion caused by anticholinergics
Sympathomimetics	↑ Bronchial relaxation
Thiazide diuretics	↑ Bioavailability of thiazide diuretics
Thioxanthines	Potentiation of anticholinergic side effects

Dosage: See individual agents. The agents are usually initiated at low dosage and increased gradually, until optimum levels have been reached. Excessive untoward reactions can often be corrected by decrease in dosage. Agent should not be discontinued abruptly, but decreased gradually while another drug with the same effect is introduced slowly.

NURSING CONSIDERATIONS

Administration/Storage

1. Cholinergic blocking agents may increase the risk of heat stroke when taken in hot weather.
2. May be given alone or with other anticholinergic agents.
3. Initial dosage of drug is usually low, and increased gradually until an optimum level is attained.
4. Review the list of drugs with which anticholinergic agents interact.
5. Clients may take the drugs before or after meals depending on their reactions.

Assessment

1. Determine if the client has any prior history of adverse reactions to anticholinergic medications.
2. Note any history of cardiac disease or respiratory problems such as asthma. Clients with these problems are at risk for adverse reactions to anticholinergic agents.
3. Check client history for evidence of glaucoma, pyloric obstruction, obstruction of the intestines or urinary tract. These are contraindications for anticholinergic medications.
4. Review the impact of Parkinson's disease on the client's ability to perform activities of daily living such as feeding, swallowing, ambulation, etc.
5. Observe and document the extent of the client's tremors, muscle weakness, muscle rigidity or akinesia. Listen to the sound of the client's voice as he/she speaks.
6. Evaluate the client's motor functioning, mental status and control of autonomic functioning.
7. Obtain complete laboratory tests including CBC, serum liver enzymes, liver and renal function studies, as well as a record of vital signs, ECG, respiratory assessment and determine bladder function prior to initiating therapy. These may be used as baseline information against which to measure medication responses.

Interventions

1. Check dosage of drugs and provide exact measurement as ordered. Some of the drugs in this category are prescribed in small amounts. Overdosage may occur easily and can lead to toxicity.
2. Note and record any complaints of epigastric distress, nausea or vomiting. These may indicate G I problems which would require a change in the drug regimen.
3. Observe clients for symptoms of biliary obstruction, such as gray stools, jaundice, or yellowing of the skin and sclera. Document and report.
4. Obese clients have more problems with the regulation of drug dosage. Monitor these clients closely and report any problems to the physician.
5. Monitor for excessive intake of foods rich in pyridoxine, such as lima beans, navy beans and kidney beans. These foods may lead to antagonism of anticholinergic drugs.
6. Be alert for drug interactions that may require a reduction in dosage of medication.

Client/Family Teaching

1. If their mouth is dry, instruct clients to practice frequent mouth care, drink cold fluids, and chew sugarless gum.
2. Review with the client and family side effects that may occur. These should be reported to the physician so that the symptoms can be alleviated either by reducing the dosage of drug or temporarily taking the client off the drug. (Sometimes clients may be expected to tolerate certain side effects such as dry mouth or blurred vision because of the beneficial effects gained from drug therapy.)

3. In clients with glaucoma that still must receive the medication, explain to the client and family the signs and symptoms that indicate the drug should be withheld. These symptoms should be reported to the physician.

4. Photophobia can be relieved by wearing dark glasses.

5. Stress the importance of maintaining the dietary regimen prescribed by the physician. Provide guidance and printed instructions to help the client understand and plan meals.

6. Some clients experience muscle weakness, elevated body temperature, sweating and disorientation. Caution clients and family concerning these potential problems and advise them to avoid excessive heat. Elderly clients may easily develop heat prostration.

7. Client should be warned to avoid taking hot baths or showers and to avoid sunlight. Anticholinergic agents diminish perspiration and predispose clients to heat exhaustion.

8. Since anticholinergic drugs can cause orthostatic hypotension, warn clients to avoid rapid changes in position or prolonged periods of standing.

9. Advise clients to have a yearly ophthalmic evaluation as a precaution against drug induced glaucoma.

10. Teach the signs and symptoms of paralytic ileus, such as persistent constipation or abdominal distention. These should be reported to the physician immediately.

11. Take medication with food or with meals to minimize gastric irritation.

12. Explain to clients who have G.I. pathology how to maintain the prescribed diet and to continue to take other medications as prescribed.

13. Discuss the need to void prior to taking each dose of medication to minimize problems of urinary hesitancy or dysuria.

14. Warn that anticholinergic agents may cause drowsiness and mental confusion. Therefore, clients should avoid activities that require mental alertness such as driving or operating equipment.

15. Emotional swings are common and explain to the family that the client has little or no control over the problem.

16. Male clients should be warned of the potential for impotence. If this develops it should be reported to the physician.

17. Stress the need for the client to remain socially active and discuss the importance of maintaining mental stimulation.

18. Antiparkinsonism drugs are not to be withdrawn abruptly. Consult prescribing physician before discontinuing drug therapy.

Evaluation

1. Assess client/family knowledge and understanding of illness, response to therapy and to teaching.

2. Observe for freedom from complications of drug therapy.

3. Compare client responses and lab data with the baseline data collected at the beginning of therapy.

BENZTROPINE MESYLATE   (bens-**TROH**-peen)

Apo-Benztropine ✳, Benzylate ✳, Cogentin, PMS Benztropine ✳ (Rx)

See also *Cholinergic Blocking Agents,* p. 942.

Classification: Antiparkinson agent, synthetic anticholinergic.

Action/Kinetics: Benztropine is a synthetic anticholinergic possessing antihistamine and local anesthetic properties. **Onset, PO:** 1–2 hr; **IM, IV:** within a few minutes. Its effects are cumulative, and it is long-acting (24 hr). Full effects are manifested in 2 to 3 days. The drug produces a low incidence of side effects.

Uses: As adjunct in the treatment of parkinsonism (all types). Used to reduce severity of extrapyramidal effects in phenothiazine or other antipsychotic drug therapy (not effective in tardive dyskinesia).

Special Concerns: Pregnancy category: C. Not recommended for children under three years of age.

Dosage: Tablets, (rarely IV or IM). *Parkinsonism:* 0.5–6 mg daily. *Drug-induced parkinsonism:* **initial,** 0.5 mg daily, increased gradually to 1–4 mg 1 or 2 times daily. *Drug-induced extrapyramidal effects:* 1–4 mg 1–2 times daily. *Acute dystonic reactions:* **IM, IV,** 1–2 mg. Patients can rarely tolerate full dosage.

NURSING CONSIDERATIONS

See also *Nursing Considerations* for *Cholinergic Blocking Agents,* p. 949.

Administration/Storage

1. When used as replacement for or supplement to other antiparkinsonism drugs, substitute or add gradually.
2. For clients who have difficulty swallowing tablets, the tablets may be crushed and mixed with a small amount of food or liquid.
3. If the drug is to be administered IV, it may be given undiluted at a rate of 1 mg/min or less.

Assessment

1. When taking the client's drug history note if phenothiazine or tricyclic antidepressants are being used. These drugs when taken with benztropine mesylate can cause a paralytic ileus.
2. Assess for any evidence of medical conditions that would preclude beginning the drug therapy.
3. Note the age of the client. Anticipate that elderly clients will require a lower dosage of the drug.

Interventions

1. If the client develops excitation or vomiting, the drug may need to be withdrawn temporarily. When treatment is resumed the dosage should be lowered.
2. Monitor intake and output. Auscultate for bowel sounds. This is especially important if the client has limited mobility.
3. Inspect the client's skin at regular intervals for any evidence of skin changes.

Client/Family Teaching

1. Review the goals of therapy and the possible side effects.
2. Use caution when performing tasks that require mental alertness as drug has a sedative effect.
3. Remind clients that it usually takes 2–3 days for the drug to have a desired effect. The drug should be taken as ordered unless side effects occur. These then should be reported to the physician before interrupting drug therapy.
4. Reassure clients that side effects usually subside with continued use of the drug.
5. Advise clients that their ability to tolerate heat will be reduced. Therefore, they should avoid heat and plan rest periods during the day.

6. Instruct clients to report any difficulty in voiding or inadequate emptying of the bladder.
7. Avoid the use of alcoholic beverages.

Evaluation

1. Review goals of therapy with the client and family and determine if attained.
2. Note any changes in the client's tremors and rigidity.

BIPERIDEN HYDROCHLORIDE   (bye-PER-ih-den)

Akineton Hydrochloride (Rx)

BIPERIDEN LACTATE   (bye-PER-ih-den LAK-tayt)

Akineton Lactate (Rx)

See also *Antiparkinson Agents,* p. 681, and *Cholinergic Blocking Agents,* p. 942.

Classification: Antiparkinson agent, synthetic anticholinergic.

Action/Kinetics: Tolerance may develop to this synthetic anticholinergic. Tremor may increase as spasticity is relieved. The drug has slight respiratory and cardiovascular effects. **Time to peak levels:** 60–90 min. **Peak levels:** 4–5 mcg/L. **$t^{1/2}$:** About 18–24 hr.

Uses: Parkinsonism, especially of the postencephalitic, arteriosclerotic, and idiopathic types. Drug-induced (e.g., phenothiazines) extrapyramidal manifestations.

Additional Contraindications: Children under the age of 3 years.

Special Concerns: Pregnancy category: C. Use with caution in older children.

Additional Side Effects: Muscle weakness, inability to move certain muscles.

Dosage: Tablets (Hydrochloride). *Parkinsonism,* **Adults:** 2 mg t.i.d.–q.i.d.; *Drug-induced extrapyramidal effects:* 2 mg 1–3 times/day. Maximum daily dose: 16 mg. **IM, Slow IV (Lactate).** *Drug-induced extrapryamidal effects:* **Adults,** 2 mg; repeat q 30 min until symptoms improve, but not more than 4 doses/day. **Pediatric:** 0.04 mg/kg (1.2 mg/m²) repeat q 30 min until symptoms improve, but not more than 4 doses/day.

NURSING CONSIDERATIONS

See also *Nursing Considerations* for *Cholinergic Blocking Agents,* p. 949.

Administration/Storage

1. Administer after meals to avoid gastric irritation.
2. Note other drugs the client is taking and compare with the list of drugs with which biperiden lactate interacts.

Assessment

Note the client's age. Older clients should receive lower doses of the medication.

Interventions

1. Keep a record of stools. Encourage the client to increase the intake of fluids and fruit juices to avoid constipation.
2. If the drug is administered IV, have the client remain recumbent during the procedure and for

15 minutes after it is completed. Once the IV is finished, assist clients to get up by having them dangle their legs at the bedside prior to standing and walking, in order to lower the potential for hypotension, syncope, and falling.

3. If the drug is administered IM, assist the client in walking because of the possibility of transient incoordination.

4. Monitor and record intake and output.

ETHOPROPAZINE HYDROCHLORIDE   (eh-thoh-**PROH**-pah-zeen)

Parsidol, Parsitan ✿ (Rx)

Classification: Antiparkinson agent, synthetic anticholinergic of the phenothiazine type.

Action/Kinetics: This synthetic anticholinergic is considered by some to be a drug of choice for treatment of major tremors of parkinsonism. Ethopropazine also manifests antihistaminic, local anesthetic, and CNS depressant effects. **Onset:** 30 min. **Duration:** 4 hr. The drug produces a high incidence of side effects.

Uses: To treat all types of parkinsonism and drug-induced extrapyramidal symptoms. *Investigational:* Congenital athetosis, heptolenticular degeneration.

Special Concerns: Safe use during pregnancy and lactation has not been established.

Additional Side Effects: Tachycardia, abnormal EEG, agranulocytosis, purpura, pancytopenia, endocrine disturbances, ocular disturbances, hallucinations, jaundice. Parkinsonian symptoms may become exacerbated.

Dosage: Tablets. Adults: initial, 50 mg 1 or 2 times a day; increase by 10 mg per dose q 2 to 3 days until optimum effect or limit of tolerance. **Maintenance:** 100–600 mg daily. Most patients, especially the elderly, cannot tolerate full therapeutic dosage.

NURSING CONSIDERATIONS

See also *Nursing Considerations* for *Cholinergic Blocking Agents* under *Antiparkinson Agents,* p. 693.

Assessment

Obtain a complete blood count and liver function studies to serve as baseline data.

Interventions

1. Monitor vital signs and observe for exacerbation of symptoms.
2. Anticipate that the dosage will be lower for elderly clients.

Evaluation

Evaluate and determine if the client is experiencing a high incidence of side effects. Document and report.

ORPHENADRINE HYDROCHLORIDE   (or-**FEN**-ah-dreen)

Disipal (Rx)

See also *Cholinergic Blocking Agents,* p. 942.

Classification: Antiparkinson agent, anticholinergic.

Action/Kinetics: Orphenadrine improves rigidity but not the tremor of parkinsonism. **Peak effect:** 2 hr. **Duration:** 4–6 hr.

Uses: Adjunct in the treatment of all types of parkinsonism. Drug-induced extrapyramidal reactions.

Additional Contraindications: Glaucoma or myasthenia gravis. Use with caution for patients with tachycardia, signs of urinary retention, or during pregnancy.

Additional Untoward Reactions: Adverse CNS manifestations (dizziness, drowsiness, increased tremor) may be present during initiation but will subside with continuation of usage or reduction in dose. Mild euphoria. Aplastic anemia occurs rarely.

Dosage: Tablets, Adults: 50 mg t.i.d. Doses of up to 250 mg daily have been used without ill effects. Lower doses may be possible in patients using other antiparkinson drugs.

NURSING CONSIDERATIONS

See also *Nursing Considerations* for *Cholinergic Blocking Agents,* p. 949.

Client/Family Teaching

1. Remind client to plan work periods so that work is avoided during the hottest part of the day.
2. Report side effects to the physician. Encourage clients to continue with the medication since side effects usually subside with continued therapy.
3. Remind clients to avoid using any other medications or over-the-counter preparations unless consent has been given by the attending physician.

Evaluation

Assess client for increased tremors or adverse CNS effects that may require decreasing the dosage of drug.

PROCYCLIDINE HYDROCHLORIDE   (pron-**SYE**-klih-deen)

Kemadrin, PMS Procyclidine ✽, Procyclid ✽ (Rx)

See also *Cholinergic Blocking Agents,* p. 942.

Classification: Antiparkinson agent, synthetic anticholinergic.

Action/Kinetics: Procyclidine, a synthetic anticholinergic, appears to be better tolerated by younger patients. It also possesses direct antispasmodic effects on smooth muscle. This drug is often more effective in relieving rigidity than tremor. **Onset:** 30–45 min. **Time to peak levels:** 1–2 hr. **Peak levels:** 80 mcg/L. **t½:** 11.5–12.6 hr. **Duration:** 4–6 hr.

Uses: Treatment of all types of parkinsonism. Drug-induced extrapyramidal symptoms. Control of sialorrhea following neuroleptic drug use.

Special Concerns: Pregnancy category: C.

Additional Drug Interaction: ↑ Effectiveness of levodopa if used together; such combined use not recommended in patients with psychoses.

Dosage: Elixir, Tablets. *Parkinsonism (for patients on no other therapy):* **initial,** 2.5 mg t.i.d. after meals; dose may be increased slowly to 4–5 mg t.i.d. and, if necessary, before bedtime.
  Parkinsonism (transferring from other therapy): substitute 2.5 mg t.i.d.; slowly increase dose of

procyclidine and decrease dose of other drug to appropriate maintenance levels. *Drug-induced extrapyramidal symptoms:* **initial,** 2.5 mg t.i.d.; increase to maintenance dose of 10–20 mg/day.

NURSING CONSIDERATIONS

See *Nursing Considerations* for *Cholinergic Blocking Agents,* p. 949.

TRIHEXYPHENIDYL HYDROCHLORIDE   (try-hex-ih-**FEN**-ih-dill)

Aparkane✣, APO-Trihex✣, Artane, Artane Sequels, Novohexidyl✣, Trihexy-2 and -5 (Rx)

See also *Cholinergic Blocking Agents,* p. 942, and *Antiparkinson Drugs,* p. 681.

Classification: Antiparkinson agent, anticholinergic.

Action/Kinetics: Synthetic anticholinergic, which relieves rigidity but has little effect on tremors. Causes a direct antispasmodic effect on smooth muscle. Has a high incidence of side effects. Small doses cause CNS depression while larger doses may result in CNS excitation. **Onset, PO:** 60 min. **Duration, PO:** 6–12 hr.

Uses: Adjunct in the treatment of all types of parkinsonism (often used as adjunct with levodopa). Drug-induced extrapyramidal symptoms. Sustained-release medication is for maintenance dosage only.

Additional Contraindications: Arteriosclerosis and hypersensitivity to drug.

Special Concerns: Pregnancy category: C.

Additional Side Effects: Serious CNS stimulation (restlessness, insomnia, delirium, agitation) and psychotic manifestations.

Additional Drug Interaction: ↑ Effectiveness of levodopa if used together; such combined use not recommended in patients with psychoses.

Dosage: Elixir, Extended-release Capsules, Tablets. *Parkinsonism:* **initial (day 1),** 1–2 mg; **then,** increase by 2 mg q 3–5 days until daily dose is 6–10 mg given in divided doses. Some patients may require 12–15 mg daily (especially those with postencephalitic parkinsonism). *Adjunct with levodopa:* 3–6 mg/day in divided doses. *Drug-induced extrapyramidal reactions:* **initial,** 1 mg daily; **then,** increase as needed to total daily dose of 5–15 mg. **Maintenance: extended-release,** 5–10 mg 1–2 times daily.

NURSING CONSIDERATIONS

See also *Nursing Considerations* for *Cholinergic Blocking Agents* under *Antiparkinson Agents,* p. 693.

Interventions

1. This drug has a high incidence of side effects; early detection and intervention are imperative.
2. Determine any added untoward CNS reactions to the drug. Note any increase in restlessness, complaints of insomnia, agitation, or psychotic manifestations. Document and notify the physician, as drug dosage may need to be adjusted.
3. Monitor and record intake and output.

Evaluation

Assess client carefully for any evidence of adverse drug effects. Document and report so that drug dosage may be evaluated and adjusted as symptoms indicate.

CHAPTER THIRTY-FIVE

Centrally Acting Skeletal Muscle Relaxants

Action/Kinetics: The centrally acting skeletal muscle relaxants decrease muscle tone and involuntary movement. Many relieve anxiety and tension as well. Although the precise mechanism of action is unknown, most of these agents depress spinal polysynaptic reflexes. Their beneficial effects may also be attributable to their antianxiety activity. Several of the drugs in this group also manifest analgesic properties.

Uses: Musculoskeletal and neurologic disorders associated with muscle spasms, hyperreflexia, and hypertonia, including parkinsonism, tetanus, tension headaches, acute muscle spasms caused by trauma, and inflammation (e.g., low back syndrome, sprains, arthritis, bursitis). They also may be useful in the management of cerebral palsy and multiple sclerosis.

Side Effects: Side effects often involve the CNS, GI system, and urinary system. Symptoms of allergy may also be manifested. For specific untoward reactions, see individual drugs.

Drug Interactions: Centrally acting muscle relaxants may increase the sedative and respiratory depressant effects of CNS depressants (e.g., alcohol, barbiturates, sedatives and hypnotics, and antianxiety agents).

Dosage: For dosage, see individual agents.

Overdosage:

Symptoms

Symptoms of overdosage are often extensions of the untoward reactions. Stupor, coma, shock-like syndrome, respiratory depression, loss of muscle tone, and impaired deep tendon reflexes may also occur.

Treatment

Symptomatic. Emesis or gastric lavage (followed by activated charcoal). If necessary, artificial respiration, oxygen administration, pressor agents, and IV fluids may be used. It may be possible to increase the rate of excretion of selected drugs by diuretics (including mannitol), peritoneal dialysis, or hemodialysis.

35

NURSING CONSIDERATIONS

Administration

1. Crush tablets or empty contents of capsules into a small amount of fruit juice if the client is unable to swallow.
2. If the skeletal muscle relaxant is to be discontinued after long-term use, the dose of drug should be tapered to prevent rebound spasticity, hallucinations or other withdrawal symptoms.
3. Review list of drug interactions.
4. The lowest possible dosage of drug should be determined and used to treat the client's symptoms.
5. Have emergency drugs, gastric lavage, oxygen, pressor agents and IV fluids available in the event of a drug overdose.

Assessment

1. Obtain a complete drug history.
2. Note any history of prior seizures. Some drugs in this category may cause deterioration of seizure control.
3. Assess the extent of the client's musculoskeletal and neurologic disorders associated with muscle spasm.
4. Conduct a thorough baseline mental status examination against which to measure subsequent examinations.

Interventions

1. Monitor blood pressure every 4 hours when therapy is initiated in a hospital setting.
2. Sedentary or immobilized clients are more prone to hypotension with these drugs, upon ambulation.
3. Note client complaints of nausea, anorexia, or changes in taste perception. Notify physician if these symptoms persist as nutritional state may become impaired.
4. Monitor the client's urinary output. Anticipate the need to use drugs to increase the rate of excretion if the output is too low.

Client/Family Teaching

1. These drugs may impair the client's state of mental alertness. Advise client not to operate dangerous machinery or drive a car when taking these drugs.
2. If the urine becomes dark, the skin or sclera appears yellow, or if the client develops pruritus, notify the physician and discontinue using the medication.
3. Advise the client to avoid using antihistamines. These drugs may produce an additive depressant effect.
4. Avoid the use of alcohol.
5. Stress the importance of reporting for all scheduled lab and medical follow-up visits so that therapy can be evaluated and drug dosage adjusted as needed.

Evaluation

1. Review the goals of the medication therapy with the client and family and determine to what extent they have been met.

2. Check the client's muscle responses and deep tendon reflexes for symptoms of drug overdosage.
3. Note the client's urinary output and potential need for the use of diuretics.

BACLOFEN   (BAK-low-fen)
Lioresal (Rx)

See also *Centrally Acting Muscle Relaxants,* p. 703.

Classification: Centrally acting muscle relaxant.

Action/Kinetics: The mechanism of action of baclofen is not fully known, but the drug is known to inhibit both mono- and polysynaptic spinal reflexes. It may also act at certain brain sites. **Peak serum levels:** 2–3 hr. **Therapeutic serum levels:** 80–400 ng/mL. **t½:** 3–4 hr. 70–80% of the drug is eliminated unchanged by the kidney.

Uses: Multiple sclerosis (flexor spasms, pain, clonus, and muscular rigidity) and diseases and injuries of the spinal cord associated with spasticity. It is not effective for the treatment of cerebral palsy, stroke, parkinsonism, or rheumatic disorders. *Investigational:* Trigeminal neuralgia, tardive dyskinesia.

Contraindications: Hypersensitivity. Rheumatic disorders, spasm resulting from Parkinson's disease, stroke, cerebral palsy.

Special Concerns: Safe use in pregnancy or for children under 12 years of age has not been established. Use with caution in impaired renal function. Geriatric patients may be at higher risk for developing CNS toxicity including mental depression, confusion, hallucinations, and significant sedation.

Side Effects: *CNS:* Drowsiness, dizziness, weakness, fatigue, confusion, headaches, insomnia. Hallucinations following abrupt withdrawal. *CV:* Hypotension. Rarely, chest pain, syncope, palpitations. *GI:* Nausea, constipation. *GU:* Urinary frequency. *Other:* Rash, pruritus, ankle edema, increased perspiration, weight gain, dyspnea, nasal congestion.

Drug Interactions: Concomitant use with CNS depressants → additive CNS depression.

Laboratory Test Interference: ↑ SGOT, alkaline phosphatase, blood glucose.

Dosage: Tablets. Adults: Initial, 5 mg t.i.d. for 3 days; **then,** 10 mg t.i.d. for 3 days, 15 mg t.i.d. for 3 days, and 20 mg t.i.d. Additional increases in dose may be required but should not exceed 20 mg q.i.d.

NURSING CONSIDERATIONS

See also *Nursing Considerations* for *Centrally Acting Skeletal Muscle Relaxants,* p. 704.

Administration/Storage

1. If beneficial effects are not noted, the drug should be slowly withdrawn.
2. Have gastric lavage equipment available in the event of drug overdosage. Maintain adequate respiratory exchange. Do not use respiratory stimulants.

Assessment

1. Assess clients with epilepsy for clinical signs and symptoms of their disease. Arrange for an EEG at regular intervals as baclofen has been associated with reduced seizure control.

2. Obtain renal function studies prior to initiating therapy.

3. Note if the client has diabetes.

Interventions

1. Note any evidence of hypersensitivity and notify the physician.

2. Notify physician of clients who require hypertonicity to stand upright, to maintain balance when walking, or to increase their function. Baclofen may be contraindicated in these instances because it interferes with this coping mechanism.

3. If clients complain of constipation, encourage an increase in fluid intake and increase the roughage in the diet.

4. Monitor urinary output and test the urine for occult blood.

5. Monitor the client's weight, reporting any evidence of edema to the physician.

6. If improvement in the client's condition does not occur within 6–8 weeks, the drug should be withdrawn gradually.

Client/Family Teaching

1. Take the medication with meals or a snack to avoid gastric irritation. If GI symptoms are severe or persistent, notify the physician.

2. Reassure the family and client that it may take several weeks of therapy before physical improvement occurs.

3. Instruct clients how to monitor their own intake and output and keep a record of the frequency and amounts of each voiding.

4. If clients have diabetes mellitus, teach them how to monitor blood glucose levels and compare them with levels obtained at the onset of therapy.

5. Advise male clients of the potential for the drug to cause impotence. If this occurs, report the problem to the physician. A change of drug or dosage may be required. Clients should be warned, however, not to discontinue taking the drug without the physician's knowledge.

Evaluation

1. Evaluate for a positive clinical response to the drug therapy.

2. Review the client's lab studies of SGOT, alkaline phosphatase and blood glucose levels to ascertain if there is any untoward effect of the drug.

3. Document any improvement in the client's muscle tone and involuntary movements.

CARISOPRODOL   (kar-eye-so-**PROH**-dohl)

Rela, Sodol, Soma, Soridol, Sporodol (Rx)

See also *Centrally Acting Muscle Relaxants,* p. 703.

Classification: Centrally acting muscle relaxant.

Action/Kinetics: Carisoprodol may produce skeletal muscle relaxation by inhibiting synaptic reflexes in the descending reticular formation and spinal cord. Its sedative effects may also be responsible for muscle relaxation. **Onset:** 30 min. **Duration:** 4–6 hr. **Peak serum levels:** 4–7 mcg/mL. **t½:** 8 hr. The drug is metabolized in the liver and excreted in the urine.

Uses: As an adjunct to treat skeletal muscle disorders including bursitis, low back disorders, contusions, fibrositis, spondylitis, sprains, muscle strains, and cerebral palsy.

Contraindications: Porphyria. Hypersensitivity to carisoprodol or meprobamate. Children under 12 years of age.

Special Concerns: Use with caution during pregnancy (category: C). The drug may cause GI upset and sedation in the infant. Use with caution in impaired liver or kidney function.

Side Effects: *CNS:* Ataxia, dizziness, drowsiness, excitement, tremor, syncope, vertigo, insomnia. *GI:* Nausea, vomiting, gastric upset, hiccoughs. *Cardiovascular:* Flushing of face, postural hypotension, tachycardia. *Allergic reactions:* Pruritis, skin rashes, erythema multiforme, eosinophilia, dizziness, angioneurotic edema, asthmatic symptoms, "smarting" of the eyes, weakness, hypotension, anaphylaxis.

Drug Interactions	
Alcohol	Additive CNS depressant effects
Antidepressants, tricyclic	↑ Effect of carisoprodol
Barbiturates	Possible ↑ effect of carisoprodol, followed by inhibition of carisoprodol
Chlorcyclizine	↓ Effect of carisoprodol
CNS depressants	Additive CNS depression
MAO inhibitors	↑ Effect of carisoprodol by ↓ breakdown by liver
Phenobarbital	↓ Effect of carisoprodol by ↑ breakdown by liver
Phenothiazines	Additive depressant effects

Dosage: Tablets. Adults: 350 mg q.i.d. (take last dose at bedtime). **Pediatric:** 6.25 mg/kg q.i.d.

NURSING CONSIDERATIONS

See *Nursing Considerations* for *Centrally Acting Muscle Relaxants*, p. 704.

Administration/Storage

1. If the client is unable to swallow tablets, mix them with syrup, chocolate or a jelly mixture.
2. Administer the drug with food if gastric upset occurs.

Assessment

1. Note any history of hypersensitivity to meprobamate or carisoprodol.
2. Record the extent of the client's skeletal muscular disorders as a baseline against which to compare the effects of the therapy.
3. Review drugs the client is currently taking to assure that there will be no drug interaction.

Interventions

1. Observe client for evidence of ataxia or tremors and report.
2. If the client develops postural hypotension or tachycardia, report to the physician. These are adverse reactions that may necessitate taking the client off of the medication.

Client/Family Teaching

1. Provide the client with a printed list of the potential side effects that should be reported to the physician, should they develop.

2. Assist the client in establishing a drug schedule so that the last dose of drug is taken at bedtime.
3. Due to the possibility of drug-induced dizziness or drowsiness, caution should be used when driving or undertaking other tasks requiring mental alertness.

CHLORPHENESIN CARBAMATE   (klor-**FEN**-eh-sin)

Maolate (Rx)

See also *Centrally Acting Muscle Relaxants,* p. 703.

Classification: Centrally-acting muscle relaxant.

Action/Kinetics: The action is thought to be due to depression of polysynaptic spinal reflexes as well as the sedative effects of the drug. **Peak serum concentration:** 1–2 hr. **Peak serum levels:** 3.8–17 mcg/mL (after 800 mg). **t½:** 4 hr. Excreted in the urine as inactive metabolites.

Uses: As an adjunct for muscle spasms and muscle pain secondary to sprains, trauma, or inflammation.

Additional Contraindications: Hypersensitivity to drug. Use in children is not recommended.

Special Concerns: Use during pregnancy only if benefits clearly outweigh risks. Use with caution in impaired hepatic function.

Side Effects: *CNS:* Confusion, dizziness, drowsiness, insomnia, increased nervousness, headache, paradoxical stimulation. *GI:* Nausea, epigastric distress. *Allergic:* Drug fever, anaphylaxis. *Hematologic (rare):* Agranulocytosis, leukopenia, pancytopenia, thrombocytopenia.

Dosage: Tablets. Adults: initial, 800 mg t.i.d.; **maintenance,** 400 mg q.i.d. Safety for use longer than 8 weeks has not been established.

NURSING CONSIDERATIONS

See also *Nursing Considerations* for *Centrally Acting Skeletal Muscle Relaxants,* p. 704.

Assessment

1. Note any history of hypersensitivity to the drug.
2. Obtain hematological studies prior to beginning drug therapy.
3. Evaluate liver function studies to detect any evidence of liver disease that would indicate that the client should not receive the drug.

Interventions

1. If any evidence of agranulocytosis, leukopenia, pancytopenia or thrombocytopenia is noted, withhold medication and report to the physician.
2. Observe closely for evidence of hepatic toxicity and report.

Client/Family Teaching

1. Drugs that are centrally acting muscular relaxants should not be used continuously for more than 3 weeks.
2. Stress the importance of taking the medication only as directed.
3. Provide printed instructions regarding adverse side effects and what to do about them.

4. Advise clients to avoid other CNS depressant drugs while they are taking skeletal muscular relaxants.

5. Warn clients to avoid driving or performing any other activities that require mental alertness, coordination or sound judgement.

6. When the drugs in this class are to be discontinued, they should be tapered gradually to minimize the risk of rebound spasticity, hallucinations or other related symptoms.

7. The drug may be taken with meals, crushed and mixed with food or liquid.

CHLORZOXAZONE (klor-ZOX-ah-zohn)

Paraflex, Parafon Forte DSC (Rx)

See also *Centrally Acting Muscle Relaxants,* p. 703.

Classification: Centrally acting muscle relaxant.

Action/Kinetics: Chlorzoxazone inhibits polysynaptic reflexes at both the spinal cord and subcortical areas of the brain. Its effect may also be due to the sedative properties of the drug. **Onset:** 1 hr. **Time to peak blood levels:** 1–2 hr. **Peak serum levels:** 10–30 mcg/mL (after 750 mg dose). **Duration:** 3–4 hr. **t½:** 1–2 hr. The drug is metabolized in the liver and inactive metabolites excreted in the urine.

Uses: As adjunct therapy for acute, painful musculoskeletal conditions (e.g., muscle spasms, sprains, muscle strain).

Special Concerns: Use during pregnancy only if benefits clearly outweigh risks.

Side Effects: *CNS:* Dizziness, drowsiness, malaise, lightheadedness, stimulation. *Dermatologic:* Skin rashes, petechiae, ecchymoses (rare). *Miscellaneous:* GI upset, angioneurotic edema, anaphylaxis (rare), discoloration of urine, liver damage.

Dosage: Tablets. Adults: 250–750 mg t.i.d.–q.i.d. with meals and at bedtime; **pediatric:** 125–500 mg t.i.d.–q.i.d. (or, 20 mg/kg in 3–4 divided doses daily).

NURSING CONSIDERATIONS

See also *Nursing Considerations* for *Centrally Acting Muscle Relaxants,* p. 704.

Administration/Storage

1. Administer the drug with meals to minimize gastric irritation.
2. The drug may be mixed with food or beverages for administration to children.

Assessment

Assure that liver function studies have been conducted to serve as a baseline against which to compare liver function after the client has been taking the drug.

Intervention

If the client develops any evidence of hepatic dysfunction, order liver function studies and compare the results with premedication studies.

Client/Family Teaching

1. The drug may cause the urine to have an orange or purple-red color when exposed to the air.
2. Advise clients not to operate dangerous machinery or drive a car as the drug causes drowsiness.

CYCLOBENZAPRINE HYDROCHLORIDE   (sye-kloh-**BEN**-zah-preen)

Flexeril (Rx)

See also *Centrally Acting Muscle Relaxants,* p. 703.

Classification: Centrally acting muscle relaxant.

Action/Kinetics: Structurally and pharmacologically, cyclobenzaprine is related to the tricyclic antidepressants and possesses both sedative and anticholinergic properties. In contrast to many skeletal muscle relaxants, cyclobenzaprine hydrochloride is thought to act mainly at the level of the brain stem (compared to the spinal cord) to inhibit reflexes by reducing tonic somatic motor activity. **Onset:** 1 hr. **Time to peak plasma levels:** 3–8 hr. **Therapeutic plasma levels:** 20–30 ng/mL. **Duration:** 12–24 hr. **t½:** 1–3 days. The drug is highly bound to plasma protein. Inactive metabolites are excreted in the urine.

Uses: Adjunct to rest and physical therapy for relief of muscle spasms associated with acute and/or painful musculoskeletal conditions. It is not indicated for the treatment of spastic diseases or for cerebral palsy.

Contraindications: Hypersensitivity. Arrhythmias, heart block, CHF, or soon after myocardial infarctions. Hyperthyroidism. Concomitant use of monoamine oxidase inhibitors.

Special Concerns: Safe use during pregnancy (category: B) and lactation and in children under age 15 has not been established. Due to atropine-like effects, use with caution in situations where cholinergic blockade is not desired. Geriatric patients may be more sensitive to cholinergic blockade.

Side Effects: Symptoms of cholinergic blockade including dry mouth, dizziness, tachycardia, blurred vision, urinary retention. Also, drowsiness, weakness, dyspepsia, paresthesia, unpleasant taste, insomnia. Since cyclobenzaprine resembles tricyclic antidepressants, untoward reactions to these drugs should also be noted.

Physostigmine salicylate, 1–3 mg IV, may be used to reverse symptoms of severe cholinergic blockade.

Drug Interactions	
Anticholinergics	Additive anticholinergic side effects
CNS depressants	Additive depressant effects
Guanethidine	Cyclobenzaprine may block effect
MAO inhibitors	Hypertensive crisis, severe convulsions
Tricyclic antidepressants	Additive side effects

Dosage: Tablets. Adults: 20–40 mg daily in 3–4 divided doses (usual: 10 mg t.i.d.), up to a maximum of 60 mg daily in divided doses.

NURSING CONSIDERATIONS

See also *Nursing Considerations* for *Tricyclic Antidepressants,* p. 666, and *Centrally Acting Muscle Relaxants,* p. 704.

Administration/Storage

1. Cyclobenzaprine should only be used for 2–3 weeks.
2. If the client has been taking a monoamine oxidase inhibitor, do not administer cyclobenzaprine for at least 2 weeks after discontinuing the MAO inhibitor.
3. Review the list of drugs with which cyclobenzaprine interacts.

Assessment

1. Take a complete drug history, noting any evidence of hypersensitivity.
2. Check the client's cardiovascular system for evidence of cardiac arrhythmias. Note if the client has a history of recent myocardial infarction.
3. Obtain a complete blood count and liver profile prior to starting therapy to serve as baseline data.
4. Document the extent of the client's acute or painful musculoskeletal condition.
5. Determine if the client has any spasticity. This drug is contraindicated in the treatment of spastic conditions.

Intervention

Should the client complain of itchy skin, or show evidence of yellow sclera or skin, withhold drug and evaluate liver function studies.

Client/Family Teaching

1. Report any unusual fatigue, unexplained fever, easy bruising or bleeding or sore throat. These symptoms could indicate a blood dyscrasia and require the discontinuation of drug therapy.
2. Advise to report nausea or abdominal pain as this could indicate hepatic toxicity and require the termination of therapy.
3. Symptoms such as dry mouth, blurred vision, dizziness, tachycardia or urinary retention should also be reported so that therapy can be evaluated.
4. Due to drug-induced drowsiness, dizziness, or blurred vision, caution should be observed if the client drives or performs other activities requiring mental alertness.
5. Advise not to extend drug therapy beyond 3 weeks. Longer periods of therapy with this drug are contraindicated.

DANTROLENE SODIUM (DAN-troh-leen)

Dantrium, Dantrium IV (Rx)

See also *Centrally Acting Muscle Relaxants,* p. 703.

Classification: Centrally acting muscle relaxant.

Action/Kinetics: Dantrolene is a hydantoin derivative and, as such, is chemically unrelated to other skeletal muscle relaxants. It acts directly on skeletal muscle, probably by dissociating the excitation-contraction coupling mechanism as a result of interference of release of calcium from the sarcoplasmic reticulum. This action results in a decreased force of reflex muscle contraction and a reduction of hyperreflexia, spasticity, involuntary movements, and clonus. Its effectiveness in malignant hyperthermia is due to an inhibition of release of calcium from the sarcoplasmic reticulum. This results in prevention or reduction of the increased myoplasmic calcium ion concentration that activates the acute catabolic processes which are associated with malignant hyperthermia. Absorption is slow and incomplete, but consistent. **Peak plasma levels:** 4–6 hr. **t½: oral,** 8.7 hr; **t½: IV,** 5 hr. There is significant plasma protein binding of the drug.

Uses: Muscle spasticity associated with severe chronic disorders, such as multiple sclerosis, cerebral palsy, spinal cord injury, and stroke. Muscle pain due to exercise. Malignant hyperthermia due to hypermetabolism of skeletal muscle. *Investigational:* Exercise-induced muscle pain, heat stroke, and neuroleptic malignant syndrome.

Contraindications: Rheumatic diseases, pregnancy, lactation, or children under 5 years of age. Acute hepatitis and cirrhosis of the liver.

Special Concerns: (Pregnancy category: C—parenteral use. Use with caution in patients with impaired pulmonary function.

Side Effects: Following PO use: Untoward reactions are dose-related and decrease with usage. Fatal and nonfatal hepatotoxicity. *CNS:* Drowsiness, dizziness, weakness, malaise, lightheadedness, headaches, insomnia, seizures, speech disturbances, fatigue, confusion, depression, nervousness. *GI:* Diarrhea (common), anorexia, gastric upset, cramps, GI bleeding. *Musculoskeletal:* Backache, myalgia. *Dermatologic:* Rashes, photosensitivity, pruritus, urticaria, hair growth, sweating. *CV:* Blood pressure changes, phlebitis, tachycardia. *GU:* Urinary retention, hematuria, crystalluria, nocturia, impotence. *Miscellaneous:* Visual disturbances, chills, fever, tearing, feeling of suffocation, pleural effusion with pericarditis.

    Following IV use: Pulmonary edema, thrombophlebitis, urticaria, erythema.

Dosage: Capsules. *Spastic conditions.* **Adults: initial,** 25 mg/day; **then,** increase to 25 mg b.i.d.–q.i.d.; dose may then be increased by 25-mg increments up to 100 mg b.i.d.–q.i.d. (doses in excess of 400 mg/day not recommended). **Pediatric: initial,** 0.5 mg/kg b.i.d.; **then,** increase to 0.5 t.i.d.–q.i.d.; dose may then be increased by increments of 0.5 mg/kg to 3 mg/kg b.i.d.–q.i.d. (doses should not exceed 400 mg/day). *Malignant hyperthermia, preoperatively.* **Adults and children, PO:** 4–8 mg/kg daily in 3–4 divided doses 1–2 days before surgery. *Post malignant hyperthermic crisis:* 4–8 mg/kg daily in four divided doses for 1–33 days.

    IV infusion. *Malignant hyperthermia, crisis treatment:* **Adults and children, initial,** 2.5 mg/kg 60 min prior to surgery and infused over 1 hr. **IV push: Initial,** At least 1 mg/kg; continue administration until symptoms decrease or a cumulative dose of 10 mg/kg has been administered.

NURSING CONSIDERATIONS

See also *Nursing Consideration for Centrally Acting Muscle Relaxants,* p. 704.

Administration/Storage

1. If the drug is to be administered IV, the powder should be reconstituted by adding 60 mL of sterile water for injection.
2. Reconstituted solutions should be protected from light and used within 6 hr.
3. When administered orally, the drug can be mixed with fruit juice or other liquid vehicle.
4. If the drug is being administered to counteract spasticity, beneficial effects may not be noted for a week. The drug should be discontinued after 6 weeks if beneficial effects are not evident.
5. Due to potential hepatotoxicity, long-term benefits must be evaluated for each client.

Assessment

1. Note the client's mental status and general appearance.
2. Obtain baseline liver function studies prior to initiating drug therapy. Impaired hepatic function is more likely to occur in women over 35 years of age.
3. Auscultate lung and heart sounds prior to beginning therapy and record these findings for use as baseline data.
4. Note any evidence of impaired pulmonary function, cardiac disorders or history of the client having either benign or malignant breast tumors. Dantrolene may increase the incidence of mammary tumors.
5. Note the extent of the client's spasticity, involuntary movements and clonus. Record these findings for use as baseline data against which to compare the results of the drug therapy.

Interventions

1. Auscultate respiratory and heart sounds at regular intervals during the therapy. Note any changes.
2. Inspect the client's skin to detect any changes.
3. Routinely perform liver function studies throughout therapy. Withhold drug and notify physician of any abnormal findings.
4. Monitor intake and output and note any evidence of blood in the urine. Document and report to the physician as drug therapy may need to be discontinued.
5. Monitor stools for the presence of blood.
6. If clients develop diplopia, reassure them that this and many of the other bothersome side effects associated with drug therapy may lessen with the continued use of the drug.

Client/Family Teaching

1. Since this drug causes drowsiness, clients should be instructed not to operate dangerous machinery or drive a car.
2. Advise the client to report any increased muscle weakness or impaired physical ability.
3. Reassure the client that several weeks of therapy may be required before improvements in the client's condition will be noted.
4. Instruct the client how to take and monitor blood pressure. Also how to check stools and urine for the presence of occult blood and to keep a record of urinary output. Advise the client to report any marked changes in BP and any evidence of blood in the urine or stool.
5. Encourage female clients to have mammograms and to do breast self-examinations to detect any occurrence of lumps since this drug has the potential to cause the development of these problems. This is especially important in women with a family history of breast tumors, malignant or benign.
6. Explain to male clients the potential for impotence. Advise the client to report this side effect to the physician.

Evaluation

1. Note if the client develops slurred speech, drooling, inability to perform usual physical functions, or enuresis. These are serious side effects and may require withdrawal of the drug.
2. Assess for evidence of reduction in spasticity and/or muscle pain.
3. Document any reduction in exercise-induced muscle pain.
4. Evaluate for evidence of rebound spasticity or hallucinations after withdrawal of the client from the drug therapy.

DIAZEPAM   (dye-**AYZ**-eh-pam)

Apo-Diazepam ✽, Diazepam Intensol, E-Pam ✽, Meval ✽, Novodipam ✽, Rival ✽, Valium, Valrelease, Vivol ✽, Zetran (C-IV, Rx)

See also *Benzodiazepines,* p. 611.

Action/Kinetics: Onset: PO, 30–60 min; **IM,** 15–30 min; **IV,** more rapid. **Peak plasma levels: PO,** 0.5–2 hr; **IM,** 0.5–1.5; **IV,** 0.25 hr. **Duration:** 3 hr. **t½:** 20–70 hr. Diazepam is broken down in the liver to the active metabolites desmethyldiazepam, oxazepam, and temazepam. Diazepam and metabolites are excreted through the urine.

Uses: Anxiety, tension (more effective than chlordiazepoxide), alcohol withdrawal, muscle relaxant, anticonvulsive agent, antipanic drug. Used prior to gastroscopy and esophagoscopy, preoperatively and prior to cardioversion. In dentistry to induce sedation. Treatment of status epilepticus. Adjunct in cerebral palsy, paraplegia, or tetanus. Relieve spasms of facial muscles in occlusion and temporomandibular joint disorders.

Additional Contraindications: Narrow-angle glaucoma, children under 6 months, and parenterally in children under 12 years. During lactation.

Special Concerns: Pregnancy category: D.

Additional Drug Interactions:

1. Diazepam potentiates antihypertensive effects of thiazides and other diuretics.
2. Diazepam potentiates muscle relaxant effects of *d*-tubocurarine and gallamine.
3. Ranitidine ↓ GI absorption of diazepam.
4. Isoniazid ↑ half-life of diazepam.
5. Fluoxetine ↑ half-life of diazepam.

Dosage: Tablets, Oral Solution. Adults: *Antianxiety, anticonvulsant, adjunct to skeletal muscle relaxants:* 2–10 mg b.i.d.–q.i.d. **Elderly, debilitated patients:** 2–2.5 mg 1–2 times daily. May be gradually increased to adult level. **Pediatric, over 6 months: initial,** 1–2.5 mg (0.04–0.2 mg/kg or 1.17–6 mg/m²) t.i.d.–b.i.d. *Alcohol withdrawal:* 10 mg t.i.d.–q.i.d. during the first 24 hr; **then,** decrease to 5 mg t.i.d.–q.i.d. as required.

Extended-release Capsules. Adults: *Antianxiety, skeletal muscle relaxant:* 15–30 mg once daily. To be used in children over 6 months of age only if the dose has been determined to be 5 mg t.i.d. (use one 15-mg capsule daily). **IM, IV. Adults: IM,** *Preoperative or diagnostic use:* 10 mg 5–30 min before procedure. *Adjunct to treat skeletal muscle spasm:* 5–10 mg initially; **then,** repeat in 3–4 hr if needed (larger doses may be required for tetanus). *Moderate anxiety:* 2–5 mg q 3–4 hr if necessary. *Severe anxiety, muscle spasm:* 5–10 mg q 3–4 hr, if necessary. *Acute alcohol withdrawal:* **initial,** 10 mg; **then,** 5–10 mg q 3–4 hr. *Preoperatively:* **IM,** 10 mg prior to surgery. *Endoscopy:* **IV,** 10 mg or less although doses up to 20 mg can be used; **IM,** 5–10 mg 30 min prior to procedure. *Cardioversion:* **IV,** 5–15 mg 5–10 min prior to procedure. *Tetanus in children,* **IM, IV, over 1 month:** 1–2 mg, repeated q 3–4 hr as necessary; **5 years and over:** 5–10 mg q 3–4 hr. **IV,** *Status epilepticus:* **Adults,** 5–10 mg initially; **then,** dose may be repeated at 10–15 min intervals up to a maximum dose of 30 mg. **Children, 1 month–5 years:** 0.2–0.5 mg q 2–5 min, up to maximum of 5 mg. Can be repeated in 2–4 hr. **5 years and older:** 1 mg q 2–5 min up to a maximum of 10 mg; dose can be repeated in 2–4 hr, if needed.

Elderly or debilitated patients should not receive more than 5 mg parenterally at any one time.

NURSING CONSIDERATIONS

See *Nursing Considerations* for *Benzodiazepines,* p. 614.

Administration/Storage

1. One 15-mg sustained-release diazepam capsule may be used if the daily dosage is 5 mg t.i.d.
2. The Intensol solution should be mixed with beverages such as water, soda, and juices, or soft foods such as applesauce or puddings. Only the calibrated dropper provided with the product should be used to withdraw the medication. Once the medication is withdrawn and mixed, it should be used immediately.
3. To reduce reactions at the site of IV administration, diazepam should be given slowly (5 mg/min). Also, small veins or intra-arterial administration should not be used.
4. When administering the drug IV, have emergency equipment and drugs available.

5. Due to the possibility of precipitation and instability, diazepam should not be infused.
6. Except for the deltoid muscle, absorption from IM sites is slow and erratic.
7. Review the drug interaction chart before administering the drug.

Assessment

1. Obtain a CBC, platelet count, liver and renal profiles as baseline data.
2. Note if the client has diabetes and the type of agent used for testing the urine as diazepam interferes with many of these agents. Have client convert to finger sticks for a more accurate blood glucose determination.

Interventions

1. Parenteral administration may cause bradycardia, respiratory or cardiac arrest. Monitor vital signs and client closely.
2. Elderly clients may experience adverse reactions more quickly than younger clients. Therefore, anticipate a lower dose of drug to be ordered in this group.

METAXALONE   (meh-**TAX**-ah-lohn)

Skelaxin (Rx)

See also *Centrally Acting Muscle Relaxants,* p. 703.

Classification: Centrally acting muscle relaxant.

Action/Kinetics: The beneficial effects of metaxalone may be due to its sedative effects. The drug resembles meprobamate. **Onset:** 1 hr. **t½:** 2–3 hr. **Time to peak levels:** 2 hr (after 800 mg). **Peak serum levels:** 205 mcg/mL. **Duration:** 4–6 hr. Metabolites are excreted in the urine.

Uses: As an adjunct for acute skeletal muscle spasm associated with sprains, strains, dislocation, and other trauma.

Contraindications: Liver disease, epilepsy, impaired renal function, history of drug-induced hemolytic or other anemias, pregnancy, children under 12 years.

Special Concerns: Safe use during lactation has not been determined.

Side Effects: *CNS:* Drowsiness, dizziness, headache, nervousness, irritability. *GI:* Nausea, vomiting, gastric upset. *Miscellaneous:* Allergic reactions, jaundice, leukopenia, hemolytic anemia.

Dosage: Tablets. Adults and children over 12 yr of age: 800 mg t.i.d.–q.i.d.

NURSING CONSIDERATIONS

See also *Nursing Considerations for Centrally Acting Muscle Relaxants,* p. 704.

Assessment

1. Obtain baseline complete blood count and liver and renal function studies.
2. Note any history of drug induced hemolytic or other type anemias.
3. Determine if client has a history of epilepsy.

Interventions

1. Note any client complaint of high fever, nausea, or diarrhea. These are early symptoms of hepatotoxicity and require the withdrawal of metaxalone.
2. Client complaints of sore throat, fever, and lassitude or of having a "cold" should be further explored as these may be symptoms of blood dyscrasias.

3. Closely observe client with a history of grand mal epilepsy. Metaxalone may precipitate seizures.

Client/Family Teaching

1. Encourage clients to avoid a dry mouth by rinsing the mouth frequently and increasing their fluid intake. Sugarless gum and hard candy may also be of some benefit.

2. Since drug causes drowsiness, clients should be instructed not to operate dangerous machinery or drive a car.

3. Report any jaundice, irritability or allergic responses. These are adverse side effects to the drug therapy and may require a readjustment of the dosage or withdrawal from the drug.

METHOCARBAMOL   (meh-thoh-**KAR**-bah-mohl)

Carbacot✿, Delaxin, Marbaxin 750, Robamol, Robaxin, Robaxin-750, Robomol-500 and -750 (Rx)

See also *Centrally Acting Muscle Relaxants,* p. 703.

Classification: Centrally acting muscle relaxant.

Action/Kinetics: The beneficial action of methocarbamol may be related to the sedative properties of the drug. Of limited usefulness. The drug may be given IM or IV in polyethylene glycol 300 (50% solution). PO therapy should be initiated as soon as possible. **Onset:** 30 min. **Peak plasma levels:** 2 hr. **t½:** 1–2 hr. Inactive metabolites are excreted in the urine.

Uses: Muscle spasms associated with sprains and/or trauma, acute back pain due to nerve irritation or discogenic disease, postoperative orthopedic procedures, bursitis, and torticollis. Acute phase muscle spasms. Adjunct in tetanus.

Contraindications: Hypersensitivity, when muscle spasticity is required to maintain upright position, pregnancy, lactation, children under 12 years. Renal disease (parenteral dosage form only).

Special Concerns: Use with caution in epilepsy.

Side Effects: *Following PO use. CNS:* Dizziness, drowsiness, lightheadedness, vertigo, lassitude, headache. *GI:* Nausea. *Miscellaneous:* Allergic symptoms including rash, urticaria, pruritus, conjunctivitis, nasal congestion, blurred vision, fever. *Following IV use (in addition to above). Cardiovascular:* Fainting, hypotension, bradycardia. *Miscellaneous:* Metallic taste, GI upset, flushing, nystagmus, double vision, thrombophlebitis, pain at injection site, anaphylaxis.

Drug Interaction: CNS depressants (including alcohol) may increase the effect of methocarbamol.

Laboratory Test Interferences: Color interference in 5-hydroxyindoleacetic acid (5-HIAA) and vanillylmandelic acid (VMA).

Dosage: Tablets. Adults, initial: 1.5 g q.i.d. for the first 2–3 days (for severe conditions, 8 g daily may be given); **maintenance:** 1 g q.i.d., 0.75 g q 4 hr, or 1.5 g t.i.d. **IM, IV: usual initial,** 1 g; in severe cases, up to 2–3 g may be necessary. **IV administration should not exceed 3 days.** *Tetanus:* **IV, Adults** 1–3 g given into tube of previously inserted indwelling needle. May be given q 6 hr (up to 24 g daily may be needed) until **PO** administration is feasible. **Children, initial:** 15 mg/kg given into tube of previously inserted indwelling needle. Dose may be repeated q 6 hr.

NURSING CONSIDERATIONS

See also *Nursing Considerations* for *Centrally Acting Muscle Relaxants,* p. 704.

Administration/Storage

1. If the drug is to be administered IV, the rate should not exceed 3 mL/min.

2. For IV drip, one ampule may be added to no more than 250 mL of sodium chloride or 5% dextrose injection.

3. Before removing IV, clamp off the tubing to prevent extravasation of the hypertonic solution, which may cause thrombophlebitis.

4. If the drug is to be administered IM, inject no more than 5 mL into each gluteal region.

5. When administering IM to an adult, select a large muscle mass. When administering the drug IM to a child, use the vastus lateralis. Document and rotate sites.

Interventions

1. If the client is to receive the drug by IV, check frequently for infiltration. Extravasation of fluid may cause sloughing or thrombophlebitis.

2. Position the client in a recumbent position during IV administration. Have client maintain this position for 10–15 min after injection to minimize the side effects of postural hypotension.

3. Have side rails in place unless the client is attended during IV administration. Observe seizure precautions.

4. Monitor BP and pulse. If the heart rate drops below 60 beats per minute, notify the physician.

5. Supervise the ambulation of elderly clients or those who have been immobilized prior to drug therapy.

Client/Family Teaching

1. Urine may turn black, brown or green while client is taking this drug. This side effect will disappear once the drug is discontinued.

2. Instruct the client to rise slowly from a recumbent position and to dangle his legs before standing up.

3. Since drug causes drowsiness, clients should be instructed not to operate dangerous machinery or to drive a car.

4. Advise client to avoid the use of alcohol.

5. Nausea, anorexia and a metallic taste may occur with drug therapy. If these symptoms become severe or interfere with nutrition notify the physician.

6. Advise the client that diplopia, blurred vision, and nystagmus may occur. These side effects usually disappear with continued use of the medication. Clients should, however, report these symptoms to the physician.

7. Report any urticaria, skin eruptions, rash or pruritus. These are allergic responses and may necessitate the withdrawal of the drug.

ORPHENADRINE CITRATE   (or-**FEN**-ah-dreen)

Banflex, Blanex, Flexagin, Flexain, Flexoject, Flexon, K-Flex, Marflex, Myolin, Myotrol, Neocyten, Noradex, Norflex, O-Flex, Orflagen, Orfro, Orphenate, Tega-Flex (Rx)

See also *Centrally Acting Muscle Relaxants,* p. 703.

Classification: Centrally acting muscle relaxant.

Action/Kinetics: Action may be related, in part, to its centrally mediated analgesic effects. It also possesses anticholinergic activity. **Onset, PO:** Within 1 hr; **IM:** 5 min; **IV:** immediate. **Peak effect:** 2 hr. **Peak serum levels:** 60–120 ng/mL (after 100 mg). **Duration:** 4–6 hr. **t½:** 14 hr. Excretion of a small amount of unchanged drug and metabolites is via both urine and feces.

Uses: Adjunct to the treatment of acute musculoskeletal disorders.

Contraindications: Angle-closure glaucoma, stenosing peptic ulcers, prostatic hypertrophy, pyloric or duodenal obstruction, cardiospasm, and myasthenia gravis. Use in children.

Special Concerns: Use with caution during pregnancy and lactation. Use with caution in cardiac disease.

Side Effects: Most side effects are anticholinergic in nature. *GI:* Dry mouth (first to appear), nausea, vomiting, constipation, gastric irritation. *CV:* Tachycardia, transient syncope, palpitation. *CNS:* Headache, dizziness, drowsiness, lightheadedness, agitation, tremor, hallucinations, weakness, confusion (in geriatric patients). *GU:* Urinary retention or hesitancy. *Ophthalmologic:* Dilated pupils, blurred vision, increased intraocular tension (especially in closed-angle glaucoma). *Miscellaneous:* Hypersensitivity reactions. Rarely, aplastic anemia, urticaria, anaphylaxis.

Drug Interactions

Anticholinergics	Additive anticholinergic effects
Contraceptives, oral	Orphenadrine ↑ breakdown by liver
Griseofulvin	Orphenadrine ↑ breakdown by liver
Propoxyphene	Concomitant use may result in anxiety, tremors, and confusion

Dosage: Extended-release Tablets. Adults: 100 mg b.i.d. in the morning and evening. **IV or IM:** 60 mg. May be repeated q 12 hr.

NURSING CONSIDERATIONS

See also *Nursing Considerations* for *Centrally Acting Muscle Relaxants,* p. 704.

Administration/Storage

1. If the drug is to be administered IV, it should be given over a period of 5 minutes. The client should be in a supine position. The client should remain supine for 5 to 10 min following IV administration.
2. Sustained-release tablets should not be chewed or crushed.

Assessment

1. Note any client history of angle-closure glaucoma. The drug is contraindicated when this condition exists.
2. Note any history of any of the disorders listed above under contraindications, document and report.

Interventions

Observe the client for the presence of dry mouth. This is an indication that the dosage of drug should be reduced.

Client/Family Teaching

1. Encourage rinsing of mouth and more fluids in diet to relieve dry mouth.
2. Since drug causes drowsiness, clients should be cautioned not to operate dangerous machinery or to drive a car.
3. Instruct client and family to report any untoward reactions to the physician immediately.

CHAPTER THIRTY-SIX
Anticonvulsants

General Statement: Anticonvulsant agents are used for the control of the chronic seizures and involuntary muscle spasms or movements characteristic of certain neurologic diseases. They are most frequently used in the therapy of epilepsy, which results from disorders of nerve impulse transmission in the brain.

Therapeutic agents cannot cure these convulsive disorders, but do control seizures without impairing the normal functions of the CNS. This is often accomplished by selective depression of hyperactive areas of the brain responsible for the convulsions. Therefore, these drugs are taken at all times (prophylactically) to prevent the occurrence of the seizures.

There are several different types of epileptic disorders, including tonic-clonic (grand mal), absence seizures (petit mal), and psychomotor epilepsy. There is no single drug that can control all types of epilepsy; thus, accurate diagnosis is important. Drugs effective against one type of epilepsy may not be effective against another.

Anticonvulsant therapy must be individualized. Therapy begins with a small dose of the drug, which is continuously increased until either the seizures disappear or drug toxicity occurs. If a certain drug decreases the frequency of seizures but does not completely prevent them, another drug can be added to the dosage regimen and administered concomitantly with the first. Often a drug is ineffective and then another agent must be given. Failure of therapy most often results from the administration of doses too small to have a therapeutic effect or from failure to use two or more drugs together.

If for any reason drug therapy is discontinued, the anticonvulsant drugs must be withdrawn

36

gradually over a period of days or weeks to avoid severe, prolonged convulsions. This guideline also applies when one anticonvulsant is substituted for another; the dosage of the second drug is slowly increased at the same time that the dosage of the first drug is being reduced.

With appropriate diagnosis and selection of drugs, four out of five cases of epilepsy can be controlled adequately, but it may take the physician some time to find the best drug or combination of drugs with which to treat the patient.

Dosage: Dosage is highly individualized. However, trauma or emotional stress may necessitate an increase in drug dosage requirements (e.g., if the patient requires surgery and starts having seizures). For details, see individual agents.

NURSING CONSIDERATIONS

Administration/Storage

1. Oral suspensions of drugs should be shaken thoroughly before pouring to ensure uniform mixing.
2. Drug therapy must be individualized according to the needs of the client.
3. Medication should not be discontinued abruptly unless the physician advises it. Withdrawal should occur over a period of days or weeks to avoid severe, prolonged convulsions.
4. If there is reason to substitute one anticonvulsant drug for another, the first drug should be withdrawn slowly at the same time the dosage of the second drug is being increased.

Assessment

1. Check the client's medical history for hypersensitivity to particular types of anticonvulsant drugs. Note the derivatives of that particular type as they should also be avoided.
2. Note the client's orientation as to time and place, affect, reflexes and vital signs and record as baseline data.
3. Check intervals of EEG for regions of abnormal spike or line flat patterns. Also examine EEG for temporal lobe foci, and for spike and dome patterns before instituting therapy.
4. Determine the frequency and severity of client's seizures.
5. Assess the condition of the client's skin and mucous membranes.
6. If the client is female and of childbearing age, determine the likelihood of pregnancy. Some of these drugs have been linked to fetal abnormalities.
7. Obtain a CBC, blood glucose level, liver and renal function studies as well as urinalysis prior to initiating therapy.

Interventions

1. Monitor blood pressure, pulse and respirations. Observe for signs and symptoms of impending seizures.
2. Note any evidence of CNS side effects, such as complaints of blurred vision, dimmed vision, slurred speech, nystagmus or confusion.
3. Observe for muscle twitching, loss of muscle tone, episodes of bizarre behavior and/or subsequent amnesia and document.
4. Check if the physician wishes the client to receive folic acid supplements to prevent megaloblastic anemia.
5. Check if the physician wishes the client to receive vitamin D supplementation to prevent hypocalcemia. The usual dose is 4,000 units of vitamin D per week.
6. Clients who are to be on prolonged therapy need to have a diet rich in vitamin D.

7. Frequently check for decreased levels of serum calcium since phenytoin can contribute to demineralization of bone. This can result in osteomalacia in adults and rickets in children. The risk is particularly great in clients who are inactive.

8. Anticipate that the physician will order vitamin K to be administered to pregnant women 1 month before delivery. This is to prevent postpartum hemorrhage and bleeding in the newborn and the mother.

9. For clients who require IV administration of anticonvulsant drugs, monitor closely for respiratory depression and cardiovascular collapse.

10. Be prepared, in case of acute oral toxicity, to assist with inducing emesis (provided the client is not comatose) and with gastric lavage, along with other supportive measures such as administration of fluids and oxygen.

11. Anticipate that peritoneal dialysis or hemodialysis may be instituted in the treatment of acute toxicity for barbiturates, hydantoins, and succinimides (hemodialysis only).

Client/Family Teaching

1. Gastrointestinal distress may be lessened by taking the drugs with large amounts of fluid or with food.

2. During the initiation of therapy the anticonvulsant drugs may cause a decrease in mental alertness, drowsiness, headache, vertigo and ataxia. CNS symptoms are often dose-related and may disappear with a change of dosage or continued therapy. Therefore, the client should be warned to avoid hazardous tasks until the drug therapy has been regulated and the symptoms disappear.

3. Individuals on anticonvulsant therapy should carry identification indicating the form of epilepsy and the drug therapy being taken.

4. Take the prescribed amount of drug ordered. The doses of anticonvulsant drugs are not to be increased, decreased, or discontinued without the physician's approval. There is a danger that convulsions may result.

5. Avoid the use of alcohol as this may interfere with the action of anticonvulsants.

6. For complaints of altered sleep patterns, explain the nature of the disturbance and suggest ways to counteract the problem.

7. For alteration in bowel habits, suggest increased fluid intake and include fruit and other foods with roughage in the diet.

8. For clients who develop gingival hyperplasia, advocate the use of intensified oral hygiene, the use of a soft tooth brush, massage of the gums, and daily use of dental floss. It is also important to have routine dental visits.

9. If slurred speech develops, advocate slowing speech patterns to avoid the problem.

10. If rash, fever, severe headaches, stomatitis, rhinitis, urethritis, or balanitis (inflammation of the glans penis) occur, instruct the client to report immediately to the physician. These are early symptoms of hypersensitivity and may require a change in medication.

11. Review the importance of avoiding fever, low glucose levels, and low sodium conditions. These conditions lower the seizure threshold.

12. Report sore throat, easy bruising, petechiae, or nosebleeds, all of which are signs of hematologic toxicity.

13. Instruct client to report jaundice, dark urine, anorexia, and abdominal pain. These may be signs of hepatotoxicity.

14. Stress the importance of monthly liver function studies so as to detect early signs of hepatitis, hepatocellular degeneration and fatal hepatocellular necrosis.

15. If the client is female and likely to become pregnant, discuss the possible effects of the medication on pregnancy.

16. If the client is a lactating mother, observe and report signs of toxicity in the nursing infant.

17. Provide a list of drug and food interactions as well as side effects associated with drug therapy. Explain what to do should these occur and when to contact the physician.

18. Remind the client of the importance of reporting for all scheduled laboratory studies including CBC, renal and liver function studies as well as drug levels on a regular basis.

19. Instruct the client to report any unusual incidents in their life to the physician. There may be a need to alter the dosage of drug, especially if the client is undergoing physical trauma or emotional distress.

Evalutaion

1. Assess for evidence of client compliance with the prescribed medication regimen.
2. Assess client report of alteration in frequency of seizures and level of seizure control.
3. Obtain serum drug levels to determine if level is therapeutic.
4. Observe for freedom from complications of drug therapy.
5. Determine the client's ability to cope with the drugs prescribed and their disability. Record and report both favorable and unfavorable observations associated with drug therapy to the physician.

HYDANTOINS

General Statement: The hydantoins currently used for the treatment of epilepsy and other convulsive disorders are phenytoin, ethotoin, and mephenytoin. Of these, phenytoin (Dilantin) is the most widely used. However, patients refractory to phenytoin may respond to one of the other hydantoins.

Action/Kinetics: Although the mechanism of action is not known completely, it is believed these drugs stabilize neuronal membranes in the cell and limit the spread of neuronal or seizure activity. In addition, the hydantoins are known to activate inhibitory pathways that extend into the cerebral cortex leading to a reduction in seizure activity.

Special Concerns: Children and young adults are more susceptible to gingival hyperplasia than older adults. Children who take higher doses of hydantoins chronically may show a decreased performance in school. Geriatric patients may metabolize hydantoins more slowly leading to the possibility of toxic serum levels. Also, a decreased protein binding may be seen in geriatric patients leading to higher amount of unbound drug and possible toxicity.

ETHOTOIN   (ETH-oh-toyn)
Peganone (Rx)

See also *Hydantoins,* p. 722 and *Phenytoin,* p. 724.

Classification: Anticonvulsant, hydantoin type.

Action/Kinetics: Ethotoin is said to be less toxic, but also less effective, than phenytoin. Serum level monitoring is necessary because serum concentrations may increase disproportionately with increasing doses. **Therapeutic plasma levels:** 15–50 mcg/mL. **t½:** 3–9 hr. Metabolized by the liver and primarily eliminated through the urine with small amounts in the feces and breast milk.

Uses: Tonic-clonic seizures; psychomotor or temporal lobe seizures. May be used with other anticonvulsant drugs (except phenacemide) for combined seizure disorders.

Contraindications: Hepatic or hematologic disorders. Treatment of absence or febrile seizures.

Special Concerns: Use during pregnancy only if essential to control seizures.

Side Effects: See *Phenytoin,* p. 724. Gum hyperplasia is less common with ethotoin as is the incidence of ataxia and excessive hair growth.

Dosage: Tablets. Adults: 0.5–1 g the first day in 4–6 divided doses; **then,** dosage is increased until control has been established. Usual **maintenance:** 2–3 g daily. Geriatric and debilitated patients may require a lower initial dose.
  Pediatric: initial, not to exceed 0.75 g/day; **maintenance:** 0.5–1 g/day (up to 2 or even 3 g may be required in some patients).

NURSING CONSIDERATIONS

See also *Nursing Considerations* for *Anticonvulsants,* p. 720, and *Phenytoin,* p. 727.

Administration/Storage

1. If the client is receiving another anticonvulsant drug, it should not be discontinued abruptly when ethotoin therapy is initiated. The dosage of the first medication should be reduced gradually and the dosage of ethotoin should be increased gradually.
2. The doses of drug should be evenly spaced throughout the day.
3. Ethotoin should be taken after meals.

Evaluation

Note any changes in the frequency of the client's tonic-clonic seizures.

MEPHENYTOIN (meh-**FEN**-ih-toyn)

Mesantoin (Rx)

See also *Hydantoins,* p. 722, *Phenytoin,* p. 724.

Classification: Anticonvulsant, hydantoin type.

Action/Kinetics: Mephenytoin is a potentially dangerous drug since it is more toxic than the other hydantoins and is to be used only for patients refractory to other anticonvulsants. Blood dycrasias, skin and mucous membrane manifestations, and central effects are more common than with other hydantoins. Also mephenytoin has a sedative effect, which phenytoin does not have. Liver function tests are indicated before initiating therapy. Rapidly absorbed from GI tract; the drug has an active metabolite (nirvanol). **Time to peak levels:** 45 min–4 hr (for active metabolite—nirvanol—16–36 hr). **Therapeutic serum levels:** 25–40 mcg/mL (includes nirvanol). **t½, mephenytoin:** 7 hr; **nirvanol:** 95–144 hr.

Uses: Tonic-clonic seizure. Psychomotor or temporal lobe seizures. Focal and jacksonian seizures in patients not responding to other less toxic anticonvulsants.

Special Concerns: Use during pregnancy only if benefits clearly outweigh risks.

Dosage: Tablets: Adults and adolescents: initial, 50–100 mg daily for the first week; **then,** increase daily dosage by 50–100 mg at a minimum of weekly intervals. Usual **maintenance, adults:** 200–600 mg in 3 to 4 divided doses. **Pediatric:** 25–50 mg daily; dose can be increased by 25–50 mg at weekly intervals until seizures are controlled. **Usual maintenance:** 100–400 mg in 3 to 4 divided doses.

NURSING CONSIDERATIONS

See also *Nursing Considerations* for *Anticonvulsants,* p. 720, and *Phenytoin,* p. 727.

Administration/Storage: The pediatric dose may be divided and should be based on age, severity of seizures, and serum levels.

Client/Family Teaching

1. Advise clients not to operate machinery since drowsiness occurs more frequently with this drug than with other hydantoins.
2. Instruct client to report any changes in skin color or unusual rashes.

PHENYTOIN (DIPHENYLHYDANTOIN) (FEN-ih-toyn, dye-FEN-ill-hy-DAN-toyn)
Dilantin Infatab, Dilantin-30 Pediatric, Dilantin-125 (Rx)

PHENYTOIN SODIUM, EXTENDED (FEN-ih-toyn)
Dilantin Kapseals (Rx)

PHENYTOIN SODIUM, PARENTERAL (FEN-ih-toyn)
Dilantin Sodium (Rx)

PHENYTOIN SODIUM, PROMPT (FEN-ih-toyn)
Diphenylan Sodium (Rx)

See also *Anticonvulsants,* p. 719, and *Antiarrhythmics,* p. 533.

Classification: Anticonvulsant, hydantoin type; antiarrhythmic (Type I).

Action/Kinetics: Phenytoin acts in the motor cortex of the brain to reduce the spread of electrical discharges from the rapidly firing epileptic foci in this area. This is accomplished by stabilizing hyperexcitable cells possibly by affecting sodium efflux. Also, phenytoin decreases activity of centers in the brain stem responsible for the tonic phase of grand mal seizures. This drug has few sedative effects.

Serum levels must be monitored because the serum concentrations of phenytoin increase disproportionately as the dosage is increased. Phenytoin extended is designed for once-a-day dosage. It has a slow dissolution rate—no more than 35% in 30 min, 30%–70% in 60 min, and less than 85% in 120 min. Absorption is variable following oral dosage. **Peak serum levels: PO,** 4–8 hr. Since the rate and extent of absorption depend on the particular preparation, the same product should be used for a particular patient. **Peak serum levels (following IM):** 24 hr (wide variation). **Therapeutic serum levels:** 10–20 mcg/mL. **t¹/₂:** 8–60 hr (average: 20–30 hr). Steady state attained 7–10 days after initiation. Phenytoin is biotransformed in the liver. Both inactive metabolites and unchanged drug are excreted in the urine.

As an antiarrhythmic, phenytoin increases the electrical stimulation threshold of heart muscle, although it is less effective than quinidine, procainamide, or lidocaine. **Onset:** 30–60 min. **Duration:** 24 hr or more. **t½:** 22–36 hr. **Therapeutic serum level:** 10–20 mcg/mL.

Uses: Chronic epilepsy, especially of the tonic-clonic, psychomotor type. Not effective against absence seizures and may even increase the frequency of seizures in this disorder. Parenteral phenytoin is sometimes used to treat status epilepticus and to control seizures during neurosurgery.

Orally for certain premature ventricular contractions and IV for premature ventricular contractions and tachycardia. The drug is particularly useful for arrhythmias produced by digitalis overdosage.

Investigational: Paroxysmal choreoathetosis; to treat blistering and erosions in patients with recessive dystrophic epidermolysis bullosa; episodic dyscontrol; trigeminal neuralgia; as a muscle relaxant in neuromyotonia, myotonia congenita, or myotonic muscular dystrophy; to treat cardiac symptoms in overdosage of tricyclic antidepressants.

Contraindications: Hypersensitivity to hydantoins or exfoliative dermatitis. Administer with extreme caution to patients with a history of asthma or other allergies, impaired renal or hepatic function, and heart disease. Should not be administered to nursing mothers.

Special Concerns: Use with caution in porphyria.

Side Effects: *CNS:* Drowsiness, incoordination, ataxia, slurred speech, dizziness, extrapyramidal reactions, paradoxical increase in motor activity, psychotomimetic effects including hallucinations and delusions, fatigue, insomnia, and apathy. *GI:* Nausea, vomiting, either diarrhea or constipation. *Dermatologic:* Various dermatoses including a measles-like rash (common), scarlatiniform, maculopapular, and urticarial rashes. Rarely, drug-induced lupus erythematosus, Stevens-Johnson syndrome, exfoliative or purpuric dermatitis, and toxic epidermal necrolysis. Skin reactions may necessitate withdrawal of therapy. *Hematopoietic:* Megaloblastic anemia, lymph node hyperplasia, thrombocytopenia, leukopenia, agranulocytosis, pancytopenia, anemias including hemolytic and aplastic. *Hepatic:* Hepatitis, jaundice *Miscellaneous:* Hyperglycemia, osteomalacia, gingival hyperplasia, hirsutism, pulmonary fibrosis, alopecia, edema, photophobia.

Rapid parenteral administration may cause serious cardiovascular effects, including hypotension, arrhythmias, cardiovascular collapse, and heart block, as well as CNS depression.

Overdosage is characterized by nystagmus, ataxia, dysarthria, coma, unresponsive pupils, and hypotension, as well as by some of the CNS effects described above.

Many patients have a partial deficiency in the ability of the liver to degrade phenytoin, and as a result, toxicity may develop after a small oral dose. Liver and kidney function tests and hematopoietic studies are indicated prior to and periodically during drug therapy.

Drug Interactions	
Alcohol, ethyl	In alcoholics, ↓ effect of phenytoin due to ↑ breakdown by liver
Allopurinol	↑ Effect of phenytoin due to ↓ breakdown in liver
Antacids	↓ Effect of phenytoin due to ↓ GI absorption
Anticoagulants, oral	↑ Effect of phenytoin due to ↓ breakdown by liver. Also, possible ↑ in anticoagulant effect due to ↓ plasma protein binding
Antidepressants, tricyclic	May ↑ incidence of epileptic seizures or ↑ effect of phenytoin
Barbiturates	Effect of phenytoin may be ↑, ↓, or not changed; possible ↑ effect of barbiturates

Drug Interactions

Benzodiazepines	↑ Effect of phenytoin due to ↓ breakdown by liver
Carbamazepine	↓ Effect of phenytoin due to ↑ breakdown by liver
Chloral hydrate	↓ Effect of phenytoin due to ↑ breakdown by liver
Chloramphenicol	↑ Effect of phenytoin due to ↓ breakdown by liver
Cimetidine	↑ Effect of phenytoin due to ↓ breakdown by liver
Contraceptives, oral	Estrogen-induced fluid retention may precipitate seizures; also, ↓ effect of contraceptives due to ↑ breakdown by liver
Corticosteroids	Effect of corticosteroids ↓ due to ↑ breakdown by liver
Cyclosporine	↓ Effect of cyclosporine due to ↑ breakdown by liver
Diazoxide	↓ Effect of phenytoin due to ↑ breakdown by liver
Dicumarol	Phenytoin ↓ effect of dicumarol
Digitalis glycosides	↓ Effect of digitalis glycosides due to ↑ breakdown by liver
Disulfiram	↑ Effect of phenytoin due to ↓ breakdown by liver
Dopamine	IV phenytoin results in hypotension and bradycardia
Doxycycline	↓ Effect of doxycycline due to ↑ breakdown by liver
Estrogens	See *Contraceptives, Oral*
Folic acid	↓ Phenytoin blood levels due to ↑ breakdown by liver
Furosemide	↓ Effect of furosemide due to ↓ absorption
Haloperidol	↓ Effect of haloperidol due to ↑ breakdown by liver
Isoniazid	↑ Effect of phenytoin due to ↓ breakdown by liver
Levodopa	Phenytoin ↓ effect of levodopa
Meperidine	↓ Effect of meperidine due to ↑ breakdown by liver
Methadone	↓ Effect of methadone due to ↑ breakdown by liver
Methotrexate	↓ Effect of phenytoin due to ↓ absorption from GI tract
Metyrapone	↓ Effect of metyrapone due to ↑ breakdown by liver
Phenacemide	↑ Effect of phenytoin due to ↓ breakdown by liver
Phenothiazines	↑ Effect of phenytoin due to ↓ breakdown by liver

Drug Interactions

Phenylbutazone	↑ Effect of phenytoin due to ↓ breakdown by liver and ↓ plasma protein binding
Primidone	Possible ↑ effect of primidone
Quinidine	↓ Effect of quinidine due to ↑ breakdown by liver
Salicylates	↑ Effect of phenytoin by ↓ plasma protein binding
Sulfonamides	↑ Effect of phenytoin due to ↓ breakdown in liver
Sulfonylureas	↓ Effect of sulfonylureas
Theophylline	↓ Effect of both drugs due to ↑ breakdown by liver
Trimethoprim	↑ Effect of phenytoin due to ↓ breakdown by liver
Valproic acid	↑ Chance of phenytoin toxicity
Vinblastine	↑ Effect of phenytoin due to ↓ breakdown by liver

Laboratory Test Interferences: Alters liver function tests, ↑ blood glucose values, and ↓ PBI values. ↑ Gamma globulins. Phenytoin ↓ immunoglobulins A and G. False + Coombs' test.

Dosage: Oral Suspension, Chewable Tablets. *Seizures.* **Adults:** 125 mg t.i.d. initially; adjust dosage at 7–10 day intervals until seizures are controlled (**usual, maintenance:** 300–400 mg/day, although 600 mg/day may be required in some). **Pediatric: initial,** 5 mg/kg/day in 2–3 divided doses; **maintenance,** 4–8 mg/kg (up to maximum of 300 mg/day). Children over 6 years may require up to 300 mg/day. **Geriatric:** 3 mg/kg initially in divided doses; **then,** adjust dosage according to serum levels and response. Once dosage level has been established, the extended capsules may be used for once-a-day dosage.

   Capsules, Extended-release Capsules. *Seizures:* **Adults, initial** 100 mg t.i.d.; adjust dose at 7–10 day intervals until control is achieved. An initial loading dose of 12–15 mg/kg divided into 2–3 doses over 6 hr followed by 100 mg t.i.d. on subsequent days may be preferred if seizures are frequent. **Pediatric:** See dose for oral suspension and chewable tablets.

   IV. *Status epilepticus:* 20 mg/kg at a rate not to exceed 50 mg/min; **then,** 100 mg q 6–8 hr at a rate not exceeding 50 mg/min. Oral administration at a dose of 5 mg/kg daily divided into 2–4 doses should begin 12–24 hr after a loading dose is given. **Pediatric:** 15–20 mg/kg given at a rate of 1 mg/kg, not to exceed 50 mg/min. **IM** dose should be 50% greater than the PO dose. *Neurosurgery:* 100–200 mg IM q 4 hr during and after surgery (during first 24 hr, no more than 1,000 mg should be administered; after first day, give maintenance dosage).

   Arrhythmias: **PO:** 200–400 mg daily. **IV:** 100 mg q 5 min up to maximum of 1 g.

   Full effectiveness of orally administered hydantoins is delayed and may take 6–9 days to be fully established. A similar period of time will elapse before effects disappear completely.

   When hydantoins are substituted for or added to another anticonvulsant medication, their dosage is gradually increased, while dosage of the other drug is decreased proportionally.

NURSING CONSIDERATIONS

See also *Nursing Considerations* for *Anticonvulsants,* p. 720, and *Antiarrhythmics,* p. 534.

Administration/Storage

1. For parenteral preparations:

- Only a clear solution of the drug may be used.
- Dilute with special diluent supplied by manufacturer.
- Shake the vials until the solution is clear. It may take about 10 min for the drug to dissolve.
- To hasten the process, warm the vial in warm water after adding the diluent.
- The drug is incompatible with acid solutions.

2. IV phenytoin may form a precipitate. Therefore flush tubing thoroughly with sodium chloride before and after IV administration. *Do not* use dextrose solutions. Use an in-line filter to collect microscopic particulate matter.

3. Following the IV administration of the drug, administer sodium chloride injection through the same needle or IV catheter to avoid local irritation of the vein. This is caused by alkalinity of the solution.

4. For treatment of status epilepticus, inject the IV slowly at a rate not to exceed 50 mg/min. If necessary, the dose may be repeated 30 min after the initial administration.

5. Avoid subcutaneous or perivascular injections. Pain, inflammation, and necrosis may be caused by the highly alkaline solutions.

6. *Do not* add phenytoin to an already running IV solution.

7. If the client is receiving tube feedings of Isocal or Osmolite there may be interference with the absorption of oral phenytoin. Therefore, do not administer them together.

Assessment

1. Note the history and nature of the client's epileptic seizures.

2. Determine if the client is hypersensitive to hydantoins or has exfoliative dermatitis.

3. If the client is female and pregnant note that she should not breast feed the baby following delivery.

4. Obtain liver and renal function studies as baseline data against which to measure alterations once therapy is initiated.

Interventions

1. Monitor serum drug levels on a routine basis.

2. Seven to 10 days may be required to achieve recommended serum levels. The drug is metabolized much more slowly by elderly clients.

3. If the client is receiving drugs that interact with hydantoins or has impaired liver function, the serum phenytoin level should be done periodically. The clinically effective range is 10–20 mcg/mL.

4. Monitor the complete blood cell count and white cell differential throughout drug therapy.

5. During the IV administration, monitor BP closely for hypotension.

6. If client complains of weakness, ease of fatigue, headaches, or feeling faint, assess for signs of folic acid deficiency. Document and report to the physician. Invite a dietitian to review food intake and diet with the client.

7. Note if the client is developing an overgrowth of hair, coarse hair or acne. Document and report these symptoms to the physician. Provide emotional support and discourage the client from discontinuing therapy because of these side effects. Consult a dermatologist as needed.

8. The drug may alter thyroid function results. If thyroid studies are conducted, for ensured accuracy, they should be repeated 10 days after therapy has been discontinued.

Client/Family Teaching

1. Review symptoms of overdose and instruct client to notify the physician should any of these occur.

2. Do not substitute phenytoin products or exchange brands, as bioavailability of phenytoin may vary. Seizure control may be lost, or toxic blood levels may develop if a substitution is made.

3. Prompt release forms of the medication cannot be substituted for another unless the dosage is also adjusted.

  • If the client is taking phenytoin extended, he should not substitute chewable tablets for capsules. The strengths of the medications are not equal.
  • Clients taking phenytoin extended should check the labels of the bottle carefully. Chewable tablets are never in the extended form.
  • Clients taking phenytoin extended should take only a single dose of medication a day. It should be taken as directed by the physician. Also, take only the brand prescribed by the physician.

4. If the client misses a dose of medication, take the dose as soon as it is remembered. Then resume the usual schedule. Do not, however, double up to make up for the missed dose of drug. If the doses of drug are scheduled throughout the day, and one of the doses is missed, take the drug as soon as it is realized that the dose has been missed unless it is within 4 hours of the next dose of drug. In that case, omit the missed dose unless otherwise instructed.

5. Take with food to minimize GI upset.

6. Avoid ingestion of alcohol.

7. Do not take any other medication without medical supervision. Hydantoins interact with many other medications, and the addition of other drugs may require adjustment of the anticonvulsant dose.

8. If the client has diabetes mellitus, blood glucose levels should be monitored frequently when initiating therapy, or if the client is having the dosage of phenytoin adjusted. It may be necessary to adjust insulin dosage and/or the client's diet.

9. Clients with diabetes should report any changes in glucose determinations with urine tests and/or finger sticks to the physician.

10. Warn that hydantoin may cause the urine to appear pink, red, or brown.

11. To minimize bleeding from the gums, practice good oral hygiene. Client should be encouraged to brush teeth with a soft toothbrush, massage the gums and floss every day.

12. Hydantoin has an androgenic effect on the hair follicle. Clients may develop acne. They should be encouraged to practice good skin care.

13. Report any excessive growth of hair on the face and trunk, and any discolorations or skin rash to the physician.

14. Stress the importance of reporting for laboratory studies as ordered including a complete blood count, drug levels, and renal and liver function studies on a regular basis.

15. Do not abruptly stop medications without physician consent.

16. Report all bothersome side effects as these effects may be dose-related.

17. Provide sexually active women of childbearing age with birth control information while receiving phenytoin therapy.

Evaluation

1. Assess client/family knowledge and understanding of illness, response to therapy and to teaching.

2. Observe for freedom from complications of drug therapy.

3. Note any evidence of noncompliance with the drug regimen and determine the cause.

4. Determine serum drug levels.

OXAZOLIDINEDIONES

Action/Kinetics: Two oxazolidinediones (paramethadione and trimethadione) are currently used for the treatment of absence seizures only. The drugs may raise the threshold for cortical seizures by decreasing projection of focal activity and reducing repetitive spinal cord transmission. Also, electroencephalograms show a decrease in the spike and wave patterns seen with absence seizures. The drugs are well absorbed from the GI tract.

Uses: Absence seizures (petit mal). Because of its toxicity, it is not the drug of choice; reserved for refractory cases.

Contraindications: Anemia, leukopenia, thrombocytopenia, renal and hepatic disease, disease of the optic nerve. Pregnancy (may be teratogenic).

Special Concerns: Use with caution during lactation. Use during pregnancy may result in "fetal trimethadione syndrome" characterized by increased frequency of congenital malformations. Exposure of these drugs prior to delivery may cause an increased risk of life-threatening hemorrhage in the neonate within the first 24 hr after birth.

Side Effects: *CNS:* May increase frequency of tonic-clonic seizures. Myasthenia gravis-like syndrome, drowsiness, irritability, insomnia, fatigue, headache, malaise, personality changes. *Hematologic:* Pancytopenia, leukopenia, thrombocytopenia, eosinophilia, agranulocytosis, neutropenia, anemia (aplastic or hypoplastic). Also, petechiae, retinal hemorrhage, bleeding from gums, nose, or vagina. *Dermatologic:* Skin rash, exfoliative dermatitis, erythema multiforme. Alopecia, pruritus. *GI:* Nausea, vomiting, abdominal distress and pain, anorexia, weight loss, hiccoughs. *Other:* Lupus erythematosus, pseudolymphomas, nephrotic symptoms (nephrosis, proteinuria), hepatitis (rare), photophobia, double vision, blood pressure changes.

Complete blood counts should be undertaken before therapy begins and at monthly intervals thereafter. Periodic ophthalmologic examinations are necessary.

Drug Interactions	
Aminosalicylic acid (PAS)	PAS ↑ CNS depressant effects of the oxazolidinediones
Anticoagulants, oral	↑ CNS depressant effects of the oxazolidinediones
Narcotic analgesics	Concomitant administration may cause severe respiratory depression, coma, and death

NURSING CONSIDERATIONS

See also *Nursing Considerations* for *Anticonvulsants,* p. 720.

Assessment

1. Note if the client has a history of blood dyscrasias. Check CBC results and evaluate before initiating therapy.
2. Determine if the client has any history of vision problems prior to initiating therapy.
3. If the client is female and of childbearing age, determine if pregnant. These drugs should not be used if the client becomes pregnant since they have been linked to fetal abnormalities.
4. Review the list of drug interactions and determine if the client is taking any drugs that may interact with this group.
5. Assess frequency and severity of client's seizures.

6. Ensure that baseline CBC, liver and renal function studies have been completed prior to initiating therapy.

Interventions

1. Note if the client develops any increase in the frequency of tonic-clonic seizures and report.
2. Observe the client for any changes in behavior, such as increased irritability or personality changes.
3. Note any evidence of unusual vaginal bleeding or excessive hair loss.
4. Clients may develop neurological reactions such as myasthenia gravis-like syndrome. These symptoms should all be reported to the physician at the first sign of the problem and either the dosage of drug will be reduced or the drug will be discontinued.

Client/Family Teaching

1. Report immediately fever, sore throat, swollen glands, joint pains. These could be symptoms of blood dyscrasias.
2. Report frequency of urination, burning on urination, cloudy urine, or the presence of edema. These may be symptoms of renal dysfunction and may require a change in medication. A urinalysis should be conducted periodically throughout therapy.
3. Instruct the client/family to report immediately any signs of jaundice.
4. Drowsiness and blurred vision may occur with the use of these drugs. Activities should be planned that minimize hazard caused by lack of alertness and coordination.
5. Day blindness should be reported. It may be relieved by wearing dark glasses.
6. Stress the importance of periodic laboratory and eye examinations during therapy.
7. Review birth control measures with women of childbearing age. Stress the importance of adhering to these measures during drug therapy.
8. Emphasize the importance of compliance with all aspects of the drug regimen and of reporting any changes that occur, however minor they may seem.

PARAMETHADIONE   (pah-rah-meth-ah-DYE-ohn)

Paradione (Rx)

See also *Anticonvulsants,* p. 719 and *Oxazolidinediones,* p. 730.

Classification: Anticonvulsant, oxazolidinedione type.

Action/Kinetics: Has greater sedative effects but is said to be less toxic and less effective than trimethadione. Toxic doses may lead to unconsciousness and respiratory depression. **t$^{1}/_{2}$:** 12–24 hr.

Special Concerns: Pregnancy category: D.

Dosage: Capsules, Oral Solution. Adults and adolescents: Initial, 300 mg t.i.d.–q.i.d.; increase by 300 mg at weekly intervals until seizures controlled or toxicity appears. **Maintenance:** 300–600 mg t.i.d.–q.i.d., not to exceed 2.4 g daily. **Pediatric, 6 years and older:** 300 t.i.d.; **2–6 years:** 200 mg t.i.d.; **up to 2 years of age:** 100 mg t.i.d.

NURSING CONSIDERATIONS

See *Nursing Considerations* for *Anticonvulsants,* p. 720 and *Oxazolidinediones,* p. 730.

Administration/Storage

The oral solution must be diluted with milk, juice, or other diluent before administration.

TRIMETHADIONE   (try-meth-ah-**DYE**-ohn)

Tridione (Rx)

See also *Anticonvulsants,* p. 719, and *Oxazolidinediones,* p. 730.

Classification: Anticonvulsant, oxazolidinedione type.

Action/Kinetics: Peak plasma levels: 30 min–2 hr. Biotransformed by the liver to the active metabolite dimethadione. **t½** (trimethadione): 12–24 hr; **t½** (dimethadione): 6–13 days. **Therapeutic serum levels of dimethadione:** 700 mcg/mL (approximate). Dimethadione is excreted unchanged by the kidney. Trimethadione does not bind significantly to plasma protein.

Dosage: Capsules, Oral Solution, Tablets. Adults and adolescents: initial, 300 mg t.i.d.–q.i.d.; increase by 300 mg at weekly intervals until seizures controlled or toxicity appears. **Maintenance:** 300–600 mg t.i.d.–q.i.d., not to exceed 2.4 g daily. **Pediatric:** 13 mg/kg (335 mg/m^2) t.i.d. Alternatively, **children, 6 years and older:** 300 mg t.i.d.–q.i.d.; **2–6 years:** 200 mg t.i.d.; **up to 2 years of age:** 100 mg t.i.d.

NURSING CONSIDERATIONS

See *Nursing Considerations* for *Anticonvulsants,* p. 720, and *Oxazolidinediones,* p. 730.

Administration/Storage

The solution can be diluted with water before administering to small children.

SUCCINIMIDES

General Statement: Three succinimide derivatives are currently used primarily for the treatment of absence seizures (petit mal): ethosuximide, methsuximide, and phensuximide. Ethosuximide is currently the drug of choice. Methsuximide should be used only when the patient is refractory to other drugs. These drugs may be given concomitantly with other anticonvulsants if other types of epilepsy are manifested with absence seizures.

Action/Kinetics: The succinimide derivatives suppress the abnormal brain wave patterns associated with lapses of consciousness in absence seizures. They apparently do so by depressing the motor cortex and by raising the threshold of the CNS to convulsive stimuli.

Uses: Primarily absence seizures (petit mal).

Contraindications: Hypersensitivity to succinimides.

Special Concerns: Safe use during pregnancy has not been established. Must be used with caution in patients with abnormal liver and kidney function.

Side Effects: *CNS:* Drowsiness, ataxia, dizziness, headaches, euphoria, lethargy, fatigue, insomnia, hyperactivity. Psychiatric or psychological aberrations such as mental slowing, hypochondriasis, sleep disturbances, inability to concentrate, depression, confusion, aggressiveness. *GI:* Nausea, vomiting, hiccoughs, anorexia, diarrhea, gastric distress and pain, cramps, constipation. *Hematologic:* Leukopenia, granulocytopenia, eosinophilia, agranulocytosis, pancytopenia, aplastic anemia, monocytosis. *Dermatologic:* Pruritus, urticaria, erythema multiforme, lupus erythematosus, Stevens-Johnson syndrome, photophobia. *Miscellaneous:* Blurred vision, alopecia, muscle weakness, hirsutism, hyperemia, hypertrophy of gums, swollen tongue, myopia, vaginal bleeding.

Drug Interactions: Succinimides may increase the effects of hydantoins by decreasing breakdown by the liver.

Dosage: *Individualized.* See individual agents. Succinimides may be given in combination with other anticonvulsants if two or more types of seizures are present.

NURSING CONSIDERATIONS

See also *Nursing Considerations* for *Anticonvulsants,* p. 720.

Client/Family Teaching

1. Report any increase in frequency of tonic-clonic (grand mal) seizures.
2. Alert the family to the possibility of transient personality changes, hypochondriacal behavior, and aggressiveness. Stress the need to report these personality changes immediately to the physician.
3. Clients should be advised to report any persistent fever, swollen glands, and bleeding gums. These may be symptoms of a blood dyscrasia.
4. Instruct the client to report for complete blood counts and liver and renal function studies on a scheduled basis.

ETHOSUXIMIDE   (eth-oh-**SUX**-ih-myd)

Zarontin (Rx)

See also *Anticonvulsants,* p. 719, and *Succinimides,* p. 732.

Classification: Anticonvulsant, succinimide type.

Action/Kinetics: Peak serum levels: 3–7 hr. **t½: adults,** 60 hr; **t½: children,** 30 hr. Steady serum levels reached in 7–10 days. **Therapeutic serum levels:** 40–100 mcg/mL. The drug is metabolized in the liver. Both inactive metabolites and unchanged drug are excreted in the urine.

Additional Drug Interactions: Both isoniazid and valproic acid may ↑ the effects of ethosuximide.

Dosage: Capsules, Syrup. Adults and children over 6 years, initial: 250 mg b.i.d.; the dose may be increased by 250 mg daily at 4–7-day intervals until seizures are controlled or until total daily dose reaches 1.5 g. **Children under 6 years, initial:** 250 mg once daily; dosage may be increased by 250 mg daily every 4–7 days until control is established or total daily dose reaches 1 g.

NURSING CONSIDERATIONS

See also *Nursing Considerations* for *Anticonvulsants,* p. 720, and *Succinimides,* p. 733.

Client/Family Teaching

Instruct the client to take medication with meals to minimize GI upset.

METHSUXIMIDE   (meth-**SUX**-ih-myd)

Celontin (Rx)

See also *Anticonvulsants,* p. 719, and *Succinimides,* p. 732.

Classification: Anticonvulsant, succinimide type.

Action/Kinetics: t½: 1–3 hr for methsuximide and 36–45 hr for the active metabolite. **Therapeutic serum levels:** 10–40 mcg/mL.

Uses: Methsuximide is used for absence seizures refractory to other drugs.

Additional Untoward Reactions: Most common are ataxia, dizziness, and drowsiness.

Additional Drug Interaction: Methsuximide may ↑ the effect of primidone.

Dosage: Capsules. Adults and children: initial, 300 mg daily for first week; **then,** increase dosage by 300 mg at weekly intervals until control established. **Maximum daily dose:** 1.2 g in divided doses.

NURSING CONSIDERATIONS

See *Nursing Considerations* for *Anticonvulsants,* p. 720, and *Succinimides,* p. 733.

PHENSUXIMIDE   (fen-**SUX**-ih-myd)

Milontin (Rx)

See also *Anticonvulsants,* p. 719, and *Succinimides,* p. 732.

Classification: Anticonvulsant, succinimide type.

Action/Kinetics: Phensuximide is said to be less effective as well as less toxic than other succinimides. May color the urine pink, red, or red-brown. **t½:** 5–12 hr. **Peak effect:** 1–4 hr.

Special Concerns: Use with caution in patients with intermittent porphyria.

Additional Side Effects: Kidney damage, hematuria, urinary frequency.

Dosage: Capsules. Adults and children, initial: 0.5 g b.i.d.; **then,** dose can be increased by 0.5 g daily at one week intervals until seizures are controlled or the daily dosage reaches 3 g. May be used with other anticonvulsants in the presence of multiple types of epilepsy.

NURSING CONSIDERATIONS

See *Nursing Considerations* for *Anticonvulsants,* p. 720, and *Succinimides,* p. 733.

MISCELLANEOUS ANTICONVULSANTS

ACETAZOLAMIDE   (ah-see-tah-**ZOHL**-ah-myd)

Acetazolam✿, AK-Zol, Apo-Acetazolamide✿, Daranide, Dazamide, Diamox, Diamox Sequels, Neptazane (Rx)

ACETAZOLAMIDE SODIUM   (ah-see-tah-**ZOHL**-ah-myd)

Diamox (Rx)

See also *Anticonvulsants,* p. 719.

Classification: Anticonvulsant (miscellaneous), diuretic (carbonic anhydrase inhibitor).

Action/Kinetics: Acetazolamide is a sulfonamide derivative possessing carbonic anhydrase inhibitor activity. As an anticonvulsant, beneficial effects may be due to inhibition of carbonic anhydrase in the CNS which increases carbon dioxide tension resulting in a decrease in neuronal conduction. Systemic acidosis may also be involved. As a diuretic, the drug inhibits carbonic anhydrase in the kidney which decreases formation of bicarbonate and hydrogen ions from carbon dioxide thus reducing the availability of these ions for active transport. Use as a diuretic is limited because the drug promotes metabolic acidosis, which inhibits diuretic activity. This may be partially circumvented by giving acetazolamide on alternate days. Acetazolamide also reduces intraocular pressure.

Absorbed from the GI tract and widely distributed throughout the body, including the CNS. Excreted unchanged in the urine. **Tablets: Onset,** 60–90 min; **peak:** 2–4 hr; **duration:** 8–12 hr. **Sustained-release capsules: Onset,** 2 hr; **peak:** 8–12 hr; **duration:** 18–24 hr. **Injection (IV): Onset,** 2 min; **peak:** 15 min; **duration:** 4–5 hr. The drug is eliminated mainly unchanged through the kidneys.

Uses: Adjunct in clonic-tonic, myoclonic seizures, absence seizures (petit mal), mixed seizures, simple partial seizure patterns. Open-angle, secondary, angle-closure, or malignant glaucoma. Prophylaxis or treatment of acute mountain sickness. *Investigational:* Hypokalemic and hyper-kalemic forms of familial periodic paralysis; to induce forced alkaline diuresis to increase excretion of certain weakly acidic drugs; prophylaxis of uric acid or cystine renal calculi.

Contraindications: Low serum levels of sodium and potassium. Renal and hepatic dysfunction. Hyperchloremic acidosis, adrenal insufficiency, hypersensitivity to thiazide diuretics. Not to be used chronically in presence of noncongestive angle-closure glaucoma.

Special Concerns: Use with caution in the presence of mild acidosis, advanced pulmonary disease, and pregnancy.

Side Effects: *Short-term therapy* (minimal adverse reactions): Anorexia, polyuria, drowsiness, confusion, paresthesia. *Long-term therapy:* Acidosis, transient myopia. *Rarely:* Urticaria, glycosuria, hepatic insufficiency, melena, flaccid paralysis, convulsions. Also, side effects similar to those produced by sulfonamides.

Drug Interactions: Also see *Diuretics,* p. 1250.

Drug Interactions	
Amphetamine	↑ Effect of amphetamine by ↑ renal tubular reabsorption
Ephedrine	↑ Effect of ephedrine by ↑ renal tubular reabsorption
Lithium carbonate	↓ Effect of lithium by ↑ renal excretion
Methotrexate	↓ Effect of methotrexate due to ↑ renal excretion
Primidone	↓ Effect of primidone due to ↓ GI absorption
Pseudoephedrine	↑ Effect of pseudoephedrine by ↑ renal tubular reabsorption
Quinidine	↑ Effect of quinidine by ↑ renal tubular reabsorption
Salicylates	↓ Effect of salicylates by ↑ renal excretion

Dosage: Extended-release Capsules, Tablets. *Seizures.* **Adults/children:** 4–30 mg/kg/day in divided doses. Optimum daily dosage: 375–1,000 mg (doses higher than 1,000 mg do not increase therapeutic effect). *If used as adjunct to other anticonvulsants:* **initial,** 250 mg once daily; dose can be increased up to 1,000 mg/day if necessary.

Glaucoma, simple open angle: 0.25–1 g daily in divided doses. *Glaucoma, closed angle prior to surgery or secondary:* 0.25 g q 4 hr, 0.25 g b.i.d., or 0.5 g followed by 0.125–0.25 g q 4 hr. **Extended release capsules:** 500 mg b.i.d. in the morning and evening. **Pediatric:** 8–30 mg/kg (usual: 10–15 mg/kg or 300–900 mg/m²) daily in divided doses.

Acute mountain sickness. 250 mg b.i.d.–q.i.d. (500 mg 1–2 times daily of extended-release capsules). During rapid ascent, 1 g daily is recommended.

NURSING CONSIDERATIONS

See also *Nursing Considerations* for *Diuretics,* p. 1250, and *Sulfonamides,* p. 207.

Administration/Storage

1. Change from other anticonvulsant therapy to acetazolamide should be gradual.
2. Use parenteral solutions within 24 hr after reconstitution.
3. IV administration is preferred; IM administration is painful due to alkalinity.
4. Reconstitute with at least 5 mL of sterile water for injection.
5. Tolerance after prolonged use may necessitate dosage increase.
6. Do not administer the sustained-release dosage form as an anticonvulsant.
7. When used for prophylaxis of mountain sickness, dosage should be initiated 1–2 days before ascent and should be continued for at least 2 days while at high altitudes.
8. Due to possible differences in bioavailability, brands should not be interchanged.

Assessment

1. Obtain a complete nursing history.
2. Evaluate laboratory findings for levels of electrolytes, uric acid and glucose. Obtain labs for and document any evidence of liver and renal dysfunction prior to administering the medication.
3. Obtain a complete client drug history to assure that the client is not receiving any drug therapy that interacts with the medication.

Client/Family Teaching

1. Taking the drug with food may decrease gastric irritation and GI upset.
2. The drug increases the frequency of voiding. Therefore, take the medication early in the day to avoid interrupting sleep.
3. Clients with diabetes should be warned that the drug may increase blood glucose levels. Therefore, they should monitor serum glucose levels carefully and report increases as the dose of hypoglycemic agent may require adjustment.
4. If nausea, dizziness, muscle weakness, or cramps occur, report these to the physician.
5. Note any changes in the color of stools and report.
6. Stress the importance of reporting for scheduled laboratory studies.

CARBAMAZEPINE (kar-bahm-**AYZ**-eh-peen)

Apo-Carbamazepine ✽, Mazepine ✽, Epitol, Novocarbamaz ✽, Tegretol, Tegretol Chewtabs ✽, Tegretol CR ✽ (Rx)

See also *Anticonvulsants,* p. 719.

Classification: Anticonvulsant, miscellaneous.

Action/Kinetics: Carbamazepine is chemically similar to the cyclic antidepressants. It also manifests antimanic, antineuralgic, antidiuretic, anticholinergic, antiarrhythmic, and antipsychotic effects. The anticonvulsant action is not known but may involve depressing activity in the nucleus ventralis anterior of the thalamus. Due to the potentially serious blood dyscrasias, a benefit-to-risk evaluation should be undertaken before the drug is instituted. **Peak serum levels:** 4–5 hr. **t¹/₂** (serum): 12–17 hr with repeated doses. **Therapeutic serum levels:** 4–12 mcg/mL. Carbamazepine is metabolized in the liver to an active metabolite (epoxide derivative) with a half-life of 5–8 hr. Metabolites are excreted through the feces and urine.

Uses: Epilepsy, especially partial seizures with simple or complex symptomatology. Clonic-tonic seizures, psychomotor epilepsy, and diseases with mixed seizure patterns. Carbamazepine is often a drug of choice due to its low incidence of side effects. To treat pain associated with tic douloureux (trigeminal neuralgia) and glossopharyngeal neuralgia. *Investigational:* Neurogenic diabetes insipidus, alcohol withdrawal, herpes zoster, selected psychiatric disorders such as resistant schizophrenia, dyscontrol syndrome with limbic system dysfunction, and bipolar disorders.

Contraindications: History of bone marrow depression. Hypersensitivity to drug or tricyclic antidepressants. Lactation. In patients taking MAO inhibitors. Should not be used to relieve general aches and pains.

Special Concerns: Safe use during pregnancy (category: C) has not been established. Safety and effectiveness have not been established in children less than 6 years of age. Use with caution in glaucoma and in hepatic, renal, and cardiovascular disease. Use with caution in patients with mixed seizure disorder that includes atypical absence seizures (carbamazepine not effective). Use in geriatric patients may cause an increased incidence of confusion, agitation, AV heart block, syndrome of inappropriate antidiuretic hormone, and bradycardia.

Side Effects: *GI:* Nausea and vomiting (common), diarrhea, constipation, abdominal pain or upset, anorexia, glossitis, stomatitis, dryness of mouth and pharynx. *Hematologic:* Aplastic anemia, leukopenia, eosinophilia, thrombocytopenia, purpura, agranulocytosis, leukocytosis, pancytopenia, bone marrow depression. *CNS:* Dizziness, drowsiness and unsteadiness (common); headache, fatigue, confusion, speech disturbances, visual hallucinations, depression with agitation, talkativeness, hyperacusis, abnormal involuntary movements, behavioral changes in children. *CV:* Congestive heart failure, hypertension, hypotension, syncope, thrombophlebitis, worsening of angina, arrhythmias (including AV block). *GU:* Urinary frequency or retention, oliguria, impotence, renal failure, azotemia, albuminuria, glycosuria, increased BUN. *Dermatologic:* Pruritus, urticaria, photosensitivity, exfoliative dermatitis, erythematous rashes, alterations in pigmentation, alopecia, sweating, purpura, aggravation of toxic epidermal necrolysis (Lyell's syndrome), Stevens-Johnson syndrome, aggravation of systemic lupus erythematosus, alopecia, erythema nodosum or multiforme. *Ophthalmologic:* Nystagmus, double vision, blurred vision, oculomotor disturbances, conjunctivitis; scattered, punctate lens opacities. *Other:* Peripheral neuritis, paresthesias, tinnitus, fever, chills, joint and muscle aches and cramps, adenopathy or lymphadenopathy, dyspnea, pneumonitis, pneumonia, inappropriate antidiuretic hormone secretion syndrome.

Drug Interactions	
Acetaminophen	↑ Breakdown of acetaminophen → ↓ effect and ↑ risk of hepatotoxicity
Anticoagulants, oral	↓ Effect of anticoagulant due to ↑ breakdown by liver
Charcoal	↓ Effect of carbamazepine due to ↓ absorption from GI tract

Drug Interactions

Cimetidine	↑ Effect of carbamazepine due to ↓ breakdown by liver
Contraceptives, oral	↓ Effect of contraceptives due to ↑ breakdown by liver
Danazol	↑ Effect of carbamazepine due to ↓ breakdown by liver
Diltiazem	↑ Effect of carbamazepine due to ↓ breakdown by liver
Doxycycline	↓ Effect of doxycycline due to ↑ breakdown by liver
Erythromycin	↑ Effect of carbamazepine due to ↓ breakdown by liver
Ethosuximide	↓ Effect of ethosuximide due to ↑ breakdown by liver
Isoniazid	↑ Effect of carbamazepine due to ↓ breakdown by liver; also, carbamazepine may ↑ risk of isoniazid-induced hepatotoxicity
Lithium	↑ CNS toxicity
MAO inhibitors	Exaggerated side effects of carbamazepine
Muscle relaxants, nondepolarizing	↓ Effect of muscle relaxants
Nicotinamide	↑ Effect of carbamazepine due to ↓ breakdown by liver
Phenobarbital	↓ Effect of carbamazepine due to ↑ breakdown by liver
Phenytoin	↓ Effect of carbamazepine due to ↑ breakdown by liver; also, phenytoin levels may ↑ or ↓
Posterior pituitary hormones	Carbamazepine ↑ effect of posterior pituitary hormones
Primidone	↓ Effect of carbamazepine due to ↑ breakdown by liver
Propoxyphene	↑ Effect of carbamazepine due to ↓ breakdown by liver
Theophyllines	Effect of both drugs may be ↓
Troleandomycin	↑ Effect of carbamazepine due to ↓ breakdown by liver
Valproic acid	↓ Effect of valproic acid due to ↑ breakdown by liver
Verapamil	↑ Effect of carbamazepine due to ↓ breakdown by liver

Dosage: Oral Suspension, Tablets, Chewable Tablets, Extended-release Tablets. *Anticonvulsant.* **Adults and children over 12 years: initial,** 200 mg b.i.d. on day 1. Increase by 200 mg/day at weekly intervals until best response is attained. Divide total dose and administer q 6–8 hr. **Maximum dose, children 12–15 years:** 1,000 mg daily; **adults and children over 15 years:** 1,200 mg daily. **Maintenance:** decrease dose gradually to 800–1,200 mg daily. **Children, 6–12 years: initial,** 100 mg b.i.d. on day 1; **then,** increase slowly, at weekly intervals, by 100 mg/day; dose is divided and given q 6–8 hr. Daily dose should not exceed 1,000 mg. **Maintenance:** 400–800 mg daily. **Children, less than 6 years of age:** 10–20 mg/kg daily in 2–3 divided doses; dose can be increased slowly in weekly increments to maintenance levels of 250–300 mg daily (not to exceed 400 mg daily).

Trigeminal neuralgia: **initial,** 100 mg b.i.d. on day 1; increase by no more than 200 mg/day, using increments of 100 mg q 12 hr as needed, up to maximum of 1,200 mg daily. **Maintenance:** *usual,* 400–800 mg daily (range: 200–1,200 mg daily). Attempt discontinuation of drug at least 1 time q 3 months.

NURSING CONSIDERATIONS

See also *Nursing Considerations* for *Anticonvulsants,* p. 720.

Administration/Storage

1. Do not administer for a minimum of 2 weeks after client has received MAO inhibitor drugs.
2. Protect tablets from moisture.
3. The drug should be taken with meals.
4. The therapy should be started gradually with the lowest doses of drug to minimize adverse reactions.
5. Carbamazepine should be added gradually to other anticonvulsant therapy. The other anticonvulsant dosage may be maintained or decreased except for phenytoin which may need to be increased.

Assessment

1. Obtain baseline hematologic, liver and renal function tests prior to beginning therapy. Do not initiate therapy until significant abnormalities have been ruled out.
2. Obtain baseline eye examinations for evidence of opacities and intraocular pressure measurement.
3. Assess if the client has a history of psychoses, as drug may activate symptoms.

Interventions

1. CNS depression may impair client functions. If the client becomes agitated, side rails should be used.
2. Blood cell evaluation should be done on a weekly basis for the first 3 months of therapy, and monthly thereafter. The following guide should be used to determine the extent of bone marrow depression:
   - Erythrocyte count less than 4 million/mm³.
   - Hematocrit less than 32%.
   - Hemoglobin less than 11 g/dL.
   - Leukocytes less than 4,000/mm³.
   - Reticulocytes less than 0.3% of erythrocytes (20,000/mm³).
   - Serum iron greater than 150 mcg%.
3. Carbamazepine should be discontinued slowly at the first sign of a blood cell disorder.
4. Monitor intake and output ratios and vital signs for evidence of fluid retention, renal failure or cardiovascular complications during the period of dosage adjustment.
5. An EEG should be obtained periodically throughout the therapy.
6. If the drug has been quickly withdrawn from a client, use seizure precautions. Quick withdrawal may precipitate status epilepticus.

Client/Family Teaching

1. Withhold drug and check with the physician if any of the following symptoms occur:
   - Fever, sore throat, mouth ulcers, easy bruising, petechial and purpuric hemorrhages. These are early signs of bone marrow depression.

- Urinary frequency, acute urinary retention, oliguria, and sexual impotence. These are early signs of GU dysfunction.
- Symptoms of congestive heart failure, syncope, collapse, edema, thrombophlebitis, or cyanosis. These are cardiovascular side effects that require immediate attention.

2. Use caution in operating an automobile or other dangerous machinery because the drug may interfere with vision and coordination.
3. Report any skin eruptions or changes in skin pigmentation. These may require withdrawal of the drug.
4. Advise clients to avoid excessive sunlight and to use appropriate sun screen because of the risk of photosensitivity.
5. Stress the importance of reporting for scheduled laboratory studies to assess for early organ dysfunction.

Evaluation

Determine if there is a reduction in seizures among clients who have been unresponsive to other drug regimens.

CLONAZEPAM   (kloh-**NAYZ**-eh-pam)

Klonopin, Rivotril ✤ (C-IV) (Rx)

See also *Anticonvulsants,* p. 719, and *Benzodiazepines,* p. 611.

Classification: Anticonvulsant, miscellaneous.

Action/Kinetics: Benzodiazepine derivative. Clonazepam increases presynaptic inhibition and suppresses the spread of seizure activity. **Peak plasma levels:** 1–2 hr. **t½:** 18–50 hr. **Peak serum levels:** 20–80 ng/mL. The drug is more than 80% bound to plasma protein; it is metabolized almost completely in the liver to inactive metabolites, which are excreted in the urine.

Even though a benzodiazepine, clonazepam is used only as an anticonvulsant. However, contraindications, untoward reactions, and so forth are similar to those for diazepam.

Uses: Absence seizures (petit mal) including Lennox-Gastaut syndrome, akinetic and myoclonic seizures. Some effectiveness in patients resistant to succinimide therapy. *Investigational:* Treatment of panic attacks.

Contraindications: Sensitivity to benzodiazepines. Severe liver disease, acute narrow-angle glaucoma. Pregnancy.

Additional Side Effects: In patients in whom different types of seizure disorders exist, clonazepam may elicit or precipitate grand mal seizures.

Drug Interactions	
CNS depressants	Potentiation of CNS depressant effect of clonazepam
Phenobarbital	↓ Effect of clonazepam due to ↑ breakdown by liver
Phenytoin	↓ Effect of clonazepam due to ↑ breakdown by liver
Valproic acid	↑ Chance of absence seizures

Dosage: Tablets. Adults: initial, 0.5 mg t.i.d. Increase by 0.5–1 mg daily q 3 days until seizures are under control or side effects become excessive; **maximum:** 20 mg/day. **Pediatric up to 10 years or 30 kg:** 0.01–0.03 mg/kg/day in 2–3 divided doses up to a maximum of 0.05 mg/kg/day. Increase by increments of 0.25–0.5 mg q 3 days until seizures are under control or maintenance of 0.1–0.2 mg/kg is attained.

NURSING CONSIDERATIONS

See *Nursing Considerations* for *Benzodiazepines,* p. 614, and *Anticonvulsants,* p. 720.

Administration/Storage

1. Approximately one-third of clients show some loss of anticonvulsant activity within 3 months; adjustment of dose may reestablish effectiveness.
2. Adding clonazepam to existing anticonvulsant therapy may increase the depressant effects.
3. The daily dose should be divided into 3 equal doses; if doses cannot be divided equally, the largest dose should be given at bedtime.

CLORAZEPATE DIPOTASSIUM (kloh-**RAYZ**-eh-payt)

Gen-Xene, Novoclopate ✳, Tranxene-SD, Tranxene-SD Half (C-IV, Rx)

See also *Benzodiazepines,* p. 611.

Classification: Antianxiety agent, benzodiazepine type; anticonvulsant.

Action/Kinetics: Peak plasma levels: 1–2 hr. **t½:** 30–100 hr. Clorazepate is hydrolyzed in the stomach to desmethyldiazepam, the active metabolite. Oxazepam is also an active metabolite. **t½, desmethyldiazepam:** 30–100 hr; **t½, oxazepam:** 5–15 hr. **Time to peak plasma levels:** 0.5–2 hr. The drug is slowly excreted by the kidneys.

Uses: Anxiety, tension. Acute alcohol withdrawal, as adjunct in treatment of seizures. Adjunct for treating partial seizures.

Additional Contraindications: Depressive patients, nursing mothers. Give cautiously to patients with impaired renal or hepatic function.

Special Considerations: Pregnancy category: D.

Dosage: Capsules/Tablets. *Anxiety:* **initial,** 7.5–15 mg b.i.d.–q.i.d.; **maintenance:** 15–60 mg/day in divided doses. **Elderly or debilitated patients: initial,** 7.5–15 mg/day. **Alternative: Single daily dosage: Adult, initial,** 15 mg; **then,** 11.25–22.5 mg once daily. *Acute alcohol withdrawal: Day 1,* **initial,** 30 mg; **then,** 15 mg b.i.d.–q.i.d. the first day; *day 2,* 45–90 mg/day; *day 3,* 22.5–45 mg/day; *day 4,* 15–30 mg/day. Thereafter, reduce to 7.5–15 mg/day and discontinue as soon as possible. *Anticonvulsant, adjunct:* **Adults and children over 12 years: initial,** 7.5 mg t.i.d.; increase no more than 7.5 mg/week to maximum of 90 mg/day. **Children (9–12 years): initial,** 7.5 mg b.i.d.; increase no more than 7.5 mg/week to maximum of 60 mg/day. Not recommended for children under 9 years of age.

NURSING CONSIDERATIONS

See *Nursing Considerations* for *Benzodiazepines,* p. 614.

DIAZEPAM (dye-AYZ-eh-pam)

Apo-Diazepam✣, Diazepam Intensol, E-Pam✣, Meval✣, Novodipam✣, Rival✣, Valium, Valrelease, Vivol✣, Zetran (C-IV, Rx)

See also *Benzodiazepines,* p. 611.

Action/Kinetics: Onset: PO, 30–60 min; **IM,** 15–30 min; **IV,** more rapid. **Peak plasma levels: PO,** 0.5–2 hr; **IM,** 0.5–1.5; **IV,** 0.25 hr. **Duration:** 3 hr. **t½:** 20–70 hr. Diazepam is broken down in the liver to the active metabolites desmethyldiazepam, oxazepam, and temazepam. Diazepam and metabolites are excreted through the urine.

Uses: Anxiety, tension (more effective than chlordiazepoxide), alcohol withdrawal, muscle relaxant, anticonvulsive agent, antipanic drug. Used prior to gastroscopy and esophagoscopy, preoperatively and prior to cardioversion. In dentistry to induce sedation. Treatment of status epilepticus. Adjunct in cerebral palsy, paraplegia, or tetanus. Relieve spasms of facial muscles in occlusion and temporomandibular joint disorders.

Additional Contraindications: Narrow-angle glaucoma, children under 6 months, and parenterally in children under 12 years. During lactation.

Special Concerns: Pregnancy category: D.

Additional Drug Interactions:

1. Diazepam potentiates antihypertensive effects of thiazides and other diuretics.
2. Diazepam potentiates muscle relaxant effects of *d*-tubocurarine and gallamine.
3. Ranitidine ↓ GI absorption of diazepam.
4. Isoniazid ↑ half-life of diazepam.
5. Fluoxetine ↑ half-life of diazepam.

Dosage: Tablets, Oral Solution. Adults: *Antianxiety, anticonvulsant, adjunct to skeletal muscle relaxants:* 2–10 mg b.i.d.–q.i.d. **Elderly, debilitated patients:** 2–2.5 mg 1–2 times daily. May be gradually increased to adult level. **Pediatric, over 6 months: initial,** 1–2.5 mg (0.04–0.2 mg/kg or 1.17–6 mg/m²) t.i.d.–b.i.d. *Alcohol withdrawal:* 10 mg t.i.d.–q.i.d. during the first 24 hr; **then,** decrease to 5 mg t.i.d.–q.i.d. as required.

    Extended-release Capsules. Adults: *Antianxiety, skeletal muscle relaxant:* 15–30 mg once daily. To be used in children over 6 months of age only if the dose has been determined to be 5 mg t.i.d. (use one 15-mg capsule daily). **IM, IV. Adults: IM,** *Preoperative or diagnostic use:* 10 mg 5–30 min before procedure. *Adjunct to treat skeletal muscle spasm:* 5–10 mg initially; **then,** repeat in 3–4 hr if needed (larger doses may be required for tetanus). *Moderate anxiety:* 2–5 mg q 3–4 hr if necessary. *Severe anxiety, muscle spasm:* 5–10 mg q 3–4 hr, if necessary. *Acute alcohol withdrawal:* **initial,** 10 mg; **then,** 5–10 mg q 3–4 hr. *Preoperatively:* **IM,** 10 mg prior to surgery. *Endoscopy:* **IV,** 10 mg or less although doses up to 20 mg can be used; **IM,** 5–10 mg 30 min prior to procedure. *Cardioversion:* **IV,** 5–15 mg 5–10 min prior to procedure. *Tetanus in children,* **IM, IV, over 1 month:** 1–2 mg, repeated q 3–4 hr as necessary; **5 years and over:** 5–10 mg q 3–4 hr. **IV,** *Status epilepticus:* **Adults,** 5–10 mg initially; **then,** dose may be repeated at 10–15 min intervals up to a maximum dose of 30 mg. **Children, 1 month–5 years:** 0.2–0.5 mg q 2–5 min, up to maximum of 5 mg. Can be repeated in 2–4 hr. **5 years and older:** 1 mg q 2–5 min up to a maximum of 10 mg; dose can be repeated in 2–4 hr, if needed.

    Elderly or debilitated patients should not receive more than 5 mg parenterally at any one time.

NURSING CONSIDERATIONS

See *Nursing Considerations* for *Benzodiazepines,* p. 614.

Administration/Storage

1. One 15-mg sustained-release diazepam capsule may be used if the daily dosage is 5 mg t.i.d.
2. The Intensol solution should be mixed with beverages such as water, soda, and juices, or soft foods such as applesauce or puddings. Only the calibrated dropper provided with the product should be used to withdraw the medication. Once the medication is withdrawn and mixed, it should be used immediately.
3. To reduce reactions at the site of IV administration, diazepam should be given slowly (5 mg/min). Also, small veins or intra-arterial administration should not be used.
4. When administering the drug IV, have emergency equipment and drugs available.
5. Due to the possibility of precipitation and instability, diazepam should not be infused.
6. Except for the deltoid muscle, absorption from IM sites is slow and erratic.
7. Review the drug interaction chart before administering the drug.

Assessment

1. Obtain a CBC, platelet count, liver and renal profiles as baseline data.
2. Note if the client has diabetes and the type of agent used for testing the urine as diazepam interferes with many of these agents. Have client convert to finger sticks for a more accurate blood glucose determination.

Interventions

1. Parenteral administration may cause bradycardia, respiratory or cardiac arrest. Monitor vital signs and client closely.
2. Elderly clients may experience adverse reactions more quickly than younger clients. Therefore, anticipate a lower dose of drug to be ordered in this group.

DIVALPROEX SODIUM   (dye-**VAL**-proh-ex)
Depakote, Epival ✳ (Rx)

See also *Valproic Acid,* p. 748.

MAGNESIUM SULFATE   (mag-**NEE**-see-um)
Epsom Salts (OTC and Rx)

See also *Anticonvulsants,* p. 719, and *Laxatives,* p. 1048.

Classification: Anticonvulsant, electrolyte, saline laxative.

Action/Kinetics: Magnesium is an important cation present in the extracellular fluid at a concentration of 1.5–2.5 mEq/L. Magnesium is an essential element for muscle contraction, certain enzyme systems, and nerve transmission.

Magnesium depresses the CNS and controls convulsions by blocking release of acetylcholine at the myoneural junction. Also, the drug decreases the sensitivity of the motor end plate to acetylcholine and decreases the excitability of the motor membrane. **Therapeutic serum levels:**

4–6 mEq/L (normal Mg levels: 1.5–3.0 mEq/L). **Onset: IM,** 1 hr; **IV,** immediate. **Duration: IM,** 3–4 hr; **IV,** 30 min. Magnesium is excreted by the kidneys.

Uses: Seizures associated with toxemia of pregnancy, epilepsy, or when abnormally low levels of magnesium may be a contributing factor in convulsions, such as in hypothyroidism or glomerulonephritis. Acute nephritis in children. Uterine tetany. Replacement therapy in magnesium deficiency. Adjunct in total parenteral nutrition (TPN). Laxative.

Contraindications: In the presence of heart block or myocardial damage.

Special Concerns: Pregnancy category: A. Use with caution in patients with renal disease because magnesium is removed from the body solely by the kidneys.

Side Effects: Magnesium intoxication. *CNS:* Depression. *CV:* Flushing, hypotension, circulatory collapse, depression of the myocardium. *Other:* Sweating, hypothermia, muscle paralysis, respiratory paralysis. Suppression of knee jerk reflex can be used to determine toxicity. Respiratory failure may occur if given after knee jerk reflex disappears.

Treatment of Magnesium Intoxication:

1. Use artificial ventilation immediately.
2. Have 5–10 mEq of calcium (e.g., 10–20 mL of 10% calcium gluconate) readily available for IV injection.

Drug Interactions	
CNS depressants (general anesthetics, sedative-hypnotics, narcotics)	Additive CNS depression
Digitalis	Heart block when Mg intoxication is treated with calcium in digitalized patients
Neuromuscular blocking agents	Possible additive neuromuscular blockade

Dosage: IM. *Anticonvulsant:* 1–5 g of a 25%–50% solution up to 6 times daily. **Pediatric:** 20–40 mg/kg using the 20% solution (may be repeated if necessary). **IV:** 1–4 g using 10%–20% solution, not to exceed 1.5 mL/min of the 10% solution. **IV infusion:** 4 g in 250 mL 5% dextrose at a rate not to exceed 3 mL/min.

Hypomagnesemia, mild, **IM:** 1 g as a 50% solution q 6 hr for 4 times (or total of 32.5 mEq/24 hr). *Severe,* **IM:** up to 2 mEq/kg over 4 hr or **IV:** 5 g (40 mEq) in 1,000 mL dextrose 5% or sodium chloride solution by **slow** infusion over period of 3 hr. *Hyperalimentation,* **adults:** 8–24 mEq/day; **infants:** 2–10 mEq/day.

Laxative. **PO. Adults:** 10–15 g; **pediatric:** 5–10 g.

NURSING CONSIDERATIONS

See also *Nursing Considerations* for *Anticonvulsants,* p. 720, and *Laxatives,* p. 1049.

Administration/Storage

1. For IV injections, administer only 1.5 mL of 10% solution per minute. Discontinue administration when convulsions cease.
2. For IV infusion, administration should not exceed 3 mL/min.
3. Dilutions for IM: deep injection of 50% concentrate is appropriate for adults. A 20% solution should be used for children. IV: dilute as specified by manufacturer.
4. When used as a laxative, dissolve in a glassful of ice water or other fluid to lessen the disagreeable taste.

Assessment

1. Obtain baseline serum magnesium levels.
2. Determine if the client has a history of kidney disease.
3. Assess ECG for evidence of any abnormality prior to administering drug IV.

Interventions

1. Check with the physician before administering magnesium if any of the following conditions exist:
   - Absent patellar reflexes or knee jerk reflex.
   - Respirations are below 16/min.
   - Urinary output less than 100 mL during the past 4 hr.
   - Early signs of hypermagnesemia: flushing, sweating, hypotension, or hypothermia.
   - The client has a past history of heart block or myocardial damage.
2. Have available IV calcium gluconate or IV calcium gluceptate to use as an antidote. Also, during IV therapy, have emergency resuscitative drugs and equipment readily available.
3. Anticipate that the dose of CNS depressants administered to the client receiving magnesium sulfate will be adjusted.
4. If the client is receiving digitalis preparations and magnesium sulfate, monitor the client closely. Toxicity treated with calcium is extremely dangerous and may result in heart block.
5. Do not administer magnesium sulfate for 2 hours preceding the delivery of a baby.
6. If a mother has received continuous IV therapy of magnesium sulfate during 24 hr prior to delivery, assess the newborn for neurologic and respiratory depression.

PARALDEHYDE   (pah-**RAL**-deh-hyd)

Paral (Rx)

See Chapter 30, p. 605.

PHENACEMIDE   (feh-**NASS**-ih-myd)

Phenurone (Rx)

Classification: Anticonvulsant, miscellaneous.

Action/Kinetics: Phenacemide reduces focal seizures of the psychomotor type; the drug also increases the anticonvulsant effect of mephenytoin, phenobarbital, and trimethadione. It is absorbed well following oral administration. **Duration:** 5 hr. It is metabolized in the liver to inactive metabolites, which are excreted in the urine.

Uses: Mixed types of psychomotor seizures refractory to other drugs. Not the drug of choice for any disorder because of its *severe toxic effects*.

Contraindications: Hypersensitivity to drug or impaired liver function.

Special Concerns: Pregnancy category: D. Use with caution in patients with history of psycho-neurosis and allergy. Safety for use during lactation is not known. Safety and effectiveness in children less than 5 years of age has not been established.

Side Effects: Phenacemide is more toxic than most other anticonvulsants and its administration requires close supervision of patient. *CNS:* Psychic changes, toxic psychoses, dizziness, fatigue, fever, sedation, drowsiness, insomnia, headache. *GI:* Anorexia, nausea, weight loss. *Hematologic:* Aplastic anemia, leukopenia. *Other:* Dermatologic manifestations, hepatitis, liver damage, nephritis, paresthesias, muscle pain, palpitations. Liver function tests and complete blood counts are indicated before and periodically after therapy has been initiated.

Drug Interactions	
Hydantoins	↑ Effect of hydantoins due to ↓ breakdown by liver
Mephenytoin	Since these anticonvulsants have similar toxic
Oxazolidinediones	effects as phenacemide, they should not be
Succinimides	used concomitantly

Dosage: Tablets. *Highly individualized.* Aim at minimum effective dosage. **Adult, initial,** 250–500 mg t.i.d. Dose may be increased at weekly intervals by 500 mg and up to a maximum of 2–5 g daily; **pediatric 5–10 years:** half of adult dose.

NURSING CONSIDERATIONS

See also *Nursing Considerations* for *Anticonvulsants,* p. 720.

Administration/Storage

1. May be used alone or in combination with other anticonvulsant drugs.
2. If phenacemide is to replace another anticonvulsant drug, the dose of the other drug should be decreased gradually as the dose of phenacemide is increased to maintenance levels.

Assessment

1. Obtain baseline complete blood count and liver and renal function studies.
2. Determine if there is any history of allergy and/or personality disorder before administering phenacemide.

Client/Family Teaching

1. Instruct the family to report any changes in the client's mental attitude, such as apathy or depression. These may indicate a severe personality change and are often followed by toxic psychoses.
2. Discontinue drug at the first sign of a rash or any other allergic manifestations and report to the physician.
3. Report any evidence of urinary frequency, burning on urination, cloudy urine and edema. These may be signs of renal dysfunction and require immediate attention. Stress the importance of periodic urinalysis.

PRIMIDONE   (PRIM-ih-dohn)

Apo-Primidone ✿, Myidone, Mysoline, Sertan ✿ (Rx)

Classification: Anticonvulsant, miscellaneous.

Action/Kinetics: Primidone is closely related to the barbiturates; however, the mechanism for its anticonvulsant effects is unknown. Primidone produces a greater sedative effect than barbiturates when used for seizure treatment. Side effects usually subside with use. **Peak plasma levels:** 3 hr.

Primidone is converted in the liver to two active metabolites, phenobarbital and phenylethyl-malonamide (PEMA). **Peak plasma levels (PEMA):** 7–8 hr. **t½ (primidone):** 3–24 hr; **t½ (PEMA):** 24–48 hr; **t½ (phenobarbital):** 72–144 hr. The appearance of phenobarbital in the plasma may be delayed several days after initiation of therapy. **Therapeutic plasma levels, primadone:** 5–12 mcg/mL; **phenobarbital,** 10–30 mcg/mL. Primidone and metabolites are excreted through the kidneys.

Uses: Psychomotor seizures, focal seizures, or refractory tonic-clonic seizures. May be used alone or with other drugs. Often reserved for patient refractory to barbiturate-hydantoin regimen. *Investigational:* Benign familial tremor.

Contraindications: Porphyria. Hypersensitivity to phenobarbital. Lactation.

Special Concerns: Safe use during pregnancy has not been determined. Use during lactation may result in drowsiness in the neonate. Children and geriatric patients may react to primidone with restlessness and excitement.

Side Effects: *CNS:* Drowsiness, ataxia, vertigo, irritability, general malaise, headache, fatigue, emotional disturbances, including mood changes and paranoia. *GI:* Nausea, vomiting, anorexia, painful gums. *Hematologic:* Megaloblastic anemia, leukopenia, thrombocytopenia. *Ophthalmologic:* Diplopia, nystagmus. *Miscellaneous:* Skin rash, edema of eyelids and legs, alopecia, or impotence. Occasionally has caused hyperexcitability, especially in children. Postpartum hemorrhage and hemorrhagic disease of the newborn. Symptoms of systemic lupus erythematosus.

Drug Interactions: See also *Barbiturates,* p. 581.

Drug Interactions	
Acetazolamide	↓ Effect of primidone
Carbamazepine	↑ Plasma levels of phenobarbital
Isoniazid	↑ Effect of primidone due to ↓ breakdown by liver
Phenytoin	↑ Effect of primidone due to ↓ breakdown by liver

Dosage: Oral Suspension, Tablets, Chewable Tablets. Adults and children over 8 years: **initial,** *in patients on no other anticonvulsant medication:* days 1–3, 100–125 mg at bedtime; days 4–6, 100–125 mg b.i.d.; days 7–9, 100–125 mg t.i.d.; **maintenance:** 250 mg t.i.d. (may be increased to 250 mg 5–6 times per day; daily dosage should not exceed 500 mg q.i.d.). **Children under 8 years: initial,** days 1–3, 50 mg at bedtime; days 4–6, 50 mg b.i.d.; days 7–9, 100 mg b.i.d.; **maintenance:** 125 mg b.i.d.–250 mg t.i.d. *If patient receiving other anticonvulsants:* **initial,** 100–125 mg at bedtime; **then,** increase to maintenance levels as other drug is slowly withdrawn (transition should take at least 2 weeks).

NURSING CONSIDERATIONS

See also *Nursing Considerations* for *Anticonvulsants,* p. 720.

Client/Family Teaching

1. Review the goals of therapy and associated side effects of drug therapy. Instruct the client/family that the following conditions should be reported to the physician:
   - Hyperexcitability in children.
   - Excessive loss of hair.
   - Edema of eyelids and legs.
   - Impotence.

2. Remind the pregnant client that the physician may order vitamin K during the last month of pregnancy. This is to prevent postpartum hemorrhage in the mother and hemorrhagic disease of the newborn.

VALPROIC ACID   (val-PROH-ik AH-sid)
Dalpro, Depa, Depakene, Myproic Acid (Rx)

Classification: Anticonvulsant, miscellaneous.

Action/Kinetics: The precise anticonvulsant action is unknown, but activity is believed to be caused by increased brain levels of the neurotransmitter gamma-amino butyric acid (GABA). Another possibility is that valproic acid acts on postsynaptic receptor sites to mimic or enhance the inhibitory effect of GABA. Absorption from the GI tract is more rapid following administration of the syrup (sodium salt) than capsules. **Peak serum levels, capsules and syrup:** 1–4 hr (delayed if the drug is taken with food); **peak serum levels, enteric-coated tablet (divalproex sodium):** 3–4 hr. **t½:** 6–16 hr. **Therapeutic serum levels:** 50–100 mcg/mL. The drug is approximately 90% bound to plasma protein. It is metabolized in the liver and inactive metabolites are excreted in the urine; small amounts of valproic acid are excreted in the feces.

Uses: Alone (preferred) or in combination with other anticonvulsants for treatment of epilepsy characterized by simple and complex absence seizures (petit mal). As an adjunct in mixed seizure patterns. *Investigational:* Alone or in combination to treat atypical absence, myoclonic, and grand mal seizures; also, atonic, complex partial, elementary partial, and infantile spasm seizures. Prophylaxis of febrile seizures in children.

Special Concerns: Safe use during pregnancy (category: D) and during lactation has not been established. Use with caution in presence of liver disease. Use with caution in children 2 years of age or less. Pediatric patients are at greater risk of developing serious or fatal hepatotoxicity. Geriatric patients should receive a lower daily dose as they may have increased free, unbound valproic acid levels in the serum.

Side Effects: *GI:* (most frequent): Nausea, vomiting, indigestion. Also, abdominal cramps, diarrhea, constipation, anorexia. *CNS:* Sedation, depression, psychoses, hyperactivity, emotional changes. *Hematologic:* Thrombocytopenia, leukopenia, eosinophilia, anemia, bone marrow suppression. *Dermatologic:* Transient alopecia, petechiae, erythema multiforme, skin rashes. *Miscellaneous:* **Hepatotoxicity.** Also weakness, skin rashes, bruising, hematoma formation, menstrual irregularities, acute pancreatitis, hyperammonemia, edema of arms and legs, increase in SGOT and serum alkaline phosphatase values.

Drug Interactions	
Alcohol	↑ Incidence of CNS depression
Aspirin	↑ Effect of valproic acid due to ↓ plasma protein binding. Also, additive anticoagulant effect
Benzodiazepines	↑ Effect of benzodiazepines due to ↓ breakdown by liver
Clonazepam	↑ Chance of absence seizures (petit mal) and ↑ toxicity due to clonazepam
CNS depressants	↑ Incidence of CNS depression

Drug Interactions (continued)

Ethosuximide	↑ Effect of ethosuximide
Phenobarbital	↑ Effect of phenobarbital due to ↓ breakdown by liver
Phenytoin	↑ Effect of phenytoin due to ↓ breakdown by liver or ↓ effect of phenytoin due to ↓ total serum phenytoin
Warfarin sodium	↑ Effect of valproic acid due to ↓ plasma protein binding. Also, additive anticoagulant effect

Laboratory Test Interference: False + for ketonuria. Altered thyroid function tests.

Dosage: Capsules, Syrup, Enteric-coated Tablets (Divalproex). Adults and adolescents: initial, monotherapy 5–15 mg/kg/day. Increase at 1-week intervals by 5–10 mg/kg/day; **maximum:** 60 mg/kg/day. If the total daily dose exceeds 250 mg, the dosage should be divided. **Pediatric, 1–12 years of age: initial, monotherapy:** 15–45 mg/kg daily; dose can be increased by 5–10 mg/kg daily at 1-week intervals. **Adults and adolescents: initial, polytherapy:** 10–30 mg/kg daily; dose can be increased by 5–10 mg/kg daily at 1-week intervals. **Pediatric, 1–12 years of age: initial, polytherapy:** 30–100 mg/kg daily; dose can be increased by 5–10 mg/kg daily at on1-week intervals.

NURSING CONSIDERATIONS

See also *Nursing Considerations* for *Anticonvulsants,* p. 720.

Administration/Storage

1. Divide daily dosage if it exceeds 250 mg/day.
2. Initiate at lower dosage level or give with food to clients who suffer from GI irritation.
3. Capsules should be swallowed whole to avoid local irritation.
4. Depakote is enteric coated and may decrease GI upset.
5. Do not administer valproic acid syrup to clients whose *sodium* intake must be restricted. Consult physician if a sodium-restricted client is unable to swallow capsules.

Client/Family Teaching

1. Advise diabetic clients on valproic acid therapy that the drug may cause a false + urine test for ketones. Review some of the symptoms of ketoacidosis (dry mouth, thirst, and dry flushed skin) so that clients can determine if they are acidotic. Instruct them to report the development of any of these symptoms to the physician.
2. Stress the importance of reporting for periodic CBC, serum ketones, and liver function studies as scheduled, throughout therapy with valproic acid.

CHAPTER THIRTY-SEVEN

Narcotic Analgesics and Antagonists

NARCOTIC ANALGESICS

General Statement: The narcotic analgesics include opium, morphine, codeine, various opium derivatives, and totally synthetic substances with similar pharmacologic properties. Of these, meperidine (Demerol) is the best known. The relative activity of all narcotic analgesics is measured against morphine.

Opium itself is a mixture of alkaloids obtained since ancient times from the poppy plant. Morphine and codeine are two of the pure chemical substances isolated from opium. Certain drugs (pentazocine, butorphanol, nalbuphine) have both narcotic agonist and antagonist properties. Such drugs may precipitate a withdrawal syndrome if given to patients dependent on narcotics.

Dependence and Tolerance

It is important to remember that all drugs of this group are addictive. Psychological and physical dependence and tolerance develop even when using clinical doses. Tolerance is characterized by the fact that the patient requires shorter periods of time between doses or larger doses for relief of pain. Tolerance usually develops faster when the narcotic analgesic is administered regularly and when the dose is large.

Effects of Narcotic Analgesics

The most important effect of the narcotic analgesics is on the CNS. In addition to an alteration of pain perception (analgesia), the drugs, especially at higher doses, induce euphoria, drowsiness, changes in mood, mental clouding, and deep sleep.

The narcotic analgesics also depress respiration. The effect is noticeable with small doses. Death by overdosage is almost always the result of respiratory arrest.

The narcotic analgesics have a nauseant and emetic effect (direct stimulation of the chemoreceptor trigger zone). They depress the cough reflex, and small doses of narcotic analgesics (codeine) are part of several antitussive preparations.

The narcotic analgesics have little effect on blood pressure when the patient is in a supine position. However, most narcotics decrease the capacity of the patient to respond to stress. Morphine and other narcotic analgesics induce peripheral vasodilation, which may result in hypotension.

Many narcotic analgesics constrict the pupil. With such drugs, pupillary constriction is the most obvious sign of dependence.

The narcotic analgesics also decrease peristaltic motility. The constipating effects of these agents (Paregoric) are sometimes used therapeutically in severe diarrhea. The narcotic analgesics also increase the pressure within the biliary tract.

Acute Toxicity

This state is characterized by profound respiratory depression, deep sleep, stupor or coma, and pinpoint pupils. The respiratory rate may be as low as 2–4 breaths/min. The patient may be cyanotic. The blood pressure falls gradually. Urine output is decreased, the skin feels clammy, and there is a decrease in body temperature. Death almost always results from respiratory depression.

Treatment of Acute Overdosage

Gastric lavage and induced emesis are indicated in case of oral poisoning. Treatment, however, is aimed at combating the progressive respiratory depression (usually artificial respiration). The narcotic antagonist naloxone (Narcan), 0.4 mg IV, is effective in the treatment of acute overdosage.

Respiratory stimulants (e.g., caffeine) should not be used to treat depression from the narcotic overdosage.

Chronic Toxicity

The problem of chronic dependence on narcotics is well known. Not only is dependence a problem of "the street" but is also found often among those who have easy access to narcotics (physicians, nurses, pharmacists). All of the principal narcotic analgesics (morphine, opium, heroin, codeine, and meperidine) are used at times for nontherapeutic purposes.

The nurse must be aware of the problem and be able to recognize signs of chronic dependence. These are constricted pupils, GI effects (constipation), skin infections, needle scars, abscesses, and itching, especially on the anterior surfaces of the body, where the patient may inject the drug.

37

Withdrawal signs appear after drug is withheld for 4–12 hr. They are characterized by intense craving for the drug, insomnia, yawning, sneezing, vomiting, diarrhea, tremors, sweating, mental depression, muscular aches and pains, chills, and anxiety. Although the symptoms of narcotic withdrawal are uncomfortable, they are rarely life-threatening. This is in contrast to the withdrawal syndrome from depressants, where the life of the individual may be endangered because of the possibility of tonic-clonic seizures.

Action/Kinetics: The narcotic analgesics attach to specific receptors located in the CNS (cortex, brain stem, and spinal cord), resulting in analgesia. Although the details are unknown, the mechanism is believed to involve decreased permeability of the cell membrane to sodium, which results in diminished transmission of pain impulses. There are five categories of opioid receptors that have been identified: mu, kappa, sigma, delta, and epsilon. Narcotic analgesics are believed to exert their activity at mu, kappa, and sigma receptors. Mu receptors are thought to mediate supraspinal analgesia, euphoria, and respiratory depression. Pentazocine-like spinal analgesia, miosis, and sedation are mediated by kappa receptors while sigma receptors mediate dysphoria, hallucinations, as well as respiratory and vasomotor stimulation (caused by drugs with antagonist activity). For kinetics, see individual agents.

Uses: Severe pain, especially of coronary, pulmonary, or peripheral origin. Hepatic and renal colic. Preanesthetic medication and adjuncts to anesthesia. Postsurgical pain. Acute vascular occlusion, especially of coronary, pulmonary, and peripheral origin. Diarrhea and dysentery. Pain from myocardial infarction, carcinoma, burns. Postpartum pain. Some members of this group are primarily used as antitussives. Methadone is used for heroin withdrawal and maintenance.

Contraindications: Asthmatic conditions, emphysema, kyphoscoliosis, severe obesity, convulsive states as in epilepsy, delirium tremens, tetanus and strychnine poisoning, diabetic acidosis, myxedema, Addison's disease, hepatic cirrhosis, and children under 6 months.

Special Concerns: To be used cautiously in patients with head injury or after head surgery because of morphine's capacity to elevate intracranial pressure and mask the pupillary response.

To be used with caution in the elderly, the debilitated, in young children, in cases of increased intracranial pressure, in obstetrics, and with patients in shock or during acute alcoholic intoxication.

Morphine should be used with extreme caution in patients with pulmonary heart disease (cor pulmonale). Deaths following ordinary therapeutic doses have been reported. Use cautiously in patients with prostatic hypertrophy, since it may precipitate acute urinary retention.

To be used cautiously in patients with reduced blood volume, such as in hemorrhaging patients who are more susceptible to the hypotensive effects of morphine.

Since the drugs depress the respiratory center, they should be given early in labor, at least 2 hr before delivery, so as to reduce the danger of respiratory depression in the newborn. When given before surgery, the narcotic analgesics should be given at least 1 to 2 hr preoperatively so that the danger of maximum depression of respiratory function will have passed before anesthesia is initiated.

These drugs should sometimes be withheld prior to diagnostic procedures so that the physician can use pain to locate dysfunction.

Side Effects: *Respiratory:* Respiratory depression, apnea. *CNS:* Dizziness, lightheadedness, sedation, lethargy, headache, euphoria, mental clouding, fainting. Idiosyncratic effects including excitement, restlessness, tremors, delirium, insomnia. *GI:* Nausea, vomiting, constipation, increased pressure in biliary tract, dry mouth, anorexia. *CV:* Flushing, changes in heart rate and blood pressure, circulatory collapse. *Allergic:* Skin rashes including pruritus and urticaria. Sweating, laryngospasm, edema.

Miscellaneous: Urinary retention, oliguria, reduced libido, changes in body temperature. Narcotics cross the placental barrier and depress respiration of the fetus or newborn.

Drug Interactions	
Alcohol, ethyl	Potentiation or addition of CNS depressant effects; concomitant use may lead to drowsiness, lethargy, stupor, respiratory collapse, coma, or death
Anesthetics, general	See *Alcohol*
Antianxiety drugs	See *Alcohol*
Antidepressants, tricyclic	↑ Narcotic-induced respiratory depression
Antihistamines	See *Alcohol*
Barbiturates	See *Alcohol*
Cimetidine	↑ CNS toxicity (e.g., disorientation, confusion, respiratory depression, apnea, seizures) with narcotics
CNS depressants	See *Alcohol*
Methotrimeprazine	Potentiation of CNS depression
Monoamine oxidase inhibitors	Possible potentiation of either monoamine oxidase inhibitor (excitation, hypertension) or narcotic (hypotension, coma) effects; death has resulted
Phenothiazines	See *Alcohol*
Sedative-hypnotics, nonbarbiturate	See *Alcohol*
Skeletal muscle relaxants (surgical)	↑ Respiratory depression and ↑ muscle relaxation

Laboratory Test Interferences: Altered liver function tests. False + or ↑ urinary glucose test (Benedict's). ↑ Plasma amylase or lipase.

Dosage: (See individual drugs.) The dosage of narcotics and the reaction of a patient to the dosage depend on the amount of pain. Two to four times the usual dose may be tolerated for relief of excruciating pain. However, the nurse should be aware that if, for some reason, the pain disappears, severe respiratory depression may result. This respiratory depression is not apparent while the pain is still present.

NURSING CONSIDERATIONS

Administration

1. Have emergency drugs and equipment readily available in the event of an overdosage. Gastric lavage equipment may be needed when the drugs have been administered orally.
2. A narcotic antagonist, such as naloxone, should be available to treat respiratory depression resulting from narcotic overdose.
3. Review the list of drugs with which narcotics are interactant and their associated effects.
4. Request that the physician rewrite the orders at timed intervals as required for continued administration.
5. Record the amount of narcotic used on the narcotic inventory sheet, indicating if it was

administered, the date, the time, the dose, and to whom, or if the drug was wasted and include an appropriate witness as necessary.

Assessment

1. Note if the client has had any prior experience such as an adverse reaction with the drug or category of drugs prescribed.
2. Determine the amount of pain and discomfort, its location and duration, frequency of occurrence, and what drug has been effective in the past. The amount and type of narcotic ordered should be individualized according to the client's response.
3. Use a pain rating scale so that clients can calculate or describe their level of pain. This may be used as a baseline against which to measure the effectiveness of drug therapy.
4. Obtain baseline vital signs prior to administering the drug. Generally, if the respiratory rate is less than 12 per minute or the systolic BP is less than 90 mm Hg a narcotic should not be administered unless there is ventilatory support or specific written guidelines by the physician with parameters for administration.
5. Note the client's weight, age, and general body size. Too large a dosage of medication for the client's weight and age can result in serious side effects. For the elderly client, the blood levels may be higher, resulting in longer periods of pain relief.
6. Note the amount of time that has elapsed between the doses, for the client to have relief from recurring pain.
7. Note precipitating factors as well as the impact of the pain on the client's ability to function.
8. Document any history of asthma, or other conditions that tend to compromise respirations.
9. If the client is of childbearing age, discuss the possibility of pregnancy. Narcotics cross the placental barrier and depress the respirations of the fetus. The drugs may be contraindicated under certain circumstances.
10. Baseline CBC, liver and renal function studies as well as electrolytes should be considered.

Interventions

1. Use supportive nursing measures such as relaxation techniques, repositioning the client, and reassurance to assist in relieving pain.
2. Explore the problem and source of the client's pain. Use nonnarcotic analgesic medications when possible.
3. Administer the medication when it is needed. Prolonging the medication until the client experiences the maximum amount of pain reduces the effectiveness of the medication.
4. Monitor vital signs and mental status.
   - Monitor the respiratory rate for signs of respiratory depression. Obtain written parameters for administration if necessary.
   - Narcotic analgesics depress the cough reflex. Therefore, turn clients every 2 hours, have them cough and take deep breaths to prevent atelectasis.
   - Monitor blood pressure. Hypotension is more apt to occur in the elderly and in those who are receiving other medications that may have hypotension as a side effect.
   - Monitor the heart rate. If the pulse drops below 60 beats per minute in the adult, or 110 bpm in an infant, withhold the drug and notify the physician.
   - Observe the client for any decrease in blood pressure, deep sleep or constricted pupils. Withhold the drug if any of these symptoms occur. Document and report to the physician.

- Note the effects of the drug on the client's mental status. A client who has experienced pain, fear or anxiety may become euphoric and excited. Record this and report.

5. Report if the client develops nausea and vomiting. If this occurs, the physician may order an anti emetic or change the medication therapy.

6. If the client is taking a narcotic medication by mouth, a snack or milk may decrease gastric irritation and lessen nausea.

7. Monitor bowel function. Narcotics, especially morphine can have a depressant effect on the GI tract. Clients may become constipated as a consequence. If their condition permits, increase the fluid intake to 2500–3000 mL per day and increase their intake of fruit juices, fruits and fiber as well as level of exercise as tolerated.

8. Narcotic drugs may cause urinary retention. Monitor the client's intake and urinary output and palpate the abdomen to detect for evidence of bladder distention. Encourage the client to attempt to empty his bladder every 3–4 hours. Question clients about difficulty voiding, pain in the bladder area, sensation of not emptying the bladder, or any unusual odors.

9. Note client complaint of difficulty with vision. Examine the client's pupillary response to light. If the client's pupils remain constricted, notify the physician and record this on the client's record.

10. If the client is bed ridden, put up side rails and provide other protective measures.

11. When administering medication, reassure client that flushing and a feeling of warmth sometimes may occur with therapeutic doses of drug.

12. Because clients may perspire profusely when receiving a narcotic, be prepared to bathe and change their linens frequently.

13. If a client is to be receiving a narcotic preparation over a period of time, monitor renal and liver function studies.

14. Assess hospitalized clients receiving around-the-clock therapy for evidence of tolerance and addiction.

15. In clients with terminal cancer, dependence to drug therapy is not considered a problem, whereas adequate pain control is of the utmost concern.

Client/Family Teaching

1. Inform the client and family that the drug may become habit-forming.

2. Review the side effects of the drug with the client and family and discuss the goals of therapy.

3. Provide the client with a printed card listing the side effects of drug therapy that may occur. Review these with the client upon discharge, and again when the client returns for a visit to the office or clinic.

4. Do not take OTC drugs without first consulting the physician. Many have small amounts of alcohol. Also, they may interact unfavorably with the prescribed medication.

5. Avoid consuming alcohol in any form.

6. For fecal impaction, explain to the client preventive actions that need to be taken such as increased fluid intake, increased use of fruit and fruit juices, and the possible need for a stool softener.

7. If the client is to go home on a narcotic medication, explain that the drug can cause drowsiness and dizziness. Therefore, client should use caution when operating a motor vehicle or performing other tasks that require mental alertness.

8. If the client is to be treated by a physician other than the one prescribing the medication, tell the physician about the drug being used and the reason for the prescribed therapy.

9. Stress the importance of storing all drugs in a safe place, out of the reach of children. Store away from the bedside to prevent accidental overdosage.

Evaluation

1. Review the anticipated goals of the therapy with the client and family and determine whether or not these have been achieved.
2. If the goals have not been achieved, determine the source of the problem and modify the next plan of action.
3. Determine the extent of the pain relief achieved with each dosage of medication (i.e. pain level decreased from a level 5 to a level 2, 20 min after administration of medication).
4. Client exhibits no symptoms of acute toxicity, tolerance or addiction.

ALFENTANIL HYDROCHLORIDE   (al-FEN-tah-nil)

Alfenta (C-II, Rx)

See also *Narcotic Analgesics,* p. 750.

Classification: Narcotic analgesic.

Action/Kinetics: Onset: Immediate. $t^{1/2}$: 1–2 hr (after IV use).

Uses: *Continuous infusion:* With nitrous oxide/oxygen to maintain general anesthesia. *Incremental doses:* As an adjunct with barbiturate/nitrous oxide/oxygen to maintain general anesthesia. *Anesthetic induction:* As primary agent when endotracheal intubation and mechanical ventilation are necessary.

Contraindications: Use during labor.

Special Concerns: Pregnancy category: C. Use in children less than 12 years of age is not recommended. Use with caution during lactation.

Additional Side Effects: Bradycardia, postoperative confusion, blurred vision, hypercapnia, shivering, and asystole hypercarbia. Neonates with respiratory distress syndrome have manifested hypotension with doses of 20 mcg/kg.

Dosage: *Continuous infusion, duration 45 min or more:* **initial for induction:** 50–75 mcg/kg; **maintenance, with nitrous oxide/oxygen:** 0.5–3 mcg/kg/min. Following the induction dose, the infusion rate requirement should be reduced by 30–50% for the first hour of maintenance.
   Induction of anesthesia, duration 45 min or more: **initial for induction:** 130–245 mcg/kg; **maintenance:** 0.5–1.5 mcg/kg/min. If a general anesthetic is used for maintenance, the concentration of inhalation agents should be reduced by 30–50% for the first hour.
   Anesthetic adjunct, 30–60 min duration: **initial for induction:** 20–50 mcg/kg; **maintenance:** 5–15 mcg/kg, up to a total dose of 75 mcg/kg.
   Anesthetic adjunct, less than 30 min duration: **initial for induction:** 8–20 mcg/kg; **maintenance:** 3–5 mcg/kg (or 0.5–1 mcg/kg/min, up to a total dose of 8–40 mcg/kg).
   If there is a lightening of general anesthesia or the patient manifests signs of surgical stress, the rate of administration of alfentanil may be increased to 4 mcg/kg/min or a bolus dose of 7 mcg/kg may be used. If the situation is not controlled following three bolus doses over 5 min, an inhalation anesthetic, a barbiturate, or a vasodilator should be used.

If signs of lightening anesthesia are noted within the last 15 min of surgery, a bolus dose of 7 mcg/kg should be given rather than increasing the infusion rate. A potent inhalation anesthetic may be used as an alternative.

NURSING CONSIDERATIONS

See also *Nursing Considerations* for *Narcotic Analgesics,* p. 753.

Administration/Storage

1. The dosage of drug must be individualized for each client and for each use.
   - For elderly or debilitated clients the dosage of drug should be reduced.
   - For obese clients who are more than 20% above their ideal body weight, the dosage should be based on lean body weight.
2. The injectable may be reconstituted with either normal saline, 5% dextrose in normal saline, lactated Ringer's solution, or 5% dextrose in water.
3. The infusion should be discontinued 10–15 minutes prior to the end of surgery.

Assessment

1. Note if the client has a history of drug sensitivity. The drug should be avoided if this is evident.
2. Determine if the client's pain is the result of a head injury. The drug is contraindicated in this instance.
3. Obtain baseline vital signs prior to administering the medication. Assisted or controlled ventilation may be required.

Interventions

Some clients may develop muscular rigidity. If this occurs, report it to the physician before proceeding with the next dose of medication.

BROMPTON'S COCKTAIL (BROMPTON'S MIXTURE) (BRAHMP-tons KOK-tayl)

(Rx)

See also *Narcotic Analgesics,* p. 750.

Action/Kinetics: Narcotic analgesic mixture.

General Statement: Brompton's Cocktail is a complex variable mixture of a narcotic analgesic (usually morphine or methadone), cocaine or a phenothiazine, alcohol (ethanol, gin, brandy, or vermouth), and flavoring agents (honey, syrups). Little tolerance to this combination occurs. Cocaine, however, is not believed to add to the effectiveness of the mixture. The alcohol increases palatability, improves mood, and enhances sedation. **Duration:** morphine, 3–4 hr; methadone, 6–8 hr.

Uses: Pain relief, especially in terminal cancer patients when use of narcotic analgesic alone has proved ineffective.

Special Concerns: Pregnancy category: C.

Dosage: The range of doses is as follows: morphine or methadone, 5–15 mg; cocaine, 5–15 mg; ethanol (90–98%), 1.25–2.5 mL. Frequency of administration must be titrated for each patient and should be on a regular schedule.

NURSING CONSIDERATIONS

See also *Nursing Considerations* for *Narcotic Analgesics,* p. 753.

Administration/Storage

1. The mixture should be discarded after 2 weeks if unused and if stability is unknown.
2. Dosage adjustments should be made every 48–72 hr and only one drug dosage varied at any given time.
3. If cocaine is used, the mixture should be swished around in the mouth before swallowing (to increase absorption through the oral mucosa).
4. Never mix with soft drinks or fruit juices; the cocktail may be served on ice.

Assessment

1. Assess the severity of the client's pain, fear, anxiety, and/or depression.
2. When working with clients who have terminal cancer, determine the ability of the client and family to utilize hospice care in conjunction with the pain medication.

Interventions

1. To maintain continuous analgesia and euphoria, administer the mixture on schedule as ordered. Assure that the client is relaxed and does not fear the return of pain.
2. Monitor the client for excessive sedation, respiratory depression, and nausea. Document and report to the physician, as these assessment data are essential for titrating the dosage according to the client's needs.

Client/Family Teaching

1. Brompton's cocktail should be administered on a regular schedule around the clock as ordered to control the client's pain as well as fears and anxiety about the return of severe pain.
2. Discuss with the family that tolerance does not usually develop and that dependence is not considered a problem in treating the client with terminal cancer. Encourage the family to assist the client to avoid the fear of dependence.
3. Explain the methods of how to monitor for excessive sedation, respiratory depression, and nausea. Emphasize the importance of reporting the data to the physician so that the dosage of medication can be properly adjusted to suit the client's needs and control discomfort and pain.
4. Show the client and family how to measure the dose of drug accurately and the appropriate method of administration.
5. If the dosage of drug seems ineffective, consult with the physician before increasing the dosage themselves.

BUPRENORPHINE HYDROCHLORIDE   (byou-preh-**NOR**-feen)

Buprenex (C-V, Rx)

See also *Narcotic Analgesics,* p. 750.

Classification: Narcotic agonist/antagonist.

Action/Kinetics: Semisynthetic opiate possessing both narcotic agonist and antagonist activity. It has limited activity at the mu receptor. **IM, onset:** 15 min; **Peak effect:** 1 hr; **Duration:** 6 hr. **t¹/₂:** 2–3 hr. May also be given IV with shorter onset and peak effect. Buprenorphine is about equipotent with naloxone as a narcotic antagonist.

Uses: Moderate to severe pain.

Special Concerns: Use during pregnancy (category: C) and lactation only if benefits outweigh risks. In children, safety and efficacy have not been established. Use with caution in patients with compromised respiratory function, in head injuries, in impairment of liver or renal function, Addison's disease, prostatic hypertrophy, biliary tract dysfunction, urethral stricture, myxedema, and hypothyroidism. Administration to individuals physically dependent on narcotics may result in precipitation of a withdrawal syndrome.

Side Effects: *CNS:* Sedation, dizziness, confusion, headache, euphoria, slurred speech, depression, paresthesia, psychosis, malaise, hallucinations, coma, dysphoria, agitation, seizures. *GI:* Nausea, vomiting, constipation, dyspepsia, loss of appetite, dry mouth. *Ophthalmologic:* Miosis, blurred vision, double vision, conjunctivitis. *CV:* Hypotension, bradycardia, tachycardia, Wenckebach block. *Respiratory:* Decreased respiratory rate, cyanosis, dyspepsia. *Dermatologic:* Sweating, rash, pruritus, flushing. *Other:* Urinary retention, chills, tinnitus.

Drug Interactions: Additive CNS depression with alcohol, general anesthetics, antianxiety agents, sedative-hypnotics, phenothiazines, and other narcotic analgesics.

Dosage: IM, Slow IV, over 13 years of age: 0.3 mg q 6 hr. Up to 0.6 mg may be given; doses greater than 0.6 mg not recommended.

NURSING CONSIDERATIONS

See also *Nursing Considerations* for *Narcotic Analgesics,* p. 753.

Administration/Storage

1. Buprenorphine may be mixed with isotonic saline, lactated Ringer's solution, and 5% dextrose and 0.9% saline.
2. Buprenorphine may be mixed with solutions containing haloperidol, glycopyrrolate, scopolamine hydrobromide, hydroxyzine chloride, or droperidol.
3. Buprenorphine should not be mixed with solutions containing diazepam or lorazepam.
4. Storage in excessive heat and light should be avoided.

Assessment

1. Determine if the client has evidence of respiratory depression and report to the physician as drug is contraindicated.
2. Note if the client has any head injuries and if so report immediately.
3. If the client has been receiving narcotics, observe for evidence of withdrawal effects and document on the chart.
4. Note any evidence of liver or renal dysfunction, diseases of the biliary tract or prostatic hypertrophy.

BUTORPHANOL TARTRATE   (byou-**TOR**-fah-nol)

Stadol (Rx)

See also *Narcotic Analgesics,* p. 750.

Classification: Narcotic analgesic—agonist-antagonist.

Action/Kinetics: Butorphanol has both narcotic agonist and antagonist properties. Its analgesic potency is said to be up to 7 times that of morphine and 30–40 times that of meperidine. Overdosage responds to naloxone. **Onset: IM,** 10 min; **IV,** rapid. **Duration:** 3–4 hr. **Peak analgesia:** 30–60 min following IM and more rapidly following IV administration. **t½:** 2.5–4 hr. Butorphanol is metabolized in the liver and excreted by the kidney. The drug has about 1/40 the narcotic antagonist activity as naloxone.

Uses: Moderate to severe pain, especially after surgery. Also as preoperative medication (as part of balanced anesthesia). Postpartum pain.

Special Concerns: Safe use during pregnancy, during labor for premature infants, or in children under 18 years not established. Use with extreme caution in patients with acute myocardial infarction, ventricular dysfunction, and coronary insufficiency (morphine or meperidine are preferred).

Additional Drug Interactions: Butorphanol may precipitate withdrawal in patients physically dependent on narcotics..

Dosage: IM: usual, 2 mg q 3–4 hr, as necessary; **range:** 1–4 mg q 3–4 hr. **IV: usual,** 1 mg q 3–4 hr; **range:** 0.5–2 mg q 3–4 hr. **Not recommended for use in children.**

NURSING CONSIDERATIONS

See also *Nursing Considerations* for *Narcotic Analgesics,* p. 753, and *Narcotic Antagonists,* p. 778.

Administration

If the drug is to be administered by direct IV infusion, it may be given undiluted. Administer it at a rate of 2 mg or less over a 3–5 min period of time.

Assessment

1. Determine if the client is likely to be dependent on narcotics. Butorphanol may precipitate withdrawal symptoms.
2. Note if the client has a history of cardiovascular problems. Document and report as morphine may be a preferred drug to use.

CODEINE PHOSPHATE   (KOH-deen FOS-fayt)

Paveral ✤ (C-II, Rx)

CODEINE SULFATE   (KOH-deen SUL-fayt)

(C-II, Rx)

See also *Narcotic Analgesics,* p. 750.

Classification: Narcotic analgesic, morphine type.

Action/Kinetics: Codeine resembles morphine pharmacologically but produces less respiratory depression, nausea, and vomiting. It is moderately habit-forming and constipating. Dosages over 60 mg often cause restlessness and excitement and irritate the cough center. However, in lower doses, it is a potent antitussive and is an ingredient in many cough syrups. **Onset:** 10–30 min. **Peak effect:** 30–60 min. **Duration:** 4–6 hr. **t½:** 3–4 hr. Codeine is 2/3 as effective orally as parenterally.

It is often used to supplement the effect of nonnarcotic analgesics such as aspirin and acetaminophen. Codeine is also found in many combination cough/cold products and analgesics.

Uses: Relief of mild to moderate pain. Antitussive.

Special Concerns: Pregnancy category: C. May increase the duration of labor.

Additional Drug Interaction: Combination with chlordiazepoxide may induce coma.

Dosage: Tablets, IM, IV, SC. *Analgesia:* **Adults:** 15–60 mg q 4–6 hr, not to exceed 120 mg a day. **Pediatric, over 1 year of age:** 0.5 mg/kg q 4–6 hr. IV should not be used in children. *Antitussive:* **Adults:** 10–20 mg q 4–6 hr, up to maximum of 120 mg/day. **Pediatric, 2–6 years:** 2.5–5 mg orally q 4–6 hr, not to exceed 30 mg/day; **6–12 years:** 5–10 mg q 4–6 hr, not to exceed 60 mg/day.

NURSING CONSIDERATIONS

See also *Nursing Considerations* for *Narcotic Analgesics,* p. 753.

Client/Family Teaching

Clients taking codeine syrup to suppress coughs should be discouraged from overuse. Productive coughing is suppressed and may result in additional congestion.

EMPIRIN WITH CODEINE   (EM-pih-rin, KOH-deen)

(C-III, Rx)

See also *Narcotic Analgesics,* p. 750, and *Aspirin,* p. 783.

Classification/Content: *Nonnarcotic analgesic:* Aspirin, 325 mg (in all tablets). *Narcotic analgesic:* Codeine, 15 mg (No. 2), 30 mg (No. 3), 60 mg (No. 4).

Uses: Relief of mild, moderate, or moderate-severe pain.

Special Concerns: Pregnancy category: C.

Dosage: PO. Individualized. Adults, usual: 1–2 tablets of No. 2 or No. 3 q 4 hr as needed; 1 tablet of No. 4 q 4 hr.

NURSING CONSIDERATIONS

See *Nursing Considerations* for *Narcotic Analgesics,* p. 753, and *Aspirin,* p. 788.

Administration/Storage

1. This product may be habit-forming.
2. Take with food, milk, or water to decrease gastric irritation.

FENTANYL CITRATE   (FEN-tah-nil SYE-trayt)

Sublimaze (C-II, Rx)

See also *Narcotic Analgesics,* p. 750.

Classification: Narcotic analgesic, morphine type.

Action/Kinetics: Similar to those of morphine and meperidine. **Onset:** 7–8 min. **Peak effect:**

Approximately 30 min. **Duration:** 1–2 hr. **t¹/₂:** 1.5–6 hr. The drug is faster-acting and of shorter duration than morphine or meperidine.

Uses: Preanesthetic medication, induction, and maintenance of anesthesia of short duration and immediate postoperative period. Supplement in general or regional anesthesia. Combined with droperidol for preanesthetic medication, induction of anesthesia, or as adjunct in maintenance of general or regional anesthesia. Combined with oxygen for anesthesia in high-risk patients such as open heart surgery, orthopedic procedures, or complicated neurological procedures.

Additional Contraindications: Myasthenia gravis and other conditions in which muscle relaxants should not be used. Patients particularly sensitive to respiratory depression. Use during labor.

Special Concerns: Pregnancy category: C. Safety and effectiveness have not been determined in children less than 2 years of age. Use with caution and at reduced dosage in poor-risk patients, children, the elderly, and when other CNS depressants are used.

Additional Side Effects: Skeletal and thoracic muscle rigidity, especially after rapid IV administration. Bradycardia, seizures, diaphoresis.

Additional Drug Interaction: ↑ Risk of cardiovascular depression when high doses of fentanyl are combined with nitrous oxide or diazepam.

Dosage: *Preoperatively:* **IM,** 0.05–0.1 mg 30–60 min before surgery. *Adjunct to anesthesia: induction,* **IV,** 0.002–0.05 mg/kg, depending on length and depth of anesthesia desired; *maintenance:* **IV, IM,** 0.025–0.1 mg/kg when indicated. *Adjunct to regional anesthesia:* **IM, IV,** 0.05–0.1 mg over 1–2 min when indicated. *Postoperatively:* **IM,** 0.05–0.1 mg q 1–2 hr for control of pain. *As general anesthetic with oxygen and a muscle relaxant:* 0.05–0.1 mg/kg (up to 0.15 mg/kg may be required).

    Pediatric, 2–12 years: *Induction and maintenance:* 1.7–3.3 mcg/kg.

NURSING CONSIDERATIONS

See also *Nursing Considerations* for *Narcotic Analgesics,* p. 753.

Administration/Storage

1. Direct IV infusions may be given, undiluted, over a period of 2–3 min.
2. After an IV injection, anticipate that the client will feel the onset of action within a few minutes and it should last for 30–60 min.
3. Clients receiving an IM injection of drug can expect to have relief within 15 min and expect a duration of 1–2 hr.
4. Protect from light.

FIORINAL   (fee-**OR**-in-al)

(Rx)

FIORINAL WITH CODEINE   (fee-**OR**-in-al, **KOH**-deen)

(C-III, Rx)

See also *Narcotic Analgesics,* p. 750, *Aspirin,* p. 783, and *Barbiturates,* p. 581.

Classification/Content: Each Fiorinal capsule or tablet contains:
    Nonnarcotic analgesic: Aspirin, 325 mg.
    Sedative barbiturate: Butalbital, 50 mg.
    CNS stimulant: Caffeine, 40 mg.

In addition to the above, Fiorinal with codeine capsules contain phosphate, 7.5 mg (No. 1), 15 mg (No. 2), or 30 mg (No. 3).

Uses: Fiorinal is indicated for tension headaches. Fiorinal with codeine is indicated as an analgesic for all types of pain.

Special Concerns: Pregnancy category: C (Fiorinal with Codeine).

Dosage: Capsules, Tablets. *Fiorinal:* 1–2 tablets or capsules q 4 hr not to exceed 6 tablets or capsules daily. *Fiorinal with Codeine.* **Initial,** 1–2 capsules; **then,** dose may be repeated, if necessary, up to maximum of 6 capsules daily.

NURSING CONSIDERATIONS

See *Nursing Considerations* for *Aspirin,* p. 788, and *Narcotic Analgesics,* p. 753.

HYDROCHLORIDES OF OPIUM ALKALOIDS (hi-droh-**KLOH**-ryds, **OH**-pee-um **AL**-ka-loyds)
Pantopon (C-II, Rx)

See also *Narcotic Analgesics,* p. 750.

Classification: Narcotic analgesic, morphine type.

Action/Kinetics: This preparation is a mixture of alkaloids obtained from opium. It is rapidly absorbed from the GI tract and has a low incidence of side effects.

Uses: Severe pain.

Additional Contraindications: Not to be given IV.

Special Concerns: Pregnancy category: C.

Dosage: IM or SC only: 5–20 mg q 4–5 hr. Each 20 mg of Pantopon is equivalent to 15 mg of morphine.

NURSING CONSIDERATIONS

See *Nursing Considerations* for *Narcotic Analgesics,* p. 753.

HYDROMORPHONE HYDROCHLORIDE (hi-droh-**MOR**-fohn)
Dilaudid, Dilaudid-HP (C-II, Rx)

See also *Narcotic analgesics,* p. 750.

Classification: Narcotic analgesic, morphine type.

Action/Kinetics: Hydromorphone is 7–10 times more analgesic than morphine, with a shorter duration of action. It manifests less sedation, less vomiting and less nausea than morphine, although it induces pronounced respiratory depression. **Onset:** 15–30 min. **Peak effect:** 30–60 min. **Duration:** 4–5 hr. **t½:** 2–3 hr. The drug can be given rectally for prolonged activity.

Uses: Analgesia for moderate to severe pain (e.g., surgery, cancer, biliary colic, burns, renal colic, myocardial infarction, bone trauma).

Additional Contraindications: Migraine headaches. Use in children. Status asthmaticus, obstetrics, respiratory depression in absence of resuscitative equipment.

Special Concerns: Pregnancy category: C.

Additional Side Effect: Nystagmus.

Dosage: Tablets. Adults: 2 mg q 4–6 hr as necessary. For severe pain, 4 or more mg q 4–6 hr. **Suppositories:** 3 mg q 6–8 hr. **SC, IM, IV:** 1–2 mg q 4–6 hr. For severe pain, 3–4 mg q 4–6 hr.

NURSING CONSIDERATIONS

See also *Nursing Considerations* for *Narcotic Analgesics,* p. 753.

Administration/Storage

1. May be administered by slow IV injection. When using this route, administer the drug slowly to minimize hypotensive effects and respiratory depression. Dilute with 5 mL of sterile water or normal saline.
2. Suppositories should be refrigerated.
3. Drug may be administered as Dilaudid brand cough syrup. Be alert to the possibility of an allergic response in people sensitive to yellow dye #5.

Assessment

Take a complete history of client response to narcotic agents. If the drug is to be administered as a cough syrup determine and record any allergies to dyes.

Interventions

Observe client closely for respiratory depression, as it is more profound with hydromorphone than with other narcotic analgesics.

LEVORPHANOL TARTRATE   (lee-**VOR**-fah-nohl)

Levo-Dromoran (C-II, Rx)

See also *Narcotic Analgesics,* p. 750.

Classification: Narcotic analgesic, morphine type.

Action/Kinetics: Levorphanol is 5 times more potent than morphine as an analgesic; respiratory depression, smooth muscle contraction, and dependence liability are increased proportionally. Levorphanol may be used safely with a wide range of anesthetics, including nitrous oxide. **Onset:** 30–90 min. **Peak effect:** 30–60 min. **Duration:** 6–8 hr. **t½:** 12–16 hr.

Uses: Moderate to severe pain. Preoperatively to reduce apprehension, to provide prolonged analgesia, and to reduce thiopental requirements and recovery time.

Additional Contraindications: Acute alcoholism, respiratory depression, increased intracranial pressure, bronchial asthma, anoxia.

Special Concerns: Pregnancy category: C.

Dosage: Tablets, SC: 2–3 mg. Give slow IV for special conditions.

NURSING CONSIDERATIONS

See *Nursing Considerations* for *Narcotic Analgesics,* p. 753.

Administration

If the drug is to be administered IV, dilute the dose of drug in 5 mL of sterile water or normal saline. Administer the drug at a rate of 3 mg or less over a 3–5 minute period.

MEPERIDINE HYDROCHLORIDE (PETHIDINE HYDROCHLORIDE) (meh-PEH-rih-deen)

Demerol Hydrochloride (C-II, Rx)

See also *Narcotic Analgesics,* p. 750.

Classification: Narcotic analgesic, synthetic.

Action/Kinetics: The pharmacologic activity of meperidine is similar to that of the opiates; however, meperidine is only one-tenth as potent an analgesic as morphine. Its analgesic effect is only one-half when given orally rather than parenterally. Meperidine has no antitussive effects and does not produce miosis. The drug does produce moderate spasmogenic effects on smooth muscle. The duration of action of meperidine is less than that of most opiates, and this must be kept in mind when a dosing schedule is being established.

Meperidine will produce both psychological and physical dependence; overdosage is manifested by severe respiratory depression (see *Morphine Overdosage,* p. 751). **Onset:** 10–45 min. **Peak effect:** 30–60 min. **Duration:** 2–4 hr. **t½:** 3–4 hr.

Uses: Any situation that requires a narcotic analgesic: severe pain, hepatic and renal colic, obstetrics, preanesthetic medication, adjunct to anesthesia. Particularly useful for minor surgery, as in orthopedics, ophthalmology, rhinology, laryngology, and dentistry, and for diagnostic procedures such as cystoscopy, retrograde pyelography, and gastroscopy. Spasms of GI tract, uterus, urinary bladder. Anginal syndrome and distress of CHF.

Additional Contraindications: Hypersensitivity to drug, convulsive states as in epilepsy, tetanus and strychnine poisoning, children under 6 months, diabetic acidosis, head injuries, shock, liver disease, respiratory depression, increased cranial pressure, and before labor during pregnancy.

Special Concerns: To be used with caution in pregnancy (pregnancy category: C), lactating mothers, and in older or debilitated patients. Use with extreme caution in patients with asthma. Meperidine has atropine-like effects that may aggravate glaucoma, especially when given with other drugs, which should be used with caution in glaucoma.

Additional Side Effects: Transient hallucinations, transient hypotension (high doses), visual disturbances. Meperidine may accumulate in patients with renal dysfunction leading to an increased risk of CNS toxicity.

Additional Drug Interactions

Antidepressants, tricyclic	Additive anticholinergic side effects
Hydantoins	↓ Effect of meperidine due to ↑ breakdown by liver
Monoamine oxidase inhibitors	↑ Risk of severe symptoms including hyperpyrexia, restlessness, hyper- or hypotension, convulsions, or coma

Dosage: Tablets, Syrup, IM, SC: *Analgesic.* **Adults:** 50–100 mg q 3–4 hr as needed; **pediatric:**

1.1–1.8 mg/kg, up to adult dosage, q 3–4 hr as needed. *Preoperatively:* **Adults: IM, SC,** 50–100 mg 30–90 min before anesthesia; **pediatric: IM, SC,** 1–2 mg/kg 30–90 min before anesthesia. *Support of anesthesia:* **IV infusion** (1 mg/mL) or **slow IV injection** (10 mg/mL) until patient needs met. *Obstetrics:* **IM, SC:** 50–100 mg q 1–3 hr.

NURSING CONSIDERATIONS

See also *Nursing Considerations* for *Narcotic Analgesics,* p. 753.

Administration/Storage

1. For repeated doses, IM administration is preferred over SC use.
2. Meperidine is more effective when given parenterally than when given orally.
3. The syrup should be taken with ½ glass of water to minimize anesthetic effect on mucous membranes.
4. If used concomitantly with phenothiazines or antianxiety agents, the dose of meperidine should be reduced by 25%–50%.
5. Meperidine for IV use is incompatible with the following drugs: aminophylline, barbiturates, heparin, iodide, methicillin, morphine sulfate, phenytoin, sodium bicarbonate, sulfadiazine, and sulfisoxazole.

Assessment

1. Note any evidence of head injury or history of epileptic seizures.
2. Record any client history of asthma or other conditions that tend to compromise respirations.

METHADONE HYDROCHLORIDE   (METH-ah-dohn)

Dolophine, Methadose (C-II, Rx)

See also *Narcotic Analgesics,* p. 750.

Classification: Narcotic analgesic, morphine type.

Action/Kinetics: Methadone produces only mild euphoria, which is the reason it is used as a heroin withdrawal substitute and for maintenance programs. Methadone produces physical dependence, but the abstinence syndrome develops more slowly upon termination of therapy; also, withdrawal symptoms are less intense but more prolonged than those associated with morphine. Methadone does not produce sedation or narcosis.

Methadone is not effective for preoperative or obstetric anesthesia. When administered orally, it is only one-half as potent as when given parenterally. **Onset:** 30–60 min. **Peak effects:** 30–60 min. **Duration:** 4–6 hr. **t½:** 15–30 hr. Both the duration and half-life increase with repeated use due to cumulative effects.

Uses: Severe pain. Drug withdrawal and maintenance of narcotic dependence.

Additional Contraindications: IV use, liver disease; give rarely, if at all, during pregnancy. Use in children. Use in obstetrics (due to long duration of action and chance of respiratory depression in the neonate).

Special Concerns: Pregnancy category: C. Use with caution during lactation.

Additional Side Effects: Marked constipation, excessive sweating, pulmonary edema, choreic movements.

Drug Interactions: Rifampin and phenytoin ↓ plasma methadone levels by ↑ breakdown by liver; thus, possible symptoms of narcotic withdrawal may develop.

Laboratory Test Interference: ↑ Immunoglobulin G.

Dosage: Tablets, Oral Solution, Oral Concentrate, IM, SC. *Analgesia:* **Adults, individualized,** 2.5–10 mg q 3–4 hr, although higher doses may be necessary for severe pain or due to development of tolerance. *Narcotic withdrawal:* **initial,** 15–20 mg/day orally (some may require 40 mg/day); **then,** depending on need of the patient, slowly decrease dosage. *Maintenance (individualized):* **PO, initial,** 20–40 mg 4–8 hr after heroin is stopped; **then,** adjust dosage as required up to 120 mg daily.

NURSING CONSIDERATIONS
See also *Nursing Considerations* for *Narcotic Analgesics,* p. 753.

Administration/Storage
1. Oral concentrations of solution should be diluted in at least 90 mL of water prior to administration.
2. If the client is taking dispersible tablets, the tablets should be diluted with 120 mL of water, orange juice, citrus flavored drink or other acidic fruit drink. Allow at least 1 minute for complete dispersion of the drug.
3. For repeated analgesic doses, IM administration is preferred over SC administration.
4. Clients receiving methadone for detoxification purposes should be on the drug no longer than 21 days. The treatment should not be repeated until 4 weeks have elapsed.

Interventions
1. Inspect the injection sites for signs of irritation.
2. If the client has nausea and vomiting as a result of the medication therapy, a lower dose of drug may relieve these symptoms.

Client/Family Teaching
1. Review side effects with the client and family. Note that if the client is ambulatory and not suffering acute pain, side effects may be more pronounced.
2. If the client is on narcotic withdrawal therapy, advise that the drug should be stored out of the reach of children.

MORPHINE SULFATE (MOR-feen)

Astramorph PF, Duramorph, Epimorph✶, Morphine H.P.✶, MS Contin, Morphitec✶, M.O.S.✶, M.O.S.-S.R.✶, MSIR, RMS, RMS Rectal Suppositories, Roxanol, Roxanol 100, Roxanol SR, Roxanol UD, Statex✶ (C-II, Rx)

See also *Narcotic Analgesics,* p. 750.

Classification: Narcotic analgesic, morphine type.

Action/Kinetics: Morphine is the prototype for opiate analgesics. **Onset:** approximately 15–60 min. **Peak effect:** 30–60 min. **Duration:** 3–7 hr. **t½:** 1.5–2 hr. Oral morphine is only one-third to one-sixth as effective as parenteral products.

Uses: Intrathecally, epidurally, orally, or by continuous IV infusion for acute or chronic pain. In low doses, morphine is more effective against dull, continuous pain than against intermittent, sharp pain. Large doses, however, will dull almost any kind of pain. Preoperative medication. To facilitate induction of anesthesia and reduce dose of anesthetic. *Investigational:* Acute left ventricular failure (for dyspneic seizures) and pulmonary edema. Morphine should not be used with papaverine for analgesia in biliary spasms but may be used with papaverine in acute vascular occlusions.

Additional Contraindications: Epidural or intrathecal morphine if infection is present at injection site, in patients on anticoagulant therapy, bleeding diathesis, if patient has received parenteral corticosteroids within the past 2 weeks.

Special Concerns: Pregnancy category: C. Morphine may increase the length of labor. Patients with known seizure disorders may be at greater risk for morphine-induced seizure activity.

Dosage: Tablets, Oral Solution, Soluble Tablets. 10–30 mg q 4 hr. **Sustained release:** 30 mg q 8–12 hr, depending on patient needs and response. **IM, SC: Adults,** 5–20 mg/70 kg q 4 hr as needed; **pediatric:** 100–200 mcg/kg up to a maximum of 15 mg. **IV infusion: Adults,** 2.5–15 mg/70 kg in 4–5 mL of water for injection (should be administered slowly over 4–5 min). **IV infusion, continuous:** 0.1–1 mg/mL in 5% dextrose in water by a controlled-infusion pump. **Rectal:** 10–20 mg q 4 hr. **Intrathecal: Adults,** 0.2–1 mg as a single daily injection. **Epidural: initial,** 5 mg daily in the lumbar region; if analgesia is not manifested in 1 hr, increasing doses of 1–2 mg can be given, not to exceed 10 mg daily. For continuous infusion, 2–4 mg daily with additional doses of 1–2 mg if analgesia is not satisfactory.

Dose may be lower in geriatric patients or those with respiratory disease.

NURSING CONSIDERATIONS

See also *Nursing Considerations* for *Narcotic Analgesics,* p. 753.

Administration/Storage

1. Controlled release tablets should not be crushed or chewed.
2. Rapid IV administration increases the risk of untoward reactions; a narcotic antagonist (e.g. naloxone) should be available at all times if morphine is given IV.
3. For intrathecal use, no more than 2 mL of the 5 mg/10 mL preparation or 1 mL of the 10 mg/10 mL product should be given.
4. Intrathecal administration should be only in the lumbar region; repeated injections are not recommended.
5. To reduce the chance of untoward reactions with intrathecal administration, a constant IV infusion of naloxone (0.6 mg/hr for 24 hr after intrathecal injection) is recommended.
6. In certain circumstances (e.g., tolerance, severe pain), the physician may prescribe doses higher than those listed above.

Interventions

1. Use an electronic infusion device for IV solutions.
2. Obtain written parameters for BP and respirations during IV infusions.

NALBUPHINE HYDROCHLORIDE   (nal-BYOU-feen)

Nubain (Rx)

See also *Narcotic Analgesics,* p. 750.

Classification: Narcotic analgesic—agonist-antagonist.

Action/Kinetics: Nalbuphine, a synthetic compound resembling oxymorphone and naloxone, is a potent analgesic with both narcotic agonist and antagonist actions. Its analgesic potency is approximately equal to that of morphine, while its antagonistic potency is approximately one-fourth that of nalorphine. **Onset: IV,** 2–3 min; **SC or IM,** less than 15 min. **Peak effect:** 30–60 min. **Duration:** 3–6 hr; **t½:** 5 hr.

Uses: Moderate to severe pain. Preoperative analgesia, anesthesia adjunct, obstetric analgesia.

Contraindications: Hypersensitivity to drug. Children under 18 years.

Special Concerns: Safe use during pregnancy (except for delivery) and lactation not established. Use with caution in presence of head injuries and asthma, myocardial infarction (if patient is nauseous or vomiting), biliary tract surgery (may induce spasms of sphincter of Oddi), renal insufficiency. Patients dependent on narcotics may experience withdrawal symptoms following use of nalbuphine.

Additional Side Effects: Even though nalbuphine is an agonist-antagonist, it may cause dependence and may precipitate withdrawal symptoms in an individual physically dependent on narcotics. *CNS:* Sedation is common. Crying, feelings of unreality, and other psychological reactions. *GI:* Cramps, dry mouth, bitter taste, dyspepsia. *Skin:* Itching, burning, urticaria, sweaty, clammy skin. *Other:* Blurred vision, difficulty with speech, urinary frequency.

Drug Interactions: Concomitant use with CNS depressants, other narcotics, phenothiazines, may result in additive depressant effects.

Dosage: SC, IM, IV. Adults: 10 mg for 70-kg patient q 3–6 hr as needed (single dose should not exceed 20 mg q 3–6 hr; total daily dose should not exceed 160 mg).

Overdosage: See *Narcotic Analgesics,* p. 750, and *Narcotic Antagonists,* p. 778.

NURSING CONSIDERATIONS

See also *Nursing Considerations* for *Narcotic Analgesics,* p. 753.

Administration

Nalbuphine hydrochloride may be administered IV, undiluted. Administer each 10 mg or less over a 3–5 minute period.

Assessment

1. Take a complete client history, noting any evidence of dependence on narcotics. Nalbuphine may precipitate withdrawal symptoms in clients with narcotic addiction.
2. Note client history of head injuries, asthma or cardiac dysfunction. The drug may be contraindicated.

Interventions

Note any client symptoms of withdrawal such as extreme restlessness, lacrimation, rhinorrhea, yawning, perspiration, and dilation of the pupils. These are indications of narcotic dependence. Document and report these symptoms to the physician.

OXYCODONE HYDROCHLORIDE   (ox-ee-**KOH**-dohn)

Roxicodone, Supeudol✹ (C-II, Rx)

OXYCODONE TEREPHTHALATE   (ox-ee-**KOH**-dohn teh-ref-**THAL**-ayt)

(C-II, Rx)

See alo *Narcotic Analgesics,* p. 750.

Classification: Narcotic analgesic, morphine type.

Action/Kinetics: A semisynthetic opiate, oxycodone produces mild sedation with little or no antitussive effect. It is most effective in relieving acute pain. **Onset:** 15–30 min. **Peak effect:** 60 min. **Duration:** 4–6 hr. Dependence liability is moderate. Oxycodone terephthalate is only available in combination with aspirin (e.g., Percodan) or acetaminophen.

Uses: Moderate to severe pain.

Additional Contraindications: Use in children.

Special Concerns: Pregnancy category: C.

Additional Drug Interactions: Patients with gastric distress, such as colitis or gastric or duodenal ulcer, and patients who have glaucoma should not receive Percodan, which also contains aspirin.

Dosage: Oral Solution, Tablets. Adults: 5 mg q 6 hr. Use in children not recommended.

NURSING CONSIDERATIONS

See also *Nursing Considerations* for *Narcotic Analgesics,* p. 753.

Client/Family Teaching

Advise client to take medication with food to minimize GI upset.

OXYMORPHONE HYDROCHLORIDE   (ox-ee-**MOR**-fohn)

Numorphan (C-I, Rx)

See also *Narcotic Anagesics,* p. 778.

Classification: Narcotic analgesic, morphine type.

Action/Kinetics: Oxymorphone, on a weight basis, is said to be 2 to 10 times more potent as an analgesic than morphine although potency depends on the route of administration. It produces mild sedation and moderate depression of the cough reflex. **Onset:** 5–10 min. **Peak effect:** 30–60 min. **Duration:** 3–6 hr.

Uses: Moderate to severe pain. Parenteral: Preoperative analgesia, to support anesthesia, obstetrics, relief of anxiety in patients with dyspnea associated with acute left ventricular failure and pulmonary edema.

Special Concerns: Pregnancy category: C.

Dosage: SC, IM. Initial: 1–1.5 mg q 4–6 hr; dose can be increased carefully until analgesic response obtained. *Analgesia during labor:* **IM,** 0.5–1.0 mg. **IV: initial,** 0.5 mg. **Suppositories:** 5 mg q 4–6 hr. **Not recommended for children under 12 years of age.**

NURSING CONSIDERATIONS

See also *Nursing Considerations* for *Narcotic Analgesics,* p. 753.

Administration/Storage

1. If the drug is to be administered IV, dilute the dosage in 5 mL of sterile water or normal saline.
2. Suppositories should be stored in the refrigerator.

Interventions

1. Encourage client to cough and breathe deeply several times each hour while awake to prevent atelectasis. Incentive spirometry may also be of some assistance.
2. Assess any client complaint of pain that resembles gallbladder pain and report to the physician. This particular drug may aggravate gallbladder pain.

PAREGORIC (CAMPHORATED TINCTURE OF OPIUM) (pah-reh-**GOR**-ik)
(C-III, Rx)

See also *Narcotic Analgesics,* p. 750.

Classification: Narcotic analgesic, morphine type.

Note: Paregoric contains 2 mg of morphine equivalent per 5 mL. The product also contains 45% alcohol. For all details, consult morphine, general statement on narcotic analgesics (Chapter 37, p. 750) and paregoric, antidiarrheal (Chapter 55, p. 1062).

Uses: Moderate to severe pain, diarrhea.

Special Concerns: Pregnancy category: C.

Dosage: Liquid. Adults: 5–10 mL (2–4 mg morphine) 1–4 times/day. **Pediatric:** 0.25–0.5 mL/kg 1–4 times/day.

NURSING CONSIDERATIONS

See *Nursing Considerations* for *Narcotic Analgesics,* p. 753, and *Antidiarrheal Agents,* p. 1062.

Assessment

Several combinations contain bismuth or other compounds. Review client sensitivity to bismuth.

PENTAZOCINE HYDROCHLORIDE WITH NALOXONE (pen-**TAY**-zoh-seen, nah-**LOX**-ohn)
Talwin NX (C-IV, Rx)

PENTAZOCINE LACTATE (pen-**TAY**-zoh-seen **LAK**-tayt)
Talwin (C-IV, Rx)

See also *Narcotic Analgesics,* p. 750.

Classification: Narcotic analgesic—agonist-antagonist.

General Statement: When administered preoperatively for pain, pentazocine is approximately one-third as potent as morphine. It is a weak antagonist of the analgesic effects of meperidine, morphine, and other narcotic analgesics. It also manifests sedative effects.

Pentazocine has been abused by combining it with the antihistamine tripelennamine (a combination known as *T's and Blues*). This combination has been injected IV as a substitute for heroin. To reduce this possibility, the oral dosage form of pentazocine has been combined with naloxone (Talwin NX), which will prevent the effects of IV administered pentazocine but will not affect the efficacy of pentazocine when taken orally.

Action/Kinetics: Pentazocine manifests both narcotic agonist and antagonist properties. **Onset: IM,** 15–20 min; **PO,** 15–30 min; **IV,** 2–3 min. **Peak effect: IM,** 15–60 min; **PO,** 60–180 min. **Duration, all routes:** 3 hr. However, onset, duration, and degree of relief depend on both dose and severity of pain. **t½:** 2–3 hr.

Uses: PO: Moderate to severe pain. **Parenteral:** Preoperative or preanesthetic medication, obstetrics, supplement to surgical anesthesia.

Additional Contraindications: Increased intracranial pressure or head injury. Not recommended for use in children under 12 years of age. Avoid using methadone or other narcotics for pentazocine withdrawal.

Special Concerns: Pregnancy category: C. Use with caution in impaired renal or hepatic function, as well as after myocardial infarction, when nausea and vomiting are present. Use with caution in women delivering premature infants.

Additional Side Effects: Edema of the face, syncope, dysphoria, nightmares, and hallucinations. Also, decreased white blood cells, paresthesia, chills. Both psychological and physical dependence are possible, although the addiction liability is thought to be no greater than for codeine.

Dosage: Tablets. *Pentazocine hydrochloride with naloxone.* **Adults,** 50 mg q 3–4 hr, up to 100 mg. Daily dose should not exceed 600 mg. **IM, IV, SC.** *Pentazocine lactate.* 30 mg q 3–4 hr; doses exceeding 30 mg IV or 60 mg IM not recommended. Total daily dosage should not exceed 360 mg. *Obstetric analgesia:* **IM,** 30 mg; **IV,** 20 mg. Dosage may be repeated 2–3 times at 2- to 3-hr intervals.

NURSING CONSIDERATIONS

See also *Nursing Considerations* for *Narcotic Analgesics,* p. 753.

Administration/Storage

1. Do not mix soluble barbiturates in the same syringe with pentazocine. It will form a precipitate.
2. IV pentazocine may be administered undiluted. However, if the drug is to be diluted, place 5 mg of drug into 5 mL of sterile water for injection. Administer each 5 mg of drug or less over a 1-min period.
3. Review the list of drugs with which the medication interacts.

PERCOCET   (PER-koh-set)

(C-II, Rx)

See also *Acetaminophen,* p. 793, and *Narcotic Analgesics,* p. 750.

Classification/Content: *Nonnarcotic analgesic:* Acetaminophen, 325 mg. *Narcotic analgesic:* Oxycodone HCl, 5 mg.

Uses: Moderate to moderately severe pain.

Special Concerns: Pregnancy category: C.

Dosage: Tablets. Adults, usual: One tablet q 6 hr as required for pain.

NURSING CONSIDERATIONS

See *Nursing Considerations* for *Narcotic Analgesics,* p. 753, and *Acetaminophen*, p. 795.

Administration/Storage

It may be necessary to increase the dose if tolerance occurs or if the pain is severe.

PERCODAN AND PERCODAN-DEMI   (PER-koh-dan, PER-koh-dan DEH-mee)
(C-II, Rx)

See also *Aspirin,* p. 783, and *Narcotic Analgesics,* p. 750.

Classification/Content: Percodan: *Nonnarcotic analgesic:* Aspirin, 325 mg. *Narcotic Analgesics:* Oxycodone HCl, 4.5 mg; Oxycodone terephthalate, 0.38 mg. Percodan-Demi contains the same amount of aspirin as Percodan but one-half the amount of oxycodone HCl and oxycodone terephthalate.

Uses: Treatment of moderate to moderately severe pain.

Special Concerns: Use during pregnancy only if benefits outweigh risks.

Dosage: Tablets. Adults, usual: One tablet q 6 hr as required for pain.

NURSING CONSIDERATIONS

See also *Nursing Considerations* for *Narcotic Analgesics,* p. 753, and *Aspirin*, p. 788.

Administration/Storage

It may be necessary to increase the dose if tolerance occurs or if the pain is severe.

PHENAPHEN WITH CODEINE NO. 2, NO. 3, AND NO. 4   (FEN-ah-fen, KOH-deen)
(C-III, Rx)

See also *Acetaminophen,* p. 793, and *Narcotic Analgesics,* p. 750.

Classification/Content: *Nonnarcotic analgesic:* Acetaminophen, 325 mg (in each strength). *Narcotic analgesic:* Codeine phosphate, 15 mg (No. 2), 30 mg (No. 3), and 60 mg (No. 4).

Uses: Mild to moderately severe pain.

Special Concerns: Pregnancy category: C.

Dosage: Capsules. Individualized. Adults, usual: 1–2 capsules of Phenaphen with Codeine No. 2 or No. 3 q 4 hr as required for pain. Or, 1 capsule of Phenaphen No. 4 q 4 hr as required for pain. **Pediatric:** Dose of codeine equivalent to 0.5 mg/kg q 4 hr as required for pain.

NURSING CONSIDERATIONS

See also *Nursing Considerations* for *Narcotic Analgesics,* p. 753, and *Acetaminophen,* p. 795.

Administration/Storage

Doses of codeine greater than 60 mg do not increase the analgesic effect but may increase the incidence of unpleasant side effects.

PROPOXYPHENE HYDROCHLORIDE   (proh-**POX**-ih-feen)

642 Tablets✤, Darvon, Dolene, Doraphen, Doxaphene, Novopropoxyn✤, Profene, Pro Pox, Propoxycon (C-IV, Rx)

PROPOXYPHENE NAPSYLATE   (proh-**POX**-ih-feen **NAP**-sih-layt)

Darvon-N (C-IV, Rx)

Classification: Analgesic, narcotic, miscellaneous.

Action/Kinetics: Propoxyphene resembles the narcotics with respect to its mechanism and analgesic effect; it is one-half to one-third as potent as codeine. It is devoid of antitussive, anti-inflammatory or antipyretic activity. When taken in excessive doses for long periods, psychological dependence, and occasionally physical dependence and tolerance, will be manifested. **Peak plasma levels:** *hydrochloride:* 2–2.5 hr; *napsylate:* 3–4 hr. **Analgesic onset:** up to 1 hr. **Peak analgesic effect:** 2 hr. **Duration:** 4–6 hr. **Therapeutic serum levels:** 0.05–0.12 mcg/mL. **$t^{1/2}$, propoxyphene:** 6–12 hr; **norpropoxyphene:** 30–36 hr. Extensive first-pass effect; metabolites are excreted in the urine.

Propoxyphene is often prescribed in combination with salicylates. In such instances, the information on salicylates should also be consulted. Propoxyphene hydrochloride is found in Darvon Compound and Wygesic, while propoxyphene napsylate is found in Darvocet-N.

Uses: To relieve mild to moderate pain. Propoxyphene napsylate has been used experimentally to suppress the withdrawal syndrome from narcotics.

Contraindications: Hypersensitivity to drug.

Special Concerns: Safe use during pregnancy has not been established. Use with caution during lactation. Safety and efficacy have not been established in children.

Side Effects: *GI:* Nausea, vomiting, constipation, abdominal pain. *CNS:* Sedation, dizziness, lightheadedness, headache, weakness, euphoria, dysphoria. *Other:* Skin rashes, visual disturbances. Propoxyphene can produce psychological dependence, as well as physical dependence and tolerance. Symptoms of overdosage are similar to those of narcotics and include respiratory depression, coma, pupillary constriction, and circulatory collapse. Treatment of overdosage consists of maintaining an adequate airway, artificial respiration, and the use of a narcotic antagonist (naloxone) to combat respiratory depression. Gastric lavage or administration of activated charcoal may be helpful.

Drug Interactions

Alcohol, antianxiety agents, antipsychotic agents, narcotics, sedative-hypnotics	Concomitant use may lead to drowsiness, lethargy, stupor, respiratory, depression, and coma

Drug Interactions

Carbamazepine	↑ Effect of carbamazepine due to ↓ breakdown by liver
CNS depressants	Additive CNS depression
Orphenadrine	Concomitant use may lead to confusion, anxiety, and tremors
Phenobarbital	↑ Effect of phenobarbital due to ↓ breakdown by liver
Skeletal muscle relaxants	Additive respiratory depression
Warfarin	↑ Hypoprothrombinemic effects of warfarin

Dosage: Capsules: (Hydrochloride). Adults, 65 mg q 4 hr, not to exceed 390 mg/day.

Oral Suspension, Tablets: (Napsylate). Adults, 100 mg q 4 hr, not to exceed 600 mg/day. Dose of propoxyphene should be reduced in patients with renal or hepatic impairment. **Not recommended for use in children.**

NURSING CONSIDERATIONS

See also *Nursing Considerations* for *Narcotic Analgesics,* p 753.

Intervention

Anticipate reduced dose with renal and liver dysfunction.

SUFENTANIL   (soo-FEN-tah-nil)

Sufenta (Rx)

See also *Narcotic Analgesics,* p. 750.

Classification: Narcotic analgesic.

Action/Kinetics: Onset, IV: 1.3–8 min. **Anesthetic blood concentration:** 8–30 mcg/kg. **t½:** 2.5 hr. Allows appropriate oxygenation of the heart and brain during prolonged surgical procedures. May be used in children.

Uses: Narcotic analgesic used as an adjunct to maintain balanced general anesthesia. To induce and maintain general anesthesia (with 100% oxygen), especially in neurosurgery or cardiovascular surgery.

Additional Contraindications: Use during labor.

Special Concerns: Pregnancy category: C. Dosage must be decreased in the obese, elderly, or debilitated patient.

Additional Side Effects: Erythema, chills, intraoperative muscle movement. Extended postoperative respiratory depression.

Dosage: IV, individualized, adults, usual initial: 1–2 mcg/kg with oxygen and nitrous oxide; **maintenance:** 10–25 mcg as required. *For complicated surgery:* 2–8 mcg/kg with oxygen and nitrous oxide; **maintenance:** 10–50 mcg. *To induce and maintain general anesthesia:* 8–30 mcg/kg with 100% oxygen and a muscle relaxant; **maintenance:** 25–50 mcg. **Pediatric, less than 12 years:** *To induce and maintain general anesthesia:* 10–25 mcg/kg with 100% oxygen;

maintenance: 25–50 mcg. *Induction and maintenance of general anesthesia in children less than 12 years of age undergoing cardiovascular surgery:* 10–25 mcg/kg with 100% oxygen; **maintenance:** 25–50 mcg.

NURSING CONSIDERATIONS

See also *Nursing Considerations* for *Narcotic Analgesics,* p. 753.

Administration/Storage

1. Dose should be reduced in the debilitated or elderly client.
2. The dose should be calculated based on lean body weight.

SYNALGOS-DC   (sih-**NAL**-gohs)

(C-III, Rx)

See also *Aspirin,* p. 783, *Narcotic Analgesics,* p. 750, and *Caffeine,* p. 854.

Classification/Content: *Nonnarcotic analgesic:* Aspirin, 356.4 mg. *Narcotic analgesic:* Dihydrocodeine bitartrate, 16 mg. *CNS stimulant:* Caffeine, 30 mg.
See also information on individual components.

Uses: Relief of moderate to moderately severe pain.

Contraindications: Safe use during pregnancy has not been established.

Dosage: Capsules. Individualized. Adults, usual: Two capsules q 4 hr as required for pain.

NURSING CONSIDERATIONS

See also *Nursing Considerations* for *Narcotic Analgesics,* p. 753, *Aspirin,* p. 788, and *Caffeine,* p. 856.

Administration/Storage

The dosage can be adjusted depending on the response of the client.

TYLENOL WITH CODEINE CAPSULES, ELIXIR, OR TABLETS   (**TIE**-leh-nol)

(tablets and capsules are C-III and elixir is C-V) (Rx)

See also *Acetaminophen,* p. 793, and *Narcotic Analgesics,* p. 750.

Classification/Content: *Nonnarcotic analgesic:* Acetaminophen 300 mg in each tablet or capsule and 120 mg/5 mL elixir. *Narcotic analgesic:* Codeine phosphate, 7.5 mg (No. 1 Tablets), 15 mg (No. 2 Tablets), 30 mg (No. 3 Tablets), 60 mg (No. 4 Tablets), 30 mg (No. 3 Capsules), 60 mg (No. 4 Capsules), 12 mg/5 mL (Elixir).

Uses: The capsules and tablets are used for mild to moderately severe pain while the elixir is used for mild to moderate pain.

Special Concerns: Pregnancy category: C.

Dosage: Tablets, Capsules. Adults, individualized, usual: 1–2 No. 1, No. 2, or No. 3 Tablets or No. 3 Capsules q 2–4 hr as needed for pain. Or, 1 No. 4 Tablet or Capsule q 4 hr as required.

Pediatric: Dosage equivalent to 0.5 mg/kg codeine. **Elixir. Adults, individualized, usual:** 15 mL q 4 hr as needed; **pediatric, 7–12 years:** 10 mL t.i.d.–q.i.d.; **3–6 years:** 5 mL t.i.d.–q.i.d. Dosage has not been established for children under 3 years of age.

NURSING CONSIDERATIONS

See also *Nursing Considerations* for *Narcotic Analgesics,* p. 753, and *Acetaminophen,* p. 795.

Administration/Storage

Doses of codeine greater than 60 mg do not provide additional analgesia but may lead to an increased incidence of side effects.

TYLOX   (TIE-lox)
(C-II, Rx)

See also *Acetaminophen,* p. 793, and *Narcotic Analgesics,* p. 750.

Classification/Content: *Nonnarcotic analgesic:* Acetaminophen, 500 mg. *Narcotic analgesic:* Oxycodone HCl, 5 mg.

Uses: Relief of moderate to moderately severe pain.

Special Concerns: Pregnancy category: C.

Dosage: Capsule. Individualized. Adults, usual: One capsule q 6 hr as required for pain.

NURSING CONSIDERATIONS

See also *Nursing Considerations* for *Narcotic Analgesics,* p. 753, and *Acetaminophen,* p. 795.

Administration/Storage

As the dose of oxycodone is increased, the incidence of side effects increases.

VICODIN   (VYE-koh-din)
(C-III, Rx)

See also *Acetaminophen,* p. 793, and *Narcotic Analgesics,* p. 750.

Classification/Content: *Nonnarcotic analgesic:* Acetaminophen, 500 mg. *Narcotic analgesic:* Hydrocodone bitartrate, 5 mg.

Uses: Moderate to moderately severe pain.

Special Concerns: Pregnancy category: C.

Dosage: Tablets. Adults, individualized, usual: One tablet q 4–6 hr as needed for pain. If pain is severe, 2 tablets may be taken q 6 hr, up to maximum of 8 tablets in 24 hr.

NURSING CONSIDERATIONS

See *Nursing Considerations* for *Acetaminophen,* p. 795, and *Narcotic Analgesics* p. 753.

NARCOTIC ANTAGONISTS

General Statement: The narcotic antagonists are able to prevent or reverse many of the pharmacologic actions of morphine-type analgesics and meperidine. For example, respiratory depression induced by these drugs is reversed within minutes. Naloxone is considered a pure antagonist in that it does not produce morphine-like effects.

The narcotic antagonists are not effective in reversing the respiratory depression induced by barbiturates, anesthetics, or other nonnarcotic agents. Narcotic antagonists almost immediately induce withdrawal symptoms in narcotic addicts and are sometimes used to unmask dependence.

Action/Kinetics: Narcotic antagonists block the action of narcotic analgesics by displacing previously given narcotics from their receptor sites or by preventing narcotics from attaching to the opiate receptors, thereby preventing access by the analgesic. This type of antagonism is competitive.

NURSING CONSIDERATIONS

Assessment

1. Determine the etiology of respiratory depression. Narcotic antagonists do not relieve the toxicity of nonnarcotic CNS depressants.
2. Assess and obtain baseline vital signs before administering any narcotic antagonist.

Interventions

1. Monitor respirations closely after the duration of action of the narcotic antagonist. Additional doses of drug may be necessary.
2. Observe for the appearance of withdrawal symptoms after administration of the narcotic antagonist. Withdrawal symptoms are characterized by restlessness, lacrimation, rhinorrhea, yawning, perspiration, and pupil dilation.
3. Have emergency drugs and equipment readily available.
4. If the client is comatose, turn frequently and position on his side to prevent aspiration.
5. Maintain a safe, protective environment. Utilize side rails and soft supports as needed.

Evaluation

1. Assess the vital signs after drug administration to determine the effectiveness of the drug.
2. Note the appearance of narcotic withdrawal symptoms after the antagonist has been administered.
3. If the narcotic antagonist is being used to diagnose narcotic use or dependence, observe the initial dilation of the client's pupils, followed by constriction.

NALOXONE HYDROCHLORIDE   (nah-**LOX**-ohn)

Narcan (Rx)

See also *Narcotic Antagonists, above.*

Classification: Narcotic antagonist.

Action/Kinetics: Naloxone, administered by itself, does not produce significant pharmacologic activity. Since the duration of action of naloxone is shorter than that of the narcotic analgesics, the respiratory depression may return when the narcotic antagonist has worn off. **Onset: IV,** 2 min; **SC, IM:** less than 5 min. **Time to peak effect:** 5–15 min. **Duration:** Dependent on dose and route of administration but may be as short as 45 min. **t½:** 60–100 min. Metabolized in the liver to inactive products which are eliminated through the kidneys.

Uses: Respiratory depression induced by natural and synthetic narcotics, including butorphanol, methadone, nalbuphine, pentazocine, and propoxyphene. Drug of choice when nature of depressant drug is not known. Diagnosis of acute opiate overdosage. Not effective when respiratory depression is induced by hypnotics, sedatives, or anesthetics and other nonnarcotic CNS depressants. *Investigational:* Refractory shock to improve circulation. Treatment of Alzheimer's dementia, alcoholic coma, and schizophrenia.

Contraindications: Sensitivity to drug. Narcotic addicts (drug may cause severe withdrawal symptoms). Not recommended for use in neonates.

Special Concern: Pregnancy category: B. Safe use during lactation and in children is not established.

Side Effects: Nausea, vomiting, sweating, hypertension, tremors, sweating due to reversal of narcotic depression. If used postoperatively, excessive doses may cause tachycardia, fibrillation, hypo- or hypertension, pulmonary edema.

Dosage: IV, IM, SC. *Narcotic overdosage:* **Initial,** 0.4–2 mg; if necessary, additional IV doses may be repeated at 2- to 3-min intervals. If no response after 10 mg, reevaluate diagnosis. *To reverse postoperative narcotic depression:* **IV, initial,** 0.1- to 0.2-mg increments at 2- to 3-min intervals; **then,** repeat at 1- to 2-hr intervals if necessary. Supplemental IM dosage increases the duration of reversal. **Pediatric.** *Narcotic overdosage:* **IV, IM, SC, initial,** 0.01 mg/kg; **then,** 0.1 mg/kg, if needed. *To reverse postoperative narcotic depression:* **initial,** increments of 0.005–0.01 mg **IV** q 2–3 min to desired effect. *To reverse narcotic depression:* **IV, IM, SC,** initial 0.01 mg/kg; may be repeated if necessary.

NURSING CONSIDERATIONS

See also *Nursing Considerations* for *Narcotic Antagonists,* p. 778.

Administration/Storage

1. If the drug is to be administered IV, 2 mg total may be added to 500 mL of normal saline or 5% dextrose to provide a concentration of 0.004 mg/mL. The rate of administration varies with the response of the client.
2. Do not mix naloxone with preparations containing bisulfite, metabisulfite, anions which are long-chain or high molecular weight, or solutions with an alkaline pH.
3. When naloxone is mixed with other solutions they should be used within 24 hr.
4. Naloxone is effective within 2 minutes after IV administration.

Interventions

1. The duration of the effects of the narcotic may exceed the effects of naloxone. Therefore, more than one dose of drug may be necessary to counteract the effects of the narcotic.
2. Monitor the client's blood pressure, pulse and respirations at 5-min intervals, then every 30 minutes once vital signs have stabilized.
3. Have emergency drugs and equipment available for resuscitation.
4. For acutely ill clients or those who are in a coma, have a suction machine immediately available. These clients additionally should be attached to a cardiac monitor.

NALTREXONE   (nal-TREX-ohn)

Trexan (Rx)

See also *Narcotic Antagonists,* p. 778.

Classification: Narcotic antagonist.

Action/Kinetics: Naltrexone binds to opiate receptors, thereby reversing or preventing the effects of narcotics. This is an example of competitive inhibition. **Peak plasma levels:** 1 hr. **Duration:** 24–72 hr. Metabolized in the liver; a major metabolite—6-β-naltrexol—is active. **Peak serum levels, after 50 mg: naltrexone,** 8.6 ng/mL; **6-β-naltrexol,** 99.3 ng/mL. **t¹/₂: naltrexone,** approximately 4 hr; **6-β-naltrexol,** 13 hr. Naltrexone and its metabolites are excreted in the urine.

Uses: To prevent narcotic use in former narcotic addicts. *Investigational:* To treat eating disorders and postconcussional syndrome not responding to other approaches.

Contraindications: Patients taking narcotic analgesics, those dependent on narcotics, those in acute withdrawal from narcotics. Liver disease, acute hepatitis.

Special Concerns: Safety during pregnancy (pregnancy category: C) and lactation and in children under 18 years of age has not been established.

Side Effects: *CNS:* Headache, anxiety, nervousness, sleep disorders, dizziness, change in energy level, depression, confusion, restlessness, disorientation, hallucinations, nightmares, paranoia, fatigue, drowsiness. *GI:* Nausea, vomiting, diarrhea, constipation, anorexia, abdominal pain or cramps, flatulence, ulcers, increased appetite, weight gain or loss, increased thirst, xerostomia. *CV:* Phlebitis, edema, increased blood pressure, changes in ECG, palpitations, epistaxis, tachycardia. *GU:* Delayed ejaculation, increased urinary frequency or urinary discomfort, changes in interest in sex. *Respiratory:* Cough, sore throat, nasal congestion, rhinorrhea, sneezing, excess secretions, hoarseness, shortness of breath, heaving breathing, sinus trouble. *Dermatologic:* Rash, oily skin, itching, pruritus, acne, cold sores, alopecia, athlete's foot. *Musculoskeletal:* Joint/muscle pain, muscle twitches, tremors, pain in legs, knees, or shoulders. *Other:* Hepatoxicity, blurred vision, tinnitus, painful ears, aching or strained eyes, chills, swollen glands, inguinal pain, cold feet, "hot" spells, "pounding" head, fever.

A severe narcotic withdrawal syndrome may be precipitated if naltrexone is administered to a dependent individual. The syndrome may begin within 5 min and last for up to 2 days.

Dosage: Tablets. *To produce blockade of opiate actions:* **Initial:** 25 mg followed by an additional 25 mg in 1 hr if no withdrawal symptoms occur. **Maintenance:** 50 mg daily. *Alternate dosing schedule:* The weekly dose of 350 mg may be given as: (a) 50 mg daily on weekdays and 100 mg on Saturday; (b) 100 mg q 48 hr; (c) 100 mg every Monday and Wednesday and 150 mg on Friday; or, (d) 150 mg q 72 hr.

NURSING CONSIDERATIONS

See also *Nursing Considerations* for *Narcotic Antagonists,* p. 778.

Administration/Storage

1. Naltrexone therapy should **never** be initiated until it has been determined that the individual is not dependent on narcotics (i.e., a naloxone challenge test should be completed).
2. The client should be opiate free for at least 7–10 days before beginning naltrexone therapy.
3. When initiating naltrexone therapy, begin with 25 mg and observe for 1 hr for any signs of narcotic withdrawal.

4. The blockade produced by naltrexone may be overcome by taking large doses of narcotics. Such doses may be fatal.

5. Clients taking naltrexone may not respond to preparations containing narcotics for use in coughs, diarrhea, or pain.

Assessment

1. Determine if the client is addicted to opiates and when he had his last dose of this drug.

2. Obtain a baseline blood pressure, pulse, respirations, and ECG prior to initiating therapy.

3. Ensure that liver function studies have been performed prior to administering drug therapy.

Interventions

1. Note client complaints of headache, restlessness and irritability. These are usually due to the effects of naltrexone.

2. Anticipate that the physician will order a naloxone challenge test prior to administration. Clients must be opiate free for 7–10 days when this drug is given.

3. Monitor blood pressure, pulse and respirations daily. If the respirations are severely lowered or if the client complains of difficulty breathing, notify the physician.

4. Routinely order liver function studies while the client is receiving drug therapy.

5. Note client complaints of abdominal pain or difficulty with bowel function. If the discomfort becomes severe, notify the physician and anticipate a reduction in the dosage of naltrexone.

Client/Family Teaching

1. Review the goals of therapy with the client and family.

2. Provide clients with printed information outlining the adverse side effects to be reported to the physician in the event that they occur.

3. Advise clients to inform health care providers that they are taking naltrexone.

4. Encourage clients to remain drug free. Provide clients with the names of health care agencies and support groups that may assist them in remaining drug free.

5. Advise clients to wear a medical identification tag or bracelet indicating that they are taking the drug naltrexone.

CHAPTER THIRTY-EIGHT

Nonnarcotic Analgesics and Antipyretics

General Statement: Drugs such as aspirin and acetaminophen are available without a prescription and are thus consumed in large quantities for the relief of pain and fever. However, if used improperly, their administration may cause serious side effects. Aspirin is responsible for accidental poisonings in small children.

In addition to their analgesic and antipyretic effects, many of the drugs of this group have specific anti-inflammatory effects and are the drugs of choice for rheumatic diseases. For these conditions the drugs are, however, prescribed at much higher dosage levels than for fever or simple analgesia.

The nonnarcotic analgesics include the salicylates, acetaminophen, nonsteroidal anti-inflammatory agents (see Chapter 39), and various miscellaneous drugs.

SALICYLATES

All general information for salicylates will be found under acetylsalicylic acid. Consult Table 12, p. 784, for information on salicylates other than acetylsalicylic acid, diflunisal, and mesalamine.

ACETYLSALICYLIC ACID   (ah-**SEE**-til-sah-lih-**SILL**-ik **AH**-sid)

Arthrinol✿, Artria S.R., A.S.A., A.S.A. Enseals, Astrin✿, Aspergum, Aspirin, Bayer Aspirin, Bayer Timed-Release Arthritic Pain Formula✿, Corphyen✿, Easprin, Ecotrin, Empirin, Entrophen✿, 8-Hour Bayer Timed-Release, Measurin, Norwich Aspirin, Novasen✿, Riphen✿, Sal-Adult✿, Sal-Infant✿, Supasa✿, Triaphen✿, ZORprin (OTC) (Easprin and ZORprin are Rx)

ACETYLSALICYLIC ACID, BUFFERED   (ah-**SEE**-til-sah-lih-**SILL**-ik **AH**-sid)

Alka-Seltzer Effervescent Pain Reliever and Antacid, APF Arthritis Pain Formula✿, Arthritis Pain Formula, Ascriptin, Ascriptin A/D, Buffaprin, Bufferin, Buffinol, Cama Arthritis Pain Formula, Magnaprin, Magnaprin Arthritis Strength, Maprin, Maprin I-B (OTC)

Classification: Nonnarcotic analgesic, antipyretic, anti-inflammatory agent.

Action/Kinetics: Aspirin manifests antipyretic, anti-inflammatory, and analgesic effects. The antipyretic effect is due to an action on the hypothalamus that results in heat loss by vasodilation of peripheral blood vessels and promoting sweating. The anti-inflammatory effects are probably mediated through inhibition of cyclo-oxygenase, which results in a decrease in prostaglandin synthesis and other mediators of the pain response. Prostaglandins have been implicated in the inflammatory process, as well as in mediation of pain. Thus, if levels are decreased, the inflammatory reaction may subside. The mechanism of action for the analgesic effects of aspirin is not known fully but is partly attributable to improvement of the inflammatory condition. Aspirin also produces inhibition of platelet aggregation by decreasing the synthesis of endoperoxides and thromboxanes—substances that mediate platelet aggregation.

Large doses of aspirin (5 g/day or more) increase uric acid secretion, while low doses (2 g/day or less) decrease uric acid secretion. However, aspirin antagonizes drugs used to treat gout.

Aspirin is rapidly absorbed after PO administration. Aspirin is hydrolyzed to the active salicylic acid, which is 70–90% protein bound. For arthritis and rheumatic disease, blood levels of 150–300 mcg/mL should be maintained. For analgesic and antipyretic, blood levels of 25–50 mcg/mL should be achieved. For acute rheumatic fever, blood levels of 150–300 mcg/mL should be achieved. **Therapeutic salicylic acid serum levels:** 150–300 mcg/mL, although tinnitus occurs at serum levels above 200 mcg/mL and serious toxicity above 400 mcg/mL. **t½:** aspirin, 15–20 min; salicylic acid, 2–20 hr, depending on the dose. Salicylic acid and metabolites are excreted by the kidney. The bioavailability of enteric-coated salicylate products may be poor.

Aspirin is found in many combination products including Darvon Compound, Empirin Compound Plain and with Codeine, Equagesic, Fiorinal Plain and with Codeine, Norgesic and Norgesic Forte, and Synalgos DC.

Uses: Pain arising from integumental structures, myalgias, neuralgias, arthralgias, headache, dysmenorrhea, and similar types of pain. Antipyretic. Anti-inflammatory agent in conditions such as arthritis, osteoarthritis, systemic lupus erythematosus, acute rheumatic fever, gout, and many other conditions. Aspirin is also used to reduce the risk of recurrent transient ischemic attacks and strokes in men. Decrease risk of death of nonfatal myocardial infarction in patients who have a history of infarction or who manifest unstable angina; aortocoronary bypass surgery. Gout. May be effective in less severe postoperative and postpartum pain; pain secondary to trauma and cancer. *Investigational:* Chronic use to prevent cataract formation; low doses to prevent toxemia of pregnancy; in pregnant women with inadequate uteroplacental blood flow.

Contraindications: Hypersensitivity to salicylates. Patients with asthma, hay fever, or nasal polyps have a higher incidence of hypersensitivity reactions. Severe anemia, history of blood coagulation defects, in conjunction with anticoagulant therapy. Salicylates can cause congestive failure when taken in the large doses used for rheumatic diseases. Vitamin K deficiency; one week before and after surgery. In pregnancy, especially the last trimester as the drug may cause problems in the

38

Table 12 Salicylates

Drug	Uses	Dosage	Remarks
Choline salicylate (Arthropan), OTC	Mild to moderate pain; anti-inflammatory for rheumatoid arthritis, osteoarthritis, rheumatic fever.	**Oral Solution. Adults and children over 12 years:** *Analgesic, antipyretic:* 435–669 mg q 3 hr; 435–870 mg q 4 hr; or, 870–1338 mg q 6 hr. Total daily dose should not exceed 5352 mg. **Pediatric, 11–12 yr:** 435–652.5 mg q 4 hr; **9–11 years:** 435–543.8 mg; **6–9 years:** 435 mg q 4 hr; **4–6 years:** 326.5 mg q 4 hr; **2–4 years:** 217.5 mg q 4 hr. *Antirheumatic:* **Adults,** 4.8–7.2 g. **Pediatric:** 107–133 mg/kg daily in divided doses.	Choline salicylate is marketed in liquid form, which contains 870 mg/5 ml. Has fewer GI side effects than aspirin. May be preferred to sodium salicylate when sodium restriction is necessary. Use should be avoided during pregnancy, especially the last trimester.
Choline and Magnesium salicylate (Trilisate) (Rx)	Analgesic; antipyretic, anti-inflammatory.	**Oral Solution, Tablets. Adults,** 0.5–1.5 g (of salicylate) b.i.d.–t.i.d.	Use should be avoided during pregnancy, especially the last trimester. Dose has not been established in children. Should be taken with food or a full glass of water. Does not have significant effects on platelet aggregation.
Magnesium salicylate (Doan's Pills, Magan, Mobidin) (Rx; Doan's Pills are OTC) Pregnancy category: C.	Mild to moderate pain; anti-inflammatory for rheumatoid arthritis, osteoarthritis, rheumatic fever.	**Tablets. Adults, initial:** 0.325–1.3 g t.i.d.–q.i.d. Dose may be increased if necessary. Dosage not established in children.	Contains no sodium and has a low incidence of GI distress. *Precautions:* 1. Use with caution in patients with renal impairment. 2. Use should be avoided during pregnancy, especially the last trimester. 3. May cause magnesium toxicity in persons with renal impairment.
Salicylamide (Uromide) OTC	Only used as an analgesic.	**Tablets. Adults** 667 mg t.i.d.–q.i.d. **Pediatric, less than 12 years:** Dose individualized by the physician.	Patients allergic to aspirin may be able to tolerate salicylamide. Is less effective than aspirin. Does not inhibit platelet aggregation.

Salsalate (Disalcid, Mono-Gesic, Salflex, Salgesic, Salsitab) (Rx) Pregnancy category: C.	Analgesic, anti-inflammatory, antipyretic, antirheumatic.	**Capsules. Adults, initial,** 1 g t.i.d.; **then,** adjust dose to patient response. **Tablets. Adults, initial,** 0.5–1 g b.i.d.–t.i.d.; **then,** adjust dose to patient response.	*Untoward reactions:* GI upset, dizziness, drowsiness. Administer after meals or with fluids to minimize gastric upset. Use should be avoided during pregnancy, especially the last trimester. Salsalate slowly releases two molecules of salicylic acid in the small intestine. The drug is not absorbed until it reaches the small intestine. Safety and efficacy have not been determined in children. Causes less GI upset than other salicylates.
Sodium salicylate (Uracel) OTC	Antipyretic, analgesic, antipyretic, antirheumatic.	**Tablets, Delayed release Tablets.** *Analgesic, antipyretic:* **Adults,** 325–650 mg q 4 hr as needed, not to exceed 4 g daily if used OTC. **Pediatric,** aged 6 years and older: 325 mg q 4 hr as needed, not to exceed 5 doses daily. *Antirheumatic:* **Adults and children** 80–100 mg/kg daily in divided doses. Up to 130 mg/kg may be required in some patients.	Use should be avoided during pregnancy, especially the last trimester. Does not affect platelet aggregation significantly. Less effective than aspirin as an analgesic or antipyretic. Patients allergic to aspirin may be able to tolerate sodium salicylate. Each g contains 6.25 mEq sodium. Contraindicated in patients with asthma (parenteral form). Use should be avoided during pregnancy, especially the last trimester. Does not significantly affect platelet aggregation.
Sodium thiosalicylate (Asproject, Rexolate, Tusal) (Rx)	Rheumatic fever, gout, analgesic for muscle pain.	**IM.** *Muscle pain:* 50–100 mg daily or on alternate days. *Acute gout:* 100 mg q 3–4 hr for 2 days; **then,** 100 mg daily. *Rheumatic fever:* 100–150 mg q 4–6 hr for 3 days; **then,** 100 mg b.i.d. until no symptoms are present.	Use should be avoided during pregnancy, especially the last trimester.

newborn child or complications during delivery. In children or teenagers with chicken pox or flu due to possibility of development of Reye's syndrome.

Controlled release aspirin is not recommended for use as an antipyretic or short-term analgesia as adequate blood levels may not be reached. Also, controlled release products are not recommended for children less than 12 years of age and in children with fever accompanied by dehydration.

Special Concerns: Pregnancy category: C. Use with caution during lactation. Salicylates are to be used with caution in the presence of gastric or peptic ulcers, in mild diabetes, erosive gastritis or bleeding tendencies, and in patients with cardiac disease. Use with caution in liver or kidney disease.

Side Effects: The toxic effects of the salicylates are dose-related. *GI:* Dyspepsia, heartburn, anorexia, nausea, occult blood loss, epigastric discomfort, massive GI bleeding, potentiation of peptic ulcer. *Allergic:* Bronchospasm, asthma-like symptoms, anaphylaxis, skin rashes, angioedema, urticaria, rhinitis, nasal polyps. *Hematologic:* Prolongation of bleeding time, thrombocytopenia, leukopenia, purpura, shortened erythrocyte survival time, decreased plasma iron levels. *Miscellaneous:* Thirst, fever, dimness of vision.

Note: Use of aspirin in children and teenagers with flu or chicken pox may result in the development of Reye's syndrome. Also, dehydrated, febrile children are more prone to salicylate intoxication.

Salicylism—mild toxicity. Seen at serum levels between 150–200 mcg/mL. *GI:* Nausea, vomiting, diarrhea, thirst. *CNS:* Tinnitus (most common), dizziness, difficulty in hearing, mental confusion, lassitude. *Miscellaneous:* Flushing, sweating, tachycardia. Symptoms of salicylism may be observed with doses used for inflammatory disease or rheumatic fever.

Severe salicylate poisoning. Seen at serum levels over 400 mcg/mL. *CNS:* Excitement, confusion, disorientation, irritability, hallucinations, lethargy, stupor, coma, respiratory failure, seizures. *Metabolic:* Respiratory alkalosis (initially), respiratory acidosis and metabolic acidosis, dehydration. *GI:* Nausea, vomiting. *Hematologic:* Platelet dysfunction, hypoprothrombinemia, increased capillary fragility. *Miscellaneous:* Hyperthermia, hyperventilation, hemorrhage, pulmonary edema, cardiovascular collapse, renal failure, tetany, hypoglycemia (late).

For treatment, see *Nursing Considerations,* on p. 790.

Drug Interactions	
Acetazolamide	↑ CNS toxicity of salicylates; also, ↑ excretion of salicylic acid if urine kept alkaline
Alcohol, ethyl	↑ Chance of GI bleeding caused by salicylates
Alteplase, recombinant	↑ Risk of bleeding
Aminosalicylic acid (PAS)	Possible ↑ effect of PAS due to ↓ excretion by kidney or ↓ plasma protein binding
Ammonium chloride	↑ Effect of salicylates by ↑ renal tubular reabsorption
Angiotensin converting enzyme (ACE) inhibitors	↓ Effect of ACE inhibitors possibly due to prostaglandin inhibition
Antacids	↓ Salicylate levels in plasma due to ↑ rate of renal excretion
Anticoagulants, oral	↑ Effect of anticoagulant by ↓ plasma protein binding and plasma prothrombin
Antirheumatics	Both are ulcerogenic and may cause ↑ GI bleeding
Ascorbic acid	↑ Effect of salicylates by ↑ renal tubular reabsorption

Drug Interactions

Beta-Adrenergic Blocking Agents	Salicylates ↓ action of beta-blockers, possibly due to prostaglandin inhibition
Charcoal, activated	↓ Absorption of salicylates from GI tract
Corticosteroids	Both are ulcerogenic; also, corticosteroids may ↓ blood salicylate levels by ↑ breakdown by liver and ↑ excretion
Dipyridamole	Additive anticoagulant effects
Furosemide	↑ Chance of salicylate toxicity due to ↓ renal excretion; also, salicylates may ↓ effect of furosemide in patients with impaired renal function or cirrhosis with ascites
Heparin	Inhibition of platelet adhesiveness by aspirin may result in bleeding tendencies
Hypoglycemics, oral	↑ Hypoglycemia due to ↓ plasma protein binding and ↓ excretion
Indomethacin	Both are ulcerogenic and may cause ↑ GI bleeding
Insulin	Salicyaltes ↑ hypoglycemic effect of insulin
Methionine	↑ Effect of salicylates by ↑ renal tubular reabsorption
Methotrexate	↑ Effect of methotrexate by ↓ plasma protein binding; also, salicylates block renal excretion of methotrexate
Nitroglycerin	Combination may result in unexpected hypotension
Nizatidine	↑ Serum levels of salicylates
Nonsteroidal anti-inflammatory drugs	Additive ulcerogenic effects; also, aspirin may ↓ serum levels of NSAIDs
Phenylbutazone	Combination may produce hyperuricemia
Phenytoin	↑ Effect of phenytoin by ↓ plasma protein binding
Probenecid	Salicylates inhibit uricosuric activity of probenecid
Sodium bicarbonate	↓ Effect of salicylates by ↑ rate of excretion
Spironolactone	Aspirin ↓ diuretic effect of spironolactone
Sulfinpyrazone	Salicylates inhibit uricosuric activity of sulfinpyrazone
Sulfonamides	↑ Effect of sulfonamides by ↑ blood levels of salicylates
Valproic acid	↑ Effect of valproic acid due to ↓ plasma protein binding

Laboratory Test Interferences: False + or ↑ : Amylase, SGOT, SGPT, uric acid, PBI, urinary VMA (most tests), catecholamines, urinary glucose (Benedict's, Clinitest), and urinary uric acid (at high doses) values. False − or ↓ : CO_2 content, glucose (fasting), potassium, urinary VMA (Pisano method) and thrombocyte values.

Dosage: Capsules, Tablets, Chewable Tablets, Chewing Gum, Tablets, Delayed-Release Tablets, Extended-Release Tablets. Adults: *Analgesic/antipyretic,* 325–500 mg q 3 hr, 325–600 mg q 4 hr, or 650–1,000 mg q 6 hr. *Arthritis/rheumatic diseases:* 3.6–5.4 g/day in divided doses. *Juvenile rheumatoid arthritis:* 80–100 mg/kg/day (alternate dose: 3 g/m^2) in divided doses q 4–6 hr.

Pediatric: *Analgesic, antipyretic:* 65 mg/kg/day (alternate dose: 1.5 g/m^2/day) in divided doses q 4–6 hr, not to exc ·ed 3.6 g/day. Alternatively, the following dosage regimen can be used: **Pediatric, 2–4 years:** 160 mg q 4 hr as needed; **4–6 years:** 240 mg q 4 hr as needed; **6–9 years:** 320–325 mg q 4 hr as needed; **9–11 years:** 320–400 mg q 4 hr as needed; **11–12 years:** 320–480 mg q 4 hr as needed.

Acute rheumatic fever: **adults, initial,** 5–8 g daily. **Pediatric, initial,** 100 mg/kg/day (3 g/m^2/day); **then,** decrease to 75 mg/kg daily for 4–6 weeks. *Inhibitor of platetlet aggregation:* 325 mg daily with the following exceptions: *Recurrent cerebral thromboembolism:* 1 g daily. *Transient ischemic attacks associated with mitral valve prolapse:* 325–1,000 mg daily. *Prophylaxis of thrombosis or occlusion of coronary bypass graft:* 325 mg 7 hr postoperative via a nasogastric tube; **then,** 325 mg t.i.d. with 75 mg daily of dipyridamole.

Note: Doses as low as 80–100 mg daily are being studied for use in unstable angina, myocardial infarction, and aortocoronary bypass surgery.

Suppositories. *Analgesic/antipyretic:* **Adults:** 325–650 mg q 4 hr as needed. **Pediatric:** See above. *Antirheumatic:* **Adults:** 3.6–5.4 g/day in divided doses. **Pediatric:** 80–100 mg/kg daily in divided doses.

NURSING CONSIDERATIONS

Administration/Storage

1. To reduce gastric irritation, administer with meals, milk or crackers.
2. If ordered by the physician, sodium bicarbonate may be given concurrently to lessen gastric irritation.
3. Enteric-coated tablets or buffered tablets are better tolerated by some clients.
4. Aspirin should be taken with a full glass of water to prevent lodging of the drug in the esophagus.
5. Individuals allergic to tartrazine should not take aspirin.
6. Have epinephrine available to counteract hypersensitivity reactions should they occur. Asthma caused by hypersensitive reaction to salicylates may be refractory to epinephrine, so antihistamines should also be available for parenteral and oral use.

Assessment

1. Take a complete drug history and note any evidence of hypersensitivity. Clients who have tolerated salicylates well for a long period of time may suddenly have an allergic or anaphylactoid reaction.
2. If aspirin is being administered for pain, determine the type of pain, the pattern of pain, if the pain is unusual, or if it is a recurring pain. Use a pain rating scale to assess the level of pain. Note the effectiveness of aspirin if used in the past for pain control.
3. Determine the precipitating factors related to the problem.
4. Note if the client has asthma, hay fever or nasal polyps.
5. If the client is a child, determine if it is possible for child to have chicken pox or the flu.
6. Note any client history of peptic ulcers or other conditions that could suggest potential problems with the use of salicylates.
7. Determine if the client is to have diagnostic tests. Many of these can be affected by the use of salicylates.

8. Determine if the client has a history of any bleeding tendencies.
9. Review the drugs the client is currently taking to determine the possibility of any drug interactions.

Interventions

1. If the client is in a hospital, administer salicylates only on an order from the physician and at the time scheduled.
2. Minimize the client's distress by assisting the client to preserve energy.
3. Provide a comforting, relaxing environment for the client.
4. When administering salicylates for antipyretic effect, assure that the physician has indicated the temperature at which the drug should be administered.
   * Monitor the client's temperature at least one hour after administering the medication.
   * Check the client for marked diaphoresis.
   * If there is marked diaphoresis, dry the client, change the linens, provide fluids, and prevent chilling.
5. Note if the client has blood in the stool or urine. Document and report to the physician.
6. Observe client receiving anticoagulant therapy for bruises, or bleeding of the mucous membranes. Large doses of salicylates may increase the prothrombin time.
7. Assess for gastric irritation and pain.

Client/Family Teaching

1. Do not take salicylates if they are off color or have a strange odor.
2. Explain that if sodium bicarbonate is to be used it should be taken only with the consent of the physician. Sodium bicarbonate may decrease the serum level of aspirin more rapidly than normal, thus reducing the effectiveness of the aspirin.
3. Discuss the toxic symptoms to be reported: ringing in the ears, difficulty hearing, dizziness or fainting spells, unusual increase in sweating, severe abdominal pain or mental confusion. The client should be instructed to call the physician if any of these symptoms occur.
4. If the client has diabetes mellitus, discuss the possibility of hypoglycemia occurring because salicylates potentiate the effects of the antidiabetic drugs. Clients should monitor their blood glucose levels carefully and contact the physician for possible adjustment in drug dosage should hypoglycemia occur.
5. In cardiac clients on large doses of drug, advise that they should be alert to symptoms of CHF and to report to the physician.
6. Remind clients to tell their dentist and other health providers that they are taking salicylates and the reasons for this therapy.
7. Before purchasing other OTC preparations, tell the physician, pharmacist or nurse that you are taking salicylates and the quantity used per day.
8. Salicylates should be administered to children only upon the recommendation of their physician.
9. If a child refuses to take the medication or vomits it, discuss with the physician the possibility of using aspirin suppositories or acetaminophen.
10. If a client is to undergo surgery consult the physician about whether to continue to take salicylates. Aspirin and other such drugs are usually discontinued a week before surgery to prevent the possibility of postoperative bleeding.
11. Warn clients to avoid indiscriminate use of salicylate drugs.

12. Parents should be advised not to give aspirin routinely to children under 12 years of age without first consulting the physician.

13. Children who are dehydrated and who have a fever are especially susceptible to aspirin intoxication from even small amounts of aspirin.

14. Report to the physician any gastric irritation and pain experienced by the child. These may be symptoms of hypersensitivity or toxicity.

Evaluation

1. Client will indicate that the drug has eliminated the discomfort.
2. Be alert to signs of infection where a fever may be masked by salicylates.
3. Observe for freedom from complications of drug therapy.

Interventions For Salicylate Toxicity:

1. If the client has had repeated administration of large doses of salicylates, note evidence of hyperventilation or client complaints of auditory or visual disturbances (symptoms of salicylism). Report these to the physician and record on the client's chart.

2. Severe salicylate poisoning, whether due to overdose or accumulation, will have an exaggerated effect on the CNS and the metabolic system.
   - Clients may develop a salicylate jag characterized by garrulous behavior. They may act as if they were inebriated.
   - Convulsions and coma may follow.

3. When working with febrile children or the elderly who have been treated with aspirin, maintain adequate fluid intake. These two categories of clients are more susceptible to salicylate intoxication if they are dehydrated.

4. Have the following emergency supplies available for treatment of acute salicylate toxicity
   - Apomorphine.
   - Emetics and equipment for gastric lavage.
   - IV equipment and solutions of dextrose, saline, potassium, and sodium bicarbonate; vitamin K.
   - Oxygen and a ventilator.
   - Short-acting barbiturates such as pentobarbital or secobarbital to treat convulsions.

DIFLUNISAL   (dye-FLEW-nih-sal)
Dolobid (Rx)

Classification: Nonsteroidal analgesic, anti-inflammatory, antipyretic.

Action/Kinetics: Diflunisal is a salicylic acid derivative although it is not metabolized to salicylic acid. Its mechanism is not known, although it is thought to be an inhibitor of prostaglandin synthetase. **Onset:** 1 hr. **Peak plasma levels:** 2–3 hr. **Peak effect:** 2–3 hr. **t½:** 8–12 hr. Ninety-nine percent protein bound. Metabolites excreted in urine.

Uses: Analgesic, rheumatoid arthritis, osteoarthritis, ankylosing spondylitis, psoriatic arthritis, musculoskeletal pain. Prophylaxis and treatment of vascular headaches.

Contraindications: Hypersensitivity to diflunisal, aspirin, or other anti-inflammatory drugs. Acute asthmatic attacks, urticaria, or rhinitis precipitated by aspirin. During lactation and in children less than 12 years of age.

Special Concerns: Pregnancy category: C. Use with caution in presence of ulcers or in patients with a history thereof; in patients with hypertension, compromised cardiac function, or in conditions leading to fluid retention. Use with caution in only first two trimesters of pregnancy. Geriatric patients may be at greater risk of GI toxicity.

Side Effects: *GI:* Nausea, dyspepsia, GI pain and bleeding, diarrhea, vomiting, constipation, flatulence, peptic ulcer, eructation, anorexia. *CNS:* Headache, fatigue, fever, malaise, dizziness, somnolence, insomnia, nervousness, vertigo, depression, paresthesias. *Dermatologic:* Rashes, pruritus, sweating, Stevens-Johnson syndrome, dry mucous membranes, erythema multiforme. *CV:* Palpitations, syncope, edema. *Other:* Tinnitus, asthenia, chest pain, hypersensitivity reactions, anaphylaxis, dyspnea, dysuria, muscle cramps, thrombocytopenia.

Drug Interactions	
Acetaminophen	↑ Plasma levels of acetaminophen
Antacids	↓ Plasma levels of diflunisal
Anticoagulants	↑ Prothrombin time
Furosemide	↓ Hyperuricemic effect of furosemide
Hydrochlorothiazide	↑ Plasma levels and ↓ hyperuricemic effect of hydrochlorothiazide
Indomethacin	↓ Renal clearance of indomethacin → ↑ plasma levels
Naproxen	↓ Urinary excretion of naproxen and metabolite

Dosage: Tablets. *Mild to moderate pain:* **initial,** 1,000 mg; **then,** 250–500 mg q 8–12 hr. *Rheumatoid arthritis, osteoarthritis:* 250–500 mg b.i.d. Doses in excess of 1,500 mg/day are not recommended. For some patients, an initial dose of 500 mg followed by 250 mg q 8–12 hr may be effective. Dosage should be reduced in patients with impaired renal function.

NURSING CONSIDERATIONS

Administration/Storage

1. When given for analgesic or antipyretic effect, expect the onset of action to occur within 20 min and to last for 4–6 hr.
2. If administering the drug to counteract the pain and swelling of arthritis, expect maximum relief to occur in 2–3 weeks.
3. Diflunisal may be given with water, milk, or meals to reduce gastric irritation.
4. Do not give acetaminophen or aspirin with diflunisal.
5. Tablets should not be crushed or chewed.
6. Serum salicylate levels are not used as a guide to dosage or toxicity as the drug is not hydrolyzed to salicylic acid.

Assessment

1. Note any client history of hypersensitivity to salicylates or other anti-inflammatory drugs.
2. Review the client's history, noting whether or not the client has had peptic ulcers, hypertension, or any evidence of compromised cardiac function.
3. If the client is female, of childbearing age and sexually active question her concerning the possibility of pregnancy. The drug should be avoided or used with extreme caution during the first two trimesters of pregnancy.

4. If the client is on anticoagulant therapy, have prothrombin and coagulation times checked prior to administering drug.

Interventions

1. Assess clients for increased tendencies of bleeding when receiving high doses of diflunisal. This drug may inhibit platelet aggregation.
2. If the client is on oral anticoagulant therapy, observe for any increase in bleeding tendencies. The prothrombin time may be increased due to drug interactions.
3. If the client is elderly, note complaints of diarrhea. This can cause an electrolyte imbalance and should be corrected. Document and report to the physician.

Client/Family Teaching

1. Antacids may lower plasma levels of diflunisal, reducing the effectiveness of the drug. Therefore, consult the physician before using an antacid to prevent gastric irritation.
2. To minimize gastric irritation, take the medication with meals, milk or a snack. If these measures do not work, consult the physician concerning the use of an antacid.
3. Taking the medication on a regular basis is necessary to sustain the anti-inflammatory effect of the drug. Therefore, compliance with the prescribed regimen is of utmost importance.
4. The medication needs to be adjusted according to the client's age, condition and changes in disease activity. Urge the client to report for medical follow-up and supervision on a regular basis.
5. The medication may cause dizziness or drowsiness. Caution client to use care when operating machinery or driving a car.
6. Advise parents to avoid aspirin or salicylates when treating children with a fever, children infected with varicella or children who have influenza-like symptoms. Stress the importance of consulting with the child's physician before administering any OTC or unprescribed drugs.

MESALAMINE (5-AMINOSALICYLIC ACID)

(mes-**AL**-a-mine, ah-mee-noh-sal-ih-**SILL**-ick)

Rowasa, Salofalk✻ (Rx)

Classification: Anti-inflammatory agent.

Action/Kinetics: Chemically, mesalamine is related to acetylsalicylic acid. Mesalamine is believed to act locally in the colon to inhibit prostaglandin synthesis, thereby reducing inflammation of colitis. Mesalamine is administered rectally; thus, it is excreted mainly in the feces. However, between 10%–30% is absorbed and is excreted through the urine as the N-acetyl-5-aminosalicylic acid metabolite. **t½, mesalamine:** 0.5–1.5 hr; **t½, n-acetyl mesalamine:** 5–10 hr.

Uses: Mild to moderate distal ulcerative colitis, proctitis, or proctosigmoiditis.

Contraindications: Lactation.

Special Concerns: Use during pregnancy (pregnancy category: B) only if benefits outweigh risks. Use with caution in patients with sulfasalazine sensitivity. Safety and efficacy have not been established in children.

Side Effects: *Sulfite sensitivity:* Hives, wheezing, itching, anaphylaxis. *Intolerance syndrome:* Acute abdominal pain, cramping, bloody diarrhea, rash, fever, headache. *GI:* Abdominal pain or discomfort, flatulence, cramps, nausea, diarrhea, hemorrhoids, rectal pain or burning, constipation. *CNS:* Headache, dizziness, insomnia, fatigue, malaise. *Miscellaneous:* Asthenia, flu-like symptoms, fever, rash, sore throat, leg or joint pain, back pain, itching, hair loss, peripheral edema, urinary burning.

Dosage: Rectal, suspension enema: 4 g in 60 mL once daily for 3–6 weeks, usually given at bedtime. For maintenance, the drug can be given on every other day or every third day at doses of 1–2 g.

NURSING CONSIDERATIONS

Administration/Storage

1. Shake the bottle well to ensure that the suspension is homogeneous.
2. Have the client lie on their left side with the lower leg extended and the upper right leg flexed forward. The knee-chest position may also be used.
3. Insert the applicator tip and squeeze the bottle steadily to allow the bottle to empty.
4. The client should retain the enema for approximately 8 hr.

Assessment

1. Prior to initiating therapy, determine if the client has a history of sulfite sensitivity.
2. Obtain baseline renal function studies.

Client/Family Teaching

1. Demonstrate the proper technique for administering the suspension enema. Have the client/family do a return demonstration to ensure that they understand the procedure.
    - Explain that prior to use, the bottle should be shaken until all contents are thoroughly mixed.
    - Review the appropriate positions that facilitate administering enemas.
    - Describe how to protect the bed linens.
2. To ensure the proper absorption of the drug it must be retained for 8 hours. This may best be accomplished by administering the enema at bedtime and retaining throughout the sleep cycle.
3. The therapy may last 3–6 weeks. Therefore, it is important to continue taking the medication therapy as prescribed.
4. If any severe abdominal pain, cramping, bloody diarrhea, rash, fever or headache occurs, discontinue the drug and report to the physician.

ACETAMINOPHEN

ACETAMINOPHEN (APAP, PARACETAMOL) (ah-see-toe-**MIN**-oh-fen)

Capsules: Anacin-3✴, Anacin-3 Extra Strength✴, Panadol, Apacet Extra Strength, Meda Cap, Ty-Tab. Granules: Snaplets-FR Granules. Oral Solution/Elixir: Aceta, Actamin, Actamin Extra, Alba-Temp 300, Apacet Oral Solution, Atasol✴, Children's Anacin-3 Elixir, Children's Genapap Elixir, Children's Panadol, Children's Tylenol Elixir, Dolanex, Dorcal Children's Fever and Pain Reducer, Genapap, Halenol Elixir, Infants' Anacin-3, Infants' Genapap, Infants' Tylenol, Liquiprin Children's Elixir, Myapap, Myapap Elixir, Oraphen-PD, Panadol, Pedric, Robigesic✴, St. Joseph Aspirin-Free Fever Reducer for Children, Tempra, Tenol, Tylenol✴, Tylenol Extra Strength, Valdol Liquid. Oral Suspension: Liquiprin Infants' Drops. Tablets: Aceta, Actamin, Actamin Extra, Aminofen, Aminofen Max, Anacin-3, Anacin-3 Extra Strength, Anacin-3 Maximum Strength Caplets, Apacet, Apacet Extra Strength, Apacet Extra Strength Caplets, Apo-Acetaminophen✴, Atasol✴, Atasol Caplets✴, Atasol Forte✴, Atasol Forte Caplets✴, Banesin,

Campain✿, Conacetol, Dapa, Datril Extra-Strength, Datril Extra-Strength Caplets, Exdol✿, Exdol Strong✿, Genapap, Genapap Extra Strength, Genapap Extra Strength Caplets, Genebs, Genebs Extra Strength, Genebs Extra Strength Caplets, Halenol, Halenol Extra Strength, Halenol Extra Strength Caplets, Meda Tab, Panadol, Panadol Caplets, Panadol Junior Strength Caplets, Panex, Panex-500, Phenaphen Caplets, Robigesic✿, Rounox✿, Tapanol, Tapanol Extra Strength, Tapanol Extra Strength Caplets, Tapar, Tenol, Tylenol, Tylenol Caplets, Tylenol Extra Strength, Tylenol Extra Strength Caplets, Tylenol Extra Strength Gelcaps, Tylenol Junior Strength Caplets, Ty-Tab, Ty-Tab Caplets, Ty-Tab Extra Strength, Valadol, Valorin, Valorin Extra. Tablets, Chewable: Children's Anacin-3, Children's Genapap, Children's Panadol, Children's Tylenol, Children's Ty-Tab, Panadol✿, St. Joseph Aspirin-Free Fever Reducer for Children, Tempra, Tempra Double Strength. Suppositories: Acephen, Children's Feverall, Junior Strength Feverall, Neopap, Suppap-120, Suppap-325, Suppap-650. Wafers: Pedric. (OTC)

ACETAMINOPHEN, BUFFERED   (ah-see-toe-**MIN**-oh-fen)

Bromo Seltzer (OTC)

Classification: Nonnarcotic analgesic, para-aminophenol type.

Action/Kinetics: The only para-aminophenol derivative currently used is acetaminophen. It decreases fever by an effect on the hypothalamus leading to sweating and vasodilation. Acetaminophen also inhibits the effect of pyrogens on the hypothalamic heat-regulating centers. It may cause analgesia by inhibiting CNS prostaglandin synthesis; however, due to minimal effects on peripheral prostaglandin synthesis, acetaminophen has no anti-inflammatory or uricosuric effects. It does not manifest any anticoagulant effect and does not produce ulceration of the GI tract. The magnitude of its antipyretic and analgesic effects is comparable to that of aspirin.

Peak plasma levels: 30–120 min. **t½:** 45 min–3 hr. **Therapeutic serum levels** (analgesia): 5–20 mcg/mL. **Plasma protein binding:** Approximately 25%. Acetaminophen is metabolized in the liver and is excreted in the urine as glucuronide and sulfate conjugates. However, an intermediate hydroxylated metabolite is hepatotoxic following large doses of acetaminophen.

Acetaminophen is often combined with other drugs, as in Darvocet-N, Parafon Forte, Phenaphen with Codeine, and Tylenol with Codeine.

The buffered product is a mixture of acetaminophen, sodium bicarbonate, and citric acid that effervesces when placed in water. This product has a high sodium content (0.76 g per ¾ capful).

Uses: Control of pain due to headache, dysmenorrhea, arthralgia, myalgia, musculoskeletal pain, immunizations, teething, tonsillectomy. To reduce fever in bacterial or viral infections. As a substitute for aspirin in upper GI disease, aspirin allergy, bleeding disorders, patients on anticoagulant therapy, and gouty arthritis. *Investigational:* In children receiving DPT vaccination to decrease incidence of fever and pain at injection site.

Contraindications: Renal insufficiency, anemia. Patients with cardiac or pulmonary disease are more susceptible to toxic effects of acetaminophen.

Special Concerns: Evidence indicates that acetaminophen may have to be used with caution in pregnancy.

Side Effects: Few when taken in usual therapeutic doses. Chronic and even acute toxicity can develop after long symptom-free usage. *Hematologic:* Methemoglobinemia, hemolytic anemia, neutropenia, thrombocytopenia, pancytopenia, leukopenia. *Allergic:* Skin rashes, fever. *Miscellaneous:* CNS stimulation, hypoglycemia, jaundice, drowsiness, glossitis.

Symptoms of Overdosage

There may be few initial symptoms. *Hepatic toxicity. CNS:* CNS stimulation, general malaise, delirium followed by depression, seizures, coma, death. *GI:* Nausea, vomiting, diarrhea, gastric upset. *Miscellaneous:* Sweating, chills, fever, vascular collapse.

Treatment of Overdosage

Initially, induction of emesis, gastric lavage, activated charcoal. Oral *N*-acetylcysteine is said to reduce or prevent hepatic damage by inactivating acetaminophen metabolites, which cause liver effects.

Drug Interactions	
Alcohol, ethyl	Chronic use of alcohol ↑ toxicity of larger therapeutic doses of acetaminophen
Anticoagulants, oral	Acetaminophen may ↑ hypoprothrombinemic effect
Barbiturates	↑ Potential of hepatotoxicity due to ↑ breakdown of acetaminophen by liver
Carbamazepine	↓ Potential of hepatotoxicity due to ↑ breakdown of acetaminophen by liver
Diflunisal	↑ Plasma levels of acetaminophen
Caffeine	↑ Analgesic effect of acetaminophen
Chloramphenicol	Acetaminophen ↑ serum chloramphenical levels
Hydantoins	↑ Potential of hepatotoxicity due to ↑ breakdown of acetaminophen by liver
Oral contraceptives	↑ Breakdown of acetaminophen by liver
Phenobarbital	↑ Potential of hepatotoxicity due to ↑ breakdown of acetaminophen by liver
Phenytoin	↑ Potential of hepatotoxicity due to ↑ breakdown of acetaminophen by liver
Sulfinpyrazone	↑ Potential of hepatotoxicity due to ↑ breakdown of acetaminophen by liver

Dosage: Capsules, Granules, Elixir, Oral Solution, Oral Suspension, Tablets, Suppositories, Wafers. Adults, 325–650 mg q 4 hr; doses up to 1 g q.i.d. may be used. Daily dosage should not exceed 4 g. **Pediatric:** Doses given 4–5 times/day. **Up to 3 months:** 40 mg/dose; **4–12 months:** 80 mg/dose; **1–2 years:** 120 mg/dose; **2–3 years:** 160 mg/dose; **4–5 years:** 240 mg/dose; **6–8 years:** 320 mg/dose; **9–10 years:** 400 mg/dose; **11–12 years:** 480 mg/dose. *Alternative pediatric dose:* 10 mg/kg/dose.

Suppositories. Adults, 650 mg q 4–6, hr not to exceed 6 suppositories per day. **Pediatric, less than 3 years:** physician should be consulted; **3–6 years:** 120 mg q 4–6 hr, not to exceed 2.6 g/day; **6–12 years:** 325 mg q 4–6 hr not to exceed 720 mg/day.

Buffered. **Adult, usual:** 1 or 2 three-quarter capfuls are placed into an empty glass; add half a glass of cool water. May be taken while fizzing or after settling. Can be repeated every 4 hr as required or directed by physician.

NURSING CONSIDERATIONS

Administration/Storage

Suppositories should be stored below 80°F (27°C).

Assessment

If the client is to receive long-term therapy, liver function studies should be conducted prior to initiating drug therapy.

Interventions

1. Note the presence of bluish color of the mucosa and fingernails, or client complaints of

dyspnea, weakness, headache or vertigo. These symptoms of methemoglobinemia are caused by anoxia and require immediate attention.

2. Observe for pallor, weakness, and complaints of heart palpitations. Document and report as these symptoms may signal the presence of hemolytic anemia.

3. To assess for evidence of nephritis, check the client's urine for occult blood and the presence of albumin on a routine basis, especially when client is receiving long-term drug therapy.

4. Clients complaining of dyspnea, rapid weak pulse, cold extremities, clammy sweat, or subnormal temperatures, are displaying symptoms of chronic poisoning and may collapse with confusion. All complaints and symptoms observed during drug therapy should be immediately reported to the physician.

5. CNS stimulation, excitement, and delirium are symptoms of toxicity. Have Mucomyst (see *Acetylcysteine,* p. 1000) available for treatment of overdosage.

Client/Family Teaching

1. Teach the client and family symptoms of acute toxicity such as nausea, vomiting and abdominal pain. Instruct them to notify the physician immediately.

2. Provide clients and families with printed information to familiarize them with the signs and symptoms of severe poisoning. Instruct them to report all such signs and symptoms.

3. Review with the client signs that may indicate possible chronic overdose of medication, such as unexplained bleeding, bruising, sore throat, malaise and fever.

4. Phenacetin, the major active metabolite of acetaminophen, may cause the urine to become dark brown or wine in color.

5. Teach clients to read the labels on all OTC preparations that they take. Many contain acetaminophen and, as a result, can produce toxic reactions if taken over a period of time with the prescribed drug.

6. Explain that so-called headache and minor pain relievers containing combinations of salicylates, acetaminophen, and caffeine may be no more beneficial than aspirin alone and that such combinations may be more dangerous. When in doubt consult pharmacist or physician.

7. Any pain or fever that persists for 3–5 days requires medical attention.

MISCELLANEOUS AGENT

METHOTRIMEPRAZINE   (meth-oh-try-**MEP**-rah-zeen)

Levoprome, Nozinan ✤ (Rx)

Classification: Analgesic, nonnarcotic, miscellaneous.

Action/Kinetics: Methotrimeprazine is a phenothiazine derivative with many pharmacologic effects, including sedation, analgesic, amnesic, antipruritic, local anesthetic, and anticholinergic effects. The effects on the CNS are thought to be due to depression of subcortical areas of the brain including the thalamus, limbic and reticular systems, and the hypothalamus all of which result in a decrease in sensory impulses, reduction of locomotor activity and subsequent sedation, and an antiemetic effect. **Peak effect:** 20–40 min after IM use. **Peak plasma levels:** 30–90 min. **Duration:** about 4 hr. **Therapeutic blood level:** 1 mg/mL. **t½:** 15–30 hr. The drug is metabolized in the liver and the metabolites (which possess minimal pharmacologic activity) are excreted in the urine and feces.

Uses: Analgesic in nonambulatory patients. Obstetric analgesia where respiratory depression is to be avoided. As preanesthetic for producing sedation and relief of anxiety and tension. Adjunct to general anesthesia to increase effects of anesthetics. Psychoses.

Contraindications: Administration with antihypertensive drugs. Overdose of CNS depressants; during coma; severe myocardial, renal, or hepatic disease; hypotension; children less than 12 years of age.

Special Concerns: Use with caution in geriatric or debilitated patients with heart disease. Use with caution during pregnancy. Children may be more prone to dystonias, especially those with chicken pox, CNS illnesses, measles, gastroenteritis, or dehydration. Geriatric patients are at greater risk to develop anticholinergic effects, sedation, and orthostatic hypotension.

Side Effects: *CV:* Orthostatic hypotension accompanied by fainting or weakness. *CNS:* Dizziness, speech problems, excess sedation, disorientation. *GI:* Nausea, vomiting, dry mouth, abdominal discomfort. *Miscellaneous:* Urinary difficulties, allergic symptoms, jaundice, agranulocytosis, chills, nasal congestion, pain at injection site.

Drug Interactions	
Alcohol, ethyl	Potentiation or addition of CNS depressant effects; concomitant use may lead to drowsiness, lethargy, stupor, respiratory depression, coma, and possibly death
Anticholinergic agents	Tachycardia, hypotension, and possibility of extrapyramidal symptoms with concomitant use
Antihypertensives	Additive hypotensive effect
(CNS depressants Antianxiety agents, barbiturates, narcotics, phenothiazines, sedative-hypnotics)	See *Alcohol, ethyl*
Guanethidine	Additive hypotensive effect
Methyldopa	Additive hypotensive effect
Phenothiazines	See *Alcohol, ethyl;* also, additive extrapyramidal effects
Reserpine	Additive hypotensive effect
Skeletal muscle relaxants, surgical	↑ Muscle relaxation

Dosage: Oral Solution, Syrup, Tablets. *Pain, psychoses:* **Adults, initial:** 6–25 mg daily in three divided doses with meals for moderate pain or psychoses to 50–75 mg daily in 2–3 divided doses with meals for severe pain or psychoses. The patients should be confined to bed for the first few days if doses of 100–200 mg daily are needed. *Presurgical sedation:* 6–25 mg daily in three divided doses with meals. **Pediatric:** *all uses,* 0.25 mg/kg daily in 2–3 divided doses with meals, not to exceed 40 mg daily in children less than 12 years of age.

IM. Adults: 10–20 mg q 4–6 hr as needed for analgesia (range: 5–40 mg at intervals of 1–24 hr). Dose should be reduced in geriatric patients: **initial,** 5–10 mg; **then,** increase gradually, if necessary. *Obstetric analgesia:* **initial,** 15–20 mg; may be repeated if necessary. *Preanesthetic medication:* 2–20 mg given 45 min to 3 hr before surgery. *Postoperative analgesia:* **initial,** 2.5–7.5 mg (due to residual effects of anesthetic); **then,** give additional dosage, as required, q 4–6 hr. **Do not administer SC or IV.**

NURSING CONSIDERATIONS

Administration/Storage

1. Administer by deep IM injection into a large muscle mass. Rotation of sites is advisable.
2. Do not administer SC, as irritation may occur.
3. Should only be mixed with either atropine or scopolamine in the same syringe.

Assessment

1. Note client drug history and determine if the client is taking any antihypertensive medications. The drug is contraindicated in such instances.
2. Review and list all drugs the client is currently taking. Compare with those with which methotrimeprazine interacts.

Interventions

1. Avoid ambulation for at least 6 hours following the initial dose of drug. Clients may develop orthostatic hypotension, fainting, and dizziness.
2. Note signs of tolerance that may occur with repeated administration of medication.

COMMONLY USED COMBINATION DRUGS

DARVOCET-N 50 AND DARVOCET-N 100   (DAR-voh-set)
(Rx)

See also *Acetaminophen,* p. 793, and *Propoxyphene,* p. 773.

Classification/Content: *Nonnarcotic analgesic:* Acetaminophen, 325 or 650 mg. *Analgesic:* Propoxyphene napsylate, 50 or 100 mg.

Uses: Mild to moderate pain.

Special Concerns: Use during pregnancy only if benefits outweigh risks.

Dosage: Tablets. Two Darvocet-N 50 tablets or one Darvocet-N 100 tablet q 4 hr. Maximum daily dose of propoxyphene napsylate should not exceed 600 mg. Total daily dose should be reduced in patients with impaired hepatic or renal function.

NURSING CONSIDERATIONS
See *Nursing Considerations* for *Acetaminophen,* p. 795.

DARVON COMPOUND AND DARVON COMPOUND 65   (DAR-von)
(Rx)

DARVON WITH A.S.A. AND DARVON-N WITH A.S.A.   (DAR-von)
(Rx)

See also *Aspirin,* p. 783, and *Propoxyphene,* p. 773.

Classification/Content: Darvon Compound: Propoxyphene HCl, 32.5 mg; aspirin, 389 mg; and, caffeine, 32.4 mg. Darvon Compound 65-Propoxyphene HCl, 65 mg; aspirin, 389 mg; and caffeine, 32.4 mg.

Darvon with A.S.A.: Propoxyphene HCl, 65 mg: aspirin, 325 mg.

Darvon-N with A.S.A.: Propoxyphene napsylate, 100 mg; aspirin, 325 mg.

Propoxyphene and aspirin are analgesics whereas caffeine is a CNS stimulant.

Uses: Mild to moderate pain, with or without accompanying fever.

Special Concerns: Use during pregnancy only if benefits outweigh risks.

Dosage: Capsules. One capsule q 4 hr of either Darvon Compound, Darvon Compound 65, Darvon with A.S.A. or Darvon-N with A.S.A. Total daily dose of propoxyphene HCl should not exceed 390 mg. Total daily dosage should be decreased in patients with hepatic or renal impairment.

NURSING CONSIDERATIONS

See *Nursing Considerations* for *Aspirin,* p. 788, and *Caffeine,* p. 858.

EQUAGESIC   (eh-kuah-**JEE**-sik)
(Rx)

See also *Aspirin,* p. 783, and *Meprobamate,* p. 625.

Classification/Content: *Nonnarcotic Analgesic:* Aspirin, 325 mg. *Antianxiety Agent:* Meprobamate, 200 mg.

Contraindications: Pregnancy.

Uses: Treatment (short-term only) of pain due to musculoskeletal disease accompanied by anxiety and tension.

Additional Contraindications: Children under 12 years of age. Use for longer than 4 months.

Dosage: Tablets. Adults: 1–2 tablets t.i.d.–q.i.d.

NURSING CONSIDERATIONS

See *Nursing Considerations for Aspirin,* p. 788, and *Benzodiazepines,* p. 614.

SOMA COMPOUND   (**SO**-mah)
(Rx)

SOMA COMPOUND WITH CODEINE   (**SO**-mah, **KOH**-deen)
(Rx, C-III)

See also *Aspirin,* p. 783, *Carisoprodol,* p. 706, and *Codeine,* p. 760.

Classification/Content: Soma Compound contains: *Nonnarcotic Analgesic:* Aspirin, 325 mg. *Centrally acting skeletal muscle relaxant:* Carisoprodol, 200 mg. In addition to the above, Soma Compound with Codeine contains: *Narcotic analgesic:* Codeine phosphate, 16 mg.

See also information on individual components.

Uses: Acute, painful musculoskeletal conditions, to treat muscle spasm, pain, and limited mobility.

Contraindication: Use in children less than 12 years of age.

Dosage: Tablets: Soma Compound and Soma Compound with Codeine: Adults, 1–2 tablets q.i.d.

Special Concerns: Pregnancy category: C.

NURSING CONSIDERATIONS

See *Nursing Considerations* for *Aspirin*, p. 788, and *Narcotic Analgesics*, p. 753.

CHAPTER THIRTY-NINE

Antirheumatic and Nonsteroidal Anti-Inflammatory Agents

General Statement: Arthritis, which means inflammation of the joints, refers to approximately 80 different conditions also called rheumatic, collagen, or connective tissue diseases. The most prominent symptoms of these conditions are painful, inflamed joints, but the cause for this joint inflammation varies from disease to disease. The joint pain of gout, for example, results from sodium urate crystals that are formed as a consequence of the overproduction or underelimination of uric acid. Osteoarthritis is caused by the degeneration of the joint; rheumatoid arthritis and systemic lupus erythematosus (SLE) are autoimmune diseases. Immune factors trigger the release of corrosive enzymes in the joints in a complex manner. Infectious arthritis is the result of rapid joint destruction by microorganisms like gonococci that invade the joint cavity. Treatment must be aimed at the cause of the particular form of arthritis, and a thorough diagnostic evaluation must therefore precede the initiation of therapy. Gout is treated with uricosuric agents, which alter uric acid metabolism (Chapter 40); infectious arthritis responds to antibiotics (Chapter 9); osteoarthritis, rheumatoid arthritis, ankylosing spondylitis, and systemic lupus erythematosus respond to anti-inflammatory drugs. Rheumatoid arthritis may also be treated with two remitting agents (gold and penicillamine) or with hydroxychloroquine sulfate (Chapter 14). Aspirin (Chapter 38) is an important agent in the treatment of all rheumatic diseases. Corticosteroids (Chapter 61) are used, preferably for short-term therapy only, for some of the more resistant cases of rheumatoid arthritis and SLE or for situations of exacerbation of these diseases. Corticosteroids also are used for intra-articular injection. Drug therapy of the arthritides must be supplemented by a physical therapy program, as well as proper rest and diet. Total joint replacement is also an important mode of therapy to correct the ravages of arthritis.

NONSTEROIDAL ANTI-INFLAMMATORY AGENTS

Action/Kinetics: Over the past decade, a growing number of nonsteroidal anti-inflammatory agents have been developed which have anti-inflammatory, analgesic, and antipyretic effects. Chemically, these drugs are related to indene, indole, or propionic acid. As in the case of aspirin, the therapeutic actions of these agents are believed to result from the inhibition of the enzyme cyclo-oxygenase which results in decreased prostaglandin synthesis. The agents are effective in reducing joint swelling, pain, and morning stiffness, as well as in increasing mobility in arthritic patients. They do not alter the course of the disease, however. Their anti-inflammatory activity is comparable to that of aspirin.

The analgesic activity is due, in part, to relief of inflammation. Also, the drugs may block generation of pain impulses and may inhibit synthesis or action of substances that sensitize pain receptors to chemical or mechanical stimuli. The antipyretic action is believed to occur by decreasing prostaglandin synthesis in the hypothalamus resulting in an increase in peripheral blood flow and heat loss as well as to promote sweating.

The nonsteroidal anti-inflammatory agents have an irritating effect on the GI tract. They differ from one another slightly with respect to their rate of absorption, length of action, anti-inflammatory activity and effect on the GI mucosa. Most are rapidly and completely absorbed from the GI tract; food delays the rate, but not the total amount, of drug absorbed. These drugs are metabolized in the kidney and are excreted through the urine, mainly as metabolites.

39

Uses: Rheumatoid arthritis (acute flares and long-term management in adults and children), osteoarthritis, anklyosing spondylitis, gout, and other musculoskeletal diseases. Treatment of nonrheumatic inflammatory conditions including bursitis, synovitis, tendinitis, or tenosynovitis. Mild to moderate pain including primary dysmenorrhea, episiotomy pain, strains and sprains, postextraction dental pain.

Contraindications: Most for children under 14 years of age. Lactation. Hypersensitivity to any of these agents or to aspirin. Patients in whom aspirin, nonsteroidal anti-inflammatory agents, or iodides have caused acute asthma, rhinitis, urticaria, nasal polyps, bronchospasm, angioedema or other symptoms of allergy or anaphylaxis.

Special Concerns: Patients intolerant to one of the nonsteroidal anti-inflammatory agents may be intolerant to others in this group. Use with caution in patients with a history of GI disease, reduced renal function and in geriatric patients.

Side Effects: *GI (most common):* Peptic or duodenal ulceration and GI bleeding, reactivation of preexisting ulcers. Heartburn, dyspepsia, nausea, vomiting, anorexia, diarrhea, constipation, increased or decreased appetite, indigestion, stomatitis, epigastric pain, abdominal cramps or pain, gastroenteritis, paralytic ileus, salivation, dry mouth, glossitis, pyrosis, icterus, ulcerative colitis, rectal bleeding, melena, perforation and hemorrhage of esophagus, stomach, duodenum or large intestine. *CNS:* Dizziness, drowsiness, vertigo, headaches, lightheadedness, paresthesia, peripheral neuropathy, excitation, tremor, seizures, myalgia, asthenia, malaise, insomnia, fatigue, drowsiness, confusion, emotional lability, depression, inability to concentrate, psychoses, hallucinations, depersonalization, amnesia, coma, syncope. *CV:* Congestive heart failure, hypotension, hypertension, arrhythmias, palpitation, tachycardia, chest pain, sinus bradycardia, peripheral vascular disease, peripheral edema. *Respiratory:* Bronchospasm, laryngeal edema, rhinitis, dyspnea, pharyngitis, hemoptysis, shortness of breath. *Hematologic:* Bone marrow depression, neutropenia, leukopenia, pancytopenia, eosinophila, thrombocytopenia, granulocytopenia, agranulocytosis, aplastic anemia, hemolytic anemia. *Ophthalmologic:* Amblyopia, visual disturbances, corneal deposits, retinal hemorrhage, scotomata, retinal pigmentation changes or degeneration, iritis, loss of color vision (reversible), optic neuritis, cataracts, swollen, dry, or irritated eyes. *Skin:* Pruritus, skin eruptions, sweating, ecchymoses, rashes, urticaria, purpura, Stevens-Johnson syndrome, exfoliative dermatitis, photosensitivity, alopecia, skin irritation, peeling, erythema multiforme, desquamation, skin discoloration. *GU:* Menometrorrhagia, menorrhagia, impotence, hematuria, cystitis, azotemia, nocturia, proteinuria, urinary tract infections, polyuria, dysuria, urinary frequency, oliguria, pyuria, anuria, renal insufficiency, nephrosis, nephrotic syndrome, glomerular and interstitial nephritis, urinary casts. *Metabolic:* Hyperglycemia, hypoglycemia, glycosuria, hyperkalemia, hyponatremia. *Other:* Tinnitus, hearing loss or disturbances, ear pain, deafness, metallic or bitter taste in mouth, thirst, chills, fever, flushing, jaundice, diabetes mellitus, sweating, gynecomastia, muscle cramps, facial edema, pain, serum sickness.

Drug Interactions	
Anticoagulants	Concomitant use results in ↑ prothrombin time
Aspirin	↓ Effect of nonsteroidal agents due to ↓ blood levels
Beta-adrenergic blocking agents	↓ Antihypertensive effect of blocking agents
Phenobarbital	↓ Effect of anti-inflammatory drug due to ↑ breakdown by liver
Phenytoin	↑ Effect of phenytoin due to ↓ plasma protein binding
Probenecid	↑ Effect of nonsteroidal agents due to ↑ plasma levels

Drug Interactions

Sulfonamides	↑ Effect of sulfonamides due to ↓ plasma protein binding
Sulfonylureas	↑ Effect of sulfonylureas due to ↓ plasma protein binding

Dosage: See individual drugs.

NURSING CONSIDERATIONS

Administration/Storage

Alcohol and aspirin should not be taken together with nonsteroidal anti-inflammatory agents.

Assessment

1. Note any history of allergic responses to aspirin or other anti-inflammatory agents. These drugs are contraindicated in this event.
2. Determine if the client has asthma. This condition may be exacerbated by the use of nonsteroidal anti-inflammatory drugs (NSAIDS).
3. Note the age of the client. Children under 14 years of age should not receive drugs in this category.
4. Determine if client is taking oral hypoglycemic agents or insulin and document this information.
5. Interview the client concerning other medications that they are currently taking. Determine if any of these drugs are on the drug interaction list and report.

Client/Family Teaching

1. Take anti-inflammatory agents with a full glass of water, milk, meals or with an antacid prescribed by the physician to reduce gastric irritation.
2. Encourage the client to comply with the drug regimen, because regular intake of drug is necessary to sustain anti-inflammatory effects.
3. Discuss the need for regular medical supervision so that dosages of drug can be adjusted based on the client's condition, age, changes in disease activity and overall drug response.
4. Report to the physician symptoms of GI irritation that are not relieved by adhering to the prescribed protocol.
5. Instruct client to report any episodes of bleeding, blurred vision or other eye symptoms, tinnitus, skin rashes, purpura, weight gain or edema.
6. Use caution in operating machinery or in driving a car because medication may cause dizziness or drowsiness.
7. If the client has diabetes mellitus, explain the possible increase in hypoglycemic effect of the drugs on hypoglycemic agents. Advise clients to pay particular attention to urine and blood testing and report any symptoms of hypoglycemica to the physician. The dosage of agent and NSAID may need to be adjusted.
8. Remind clients to tell other physicians and health care providers of the medication being taken to avoid having prescriptions written for drugs that would interact with NSAID.

CARPROFEN (kar-PROH-fen)

Rimadyl (Rx)

See also *Nonsteroidal Anti-Inflammatory Agents,* p. 801.

Classification: Anti-inflammatory, nonsteroidal analgesic.

Action/Kinetics: $t^1/2$: 6–17 hr. **Time to peak levels:** 1 hr.

Uses: Acute and chronic rheumatoid arthritis and osteoarthritis; acute gouty arthritis.

Special Concerns: Pregnancy category: C.

Additional Side Effects: Compared with other nonsteroidal anti-inflammatory agents, carprofen causes increased incidence of rashes, lower urinary tract symptoms, and leukopenia. Also, there is a greater incidence of abnormalities in levels of transaminase and alkaline phosphatase.

Dosage: PO. *Chronic rheumatoid arthritis and osteoarthritis:* Not to exceed 150 mg b.i.d. or 100 mg t.i.d. *Acute gouty arthritis:* 600 mg daily in divided doses for 3–10 days. If ineffective after 2 days, the drug should be discontinued and other treatment started.

NURSING CONSIDERATIONS

See also *Nursing Considerations* for *Nonsteroidal Anti-Inflammatory Agents,* p. 803.

Administration/Storage

1. When the client is to use the drug to treat chronic conditions, attempts should be made to reduce the dosage of drug after taking it for several weeks.
2. Lower doses of medication should be used for elderly clients and those with renal disease.
3. The maximum recommended dose is 300 mg daily.

Assessment

Determine that baseline transaminase, alkaline phosphatase and renal function studies have been completed.

Interventions

1. Note if the client develops a rash during drug therapy and document and report to the physician.
2. Observe clients for evidence of lower urinary tract symptoms such as cystitis, nocturia, oliguria, anuria or urinary frequency and report.

Client/Family Teaching

1. Notify the physician if there are no improvements noted after 2 days of therapy.
2. Provide a list of side effects such as GU reactions and rashes which should be reported to the physician immediately.
3. Provide the client and family with the names and addresses or phone numbers of local support groups that may assist them in understanding and coping with chronic disorders.

DICLOFENAC SODIUM (dye-KLOH-fen-ack)

Voltaren, Voltaren SR (Rx)

See also *Nonsteroidal Anti-Inflammatory Agents,* p. 801.

Classification: Nonsteroidal anti-inflammatory analgesic.

Action/Kinetics: Diclofenac sodium is a phenylacetic acid derivative. **Peak plasma levels:** 2–3 hr. **t½:** 2 hr. Food will affect the rate, but not the amount, of drug absorbed from the GI tract. The drug is metabolized in the liver and excreted by the kidneys.

Uses: Rheumatoid arthritis, osteoarthritis, ankylosing spondylitis. *Investigational:* Mild to moderate pain, juvenile rheumatoid arthritis, acute painful shoulder, sunburn.

Special Concerns: Pregnancy category: B. Use with caution during lactation.

Dosage: Delayed-release Tablets. *Rheumatoid arthritis:* 150–200 mg daily in 2–4 divided doses. *Osteoarthritis:* 100–150 mg daily in 2–3 divided doses. *Ankylosing spondylitis:* 25 mg q.i.d. with an extra 25 mg dose at bedtime, if necessary.

NURSING CONSIDERATIONS

See *Nursing Considerations* for *Nonsteroidal Anti-Inflammatory Agents,* p. 803.

Administration/Storage

1. May be taken with meals, a full glass of water or milk if GI upset occurs.
2. Up to 3 weeks may be required for beneficial effects to be realized when used for rheumatoid arthritis or osteoarthritis.
3. The delayed-release tablets should not be crushed or chewed.

Interventions

Monitor liver and renal function studies on a routine basis.

FENOPROFEN CALCIUM   (fen-oh-**PROH**-fen)

Nalfon (Rx)

See also *Nonsteroidal Anti-Inflammatory Agents,* p. 801.

Classification: Nonsteroidal anti-inflammatory analgesic.

Action/Kinetics: Peak serum levels: 1–2 hr; **t½:** 2–3 hr. Ninety-nine percent protein bound. Food (but not antacids) delays absorption and decreases the total amount absorbed. When used for arthritis, onset of action is within 2 days but 2–3 weeks may be necessary to assess full therapeutic effects. Safety and efficacy in children have not been established.

Uses: Rheumatoid arthritis, osteoarthritis, mild to moderate pain. *Investigational:* Juvenile rheumatoid arthritis, migraine, sunburn.

Additional Contraindications: Renal dysfunction.

Special Concerns: Dosage has not been determined in children.

Additional Side Effects: *GU:* Dysuria, hematuria, cystitis, interstitial nephritis, nephrotic syndrome. Overdosage has caused tachycardia and hypotension.

Dosage: Capsules, Tablets. *Rheumatoid and osteoarthritis:* 300–600 mg t.i.d.–q.i.d. Adjust dose according to response of patient. *Mild to moderate pain:* 200 mg q 4–6 hr. Maximum daily dose for all uses: 3,200 mg.

NURSING CONSIDERATIONS

See also *Nursing Considerations* for *Nonsteroidal Anti-Inflammatory Agents,* p. 803.

Administration/Storage

1. Give the drug 30 min before or 2 hr after meals. Food decreases the rate and extent of absorption of fenoprofen.
2. Expect the peak effect to be realized in 2–3 hr and to last for 4–6 hr.
3. Two to 3 weeks may be required before a beneficial effect is seen.
4. Elderly clients over 70 years of age usually require half the usual adult dose of fenoprofen.
5. The drug is not recommended for children under 12 years of age or for pregnant women.
6. For clients who have difficulty swallowing, the tablets can be crushed and the contents mixed with applesauce or other similar foods.
7. If fenoprofen is given chronically, auditory tests should be performed periodically.

Assessment

1. Note the drugs the client is currently taking to assure that there is no potential drug interactions.
2. Obtain a baseline ophthalmic and auditory examination against which to measure any auditory or visual changes once drug therapy begins.
3. Obtain baseline liver and renal function studies.

Interventions

1. Note client complaints of headache, sleepiness, dizziness, nervousness, weakness or fatigue. These may be drug side effects and should be documented and reported to the physician.
2. Monitor intake and output. If the client is vomiting or has diarrhea, also monitor client's weight.
3. Perform a routine urinalysis, serum electrolytes, BUN and creatinine to detect evidence of renal failure and nephrotic syndrome.
4. Note evidence of easy bruising, prolonged bleeding times or anemia. Inspect the client for petechiae, oozing of blood from the gums, nosebleeds, sore throat and fever. Report these to the physician.
5. Monitor CBC with differential, platelet counts and bleeding times during therapy.
6. Assess clients for the development of jaundice, right upper quadrant abdominal pain, or a change in the color and consistency of stools. Document and report to the physician.

Client/Family Teaching

1. Remind the clients to take the medication as ordered.
2. Explain that it takes 2–3 weeks of therapy to realize improvement in arthritic conditions.

FLURBIPROFEN   (flur-bih-**PROH**-fen)

Ansaid, Froben✤ (Rx)

FLURBIPROFEN SODIUM   (flur-bih-**PROH**-fen)

Ocufen (Rx)

Classification: Nonsteroidal anti-inflammatory agent, ophthalmic and systemic use.

Action/Kinetics: By inhibiting prostaglandin synthesis, flurbiprofen reverses prostaglandin-induced vasodilation, leukocytosis, increased vascular permeability, and increased intraocular pressure. The drug also inhibits miosis, which occurs during cataract surgery. **PO form, time to peak levels:** 1.5 hr; **t½:** 5.7 hr.

Uses: Prevention of intraoperative miosis, rheumatoid arthritis, osteoarthritis. *Investigational:* Inflammation following cataract surgery, uveitis syndromes. Topically to treat cystoid macular edema. Mild to moderate pain, primary dysmenorrhea, sunburn.

Contraindications: Dendritic keratitis.

Special Concerns: Pregnancy category: B for flurbiprofen and C for flurbiprofen sodium. Use with caution in patients hypersensitive to aspirin or other nonsteroidal anti-inflammatory agents. Use with caution during lactation. Safety and efficacy in children have not been established.

Additional Side Effects: *Ophthalmic:* Ocular irritation, transient stinging or burning following use, delay in wound healing.

Dosage: *Ophthalmic:* Beginning 2 hr before surgery, instill 1 drop every 30 min (i.e., total of 4 drops of 0.03% solution). **Tablets.** *Rheumatoid arthritis, osteoarthritis:* **initial,** 200–300 mg daily in divided doses b.i.d.–q.i.d.; **then,** adjust dose to patient response. Doses greater than 300 mg daily are not recommended. *Dysmenorrhea:* 50 mg q.i.d.

NURSING CONSIDERATIONS

See also *Nursing Considerations* for *Nonsteroidal Anti-Inflammatory Agents,* p. 803.

Administration/Storage

The maximum dose of 300 mg should be used only for initiating therapy or for treating acute exacerbations of the disease.

Interventions

1. Assess and report any delays in wound healing.
2. Prior to surgery, carefully follow the administration regimen established.

Client/Family Teaching

1. Instruct client and family in the appropriate method of administering the eye medication.
2. Advise clients to avoid rubbing the eyes after the medication has been administered.
3. Instruct the client to report any stinging, burning, or irritation immediately to the physician.

IBUPROFEN   (eye-byou-**PROH**-fen)

Rx: Apo-Ibuprofen✿, Amersol✿, Children's Advil, Dolgesic, Ibren, Ibumed, Ibupro-600, Ifen, Motrin, Novoprofen✿, Pedia Profen, Ro-Profen, Rufen. OTC: Aches-N-Pain, Advil, Genpril, Haltran, Ibuprin, Medipren, Midol 200, Motrin-IB, Nuprin, Pamprin-IB, Trendar

See also *Nonsteroidal Anti-Inflammatory Agents,* p. 801.

Classification: Anti-inflammatory, nonsteroidal analgesic.

Action/Kinetics: Onset: 30 min for analgesia and approximately 1 week for anti-inflammatory effect. **Peak serum levels:** 1–2 hr. **t½:** 2 hr. **Duration:** 4–6 hr for analgesia and 1–2 weeks for anti-inflammatory effect. Food delays absorption rate but not total amount of drug absorbed.

The OTC products each contain 200 mg of ibuprofen.

Uses: Analgesic for mild to moderate pain. Primary dysmenorrhea, rheumatoid arthritis and osteoarthritis, antipyretic. *Investigational:* Resistant acne vulgaris (with tetracyclines); inflammation due to ultraviolet-B exposure (sunburn), migraine.

Contraindications: Use of ibuprofen is not recommended during pregnancy, especially during the last trimester.

Special Concerns: The dosage must be individually determined for children less than 12 years of age.

Additional Side Effects: Dermatitis (maculopapular type), rash.

Additional Drug Interactions

Furosemide	Ibuprofen ↓ diuretic effect of furosemide due to ↓ renal prostaglandin synthesis
Lithium	Ibuprofen ↑ plasma levels of lithium
Thiazide diuretics	Ibuprofen ↓ diuretic effect of furosemide due to ↓ renal prostaglandin synthesis

Dosage: Tablets. *Rheumatoid arthritis, osteoarthritis:* Either 300 mg q.i.d. or 400, 600, or 800 mg t.i.d.–q.i.d.; adjust dosage according to patient response. Full therapeutic response may not be noted for 2 or more weeks. *Juvenile arthritis:* 30–40 mg/kg daily in 3–4 divided doses. *Mild to moderate pain:* 400 mg q 4–6 hr. *Antipyretic:* **Pediatric:** 5 mg/kg if baseline temperature is 102.5°F or below or 10 mg/kg if baseline temperature is greater than 102.5°F. *Dysmenorrhea:* 400 mg q 4 hr. **OTC use:** *Mild to moderate pain, antipyretic, dysmenorrhea:* 200 mg q 4–6 hr, not to exceed 1,200 mg daily.

NURSING CONSIDERATIONS

See also *Nursing Considerations* for *Nonsteroidal Anti-Inflammatory Agents,* p. 803.

Administration/Storage

1. Ibuprofen purchased OTC should not be used as an antipyretic for more than 3 days.
2. This drug should not be used as an analgesic for more than 10 days unless approved by a physician.
3. Anticipate an onset of action in 30 min and that the effect will last 4–6 hr.

Assessment

1. Take a complete drug history, noting if the client is currently taking any of the drugs with which ibuprofen interacts unfavorably.
2. Note the age of the client, and if female determine if sexually active and potentially pregnant. The drug is contraindicated in pregnancy.
3. Obtain a baseline eye examination prior to initiating drug therapy.

Client/Family Teaching

1. Remind the client to take the medication only as ordered.
2. Provide the client with a printed list of adverse side effects. Encourage the client to report these to the physician.
3. Take the medication with a snack, milk, antacid or meals to decrease GI upset. If nausea, vomiting, diarrhea or constipation persist, report to the physician as the drug may need to be discontinued.

4. In clients with a history of congestive heart failure or compromised cardiac function, instruct them to carefully record weight and to report any evidence of edema. Records of BP and intake and output may be requested with some individuals.

5. Instruct clients to report any evidence of blurred vision. Periodic eye examinations should be performed on clients undergoing long-term therapy.

6. Remind the client that it may take 2–3 weeks of therapy to realize an improvement in arthritic pain. Therefore, the client should remain on the drug unless side effects occur.

7. Stress the importance of reporting for scheduled lab tests including BUN, serum electrolytes, creatinine, and urinalysis.

INDOMETHACIN   (in-doh-**METH**-ah-sin)

Indameth, Indocid✽, Indocin, Indocin SR, Indo-Lemmon, Novomethacin✽ (Rx)

INDOMETHACIN SODIUM TRIHYDRATE   (in-doh-**METH**-ah-sin)

Indocin I.V. (Rx)

See also *Nonsteroidal Anti-Inflammatory Agents,* p. 801.

Classification: Anti-inflammatory, analgesic, antipyretic.

Action/Kinetics: Indomethacin is not considered to be a simple analgesic and should only be used for the conditions listed. **PO. Onset:** 1–2 hr for analgesia and up to 1 week for anti-inflammatory effect. **Peak plasma levels:** 30–120 min. **Duration:** 4–6 hr for analgesia and 1–2 weeks for anti-inflammatory effect. **Therapeutic plasma levels:** 10–18 mcg/mL. **t½:** Approximately 5 hr. **Plasma t½ following IV in infants:** 12–20 hr, depending on age and dose. Approximately 90% plasma protein bound. The drug is metabolized in the liver and excreted in both the urine and feces.

Uses: Moderate to severe rheumatoid arthritis, osteoarthritis, ankylosing spondylitis (drug of choice). Acute gouty arthritis, tendinitis, bursitis, acute painful shoulder. *IV:* Pharmacologic closure of persistent patent ductus arteriosus in premature infants. *Investigational:* Topically to treat cystoid macular edema (0.5% and 1% drops), sunburn, primary dysmenorrhea.

Additional Contraindications: Pregnancy. Oral indomethacin in children under 14 years of age. GI lesions. *IV use:* GI or intracranial bleeding, thrombocytopenia, renal disease, defects of coagulation, necrotizing enterocolitis. *Suppositories:* recent rectal bleeding, history of proctitis.

Special Concerns: Use in children should be restricted to patients unresponsive to or intolerant of other anti-inflammatory agents. Geriatric patients are at greater risk of developing CNS side effects, especially confusion. To be used with caution in patients with history of epilepsy, psychiatric illness, parkinsonism, and in the elderly. Indomethacin should be used with extreme caution in the presence of existing, controlled infections.

Additional Side Effects: Reactivation of latent infections may mask signs of infection. More marked CNS manifestations than for other drugs of this group.

Additional Drug Interactions

Captopril	Indomethacin ↓ effect of captopril, probably due to inhibition of prostaglandin synthesis
Diflunisal	↑ Plasma levels of indomethacin; also, possible fatal GI hemorrhage

---

Additional Drug Interactions

Diuretics (loop, potassium-sparing, thiazide)	Indomethacin may reduce the antihypertensive and natriuretic action of diuretics
Lisinopril	Possible ↓ effect of lisinopril
Prazosin	Indomethacin ↓ antihypertensive effects of prazosin

Dosage: Capsules, Oral Suspension. *Moderate to severe arthritis, osteoarthritis, ankylosing spondylitis:* **Initial:** 25 mg b.i.d.–t.i.d.; may be increased by 25–50 mg at weekly intervals, according to condition, until satisfactory response is obtained. **Maximum daily dosage:** 150–200 mg. In acute flares of chronic rheumatoid arthritis, the dose may need to be increased by 25–50 mg daily until the acute phase is under control. *Gouty arthritis:* **Initial:** 100 mg; **then,** 50 mg t.i.d. for 3–5 days. Reduce dosage rapidly until drug is withdrawn. *Bursitis/tendinitis:* 75–150 mg/day in 3–4 divided doses for 1–2 weeks. **Extended-release Capsules.** *Antirheumatic, anti-inflammatory:* **Adults:** 75 mg, of which 25 mg is released immediately, 1–2 times daily.

Suppositories. *Anti-inflammatory, antirheumatic, antigout:* **Adults:** 50 mg up to q.i.d. **Pediatric:** 1.5–2.5 mg/kg daily in 3–4 divided doses (up to a maximum of 4 mg/kg or 250–200 mg daily, whichever is less).

IV only. *Patent ductus arteriosus:* 3 IV doses, depending on age of the infant, are given at 12- to 24-hr intervals. **Infants less than 2 days:** first dose, 0.2 mg/kg, followed by 2 doses of 0.1 mg/kg each; **infants 2–7 days:** 3 doses of 0.2 mg/kg each; **infants more than 7 days:** first dose, 0.2 mg/kg, followed by 2 doses of 0.25 mg/kg each. If patent ductus arteriosus reopens, a second course of 1–3 doses may be given. Surgery may be required if there is no response after 2 courses of therapy.

NURSING CONSIDERATIONS

See also *Nursing Considerations* for *Nonsteroidal Anti-Inflammatory Agents,* p. 803.

Administration/Storage

1. Store in amber-colored containers.
2. The IV solution should be prepared with sodium chloride injection or water for injection. Diluent should not contain preservatives.
3. IV solutions should be freshly prepared prior to use.
4. The IV solution should be given over 5–10 sec.
5. Up to 100 mg of the total daily dose can be given at bedtime for clients with night pain or morning stiffness.
6. The sustained-release form should not be crushed and should not be used in clients with acute gouty arthritis.
7. If the client has difficulty swallowing capsules, the contents may be emptied into applesauce, food or liquid to assure that the client receives the prescribed dose.
8. Suppositories (50 mg) may be used in clients unable to take oral medication.
9. Anticipate a peak action of drug to occur in 24–36 hr in clients taking the medication for gout.
10. Peak drug activity in clients taking the medication for anti-rheumatic effect will occur in about 4 weeks.
11. The smallest effective dose of the drug should be administered, based on individual need. Adverse reactions are dose related.

Interventions

1. Monitor intake and output. If clients are experiencing nausea or vomiting, monitor and record their weight also.
2. Inspect the urine for signs of hematuria. Also monitor the client for signs and symptoms of anemia and report these to the physician.
3. If any adverse reactions to the drug occur, withhold the drug and report to the physician. Any of the adverse responses may be serious enough to take the client off the medication.
4. Indomethacin masks infections. Therefore, assess clients carefully, reporting any incidence of fever.

Client/Family Teaching

1. Report for scheduled ophthalmologic examinations and lab studies, especially if the client is receiving long-term therapy.
2. Use caution when operating potentially hazardous equipment, because of possible lightheadedness and decreased alertness.
3. Take the medication with food or milk, to decrease GI upset.
4. Take medication only as prescribed by the physician.
5. Remind clients that it will take from 2–4 weeks of therapy before they will see significant improvement in arthritic conditions. Therefore they should follow the prescribed drug regimen carefully and refrain from becoming discouraged.
6. Stress the importance of reporting any side effects from drug therapy immediately to the physician.

KETOPROFEN   (kee-toe-PROH-fen)

Orudis, Orudis-E✦ (Rx)

See also *Nonsteroidal Anti-Inflammatory Agents,* p. 801.

Classification: Nonsteroidal anti-inflammatory agent.

Action/Kinetics: The drug possesses anti-inflammatory, antipyretic, and analgesic properties. It is known to inhibit both prostaglandin and leukotriene synthesis, to have antibradykinin activity, and to stabilize lysosomal membranes. **Peak plasma levels:** 0.5–2 hr. **t½:** 2–4 hr. The t½ is increased to approximately 5 hr in geriatric patients. Ketoprofen is 99% bound to plasma proteins. Food does not alter the bioavailability; however, the rate of absorption is reduced.

Uses: Acute or chronic rheumatoid arthritis and osteoarthritis. Primary dysmenorrhea. Analgesic for mild to moderate pain. *Investigational:* Juvenile rheumatoid arthritis, sunburn.

Contraindications: Should not be used during late pregnancy. Use should be avoided during lactation and in children.

Special Concerns: Pregnancy category: B (use only if benefits outweigh risks). Dosage has not been established in children. Geriatric patients may manifest increased and prolonged serum levels due to decreased protein binding and clearance. Use with caution in patients with a history of GI tract disorders, in fluid retention, hypertension, and heart failure.

Additional Side Effects: *GI:* Peptic ulcer, GI bleeding, dyspepsia, nausea, diarrhea, constipation, abdominal pain, flatulence, anorexia, vomiting, stomatitis. *CNS:* Headache. *CV:* Peripheral edema, fluid retention.

Additional Drug Interactions

Acetylsalicylic acid	↑ plasma ketoprofen levels due to ↓ Plasma protein binding
Hydrochlorothiazide	↓ Chloride and potassium excretion
Methotrexate	Concomitant use → toxic plasma levels of methotrexate
Probenecid	↓ Plasma clearance of ketoprofen and ↓ plasma protein binding
Warfarin	Additive effect to cause bleeding

Dosage: Capsules. *Rheumatoid arthritis, osteoarthritis:* **Initial:** 75 mg t.i.d. or 50 mg q.i.d. Dose may be increased to 300 mg daily in divided doses, if necessary; doses above 300 mg daily are not recommended. Dosage should be decreased by one-half to one-third in patients with impaired renal function or in geriatric patients. *Analgesia, dysmenorrhea:* 25–50 mg q 6–8 hr as required, not to exceed 300 mg daily. Dosage should be reduced in geriatric patients and in patients with liver or renal dysfunction.

NURSING CONSIDERATIONS

See also *Nursing Considerations* for *Nonsteroidal Anti-Inflammatory Agents,* p. 803.

Administration/Storage

1. GI side effects may be minimized by taking ketoprofen with antacids, milk, or food.
2. The onset of action takes 15–30 minutes and lasts from 4–6 hours.

Assessment

1. Note any client history of GI disorders, cardiac failure, hypertension or fluid retention.
2. Note if the client is pregnant.
3. Determine age, as the drug is not recommended for children under 12 years of age.
4. Obtain baseline bleeding profiles, liver and renal function studies.

Interventions

1. Anticipate a reduced dosage of drug in elderly clients and those with impaired renal function.
2. Monitor bleeding time and prothrombin time. The drug may prolong bleeding times by decreasing platelet aggregation.
3. Inspect the client periodically for petechiae, unexplained bruising, bleeding from the gums or nose bleeds. Document and report these to the physician.
4. Monitor urine and stools for occult blood and report positive findings to the physician.
5. Inspect clients for evidence of liver dysfunction such as jaundice, upper right quadrant pain, clay colored stools or yellowing of the skin and sclera. Document findings, request a liver profile and report to the physician.

Client/Family Teaching

1. Advise client to avoid ingesting alcoholic beverages.
2. Instruct client not to take any aspirin during therapy unless physician prescribed.

3. Report any new symptoms to the physician, such as rash, headaches, black stools, or disturbances in vision.

4. Provide a printed list of drug side effects, which should be reported to the physician should they occur.

5. Stress the importance of reporting for scheduled lab studies and eye exams throughout therapy.

KETOROLAC TROMETHAMINE   (KEE-toe-roh-lack)

Toradol (Rx)

See also *Nonsteroidal Anti-inflammatory Agents,* p. 801.

Classification: Nonsteroidal anti-inflammatory agent.

Action/Kinetics: Ketorolac is a parenterally administered nonsteroidal anti-inflammatory agent. The drug has no opiate-like activity. **Time to peak plasma levels:** 30–60 min. **Peak plasma levels:** 1–1.4 mcg/mL after 15 mg, 2–2.3 mcg/mL after 30 mg, and 4–4.5 mcg/mL after 60 mg. **t½, terminal:** 3.8–6.3 hr for young adults and 4.7–8.6 hr in geriatric patients. Over 99% bound to plasma protein. Metabolized in the liver, with over 90% excreted through the urine.

Uses: Short-term use for pain including dentistry.

Contraindications: Nasal polyps (complete or partial syndrome), angioedema, allergy to aspirin or other nonsteroidal anti-inflammatory agents. Not recommended for use during labor and delivery.

Special Concerns: Pregnancy category: B. Use with caution during lactation. Safety and efficacy have not been determined in children. Use with caution in patients with impaired renal or hepatic function, with cardiac decompensation or hypertension, and in geriatric patients. Carefully observe patients who have coagulation disorders or who are on anticoagulant drug therapy.

Side Effects: Short-term use of ketorolac is not associated with significant side effects; however, chronic use may cause similar side effects as chronic use of aspirin. *GI:* Nausea, GI pain, dyspepsia, diarrhea, constipation, GI fullness, dry mouth, excessive thirst, flatulence, peptic ulcer, rectal bleeding, vomiting, stomatitis, melena. *CNS:* Drowsiness (most common), dizziness, sweating, headache, paresthesia, depression, euphoria, insomnia, inability to concentrate, vertigo, stimulation. *CV:* Pallor, vasodilation, edema. *Dermatologic:* Pruritus, urticaria. *Urogenital:* Increased urinary frequency, oliguria. *Miscellaneous:* Asthenia, myalgia, liver function abnormalities, purpura, asthma, dyspnea, abnormal taste, abnormal vision.

Drug Interactions	
Lithium	Possibly ↑ lithium levels
Methotrexate	↑ Risk of methotrexate toxicity due to ↓ clearance
Salicylates	↑ Effect of ketorolac due to ↓ plasma protein binding
Warfarin	Slight ↓ in plasma protein binding of warfarin

Dosage: Parenteral: IM. Adults, initial: 30–60 mg as a loading dose followed by 15–30 mg q 6 hr as needed to control pain. Maximum dose for day 1 is 150 mg and for subsequent days 120 mg.

NURSING CONSIDERATIONS

See also *Nursing Considerations* for *Nonsteroidal Anti-Inflammatory Agents,* p. 803.

Administration/Storage

1. If pain returns within 3–5 hr, the next dose can be increased by 50% (based on the t½).
2. If analgesia is inadequate with the dose used, meperidine or morphine can be used concomitantly.
3. If pain does not return for 8–12 hr, the next dose can either be decreased by 50% or the dosage interval can be increased to q 8–12 hr.
4. Lower doses should be administered to geriatric clients, clients with impaired renal function, and individuals weighing less than 50 kg.
5. The drug should be protected from light.

Assessment

1. Take a complete drug history, noting if the client is currently taking any of the drugs with which ketorolac interacts unfavorably.
2. Determine age and weight of client as these may affect dosage requirements.
3. Note any client history of impaired renal or hepatic function, cardiac decompensation, hypertension, or coagulation disorders.
4. Obtain baseline liver and renal function studies.

Client/Family Teaching

1. Provide a printed list of side effects associated with drug therapy that should be reported to the physician, should they occur.
2. Advise client to use caution when operating equipment or driving a car as the drug may cause drowsiness or dizziness.
3. Instruct client to take medication with a snack, meals or glass of milk to decrease GI upset.
4. Stress the importance of reporting for all scheduled visits and lab studies so that drug effectiveness can be evaluated.

MECLOFENAMATE SODIUM   (meh-kloh-FEN-ah-mayt)

Meclofen, Meclomen (Rx)

See also *Nonsteroidal Anti-Inflammatory Agents,* p. 801.

Classification: Anti-inflammatory, nonsteroidal, analgesic.

Action/Kinetics: Peak plasma levels: 30–60 min. **t½:** 2–3.3 hr. Peak anti-inflammatory activity may not be observed for 2–3 weeks. Excreted through urine and feces.

Uses: Acute and chronic rheumatoid arthritis and osteoarthritis. Not indicated as the initial drug for rheumatoid arthritis due to GI side effects. Has been used in combination with gold salts or corticosteroids. Mild to moderate pain. *Investigational:* Menorrhagia, sunburn.

Additional Contraindications: Not recommended for use during pregnancy or lactation.

Special Concerns: Safe use during lactation and in children under 14 years not established. Safety and efficacy not established in functional class IV rheumatoid arthritis.

Additional Side Effects: Severe diarrhea, nausea, headache, rash, dermatitis, abdominal pain, pyrosis, flatulence, malaise, fatigue, paresthesia, insomnia, depression, taste disturbances, nocturia, blood loss (through feces: 2 mL/day).

Drug Interactions

Aspirin	↓ Plasma levels of meclofenamate
Warfarin	↑ Effect of warfarin

Laboratory Test Interferences: ↑ Serum transaminase, alkaline phosphatase; rarely, ↑ serum creatinine or BUN.

Dosage: Capsules. *Rheumatoid arthritis, osteoarthritis:* **usual,** 200–400 mg/day in 3–4 equal doses. Initiate at lower dose and increase to maximum of 400 mg daily if necessary. After initial satisfactory response, lower dosage to decrease severity of side effects. *Mild to moderate pain:* 50 mg q 4–6 hr (100 mg may be required in some patients), not to exceed 400 mg daily.

NURSING CONSIDERATIONS

See also *Nursing Considerations* for *Nonsteroidal Anti-Inflammatory Agents,* p. 803.

Client/Family Teaching

1. Instruct the client to continue to take the drug as ordered and not to become discouraged. Beneficial effects are not readily evident and it may take 2–3 weeks to see improvement in arthritic conditions.
2. May be administered with milk to diminish GI effects.

MEFENAMIC ACID   (meh-fen-**NAM**-ick **AH**-sid)

Ponstan✶, Ponstel (Rx)

See also *Nonsteroidal Anti-Inflammatory Agents,* p. 801.

Classification: Nonsteroidal, anti-inflammatory analgesic.

Action/Kinetics: Mefenamic acid inhibits prostaglandin synthesis. It possesses anti-inflammatory, antipyretic, and analgesic effects. **Peak plasma levels:** 2–4 hr; **t½:** 2–4 hr; **duration:** 4–6 hr. The drug is slowly absorbed from the GI tract, metabolized by the liver, and excreted in the urine and feces.

Uses: Short-term relief (less than one week) of mild to moderate pain (e.g., pain associated with tooth extraction and musculoskeletal disorders). Primary dysmenorrhea. *Investigational:* Premenstrual syndrome, sunburn.

Contraindications: Ulceration or chronic inflammation of the GI tract, pregnancy or possibility thereof, children under 14, and hypersensitivity to the drug.

Special Concerns: Pregnancy category: C. Dosage has not been established in children less than 14 years of age. Use with caution in patients with impaired renal or hepatic function, asthma, or patients on anticoagulant therapy.

Additional Side Effects: Autoimmune hemolytic anemia if used more than 12 months. Diarrhea may be significant. Rash (maculopapular type).

Drug Interactions	
Anticoagulants	↑ Hypoprothrombinemia due to ↓ plasma protein binding
Insulin	↑ Insulin requirement
Lithium	↑ Plasma levels of lithium

Laboratory Test Interference: False + test for urinary bile using diazo tablets.

Dosage: Capsules. *Analgesia, primary dysmenorrhea.* **Adults and children over 14 years of age: initial,** 500 mg; **then,** 250 mg q 6 hr.

NURSING CONSIDERATIONS

See also *Nursing Considerations* for *Nonsteroidal Anti-inflammatory Agents,* p. 803.

Administration/Storage

1. Give with food.
2. The drug should not be used for more than a week at a time.

Interventions

1. Withhold the drug and report if the client develops a rash or diarrhea.
2. Assess the client for any signs of bleeding, as drug lowers the prothrombin time. Monitor prothrombin values.
3. Inspect the client's skin for rashes, urticaria and increased sweating. Document and report these findings to the physician.

Client/Family Teaching

1. Advise the client to use caution when operating potentially hazardous machinery, as in driving, because drug may cause dizziness, lightheadedness, or confusion.
2. Review anticipated benefits and possible side effects that may be associated with drug therapy.
3. Remind clients to report any side effects that may develop to the physician as therapy may need to be altered.

NAPROXEN   (nah-**PROX**-en)

Apo-Naproxen ✿, Naprosyn, Naxen ✿, Novonaprox ✿ (Rx)

NAPROXEN SODIUM   (nah-**PROX**-en)

Anaprox, Anaprox DS (Rx)

See also *Nonsteroidal Anti-Inflammatory Agents,* p. 801.

Classification: Nonsteroidal, anti-inflammatory analgesic.

Action/Kinetics: Peak serum levels of naproxen: 2–4 hr; **for sodium salt:** 1–2 hr. **t½ for naproxen:** 12–15 hr; **for sodium salt:** 12–13 hr. **Duration, analgesia:** Approx. 7 hr. The onset of anti-inflammatory effects may take up to 2 weeks and may last 2–4 weeks. Naproxen is more than 90% bound to plasma protein. Food delays the rate but not the amount of drug absorbed. Clinical improvement for inflammatory disease may not be observed for 2 weeks.

Uses: Mild to moderate pain. Musculoskeletal and soft tissue inflammation including rheumatoid arthritis, osteoarthritis, bursitis, tendinitis, ankylosing spondylitis. Primary dysmenorrhea, acute gout. Juvenile rheumatoid arthritis (naproxen only). *Investigational:* Antipyretic in cancer patients, sunburn, migraine (sodium salt only), premenstrual syndrome (sodium salt only).

Contraindications: Use of naproxen and naproxen sodium simultaneously.

Special Concerns: Pregnancy category: B. Safety and effectiveness of naproxen have not been determined in children less than 2 years of age; the safety and effectiveness of naproxen sodium have not been established in children. Geriatric patients may manifest increased total plasma levels of naproxyn.

Drug Interactions	
Methotrexate	Possibility of a fatal interaction
Probenecid	↓ Plasma clearance of naproxen

Laboratory Test Interferences: Naproxen may increase urinary 17-ketosteroid values. Both forms may interfere with urinary assays for 5-hydroxyindoleacetic acid.

Dosage: Naproxen: Oral Suspension, Tablets. *Antirheumatic (rheumatoid arthritis, osteoarthritis, ankylosing spondylitis):* **Adults, individualized. Usual:** 250, 375, or 500 mg b.i.d. in the morning and evening. Improvement should be observed within 2 weeks; if no improvement is seen, an additional 2 week course of therapy should be considered. May increase to 1.5 g for short periods of time. *Acute gout:* **initial,** 750 mg; **then,** 250 mg naproxen q 8 hr until symptoms subside. *Pain, dysmenorrhea, bursitis, tendinitis:* **initial,** 500 mg; **then,** 250 mg q 6–8 hr. Total daily dosage should not exceed 1,250 mg. *Juvenile rheumatoid arthritis:* Naproxen only, 10 mg/kg daily in 2 divided doses. If the suspension is used, the following dosage can be used: **13 kg:** 2.5 mL b.i.d.; **25 kg:** 5 mL b.i.d.; **38 kg:** 7.5 mL b.i.d.

Naproxen Sodium: Tablets. Adults: *Antirheumatic,* 275 mg b.i.d. in the morning and evening (alternate dosage: 275 mg in the morning and 550 mg at night). *Acute gout:* **initial,** 825 mg; **then,** 275 mg q 8 hr until symptoms subside. *Pain, dysmenorrhea:* **initial,** 550 mg; **then,** 275 mg q 6–8 hr as needed. Total daily dose should not exceed 1,375 mg.

NURSING CONSIDERATIONS

See also *Nursing Considerations* for *Nonsteroidal Anti-Inflammatory Agents,* p. 803.

Administration/Storage

1. The onset of action is 1–2 hours. The duration of action is 7 hours.
2. It is recommended that the medication be taken in the morning and in the evening. The doses do not have to be equal.
3. Naproxen sodium should not be administered to children.

Assessment

1. Note any client history of hypersensitivity to naproxen or other NSAIDs.
2. Review the client's medical history. The drug is contraindicated for persons with GI bleeding or ulcers.

Client/Family Teaching

Instruct the client to report any persistent abdominal pain or dark colored stools to the physician immediately.

PIROXICAM (pih-**ROX**-ih-kam)

Apo-Piroxicam ❀, Feldene, Novopirocam ❀ (Rx)

See also *Nonsteroidal Anti-Inflammatory Agents,* p. 801.

Classification: Nonsteroidal anti-inflammatory, analgesic, antipyretic.

Action/Kinetics: Piroxicam may inhibit prostaglandin synthesis. **Peak plasma levels:** 1.5–2 mcg/mL after 3–5 hr (single dose). **Steady-state plasma levels** (after 7–12 days): 3–8 mcg/mL. **t½:** 50 hr. **Analgesia, onset:** 1 hr; **duration:** 2–3 days. **Anti-inflammatory activity, onset:** 7–12 days; **duration:** 2–3 weeks. Metabolites and unchanged drug excreted in urine and feces.

The effect of piroxicam is comparable to that of aspirin, but with fewer GI side effects and less tinnitus. May be used with gold, corticosteroids, and antacids.

Uses: Acute and chronic treatment of rheumatoid arthritis and osteoarthritis. *Investigational:* Juvenile rheumatoid arthritis, primary dysmenorrhea, sunburn.

Contraindications: Safe use during pregnancy has not been determined. Lactation.

Special Concerns: Safety and efficacy have not been established in children. Increased plasma levels and elimination half-life may be observed in geriatric patients (especially females).

Laboratory Test Interference: Reversible ↑ BUN.

Dosage: Capsules. Adults: *Anti-inflammatory, antirheumatic,* 20 mg daily in 1 or more divided doses. Effect of therapy should not be assessed for 2 weeks.

NURSING CONSIDERATIONS

See also *Nursing Considerations* for *Nonsteroidal Anti-Inflammatory Agents,* p. 803.

Administration/Storage

1. Steady-state plasma levels may not be reached for 2 weeks.
2. Clients over 70 years of age usually require ½ the usual adult dose of medication.
3. The drug is not recommended for children under 14 years of age.
4. Review the list of drugs with which piroxicam interacts.

Client/Family Teaching

1. Remind client that the therapeutic effects of the medication cannot be evaluated fully for at least 2 weeks after beginning treatment with piroxicam.
2. Aspirin decreases the effectiveness of piroxicam and may increase the occurrence of side effects. Therefore, avoid taking aspirin while receiving piroxicam.
3. Report any increased abdominal pain or changes in the color of the stool to the physician.

SULINDAC (su-**LIN**-dak)

Clinoril, Novo-Sundac ❀ (Rx)

See also *Nonsteroidal Anti-Inflammatory Agents,* p. 801.

Classification: Antirheumatic, analgesic.

Action/Kinetics: Sulindac is biotransformed in the liver to a sulfide, the active metabolite. **Peak**

plasma levels of sulfide: after fasting, 2 hr; after food, 3–4 hr. **Onset, anti-inflammatory effect:** within 1 week; **duration, anti-inflammatory effect:** 1–2 wk. **t½,** of sulindac: 7.8 hr; of metabolite: 16.4 hr. Excreted in both urine and feces.

Uses: Acute and chronic treatment of rheumatoid arthritis, osteoarthritis, ankylosing spondylitis, acute gouty arthritis; acute, painful shoulder; tendinitis, bursitis. *Investigational:* Juvenile rheumatoid arthritis, sunburn.

Special Concerns: Safety and efficacy have not been established for children. Safe use during pregnancy has not been established. Use with caution during lactation.

Additional Side Effects: Hypersensitivity, pancreatitis, GI pain (common), rash, dermatitis.

Additional Drug Interactions: Sulindac ↑ effect of warfarin due to ↓ plasma protein binding.

Dosage: Tablets. Adults: *Osteoarthritis, rheumatoid arthritis, ankylosing spondylitis:* 150 or 200 mg b.i.d. *Acute painful shoulder, acute gouty arthritis:* 200 mg b.i.d. for 7–14 days. *Antigout:* 200 mg b.i.d. for 7 days.

NURSING CONSIDERATIONS

See also *Nursing Considerations* for *Nonsteroidal Anti-Inflammatory Agents,* p. 803.

Administration/Storage

1. When used for arthritis, a favorable response usually occurs within one week.
2. For acute conditions, reduce dosage when satisfactory response is attained.

Interventions

If intake and output or laboratory studies indicate renal dysfunction, anticipate a reduction in dosage of drug.

Client/Family Teaching

1. Advise clients not to take aspirin while taking sulindac. Plasma levels of sulindac would be reduced.
2. Instruct clients to report any incidence of unexplained bleeding such as oozing of blood from the gums, nosebleeds, or excessive bruising.

SUPROFEN   (soo-**PROH**-fen)

Profenal (Rx)

See also *Nonsteroidal Anti-Inflammatory Agents,* p. 801.

Classification: Nonsteroidal anti-inflammatory agent, ophthalmic use.

Action/Kinetics: By inhibiting prostaglandin synthesis, suprofen reverses prostaglandin-induced vasodilation, leukocytosis, increased vascular permeability, and increased intraocular pressure. The drug also inhibits miosis, which occurs during cataract surgery.

Uses: Inhibition of intraoperative miosis.

Contraindications: Dendritic keratitis.

Special Concerns: Pregnancy category: C. Use with caution in patients sensitive to aspirin and other nonsteroidal anti-inflammatory agents. Use with caution in surgical patients with a history of bleeding tendencies or who are on drugs that prolong bleeding time. Use with caution during lactation. Safety and efficacy have not been established in children.

Side Effects: *Ophthalmic:* Ocular irritation, transient burning and stinging upon installation.

Drug Interactions: Acetylcholine and carbachol may be ineffective if used in combination with suprofen.

Dosage: Ophthalmic. *Day before surgery:* 2 gtt into the conjunctival sac q 4 hr during waking hours. *Day of surgery:* 2 gtt into the conjunctival sac 3, 2, and 1 hr prior to surgery.

NURSING CONSIDERATIONS

See also *Nursing Considerations* for *Nonsteroidal Anti-Inflammatory Agents,* p. 803.

Administration

For best results, follow administration guidelines carefully.

TOLMETIN SODIUM   (TOHL-met-in)

Tolectin ✹, Tolectin 200, Tolectin DS (Rx)

See also *Nonsteroidal Anti-Inflammatory Agents,* p. 801.

Classification: Nonsteroidal, anti-inflammatory, analgesic.

Action/Kinetics: Peak plasma levels: 30–60 min. **t½:** 1 hr. **Therapeutic plasma levels:** 40 mcg/mL. **Onset, anti-inflammatory effect:** within 1 week; **duration, anti-inflammatory effect:** 1–2 weeks. Inactivated in liver and excreted in urine.

Uses: Acute and chronic treatment of rheumatoid arthritis and osteoarthritis. Juvenile rheumatoid arthritis. *Investigational:* Sunburn.

Special Concerns: Pregnancy category: C. Use with caution during lactation. Dosage has not been determined in children less than 2 years of age.

Laboratory Test Interference: Tolmetin metabolites give a false + test for proteinuria using sulfosalicylic acid.

Dosage: Capsules, Tablets. Adults: *Rheumatoid arthritis, osteoarthritis:* **Adults:** 400 mg t.i.d. (one dose on arising and one at bedtime); adjust dosage according to patient response. **Maintenance:** *rheumatoid arthritis,* 600–1,800 mg daily in 3–4 divided doses; *osteoarthritis,* 600–1,600 mg daily in 3–4 divided doses. Doses larger than 2,000 mg/day for rheumatoid arthritis and 1,600 mg/day for osteoarthritis are not recommended. *Juvenile rheumatoid arthritis:* **2 years and older, initial:** 20 mg/kg/day in 3–4 divided doses to start; **then,** 15–30 mg/kg/day. Doses higher than 30 mg/kg daily are not recommended. Beneficial effects may not be observed for several days to a week.

NURSING CONSIDERATIONS

See also *Nursing Considerations* for *Nonsteroidal Anti-Inflammatory Agents,* p. 803.

Administration/Storage

1. Doses of medication should be spaced so that one dose is taken in the morning upon arising, one during the day, and one at bedtime.

2. If the client develops symptoms of gastric irritation, administer the drug with meals, milk, a full glass of water or antacids (other than sodium bicarbonate).

3. Elderly clients are particularly susceptible to gastric irritation. Therefore, they should receive their medication with milk, meals or with an antacid.
4. Never administer the medication with sodium bicarbonate.

PYRAZOLONE DERIVATIVE

PHENYLBUTAZONE   (fen-ill-**BYOU**-tah-zohn)

Alka-Butazolidin🍁, Alkabutazone🍁, Alka-Phenylbutazone🍁, Apo-Phenylbutazone🍁, Butazolidin, Butazone, Intrabutazone, Novobutazone🍁, Phenylone Plus🍁 (Rx)

Classification: Anti-inflammatory, pyrazolone derivatives.

Action/Kinetics: Phenylbutazone possesses antipyretic, analgesic, anti-inflammatory, and weak uricosuric effects. The anti-inflammatory effects are believed to result from a combination of the inhibition of prostaglandin synthesis, leukocyte migration, and release of lysosomal enzymes. **Onset:** 30–60 min, **peak plasma levels, phenylbutazone:** 2.5 hr; **duration:** 3–5 days. **t½, phenylbutazone:** 77 hr; **t½, oxyphenbutazone:** 72 hr. **Plasma protein binding:** 98%. Phenylbutazone is metabolized to oxyphenbutazone, which is the active metabolite.

Uses: Acute gouty arthritis, active rheumatoid arthritis, degenerative joint disease of the hips and knees, ankylosing spondylitis, painful shoulder. Due to the possibility of severe toxic effects, phenylbutazone should be used only as a last resort when other therapy has proven unsuccessful.

Contraindications: History of peptic ulcer disease, cardiac failure, pancreatitis, senility, children under 14 years of age, hypertension, thyroid disease, blood dyscrasias, edema, arteritis, drug allergy, stomatitis, parotiditis. Severe cardiac, renal, or hepatic disease. Concomitantly with drugs causing similar untoward reactions. Pregnancy and lactation.

Special Concerns: Pregnancy category: C. Use in children less than 15 years of age is not recommended. In geriatric patients 60 years and older, therapy should be restricted to no more than 1 week due to the increased risk of severe, possibly fatal, side effects.

Side Effects: The most serious toxic reactions are blood dyscrasias, including agranulocytosis, leukopenia, aplastic anemia, and thrombocytopenia. The untoward reactions are of a hypersensitivity nature and are not necessarily dose-related. The effects can be developed by persons who have taken these drugs without ill effects for a number of years. Patients should be monitored carefully. *GI:* Vomiting, diarrhea, constipation, flatulence, gastritis, gastric upset, stomatitis, enlargement of salivary glands, ulceration and perforation of the GI tract, development or reactivation of peptic ulcer, GI hemorrhage, hematemesis. *CNS:* Headache, weakness, drowsiness, confusion, numbness, tremors, lethargy, agitation. *Hematologic:* Thrombocytopenia, pancytopenia, agranulocytosis, aplastic anemia, generalized bone marrow depression, hemolytic anemia, leukopenia, anemia, leukemia. *CV:* Edema, congestive heart failure, hypertension, interstitial myocarditis, pericarditis. *Metabolic:* Metabolic acidosis, respiratory alkalosis, hyperglycemia, thyroid hyperplasia, goiter associated with hyperthyroidism or hypothyroidism, pancreatitis. *Allergic:* Urticaria, rashes, fever, polyarteritis, vasculitis, Stevens-Johnson syndrome, anaphylaxis, exacerbation of lupus erythematosus, serum sickness, arthralgia. *Renal:* Glomerulonephritis, necrosis (cortical and acute tubular), obstruction, nephrotic syndrome, hematuria, proteinuria, anuria, oliguria, renal stones, azotemia with renal failure. *Ophthalmologic:* Blurred vision, double vision, detached retina, optic neuritis, hemorrhage of retina, toxic amblyopia, oculomotor palsy, scotomata. *Dermatologic:* Purpura, pruritus, erythema nodosum, erythema multiforme. *Other:* Hepatitis, cholestasis, hearing loss, tinnitus, lymphadenopathy.

Drug Interactions

Alcohol	Impairment of psychomotor skills
Anabolic steroids	Certain androgens ↑ effect of phenylbutazone
Anti-inflammatory drugs	↑ Effect of anti-inflammatory agents due to ↓ plasma protein binding
Anticoagulants, oral	Additive hypoprothrombinemic effects; phenylbutazone may also produce GI ulceration and therefore ↑ chance of bleeding
Antidiabetic agents	↑ Hypoglycemic response due to ↓ renal clearance
Barbiturates	↓ Effect of phenylbutazone due to ↑ breakdown by liver
Cholestyramine	↓ Effect of phenylbutazone due to ↓ absorption from GI tract
Chlorpheniramine	↓ Effect of phenylbutazone due to ↑ breakdown by liver
Corticosteroids	↓ Effect of phenylbutazone due to ↑ breakdown by liver
Dicumarol	↓ Effect of phenylbutazone due to ↑ breakdown by liver
Digitalis glycosides	↓ Effect of phenylbutazone due to ↑ breakdown by liver
Insulin	↑ Effect of insulin
Lithium	↑ Effect of lithium due to ↑ reabsorption by kidney tubules
Methotrexate	↑ Effect of methotrexate
Phenytoin	↑ Effect of phenytoin due to ↓ breakdown by liver; also, ↑ effect of phenytoin due to ↓ plasma protein binding
Rifampin	↓ Effect of phenylbutazone due to ↑ breakdown by liver
Salicylates	Phenylbutazone inhibits uricosuric activity of salicylates
Sulfonamides	↑ Effect of sulfonamides due to ↓ plasma protein binding

---

Laboratory Test Interferences: May alter liver function tests. False + Coombs test. ↑ Prothrombin time.

Dosage: Tablets, Delayed-release Tablets. *Rheumatoid arthritis, degenerative joint disease, ankylosing spondylitis:* **Adults,** 300–600 mg/day in 3 to 4 doses; **maintenance:** 100–200 mg/day, not to exceed 400 mg/day. *Acute gouty arthritis:* **initial,** 400 mg; **then,** 100 mg q 4 hr for 4–7 days.

NURSING CONSIDERATIONS

Administration/Storage

1. Administer before or after meals with a glass of milk to minimize gastric irritation.
2. If a favorable response is not seen after one week, therapy should be discontinued.
3. The dose should be discontinued in clients over 60 years of age as soon as possible after 7 days of therapy. This is due to the increased risk of severe untoward reactions in this group of clients.
4. Hemogram tests and urinalysis should be done prior to and at 1–2 week intervals during therapy.

Assessment

1. Determine if the client has a history of peptic ulcer disease, has had cardiac failure, or pancreatitis.
2. Note the mental ability of the client. The drug is contraindicated for use in clients who are senile.
3. If the client is currently taking any medications, determine if they interact unfavorably with phenylbutazone.
4. Obtain a baseline eye examination prior to beginning drug therapy.

Interventions

1. If the client develops any allergic manifestations such as a rash, edema, or wheezing, discontinue the medication and notify the physician.
2. Be prepared to treat clients exhibiting signs of toxicity with oxygen, blankets for warmth and gastric lavage equipment.
3. Order routine hematological examinations (CBC with differential, bleeding times, platelet count). If agranulocytosis is severe, be prepared to practice reverse isolation techniques.
4. Weigh the client daily, record and report unusual weight gain to the physician.
5. Inspect the client for evidence of petechiae, bruises, rash, the development of a sore throat, and pruritus and if evident, report to the physician.
6. If the client is to remain on the therapy for longer than 2 weeks, monitor closely for jaundice, client complaint of right upper quadrant pain and changes in the color of the stools.
7. Positive results of the treatment should be achieved by the third to fourth day. Trial therapy is not usually continued beyond 1 week in the absence of favorable results.

Client/Family Teaching

1. To minimize gastric upset, take the medication with food, large volumes of water, snacks or with milk.
2. Take only the dose of drug prescribed. Do not increase the amount or frequency of medication unless instructed to do so by the physician.
3. Provide the client with a printed list of high sodium foods to avoid. Teach the client how to restrict sodium intake so as to minimize edema.
4. Instruct the client to keep a written record of their daily intake and output and to report any decrease in urinary output to the physician.
5. Show the client how to determine if edema is present.

6. Advise clients to weigh themselves each morning before breakfast, wearing the same type of clothing. Record this weight and report any progressive weight gain to the physician.

7. Instruct clients that if skin rashes occur, if a fever develops, or if they have malaise, a sore throat or ulcers along their mucous membranes, to report this to physician immediately. These are symptoms of agranulocytosis and demand immediate attention.

8. Caution the clients to notify the physician if there are any changes in vision or if they develop headaches, sleepiness, dizziness, nervousness, weakness, paresthesias or tremors.

9. Stress the importance of reporting for scheduled lab studies, especially for complete blood counts.

10. Advise clients to have periodic eye examinations.

REMITTING AGENTS

AURANOFIN   (or-AN-oh-fin)

Ridaura (Rx)

Classification: Oral gold compound for arthritis.

Action/Kinetics: Auranofin is a gold-containing (29%) compound that was developed for oral administration. The oral drug has fewer side effects than injectable gold products. Although the mechanism is not known, auranofin will improve symptoms of rheumatoid arthritis; it is most effective in the early stages of active synovitis and may act by inhibiting sulfhydryl systems. Other possible mechanisms include inhibition of phagocytic activity of macrophages and polymorphonuclear leukocytes, alteration of biosynthesis of collagen, and alteration of the immune response. Gold will not reverse damage to joints caused by disease. Approximately 25% of an oral dose is absorbed. **Plasma t½ of auranofin gold:** 26 days. **Onset:** 3–4 months (up to 6 months in certain patients). Approximately 3 months are required for steady state blood levels to be achieved. The drug is metabolized and excreted in both the urine and feces.

Uses: Adults and children with rheumatoid arthritis that have not responded to other drugs. Up to 6 months may be required for beneficial effects to occur. Auranofin should be part of a total treatment regimen for rheumatoid arthritis, including nondrug treatments.

Contraindications: History of gold-induced disorders including necrotizing enterocolitis, pulmonary fibrosis, exfoliative dermatitis, bone marrow aplasia, or other hematologic disorders. Use during lactation.

Special Concerns: Pregnancy category: C. Use with caution in renal or hepatic disease, skin rashes, or history of bone marrow depression. Although used in children, a recommended dosage has not been established.

Side Effects: *GI:* Nausea, vomiting, diarrhea (common), abdominal pain, metallic taste, stomatitis, glossitis, gingivitis, anorexia, constipation, flatulence, dyspepsia, dysgeusia. Rarely, melena, GI bleeding, dysphagia, ulcerative enterocolitis. *Dermatologic:* Skin rashes, pruritus, alopecia, urticaria, angioedema. *Hematologic:* Leukopenia, anemia, thrombocytopenia, hematuria, neutropenia, agranulocytosis. *Renal:* Proteinuria, hematuria. *Other:* Conjunctivitis, cholestatic jaundice, fever, interstitial pneumonia and fibrosis, peripheral neuropathy.

Laboratory Test Interference: ↑ Liver enzymes.

Dosage: Capsules. Adults: initial, either 6 mg once daily or 3 mg b.i.d. If response is unsatisfactory after 6 months, increase to 3 mg t.i.d. If response is still inadequate after 3 additional months, the drug should be discontinued. Dosages greater than 9 mg daily are not recommended. *Transfer from injectable gold:* Discontinue injectable gold and begin auranofin at a dose of 6 mg daily.

NURSING CONSIDERATIONS

Administration

1. This is the only gold compound administered orally.
2. A positive response should be noted after 6 months of therapy.

Assessment

1. Review client medical history and note any other severe systemic diseases such as renal disease, history of hepatic infections or heart disease.
2. Note the extent of the client's debilitation.
3. Inspect the client's skin prior to initiating therapy to determine if there are any skin eruptions.
4. Assess the client's gums and oral mucosa prior to therapy, noting any lesions or need for treatment of oral problems.

Interventions

1. Monitor and record intake and output and daily weights.
2. If the client complains of diarrhea, monitor electrolytes and report any evidence of abnormality to the physician.
3. Monitor liver and renal function studies. Send urine to test for evidence of protein and blood. Document and report results to the physician.
4. Observe client for the presence of peripheral neuropathy.
5. To encourage client to return for appropriate follow-up evaluation, only provide the client with a 2-week supply of medications.

Client/Family Teaching

1. Instruct clients to report any skin lesions or changes in the mucous membranes immediately to their physician.
2. Advise clients to avoid sunlight. If clients go out in the sun, instruct them to wear long sleeves, a hat, keep their legs covered and apply sun screen.
3. Teach clients to inspect their mouths regularly. Advise clients on a regular program of oral hygiene. This should include regular brushing of the teeth, daily flossing, and the proper mouth washes, avoiding those with alcohol or other drying ingredients.
4. Provide the client with a list of the signs of toxicity that require immediate reporting and attention by the physician. Remind clients that side effects can occur at any time and must be reported.
5. Advise the client that it may take several weeks of therapy before improvement will be noticed.
6. Women of childbearing age who are sexually active may wish to use some form of birth control while they are receiving gold therapy.

AUROTHIOGLUCOSE SUSPENSION   (or-oh-thigh-oh-**GLOO**-kohz)

Solganol (Rx)

Classification: Antirheumatic agent.

Note: For additional information regarding aurothioglucose, see *Gold Sodium Thiomalate,* below.

Special Concerns: Pregnancy category: C.

Dosage: IM only. Adults: *week 1:* 10 mg; *weeks 2 and 3:* 25 mg; **then,** 25–50 (maximum) mg weekly until a total of 0.8–1 g has been administered. If patient tolerates the dose and has improved, 50 mg may be given q 3–4 weeks for several months. **Pediatric, 6–12 years:** *week 1:* 2.5 mg; *weeks 2 and 3:* 6.25 mg; **then,** 12.5 mg q week until a total dose of 200–250 mg has been administered. **Maintenance:** 6.25–12.5 mg q 3–4 weeks.

NURSING CONSIDERATIONS

See also *Nursing Considerations* for *Gold Sodium Thiomalate,* below.

Administration/Storage:

1. The client should remain supine for 10 min after the injection and should be observed for 15 min following drug administration.
2. IM injections should be made only in the upper outer quadrant of the gluteal region; an 18-gauge, 1½ inch needle (or 2 inches for obese clients) should be used.
3. To obtain a uniform suspension, the vial should be shaken carefully before the dose is withdrawn.
4. Both the syringe and needle used to withdraw the dose should be dry.
5. The vial can be immersed in warm water in order to assist with withdrawing the appropriate dose of the suspension.

GOLD SODIUM THIOMALATE   (gold **SO**-dee-um **THIGH**-oh-mal-ayt)

Myochrysine (Rx)

Classification: Antirheumatic.

Action/Kinetics: Although the exact mechanism is not known, gold salts may inhibit lysosomal enzyme activity in macrophages and decrease macrophage phagocytic activity. Other mechanisms may include alteration of the immune response and alteration of biosynthesis of collagen. Gold salts suppress, but do not cure, arthritis and synovitis. The beneficial effects may not be seen for 3–12 months. Most patients experience transient side effects, although serious effects may be manifested in some. **Peak blood levels (IM):** 4–6 hr. **t½:** increases with continued therapy. Gold may accumulate in tissues and persist for years. Significantly bound to plasma proteins. The drug is eliminated slowly through both the urine (60–90%) and feces (10–40%). This preparation contains 50% gold.

Uses: Adjunct to the treatment of rheumatoid arthritis (active and progressive stages) in children and adults. It is most effective in the early stages of the disease.

Contraindications: Hepatic disease, cardiovascular problems such as hypertension or congestive heart failure, severe diabetes, debilitated patients, renal disease, blood dyscrasias, agranulocytosis, hemorrhagic diathesis, patients receiving radiation treatments, colitis, lupus erythematosus, pregnancy, lactation, children under 6 years of age. Patients with eczema or urticaria.

Special Concerns: Pregnancy category: C.

Side Effects: *Skin:* Dermatitis (most common), pruritus, erythema, dermatoses, gray to blue pigmentation of tissues, alopecia, loss of nails. *GI:* Stomatitis (second most common), metallic taste, gastritis, colitis, gingivitis, glossitis, nausea, vomiting, diarrhea (may be persistent), colic, anorexia, cramps, enterocolitis. *Hematologic:* Anemia, thrombocytopenia, granulocytopenia, leukopenia, eosinophilia, hemorrhagic diathesis. *Allergic:* Flushing, fainting, sweating, dizziness, anaphylaxis, syncope, bradycardia, angioneurotic edema, respiratory difficulties. *Other:* Interstitial pneumonitis, pulmonary fibrosis, nephrotic syndrome, glomerulitis (with hematuria), proteinuria, hepatitis, fever, headache, arthralgia, ophthalmologic problems including corneal ulcers, iritis, gold deposits, EEG abnormalities, peripheral neuritis.

Corticosteroids may be used to treat symptoms such as stomatitis, dermatitis, GI, renal, hematologic, or pulmonary problems. Also, if symptoms are severe and do not respond to corticosteroids, a chelating agent such as dimercaprol may be used. Patients should be monitored carefully.

Drug Interactions: Concomitant use contraindicated with drugs known to cause blood dyscrasias (e.g., antimalarials, cytotoxic drugs, pyrazolone derivatives, immunosuppressive drugs).

Laboratory Test Interference: Alters liver function tests. Urinary protein and RBCs, altered blood counts (indicative of toxic effect of drug).

Dosage: IM. *Rheumatoid arthritis.* **Adults,** week 1: 10 mg as a single injection; week 2: 25 mg as a single dose. Thereafter, 25–50 mg/week until 0.8–1 g total has been given. Thereafter according to individual response. *Usual maintenance:* 25–50 mg every other week for up to 20 weeks. If condition remains stable, the dose can be given every third or fourth week indefinitely. **Pediatric: initial,** *week 1:* 10 mg; **then,** usual dose is 1 mg/kg, not to exceed 50 mg/injection using the same spacing of doses as for adults.

NURSING CONSIDERATIONS

Administration/Storage

1. Shake vial well to ensure uniformity of suspension before withdrawing medication.
2. Inject into gluteus maximus.
3. Gold therapy may be reinstituted following mild toxic symptoms but not after severe symptoms.
4. Geriatric clients manifest a lower tolerance to gold.

Interventions

1. Have the client remain in a recumbent position for at least 20 min after the injection to prevent falls resulting from transient vertigo or giddiness.
2. Have dimercaprol (BAL) readily available to use as an antidote in case of severe toxicity.

Client/Family Teaching

1. Explain to client and family that close medical supervision is required during gold therapy.
2. Do not become discouraged. Stress that beneficial effects are slow to appear but that therapy may be continued for up to 12 months in anticipation of relief.

PENICILLAMINE   (peh-nih-**SIL**-ah-meen)

Cuprimine, Depen (Rx)

Classification: Antirheumatic, heavy metal antagonist, to treat cystinuria.

Action/Kinetics: Penicillamine, a degradation product of penicillin, is a chelating agent for mercury, lead, iron, and copper thus decreasing toxic levels of the metal (e.g. copper in Wilson's disease). The anti-inflammatory activity of penicillamine may be due to its ability to inhibit T-lymphocyte function and therefore decrease cell-mediated immune response. It may also protect lymphocytes from hydrogen peroxide generated at the site of inflammation by inhibiting release of lysosomal enzymes and oxygen radicals. In cystinuria, penicillamine is able to reduce excess cystine excretion, probably by disulfide interchange between penicillamine and cystine. This results in penicillamine-cysteine disulfide, which is a complex that is more soluble than cystine and is thus readily excreted. Penicillamine is well absorbed from the GI tract and is excreted in urine. **Peak plasma levels:** 1–3 hr. About 80% is bound to plasma albumin. **t½:** Approximately 2 hr. Metabolites are excreted through the urine. **It may take 2–3 months for positive responses to become apparent when treating rheumatoid arthritis.**

Uses: Wilson's disease, cystinuria, and rheumatoid arthritis—severe active disease that does not respond to conventional therapy. Heavy metal antagonist. *Investigational:* Primary biliary cirrhosis. Rheumatoid vasculitis, Felty's syndrome.

Contraindications: Pregnancy, lactation, penicillinase-related aplastic anemia or agranulocytosis, hypersensitivity to drug. Patients allergic to penicillin may cross-react with penicillamine. Renal insufficiency or history thereof.

Special Concerns: The use of penicillamine for juvenile rheumatoid arthritis has not been established. Patients older than 65 years may be at greater risk of developing hematologic side effects.

Side Effects: This drug manifests a large number of potentially serious side effects. Patients should be carefully monitored. *GI:* Altered taste perception (common), nausea, vomiting, diarrhea, anorexia, GI pain, stomatitis, oral ulcerations, reactivation of peptic ulcer, glossitis, cheilosis, colitis. *Hematologic:* Thrombocytopenia, leukopenia, agranulocytosis, aplastic anemia, eosinophilia, monocytosis, red cell aplasia, thrombocytopenia, hemolytic anemia, leukocytosis, thrombocytosis. *Renal:* Proteinuria, hematuria, nephrotic syndrome, Goodpasture's syndrome (a severe and ultimately fatal glomerulonephritis). *Allergic:* Rashes (common), lupus-like syndrome, pruritus, pemphigoid-type symptoms (e.g., bullous lesions), drug fever, arthralgia, lymphadenopathy, dermatoses, urticaria, obliterative bronchiolitis, thyroiditis, hypoglycemia, migratory polyarthralgia, polymyositis, allergic alveolitis. *Other:* Tinnitus, optic neuritis, neuropathy, thrombophlebitis, alopecia, precipitation of myasthenia gravis, increased body temperature, pulmonary fibrosis, pneumonitis, bronchial asthma, renal vasculitis (may be fatal), hot flashes, increased skin friability, pancreatitis, hepatic dysfunction, intrahepatic cholestasis.

Drug Interactions	
Antacids	↓ Effect of penicillamine due to ↓ absorption from GI tract
Digoxin	Penicillamine ↓ effect of digoxin
Iron salts	↓ Effect of penicillamine due to ↓ absorption from GI tract
Antimalarials, cytotoxic drugs, gold therapy, oxyphenbutazone, phenylbutazone	↑ Risk of blood dyscrasias and adverse renal effects

Laboratory Test Interferences: ↑ Serum alkaline phosphatase, LDH + thymol turbidity test and cephalin flocculation test.

Dosage: Capsules, Tablets. *Wilson's disease:* Dosage is usually calculated on the basis of the urinary excretion of copper. One gram of penicillamine promotes excretion of 2 mg of copper. **PO, adults and adolescents:** *usual, initial,* 250 mg q.i.d. Dosage may have to be increased to 2 g daily. A further increase does not produce additional excretion. **Pediatric, 6 months—young children:** 250 mg as a single dose given in fruit juice.

Antidote for heavy metals: **Adults,** 0.5–1.5 g daily for 1–2 months; **pediatric:** 30–40 mg/kg daily (600–750 mg/m² daily) for 1–6 months.

Cystinuria: individualized and based on excretion rate of cystine (100–200 mg/day in patients with no history of stones, below 100 mg with patients with history of stones or pain). Initiate at low dosage (250 mg/day) and increase gradually to minimum effective dosage. **Adult:** *Usual,* 2 g/day (range: 1–4 g/day); **pediatric:** 7.5 mg/kg q.i.d. If divided in fewer than 4 doses, give larger dose at night.

Rheumatoid arthritis: **PO, individualized: initial,** 125–250 mg/day. Dosage may be increased at 1- to 3-month intervals by 125- to 250-mg increments until adequate response is attained. **Maximum:** 500–750 mg/day. Up to 500 mg/day can be given as a single dose; higher dosages should be divided. **Maintenance:** Individualized. **Range:** 500–750 mg daily.

Primary biliary cirrhosis: 600–900 mg daily.

NURSING CONSIDERATIONS

Administration/Storage

1. Give penicillamine on an empty stomach 1 hr before or 2 hr after meals. Also wait 1 hr after ingestion of any other food, milk, or drug.
2. If client cannot tolerate dosage for cystinuria, the bedtime dosage should be larger and should be continued.
3. For treatment of cystinuria, the client should be advised to consume large amounts of fluid (e.g., 1 pint at bedtime and another pint during the night, since the urine is more concentrated and more acidic during the night).
4. Administer the contents of the capsule in 15–30 mL of chilled juice or pureed fruit if client is unable to swallow capsules or tablets.
5. The drug should be discontinued if doses of penicillamine up to 1.5 g/day for 2–3 months do not produce improvement when treating rheumatoid arthritis.

Assessment

1. Determine if the client has any allergies to penicillin. Document and report to the other health care providers.
2. Obtain baseline CBC, platelet count, and urinalysis prior to beginning therapy.
3. Assure that liver function tests are conducted prior to the start of therapy.
4. Determine if the client is taking any medication with which penicillamine will unfavorably interact.
5. Assess the client's hearing to detect any evidence of hearing loss and to serve as a baseline for further auditory testing throughout drug therapy.
6. Women of childbearing age, who are sexually active should be tested for pregnancy. Penicillamine is contraindicated during pregnancy because it can cause fetal damage.

Interventions

1. Monitor for changes in hearing and assess clients for alterations in vision.

2. Note client complaints of nausea, vomiting or diarrhea. Check for any alterations in taste. Monitor weight, intake and output and report persistent side effects to the physician.

3. Inspect the client's mucosal surfaces at regular intervals throughout the therapy. If ulcers appear and are severe or persistent, it may be necessary for the physician to reduce the dose of the drug.

4. Inspect the skin routinely. If skin changes occur these should be reported to the physician.

5. Routinely monitor the client's WBC and platelet counts. If the WBC count falls below 3,500/mm^3 or the platelet count falls below 100,000/mm^3, withhold the penicillamine and report these findings to the physician. If the counts are low for 3 successive laboratory tests, a temporary interruption of therapy is indicated.

6. Monitor liver function studies, especially if the client develops jaundice or demonstrates other signs of hepatic dysfunction.

7. White papules appearing at the site of venipuncture or at surgical sites may indicate sensitivity to penicillamine or the presence of infection. Check for signs of infection.

8. If the client is to undergo surgery, anticipate that the dosage of medication will be reduced to 250 mg/day until wound healing is complete. Anticipate that the physician may order vitamin B$_6$ prophylactically prior to and following surgery.

9. Clients may develop symptoms that suggest an antinuclear antibody test be conducted. A positive test indicates that the client may develop a lupus-like syndrome in the future. The drug need not be discontinued. Rather, the nurse needs to be aware of the potential and report any symptoms to the physician should they occur.

10. Penicillamine increases the body's need for pyridoxine. Therefore, pyridoxine should be ordered as a supplement.

11. If the client develops cystinuria, encourage a high fluid intake throughout the day and at bedtime.

12. For clients being treated for Wilson's disease, avoid multivitamin preparations containing copper.

Client/Family Teaching

1. Review with the client and family the goals of the therapy, the anticipated benefits, and provide them with a list of possible side effects.

2. Instruct clients to take their temperature nightly during the first few months of therapy. If a fever develops it may indicate a hypersensitivity reaction. Stress that the physician should be notified.

3. Any incidents of fever, sore throat, chills, bruising or bleeding need to be reported to the physician immediately. These are early symptoms of granulocytopenia.

4. If stomatitis occurs, it needs to be reported immediately and the drug discontinued. Instruct the client on oral hygiene such as brushing the teeth with a soft tooth brush, flossing daily and using mouth rinses free of alcohol.

5. Taste perception may become blurred. This may last for 2 or more months. Encourage the client to maintain adequate nutrition throughout, noting that nutrition is important and that the condition is usually self-limiting.

6. If the client is to receive an oral iron preparation, at least 2 hr should elapse between ingestion of penicillamine and the dose of therapeutic iron. Iron decreases the cupruretic effects of penicillamine.

7. The skin of clients taking penicillamine tends to become friable and susceptible to injury. Caution clients to avoid activities that could injure the skin. When working with elderly clients teach them how to avoid excessive pressure on the shoulders, elbows, knees, toes, and buttocks. Instruct clients to report all skin changes to the physician for evaluation.

8. Advise clients to report cloudy urine, or urine that is smoky brown in color. These are signs of proteinuria and hematuria and may require withdrawal of the drug.

9. Women of childbearing age should be instructed to practice a safe form of birth control. If the client misses a menstrual period or has other symptoms of pregnancy, it should be reported to the physician.

10. If the drug is used to treat clients with Wilson's disease they should be advised as follows:
   - Eat a diet low in copper. Exclude foods such as chocolate, nuts, shellfish, mushrooms, liver, molasses, broccoli, and copper-enriched cereals.
   - Use distilled or demineralized water if the drinking water contains more than 0.1 mg/L copper.
   - Unless the client is taking iron supplements, take sulfurated potash or Carbo-Resin with meals to minimize the absorption of copper.
   - It may take 1–3 months for neurologic improvements to occur. Therefore, continue the therapy even if no improvements seem evident.
   - Check any vitamin preparations being used to ensure that they do not contain copper.

11. If a client develops cystinuria advise the following:
   - Drink large amounts of fluid to prevent the formation of renal calculi. Drink 500 ml of fluid at bedtime, and another pint during the night, when the urine tends to be the most concentrated and most acidic.
   - Teach client how to measure specific gravity and determine pH. The urine specific gravity should be maintained at less than 1.010 and the pH maintained at 7.5–8.0.
   - Advise clients to have a yearly x-ray of the kidneys to detect the presence of renal calculi.
   - Eat a diet low in methionine, a major precursor of cystine. Exclude from the diet foods high in cystine such as, rich meat soups and broths, milk, eggs, cheeses, and peas.
   - If the client is pregnant or is a child, a diet low in methionine is also low in calcium. Therefore, such a diet is contraindicated in these instances.

12. If the client has rheumatoid arthritis, advise them to continue using other approaches to achieve relief from their symptoms since penicillamine may take up to 6 months to have a therapeutic effect.

Evaluation

1. Review with the client the goals of therapy and assess the progress with this drug therapy.
2. Observe for freedom from complications of drug therapy.
3. Note even small improvements in the client's condition and offer continued encouragement and support.
4. Review the prescribed therapeutic regimen and assess client compliance. Stress the need to adhere to all aspects of the program in order to obtain a positive clinical response.

MISCELLANEOUS AGENT

HYDROXYCHLOROQUINE SULFATE   (hi-**DROX**-ee-**KLOR**-oh-kwin)

Plaquenil (Rx)

See also *4-Aminoquinolines,* p. 241.

Classification: 4-Aminoquinoline, antimalarial and antirheumatic.

Action/Kinetics: Hydroxychloroquine is not a drug of choice for rheumatoid arthritis and should be discontinued after 6–12 months if no beneficial effects are noted. It is thought to act by suppression of formation of antigens, which leads to hypersensitivity reactions. These reactions cause the symptoms of the disease.

Peak plasma levels: 1–3 hr. Unchanged drug is excreted in the urine. Excretion may be enhanced by acidifying the urine and decreased by alkalinizing the urine.

Patients on long-term therapy should be examined thoroughly at regular intervals for knee and ankle reflexes and hematopoietic studies. *Drug may cause retinopathy;* thus, baseline ophthalmologic examinations, repeated at 3-month intervals, must be performed and the drug discontinued in the event of ophthalmic damage, impaired reflexes, and blood dyscrasias.

Treatment of toxic symptoms: Administration of 8 g ammonium chloride in divided doses 3 to 4 times/week for several months to improve residual excretion of drug.

Uses: Antimalarial, antirheumatic, discoid and lupus erythematosus. Not used as a first line of therapy.

Additional Contraindications: Long-term therapy in children, ophthalmologic changes due to 4-aminoquinolines.

Special Concerns: Use with caution in alcoholism or liver disease.

Additional Side Effects: The appearances of skin eruptions or of misty vision and visual halos are indications for withdrawal.

Drug Interaction	
Digoxin	Hydroxychloroquine ↑ serum digoxin levels
Gold salts	Dermatitis and ↑ risk of severe skin reactions
Phenylbutazone	Dermatitis and ↑ risk of severe skin reactions

Dosage: Tablets. *Acute malarial attack:* **Adults, initial,** 800 mg; **then,** 400 mg after 6–8 hr and 400 mg/day for next 2 days. **Children:** A total of 32 mg/kg given over a three day period as follows: **initial,** 12.9 mg/kg (not to exceed a single dose of 800 mg); **then,** 6.4 mg/kg (not to exceed a single dose of 400 mg) 6, 24, and 48 hr after the first dose. *Suppression of malaria:* **Adults,** 400 mg q 7 days. If therapy has not been initiated 14 days prior to exposure, an initial loading dose of 800 mg may be given in 2 divided doses 6 hr apart. **Children:** 6.4 mg/kg (not to exceed the adult dose) q 7 days. If therapy has not been initiated 14 days prior to exposure, an initial loading dose of 12.9 mg/kg may be given in 2 doses 6 hr apart.

Rheumatoid arthritis: **Adults,** 400–600 mg daily taken with milk or meals; *maintenance* (usually after 4–12 weeks): 200–400 mg daily. (*Note:* Several months may be required for a beneficial effect to be seen). *Lupus erythematosus:* **Adults, usual,** 400 mg once or twice daily; **prolonged maintenance:** 200–400 mg daily.

NURSING CONSIDERATIONS

See also *Nursing Considerations* for *4-Aminoquinolines,* p. 242, and *General Nursing Considerations for All Anti-Infectives* under *Penicillins,* p. 140.

Assessment

1. Note if the client is receiving gold therapy. Hydroxychloroquine increases the incidence of skin reactions when administered in conjunction with gold therapy.
2. Obtain a baseline neurological examination and determine the client's mental status prior to initiating therapy.

3. Determine any evidence of muscular or tendon weakness before instituting therapy.

4. Obtain audiometric and ophthalmic examinations prior to beginning therapy.

5. Note the medications the client is currently receiving and determine if any of these medications interact unfavorably with hydroxychloroquine.

Interventions

1. Repeat audiometric and ophthalmic examinations routinely throughout drug therapy. Changes should be recorded and reported to the physician.

2. Note any client complaints of nausea, vomiting or persistent diarrhea. Gastric irritation may be relieved by administering the medication with a glass of milk or with meals. However, if the problems persist, notify the physician and anticipate that the dosage of drug may be changed.

3. Reassure the client and indicate that benefits from the medication may not occur until 6 to 12 months after initiation of therapy.

4. Side effects may necessitate a reduction of therapy. After 5 to 10 days of reduced dosage of medication, the amount may be increased gradually to the desired level.

5. Once the desired response has been obtained, the dosage of drug will likely be reduced. This enables the drug to be effective at a later date, if the conditions recurs.

6. The physician may use corticosteroids and salicylates concomitantly.

7. Monitor the clients muscle strength and tendon reflexes at regular intervals. Record the results and report them as well as any other signs of weakness to the physician.

8. When the drug is being administered for lupus erythematosus, administer it with the evening meal.

9. When the drug is being used to suppress malaria, therapy should be initiated 2 weeks prior to exposure and should be continued for 6 to 8 weeks after leaving the endemic area. If the therapy is not started prior to exposure, the initial loading dose should be doubled. Adults should receive 620 mg as the base. Children should receive 10 mg/kg as the base. The doses of medication are given in 2 doses, 6 hours apart.

Client/Family Teaching

1. Advise clients to report any changes in vision to the physician.

2. Instruct clients to report any skin changes or pruritus to the physician.

3. Discuss the potential for developing photosensitivity. Advise the client to avoid undue exposure to the sun, to wear protective clothing and to apply sunscreens if exposure is necessary.

CHAPTER FORTY

Antigout Agents

General Statement: Gout or gouty arthritis is characterized by an excess of uric acid in the body. This excess results either from an overproduction of uric acid or from a defect in its breakdown or elimination.

When the concentration of sodium urate in the blood exceeds a certain level (6 mg in 100 mL), it may start to form fine, needle-like crystals that can become deposited in the joints and cause an acute inflammatory response in the synovial membrane. Hyperuricemia may also accompany other diseases such as leukemia or lymphomas. High levels of uric acid may also accompany treatment with certain antineoplastic agents or thiazide diuretics. High uric acid levels in the kidney may lead to precipitation of uric acid crystals, which can cause kidney damage.

Therapy is aimed at reducing the uric acid level of the body to normal or near-normal levels. Drugs used for the treatment of gout or hyperuricemia either promote the excretion of uric acid by the kidney or reduce the amount of uric acid formed. These drugs, however, have no analgesic or anti-inflammatory properties although colchicine will decrease urate crystal-induced inflammation.

Previously, gout was often treated by dietary measures—reduced intake of purine-rich foods such as meat. Dietary restrictions are seldom prescribed today, except for organ meats, which have a high purine content.

Acute gout. As opposed to other forms of arthritis, acute gout has a dramatic onset. Maximum pain, joint swelling, and joint tenderness are reached within hours. An acute attack of gout is often accompanied by a low-grade fever and an increase in the WBC count.

In between attacks the patient with hyperuricemia is usually symptom-free; however, since acute attacks usually recur in patients with hyperuricemia, patients are often kept on a maintenance dose of a uricosuric agent.

ALLOPURINOL   (al-low-**PYOUR**-ih-nol)

Alloprin ✿, Apo-Allopurinol ✿, Lopurin, Novopurol ✿, Purinol ✿, Zurinol, Zyloprim (Rx)

Classification: Antigout agent.

Action/Kinetics: Allopurinol and its major metabolite, oxipurinol, are potent inhibitors of xanthine oxidase, an enzyme involved in the synthesis of uric acid, without disrupting the biosynthesis of essential purine. This results in decreased levels of uric acid. The drug also increases reutilization of xanthine and hypoxanthine for synthesis of nucleotide and nucleic acid synthesis by acting on the enzyme hypoxanthine-guanine phosphoribosyltransferase. The resultant increases in nucleotides cause a negative feedback to inhibit synthesis of purines and a decrease in uric acid levels. **Peak plasma levels:** 2–6 hr for oxipurinol. **Onset:** 2–3 days. $t\frac{1}{2}$ (allopurinol); 1–3 hr; $t\frac{1}{2}$ (oxipurinol): 12–30 hr. **Peak serum levels, allopurinol:** 2–3 mcg/mL; **oxipurinol:** 5–6.5 mcg/mL (up to 50 mcg/mL in patients with impaired renal function). **Maximum therapeutic**

effect: 1–3 weeks. Well absorbed from GI tract, metabolized in liver, excreted in urine.

Uses: Not useful for the treatment of *acute* gout, but is the drug of choice for *chronic* gouty arthritis. Gout, hyperuricemia associated with polycythemia vera, myeloid metaplasia or other blood dyscrasias, and certain cases of primary and secondary renal disease. Prophylaxis in hyperuricemia and as an adjunct in some antineoplastic therapy. Recurrent calcium oxalate calculi.

Allopurinol is sometimes administered concomitantly with uricosuric agents in patients with severe tophaceous gout. (A tophus is a deposit of sodium urate.)

Contraindications: Hypersensitivity to drug. Patients with idiopathic hemochromatosis or relatives of patients suffering from this condition. Children except as an adjunct in treatment of neoplastic disease. Severe skin reactions on previous exposure.

Special Concerns: Pregnancy category: C. Use with caution in patients with liver or renal disease. Use with caution during lactation. In children use has been limited to rare inborn errors of purine metabolism or hyperuricemia as a result of malignancy or cancer therapy.

Side Effects: *Dermatologic* (most frequent): Pruritic maculopapular skin rash (may be accompanied by fever and malaise). Exfoliative urticarial, purpura-type dermatitis and alopecia. Stevens-Johnson syndrome. Skin rash has been accompanied by hypertension and cataract development. *Allergy:* Fever, chills, leukopenia, eosinophilia, arthralgia, skin rash, pruritus, nausea, vomiting, nephritis.

Drug Interactions	
Ampicillin	Concomitant use may result in skin rashes
Anticoagulants, oral	↑ Effect of anticoagulant due to ↓ breakdown by liver
Azathioprine	↑ Effect of azathioprine due to ↓ breakdown by liver
Iron preparations	Allopurinol ↑ hepatic iron concentrations
Mercaptopurine	↑ Effect of mercaptopurine due to ↓ breakdown by liver
Theophylline	Allopurinol ↑ plasma theophylline levels

Laboratory Test Interferences: Alters liver function test. ↑ Serum cholesterol. ↓ Serum glucose levels.

Dosage: Tablets. *Gout/hyperuricemia:* **Adults,** 200–600 mg/day, depending on severity (minimum effective dose: 100–200 mg/day). *Prevention of uric acid nephropathy during treatment of neoplasms:* 600–800 mg/day for 2–3 days (with high fluid intake). *Prophylaxis of acute gout:* **initial,** 100 mg/day; increase by 100 mg at weekly intervals until serum uric acid level of 6 mg/100 mL or less is reached. **Pediatric,** *Hyperuricemia associated with malignancy,* **6–10 years of age:** 300 mg/day either as a single dose of 100 mg t.i.d.; **under 6 years of age:** 150 mg/day in 3 divided doses. *Recurrent calcium oxalate calculi:* 200–300 mg daily in one or more doses (dose may be adjusted according to urinary levels of uric acid).

Transfer from colchicine, uricosuric agents and/or anti-inflammatory agents to allopurinol should be made gradually by decreasing the dosage of the above agents and increasing the dosage of allopurinol.

NURSING CONSIDERATIONS

Administration/Storage

1. Administer with food or immediately after meals to lessen potential gastric irritation.

40

2. At least 10–12 eight-ounce glasses of fluid should be taken each day.

3. To prevent the formation of uric acid stones, the urine should be kept slightly alkaline.

Assessment

1. Take a complete drug history, noting any medications that might interact with allopurinol.

2. Review client orders; determine if the client is scheduled for diagnostic tests with which allopurinol would interact.

3. If the client is female and of childbearing age and sexually active, or if the woman is nursing, allopurinol is contraindicated.

Interventions

1. If the client has been taking a uricosuric agent and is to be placed on allopurinol, anticipate that the dosage of the uricosuric agent will be gradually decreased as the dosage of allopurinol is gradually increased.

2. Assess the client for changes in vision. If such changes occur, advise the client to have an ophthalmologic exam.

3. Monitor the CBC with differential, platelet count, liver and renal function studies and serum uric acid on a routine basis during therapy.

4. Dosage should be decreased with renal impairment.

Client/Family Teaching

1. Advise clients to monitor their weight if they are experiencing nausea and vomiting or other signs of gastric irritation. If the condition persists and the client notes weight loss, report to the physician.

2. If a skin rash occurs, report to the physician. Skin rashes may start after months of drug therapy. If they are caused by allopurinol, the drug needs to be discontinued.

3. Unless otherwise indicated, advise clients to maintain a fluid intake that will result in a minimum excretion of 2 L of urine daily. This will assist to prevent kidney damage.

4. Advise clients not to take iron salts while they are taking allopurinol. High concentrations of iron may occur in the liver.

5. Avoid excessive intake of vitamin C, which may lead to increased potential for the formation of kidney stones.

6. Avoid alcoholic beverages. These decrease the effect of allopurinol.

7. Take medication at or following meal time to decrease GI upset.

8. Provide the client with a printed list of foods to avoid.

COLCHICINE   (KOHL-chih-seen)

(Rx)

Classification: Antigout agent.

Action/Kinetics: Colchicine, an alkaloid, does not increase the excretion of uric acid (not uricosuric), but it is believed to reduce the crystal-induced inflammation by reducing lactic acid production by leukocytes (resulting in a decreased deposition of sodium urate), by inhibiting leukocyte migration, and by reducing phagocytosis. The drug may also inhibit the synthesis of kinins and leukotrienes. $t\frac{1}{2}$, (IV, biphasic), initial: 20 min; final (in leukocytes): 60 hr. **Onset, IV:** 6–12 hr; **PO:** 12 hr. **Time to peak levels, PO:** 0.5–2 hr. Colchicine is metabolized in liver and mainly excreted in the feces with 10–20% excreted through the urine.

Uses: Prophylaxis and treatment of acute attacks of gout, either spontaneous or induced by allopurinol or uricosuric agents. Diagnosis of gout. *Investigational:* Amyloidosis, Paget's disease, dermatitis herpetiformis. Prophylaxis and treatment of acute, familial Mediterranean fever.

Special Concerns: Pregnancy category: D. Use with caution during lactation. Dosage has not been established for children. Geriatric patients may be at greater risk of developing cumulative toxicity. Use with extreme caution for elderly, debilitated patients, especially in the presence of chronic renal, hepatic, GI, or cardiovascular disease.

Side Effects: The drug is toxic; thus patients must be carefully monitored. Nausea, vomiting, diarrhea, abdominal cramping (discontinue drug at once and wait at least 48 hr before reinstating drug therapy). Prolonged administration can cause bone marrow depression, thrombocytopenia and aplastic anemia, peripheral neuritis, and liver dysfunction.

Acute colchicine intoxication is characterized at first by violent GI tract symptoms such as nausea, vomiting, abdominal pain, and diarrhea. The latter may be profuse, watery, bloody, and associated with severe fluid and electrolyte loss. Also, burning of throat and skin, hematuria and oliguria, rapid and weak pulse, general exhaustion, muscular depression, and CNS involvement. Death is usually caused by respiratory paralysis. Treatment of acute poisoning involves gastric lavage, symptomatic support, including atropine and morphine, artificial respiration, hemodialysis, peritoneal dialysis, and treatment of shock.

Drug Interactions	
Acidifying agents	Inhibit the action of colchicine
Alkalinizing agents	Potentiate the action of colchicine
CNS depressants	Patients on colchicine may be more sensitive to CNS depressant effect of these drugs
Sympathomimetic agents	Enhanced by colchicine
Vitamin B_{12}	Colchicine may interfere with absorption from the gut

Laboratory Test Interferences: Alters liver function tests. ↑ Alkaline phosphatase. False + for hemoglobin or red blood cells in urine.

Dosage: Tablets. Adults: *Acute attack of gout,* 0.5–1.2 mg followed by 0.5–1.3 mg initially q 1–2 hr until pain is relieved or nausea, vomiting, or diarrhea occurs. **Total amount required:** 4–8 mg. *Prophylaxis for gout:* 0.5–0.65 mg t.i.d. *Prophylaxis for surgical patients:* 0.5–0.65 mg t.i.d. for 3 days before and 3 days after surgery.

IV: Adults, initial, *acute attack of gout:* 2 mg; **subsequently,** 0.5 mg q 6 hr until pain is relieved; give up to 4 mg. (Some physicians recommend a single IV dose of 3 mg.) *Prophylaxis:* **PO:** 0.5–1 mg 1–2 times daily for 3–4 days/week. Usually, oral route is used exclusively.

NURSING CONSIDERATIONS

Administration/Storage

1. Store in tight, light-resistant containers.
2. Parenteral administration is only to be by IV route. Drug would cause severe local irritation if given SC or IM.

Assessment

1. Note age and general physical condition of the client.
2. Obtain baseline hepatic studies, prior to initiating therapy.

Interventions

1. If the client develops nausea, vomiting, or diarrhea, notify the physician and discontinue the drug. These are early signs of toxicity.
2. If severe diarrhea occurs, anticipate the use of paregoric.
3. If the drug is administered IV, have atropine readily available to counteract adverse effects.
4. Assess the client for evidence of liver damage such as jaundice and a change in stool color. Monitor liver function studies and report any abnormal results.

Client/Family Teaching

1. If the physician has prescribed colchicine for use in acute attacks of gout, instruct the client to always have colchicine available.
2. Start or increase the dosage of colchicine as ordered at the first sign of joint pain or any other symptom of an impending attack of gout.

PROBENECID   (proh-**BEN**-ih-sid)

Benemid, Benuryl✸, Parbenem, Probalan (Rx)

Classification: Antigout agent, uricosuric agent.

Action/Kinetics: Probenecid, a uricosuric agent, increases the excretion of uric acid by inhibiting the tubular reabsorption of uric acid; this action results in a decreased serum level of uric acid. Probenecid also inhibits the renal secretion of penicillins and cephalosporins; this effect is often taken advantage of in the treatment of infections, since concomitant administration of probenecid will increase plasma levels of antibiotics. **Peak plasma levels:** 2–4 hr. **Time to peak effect, uricosuric:** 0.5 hr; **for suppression of penicillin excretion:** 2 hr. **Therapeutic plasma levels for inhibition of antibiotic secretion:** 40–60 mcg/mL; **therapeutic plasma levels for uricosuric effect:** 100–200 mcg/mL. **t½:** 8–10 hr. **Duration for inhibition of penicillin excretion:** 8 hr. Probenecid is metabolized in the liver and is excreted in urine (5%–10% unchanged). Excretion is increased in alkaline urine.

Uses: Hyperuricemia in chronic gout and gouty arthritis. Adjunct in therapy with penicillins or cephalosporins to elevate and prolong plasma antibiotic levels.

Contraindications: Hypersensitivity to drug, blood dyscrasias, uric acid, and kidney stones. Use for hyperuricemia in neoplastic disease or its treatment. Not recommended for use in children less than 2 years of age.

Special Concerns: Use during pregnancy only if benefits clearly outweigh risks. Administer with caution to patients with renal disease. Use with caution in porphyria, glucose-6-phosphate dehydrogenase deficiency, and peptic ulcer.

Side Effects: *CNS:* Headaches, dizziness. *GI:* Anorexia, nausea, vomiting, diarrhea, constipation, and abdominal discomfort. *Allergic:* Skin rash or drug fever, and rarely anaphylactoid reactions. *Miscellaneous:* Flushing, hemolytic anemia, nephrotic syndrome, sore gums.
   Initially, the drug may increase frequency of acute gout attacks due to mobilization of uric acid.

Drug Interactions

Acyclovir	Probenecid ↓ renal excretion of acyclovir
Aminosalicylic acid (PAS)	↑ Effects of PAS due to ↓ excretion by kidney
Captopril	↑ Effect of captopril due to ↓ excretion by kidney
Cephalosporins	↑ Effect of cephalosporins due to ↓ excretion by kidney
Ciprofloxacin	50% ↑ in systemic levels of ciprofloxacin
Clofibrate	↑ Effect of clofibrate due to ↓ excretion and ↓ plasma protein binding
Dyphylline	↑ Effect of dyphylline due to ↓ excretion by kidney
Indomethacin	↑ Effect of indomethacin due to ↓ excretion by kidney
Methotrexate	↑ Effect of methotrexate due to ↓ excretion by kidney
Naproxen	↑ Effect of naproxen due to ↓ excretion by kidney
Penicillins	↑ Effect of penicillins due to ↓ excretion by kidney
Pyrazinamide	Probenecid inhibits hyperuricemia produced by pyrazinamide
Rifampin	↑ Effect of rifampin due to ↓ excretion by kidney
Salicylates	Salicylates inhibit uricosuric activity of probenecid
Sulfinpyrazone	↑ Effect of sulfinpyrazone due to ↓ excretion by kidney
Sulfonamides	↑ Effect of sulfonamides due to ↓ plasma protein binding
Sulfonylureas, oral	↑ Action of sulfonylureas → hypoglycemia
Thiopental	↑ Effect of thiopental

Dosage: Tablets. Adults: *Gout,* **PO, initial:** 250 mg b.i.d. for 1 week. **Maintenance:** 500 mg b.i.d. Dosage may have to be increased further (by 500 mg daily q 4 weeks to maximum of 2 g) until urate excretion is less than 700 mg in 24 hr. *Adjunct to penicillin or cephalosporin therapy:* 500 mg q.i.d. Dosage is decreased for elderly patients with renal damage. **Pediatric, 2–14 years, initial:** 25 mg/kg (or 700 mg/m^2); **maintenance,** 10 mg/kg q.i.d. (or 300 mg/m^2 q.i.d.). **For children 50 kg or more:** give adult dosage. Colbenemid, a combination tablet containing colchicine (0.5 mg) and probenecid (500 mg), is available. *Gonorrhea:* **Adults:** 1 g (as a single dose) 30 min before penicillin; **pediatric, less than 45 kg:** 25 mg/kg (up to a maximum of 1 g) with appropriate antibiotic therapy.

NURSING CONSIDERATIONS

Assessment

Note if the client has diabetes mellitus. There may be false-positive urine tests if cupric sulfate reagents such as Benedict's Qualitative Reagent are used.

Interventions

1. Anticipate that sodium bicarbonate may be used to maintain an alkaline urine to prevent urates from crystallizing and forming kidney stones.
2. Use Tes-Tape for urine tests in those clients who have diabetes mellitus.
3. For accurate blood glucose level determinations, finger sticks may be indicated for clients with diabetes.
4. Promptly report any gastric intolerance so that dosage may be corrected without loss of therapeutic effect.
5. Be alert to hypersensitivity reactions that occur more frequently with intermittent therapy.
6. Assess for toxic plasma levels in clients whose excretion is inhibited by probenecid. Make appropriate dosage adjustments.
7. Observe client for skin rash, flushing or client complaints of increased sweating, headaches or dizziness. Document and report to the physician.
8. Monitor CBC, liver and renal function studies on a regular basis. Report any abnormal findings to the physician.

Client/Family Teaching

1. Take the drug with food to minimize gastric irritation.
2. Take a liberal amount of fluid to prevent the formation of sodium urate stones.
3. Note if there is any increase in the number of acute attacks of gout at the initiation of therapy. The physician may decide to add colchicine to the regimen.
4. Continue to take probenecid during acute attacks along with colchicine, as ordered, unless specifically told by the physician to discontinue the use of probenecid.
5. Do not take salicylates during uricosuric therapy. Acetaminophen preparations may be used for analgesic purposes.

SULFINPYRAZONE (sul-fin-PIE-rah-zohn)

Antazone ✤, Anturane, Apo-Sulfinpyrazone ✤, Novopyrazone ✤, (Rx)

Classification: Antigout agent, uricosuric.

Action/Kinetics: Sulfinpyrazone inhibits the tubular reabsorption of uric acid, thereby increasing its excretion. Sulfinpyrazone also manifests antithrombotic and platelet inhibitory actions. **Peak plasma levels:** 1–2 hr. **Therapeutic plasma levels:** Up to 160 mcg/mL following 800 mg daily for uricosuria. **Duration:** 4–6 hr (up to 10 hr in some). **t½:** 3–8 hr. Sulfinpyrazone is metabolized by the liver. Approximately 45% of the drug is excreted unchanged by the kidney, and a small amount is excreted in the feces.

Uses: Chronic gouty arthritis to reduce frequency and intensity of acute attacks of gout; hyperuricemia. Sulfinpyrazone is not effective during acute attacks of gout and may even increase the frequency of acute episodes during the initiation of therapy. However, the drug should not be discontinued during acute attacks. Concomitant administration of colchicine during initiation of therapy is recommended. *Investigational:* To decrease sudden death during first year after myocardial infarction.

Contraindications: Active peptic ulcer. Blood dyscrasias. Sensitivity to phenylbutazone.

Special Concerns: Use with caution in pregnant women. Dosage has not been established in children. Use with extreme caution in patients with impaired renal function and in those with a history of peptic ulcers.

Side Effects: *GI:* Nausea, vomiting, abdominal discomfort. May reactivate peptic ulcer. *Hematologic:* Leukopenia, agranulocytosis, anemia, thrombocytopenia. *Miscellaneous:* Skin rash, which usually disappears with usage.

Acute attacks of gout may become more frequent during initial therapy. Give concomitantly with colchicine at this time.

Drug Interactions	
Anticoagulants	↑ Effect of anticoagulants due to ↓ plasma protein binding
Insulin	Potentiation of hypoglycemic effect
Probenecid	↑ Effect of sulfinpyrazone due to ↓ excretion by kidney
Salicylates	Inhibit uricosuric effect of sulfinpyrazone
Sulfonamides	↑ Effect of sulfonamides by ↓ plasma protein binding
Sulfonylureas, oral	Potentiation of hypoglycemic effect

Dosage: Capsules, Tablets. Adults: initial, 200–400 mg/day in 2 divided doses with meals. Patients who are transferred from other uricosuric agents can receive full dose at once. **Maintenance:** 100–400 mg b.i.d. Maintain full dosage without interruption even during acute attacks of gout. *Following myocardial infarction:* 200 mg q.i.d.

NURSING CONSIDERATIONS

Administration/Storage

1. At least 10–12 eight-ounce glasses of fluid should be taken daily.
2. Acidification of the urine may cause formation of uric acid stones.

Client/Family Teaching

1. Advise clients to take a liberal amount of fluid to prevent the formation of uric acid stones.
2. Explain that sodium bicarbonate may be ordered to alkalinize the urine. This is to prevent urates from crystallizing in acid urine and forming kidney stones.
3. Take the drug with meals, milk or with an antacid to minimize gastric irritation.

CHAPTER FORTY-ONE

Anorexiants, Analeptics, and Agents for Attention Deficit Disorders

General Statement: It is difficult to separate the CNS stimulants into rigid pharmacologic classes because their effect is dose-dependent. For example, any agent with primarily cerebral action will stimulate respiration, because respiratory control centers are located in the brain stem. Moreover, they can induce paradoxical reactions that are taken advantage of pharmacologically. For example, certain CNS stimulants have a quieting effect on children who suffer from hyperkinesia or other behavior problems of neurologic rather than psychologic origin. (These conditions are called attention deficit disorders.) These agents and other CNS stimulants can be beneficial for patients suffering from extrapyramidal motor symptoms and spasticity.

The effect of these drugs is often not limited to the CNS. For example, the cardiovascular and autonomic nervous systems may also be affected; such effects are unwanted when the primary goal is stimulation of the CNS.

Even though there is a great deal of overlap among the indications for the various CNS stimulants, they have been divided according to their main clinical uses or pharmacologic action into *Anorexiants, Analeptics,* and *Agents for Attention Deficit Disorders.* Spinal cord stimulants cause convulsions and are not used clinically; thus, they are not discussed.

ANOREXIANTS, AMPHETAMINES, AND DERIVATIVES

Action/Kinetics: Response to amphetamines is individualized. Psychic stimulation is often followed by a rebound effect manifested as fatigue. Tolerance will develop to all drugs of this class. The slight differences in the pharmacologic and untoward reactions of the different anorexiants (appetite suppression, respiratory stimulation, length of action) dictate their principal use.

These drugs are thought to act on the cerebral cortex and reticular activating system (including the medullary, respiratory, and vasomotor centers) by releasing norepinephrine from adrenergic neurons, blocking reuptake from the synapse, and inhibiting the activity of monoamine oxidase. The stimulatory effect on the CNS causes an increase in motor activity and mental alertness, a mood-elevating effect, a slight euphoric effect, and an anorexigenic effect. The anorexigenic effect is thought to be produced by direct stimulation of the satiety center in the limbic and hypothalamic areas of the brain. Amphetamines are readily absorbed from the GI tract and are distributed throughout most tissues, with the highest concentrations in the brain and CSF. Duration of anorexia (PO): 3–6 hr. Metabolized in liver and excreted by kidneys.

Uses: See individual drugs.

Contraindications: Hyperthyroidism, nephritis, diabetes mellitus, hypertension, narrow-angle glaucoma, angina pectoris, cardiovascular disease, and patients with hypersensitivity to these drugs. Use in emotionally unstable persons susceptible to drug abuse. Psychotic children. Appetite suppressants in children less than 12 years of age.

Special Concerns: Pregnancy category, amphetamines: C. To be used with caution in patients suffering from hyperexcitability states; in elderly, debilitated, or asthenic patients; and in patients with psychopathic personality traits or a history of homicidal or suicidal tendencies.

Side Effects: *CNS:* Nervousness, dizziness, depression, headache, insomnia, euphoria, symptoms of excitation. Rarely, psychoses. In children, manifestation of vocal and motor tics and Tourette's syndrome. *GI:* Nausea, vomiting, cramps, diarrhea, dry mouth, constipation, metallic taste, anorexia. *CV:* Arrhythmias, palpitations, dyspnea, pulmonary hypertension, peripheral hyper- or hypotension, precordial pain, fainting. *Dermatologic:* Symptoms of allergy including rash, urticaria, erythema, burning. Pallor. *GU:* Urinary frequency, dysuria. *Ophthalmologic:* Blurred vision, mydriasis. *Hematologic:* Agranulocytosis, leukopenia. *Endocrine:* Menstrual irregularities, gynecomastia, impotence, and changes in libido. *Miscellaneous:* Alopecia, increased motor activity, fever, sweating, chills, muscle pain, chest pain.

Long-term use results in psychic dependence, as well as a high degree of tolerance.

Toxic Reactions

There is a relatively wide margin of safety between the therapeutic and toxic doses of amphetamines. However, amphetamines can cause both acute and chronic toxicity. Amphetamines are excreted slowly (5 to 7 days), and cumulative effects may occur with continued administration.

Acute toxicity (overdosage) is characterized by cardiovascular symptoms (flushing, pallor, palpitations, labile pulse, changes in BP, heart block, or chest pains), hyperpyrexia, mental disturbances (confusion, delirium, acute psychoses, disorientation, delusions and hallucinations, panic states, paranoid ideation).

Death usually results from cardiovascular collapse or convulsions.

Chronic toxicity due to abuse is characterized by emotional lability, loss of appetite, somnolence, mental impairment, occupational deterioration, a tendency to withdraw from social contact, teeth grinding, continuous chewing, and ulcers of the tongue and lips.

Prolonged use of high doses can elicit symptoms of paranoid schizophrenia, including auditory and visual hallucinations and paranoid ideation.

41

Treatment of Acute Toxicity (Overdosage): Symptomatic treatment. After oral ingestion, induce emesis or perform gastric lavage, followed by use of activated charcoal. Adequate circulation and respiration should be maintained. Hyperpyrexia and other CNS symptoms may be treated with chlorpromazine. Diazepam or a barbiturate may be given for sedation. Phentolamine may be used for hypertension, while hypotension may be reversed by IV fluids and possibly vasopressors (used with caution). Stimuli should be reduced and the patient is maintained in a quiet, dim environment. Patients who have ingested an overdose of long-acting products should be treated for toxicity until all symptoms of overdosage have disappeared.

Drug Interactions	
Acetazolamide	↑ Effect of amphetamine by ↑ renal tubular reabsorption
Ammonium chloride	↓ Effect of amphetamine by ↓ renal tubular reabsorption
Anesthetics, general	↑ Risk of cardiac arrhythmias
Antihypertensives	Amphetamines ↓ effect of antihypertensives
Ascorbic acid	↓ Effect of amphetamine by ↓ renal tubular reabsorption
Furazolidone	↑ Toxicity of anorexiants
Guanethidine	↓ Effect of guanethidine by displacement from its site of action
Haloperidol	↓ Effect of amphetamine by ↓ uptake of drug at its site of action
Insulin	Amphetamines alter insulin requirements
MAO inhibitors	All peripheral, metabolic, cardiac, and central effects of amphetamine are potentiated for up to 2 weeks after termination of MAO inhibitor therapy (symptoms include hypertensive crisis with possible intracranial hemorrhage, hyperthermia, convulsions, coma); death may occur. ↓ Effect of amphetamine by ↓ uptake of drug into its site of action
Methyldopa	↓ Hypotensive effect of methyldopa by ↑ sympathomimetic activity
Phenothiazines	↓ Effect of amphetamine by ↓ uptake of drug at its site of action
Sodium bicarbonate	↑ Effect of amphetamine by ↑ renal tubular reabsorption
Thiazide diuretics	↑ Effect of amphetamine by ↑ renal tubular reabsorption

Laboratory Test Interference: ↑ Urinary catecholamines.

Dosage: Individualized. Many compounds are timed-release preparations.

NURSING CONSIDERATIONS

Administration/Storage

1. If the drug is prescribed to suppress the appetite, administer 30 minutes before meals.
2. The initial dose should be small, then increased gradually as necessary, for the individual.

3. Unless otherwise ordered by the physician, the last dose of drug for the day should be administered at least 6 hours before the client retires.

Assessment

1. Obtain a complete drug history. Identify the medications the client is currently taking, the reasons, and the effectiveness of these medications in treating the problem.
2. Note any physical conditions that would contraindicate the client receiving drugs in this category.
3. Note the client's age and whether he/she is debilitated.
4. Drugs in this category are under the Controlled Substances Act. Therefore, follow appropriate policy for handling amphetamines to restrict availability and discourage abuse.

Interventions

1. Note if the client appears agitated or complains of sleeplessness. Notify the physician and anticipate a reduction in the dosage of drug.
2. Clients who have been receiving MAO inhibitors or who have received them 7–14 days before starting amphetamine therapy are susceptible to hypertensive crisis. Monitor such clients closely. If the client develops fever, marked sweating, excitation, delirium, tremors, or twitching document and report to the physician immediately. If the client is in the hospital, pad the side rails, and have a suction machine available at the bedside.
3. Monitor vital signs and blood pressure. Assess for evidence of arrhythmias, tachycardia or hypertension. Cardiovascular changes accompanied by psychotic syndrome usually indicate acute toxicity.
4. If the client complains of loss of appetite, somnolence, appears mentally impaired, and experiences occupational impairment, the drug should be discontinued.
5. Observe for signs of psychological dependence and drug tolerance as the drug should be discontinued.
6. At least once a week weigh the client to detect weight loss. Clients receiving amphetamines may become anorexic. Severe and persistent weight loss should be reported to the physician. The dosage of drug may need to be adjusted or the drug therapy may need to be changed.

Client/Family Teaching

1. When anorexiants are used for weight reduction, their effect lasts only 4 to 6 weeks. Therefore, clients need to follow a dietary and exercise regimen established by the physician to maintain weight loss.
2. Have a dietician discuss a weight control diet with the client and assist them with meal planning.
3. Drug tolerance develops rapidly. Provide the client with a printed list of the symptoms of tolerance. If tolerance develops, notify the physician and begin decreasing the dose of medication.
4. Warn that amphetamines may mask extreme fatigue, which can impair ability to perform potentially hazardous tasks, such as operating a machine or an automobile. Using amphetamines to treat fatigue is inappropriate as rebound effects may be severe.
5. Advise clients that they should seek medical assistance if they experience extreme fatigue and depression once the drug is discontinued.
6. Amphetamines may alter insulin and dietary requirements. Therefore, clients with diabetes mellitus need to be warned to monitor their blood sugar closely. Changes may require a change in the dose of insulin, oral hypoglycemic agent and/or diet.

7. Advise clients to take medication only as prescribed and remind them of the importance of keeping all appointments for regular medical follow-up.

8. Store all medications safely out of the reach of children.

AMPHETAMINE COMPLEX   (am-FET-ah-meen)

Biphetamine 12½ and 20 (C-II) (Rx)

See also *Anorexiants,* p. 843, *Amphetamine sulfate,* p. 846, and *Dextroamphetamine sulfate,* p. 848.

Classification: Central nervous system stimulant, anorexiant.

Action/Kinetics: This product is a resin complex of amphetamine and dextroamphetamine. Biphetamine 12½ is equivalent to 10 mg dextroamphetamine while Biphetamine 20 is equivalent to 15 mg dextroamphetamine.

Contraindications: Safe use during pregnancy has not been established.

Uses: Attention deficit disorders in children, obesity.

Dosage: Capsules. *Obesity:* 1 capsule (either 12½ or 20) daily. *Attention deficit disorders in children:* Initial therapy should begin with dextroamphetamine; once the appropriate dosage level is established, amphetamine complex can be given, once daily, at the established dosage.

NURSING CONSIDERATIONS

See also *Nursing Considerations* for *Anorexiants, Amphetamines and Derivatives,* p. 844.

Administration/Storage

Administer 10–14 hours before bedtime.

AMPHETAMINE SULFATE   (am-FET-ah-meen)

(C-II) (Rx)

See also *Anorexiants, Amphetamines and Derivatives,* p. 843.

Classification: Central nervous system stimulant.

Action/Kinetics: After PO administration, completely absorbed in 3 hr. **Duration: PO,** 4–24 hr; **t½:** 10–30 hr, depending on urinary pH. Excreted in urine. Acidification will increase excretion, while alkalinization will decrease it. For every one unit increase in pH, the plasma half-life will increase by 7 hr.

Uses: Attention deficit disorders in children, narcolepsy.

Special Concerns: Pregnancy category: C. Use is not recommended in children less than 3 years of age for attention deficit disorders and in children less than 6 years of age for narcolepsy. Use is no longer recommended as an appetite suppressant.

Dosage: Tablets. *Narcolepsy:* **Adults,** 5–20 mg 1–3 times daily. **Children over 12 years, initial:** 5 mg b.i.d.; increase in increments of 10 mg/day at weekly intervals until optimum dose is reached. **Children, 6–12 years of age, initial:** 2.5 mg b.i.d.; increase in increments of 5 mg at weekly intervals until optimum dose is reached (maximum is 60 mg daily). *Attention deficit disorders in children:* **3–6 years of age, initial:** 2.5 mg/day; increase by 2.5 mg/day at weekly intervals until optimum dose is achieved (usual range 0.1–0.5 mg/kg/dose each morning). **6 years and older,**

initial: 5 mg 1–2 times/day; increase in increments of 5 mg weekly until optimum dose is achieved (rarely over 40 mg/day).

NURSING CONSIDERATIONS

See also *Nursing Considerations* for *Anorexiants, Amphetamines and Derivatives,* p. 844.

Administration/Storage

1. When used as an anorexiant, the drug should be used only for short-term therapy.
2. When used for attention deficit disorders or narcolepsy, the first dose should be given on awakening with additional one or two doses given at intervals of 4–6 hr.
3. The last dose of medication should be given 6 hr before bedtime.
4. The peak effects of the drug are observed 2–3 hr after administration. The effects last from 4–24 hr.

Assessment

1. Take a complete nursing and drug history.
2. Obtain a baseline assessment of the CNS prior to initiating therapy.
3. Obtain a baseline ECG before starting therapy.
4. Note the client's age. If the client is of childbearing age and is sexually active, determine the possibility of pregnancy, as amphetamines are contraindicated.

Interventions

1. Monitor vital signs as well as the client's weight, CNS status and ECG throughout the therapy. Record favorable responses and any side effects on the chart.
2. Note any symptoms of impaired mental processes or emotional liability. Document and report to the physician.
3. If children are receiving amphetamines, assess the child's growth. Children may have their growth retarded as a result of the medication. Children should periodically have the drug discontinued to allow growth to proceed normally and to determine if the drug therapy needs to be continued.

Client/Family Teaching

1. Advise the client and family to report any noted changes in mood or affect to the physician.
2. Caution client not to use caffeine or caffeine-containing beverages. Provide the client with a printed list of such products.
3. Instruct the client to avoid taking OTC preparations that contain caffeine, phenylpropanolamine and other drugs that can affect the cardiovascular system.
4. Advise clients to avoid using heavy machinery or driving the car until the effects of the medication can be evaluated.
5. Advise clients to monitor their weight and to maintain a written record to show the health care provider at each client visit.
6. To prevent constipation, instruct clients to drink at least 2500 mL of fluid daily and to increase the amount of high fiber foods, including fruits, in their daily diet.
7. Advise clients who have a dry mouth to chew hard, sugarless candies and to rinse the mouth frequently with nonalcoholic mouth rinses.

Evaluation

Review with the client and family the goals of therapy and assess any changes in behavior if noted.

BENZPHETAMINE HYDROCHLORIDE   (bens-FET-ah-meen)

Didrex (C-III) (Rx)

See also *Anorexiants,Amphetamines and Derivatives,* p. 843.

Classification: Anorexiant.

Action/Kinetics: t½: 6–12 hr.

Use: Short-term (8–12 weeks) treatment of exogenous obesity in conjunction with a weight reduction regimen such as exercise, restriction of calories, and behavior modification.

Additional Contraindication: Use in pregnancy (category: X).

Dosage: Tablets. Adults: initial, 25–50 mg once daily; **then,** increase dose according to response (dose ranges from 25–50 mg 1–3 times daily 1 hr before meals).

NURSING CONSIDERATIONS

See also *Nursing Considerations* for *Anorexiants,Amphetamines and Derivatives,* p. 844.

Administration/Storage

1. It is preferable to administer a single dose in mid-morning or mid-afternoon, depending on the eating habits of the client.
2. Anorexiant effects occur within 1–2 hr and last approximately 4 hr.

Assessment

1. Note any history of glaucoma, advanced arteriosclerosis, cardiac disease, or mental instability. The drug is contraindicated in these instances.
2. Determine the possibility of the client being pregnant. Benzphetamine is toxic to the fetus and should not be administered to pregnant women or nursing mothers.

DEXTROAMPHETAMINE SULFATE   (dex-troh-am-FET-ah-meen)

Dexedrine, Ferndex, Oxydess II, Spancap No. 1 (C-II) (Rx)

See also *Anorexiants, Amphetamines and Derivatives,* p. 843.

Classification: Central nervous system stimulant, amphetamine type.

Action/Kinetics: Dextroamphetamine has stronger CNS effects and weaker peripheral action than does amphetamine; thus, dextroamphetamine manifests fewer undesirable cardiovascular effects. After PO administration, completely absorbed in 3 hr. **Duration: PO,** 4–24 hr; **t½, adults:** 10–12 hr; **children:** 6–8 hr. Excreted in urine. Acidification will increase excretion, while alkalinization will decrease it.

Uses: Attention deficit disorders in children, narcolepsy.

Additional Contraindications: Lactation. Use for obesity.

Special Concerns: Use in pregnancy only if benefits outweigh risks (pregnancy category: C). Use of extended-release capsules for attention deficit disorders in children less than 6 years of age and the elixir or tablets for attention deficit disorders in children less than 3 years of age is not recommended. Dosage for narcolepsy has not been determined in children less than 6 years of age.

Dosage: Elixir, Tablets. *Attention deficit disorders in children:* **3–5 years of age, initial:** 2.5 mg/day; increase by 2.5 mg /day at weekly intervals until optimum dose is achieved (usual range 0.1–0.5 mg/kg/dose each morning). **6 years and older, initial:** 5 mg 1–2 times/day; increase in increments of 5 mg weekly until optimum dose is achieved (rarely over 40 mg/day). *Narcolepsy:* **Adults:** 5–60 mg in divided doses daily. **Children over 12 years, initial:** 10 mg daily; increase in increments of 10 mg/day at weekly intervals until optimum dose is reached. **Children, 6–12 years of age, initial:** 5 mg daily; increase in increments of 5 mg at weekly intervals until optimum dose is reached (maximum is 60 mg daily).

   Extended-release Capsule. *Narcolepsy:* **Adults:** 5–30 mg once daily. **Children, 6–12 years of age:** 5–15 mg once daily; **12 years and older:** 10–15 mg once daily. *Attention deficit disorders:* **Children, 6 years and older:** 5–15 mg once daily.

NURSING CONSIDERATIONS

See also *Nursing Considerations* for *Anorexiants, Amphetamines and Derivatives,* p. 844.

Administration/Storage

1. Long-acting products may be used for once-a-day dosing in attention deficit disorders and narcolepsy.
2. When tablets or the elixir are used for attention deficit disorders or narcolepsy, the first dose should be given on awakening with additional one or two doses given at intervals of 4–6 hr. If possible, the last dose should be given 6 hr before bedtime.
3. If the client is already receiving an MAO inhibitor, a period of at least 14 days should elapse before dextroamphetamine is initiated.

DIETHYLPROPION HYDROCHLORIDE   (dye-eth-ill-**PROH**-pee-on)

M-Orexic, Nobesine✿, Tenuate, Tenuate Dospan, Tepanil, Tepanil Ten-Tab (C-IV) (Rx)

See also *Anorexiants, Amphetamines and Derivatives,* p. 843.

Classification: Anorexiant.

Action/Kinetics: Duration, tablets: 4 hr; **extended-release tablets:** 12 hr.

Use: Short-term (8–12 weeks) treatment of exogenous obesity in conjunction with a weight reduction regimen including exercise, reduced caloric intake, and behavior modification.

Special Concerns: Pregnancy category: B. Use with caution during lactation.

Additional Side Effects: May cause increased risk of seizures in epileptics.

Dosage: Tablets. Adults: 25 mg t.i.d. 1 hr before meals.**Extended-release Tablets. Adults:** 75 mg at midmorning.

NURSING CONSIDERATIONS

See also *Nursing Considerations* for *Anorexiants, Amphetamines and Derivatives,* p. 844.

Administration/Storage

1. Give extended-release tablets in the mid-morning.
2. The drug may be taken in the mid-evening to reduce night hunger.

FENFLURAMINE   (fen-FLEW-rah-meen)
Ponderal✿, Pondimin (C-IV) (Rx)

See also *Anorexiants, Amphetamines and Derivatives,* p. 843.

Classification: Anorexiant.

Action/Kinetics: This drug produces more CNS depression and less stimulation than does amphetamine. It may exert its activity by affecting turnover of serotonin in the brain or to increased use of glucose. The abuse potential of fenfluramine appears to be different from other anorexiants in that it produces euphoria, derealization, and perceptual changes with doses of 80–400 mg. **Onset:** 1–2 hr. **Maximum effect:** 2–4 hr. **Duration:** 4–6 hr. **t½:** 11–30 hr. Excretion is pH dependent and is through the urine (alkaline urine decreases excretion).

Uses: Short-term treatment (8–12 weeks) of exogenous obesity in conjunction with a weight reduction program including reduced caloric intake, exercise, and behavior modification. To treat autistic children with high serotonin levels.

Additional Contraindication: Alcoholism.

Special Concerns: Pregnancy category: C.

Additional Side Effects: Hypoglycemia, CNS depression, impotence, drowsiness. Following long-term use (1 month), withdrawal symptoms have been observed including: tremor, ataxia, loss of sense of reality, visual hallucinations, depression, disturbed concentration and memory, suicidal feelings.

    Symptoms of overdose: *CNS:* Agitation, drowsiness, confusion, convulsions, coma. *Musculoskeletal:* Tremor, shivering, increased or decreased reflexes. *CV:* Tachycardia, ventricular extrasystoles, culminating in ventricular fibrillation and cardiac arrest (at high doses). *Miscellaneous:* Flushing, fever, sweating, abdominal pain, hyperventilation, rotary nystagmus, dilated nonreactive pupils. Treatment should be symptomatic and supportive; however, emesis should not be induced due to the depressant effects of the drug.

Additional Drug Interactions: Fenfluramine may ↑ effect of alcohol, CNS depressants, guanethidine, methyldopa, reserpine, thiazide diuretics, and tricyclic antidepressants.

Dosage: Tablets. Adults: 20 mg t.i.d. 30–60 min before meals. May be increased weekly to a maximum of 40 mg t.i.d. If initial dose is not well tolerated, reduce to 40 mg daily and increase gradually. Total daily dose should not exceed 120 mg.

    Extended-release Capsules. Adults: 60 mg once daily; the dose may be increased to a maximum of 120 mg daily, if needed.

NURSING CONSIDERATIONS

See also *Nursing Considerations* for *Anorexiants, Amphetamines and Derivatives,* p. 844.

Administration/Storage

1. Anticipate the drug will produce anorexiant effects within 1–2 hr after ingestion.
2. The effects of the drug should last approximately 4–6 hr.
3. The drug should not be abruptly withdrawn since depression can occur.

MAZINDOL   (MAY-zin-dol)
Mazanor, Sanorex (C-IV) (Rx)

See also *Anorexiants, Amphetamines and Derivatives,* p. 843.

Classification: Anorexiant.

Action/Kinetics: Onset: 30–60 min; **duration:** 8–15 hr. **t¹/₂:** Less than 24 hr. **Therapeutic blood levels:** 0.003–0.012 mcg/mL. Excreted in urine partially unchanged.

Use: Short-term (8–12 weeks) treatment of exogenous obesity in conjunction with a weight reduction program including exercise, reduced caloric intake, and behavior modification.

Special Concerns: Pregnancy category: C.

Additional Side Effects: Testicular pain.

Dosage: Tablets. Adults, initial: 1 mg once daily 1 hr before the first meal of the day; **then,** dose can be increased to 1 mg t.i.d. or 2 mg once daily 1 hr before lunch.

NURSING CONSIDERATIONS

See also *Nursing Considerations* for *Anorexiants, Amphetamines and Derivatives,* p. 844.

Administration/Storage

Clients may take the medication with meals if they experience GI distress.

METHAMPHETAMINE HYDROCHLORIDE (meth-am-**FET**-ah-meen)
Desoxyn, (C-II) (Rx)

See also *Anorexiants, Amphetamines and Derivatives,* p. 843.

Classification: CNS stimulant, amphetamine-type.

Action/Kinetics: t¹/₂: 4–5 hr, depending on urinary pH.

Uses: Attention deficit disorders in children over 6 years of age.

Contraindications: Use for obesity. Attention deficit disorders in children less than 6 years of age.

Special Concerns: Use during pregnancy only when benefits clearly outweigh risks (pregnancy category: C).

Dosage: Tablets. *Attention deficit disorders in children, 6 years and older:* **initial,** 5 mg 1–2 times daily; increase in increments of 5 mg daily at weekly intervals until optimum dose is reached (usually 20–25 mg daily).
   Extended-release Tablets. *Attention deficit disorders in children, 6 years and older:* 20–25 mg once daily.

NURSING CONSIDERATIONS

See also *Nursing Considerations* for *Anorexiants, Amphetamines and Derivatives,* p. 844.

Administration/Storage

1. When used to facilitate verbalization during psychotherapeutic interview, give second dose only if the first dose has proven effective.
2. When used for attention deficit disorders, the total daily dose can be given in 2 divided doses or once a day using the long-acting product. The long-acting product should not be used to initiate therapy.

Interventions

When used to treat attention deficit disorders, evaluate the therapy periodically to determine the need for continued treatment.

PHENDIMETRAZINE TARTRATE   (fen-dye-**MEH**-trah-zeen)

Adphen, Anorex, Bacarate, Bontrol PDM and Slow-Release, , Dital, Dyrexan-OD, Marlibar A, Melfiat-105 Unicelles, Metra, Neocurab, Obalan, Obe-Del, Obeval, Obezine, Panrexin M, Panrexin MTP, Parzine, Phendiet, Phendiet-105, Phendimet, Phentra, Phenzine, Plegine, Prelu-2, PT 105, Rexigen, Rexigen Forte, Slyn-LL, Statobex, Tega-Nil, Trimcaps, Trimstat, Trimtabs, Uni Trim, Wehless Timecelles, Weightrol, Wescoid, X-Trozine, X-Trozine LA (C-III) (Rx)

See also *Anorexiants, Amphetamines and Derivatives,* p. 843.

Classification: Anorexiant.

Action/Kinetics: Duration, tablets: 4 hr. **t½:** 5.5 hr (average).

Use: Short-term (8–12 weeks) treatment of exogenous obesity in conjunction with a weight reduction program including exercise, reduced caloric intake, and behavior modification.

Special Concerns: Pregnancy category: C.

Dosage: Capsules, Tablets. Adults: 17.5–35 mg 2–3 times daily 1 hr before meals. **Maximum daily dose:** 70 mg t.i.d. **Extended-release Capsules, Extended-release Tablets. Adults:** 105 mg once daily 30–60 min before the morning meal.

NURSING CONSIDERATIONS

See *Nursing Considerations* for *Anorexiants, Amphetamines and Derivatives,* p. 844.

PHENMETRAZINE   (fen-**MEH**-trah-zeen)

Preludin Endurets (C-II) (Rx)

See also *Anorexiants, Amphetamines and Derivatives,* p. 843.

Classification: Anorexiant.

Action/Kinetics: Duration: 4 hr for regular tablets and 12 hr for sustained-release.

Use: Short-term (8–12 weeks) treatment of exogenous obesity in conjunction with a weight reduction program including reduced caloric intake, exercise, and behavior modification.

Special Concerns: Pregnancy category: C.

Dosage: Extended-release Tablets. Adults: 75 mg in the morning or when the anorectic effect is desired.

NURSING CONSIDERATIONS

See *Nursing Considerations* for *Anorexiants, Amphetamines and Derivatives,* p. 844.

PHENTERMINE   (**FEN**-ter-meen)

Adipex-P, Anoxine-AM, Dapex-37.5, Fastin, Obe-Mar, Obe-Nix 30, Obephen, Obermine, Obestin-30, Oby-Trim, Panshape, Parmine, Phentercot, Phenterxene, Phentride, Phentrol, Phentrol 2, 4, and 5, Span-RD, T-Diet, Teramin, Wilpowr, Zatryl (C-IV) (Rx)

PHENTERMINE RESIN   (FEN-ter-meen)

Ionamin (C-IV) (Rx)

See also *Anorexiants, Amphetamines and Derivatives,* p. 843.

Classification: Anorexiant.

Action/Kinetics: Duration, 8 mg tablets: 4 hr; **duration, 30 mg capsules, 37.5 mg tablets, resin:** 12–14 hr.

Use: Short-term (8–12 weeks) treatment of exogenous obesity in conjunction with a weight reduction program including exercise, reduced caloric intake, and behavior modification.

Special Concerns: Pregnancy category: C.

Dosage: Capsules, Tablets. Adults: 15–37.5 mg once daily either before breakfast, 1–2 hr after breakfast, or in divided doses 30 min before meals.
  Resin Capsules. Adults: 15–30 mg once daily before breakfast.

NURSING CONSIDERATIONS

See *Nursing Considerations* for *anorexiants, Amphetamines and Derivatives,* p. 844.

PHENYLPROPANOLAMINE HYDROCHLORIDE   (fen-ill-proh-pah-**NOHL**-ah-meen)

Acutrim 16 Hour, Acutrim Late Day, Acutrim II Maximum Strength, Control, Dex-A-Diet Maximum Strength and Maximum Strength Caplets, Dexatrim, Dexatrim Maximum Strength and Maximum Strength Caplets, Dexatrim Maximum Strength Pre-Meal Caplets, Efed II Yellow, Maigret-50, Phenyldrine, Prolamine, Propagest, Rhindecon, Unitrol (OTC except Maigret-50 and Rhindecon)

See also *Anorexiants, Amphetamines and Derivatives,* p. 843, and *Sympathomimetics,* p. 883.

Classification: Decongestant, appetite suppressant.

Action/Kinetics: Phenylpropanolamine is thought to stimulate both alpha and beta receptors, as well as to act indirectly through release of norepinephrine from storage sites. Increases in blood pressure are due mainly to increased cardiac output rather than to vasoconstriction; has minimal CNS effects. The drug acts on alpha-adrenergic receptors to produce a decongestant effect in the nasal mucosa. **Onset, decongestant:** 15–30 min; **peak plasma levels:** 1–2 hr; **duration, capsules and tablets:** 3 hr; **extended-release tablets:** 12–16 hr. **Peak plasma levels:** 100 ng. **t½:** 3–4 hr. 80%–90% excreted in the urine unchanged.

Uses: Nasal congestion due to colds, hay fever, allergies. Short-term (8–12 weeks) treatment of exogenous obesity in conjunction with a weight reduction program including reduced caloric intake, exercise, and behavior modification. *Investigational:* Mild to moderate stress incontinence in women.

Contraindications: Arteriosclerosis, depression, glaucoma, hypertension, diabetes, kidney disease, hyperthyroidism, during or within 14 days of use of MAO inhibitors, hypersensitivity to sympathomimetics. Not recommended as an anorexiant for children less than 12 years of age.

Special Concerns: Safety and efficacy during pregnancy and lactation and for children not established. Children less than 6 years of age may be at greater risk for developing psychiatric disorders when using phenylpropanolamine. The anorexiant dose must be individualized for children between 12–18 years of age.

Side Effects: *CNS:* Dizziness, headache, insomnia, restlessness, bizarre behavior. Serious effects due to abuse include: agitation, tremor, increased motor activity, hallucinations, seizures, stroke, and death. *CV:* Palpitations, hypertension (may be severe and lead to crisis), tachycardia. *Miscellaneous:* Dry mouth, dysuria, renal failure, nausea, nasal dryness.

Drug Interactions	
Furazolidone	Possibility of hypertensive crisis and intracranial hemorrhage
Guanethidine	Phenylpropanolamine ↓ hypotensive effect
Indomethacin	Possibility of severe hypertensive episode
MAO Inhibitors	Possibility of hypertensive crisis and intracranial hemorrhage

Dosage: Capsules, Tablets. *Decongestant:* **Adults,** 25 mg q 4 hr or 50 mg q 6–8 hr (not to exceed 150 mg/day); **Children, 2–6 years:** 6.25 mg q 4 hr, not to exceed 37.5 mg in 24 hr; **6–12 years:** 12.5 mg q 4 hr, not to exceed 75 mg in 24 hr. *Anorexiant:* **Adults,** 25 mg t.i.d. 30 min before meals, not to exceed 75 mg in 24 hr.

Extended-release Capsules, Extended-release Tablets. *Decongestant:* **Adults,** 75 mg q 12 hr. *Anorexiant:* **Adults,** 75 mg once daily in the morning.

NURSING CONSIDERATIONS

See also *Nursing Considerations* for *Anorexiants, Amphetamines and Derivatives,* p. 844, and *Sympathomimetics,* p. 887.

Client/Family Teaching

Caution older men to report difficulties in voiding, because they are more susceptible to drug-induced urinary retention. Ensure that these clients understand the importance of taking the medication only as directed.

MISCELLANEOUS AGENTS

CAFFEINE   (KAH-feen)

Caffedrine, Dexitac, No Doz, Quick Pep, Tirend, Vivarin (OTC)

CAFFEINE AND SODIUM BENZOATE INJECTION   (KAH-feen)

(Rx)

CAFFEINE, CITRATED   (KAH-feen)

(OTC)

Classification: CNS stimulant, miscellaneous.

Note: Caffeine is found in a number of widely used combination drugs, including Fiorinal Plain and with Codeine, and Synalgos DC.

Action/Kinetics: Caffeine stimulates all levels of the CNS (cerebral cortex, medulla, and spinal cord). The mechanism of action includes competitive antagonism of central adenosine receptors. Caffeine is often used as an adjunct to analgesics used for headaches; the mechanism is thought to be due to constriction of blood vessels in the brain leading to a decrease in cerebral blood flow and oxygen tension of the brain. Caffeine may also help to relieve headache by enhancing the onset and effect of analgesics. Caffeine also possesses other pharmacologic activity, including dilation of coronary and peripheral blood vessels, constriction of cerebral blood vessels, increase in heart rate, stimulation of skeletal muscle, increased gastric acid secretion, and diuresis. **Peak plasma levels:** 15–45 min. **Therapeutic plasma levels:** 6–13 mcg/mL. **Levels above 20 mcg/mL produce toxic effects. t$^{1}/_{2}$, distribution:** 3.5 hr; **elimination:** 6 hr. The t$^{1}/_{2}$ is increased during pregnancy and during use of oral contraceptives. Approximately 17% bound to plasma protein. Metabolized primarily in liver and excreted by the kidneys. Sodium benzoate and citric acid increase the water solubility of caffeine.

Uses: Adjunct with nonnarcotic and narcotic analgesics to enhance pain relief; increased wakefulness by increasing mental alertness; adjunct in migraine headache therapy. Neonatal apnea. Although caffeine has been used to overcome hangover effects occurring during arousal from drug-induced coma such as that from intoxication with morphine, barbiturates, alcohol, and other CNS depressants, the use of caffeine for this purpose is neither advisable nor logical.

Contraindications: Use with caution in cardiovascular, renal, and ulcer disease, and in depression. Caffeine and sodium benzoate injection is not recommended for neonatal apnea due to the sodium benzoate content.

Special Concerns: Safety not established during pregnancy. Use with caution during lactation. Children are especially sensitive to the effects of caffeine, especially side effects; thus, use to relieve drowsiness is not recommended in children less than 12 years of age.

Side Effects: *CNS:* Symptoms of overexcitation including insomnia, nervousness, lightheadedness, restlessness, headaches. *GI:* Nausea, vomiting, diarrhea, gastric upset. *GU:* Diuresis. **Note:** Large doses may cause anxiety neurosis with sensory disturbances, palpitations, tremors, arrhythmias, flushing, and other symptoms mentioned above. *Following abrupt withdrawal after use of 500–600 mg daily:* Withdrawal symptoms including anxiety, headache, muscle tension.

Drug Interactions	
Cimetidine	↑ Effect of caffeine due to ↓ breakdown by liver
MAO inhibitors	Excessive caffeine may cause hypertensive crisis; reduce intake of caffeine containing medication
Oral contraceptives	↑ Effect of caffeine due to ↓ breakdown by liver
Propoxyphene	Caffeine given to patients taking large doses of propoxyphene may cause convulsions
Tobacco	↑ Excretion of caffeine

Laboratory Test Interference: ↑ Urinary catecholamines.

Dosage: *Caffeine.* **Tablets.** *CNS Stimulant:* **Adults,** 100–200 mg q 3–4 hr. **Extended-release Capsules: Adults,** 200–250 mg no more often than q 3–4 hr. *Neonatal apnea:* **Initial,** 10 mg/kg; **maintenance:** 2.5 mg/kg daily beginning 48–72 hr after the initial dose. Dose may be increased as required up to 6 mg/kg b.i.d. to achieve a serum level of 8–20 mg/L.

Caffeine and sodium benzoate. **IM, IV.** *CNS Stimulant:* **Adults,** Up to a maximum of 500 mg (250 mg anhydrous caffeine and 250 mg of sodium benzoate) per dose. Maximum daily dose: 1.25 g anhydrous caffeine and 1.25 g sodium benzoate.

Caffeine citrated. **Tablets.** *CNS Stimulant:* **Adults, initial** 65–325 mg (32–162 mg anhydrous caffeine) t.i.d. Up to 1 g anhydrous caffeine daily may be used. **Oral Solution, IV Injection.** *Neonatal apnea:* **Initial,** 20 mg (10 mg anhydrous caffeine and 10 mg anhydrous citric acid)/kg. **Maintenance:** 5 mg (2.5 mg anhydrous caffeine and 2.5 mg anhydrous citric acid)/kg beginning 48–72 hr after the initial dose; dose may be increased to 12 mg/kg b.i.d. to achieve a serum level of 8–20 mg/L.

NURSING CONSIDERATIONS

Administration/Storage

For neonatal apnea, caffeine tablets may be crushed and made into an oral suspension.

Interventions

1. Assess for high caffeine intake, manifested by insomnia, irritability, tremors, cardiac irregularities, and gastritis.
2. Monitor intake, output, weight and blood pressure. Document and report any unusual changes.

Client/Family Teaching

Avoid additional sources of caffeine such as coffee, tea, cocoa and colas.

ANALEPTICS

DOXAPRAM HYDROCHLORIDE   (DOX-ah-pram)

Dopram (Rx)

Classification: CNS stimulant, analeptic.

Action/Kinetics: Doxapram increases the rate and depth of respiration by stimulating carotid chemoreceptors. Higher doses also stimulate respiratory centers in the medulla with progressive stimulation of other CNS centers as well (toxic doses may induce tonic-clonic convulsions). An increase in blood pressure may also occur due to increased cardiac output. The drug will antagonize respiratory depression, but not analgesia, induced by narcotics. An increased salivation and release of both gastric acid and catecholamines may be seen. **Onset** (after IV): 20–40 sec. **Peak effect:** 1–2 min. **Duration:** 5–12 min. **t½:** Approximately 2.5–4 hr. Doxapram is metabolized in the liver and is excreted in the urine.

Uses: Respiratory stimulant in mild to moderate drug overdose, drug-induced postanesthetic respiratory depression, apnea not associated with muscle relaxants, acute respiratory insufficiency in chronic obstructive pulmonary disease (used for 2 hr).

The analeptic agents are no longer considered drugs of choice in the treatment of CNS depression caused by a severe overdosage of sedatives and hypnotics. Current therapy for overdose of sedative-hypnotics relies largely on supportive therapy, such as establishing a patent airway, administering oxygen, assisting or controlling respiration when necessary, and maintaining blood pressure and blood volume.

Contraindications: Epilepsy, convulsive states, respiratory incompetence due to muscle paresis, flail chest, pneumothorax, pulmonary fibrosis, acute bronchial asthma, extreme dyspnea, severe hypertension, and cerebrovascular accidents. Hypersensitivity. Use in newborns or immature infants (the benzoyl alcohol present may cause a fatal toxic reaction).

Special Concerns: Pregnancy category: B. Use with caution during lactation. Safety and efficacy have not been established in children less than 12 years of age. Use with caution in patients with cerebral edema, asthma, severe cardiovascular disease, hyperthyroidism and pheochromocytoma (cancer of adrenals), peptic ulcer, or gastric surgery.

Side Effects: *CNS:* Excess stimulation including hyperactivity, clonus, convulsions. Headache, apprehension, dizziness, disorientation. *Autonomic:* Flushing, sweating, paresthesia, feeling of warmth, burning, or hot sensation in area of perineum and genitalia, mydriasis. *GI:* Nausea, vomiting, diarrhea, urge to defecate. *Respiratory:* Bronchospasm, dyspnea, cough, hiccoughs, rebound hypoventilation, laryngospasm, tachypnea. *CV:* Arrhythmias, abnormal ECG, tightness in chest or chest pain, phlebitis, change in heart rate, increase in blood pressure. *GU:* Spontaneous micturition, urinary retention, proteinuria. *Miscellaneous:* Muscle spasms, involuntary movements, pruritus, increased deep tendon reflexes, pyrexia.

Overdosage

Characterized by respiratory alkalosis and by hypocapnia (too little CO_2 in blood) with tetany and apnea. Also excessive stimulation of CNS, which may result in convulsions.

Drug Interactions	
Anesthetics, general	Since doxapram increases epinephrine release, do not give until 10 min after anesthetic discontinued if halothane, cyclopropane, or enflurane used in order to minimize cardiac arrhythmias
MAO inhibitors	Additive pressor effects
Muscle relaxants	Doxapram may mask effects of muscle relaxants
Sympathomimetic amines	Additive pressor effects

Laboratory Test Interferences: ↓ Hemoglobin, hematocrit, RBCs. ↑ BUN, proteinuria.

Dosage: IV. *After anesthesia:* **Single IV injection:** 0.5–1.0 mg/kg, not to exceed 1.5–2.0 mg/kg; may be given in several injections at 5-min intervals. **IV infusion:** 1 mg/mL of dextrose or saline solution, initially at a rate of 5 mg/min; **then,** 1–3 mg/min. Total recommended dose: 4 mg/kg (approximately 300 mg). *Chronic obstructive lung disease with acute hypercapnia:* **IV infusion,** 1–2 mg/min up to maximum of 3 mg/min for no longer than 2 hr. *Drug-induced CNS depression:* **IV injection, initial:** 1–2 mg/kg as a single dose; repeat in 5 min and every 1–2 hr to a maximum of 3 g daily. **Intermittent IV infusion, initial:** 2 mg/kg; **then,** if patient not responsive, continue supportive treatment for 1–2 hr and repeat doxapram dose to a maximum of 3 g daily. If response occurs, infuse 1 mg/mL at a rate of 1–3 mg/min. The infusion should be discontinued at the end of 2 hr or if the patient awakens.

NURSING CONSIDERATIONS

Administration/Storage

1. Allow a minimum of 10 min between the discontinuation of anesthetic and the administration of doxapram.

2. Children under 12 years of age should not receive doxapram.

3. In the event of drug overdose, have short-acting barbiturates, oxygen and resuscitative equipment available.

Assessment

1. Note any client history of epilepsy or other convulsive disorders.

2. Obtain a complete baseline assessment of the CNS and ECG prior to the client receiving therapy.

3. Note the age of clients. Elderly people and debilitated clients may be unable to tolerate the increase in respirations caused by doxapram.

4. Obtain baseline arterial blood gases, BP, heart rate and deep tendon reflexes.

5. Review drugs the client is taking that may interact with doxapram and record on the client's record.

Interventions

1. Drug should only be administered in a closely monitored environment.

2. Frequently assess the client's responses to doxapram as compared with their baseline parameters to detect signs of overdosage and to provide a guide for adjusting the rate of infusion.

3. For at least ½–1 hr after the client is alert, assess them for possible poststimulation respiratory depression.

4. Position clients so that, in the event of vomiting, they will not aspirate.

5. Monitor intake and output. If the client has not voided in 2–4 hr, palpate the bladder to detect urinary retention. Catheterization may be required.

6. If the client has persistent diarrhea or vomiting, notify the physician.

7. Ensure a patent airway. Administer oxygen along with the drug to clients suffering from chronic pulmonary insufficiency.

8. Follow seizure precautions after administration of drug. Have available IV diazepam.

AGENTS FOR ATTENTION DEFICIT DISORDERS

General Statement: Several CNS stimulants are currently used for the treatment of children suffering from hyperkinesia and other behavior problems stemming from neurologic and not psychologic causes. Before drug therapy of this ill-defined condition is undertaken in children, the child must undergo extensive evaluation including medical and psychological tests. These drugs have also been used to treat a decline in mental capacity in geriatric patients.

ERGOLOID MESYLATES (DIHYDROGENATED ERGOT ALKALOIDS) (ER-go-loyd MES-ill-ayts)

Hydergine, Hydergine LC, Niloric (Rx)

Classification: Agent for attention deficit disorders.

Action/Kinetics: This combination of equal proportions of the mesylate salts of dihydroergocornine, dihydroergocristine, and dihydroergocryptine. Although the mechanism is not known, the drug may act by increasing cerebral blood flow. Ergoloid mesylates also act on the CNS to decrease vascular tone and slow the heart rate; peripherally, the drug blocks alpha-adrenergic receptors. **Peak plasma levels:** 1–2 hr. $t^{1}/_{2}$: Approximately 3.5 hr. Oral products are rapidly but incompletely absorbed from the GI tract; significant first-pass effect after oral use.

Uses: Primary progressive dementia, Alzheimer's dementia, multi-infarct dementia. Careful diagnosis should be undertaken prior to use to rule out other causes of symptoms being manifested.

Contraindications: Any type of acute or chronic psychosis. Patients with tartrazine sensitivity. Use with caution in porphyria.

Special Concerns: Geriatric patients may be at greater risk of developing hypothermia.

Side Effects: Acute intermittent porphyria in susceptible patients. Sublingual use: irritation, nausea, heartburn.

Dosage: Capsules, Oral Solution, Sublingual Tablets, Tablets. Adults: 1–2 mg t.i.d. Doses up to 12 mg daily may be necessary. Beneficial effects may not be seen for 3 to 4 weeks and up to six months therapy may be required to determine if the drug is effective.

NURSING CONSIDERATIONS

Administration/Storage

1. Client should be sure the sublingual tablet dissolves completely under the tongue.
2. Sublingual tablets should not be crushed or chewed.

Assessment

Determine that a complete neurological workup has been done prior to initiating therapy.

Client/Family Teaching

1. Report any severe abdominal pain or bothersome side effects.
2. Stress the importance of taking the medication only as prescribed.
3. Advise clients that it may take up to one month for the effects of the medication to become evident.

METHYLPHENIDATE HYDROCHLORIDE   (meth-ill-**FEN**-ih-dayt)

Ritalin, Ritalin-SR (C-II) (Rx)

Classification: CNS stimulant.

Action/Kinetics: The mechanism of action of methylphenidate is not known with certainty although it may act by blocking the reuptake mechanism of dopaminergic neurons. In children with attention deficit disorders, methylphenidate causes decreases in motor restlessness with an increased attention span. In narcolepsy the drug acts on the cerebral cortex and subcortical structures (e.g., thalamus) to increase motor activity and mental alertness and decrease fatigue. **Peak blood levels, children:** 1.9 hr for tablets and 4.7 hr for extended-release tablets. **Duration:** 4–6 hr. $t^{1}/_{2}$: 1–3 hr. The drug is metabolized by the liver and excreted by the kidney.

Uses: Attention deficit disorders in children as part of overall treatment regimen. Narcolepsy.

Contraindications: Marked anxiety, tension and agitation, glaucoma. Severe depression, use for preventing normal fatigue. Tourette's syndrome, motor tics. Should not be used in children who manifest symptoms of primary psychiatric disorders (psychoses) or acute stress.

Special Concerns: Use during pregnancy only if benefits clearly outweigh risks. Use with caution during lactation. Safety and efficacy in children less than 6 years of age have not been established. Use with great caution in patients with history of hypertension or convulsive disease.

Side Effects: *CNS:* Nervousness, insomnia, headaches, dizziness, drowsiness, chorea. Toxic psychoses, dyskinesia, Tourette's syndrome. Psychological dependence. *CV:* Palpitations, tachycardia, angina, arrhythmias, hyper- or hypotension. *GI:* Nausea, anorexia, abdominal pain, weight loss (chronic use). *Allergic:* Skin rashes, fever, urticaria, arthralgia, dermatoses, erythema. *Hematologic:* Thrombocytopenic purpura, leukopenia, anemia. *Miscellaneous:* Hair loss.

In children, the following untoward reactions are more common: anorexia, abdominal pain, weight loss (chronic use), tachycardia, insomnia.

Overdosage

Characterized by cardiovascular symptoms (hypertension, cardiac arrhythmias, tachycardia), mental disturbances, agitation, headaches, vomiting, hyperreflexia, hyperpyrexia, convulsions, and coma.

Treatment of Overdosage

Symptomatic. Excess CNS stimulation may be treated by keeping the patient in quiet, dim surroundings. A short-acting barbiturate may be used. Emesis or gastric lavage should be undertaken if the patient is conscious. Adequate circulatory and respiratory function must be maintained. Hyperpyrexia may be treated by cooling the patient (e.g., cool bath).

Drug Interactions	
Anticoagulants, oral	↑ Effect of anticoagulants due to ↓ breakdown by liver
Anticonvulsants (phenobarbital, phenytoin, primidone)	↑ Effect of anticonvulsants due to ↓ breakdown by liver
Guanethidine	↓ Effect of guanethidine by displacement from its site of action
MAO inhibitors	Possibility of hypertensive crisis, hyperthermia, convulsions, coma
Phenylbutazone	↑ Effect of phenylbutazone due to ↓ breakdown by liver
Tricyclic antidepressants	↑ Effect of antidepressants due to ↓ breakdown by liver

Laboratory Test Interference: ↑ Urinary excretion of epinephrine.

Dosage: Tablets. Adults: 5–20 mg b.i.d.–t.i.d. preferably 30–45 min before meals. *Attention deficit disorders,* **children, 6 years and older: initial,** 5 mg b.i.d. before breakfast and lunch; **then,** increase by 5–10 mg/week to a maximum of 60 mg daily.

Extended-release Tablets. Adults: 20 mg 1–3 times daily q 8 hr, preferably on an empty stomach. *Attention deficit disorders,* **children, 6 years and older:** 20 mg 1–3 times daily.

NURSING CONSIDERATIONS

Administration/Storage

1. Administer the drug before breakfast and lunch to avoid interference with sleep.

2. If the client is receiving the medication for attention deficit disorders and no improvement is noticed in 1 month, or if stimulation occurs, discontinue the medication.

3. The drug should be discontinued periodically to assess the condition of the client, as drug therapy is not considered to be indefinite. Drug therapy should be terminated at the time of puberty.

4. Sustained release tablets are effective for 8-hr and may be substituted for regular release tablets if the 8-hr dosage of the sustained release tablets is the same as the titrated 8 hr dosage of regular tablets.

Assessment

1. Obtain baseline CNS evaluation and ECG prior to starting therapy.
2. Note other drugs the client is taking that may interact with methylphenidate.

Interventions

1. Monitor BP and pulse b.i.d., to detect any changes that may occur.
2. Weigh the client 2 times per week. Clients tend to lose weight while they are taking the medication.
3. Children who do respond to the therapy should have the therapy interrupted every few months to determine if the drug therapy is still necessary.
4. Note any changes in client mood and report to the physician.
5. Monitor the client for skin rashes, exfoliative dermatitis, fever, or pain in the joints. Report any such symptoms to the physician as they may signal the development of Stevens-Johnson syndrome.
6. Have emergency resuscitative equipment available in case of overdosage. Protect the client from self-injury. Reduce external stimuli as much as possible. Provide cooling procedures in event of hyperpyrexia associated with drug overdosage.

Client/Family Teaching

Advise that caution must be used when driving or when operating hazardous machinery during methylphenidate therapy. Drug may mask fatigue and/or cause physical incoordination, dizziness, or drowsiness.

PEMOLINE   (PEH-moh-leen)
Cylert, Cylert Chewable (C-IV) (Rx)

Classification: CNS stimulant.

Action/Kinetics: Although pemoline resembles amphetamine and methylphenidate pharmacologically, its mechanism of action is not fully known. Pemoline is believed to act by dopaminergic mechanisms. The drug will result in a decrease in hyperactivity and a prolonged attention span in children. **Peak serum levels:** 2–4 hr. $t^{1}/_{2}$: 12 hr. Steady state reached in 2–3 days, and beneficial effects may not be noted for 3–4 weeks. Approximately 50% is bound to plasma protein. Pemoline is metabolized by the liver, and approximately 50% is excreted unchanged by the kidneys.

Uses: Attention deficit disorders. *Investigational:* Narcolepsy.

Contraindications: Hypersensitivity to drug. Tourette's syndrome. Children under 6 years of age.

Special Concerns: Pregnancy category: B. Safe use during lactation has not been established. Use with caution in impaired renal or kidney function. Chronic use in children may cause growth suppression.

Side Effects: *CNS:* Insomnia (most common). Dyskinesia of the face, tongue, lips, and extremities; precipitation of Tourette's syndrome. Mild depression, headache, nystagmus, dizziness, hallucinations, irritability, seizures. Exacerbation of behavior disturbances and thought disorders in psychotic children. *GI:* Transient weight loss, gastric upset, nausea. *Miscellaneous:* Skin rash.

For treatment of overdosage, see methylphenidate, p. 860.

Laboratory Test Interference: ↑ SGPT, SGOT, serum LDH.

Dosage: Tablets, Chewable Tablets. Children, 6 years and older, initial: 37.5 mg/day as a single dose in the morning; increase at 1-week intervals by 18.75 mg until desired response is attained up to maximum of 112.5 mg/day. **Usual maintenance:** 56.25–75 mg daily. *Narcolepsy:* 50–200 mg/day in 2 divided doses.

NURSING CONSIDERATIONS

Administration/Storage

1. Administer as a single dose in the morning.
2. Interrupt treatment 1 or 2 times annually to determine whether behavioral symptoms still necessitate therapy.
3. Anticipate the drug will reach peak activity in 2–4 hours, and last up to 8 hours.

Client/Family Teaching

1. Measure the height of the child every month, and weigh child twice a week. Record all measurements on a chart, and bring this chart to each follow-up medical visit so the physician can evaluate the child's growth pattern.
2. Report any noted weight loss or failure to grow to the physician.
3. Administer the drug early in the morning to minimize insomnia associated with drug therapy.
4. Advise family to continue with therapy, because behavioral changes take 3 to 4 weeks to occur.
5. Instruct the family when to interrupt drug administration, as recommended by the physician. Then, to observe behavior without the medication, to help the physician decide whether therapy should be resumed.
6. Stress the importance of bringing the child in periodically for liver function tests. This is to detect adverse reactions that would necessitate withdrawal of pemoline.
7. Provide a printed list of drug side effects. Instruct family to note signs of overdosage, such as agitation, restlessness, hallucinations, and tachycardia. If these symptoms occur, instruct parents to withhold the drug, to give supportive care, and to report immediately to the physician.

CHAPTER FORTY-TWO

Anesthetics

General Statement: Since local and general anesthetics are often administered to patients, they are reviewed here briefly in tabular form. Note their duration of action and other characteristics, since they may interfere with the other drugs a patient is receiving.

LOCAL ANESTHETICS

Action/Kinetics:: Local anesthetics decrease the nerve membrane's permeability to sodium ions. This effect stabilizes the nerve membrane and thus prevents the initiation and transmission of impulses leading to the anesthetic action. The use of epinephrine in conjunction with local anesthetics decreases systemic absorption and prolongs the duration of action of the anesthetic.

Use: General uses of local anesthetics include local or regional anesthesia prior to surgical or dental procedures and obstetrics. Topical local anesthetics are used to treat minor skin disorders such as sunburn, other minor burns, insect bites, minor wounds, and contact dermatoses (e.g., poison ivy, poison oak, poison sumac). See Table 13, p. 864, for uses of specific drugs.

Contraindications: Hypersensitivity. Large doses should not be used in patients with heart block. **Preparations containing preservatives should not be used for spinal or epidural anesthesia.**

Table 13 Local Anesthetics

Drug	Duration of Action (hr)	Indications/Concentration
Benzocaine **Dental Jelly:** Baby Anbesol, Baby Orajel, Maximum Strength Orajel, Orabase-O, Orajel, Rid-A-Pain. **Dental Paste:** Orabase-B. **Lozenges:** Children's Chloraseptic, Spec-T, T-Caine, Tyrobenz. **Rectal Ointment:** Americaine. **Topical Aerosol:** Americaine, Hurricane. **Topical Cream:** (generic only). **Topical Gel:** Americaine Anesthetic Lubricant, Hurricane. **Topical Ointment:** Americaine, Benzocol. **Topical Solution:** Hurricane.	0.5–1	*Dental:* 10 or 20% jelly, 20% paste, and 5 or 10 mg lozenge applied to affected area as needed. *Rectal:* 20% ointment in the a.m. and p.m. and after each bowel movement. *Topical:* 20% gel, aerosol, or solution applied to area with a cotton applicator or sprayed as needed. Used to suppress gag reflex, as a lubricant and anesthetic for pharyngeal and nasal airways, prior to intratracheal and urinary catheters; prior to proctoscopes, laryngoscopes, sigmoidoscopes, vaginal specula. *Cutaneous:* 5% cream, 5% or 20% ointment, 20% topical aerosol for pain, itching, and inflammation caused by burns, sunburn, insect bites, contact dermatitis (poison ivy, oak, or sumac), cuts and scratches.
Benzocaine, Butamben, and Tetracaine **Gel, Ointment, Topical Aerosol, Topical Solution:** Cetacaine	1	*Topical:* Gel, ointment, topical aerosol, and topical solution contain 14% benzocaine, 2% butamben, and 2% tetracaine. For use on mucous membranes prior to examination, instrumentation, or other procedures of the esophagus, larynx, nasal cavity, pharynx, throat, rectum, trachea, respiratory tract, and vagina (gel only). Also for dental procedures and oral surgery.
Bupivicaine Hydrochloride **Injection:** Marcaine, Sensorcaine. **Injection with Epinephrine:** Marcaine, Sensorcaine. **Injection with Dextrose:** Marcaine Spinal, Sensorcaine Spinal.	2–5	*Injection:* caudal anesthesia (0.25%, 0.5%); epidural anesthesia (0.25%, 0.5%, 0.75%); local infiltration (0.25%), peripheral nerve block (0.25%, 0.5%), retrobulbar block (0.75%), sympathetic block (0.25%). *Injection with Epinephrine:* Dental for infiltration and nerve block in maxillary and mandibular area (0.5% with 1:200,000 epinephrine/site). Used for same purposes and at same concentrations as the injection.

Table 13 (*continued*)

Drug	Duration of Action (hr)	Indications/Concentration
		Injection with Dextrose: Hyperbaric spinal anesthesia: normal vaginal delivery and cesarean section (0.75%); surgical anesthesia for lower extremity, perineal procedures, lower abdominal procedures (0.75%).
Butacaine **Ointment:** Butyn dental	1	Relief of pain associated with appliances (4%).
Butamben Picrate **Ointment:** Butesin Picrate		*Cutaneous:* 1% ointment. See Benzocaine, above.
Chlorprocaine hydrochloride **Injection:** Nescaine, Nescaine-CE♣, Nescaine-MPF.	0.25–1.5	*Injection:* caudal anesthesia (2%, 3%); epidural anesthesia for lumbar and sacral areas (2%, 3%); nerve block: brachial plexus (2%), digital (1%), infraorbital (2%), mandibular (2%); obstetrics: paracervical block (1%), pudendal block (2%).
Cocaine Hydrochloride (C-II) **Crystals, Flakes, Tablets:** To make appropriate solutions. **Topical Solution:** (generic).	0.5–1	*Mucous Membranes:* 1%–4% solution for anesthesia in the oral, nasal, and laryngeal cavities before surgery or instrumentation.
Dibucaine Hydrochloride **Topical Cream, Topical Ointment, Rectal Ointment:** Nupercainal.	2–4	*Cutaneous:* 0.5% cream or 1% ointment. See Benzocaine, above. *Rectal:* 1% ointment in the a.m. and p.m. and after each bowel movement.
Dicylonine Hydrochloride **Lozenges:** Children's Sucrets, Sucrets Maximum Strength. **Oral Topical Solution:** Sucrets Maximum Strength. **Topical Solution:** Dyclone.	Less than 1	*Lozenges:* 3 mg dissolved slowly in the mouth. *Oral Topical Solution:* 0.1% solution used in the oral or pharyngeal mucosa. 0.5% or 1% for pain caused by esophageal lesions. *Topical Solution:* 1% for mucous membrane anesthesia;
Etidocaine Hydrochloride **Injection and Injection with Epinephrine:** Duranest.	2–5	*Injection with or without Epinephrine:* caudal anesthesia (0.5%, 1%); lumbar peridural anesthesia: cesarean section, intra-abdominal or pelvic surgery, lower-limb surgery (1%); gynecological procedures (0.5%, 1%); peripheral nerve block (0.5%,1%); percutaneous infiltration (0.5%). *Injection with Epinephrine:* Dental nerve block or infiltration (1.5%).

Table 13 (*continued*)

Drug	Duration of Action (hr)	Indications/Concentration
Lidocaine **Topical Aerosol, Ointment, Solution:** Xylocaine.	0.5–1	*Mucous membranes:* topical aerosol (10%) for gingival and oral mucous membranes; ointment (5%) for use in dentistry; topical solution (5%) for oral mucosa. Also topical ointment is used for the oropharynx.
Lidocaine Hydrochloride **Injection:** Dalcaine, Dilocaine, L-Caine, Lidoject-1 and -2, Nulicaine, Xylocaine. **Injection with Dextrose:** Xylocaine, Xylocaine with Glucose. **Injection with Epinephrine:** Octocaine, Octocaine-50 and -100♣, Xylocaine. **Jelly:** Xylocaine. **Ointment:** (generic) **Oral Topical Solution:** Xylocaine Viscous. **Topical Solution:** Anestacon, Xylocaine.	0.5–1	*Injection:* caudal anesthesia: obstetrical (1%), surgical (1.5%); lumbar epidural analgesia (1%) or anesthesia (1.5%, 2%); thoracic anesthesia (1%); IV regional infiltration (0.5%); percutaneous infiltration (0.5%, 1%); peripheral nerve block: brachial (1.5%), dental (2%), intercostal (1%), paracervical (1%), paravertebral (1%), pudendal (4%); retrobulbar (4%); cervial or lumbar sympathetic nerve block (1%); transtracheal (4% along with 4% topical solution). *Injection with Dextrose:* low spinal saddle block for obstetrics (1.5%, 5%); cesarean section (5%); abdominal surgical anesthesia (5%). *Injection with Epinephrine:* See information under Injection. *Jelly:* 2% for mucous membrane anesthesia of the esophagus, larynx, trachea; 2% for urinary tract for urethral examination or prior to cystoscopy (in males). *Oral Topical Solution:* 15 mL (300 mg) in the mouth or as a gargle for pharyngeal pain. *Topical Solution:* 4% for mucous membrane anesthesia of the oral or nasal cavities, esophagus; 2% for urinary tract for examination of the urethra or painful urethritis. *Ointment:* 5% for cutaneous use to relieve pain, itching, or inflammation due to burns, insect bites, sunburn, contact dermatitis, or cuts and scratches.

Table 13 (*continued*)

Drug	Duration of Action (hr)	Indications/Concentrations
Mepivacaine Hydrochloride **Injection:** Carbocaine, Isocaine, Isocaine 3% ♣, Polocaine.	0.5–3	*Injection:* brachial, cervical, intercostal, pudendal, nerve block (1%); caudal and lumbar epidural block (1%, 1.5%); dental infiltration and nerve block of oral cavity, single site in upper or lower jaw (3%); local infiltration other than dentistry (0.5%, 1%), paracervical block (1%); block for pain management (1%, 2%); paracervical plus pudendal block (1%).
Pramoxine Hydrochloride **Rectal Aerosol Foam:** ProctoFoam. **Rectal Cream:** Tronolane, Tronothane. **Rectal Ointment:** Fleet Relief. **Rectal Suppositories:** **Topical Cream:** Prax, Tronothane. **Topical Lotion:** Prax.	Less than 1	*Rectal use:* 1% aerosol foam, cream, or ointment for anorectal disorders including hemorrhoids, inflammation, anogential pain, anogenital pruritus. 1% suppository for hemorrhoids, anorectal inflammation. *Cutaneous:* 1% cream or lotion for minor skin disorders Tronolane. including pain from burns, insect bites, sunburn, poison ivy, poison sumac, poison oak, minor wounds.
Prilocaine Hydrochloride **Injection:** Citanest. **Injection with** **Epinephrine:** Citanest Forte.	0.5–3	*Injection and Injection with Epinephrine:* 4% for dental infiltration and nerve block.
Procaine Hydrochloride **Injection:** Novocain	0.25–1.5	*Injection:* Infiltration (0.25%, 0.5%); peripheral nerve block (0.5%, 1%, 2%); subarachnoid: perineum, perineum and lower extremities (10%).
Proparacaine Hydrochloride **Ophthalmic Solution:** AK-Taine, Alcaine, Kainair, Ocu-Caine, Ophthaine, Ophthetic. conjunctival and corneal	0.25	*Ophthalmic:* Local anesthesia of short duration for tonometry, removal of sutures and foreign bodies, scraping in diagnosis and gonioscopy.
Propoxycaine and Procaine **Injection with** **Levonordefrin:** Ravocaine and Novocain with Neo- Cobefrin. **Injection with** **Norepinephrine Bitartrate:** Ravocaine and Novocaine with Levophed.		*Injections:* Both for dental infiltration and nerve block: 0.4% propoxycaine and 2% procaine.

Table 13 (*continued*)

Drug	Duration of Action (hr)	Indications/Concentration
Tetracaine Hydrochloride **Injection, Sterile Injection, and Injection with Dextrose:** Pontocaine. **Ophthalmic Ointment or Solution:** Pontocaine. **Rectal Cream:** Pontocaine Cream **Topical Ointment with Menthol:** Pontocaine Ointment. **Topical Solution:** Pontocaine.	0.5–3	*Injection:* saddle block anesthesia for vaginal delivery (1%); spinal anesthesia: perineum, perineum and lower extremities, up to costal margin (1%). *Sterile Injection:* saddle block for vaginal delivery (2–5 mg); spinal anesthesia: perineum (5 mg); perineum and lower extremities (10 mg); up to costal margin (15–20 mg). *Injection with dextrose:* saddle block (0.2%); spinal anesthesia: lower or upper abdomen, perineal (0.3%). *Ophthalmic:* 0.5% ointment or solution for local anesthesia of short duration for tonometry, removal of sutures or foreign bodies, and conjunctival and corneal scraping in diagnosis and gonioscopy. *Rectal:* 1% cream or 0.5% ointment for anorectal disorders including hemorrhoids, pain, inflammation, or pruritus. *Mucous membranes:* 0.25% or 0.5% topical solution for anesthesia of the larynx, trachea, or esophagus prior to procedures; 0.5% nebulized for oral inhalation. *Cutaneous:* 0.5% ointment or 1% cream to relieve pain from minor skin disorders including burns, sunburn, insect bites, poison ivy, poison oak, poison sumac, minor wounds.

Special Concerns: Pediatric and geriatric patients are more likely to experience systemic toxicity.

Side Effects: Swelling and paresthesia of lips and oral tissue. Systemic reactions occur when plasma levels are high, and in rare cases such reactions can be fatal. Systemic symptoms include CNS excitation with tremors, shivering, and convulsions; cardiovascular effects, including hypotension, intraventricular conduction defect, or A-V block, which may lead to cardiac and respiratory arrest; eczematoid dermatitis.

Epinephrine in local anesthetic preparations may result in anginal pain, tachycardia, tremors, headache, restlessness, palpitations, dizziness, and hypertension.

Drug Interactions

Local anesthetics containing vasoconstrictors with MAO inhibitors, tricyclic antidepressants, phenothiazines	Severe hypo- or hypertension
Local anesthetics containing vasoconstrictors and oxytocic drugs	Excess hypertensive response
Local anesthetics containing vasoconstrictors and chloroform, halothane, cyclopropane, trichloroethylene	↑ Chance of cardiac arrhythmias

Dosage: The dosage of the various local anesthetics varies over a wide range depending on the route of administration and specific use.

NURSING CONSIDERATIONS

Administration/Storage

1. Do not use preparations of local anesthetics containing preservatives for spinal or epidural anesthesia.
2. Store local anesthetics containing *epinephrine* separately from those that do not.
3. Store local anesthetics containing *preservatives* separately from those that do not.
4. Clearly mark each container indicating exactly which local anesthetics are stored in the compartment.
5. Autoclave vials of anesthetics that are not destroyed by heat for sterile handling.
6. Use antiseptic or detergent with dye as a solution in which to store anesthetics that cannot be autoclaved but that must be sterile and ready for use. The dye will indicate if there is a crack in the vial and if the sterilizing solution is seeping into the anesthetic.
7. Read the label three times to ascertain that the correct local anesthetic is being prepared or provided to the doctor for administration.
8. Discard the remainder of preparations without preservatives following initial use.
9. *Do not use epinephrine* in nerve block of digits, because blood supply can be compromised and tissue damage can result.
10. Have emergency drugs and resuscitative equipment readily available whenever local anesthetics are used.
11. Have ultrashort-acting barbiturates such as thiopental or thiamylal, and short-acting barbiturates such as secobarbital and pentobarbital to treat clients with convulsions.
12. If the client has cardiac or respiratory depression, CNS depressants should be avoided. Have a short acting muscle relaxant such as IV succinylcholine readily available.

Assessment

1. A careful drug history should be taken prior to the administration of any local anesthetic to determine any drug sensitivities.
2. Assess the client's vital signs, reflexes, sensation, and orientation as to time and place and document.
3. Note client's bowel sounds, any urinary tract problems and the status of the client's cardiovascular system.
4. During the nursing history, note any special conditions which may interfere with the intended

drug effects. Special care should be taken when administering lidocaine to elderly clients, clients who have respiratory depression, shock or myasthenia gravis.

5. The preoperative medications are an important part of the client's preparation for surgery. Administer all medications as ordered, noting the client's condition and response to the medication.

Interventions

1. When a client receives local anesthesia, he/she is awake. Minimize anxiety by limiting conversation and noise.

2. Closely monitor the client for symptoms of CNS excitation. Nervousness, complaints of dizziness, blurred vision, and tremors are frequent symptoms of this occurrence.

3. Note symptoms of CNS depression. These may include drowsiness, respiratory distress, convulsions, and loss of consciousness. Document the time and extent of these symptoms and report to the physician.

4. Monitor vital signs. Assess the client for symptoms of a cardiac depressant reaction. This is characterized by hypotension, myocardial depression, bradycardia, and possibly cardiac arrest. Therefore, assess BP, pulse rate, ECG, and appearance of client frequently.

5. Support the client's respiratory efforts by maintaining a patent airway. Supply oxygen as needed by assisted or controlled ventilatory methods.

6. Observe client for allergic reactions characterized by cutaneous lesions, urticaria, edema, or anaphylaxis. Have oxygen, epinephrine, corticosteroids, and antihistamines readily available for treatment of an allergic reaction.

7. Note client complaints of local burning, tenderness, swelling, and any evidence of tissue irritation, sloughing, or tissue necrosis. These are local reactions that should be reported immediately to the physician so that appropriate therapy can be implemented.

Anesthesia for the Eye

Interventions

The following guidelines should be followed when administering eye medications (see also Chapter 6, p. 38).

1. Do not allow the dropper to come in contact with the eyelid and surrounding tissue during the administration of eye drops.

2. Administer precisely the number of drops ordered since excess dosage causes serious side effects and retards wound healing in surgical conditions of the eye.

3. Rinse tonometer (instrument used for measuring intraocular pressure) with sterile distilled water prior to use to avoid introducing foreign bodies into the anesthetized eye.

4. Protect the eye from irritating chemicals, foreign bodies, and rubbing (of eye by client) while the eye is anesthetized.

5. Cover the anesthetized eye with a patch following the procedure because the blink reflex is temporarily absent.

6. Remind the client not to touch or rub their anesthetized eye.

Anesthesia for the Nasopharynx

Advise the client not to eat food or drink fluids for at least 1 hour following the use of topical anesthesia. Second stage swallowing (pharyngeal) is impaired and the client may aspirate.

Anesthesia for the Rectum and Anus

Intervention

If the client complains of itching and burning, examine the anal area for any evidence of a break in the skin.

Client/Family Teaching

1. Advise the client to use the lowest possible dose of medication to minimize systemic toxicity.
2. Stress the need to wash the hands before and after applying the medication.

Anesthesia by Nerve Block

Oral Cavity Block

Client/Family Teaching

1. Advise client not to eat food for at least 1 hour after injection, because the swallowing reflex is depressed and aspiration may occur. Loss of sensation in the tongue or cheek may result in injury during chewing.
2. Observe for swelling of lips and oral tissue. This may necessitate the use of cold compresses for comfort and to reduce swelling.

Pudendal Block

Interventions

1. Note the level of the client's apprehension, anxiety, and fear. This may indicate the effectiveness of the block.
2. Observe for the formation of hematoma or rectal puncture (blood flow through rectum) following a block, which would indicate complications. Document and report these findings to the physician.

Epidural Block

Interventions

1. Observe the client for evidence of diminished cardiac and respiratory function. This may occur as a result of the anesthesia.
2. Monitor pulse, BP, and skin color. If hypotension develops, summon assistance, elevate the client's legs, turn the client onto left side, administer oxygen, and increase the rate of the IV flow.
3. If the anesthesia is being administered to a woman in labor, monitor the client's contractions. The client has a diminished sensation of contractions.
4. Monitor intake and output. If the client has difficulty voiding or voids small amounts that are out of proportion to the intake, palpate the bladder for urinary retention. Catheterization may be necessary.
5. Check the client for fecal incontinence. Cleanse the perineal area as necessary while the client is in labor.
6. Monitor the fetal heart beat for signs of fetal distress. Local drugs may cross the placental barrier, depressing the fetus.

Caudal Block

Interventions

1. Monitor the client closely for indications of excessively high levels of anesthesia. The major symptom is diminished cardiac and respiratory function.

2. Note any increase in restlessness, anxiety, tremors or twitching. These are early signs of impending convulsions due to absorption of local anesthetic into the bloodstream. Use appropriate seizure precautions.

3. Observe the client for cessation of sweating and in lower extremities for a pronounced vasodilatation. These are both early signs of effective anesthesia. Do not change the client's position during the early stages of anesthesia without the consent of the physician.

4. If the client is in labor, constantly monitor the progress of labor since the client will have diminished sensation of contractions.

5. Note signs of urinary retention. Palpate bladder and catheterize the client if indicated.

6. Check for fecal incontinence and cleanse the perineal area as necessary while the woman is in labor.

Paracervical Block

Intervention

Using a fetal monitor, closely monitor the fetal heart beat. Local anesthesia by paracervical block may cause fetal bradycardia and acidosis.

Spinal Anesthesia

Interventions

1. Maintain client in a supine position 8–12 hr after anesthesia to reduce occurrence of headache.

2. Apply ice bag to head if headache occurs. A pressure dressing applied to tap site may also assist with headache control.

3. Protect client from injury and burns because client's bodily sensations are absent.

4. Reassure client that this sensation is only temporary and that their baseline normal sensations will return.

5. Chart when motion and sensation are recovered. When client can move toes, sensation is completely recovered.

6. Provide prescribed analgesics and sedatives as needed.

7. Offer fluids frequently and hydrate adequately to prevent hypotension.

8. Assist in exercising lower limbs as necessary to prevent thrombophlebitis.

9. Clients should be advised that transient nerve palsies may occur about 2 weeks after spinal anesthesia. Should this occur, the client should notify the physician immediately.

GENERAL ANESTHETICS

The objectives of general anesthesia are to produce (1) a state of unconsciousness and amnesia, (2) analgesia, (3) hyporeflexia, and (4) skeletal muscle relaxation.

There are two types of general anesthetics: inhalation anesthetics that include gases, such as nitrous oxide and highly volatile liquids, such as halothane and related drugs; and IV, or fixed-dose, anesthetics. This group includes the ultrashort-acting barbiturates, such as methohexital, thioamylal, and thiopental.

Since general anesthetics should be used only by those with specialized training and experience, only general information on special uses, advantages, and disadvantages of general anesthetics currently in use will be presented. Since the nurse is largely responsible for patient care after anesthesia, extensive nursing implications have been included.

Action/Kinetics: General anesthetics probably interfere with functioning of nerve cell membranes in the CNS by an action at the lipid membrane of the cell. Most general anesthetics are excreted unchanged through the lungs. However, agents such as halothane, enflurane, methoxyflurane, and isoflurane are metabolized by the liver. Biotransformation of enflurane, methoxyflurane, and isoflurane releases flouride ion, which may cause renal toxicity (see Table 14).

Uses: See Table 14 for uses as well as advantages and disadvantages of the various general anesthetics.

Special Concerns: The minimum alvelolar concentration (MAC) of inhalation anesthetics is higher in children (especially young children) than in adults. Geriatric patients may be more at risk of developing hypotension and depression of the circulatory system following general anesthesia.

NURSING CONSIDERATIONS

In the Operating Room

Interventions

1. To prevent fire and explosions, follow the institution protocols for safety and prevention where general anesthesia is used.
2. Review which gases are explosive.
3. Avoid using explosive gases when electrocautery and electric desiccation are used.
4. Wear conductive shoes or boots.
5. Do not wear nylon uniforms where anesthetic gases are used.
6. Do not use woolen blankets in the area.
7. If sweaters must be worn, wear cotton sweaters.
8. Assure that all electrical equipment has been checked and is adequately grounded.
9. Before activating any electrical equipment, check with the anesthesiologist.
10. Do not use matches in the operating room.
11. Ensure that the preventive maintenance program is current and that the equipment is approved prior to use and checked on a continuing basis.

Postoperatively

Interventions

1. Obtain a complete report of the client's diagnosis, surgery, or procedures performed, anesthetic administered, and time of administration, the response of the client to surgery, current condition, and level of consciousness before accepting responsibility for the client from the anesthetist.
2. Assess for adequate airway. If the endotracheal tube is still in place, attach to the ventilator and adjust as ordered to maintain adequate ventilation. Monitor arterial blood gases as indicated. Assess carefully for any respiratory obstruction, hemorrhage, or postprocedural shock.
3. Perform a quick system-by-system initial baseline assessment and document findings. Evaluate fluid status, and review estimated blood loss.
4. Determine presence and ensure proper functioning of all postprocedure devices and equipment (i.e., endotracheal tube, IVs, chest tubes, arterial lines, Swan-Ganz catheters, Jackson-Pratts, Penrose drains, hemovacs, shunts, IABP, packing, etc).
5. Check all dressings and drainage apparatus for proper position and function. Document presence and amount of drainage as a baseline.
6. To prevent aspiration of secretions and vomitus, keep the client positioned comfortably on the side until conscious, unless contraindicated.

Table 14 General Anesthetics

Generic/ Trade Name	Uses	Advantages *Volatile Liquids*	Disadvantages	Additional Nursing Considerations
Enflurane (Ethrane) (Rx)	Induction and maintenance of general anesthesia (widely used). Analgesic for obstetrics for vaginal delivery and as a supplement to other general anesthetics used for cesarean section. 2%–4.5% produces anesthesia in 7–10 min.	Induction and recovery are rapid. No significant stimulation of salivation, bronchial secretions, or bronchomotor tone. Usually provides sufficient muscle relaxation for abdominal surgery. No significant bradycardia. Less chance to cause renal problems due to release of free flouride ion. Heart rate remains constant.	As depth of anesthesia increases, hypotension increases. High concentrations may cause uterine relaxation and increased uterine bleeding. High levels accompanied by hypercapnia may cause seizures.	Monitor cardiac function more closely if epinephrine is administered, because arrhythmias are more likely to occur.
Halothane (Fluothane, Somnothane✸) (Rx)	Induction and maintenance of general anesthesia. May be given with oxygen or a mixture of oxygen and nitrous oxide. Maintenance: 0.5%–1.5%.	Rapid, pleasant induction and recovery. Little nausea/vomiting. Nonexplosive. Not an irritant to respiratory tract; thus there is no increase in secretions. Hepatic toxicity does not appear to occur in children.	Hypoxia, acidosis, or apnea may occur during deep anesthesia. Sensitizes heart to epinephrine with possible serious arrhythmias. Bradycardia. Has been said to cause hepatic damage with repeated doses. Produces only moderate muscle relaxation. Assisted or controlled ventilation may be required. May produce hypotension or malignant hyperthermia.	Anticipate shivering during recovery period.

| Isoflurane (Forane) (Rx) | Induction and maintenance of general anesthesia. Concentrations of 1.5%–3% produce surgical anesthesia in 7–10 min. Nitrous oxide at levels of 1%–2.5% sustain surgical levels of anesthesia when used with isoflurane. | Induction and recovery are rapid. Less toxicity due to flouride ion. Does not sensitize the myocardium to epinephrine. Good skeletal muscle relaxation when used alone. Pharyngeal and laryngeal reflexes are reduced. No excessive salivation or tracheobronchial secretions. Cardiac output is maintained through an increase in heart rate. | Causes significant respiratory depression. Pungent odor. Less smooth induction than halothane. Profound peripheral dilation may cause a decrease in blood pressure and increase in heart rate. May cause malignant hyperthermia. | |
| Methoxyflurane (Penthrane) (Rx) | Induction and maintenance of general anesthesia. May be combined with nitrous oxide and oxygen for surgery expected to last 4 hr or less. Also may be used alone or in combination with nitrous oxide for analgesia in obstetrics or minor surgery. 2% used for induction; 0.3%–0.8% used for analgesia and anesthesia. Maintenance: 0.1%–0.2% when given with oxygen and 50% nitrous oxide. | Analgesia and drowsiness persist so need for narcotics during immediate postoperative period reduced. Nonexplosive. Less incidence of laryngeal spasm or bronchoconstriction. Pleasant odor with minimal respiratory tract irritation. No significant sensitization of myocardium to catecholamines. Pleasant odor with minimal respiratory tract irritation. | Induction and recovery are slow. Metabolized to free flouride ion, which may cause renal damage or failure. May cause malignant hyperthermia. Minimal skeletal muscle relaxation when used alone. | Anticipate prolonged drowsiness and the effects of anesthesia postoperatively; effect may be reversed by hyperventilation. |

Table 14 (continued)

Generic/ Trade Name	Uses	Advantages	Disadvantages	Additional Nursing Considerations
		Gases		
Nitrous oxide (Rx)	Adjunct with other anesthetics, antianxiety agents, narcotics, or muscle relaxants. Dentistry. Analgesic. In combination with halothane to reach equilibrium of halothane more rapidly.	Rapid, pleasant induction and recovery. Nonexplosive gas. No significant effects on hepatic, renal, or autonomic nervous systems.	With 100% gas, which is necessary for anesthesia, hypoxia and anoxia occur; with 80% gas and 20% oxygen, produce good analgesia but poor anesthesia. Does not cause skeletal muscle relaxation. May cause malignant hyperthermia. May cause accumulation of pressure in the middle ear, bowel, and lungs. Known to cause vomiting, respiratory depression, and death. Abuse and dependence have been documented.	Dental personnel may show an increased risk of peripheral neuropathy and renal and hepatic diseases if exposed chronically to nitrous oxide. Effect can be rapidly reversed by hyperventilation.

7. Note excessive mucus in the nasopharynx and oral cavity and suction as needed.

8. Monitor BP, pulse rate, and respirations. Note the client's general appearance and document. The frequency of assessments may decrease as vital signs become stable.

9. Note which anesthetic the client received and whether a short or long recovery to consciousness is anticipated. Plan care accordingly.

10. Monitor and record parameters of CVP, ICP, arterial pressures, pulmonary artery pressures, cardiac output, cardiac monitor, and urinary output as ordered.

11. Assess and document the client's recovery utilizing a complete body systems format (e.g., neurological, respiratory, cardiovascular, GI, GU).

12. Hearing is the first sense to return when a client regains consciousness. It is important to minimize conversation and to prevent anxiety-provoking noise as much as possible. Provide orientation and positive encouragement. Assist the client to reestablish normal physiologic balance with the least anxiety possible.

13. Administer analgesics for pain as ordered, after exhalation of the anesthetic, and as all other parameters permit.

14. Note that the client's pain can cause hypotension. If this combination occurs, report it to the physician to determine whether an analgesic should be administered.

15. Cover the client to prevent vasodilation and subsequent heat loss, which tends to occur after administering anesthetic agents. Heated or warmed covers may assist with rewarming the client.

16. Note that temperature is not a reliable vital sign for 1–2 hr after surgery, because the client is adjusting to different environmental conditions and body temperature may fluctuate as a direct result.

MISCELLANEOUS GENERAL ANESTHETICS AND ADJUNCTS

ETOMIDATE   (eh-TOM-ih-dayt)

Amidate (Rx)

Classification: General anesthetic and adjunct to general anesthesia.

Action/Kinetics: Etomidate is actually a hypnotic without any analgesic activity. The drug seems to act like gamma-aminobutryic acid (GABA) and is thought to exert its mechanism by depressing the activity of the brain stem reticular system. It has minimal cardiovascular and respiratory depressant effects. **Onset:** 1 min. **Duration:** 3–5 min. $t^{1}/_{2}$: 75 min. Rapidly metabolized in the liver with inactive metabolites excreted mainly through the urine.

Uses: Induction of general anesthesia. As a supplement to nitrous oxide during short surgical procedures.

Special Concerns: Pregnancy category: C. Use with caution during lactation. Safety and efficacy have not been established in children less than 10 years of age.

Side Effects: *Skeletal muscle:* Myoclonic skeletal muscle movements, tonic movements. *Respiratory:* Apnea, hyperventilation or hypoventilation, laryngospasm. *Cardiovascular:* Either hypertension or hypotension; tachycardia or bradycardia; arrhythmias. *GI:* Nausea, vomiting. *Miscellaneous:* Eye movements (common), hiccoughs, snoring.

Dosage: IV only. *Induction of anesthesia:* **Adults and children over 10 years of age,** 0.2–0.6 mg/kg (usual: 0.3 mg/kg) injected over 30–60 sec.

NURSING CONSIDERATIONS

See also *Nursing Considerations* for *General Anesthetics,* p. 873.

Administration/Storage

1. Lower doses of etomidate may be used as adjuncts to supplement less potent general anesthetics such as nitrous oxide.
2. Etomidate may be used following preanesthetic medications.
3. The drug should be protected from extreme heat and freezing.

Interventions

1. Nausea and vomiting are likely to occur postoperatively. Have essential equipment available to counteract the problem.
2. Monitor during the immediate postoperative period, for both hypotension and hypertension, tachycardia and bradycardia. Document and report to the physician.

FENTANYL CITRATE AND DROPERIDOL   (FEN-tah-nil, droh-PER-ih-dol)

Innovar (Rx) (C-II)

See also Chapter 37, p. 761, for information on fentanyl citrate and Chapter 32, p. 646, for information on droperidol.

Classification: Agent for neuroleptanalgesia.

Action/Kinetics: The effect of combining a narcotic analgesic (fentanyl) and an antipsychotic (droperidol) is referred to as neuroleptanalgesia which is characterized by excellent analgesia, decreased motor activity, and overall quiet behavior. Complete loss of consciousness usually does not occur.

Uses: Tranquilization and analgesia for surgical or diagnostic procedures; premedication for anesthesia; induction of anesthesia; adjunct in maintenance of general and regional anesthesia.

Dosage: Dosage depends on the use and the characteristics of the patient. The package insert should be consulted prior to administration of this drug.

NURSING CONSIDERATIONS

See also *Nursing Considerations* for *General Anesthetics,* p. 873.

Administration

CNS depressants should be reduced by ⅓–½ of the normal dose, up to 8 hours postanesthesia.

KETAMINE HYDROCHLORIDE   (KEE-tah-mean)

Ketalar (Rx)

Classification: General anesthetic.

Action/Kinetics: Ketamine is rapid-acting and produces good analgesia. The drug blocks afferent impulses associated with pain perception, depresses spinal cord activity, and affects transmitter systems in the CNS. There is no effect on the pharyngeal-laryngeal reflexes. There is, however, slightly enhanced skeletal muscle tone and cardiovascular and respiratory stimulation. **Onset, IV:** 30 sec following a dose of 2 mg/kg; **onset, IM:** 3–4 min. **Duration, IV:** 5–10 min following a dose of 2 mg/kg; **duration, IM:** 12–25 min following a dose of 10 mg/kg. **t¹/₂:** 7–11 min (distribution) and 2–3 hr (elimination). The anesthetic effect is terminated by redistribution to other tissues from the brain and by liver metabolism (the major metabolite is ⅓ as active as ketamine).

Uses: For procedures in which skeletal muscle relaxation is not required. Induction of anesthesia before use of other general anesthetics. As a supplement to nitrous oxide anesthesia. *Investigational:* Adjunct to local anesthesia, to produce sedation and analgesia.

Contraindications: Schizophrenia, acute psychoses, hypertension (or in patients in whom a rise in blood pressure would be dangerous).

Special Concerns: Safe use during pregnancy has not been determined. Use with caution in the chronic alcoholic or if an individual is intoxicated with alcohol.

Side Effects: *Respiratory:* Apnea or severe respiratory depression following rapid IV administration, laryngospasm. *GI:* Nausea, vomiting, anorexia, increased salivation. *CV:* Increased blood pressure and pulse rate, bradycardia, hypotension, arrhythmias. *Skeletal muscle:* Tonic and clonic movements resembling seizures. *CNS:* Emergence reactions including dream-like states, hallucinations, delirium, vivid imagery, confusion, irrational behavior, excitement. *Ophthalmologic:* Increased intraocular pressure (slight), double vision, nystagmus. *Miscellaneous:* Morbilliform rash, transient erythema.

Drug Interactions	
Barbiturates	↑ Recovery time from ketamine
Halothane	↓ Pulse rate, blood pressure and cardiac output
Muscle relaxants, nondepolarizing	↑ Neuromuscular effects → respiratory depression
Narcotic analgesics	↑ Recovery time from ketamine
Thyroid hormones	Tachycardia and hypertension
Tubocurarine	↑ Neuromuscular effects → respiratory depression

Dosage: IV. Individualized. *Induction,* **initial:** 1–2 mg/kg (of the base) at a rate of 0.5 mg/kg/min. **Maintenance:** 0.01–0.05 mg/kg by continuous infusion at a rate of 1–2 mg/min. *Adjunct to local anesthesia:* 5–30 mg (of the base) before giving the local anesthetic. *Sedation and analgesia:* 0.2–0.75 mg/kg (of the base) given over 2–3 min; **then,** 0.005–0.02 mg/kg (of the base) per min as a continuous IV infusion.

IM. *Induction,* **initial:** 5–10 mg/kg (of the base). Doses from one-half to the full amount of the induction dose may be used to maintain anesthesia. *Maintenance of ketamine used with diazepam:* 0.1–0.5 mg/min ketamine with 2–5 mg diazepam IV as required. *Sedation and analgesia:* 2–4 mg/kg (of the base); **then,** 0.005–0.2 mg/kg (of the base) per min by continuous IV infusion.

NURSING CONSIDERATIONS

Administration/Storage:

1. The dose should be administered slowly over a 60-sec period in order to reduce respiratory depression and hypertension.

2. Vials containing 100 mg/mL should always be diluted first with an equal volume of sterile water for injection, normal saline, or 5% dextrose in water.

3. A precipitate will form if ketamine is combined with a barbiturate; thus, they should not be mixed in the same syringe.

4. Diazepam and ketamine should not be mixed in the same syringe or infusion flask.

5. Maintenance doses must be determined individually and are dependent, in part, on which additional anesthetic is used.

6. Tonic-clonic movements may occur during anesthesia; if manifested, they are not an indication for additional ketamine.

Interventions

1. To prevent dreams that are likely to occur with ketamine, place client in a quiet area after anesthesia.

2. Take vital signs gently. Avoid making noises, bumping bed, and vigorously rousing or stimulating the client. Keep side rails up.

3. If the client is excessively active during the recovery phase, anticipate that a low dose of a barbiturate sedative may be required. This may prolong recovery time.

PART SEVEN

Drugs Affecting the Autonomic Nervous System

CHAPTER FORTY-THREE

Introduction to the Autonomic Nervous System

The system that involuntarily regulates the basic physiologic functions of the body is called the autonomic nervous system (ANS).

Among the important functions regulated by the ANS are respiration, perspiration, body temperature, carbohydrate metabolism, digestion, bowel motility, pupil size, blood pressure, heart rate, and glandular secretions such as salivation.

The autonomic nervous system is a composite of two opposing subsystems—the sympathetic and the parasympathetic divisions—that interact with one another to maintain the body in physiologic equilibrium. Even though it is difficult to separate the precise functions of the sympathetic and the parasympathetic systems, since both play a role in all major physiologic processes, the sympathetic system is more closely associated with the quick regulation of the expenditure of energy during emergencies (fight or flight response), whereas the parasympathetic system is more directly involved in the storage and conservation of energy (e.g., digestion and absorption of food).

The manner in which the two divisions of the ANS work together can best be illustrated by looking at a major organ like the heart. Impulses transmitted via the *sympathetic* division will have a tendency to *increase* the heart rate, the contractibility of the muscle, and the speed at which the impulse is transmitted. The *parasympathetic* system will *decrease* the rate of contractibility and conduction.

Normally the two divisions of the ANS are in balance. In an emergency situation, however, when there is an increased need for rapidly circulating blood, the sympathetic system dominates. Impulses are sent that increase the rate of the heart. Blood pressure rises. The small arterioles that supply the skin and outlying parts of the body constrict, and blood supply to the GI tract decreases. When the situation returns to normal the parasympathetic division returns the body to more normal housekeeping functions.

Each nerve pathway in the ANS is composed of two nerve cells. The preganglionic cell is located in the spinal cord, and the axon of this cell (preganglionic fiber) travels to a nerve cell outside the cord where there is a neurojunction, or synapse. This nerve cell outside the cord is in a nerve ganglion and the neurojunction is the ganglionic synapse. Most of the sympathetic ganglia are located in the paravertebral ganglionic chain. The parasympathetic ganglia are located near the effector organ. The axon of the ganglionic cell (postganglionic fiber) then travels to the effector organ, where there is a second synapse at the organ, or effector, structure.

When a nerve impulse reaches any of these synapses, it releases the chemical mediator, a neurohormone, from special storage sites in the nerve terminal. The chemical mediator flows across the synapse and combines with a part of the cell called a receptor site. This then initiates a specific response of the effector organ. Once this is accomplished (the entire sequence of events is almost instantaneous), the remaining hormone is either destroyed by a specific enzyme or taken back up into the special storage sites of the cell. Also, a small amount of the hormone is carried away in the blood. Then the entire system is ready to respond again.

Three neurohormones are known to transmit the nerve impulse at the synapses of the ANS: *acetylcholine, epinephrine* (also known as Adrenalin, which is also found in the adrenal gland) and *norepinephrine* (levarterenol).

Acetylcholine is found at both *synapses* (preganglionic and postganglionic) of the *parasympathetic* nervous system as well as in the ganglionic synapses of the *sympathetic* nervous system. Drugs whose actions reinforce or mimic acetylcholine are called cholinergic, or parasympathomimetic. Furthermore, drugs that act at the junction of the postganglionic fiber and effector organ are called muscarinic, while drugs that act at the ganglia are called nicotinic.

Norepinephrine and/or epinephrine (adrenalin) are the chemical mediators at the postganglionic sympathetic nerve endings (junction at the effector organ). Norepinephrine combines with sites called *alpha* receptors. Epinephrine combines with *alpha* and *beta* receptors. It is now known that subtypes of both alpha and beta receptors exist. Alpha$_1$ receptors are located at postsynaptic sites in blood vessels, the eye, urinary bladder, uterus, and liver whereas alpha$_2$ receptors are known to exist at both presynaptic (thought to control the amount of neurotransmitter released) and postsynaptic sites (such as the GI tract). Beta$_1$ are located mainly in the cardiac muscle whereas beta$_2$ receptors are found in the bronchial and vascular musculature. Drugs whose actions reinforce or mimic these chemical mediators are called adrenergic or sympathomimetic.

Drugs that interfere with the enzymes that destroy the excess neurohormone after it is released from its storage vessels also increase the effectiveness of the neurohormones. Such drugs are also called *cholinergic* or *adrenergic*.

The other types of drugs that act on the ANS interfere with or block ANS nerve transmission. They are referred to as cholinergic blocking agents (*parasympatholytic*) and adrenergic blocking agents (*sympatholytic*). In recent years, adrenergic blocking agents have been developed which have specific blocking properties against beta$_1$-adrenergic receptors although most beta-adrenergic blocking drugs block both beta$_1$ and beta$_2$ receptors.

From an anatomic point of view, the sweat glands and some of the salivary glands belong to the sympathetic system. However, since acetylcholine is found at both their neurojunctions, they respond to some of the drugs effective for the parasympathetic system.

CHAPTER FORTY-FOUR

Sympathomimetic (Adrenergic) Drugs

44

SYMPATHOMIMETIC DRUGS

General Statement: The adrenergic drugs supplement, mimic, and reinforce the messages transmitted by the natural neurohormones—norepinephrine and epinephrine. These hormones are responsible for transmitting nerve impulses at the postganglionic neurojunctions of the sympathetic nervous system. The adrenergic drugs work in two ways: (1) by mimicking the action of norepinephrine or epinephrine (directly acting sympathomimetics) or (2) by causing or regulating the release of the natural neurohormones from their storage sites at the nerve terminals (indirectly acting sympathomimetics). Some drugs exhibit a combination of effects 1 and 2.

The myoneural junction is equipped with special receptors for the neurohormones. These receptors have been classified into two types: alpha (α) and beta (β), according to whether they respond to norepinephrine, epinephrine, or isoproterenol and to certain blocking agents. Alpha-adrenergic receptors are blocked by phenoxybenzamine and phentolamine, whereas beta-adrenergic receptors are blocked by propranolol and similar drugs.

Both alpha and beta receptors have been divided into subtypes. Thus adrenergic stimulation of receptors will manifest the following general effects:

Drug Interactions

$Alpha_1$-adrenergic:	Vasoconstriction, decongestion, constriction of the pupil of the eye, contraction of splenic capsule, contraction of the trigone-sphincter muscle of the urinary bladder.
$Alpha_2$-adrenergic:	Presynaptic to regulate amount of transmitter released; decrease tone, motility, and secretory activity of the GI tract (possibly involved in hypersecretory response also); decrease insulin secretion.
$Beta_1$-adrenergic:	Myocardial contraction (inotropic), regulation of heartbeat (chronotropic), improved impulse conduction, increase lipolysis.
$Beta_2$-adrenergic:	Peripheral vasodilation, bronchial dilation; decrease tone, motility, and secretory activity of the GI tract; increase renin secretion.

In addition, adrenergic agents affect the exocrine glands, the salivary glands, and the CNS. The adrenergic stimulants discussed in this section act preferentially on one or more of the above receptor subtypes; their pharmacologic effect must be carefully monitored and balanced.

Uses: Sympathomimetic agents are mainly used for the treatment of shock induced by sudden cardiac arrest, decompensation, myocardial infarction, trauma, bronchodilation, acute renal failure, drug reactions, anaphylaxis. Adrenergic drugs are also used to reverse bronchospasm caused by bronchial asthma, emphysema, chronic bronchitis, and other respiratory disorders. Sympathomimetic drugs having predominantly alpha-receptor activity are used for the relief of nasal and nasopharyngeal congestion due to rhinitis, sinusitis, head colds. See also individual drugs and the information in Table 15, p. 885.

Contraindications: Tachycardia due to arrhythmias or digitalis toxicity.

Special Concerns: Use with caution in hyperthyroidism, diabetes, prostatic hypertrophy, seizures, degenerative heart disease, especially in geriatric patients or patients with asthma, emphysema, or psychoneuroses. Also, use with caution in patients with coronary insufficiency, coronary artery disease, hypertension, or history of stroke.

Side Effects: *CV:* Tachycardia, arrhythmias, palpitations, blood pressure changes, anginal pain, precordial pain, pallor, cerebral hemorrhage. *GI:* Nausea, vomiting, heartburn, anorexia, altered taste. *CNS:* Restlessness, anxiety, tension, insomnia, hyperkinesis, drowsiness, vertigo, irritability, dizziness, headache, tremors. *Other:* Pulmonary edema, respiratory difficulties, muscle cramps, coughing, bronchospasms, irritation of oropharynx.

Table 15   Overview of Effects of Adrenergic Drugs*

Action	Therapeutic Use
Heart Excitation resulting in increase in heart rate and force of contraction. Dilation or constriction of coronary vessels. Results in increase in stroke volume and cardiac output, strengthening of pulse.	Cardiogenic shock, heart block, Stokes-Adams disease, cardiac slowing (bradycardia), resuscitation.
Blood vessels, systemic vasoconstriction Blood supply to abdominal viscera, cerebrum, skin, and mucosa sharply reduced (vasoconstriction of peripheral blood circulation). BP in large vessels increased (pressor effect) and regulated.	Increase in BP in drug-induced acute hypotension during anesthesia or after myocardial infarction or hemorrhage. Isoproterenol causes vasodilation of vessels in skeletal muscle accompanied by increase in cardiac output. Increased blood flow. Nasal decongestion, certain dermatoses, nosebleeds, migraine headaches, all types of allergic reactions, anaphylactic reaction.
GI and GU tracts Inhibition of glandular secretion. Constriction of sphincters. Decrease of muscle tone and motility in GI tract, urinary bladder. Increase of muscle tone and motility in ureter.	To relieve spasms during ureteral and biliary colic, dysmenorrhea, and labor. Enuresis.
Lungs Relaxation of muscles of bronchial tree.	Acute and chronic asthma, pulmonary emphysema and fibrosis, chronic bronchitis.
Eyes Dilates iris, increases ocular pressure, relaxes ciliary muscle.	
CNS stimulation Excitory action, respiratory stimulation, wakefulness.	Appetite control, overdosage with CNS depressant drugs, narcolepsy.
Metabolism Increase in glycogenesis (sugar metabolism). Increase in lipolysis (release of free fatty acids).	
Miscellaneous Stimulation of salivary glands.	
Sex organs Ejaculation	

*Not all drugs are useful under all circumstances.

Drug Interactions

Beta-adrenergic blocking agents	Inhibit adrenergic stimulation of the heart and bronchial tree; cause bronchial constriction; hypertension, asthma, not relieved by adrenergic agents
Ammonium chloride	↓ Effect of sympathomimetics due to ↑ excretion by kidney
Anesthetics	Halogenated anesthetics sensitize heart to adrenergics—causes cardiac arrhythmias
Anticholinergics	Concomitant use aggravates glaucoma
Antidiabetics	Hyperglycemic effect of epinephrine may necessitate ↑ in dosage of insulin or oral hypoglycemic agents
Corticosteroids	Chronic use with sympathomimetics may result in or aggravate glaucoma; aerosols containing sympathomimetics and corticosteroids may be lethal in asthmatic children
Digitalis glycosides	Combination may cause cardiac arrhythmias
Furazolidone	Furazolidone ↑ alpha-adrenergic effects of sympathomimetics
Guanethidine	Direct-acting sympathomimetics ↑ effects of guanethidine, while indirect-acting sympathomimetics ↓ effects of guanethidine
MAO inhibitors	All effects of sympathomimetics are potentiated; symptoms include hypertensive crisis with possible intracranial hemorrhage, hyperthermia, convulsions, coma; death may occur
Methyldopa	↑ Effects of sympathomimetics
Methylphenidate	Potentiates pressor effect of sympathomimetics; combination hazardous in glaucoma
Oxytocics	↑ Chance of severe hypertension
Phenothiazines	↑ Risk of cardiac arrhythmias
Reserpine	↑ Risk of hypertension following use of direct-acting sympathomimetics and ↓ effect of indirect-acting sympathomimetics
Sodium bicarbonate	↑ Effect of sympathomimetics due to ↓ excretion by kidney
Thyroxine	Potentiation of pressor response of sympathomimetics
Tricyclic antidepressants	↑ Effect of direct-acting sympathomimetics and ↓ effect of indirect-acting sympathomimetics

NURSING CONSIDERATIONS

Administration/Storage

1. Review the list of drugs with which adrenergic agents interact.
2. Discard colored solutions.
3. When administering IV infusions of adrenergic drugs, use an electronic infusion device.
4. Administer adrenergic drugs in a monitored environment.

Assessment

1. Determine if the client has any history of sensitivity to adrenergic drugs.
2. In taking the nursing history, note especially if the client has a history of tachycardia, endocrine disturbances, or respiratory tract problems and document.
3. Obtain baseline data regarding the client's general physical condition.

Interventions

1. During the period of dosage adjustment, closely monitor and record blood pressure and pulse.
2. Monitor intake and output and vital signs throughout therapy.

Client/Family Teaching

1. Discuss prescribed drug and provide printed material regarding potential side effects of this drug therapy.
2. Explain the adverse side effects of the drugs and the need to report all side effects to the physician.
3. Instruct the client not to increase the dosage of medication and not to take the medication more frequently than prescribed while on maintenance doses. If symptoms become more severe, they should consult the physician.
4. Advise the client to take the medication early in the day because these drugs may cause insomnia.

Special Nursing Considerations for Adrenergic Bronchodilators:

Assessment

1. Obtain a full baseline client history prior to starting the drug therapy.
2. Review the contraindications for adrenergic bronchodilators.
3. Assess and record the client's vital signs prior to administering the medication.
4. Obtain arterial blood gases as a baseline against which to measure the influence of medication once therapy begins.

Interventions

1. Monitor BP and pulse after therapy begins to assess cardiovascular response of the client.
2. Observe the effects of the drug on the client's CNS. If the effects on the CNS are pronounced, adjust the dosage of medication and the frequency of administration.
3. If the client has status asthmaticus and abnormal levels of arterial blood gases, continue to provide oxygen mixture and ventilating assistance even though the symptoms appear to be relieved by the bronchodilator.

4. To prevent depression of respiratory effort, administer oxygen on the basis of the evaluation of the client's clinical symptoms and the arterial blood gases.

5. If 3–5 aerosol treatments of the same agent has been administered within the last 6–12 hrs, with only minimal relief, further treatment is not advised.

6. If the client's dyspnea worsens after repeated excessive use of the inhaler, paradoxical airway resistance may occur. Be prepared to assist with alternative therapy.

Client/Family Teaching

1. To improve lung ventilation and reduce fatigue that occurs when eating, start inhalation therapy upon arising in the morning and before meals.

2. A single aerosol treatment is usually enough to control an asthma attack.

3. Increased fluid intake aids in liquefying secretions.

4. If more than 3 aerosol treatments in a 24-hr period are required for relief, contact the physician.

5. Overuse of adrenergic bronchodilators may result in reduced effectiveness, possible paradoxical reaction, and cardiac arrest.

6. If there is dizziness, chest pain, or if there is no relief when the usual dose of medication is used, consult the physician.

7. Other adrenergic medications are not to be taken unless expressly ordered by the physician.

8. Advise the client that regular, consistent use of medication is essential for maximum benefit.

9. Demonstrate how to accomplish postural drainage. Explain how to cough productively and vibrate the chest to promote good respiratory hygiene.

10. Explain the appropriate technique for use and care of prescribed inhalers and respiratory equipment.

SYMPATHOMIMETIC DRUGS

ALBUTEROL   (al-BYOU-teh-rol)

Proventil, Ventolin (Rx)

See also *Sympathomimetic Drugs,* p. 883.

Classification: Direct-acting adrenergic (sympathomimetic) agent.

Action/Kinetics: Albuterol stimulates beta$_2$ receptors of the bronchi, leading to bronchodilation. Causes less tachycardia and is longer-acting than isoproterenol. Has minimal beta$_1$ activity. **Onset, PO:** 15–30 min.; **inhalation,** 5–15 min. **Peak effect, PO:** 2–3 hr; **inhalation,** 60–90 min (after two inhalations). **Duration, PO:** 8 hr (up to 12 for extended-release); **inhalation,** 3–6 hr. Metabolites and unchanged drug excreted in urine and feces. **Tablets not to be used in children less than 12 years of age.**

Use: Bronchial asthma; bronchospasm due to bronchitis or emphysema; bronchitis; obstructive pulmonary disease; exercise-induced bronchospasm. Prophylaxis of bronchial asthma or bronchospasms. Parenteral for treatment of status asthmaticus.

Special Concerns: Pregnancy category: C. Dosage has not been established for inhalation products for children less than 12 years of age. Dosage has not been established for the syrup in children less than 2 years of age, for tablets in children less than 6 years of age, and for extended-release tablets in children less than 12 years of age.

Dosage: Aerosol for Inhalation. Adults: *Bronchodilation:* 0.18–0.2 mg (2 inhalations) q 4–8 hr. *Prophylaxis of exercise-induced bronchospasm:* 0.18–0.2 mg (2 inhalations) 15 min before exercise. **Solution for Inhalation. Adults:** *Bronchodilation:* 1.25–5 mg (of the base) in 2–5 mL of sterile 0.9% sodium chloride or sterile water for inhalation administered by intermittent positive pressure breathing or nebulization. **Capsule for Inhalation. Adults:** *Bronchodilation:* 0.2–0.4 mg q 4–6 hr (for prophylaxis of exercise-induced bronchospasm, give 15 min before exercise).

   Oral Syrup, Tablets. *Bronchodilation:* **Adults, initial** 2–6 mg (of the base) t.i.d.–q.i.d.; **then,** increase dose as needed up to a maximum of 8 mg q.i.d. **Children, 6–14 years, initial:** 2 mg (base) t.i.d.–q.i.d.; **then,** as necessary to a maximum of 24 mg daily in divided doses. **Children, 2–6 years, initial:** 0.1 mg/kg t.i.d.; **then,** increase as necessary up to 0.2 mg/kg, not to exceed 4 mg t.i.d. **Extended-release Tablets. Adults:** *Bronchodilation,* 4 or 8 mg (of the base) q 12 hr up to a maximum of 32 mg daily.

NURSING CONSIDERATIONS

See also *Nursing Considerations* for *Sympathomimetic Drugs,* p. 887.

Administration/Storage

1. Do not exceed the recommended dose.
2. If the dose of drug used previously does not provide relief, contact the physician immediately.
3. When using albuterol inhalers, do not use other inhalation medication unless prescribed by the physician.
4. The contents of the container are under pressure. Therefore, do not store near heat or open flames and do not puncture the container.
5. When given by nebulization, either a face mask or mouthpiece may be used. Compressed air or oxygen with a gas flow of 6–10 L/min should be employed with a single treatment lasting from 5–15 min.
6. When given by IPPB, the inspiratory pressure should be from 10–20 cm water with the duration of treatment ranging from 5–20 min depending on the client and instrument control.

Assessment

1. Obtain a baseline history and assess client's CNS before initiating therapy.
2. Note evidence of client anxiety as this may contribute to air hunger.
3. Determine if the client is able to self-administer the medication.

Interventions

1. If the client appears anxious, maintain a calm, reassuring attitude. If the client is acutely ill, do not leave unattended.
2. Monitor the client's CNS for effects of the therapy, adjusting the dose or frequency of medication if needed.
3. Observe the client for evidence of allergic responses.

BITOLTEROL MESYLATE   (bye-**TOHL**-ter-ohl)

Tornalate Aerosol (Rx)

See also *Sympathomimetic Drugs,* p. 883.

Classification: Bronchodilator.

Action/Kinetics: Bitolterol is considered a prodrug in that it is converted by esterases in the body to the active colterol. Colterol is said to combine with beta$_2$-adrenergic receptors, producing dilation of bronchioles. **Onset following inhalation:** 3–4 min. **Time to peak effect:** 30–60 min. **Duration:** 6–7 hr.

Uses: Prophylaxis and treatment of bronchial asthma and bronchospasms. Treatment of bronchitis, emphysema, bronchiectasis, and chronic obstructive pulmonary disease. May be used with theophylline and/or steroids.

Special Concerns: Safety has not been established for use during pregnancy (pregnancy category: C) and lactation and in children less than 12 years of age. Use with caution in ischemic heart disease, hypertension, hyperthyroidism, diabetes mellitus, cardiac arrhythmias, seizure disorders, or in those who respond unusually to beta-adrenergic agonists. There may be decreased effectiveness in steroid-dependent asthmatic patients.

Side Effects: *CNS:* Tremors, dizziness, lightheadedness, nervousness, headache, insomnia. *CV:* Palpitations, tachycardia, premature ventricular contractions, flushing. *Respiratory:* Cough, dyspnea, tightness in chest, bronchospasm. *Other:* Nausea, throat irritation.

Drug Interactions: Additive effects with other beta-adrenergic bronchodilators.

Laboratory Test Interference: ↑ SGOT. ↓ Platelets, WBCs. Proteinuria.

Dosage: Inhalation Aerosol. *Bronchodilation.* **Adults and children over 12 years,** 2 inhalations at an interval of 1–3 min q 8 hr (if necessary, a third inhalation may be taken). The dose should not exceed 3 inhalations q 6 hr or 2 inhalations q 4 hr. *Prophylaxis of bronchospasm.* **Inhalation:** 2 inhalations q 8 hr.

NURSING CONSIDERATIONS

See also *Nursing Considerations* for *Sympathomimetic Drugs,* p. 887.

Administration/Storage

1. Bitolterol is available in a metered dose inhaler. With the inhaler in an upright position, the client should breathe out completely in a normal fashion. As the client is breathing in slowly and deeply, the canister and mouthpiece should be squeezed between the thumb and forefinger, activating the medication. The breath should be held for 10 sec and then slowly exhaled.
2. The medication should not be stored above 120°F.

DOBUTAMINE HYDROCHLORIDE   (doh-**BYOU**-tah-meen)

Dobutrex (Rx)

See also *Sympathomimetic Drugs,* p. 883.

Classification: Direct-acting adrenergic (sympathomimetic) agent, cardiac stimulant.

Action/Kinetics: Stimulates beta$_1$-receptors (in the heart), increasing cardiac function, cardiac output, and stroke volume, with minor effects on heart rate. The drug decreases afterload reduction although systolic blood pressure and pulse pressure may remain unchanged or increase (due to increased cardiac output). Dobutamine also decreases elevated ventricular filling pressure and helps AV node conduction. **Onset:** 1–2 min. **Peak effect:** 10 min. **t½:** 2 min. **Therapeutic plasma levels:** 40–190 ng/mL. Metabolized by the liver and excreted in urine.

Uses: Short-term treatment of cardiac decompensation secondary to depressed contractility due to organic heart disease or cardiac surgical procedures.

Contraindications: Idiopathic hypertrophic subaortic stenosis.

Special Concerns: Safe use during pregnancy, childhood, or after acute myocardial infarction not established.

Side Effects: *CV:* Marked increase in heart rate, BP, and ventricular ectopic activity. Anginal and nonspecific chest pain, palpitations. *Other:* Nausea, headache, and shortness of breath.

Additional Drug Interactions: Concomitant use with nitroprusside causes ↑ cardiac output and ↓ pulmonary wedge pressure.

Dosage: IV infusion: *individualized,* **usual,** 2.5–15 mcg/kg/min (up to 40 mcg/kg/min). Rate of administration and duration of therapy are dependent on response of patient, as determined by heart rate, presence of ectopic activity, BP, and urine flow.

NURSING CONSIDERATIONS

See *Nursing Considerations for Sympathomimetic Drugs,* p. 887.

Administration/Storage

1. Reconstitute solution according to directions provided by manufacturer. Dilution process takes place in two stages.
2. The more concentrated solution may be stored in refrigerator for 48 hr and at room temperature for 6 hr.
3. Before administration, the solution is diluted further according to the fluid needs of the client. This more dilute solution should be used within 24 hr.
4. Dilute solutions of dobutamine may darken. This does not affect the potency of the drug when used within the time spans detailed above.
5. The drug is incompatible with alkaline solutions.
6. Have available IV equipment to infuse volume expanders before therapy with dobutamine is started.

Interventions

1. Be prepared to monitor central venous pressure in order to assess vascular volume and efficiency of cardiac pumping on the right side of the heart. The normal range is 5–10 cm water.
2. An elevated central venous pressure is generally indicative of disruption of cardiac output, as in pump failure or pulmonary edema. A low central venous pressure may be indicative of hypovolemia.
3. Be prepared to monitor pulmonary artery wedge pressure to determine the pressures in the left atrium and left ventricle and to measure the efficiency of cardiac output. The usual accepted wedge pressure range is 4–12 mm Hg.
4. Monitor ECG and blood pressure continuously during drug administration.
5. Obtain written parameters for systolic blood pressure and titrate infusion as ordered.
6. Monitor intake and output.
7. Medication should be administered utilizing an electronic infusion device. Carefully reconstitute and calculate dosage according to the client's weight.

DOPAMINE HYDROCHLORIDE   (DOH-pah-meen)

Intropin, Revimine ✢ (Rx)

See also *Sympathomimetic Drugs,* p. 883.

Classification: Direct and indirect-acting adrenergic (sympathomimetic) agent, cardiac stimulant and vasopressor.

Action/Kinetics: Dopamine is the immediate precursor of epinephrine in the body. Exogenously administered, dopamine produces direct stimulation of beta$_1$-receptors and variable (dose-dependent) stimulation of alpha receptors (peripheral vasoconstriction). Also, dopamine will cause a release of norepinephrine from its storage sites. These actions result in increased myocardial contraction, cardiac output, and stroke volume, as well as increased renal blood flow and sodium excretion. Exerts little effect on diastolic BP and induces fewer arrhythmias than are seen with isoproterenol. **Onset:** 5 min. **Duration:** 10 min. **t½:** 2 min. Metabolized in liver and excreted in urine.

Uses: Cardiogenic shock, especially in myocardial infarctions associated with severe CHF. Also shock associated with trauma, septicemia, open heart surgery, renal failure, and congestive heart failure. Especially suitable for patients who react adversely to isoproterenol. Poor perfusion of vital organs; hypotension due to poor cardiac output. Congestive heart failure in patients refractory to digitalis and diuretics.

Cardiac output may be increased if dopamine is combined with dobutamine, isoproterenol, or sodium nitroprusside.

Additional Contraindications: Pheochromocytoma, uncorrected tachycardia or arrhythmias. Pediatric patients.

Special Concerns: Use in pregnancy only if benefits outweigh risks (pregnancy category: C). Dosage has not been established in children. Dosage may have to be adjusted in geriatric patients with occlusive vascular disease.

Additional Side Effects: *CV:* Ectopic heartbeats, tachycardia, anginal pain, palpitations, vasoconstriction, hypotension, hypertension. *Other:* Dyspnea, headache, mydriasis.

Additional Drug Interactions	
Diuretics	Additive or potentiating effect
Phenytoin	Hypotension and bradycardia
Propranolol	↓ Effect of dopamine

Dosage: IV infusion: Initial, 1–5 mcg/kg/min; **then,** increase in increments of 1–4 mcg/kg/min at 10–30 min intervals until desired response is obtained. *Severely ill patients:* **initial,** 5 mcg/kg/min; **then,** increase rate in increments of 5–10 mcg/kg/min up to 20–50 mcg/kg/min as needed.

NURSING CONSIDERATIONS

See also *Nursing Considerations* for *Sympathomimetics,* p. 887.

Administration/Storage

1. Drug must be diluted before use—see package insert.
2. Dilute solution is stable for 24 hr. Protect from light.
3. In order not to overload system with excess fluid, clients receiving high doses of dopamine may receive more concentrated solutions than average.

Interventions

1. Monitor blood pressure and ECG continuously during drug administration.
2. Obtain written parameters for systolic blood pressure and titrate the infusion as ordered.
3. Monitor intake and output. If medication is being administered for renal perfusion, infuse as ordered, usually less than 5 mcg/kg/min.
4. Be prepared to monitor central venous pressure and pulmonary artery wedge pressures.
5. Monitor the client for ectopic heart beats, palpitations, anginal pain or vasoconstriction. If these side effects occur, document and report them to the physician.
6. Check infusion site frequently for extravasation. Sloughing and necrosis may occur. If extravasation occurs, local subcutaneous administration of diluted phentolamine may decrease the sloughing (see package insert).
7. Medication should be administered utilizing an electronic infusion device. Carefully reconstitute and calculate dosage according to the client's weight.

EPHEDRINE SULFATE   (eh-**FEH**-drin)

Nasal decongestants: Efedron Nasal, Vatronol Nose Drops (OTC). Systemic: Ephed II (Rx: Injection; OTC: Oral dosage forms)

See also *Sympathomimetic Drugs*, p. 883, and *Nasal Decongestants*, p. 909.

Classification: Direct- and indirect-acting adrenergic agent.

Action/Kinetics: Releases norepinephrine from synaptic storage sites. Has direct effects on alpha, $beta_1$-, and $beta_2$-receptors, causing increased blood pressure due to arteriolar constriction and cardiac stimulation, bronchodilation, relaxation of GI tract smooth muscle, nasal decongestion, mydriasis, and increased tone of the bladder trigone and vesicle sphincter. It may also increase skeletal muscle strength, especially in myasthenia patients. Ephedrine is more stable and longer-lasting than epinephrine. **Onset, IM:** 10–20 min; **PO:** 15–60 min. **Duration, IM, SC, IV:** 30–60 min; **PO:** 3–5 hr. Excreted mostly unchanged through the urine (rate dependent on urinary pH—increased in acid urine).

Uses: Bronchial asthma and reversible bronchospasms associated with obstructive pulmonary diseases; narcolepsy, angioneurotic edema, hay fever. Enuresis and myasthenia gravis (has been replaced by more effective agents). Topically as a nasal decongestant. Parenterally as a vasopressor.

Special Concerns: Use during pregnancy only if clearly needed (pregnancy category: C). Geriatric patients may be at higher risk to develop prostatic hypertrophy.

Additional Side Effects: Precordial pain, urinary retention, painful urination, decrease in urine formation, pallor, respiratory difficulty.

Drug Interactions

Dexamethasone	Ephedrine ↓ effect of dexamethasone
Diuretics	Diuretics ↓ response to sympathomimetics
Guanethidine	↓ Effect of guanethidine by displacement from its site of action
Methyldopa	Effect of ephedrine ↓ in methyldopa-treated patients

Dosage: Capsules, Syrup, Tablets. *Bronchodilator, systemic nasal decongestant, CNS stimulant:* **Adults:** 25–50 mg q 3–4 hr. **Pediatric:** 3 mg/kg (100 mg/m^2) daily in 4–6 divided doses. *Enuresis:* 25–50 mg at bedtime. *Myasthenia gravis:* 25 mg t.i.d.–q.i.d.

SC, IM, slow IV. *Bronchodilator:* **Adult:** 12.5–25 mg; subsequent doses determined by patient response. *Vasopressor:* **Adults:** 25–50 mg (IM or SC) or 5–25 mg (IV) repeated in 5 min if necessary. **Pediatric (SC, IM, IV):** 3 mg/kg (100 mg/m^2) daily in 4–6 divided doses. **Topical** (0.5% drops, 0.5% jelly): **Adults and children over 6 years:** 2–3 drops of solution or small amount of jelly in each nostril q 4 hr. Should not be used topically for more than 3 or 4 consecutive days. Not to be used in children under 6 years of age unless so ordered by physician.

NURSING CONSIDERATIONS

See also *Nursing Considerations* for *Sympathomimetic Drugs,* p. 887, and *Nasal Decongestants,* p. 909.

Assessment

1. Conduct a careful examination of the client's mental status and document prior to beginning drug therapy.
2. Take a baseline BP and pulse before initiating therapy. If the drug is being administered for hypotension, monitor frequently until the blood pressure has stabilized.

Interventions

1. If the client has used ephedrine for prolonged periods of time, observe the client for drug resistance. Allow the client to rest without medication for 3–4 days, then resume drug therapy. The client will usually respond to the drug again. If there is no further response, document and report the incident to the physician.
2. Monitor the client's mental status regularly. Note any signs of depression, lack of interest in personal appearance, or client complaints of insomnia or anorexia. Report these symptoms to the physician.
3. Monitor intake and output. Elderly men may have difficulty and pain on urination. Be alert for urinary retention and report any difficulty in voiding to the physician.

Client/Family Teaching

1. Teach the client and family how to take and record a radial pulse. Instruct the client to report to the physician an elevated or irregular pulse rate.
2. If the client is male, advise him to report any difficulty with voiding. This may be caused by drug-induced urinary retention.

EPINEPHRINE   (ep-ih-**NEF**-rin)

Adrenalin Chloride Solution, Bronkaid Mist, Primatene Mist Solution, Sus-Phrine (Both Rx and OTC)

EPINEPHRINE BITARTRATE   (ep-ih-**NEF**-rin)

Asthmahaler, Bronitin Mist, Bronkaid Mist Suspension, Epitrate, Medihaler-Epi, Primatene Mist Suspension (OTC)

EPINEPHRINE BORATE   (ep-ih-**NEF**-rin)

Epinal Ophthalmic, EPPY/N 1/2%, 1%, 2% Ophthalmic Solutions (Rx)

EPINEPHRINE HYDROCHLORIDE   (ep-ih-**NEF**-rin)

Adrenalin Chloride, Asthma Nefrin, Dey-Dose Epinephrine, Epifrin, Glaucon, Micro Nefrin, S-2 Inhalant, Vaponefrin (Both Rx and OTC)

See also *Sympathomimetic Drugs,* p. 883, and *Nasal Decongestants,* p. 909.

Classification: Direct-acting adrenergic agent.

Action/Kinetics: Epinephrine, a natural hormone produced by the adrenal medulla, induces marked stimulation of alpha, beta$_1$-, and beta$_2$-receptors, causing sympathomimetic stimulation, pressor effects, cardiac stimulation, bronchodilation, and decongestion. **Extreme caution must be taken never to inject 1:100 solution intended for inhalation—injection of this concentration has caused death. SC: Onset,** 6–15 min; **duration:** less than 1–4 hr. **Inhalation: Onset,** 3–5 min; **duration:** 1–3 hr. **IM: Onset,** variable; **duration:** less than 1–4 hr. Epinephrine is ineffective when given orally.

Uses: Cardiac arrest, Stokes-Adams syndrome, low cardiac output following extracorporeal cardiopulmonary bypass. To prolong the action of local anesthetics. As a hemostatic during ocular surgery; treatment of conjunctival congestion during surgery; to induce mydriasis during surgery; treat ocular hypertension during surgery. Topically to control bleeding. Acute bronchial asthma, bronchospasms due to emphysema, chronic bronchitis, or other pulmonary diseases. Treatment of anaphylaxis, angioedema, anaphylactic shock, drug-induced allergic reactions, transfusion reactions, insect bites or stings. As an adjunct in the treatment of open-angle glaucoma. To produce mydriasis, to treat conjunctivitis.

Additional Contraindications: Narrow-angle glaucoma. Lactation.

Special Concerns: Pregnancy category: C (may cause anoxia in the fetus). Administer parenteral epinephrine to children with caution. Syncope may occur if epinephrine is given to asthmatic children.

Additional Side Effects: *CV:* Fatal ventricular fibrillation, cerebral or subarachnoid hemorrhage, obstruction of central retinal artery. *GU:* Decreased urine formation, urinary retention, painful urination. *At injection site:* Bleeding, urticaria, wheal formation. *Ophthalmic:* Transient stinging when administered, conjunctival hyperemia, brow ache, headache, blurred vision, photophobia, poor night vision, eye ache, eye pain. Prolonged ophthalmic use may cause deposits of pigment in the cornea, lids, or conjunctiva.

Additional Drug Interaction: Epinephrine, 1:100, will inactivate chymotrypsin in 60 min.

Laboratory Test Interferences: False + or ↑ BUN, fasting glucose, lactic acid, urinary catecholamines, glucose (Benedict's), ↓ coagulation time. The drug may affect electrolyte balance.

Dosage: Inhalation Aerosol, Bitartrate Inhalation Aerosol. Adults and children over 4 years of age: *Bronchodilation,* 0.2–0.275 mg (1 inhalation) of the Aerosol or 0.16 mg (1 inhalation) of the Bitartrate Aerosol; may be repeated after 1–2 min if needed. At least 3 hr should elapse before subsequent doses. Dosage not established in children less than 4 years of age. **Inhalation Solution. Adults and children over 6 years of age:** *Bronchodilation,* 1 inhalation of the 1% solution (of the base); may be repeated after 1–2 min.

Injection: IM, IV, SC. *Bronchodilation:* **Adults:** 0.2–0.5 mg SC repeated q 20 min–4 hr as needed; dose may be increased to 1 mg/dose. **Pediatric:** 0.01 mg/kg (0.3 mg/m^2) SC up to a maximum of 0.5 mg per dose; may be repeated q 15 min for 2 doses and then q 4 hr as needed. *Anaphylaxis:* **Adults:** 0.2–0.5 mg SC q 10–15 min as needed, up to a maximum of 1 mg/dose if needed. **Pediatric:** 0.01 mg/kg (0.3 mg/m^2) up to a maximum of 0.5 mg/dose; may be repeated q 15 min for 2 doses and then q 4 hr as needed. *Vasopressor:* **Adults, IM or SC, initial:** 0.5 mg repeated q 5 min if needed; **then,** give 0.025–0.050 mg IV q 5–15 min as needed. **Adults, IV, initial:** 0.1–0.25 mg given slowly. May be repeated q 5–15 min as needed. Or, use IV infusion beginning with 0.001 mg/min and increasing the dose to 0.004 mg/min if needed. **Pediatric, IM, SC:** 0.01 mg/kg, up to a maximum of 0.3 mg repeated q 5 min if needed. **Pediatric, IV:** 0.01 mg/kg q 5–15 min if an inadequate response to IM or SC administration is observed. *Cardiac stimulant:* **Adults, intracardiac or IV:** 0.1–1 mg repeated q 5 min if needed. **Pediatric, intracardiac or IV:** 0.005–0.01 mg/kg (0.15–0.3 mg/m^2) repeated q 5 min if needed; this may be followed by IV infusion beginning at 0.0001 mg/kg/min and increased in increments of 0.0001 mg/kg/min up to a maximum of 0.0015 mg/kg/min. *Adjunct to local anesthesia:* **Adults and children:** 0.1–0.2 mg in a 1:200,000–1:20,000 solution. *Adjunct with intraspinal anesthetics:* **Adults:** 0.2–0.4 mg added to the anesthetic spinal fluid. *Antihemorrhagic, mydriatic, decongestant:* **Adults and children, intracameral or subconjunctival:** 0.01–0.1% solution. *Topical antihemorrhagic:* **Adults and children:** 0.002–0.1% solution.

    Sterile Suspension. *Bronchodilation:* **Adults, SC, initial:** 0.5 mg; **then,** 0.5–1.5 mg no more often than q 6 hr. **Pediatric, SC, initial:** 0.025 mg/kg (0.625 mg/m^2); dose may be repeated but no more often than q 6 hr.

    Ophthalmic Solution, Bitartrate Ophthalmic Solution, Borate Ophthalmic Solution. Adults: 1 drop up to 2 times daily. Dosage has not been established in children.

NURSING CONSIDERATIONS

See also *Nursing Considerations* for *Sympathomimetic Drugs,* p. 887, and *Nasal Decongestants,* p. 909.

Administration/Storage

1. *Never administer* 1:100 solution IV. Use 1:1,000 solution for IV administration.
2. Preferably use a tuberculin syringe to measure epinephrine, as the parenteral doses are small and the drug is potent. An error in measurement may be disastrous.
3. Administer epinephrine IV by a double bottle setup (piggyback) so that the rate of administration may be easily adjusted.
4. For IV administration to adults, the drug must be well diluted as a 1:1,000 solution and quantities of 0.05 to 0.1 mL of solution should be injected cautiously and slowly, taking about one minute for each injection, noting the response of the client (BP and pulse). Dose may be repeated several times if necessary.
5. Administer infusions with an electronic infusion device for safety and accuracy.
6. Briskly massage site of SC or IM injection to hasten the action of the drug. Do not expose epinephrine to heat, light, or air, as this causes deterioration of the drug.
7. Discard if solution is reddish-brown in color and after expiration date.
8. Because of the presence of sodium bisulfite as a preservative in the topical preparation, there may be slight stinging after administration.
9. The topical preparation should not be used in children under 6 years of age.

Assessment

Obtain baseline recordings of client blood pressure and pulse rate prior to beginning drug therapy.

Interventions

1. Closely monitor the client receiving solutions of IV epinephrine. Keep the environment as peaceful as possible.
2. Monitor the client's blood pressure and pulse every minute until the desired effect from the

drug has been achieved. Then take it every 2 to 5 minutes until the client's condition has stabilized. Once stable, monitor BP every 15 to 30 min as indicated.

3. Note if the client has any evidence of shock such as cold, clammy skin, cyanosis, and loss of consciousness.

4. If the client goes into hypovolemic shock, be prepared to assist with administering additional IV fluids.

ETHYLNOREPINEPHRINE HYDROCHLORIDE (eth-ill-nor-ep-ih-**NEF**-rin)
Bronkephrine (Rx)

See also *Sympathomimetic Drugs,* p. 883.

Classification: Direct-acting adrenergic agent.

Action/Kinetics: Ethylnorepinephrine stimulates beta$_1$ and beta$_2$ receptors similarly to epinephrine with minor effects on alpha receptors. Has little effect on BP and may be safer than epinephrine. Especially suitable for children, for diabetic asthmatics, and for patients refractory to isoproterenol or epinephrine. **Onset, SC or IM:** 6–12 min. **Duration:** 1–2 hr.

Uses: Treatment of bronchial asthma, bronchospasms due to emphysema or bronchitis, bronchiectasis, obstructive pulmonary disease.

Special Concerns: Pregnancy category: C.

Dosage: IM, SC. Adults: 1–2 mg (0.5–1 mL of 0.2% solution); **pediatric:** 0.2–1 mg (0.1–0.5 mL of 0.2% solution).

NURSING CONSIDERATIONS
See *Nursing Considerations* for *Sympathomimetic Drugs,* p. 887.

ISOETHARINE HYDROCHLORIDE (eye-so-**ETH**-ah-reen)
Arm-a-Med Isoetharine HCl, Bronkosol, Dey-Dose Isoetharine HCl, Dey-Dose Isoetharine S/F, Dey-Lute Isoetharine, Dey-Lute Isoetharine S/F, Dispos-a-Med Isoetharine (Rx)

ISOETHARINE MESYLATE (eye-so-**ETH**-ah-reen)
Bronkometer (Rx)

See also *Sympathomimetic Drugs,* p. 883.

Classification: Adrenergic agent, bronchodilator.

Action/Kinetics: Isoetharine has a greater stimulating activity on beta$_2$-receptors of the bronchi than on beta$_1$-receptors of the heart. Causes relief of bronchospasms. **Inhalation: Onset,** 1–6 min; **peak effect:** 15–60 min; **duration:** 1–4 hr. Partially metabolized; excreted in urine.

Special Concerns: Pregnancy category: C.

Uses: Bronchial asthma, bronchospasms due to chronic bronchitis or emphysema, bronchiectasis, pulmonary obstructive disease.

Special Concerns: Dosage has not been established in children.

Dosage: Inhalation Solution. Adults: *Hand nebulizer:* 3–7 inhalations (use undiluted) of the 0.5 or 1% solution. *Oxygen aerosolization or IPPB:* Dose depends on strength of solution used (range: 0.062%–1%) and whether the solution is used undiluted or diluted 1:3 according to the following: **0.5–1%:** 0.5–1 mL of 1:3 solution; **0.2–0.2%:** 2–2.5 mL used undiluted; **0.1–0.167%:** 2.5–4 mL used undiluted; **0.062 or 0.08%:** 3–4 mL used undiluted.

Mesylate Inhalation Aerosol. Adults: 0.34 mg (1 inhalation) repeated after 1–2 min if needed; **then,** dose may be repeated q 4 hr.

NURSING CONSIDERATIONS

See *Special Nursing Considerations For Adrenergic Bronchodilators* under *Sympathomimetics,* p. 887.

Administration/Storage

1. One or two inhalations are usually sufficient. Wait 1 min after giving initial dose to ensure necessity of another dose.
2. Treatment usually does not need to be repeated more than q 4 hr.
3. Do not use if solution contains a precipitate or is brown.

ISOPROTERENOL HYDROCHLORIDE   (eye-so-proh-**TER**-ih-nohl)

Aerolone, Dey-Dose Isoproterenol HCl, Dispos-a-Med Isoproterenol HCl, Isuprel, Isuprel Mistometer, Medihaler-Iso, Norisodrine Aerotrol (Rx)

ISOPROTERENOL SULFATE   (eye-so-proh-**TER**-ih-nol)

Medihaler-Iso (Rx)

See also *Sympathomimetic Drugs,* p. 883.

Classification: Direct-acting sympathomimetic agent.

Action/Kinetics: Isoproterenol produces pronounced stimulation of both $beta_1$- and $beta_2$-receptors of the heart, bronchi, skeletal muscle vasculature, and the GI tract. In contrast to other sympathomimetics, isoproterenol produces a drop in BP. It also causes less hyperglycemia than epinephrine, but produces bronchodilation and the same degree of CNS excitation. **Inhalation: Onset,** 2–5 min; **peak effect:** 3–5 min; **duration:** 30–120 min. **IV: Onset,** immediate; **duration:** less than 1 hr. **Sublingual: Onset,** 15–30 min; **duration:** 1–2 hr. **Rectal: Onset,** 30 min; **duration:** 2–4 hr. Partially metabolized; excreted in urine.

Uses: Bronchodilator in asthma, chronic pulmonary emphysema, bronchiectasis, bronchitis, and other conditions involving bronchospasms. Treat bronchospasms during anesthesia. Cardiac arrest, heart block, syncope due to complete heart block, Adams-Stokes syndrome. Certain cardiac arrhythmias including ventricular tachycardia, ventricular arrhythmias; syncope due to carotid sinus hypersensitivity. Hypoperfusion shock syndrome.

Special Concerns: Pregnancy category: C. Use with caution in the presence of tuberculosis.

Additional Side Effects: Flushing, sweating, swelling of the parotid gland. Excessive inhalation causes refractory bronchial obstruction. Sublingual administration may cause buccal ulceration. Side effects of drug are less severe after inhalation.

Drug Interaction: Beta-adrenergic blocking agents reverse the effects of isoproterenol.

Dosage: *Isoproterenol hydrochloride. Shock:* **IV Infusion,** 0.5–5 mcg/min (0.25–2.5 mL of 1:500,000 diluted solution). *Cardiac standstill and cardiac arrhythmias:* **Adults, IM, SC:** 1 mL (0.2 mg) of 1:5,000 solution (range: 0.02–1 mg); **IV:** 1–3 mL (0.02–0.06 mg) of 1:50,000 solution (range: 0.01–0.2 mg); **IV infusion:** 5 mcg/min (1.25 mL of 1:250,000 solution/min); **Intracardiac (in extreme emergencies):** 0.1 mL of 1:5,000 solution. *Heart block:* **IV, SC, IM:** as above.

Acute bronchial asthma: **Hand bulb nebulizer:** 5–15 deep inhalations of 1:200 solution (or, in adults, 3–7 inhalations of the 1:100 solution); repeat once more if relief not obtained after 5–10 min. **Metered-dose inhaler: Usual,** one inhalation; if relief not obtained after 2–5 min, administer again. **Maintenance:** 1–2 inhalations 4–6 times/day (**Note:** No more than 2 inhalations should be taken at once and no more than 6 in one hr.) *Chronic obstructive lung disease (bronchospasm):* **Hand bulb nebulizer:** 5–15 deep inhalations of 1:200 solution (or 3–7 inhalations of 1:100 solution) q 3–4 hr. **Nebulization by IPPE:** Dilute 0.5 mL of 1:200 solution in 2–2.5 mL diluent (to achieve concentration of 1:800–1:1,000) and deliver over 10–20 min. Can be repeated 5 times/day. **Metered-dose inhaler:** 1–2 inhalations q 3–4 hr. **Sublingual: Adults,** 10–20 mg depending on response (not to exceed 60 mg daily). **Pediatric:** 5–10 mg up to a maximum of 30 mg daily. Should not be given more than t.i.d. *Bronchospasms during anesthesia:* **IV,** 0.01–0.02 mg as required (1 mL of a 1:5,000 solution diluted to 10 mL with sodium chloride or dextrose injection).

Isoproterenol sulfate. Dispensed from metered aerosol inhaler for bronchospasms. See dosage above for *Hydrochloride.*

NURSING CONSIDERATIONS

See also *Special Nursing Considerations For Adrenergic Bronchodilators* under *Sympathomimetics,* p. 887.

Administration/Storage

1. Administration to children, except where noted, is the same as that for adults, because a child's smaller ventilatory exchange capacity will permit a proportionally smaller aerosol intake. For acute bronchospasms in children, use 1:200 solution.
2. In children, no more than 0.25 mL of the 1:200 solution should be used for each 10–15 minutes of programmed treatment.
3. Elderly clients usually receive a lower dose.

Interventions

Observe and report respiratory problems that seem to worsen after the administration of isoproterenol. Refractory reactions may necessitate withdrawal of the drug.

Client/Family Teaching

1. Advise the client to rinse his mouth with water to remove any drug residue and to minimize dryness, after inhalation therapy.
2. Warn the client that the sputum and saliva may appear pink after inhalation therapy. This is due to the drug and the client should not become alarmed.
3. Advise client not to use inhalation therapy more frequently than prescribed by the physician. Excessive use can cause severe cardiac and respiratory problems.
4. Show the client where his parotid gland is located. Instruct him to withhold the drug if his parotid gland becomes enlarged. Report this finding immediately to the physician and anticipate that the drug will be discontinued.

LEVARTERENOL BITARTRATE (NOREPINEPHRINE) (lev-ar-TER-ih-nohl)

Levophed (Rx)

See also *Sympathomimetic Drugs,* p. 883.

Classification: Direct-acting adrenergic agent, vasopressor.

Action/Kinetics: Levarterenol produces vasoconstriction (increase in BP) by stimulating alpha-adrenergic receptors. Also causes a moderate increase in contraction of heart by stimulating beta$_1$ receptors. Minimal hyperglycemic effect. **Onset:** immediate; **duration:** 1–2 min. Metabolized in liver and other tissues by the enzymes monoamine oxidase and catechol-O-methyltransferase; however, the pharmacologic activity is terminated by uptake and metabolism in sympathetic nerve endings. Metabolites excreted in urine.

Uses: Hypotensive states caused by trauma, septicemia, blood transfusions, drug reactions, spinal anesthesia, poliomyelitis, central vasomotor depression, and myocardial infarctions. Adjunct to treatment of cardiac arrest and profound hypotension.

Additional Contraindications: Hypotension due to blood volume deficiency (except in emergencies), mesenteric or peripheral vascular thrombosis, in halothane or cyclopropane anesthesia (due to possibilities of fatal arrhythmias). Pregnancy (may cause fetal anoxia or hypoxia).

Special Concerns: Use with caution in patients taking MAO inhibitors or tricyclic antidepressants.

Additional Untoward Reactions: Drug may cause bradycardia that can be abolished by atropine.

Dosage: IV infusion only (effect on BP determines dosage): initial, 8–12 mcg/min or 2–3 mL of a 4 mcg/mL solution/min; **maintenance,** 2–4 mcg/min with the dose determined by patient response.

NURSING CONSIDERATIONS

See also *Nursing Considerations* for *Sympathomimetic Drugs,* p. 887.

Administration/Storage

1. Discard solutions that are brown or that have a precipitate.
2. Do not administer through the same tube as blood products.
3. The infusion should be continued until blood pressure is maintained without therapy. Abrupt withdrawal of levarterenol should be avoided.
4. Levarterenol should be diluted in either 5% dextrose in distilled water or 5% dextrose in saline.
5. For IV administration, a large vein should be used, preferably the antecubital or subclavian. Veins with poor circulation should be avoided.
6. Administer IV solutions with an electronic infusion device. Monitor the rate of flow constantly.
7. Have phentolamine available for use at the site of extravasation to dilate local blood vessels and to minimize local necrosis.

Assessment

Obtain a baseline CBC, blood pressure and pulse recording prior to initiating therapy.

Interventions

1. During the administration of levarterenol, the client should be in a closely monitored environment.
2. Monitor the blood pressure frequently during therapy. An arterial line or Dinemapp for continuous BP determinations may be of some value.

3. Monitor the pulse frequently, noting any signs of bradycardia. Have atropine available for treatment of bradycardia.

4. Observe the IV infusion site frequently for evidence of extravasation, as ischemia and sloughing may occur.

5. Check the area for blanching along the course of the vein. This could indicate permeability of the vein wall which could allow leakage to occur. As a result, the IV site would need to be changed and phentolamine administered to the site of the extravasation.

6. The drug should be gradually withdrawn. Avoid an abrupt withdrawal. Clients may experience an initial rebound drop in blood pressure.

7. Extra fluids parenterally may diminish rebound hypotension and help stabilize BP during withdrawal of the drug.

MEPHENTERMINE SULFATE   (meh-FEN-ter-meen)
Wyamine (Rx)

See also *Sympathomimetic Drugs,* p. 883

Classification: Indirect-acting adrenergic agent, vasopressor.

Action/Kinetics: Mephentermine acts by releasing norepinephrine from its storage sites. It has slight effects on alpha and beta$_1$ receptors and moderate effects on beta$_2$ receptors mediating vasodilation. The drug causes increased cardiac output; also elicits slight CNS effects. **IV: Onset,** immediate; **duration:** 15–30 min. **IM: Onset,** 5–15 min; **duration:** 1–4 hr. Metabolized in liver. Excreted in urine within 24 hr (rate increased in acidic urine).

Uses: Hypotension due to anesthesia, ganglionic blockade, or hemorrhage (only as emergency treatment until blood or blood substitutes can be given).

Additional Contraindications: Hypotension due to phenothiazines; in combination with MAO inhibitors.

Special Concerns: Safe use during pregnancy has not been established.

Additional Drug Interactions: Mephentermine will potentiate hypotensive effects of phenothiazines.

Dosage: Injection. *Hypotension during spinal anesthesia:* **IV,** 30–45 mg; 30-mg doses may be repeated as required; or, **IV infusion:** 0.1% mephentermine in dextrose 5% in water with the rate of infusion and duration dependent on patient response. *Prophylaxis of hypotension in spinal anesthesia:* **IM,** 30–45 mg 10–20 min before anesthesia. *Shock following hemorrhage:* Not recommended, but IV infusion of 0.1% in dextrose 5% in water may maintain BP until blood volume is replaced. **Pediatric, IM, IV:** 0.4 mg/kg (12 mg/m^2) as a single dose; may be repeated if needed. **Pediatric, IV infusion:** 0.1% solution in 5% dextrose in water with the rate of infusion and duration dependent on patient response.

NURSING CONSIDERATIONS
See also *Nursing Considerations* for *Sympathomimetics,* p. 887.

Interventions

Take an initial reading of clients BP and pulse before initiating therapy. Then, take a reading every 5 min until stable. Once BP has stabilized, take a reading every 15–30 min beyond the duration of the drug's action. This is to ensure that BP has stabilized at a satisfactory level.

METAPROTERENOL SULFATE (ORCIPRENALINE SULFATE) (met-ah-proh-**TER**-ih-nohl)

Alupent, Arm-A-Med Metaproterenol, Dey-Dose Metaproterenol, Dey-Lute Metaproterenol, Metaprel (Rx)

See also *Sympathomimetic Drugs,* p. 883.

Classification: Direct-acting adrenergic agent, bronchodilator.

Action/Kinetics: Metaproterenol markedly stimulates beta$_2$ receptors, resulting in relaxation of smooth muscles of the bronchial tree, as well as peripheral vasodilation. It is similar to isoproterenol, but it has a longer duration of action and fewer side effects. Has minimal beta$_1$ activity. **Onset: Inhalation aerosol,** within 1 min; **peak effect:** 1 hr; **duration:** 1–5 hr. **Onset, hand-bulb nebulizer or IPPB:** 5–30 min; **duration:** 4–6 hr after repeated doses. **PO: Onset,** 15–30 min; **Peak effect:** 1 hr. **Duration:** 4 hr. Oral administration produces a marked first-pass effect. Metabolized in the liver and excreted through the kidney.

Uses: Bronchodilator in asthma, bronchitis, emphysema, and other conditions associated with reversible bronchospasms.

Contraindications: Inhalation for children under the age of 12 years.

Special Concerns: Safe use during pregnancy not established (pregnancy category: C). Dosage of syrup or tablets not determined in children less than 6 years of age. Inhalation not recommended for children under 12 years of age.

Drug Interactions: Possible potentiation of adrenergic effects if used before or after other sympathomimetic bronchodilators.

Dosage: Syrup, Tablets. Adults and children over 27.3 kg: 20 mg t.i.d.–q.i.d.; **children under 27.3 kg or 6–9 years of age:** 10 mg t.i.d.–q.i.d.
  Inhalation. Hand nebulizer: single dose, 10 inhalations of undiluted 5% solution. **Intermittent positive pressure breathing (IPPB):** 0.3 mL of 5% solution diluted to 2.5 mL saline or other diluent. **Metered-dose inhaler:** 2–3 inhalations (1.30–2.25 mg) q 3–4 hr. Total daily dose should not exceed 12 inhalations (9 mg). For acute bronchospasms, administer metaproterenol every 4 hr. For chronic bronchospasms (pulmonary disease), administer 3–4 times/day.

NURSING CONSIDERATIONS

See *Special Nursing Considerations for Adrenergic Bronchodilators* under *Sympathomimetics,* p. 887.

Administration/Storage

1. Instruct client to shake the container.
2. Unit dose vials should be refrigerated at 2°–8°C (35°–46°F).
3. The inhalant solution can be stored at room temperature, but excessive heat and light should be avoided.
4. The solution should not be used if it is brown or shows a precipitate.

METARAMINOL BITARTRATE   (met-ahr-**AM**-ih-nohl)

Aramine (Rx)

See also *Sympathomimetic Drugs,* p. 883.

Classification: Direct-acting adrenergic agent, vasopressor.

Action/Kinetics: Metaraminol indirectly releases norepinephrine from storage sites and directly stimulates primarily alpha receptors and, to a slight extent, beta$_1$ receptors. The drug causes marked increases in BP due primarily to vasoconstriction and to a slight increase in cardiac output. Reflex bradycardia is also manifested. CNS stimulation usually does not occur. **Onset: IV:** 1–2 min; **IM:** 10 min; **SC:** 5–20 min. **Duration, IV:** 20 min; **IM, SC:** About 60 min. Metabolized in the liver and excreted through the urine and feces. Urinary excretion of unchanged drug can be enhanced by acidifying the urine.

Uses: Hypotension associated with surgery, spinal anesthesia, hemorrhage, trauma, infections, and adverse drug reactions. Adjunct to the treatment of either septicemia or cardiogenic shock. *Investigational:* Injected intracavernosally to treat priapism due to phentolamine, papaverine, or other causes.

Additional Contraindications: As a substitute for blood or fluid replacement.

Special Concerns: Pregnancy category: C. Use with caution in cirrhosis and malaria. Hypertension and ischemic electrocardiographic changes may occur when used to treat priapism.

Dosage: Injection: IM, SC, IV. *Prophylaxis of hypotension:* **IM, SC,** 2–10 mg; **pediatric:** 0.01 mg/kg (3 mg/m^2). *Treatment of hypotension:* **IV infusion,** 15–100 mg in 500 mL of 0.9% sodium chloride injection or 5% dextrose injection given at a rate to maintain desired blood pressure (up to 500 mg/500 mL has been used). **Pediatric: IV infusion,** 0.4 mg/kg (12 mg/m^2) in a solution containing 1 mg/25 mL 0.9% sodium chloride injection or 5% dextrose injection. *Severe shock:* **Direct IV,** 0.5–5.0 mg followed by **IV infusion** of 15–100 mg in 500 mL fluid. **Pediatric, direct IV:** 0.01 mg/kg (0.3 mg/m^2).

NURSING CONSIDERATIONS

See also *Nursing Considerations* for *Sympathomimetic Drugs,* p. 887.

Administration/Storage

Do not inject IM in areas that seem to have poor circulation, as sloughing has occurred with extravasation.

Interventions

1. Take BP at frequent intervals throughout the therapy. Obtain written parameters for maintaining the systolic pressure.
2. Frequently assess the site of administration, as extravasation of drug may result in sloughing.
3. Use an electronic infusion device when administering IV drug therapy for more adequate control and titration of drug.

PHENYLEPHRINE HYDROCHLORIDE (fen-ill-EF-rin)

Nasal: Alconefrin 12, 25, and 50, Doktors, Duration, Neo-Synephrine Jelly and Solution, Nostril, Rhinall, Rhinall-10, Children's Flavored Nose Drops, St. Joseph, Vicks Sinex. Ophthalmic: AK-Dilate, AK-Nefrin, Dilatari, I-Phrine, Isopto Frin, Mydfrin, Neo-Synephrine, Ocugestrin, Ocu-Phrin, Prefrin Liquifilm, Relief. Systemic: Neo-Synephrine. (Rx: Injection and Ophthalmic Solutions 2.5% or greater; OTC: Nasal products and ophthalmic solutions 0.12% or less)

See also *Sympathomimetics,* p. 883, and *Nasal Decongestants,* p. 909.

Classification: Alpha-adrenergic agent.

Action/Kinetics: Phenylephrine stimulates alpha-adrenergic receptors, producing pronounced vasoconstriction and hence an increase in both systolic and diastolic blood pressure; reflex bradycardia results from increased vagal activity. The drug also acts on alpha receptors producing vasoconstriction in the skin, mucous membranes, and the mucosa as well as mydriasis by contracting the dilator muscle of the pupil. It resembles epinephrine, but it has more prolonged action and few cardiac effects. **IV: Onset,** immediate; **duration:** 15–20 min. **IM. SC: Onset,** 10–15 min; **duration:** ½–2 hr for IM and 50–60 min for SC. *Nasal decongestion (topical):* **Onset:** 15–20 min; **duration:** 30 min–4 hr. *Ophthalmic:* **Time to peak effect for mydriasis,** 15–60 min for 2.5% solution and 10–90 min for 10% solution. **Duration:** 3 hr for 2.5%; 3–7 hr with 10%. Excreted in urine.

Phenylephrine is also found in Chlor-Trimetron Expectorant, Naldecon, Dimetane, and Dimetapp.

Uses: Systemic: Acute hypotensive states caused by peripheral circulatory collapse. To maintain blood pressure during spinal anesthesia; to prolong spinal anesthesia. Paroxysmal supraventricular tachycardia. **Nasal:** Nasal congestion due to allergies, sinusitis, common cold, or hay fever. **Ophthalmologic: 0.08–0.12%:** Temporary relief of redness of the eye associated with colds, hay fever, wind, dust, sun, smog, smoke, contact lens. **2.5%:** Produce mydriasis for refraction, retinoscopy, blanching test, and ophthalmoscopy. **2.5% and 10%:** Treatment of uveitis with posterior synechiae, prophylaxis of posterior synechiae, preoperative mydriasis.

Special Concerns: Use with caution in geriatric patients, severe arteriosclerosis, and during pregnancy (pregnancy category: C) and lactation. Nasal and ophthalmic use of phenylephrine may be systemically absorbed. Use of the 2.5% or 10% ophthalmic solutions in children may cause hypertension and irregular heart beat. In geriatric patients, chronic use of the 2.5% or 10% ophthalmic solutions may cause rebound miosis and a decreased mydriatic effect.

Side Effects: Reflex bradycardia. Overdosage may cause ventricular extrasystoles and short paroxysm or ventricular tachycardia, tingling of the extremities and a sensation of heavy head. *Ophthalmologic:* Rebound miosis and decreased mydriatic response in geriatric patients, blurred vision.

Dosage: Injection: IM, IV, SC. *Vasopressor, mild–moderate hypotension:* **Adults, IM, SC,** 2–5 mg repeated no more often than q 10–15 min. **IV,** 0.2 mg repeated no more often than q 10–15 min. **Pediatric, IM, SC:** 0.1 mg/kg (3 mg/m²) repeated in 1–2 hr if needed. *Vasopressor, severe hypotension and shock:* **Adults, IV infusion,** 10 mg in 500 mL 5% dextrose injection or 0.9% sodium chloride injection given at a rate of 0.1–0.18 mg/min initial; **then,** give at a rate of 0.04–0.06 mg/min. *Prophylaxis of hypotension during spinal anesthesia:* **Adults, IM, SC,** 2–3 mg 3–4 min before anesthetic given; **pediatric, IM, SC:** 0.044–0.088 mg/kg. *Hypotensive emergencies during spinal anesthesia:* **Adults, IV, initial,** 0.2 mg; dose can be increased by no more than 0.2 mg for each subsequent dose not to exceed 0.5 mg/dose.

Nasal Jelly. Adults: small amount of 0.5% jelly inserted into the nostril and sniffed well back into the nasal passages q 3–4 hr as necessary. Use not recommended in children. **Nasal Solution. Adults, Drops:** 2–3 drops of the 0.25–0.5% solution into each nostril q 3–4 hr as needed. **Spray:** 1–2 sprays of the 0.25–0.5% solution into each nostril; blow nose after 3–5 min and repeat dose; then, repeat dose q 3–4 hr. **Pediatric, infants and children up to 2 years:** 2–3 drops of the 0.125% solution q 3–4 hr as needed. **2–6 years of age:** 2–3 drops of the 0.125% or 0.167% solution into each nostril q 4 hr as needed. **6–12 years of age:** 2–3 drops or 1–2 sprays of the 0.25% solution into each nostril q 3–4 hr as needed.

Ophthalmic Solution. *Mydriasis, vasoconstriction, uveitis, preoperative mydriasis:* **Adults,** 1 drop of the 2.5% or 10% solution (for children use 1 drop of the 2.5% solution). *Mydriasis in diagnostic procedures:* **Adults and children,** 1 drop of the 2.5% solution. *Refraction:* **Adults,** 1 drop of a cycloplegic followed in five min by one drop of the 2.5% solution of phenylephrine and in ten min another drop of cycloplegic (eyes are ready for refraction in 50–60 min). **Pediatric:** 1 drop of a 1% solution of atropine followed in 10–15 min by 1 drop of 2.5% phenylephrine and in 5–10 min by another drop of 1% atropine solution (eyes are ready for refraction in 1–2 hr).

NURSING CONSIDERATIONS

See also *Nursing Considerations* for *Sympathomimetics,* p. 887, and *Nasal Decongestants,* p. 909.

Administration/Storage

1. Store drug away from light in a brown bottle.
2. Anticipate that before administering Neo-Synephrine Ophthalmic Solution, instillation of a drop of local anesthetic will be necessary.
3. When the drug is used as a nasal decongestant, instruct the client to blow their nose before administration.

Client/Family Teaching

1. Using ophthalmic instillations and nasal decongestants may produce systemic sympathomimetic effects. Provide the client with printed material explaining how to identify these effects, and instruct the client to notify the physician should they occur.
2. When using ophthalmic solution, if there is no relief of symptoms within 2 days, notify the physician.
3. When using the drug for nasal decongestion, if there is no relief of symptoms within 3 days, notify the physician.

PHENYLPROPANOLAMINE HYDROCHLORIDE   (fen-ill-proh-pah-**NOHL**-ah-meen)

Acutrim 16 Hour, Acutrim Late Day, Acutrim II Maximum Strength, Control, Dex-A-Diet Maximum Strength and Maximum Strength Caplets, Dexatrim, Dexatrim Maximum Strength and Maximum Strength Caplets, Dexatrim Maximum Strength Pre-Meal Caplets, Efed II Yellow, Maigret-50, Phenyldrine, Prolamine, Propagest, Rhindecon, Unitrol (OTC except Maigret-50 and Rhindecon)

See also *Anorexiants, Amphetamines and Derivatives,* p. 843, and *Sympathomimetics,* p. 883.

Classification: Decongestant, appetite suppressant.

Action/Kinetics: Phenylpropanolamine is thought to stimulate both alpha and beta receptors, as well as to act indirectly through release of norepinephrine from storage sites. Increases in blood pressure are due mainly to increased cardiac output rather than to vasoconstriction; has minimal CNS effects. The drug acts on alpha-adrenergic receptors to produce a decongestant effect in the nasal mucosa. **Onset, decongestant:** 15–30 min; **peak plasma levels:** 1–2 hr; **duration, capsules and tablets:** 3 hr; **extended-release tablets:** 12–16 hr. **Peak plasma levels:** 100 ng. **t^{1}/₂:** 3–4 hr. 80%–90% excreted in the urine unchanged.

Uses: Nasal congestion due to colds, hay fever, allergies. Short-term (8–12 weeks) treatment of exogenous obesity in conjunction with a weight reduction program including reduced caloric intake, exercise, and behavior modification. *Investigational:* Mild to moderate stress incontinence in women.

Contraindications: Arteriosclerosis, depression, glaucoma, hypertension, diabetes, kidney disease, hyperthyroidism, during or within 14 days of use of MAO inhibitors, hypersensitivity to sympathomimetics. Not recommended as an anorexiant for children less than 12 years of age.

Special Concerns: Safety and efficacy during pregnancy and lactation and for children not established. Children less than 6 years of age may be at greater risk for developing psychiatric disorders when using phenylpropanolamine. The anorexiant dose must be individualized for children between 12–18 years of age.

Side Effects: *CNS:* Dizziness, headache, insomnia, restlessness, bizarre behavior. Serious effects due to abuse include: agitation, tremor, increased motor activity, hallucinations, seizures, stroke, and death. *CV:* Palpitations, hypertension (may be severe and lead to crisis), tachycardia. *Miscellaneous:* Dry mouth, dysuria, renal failure, nausea, nasal dryness.

Drug Interactions

Furazolidone	Possibility of hypertensive crisis and intracranial hemorrhage
Guanethidine	Phenylpropanolamine ↓ hypotensive effect
Indomethacin	Possibility of severe hypertensive episode
MAO Inhibitors	Possibility of hypertensive crisis and intracranial hemorrhage

Dosage: Capsules, Tablets. *Decongestant:* **Adults,** 25 mg q 4 hr or 50 mg q 6–8 hr (not to exceed 150 mg/day); **Children, 2–6 years:** 6.25 mg q 4 hr, not to exceed 37.5 mg in 24 hr; **6–12 years:** 12.5 mg q 4 hr, not to exceed 75 mg in 24 hr. *Anorexiant:* **Adults,** 25 mg t.i.d. 30 min before meals, not to exceed 75 mg in 24 hr.

Extended-release Capsules, Extended-release Tablets. *Decongestant:* **Adults,** 75 mg q 12 hr. *Anorexiant:* **Adults,** 75 mg once daily in the morning.

NURSING CONSIDERATIONS

See also *Nursing Considerations* for *Anorexiants, Amphetamines and Derivatives,* p. 844, and *Sympathomimetics,* p. 887.

Client/Family Teaching

Caution older men to report difficulties in voiding, because they are more susceptible to drug-induced urinary retention. Ensure that these clients understand the importance of taking the medication only as directed.

PIRBUTEROL ACETATE   (peer-**BYOU**-ter-ohl **AH**-seh-tayt)

Maxair (Rx)

See also *Sympathomimetic Drugs,* p. 883.

Classification: Sympathomimetic, bronchodilator.

Action/Kinetics: Pirbuterol causes bronchodilation by stimulating beta$_2$-adrenergic receptors. The drug also inhibits histamine release from mast cells, causes vasodilation, and increases ciliary motility. It has minimal beta$_1$ activity. **Onset, inhalation:** Approximately 5 min. **Time to peak effect:** 30–60 min. **Duration:** 5 hr.

Uses: Alone or with theophylline or steroids, for prophylaxis and treatment of bronchospasm in asthma and other conditions with reversible bronchospasms, including bronchitis, emphysema, bronchiectasis, obstructive pulmonary disease.

Contraindications: Cardiac arrhythmias due to tachycardia; tachycardia caused by digitalis toxicity.

Special Concerns: Pregnancy category: C.

Dosage: Inhalation Aerosol. Adults and children over 12 years of age: 0.2–0.4 mg (1–2 inhalations) q 4–6 hr, not to exceed 12 inhalations (2.4 mg) daily.

NURSING CONSIDERATIONS

See also *Nursing Considerations* for *Sympathomimetic Drugs,* p. 887, and *Special Nursing Considerations for Adrenergic Bronchodilators* under *Sympathomimetic Drugs,* p. 887.

Client/Family Teaching

Contact the physician immediately if the client does not obtain relief with doses of medication that have previously been effective.

PSEUDOEPHEDRINE HYDROCHLORIDE   (soo-doh-eh-**FEH**-drin)

Cenafed, Children's Sudafed Liquid, Congestac N.D. Caplets✤, Decofed, DeFed 60, Dorcol Children's Decongestant Liquid, Eltor 120✤, Genaphed, Halofed, Halofed Adult Strength, Maxenal✤, Myfedrine, NeoFed, Novafed, Ornex Cold✤, Otrivin✤, PediaCare Infants' Oral Decongestant Drops, Pseudo, Pseudofrin✤, Pseudogest, Robidrine✤, Sudafed, Sudafed 12 Hour, Sudafed 60, Sudrin, Sufedrin (OTC)

PSEUDOEPHEDRINE SULFATE   (soo-doh-eh-**FEH**-drin)

Afrinol (OTC)

See also *Sympathomimetics,* p. 883.

Classification: Direct- and indirect-acting sympathomimetic, nasal decongestant.

Action/Kinetics: Pseudoephedrine produces direct stimulation of both alpha- (pronounced) and beta-adrenergic receptors, as well as indirect stimulation through release of norepinephrine from storage sites. These actions produce a decongestant effect on the nasal mucosa. Systemic administration eliminates possible damage to the nasal mucosa. **Onset:** 15–30 min. **Time to peak effect:** 30–60 min. **Duration:** 3–4 hr. **Extended-release: duration,** 8–12 hr. Urinary excretion slowed by alkalinization, causing reabsorption of drug.

Pseudoephedrine is also found in Actifed, Chlor-Trimeton, and Drixoral.

Uses: Nasal congestion associated with sinus conditions, otitis, allergies.

Additional Contraindications: Lactation.

Special Concerns: Use during pregnancy only if benefits clearly outweigh risks (pregnancy category: B). Use with caution in newborn and premature infants due to a higher risk of side effects. Geriatric patients may be more prone to age-related prostatic hypertrophy.

Dosage: Hydrochloride: Capsules, Oral Solution, Syrup, Tablets. Adults: 60 mg q 4–6 hr not to exceed 240 mg in 24 hr. **Pediatric, 6–12 years of age:** 30 mg using the oral solution or syrup q 4–6 hr not to exceed 120 mg in 24 hr; **2–6 years:** 15 mg using the oral solution or syrup q 4–6 hr not to exceed 60 mg in 24 hr. For children less than 2 years of age, the dose must be individualized.

    Hydrochloride: Extended-release Capsules. Adults and children over 12 years: 120 mg q 12 hr or 240 mg q 24 hr. Use is not recommended for children less than 12 years of age.

    Sulfate: Extended-release Tablets. Adults and children over 12 years: 120 mg q 12 hr or 240 mg q 24 hr. Use is not recommended for children less than 12 years of age.

NURSING CONSIDERATIONS

See also *Nursing Considerations* for *Sympathomimetics,* p. 887.

Client/Family Teaching

1. Advise client to avoid taking the drug at bedtime. Pseudoephedrine causes stimulation that can produce insomnia.
2. If clients have hypertension, advise them to report to the physician symptoms such as headache or dizziness. These symptoms may be drug-related and could indicate an elevation of blood pressure.

TERBUTALINE SULFATE (ter-BYOU-tah-leen)
Brethaire, Brethine, Bricanyl (Rx)

See also *Sympathomimetics,* p. 883.

Classification: Direct-acting adrenergic agent, bronchodilator.

Action/Kinetics: Terbutaline is specific for stimulating beta$_2$ receptors, resulting in bronchodilation and relaxation of peripheral vasculature. Minimum beta$_1$ activity. Drug action resembles that of isoproterenol. **PO: Onset:** 60–120 min; **maximum effect:** 2–3 hr; **duration:** 4–8 hr. **SC: Onset,** 6–15 min; **maximum effect:** 30 min—1 hr; **duration:** 1.5–4 hr. **Inhalation: Onset,** 5–30 min; **time to peak effect:** 1–2 hr; **duration:** 3–6 hr.

Uses: Bronchodilator in asthma, bronchitis, emphysema, bronchiectasis, pulmonary obstructive disease and other conditions associated with reversible bronchospasms. *Investigational:* Inhibit premature labor.

Special Concerns: Safe use during pregnancy (pregnancy category: B) or in children less than 12 years of age not established. Use with caution during lactation.

Dosage: Tablets. *Bronchodilation:* **Adults,** 2.5–5 mg t.i.d. q 6 hr during waking hours, not to exceed 15 mg/24 hr. If disturbing side effects are observed, dose can be reduced to 2.5 mg t.i.d. without loss of beneficial effects. Anticipate use of other therapeutic measures if patient fails to respond after second dose. **Children 12–15 years:** 2.5 mg t.i.d., not to exceed 7.5 mg/24 hr. *Premature labor:* 2.5 mg q 4–6 hr until term.

SC. *Bronchodilation:* **Adults,** 0.25 mg. May be repeated 1 time after 15–30 min if no significant clinical improvement is noted. Dose should not exceed 0.5 mg over 4 hr. *Premature labor:* **IV infusion,** 0.10 mg/min initially; **then,** increase rate by 0.005 mg/min q 10 min until contractions cease or a maximum dose of 0.08 mg/min is reached. The minimum effective dose should be continued for 4–8 hr after contractions cease.

    Inhalation Aerosol. Adults and children over 12 years: 0.2–0.5 mg (1–2 inhalations) q 4–6 hr. Inhalations should be separated by 60-second intervals. Dosage may be repeated q 4–6 hr.

NURSING CONSIDERATIONS

See also *Nursing Considerations* for *Sympathomimetics,* p. 887.

Client/Family Teaching

Instruct client to report any bothersome side effects to the physician. The drug dose and administration times may need to be adjusted.

THEOPHYLLINE DERIVATIVES

Theophylline derivatives are used for the treatment of asthma. Thus, they are discussed in Chapter 49, *Antiasthmatic Drugs,* p. 976.

NASAL DECONGESTANTS

Action/Kinetics: The most commonly used agents for relief of nasal congestion are the adrenergic drugs. They act by stimulating alpha-adrenergic receptors, thereby constricting the arterioles in the nasal mucosa; this reduces blood flow to the area, decreasing congestion. Both topical (sprays, drops) and oral agents may be used.

Uses: PO. Nasal congestion due to hay fever, common cold, allergies, or sinusitis. To help sinus or nasal drainage. To relieve congestion of eustachian tubes. **Topical.** Nasal and nasopharyngeal mucosal congestion due to hay fever, common cold, allergies, or sinusitis. With other therapy to decrease congestion around the eustachian tubes. Relieve ear block and pressure pain during air travel.

Contraindications: Severe hypertension, coronary artery disease.

Special Concerns: Use with caution in hyperthyroidism, arteriosclerosis, increased intraocular pressure, prostatic hypertrophy, angina, diabetes, ischemic heart disease, hypertension. Also, patients receiving MAO inhibitors may manifest hypertensive crisis following the use of oral nasal decongestants. Use with caution in geriatric patients and during pregnancy and lactation.

Side Effects: *Topical use:* Stinging and burning, mucosal dryness, sneezing, local irritation, rebound congestion (rhinitis medicamentosa). Systemic use may produce the following symptoms. *CV:* Cardiovascular collapse with hypotension, arrhythmias, palpitations, precordial pain, tachycardia, transient hypertension, bradycardia. *CNS:* Anxiety, dizziness, headache, fear, restlessness, tremors, insomnia, tenseness, lightheadedness, drowsiness, psychological disturbances, weakness, psychoses, hallucinations, seizures, depression. *GI:* Nausea, vomiting, anorexia. *Ophthalmologic:* Irritation, photophobia, tearing, blurred vision, blepharospasm. *Other:* Dysuria, sweating, pallor, breathing difficulties, orofacial dystonia.

Note: Ephedrine may also produce anorexia and urinary retention in males with prostatic hypertrophy.

Dosage: See individual drugs, Table 16, p. 910.

NURSING CONSIDERATIONS

Administration/Storage

1. Most nasal decongestants are used topically in the form of sprays, drops, or solutions.
2. Solutions of topical nasal decongestants may become contaminated with use and result in the growth of bacteria and fungi. Thus, the dropper or spray tip should be rinsed in hot water after each use and covered.
3. Have facial tissues and a receptacle available for used tissues during administration.

Interventions

1. Use separate equipment for each client to prevent the spread of infection. If only one container of medication is available, use an individual dropper for each client.

Table 16   Topical Nasal Decongestants

Drug	Dosage	Remarks
Ephedrine hydrochloride (Efedron Nasal) (OTC) Ephedrine sulfate (Vatronol Nose Drops) (OTC)	**Adults and children over 6 years:** 2–3 gtt or small amount of jelly in each nostril 2–3 times daily. Not to be used for more than 3–4 consecutive days.	Available as 0.5% drops and 0.5% jelly.
Epinephrine hydrochloride (Adrenalin Chloride) (OTC)	**Adults and children over 6 years:** 1–2 gtt in each nostril q 4–6 hr. Can be applied as drops or spray or with a sterile swab.	1. Available as a 0.1% aqueous solution. 2. Because of presence of sodium bisulfite as a preservative, there may be a slight stinging after administration. 3. Not to be used in children under 6 years of age.
Naphazoline hydrochloride (Albalon Liquifilm✤, Degest-2✤, Naphcon-Forte✤, Opcon✤, Privine) (OTC)	**Adults and children over 6 years:** 2 gtt or sprays in each nostril no more than q 3 hr for the drops and q 4–6 hr for the spray.	1. Available as 0.05% drops and spray. 2. Contraindicated in children less than 12 years of age.
Oxymetazoline HCl (4-Way Long-Acting Nasal, Afrin Children's Strength 12 Hour Nose Drops and Regular Drops, Afrin 12 Hour Nasal Spray, Afrin 12 Hour Nose Drops, Afrin Menthol Nasal Spray, Afrin Nasal Spray, Afrin Nose Drops, Coricidin Nasal Mist, Dristan Long Lasting Nasal Spray, Duramist Plus, Duration 12 Hour Nasal Spray✤, Nafrine Decongestant Nasal Drops and Spray, Neo-Synephrine 12 Hour Spray and Drops, Nostrilla 12 Hour Nasal Decongestant, Nostril Nasal Decongestant Mild and Regular, NTZ Long Acting Decongestant Nose Drops and Spray, Sinarest 12 Hour Nasal Spray, Vicks Sinxex 12-Hour Spray) (OTC)	**Intranasal. Adults and children over 6 yr:** 2–3 sprays or 2–4 drops of 0.05% solution in each nostril in AM and PM. **Pediatric, 2–6 yr:** 2–3 gtt of 0.025% solution in each nostril in AM and PM.	Available as 0.025% solution for pediatric use and 0.05% spray (regular or menthol) and drops for adult use.

Table 16 *(Continued)*

Drug	Dosage	Remarks
Phenylephrine HCl (Alconefrin 12, 25, and 50; Doktors, Duration, Neo-Synephrine, Nostril, Rhinall, Rhinall-10 Children's Flavored Nose Drops, St. Joseph, Vicks Sinex) (OTC)	**Drops. Adults:** 2–3 gtt of a 0.25%–0.5% solution in each nostril q 3–4 hr. **Pediatric, 6–12 years:** 2–3 gtt of a 0.25% solution in each nostril q 3–4 hr; **2–6 years:** 2–3 gtt of a 0.125% solution in each nostril q 3–4 hr or 2–3 gtt of a 0.167% solution in each nostril q 4 hr; **less than 2 years:** 2–3 gtt of a 0.125% solution in each nostril q 3–4 hr. **Spray. Adults:** 1–2 sprays of 0.25%–0.5% solution in each nostril; after 3–5 min, repeat dose; subsequent doses can be given q 3–4 hr. **Pediatric, 6–12 years:** Use 0.25% solution. **Jelly. Adults:** Small amount of 0.5% jelly into each nostril and sniff well back into nasal passages q 3–4 hr.	1. Available as a 0.125%, 0.16%, 0.2%, 0.25%, 0.5%, or 1% drops; as a 0.125%, 0.25%, 0.5%, or 1% spray; or as a 0.5% nasal jelly. 2. The appropriate concentration should be used, depending on the age of the patient. 3. Children are particularly sensitive to nasal absorption resulting in systemic side effects.
Propylhexedrine (Benzedrex Inhaler) (OTC)	**Inhaler.** Inhale through nostril with the other nostril blocked.	1. Excessive use should be avoided. 2. Propylhexedrine has been abused by extraction from inhalers and injected IV as an amphetamine substitute. 3. Chronic abuse has resulted in pulmonary hypertension, foreign body emboli, severe left and right ventricular failure, and sudden death.
Tetrahydrozoline HCl (Tyzine Drops, Tyzine Pediatric Nasal Drops) (OTC)	**Solution. Adults and children over 5 years:** 2–4 gtt of 0.1% solution in each nostril no more than q 3 hr. **2–6 years:** 2–3 gtt of 0.05% solution in each nostril no more than q 3 hr.	1. Available as 0.05% pediatric solution and as a 0.1% solution for adults and children over 6 years of age. 2. Not recommended for children less than 2 years of age.
Xylometazoline HCl (Chlorohist-LA, Neo-Synephrine II Long Acting Spray or Drops, Otrivin Nasal Drops or Spray, Otrivin Pediatric Nasal Drops, Otrivin with M-D Pump♣, Sinutab Sinus Spray♣).	**Drops, Spray. Adults and children over 12 years:** 2–3 gtt of 0.1% solution in each nostril or 1–2 inhalations of 0.1% spray q 8–10 hr; **pediatric (2–12 years):** 2–3 gtt of 0.05% solution in each nostril q 8–10 hr.	1. Available as a 0.05% pediatric solution and as a 0.1% solution for drops and spray 2. Should not be used in atomizers made of aluminum. 3. The nasal spray is more effective and more likely to cause systemic side effects.

2. Instruct the client to blow the nose gently before administering therapy. If the client is unable to blow the nose, clear the nasal passages with a bulb-type aspirator.

3. After completing the treatment, rinse the dropper or tip of spray container, dry with a tissue and cover. Be careful not to introduce water into the spray container. Wipe the tip of the nasal jelly tube with a damp tissue and replace the cap.

Client/Family Teaching

1. Instruct the client in the appropriate technique for preparing the nasal passages.
2. Review the method of administration of the prescribed medication, whether drops, spray, or jelly.
3. Discuss and demonstrate the proper use and care of equipment.

CHAPTER FORTY-FIVE
Adrenergic Blocking (Sympatholytic) Drugs

General Statement: As their name implies, the adrenergic blocking agents (sympatholytics) reduce or prevent the action of the sympathomimetic agents. They do this by competing with norepinephrine or epinephrine (the neurotransmitters) for the various subtypes of either alpha-adrenergic or beta-adrenergic receptor sites. For example, alpha-adrenergic blocking agents prevent the smooth muscles surrounding the arterioles from contracting, while beta-adrenergic blocking agents prevent the excitatory effect of the neurotransmitters on the heart. It should also be noted that several antihypertensive agents act by blocking alpha (especially in the CNS) or beta receptors.

Some of the adrenergic blocking agents also have a direct systemic cardiac effect in addition to their peripheral vasodilating effect. The fall in blood pressure that accompanies their administration may trigger a compensatory tachycardia (reflex stimulation). The cardiac blood vessels of a patient with arteriosclerosis may be unable to dilate rapidly enough to accommodate these changes in blood volume, and the patient may experience an acute attack of angina pectoris or even cardiac failure.

Adrenergic blocking agents have many undesirable effects which, although not toxic, limit their use. Treatment should always be started at low doses, to be increased gradually.

Alpha-Adrenergic Blocking Agents

These drugs reduce the tone of muscles surrounding peripheral blood vessels and consequently increase peripheral blood circulation and decrease blood pressure.

Beta-Adrenergic Blocking Agents

These drugs block the nerve impulse transmission to the beta receptors of the sympathetic division of the ANS. These receptors are particularly numerous at the postjunctional terminals of the nerve fibers that control the heart muscle and reduce muscle tone. These drugs include atenolol, carteolol, metoprolol, nadolol, penbutolol, pindolol, propranolol, and timolol. These agents are discussed in Chapter 26, *Antihypertensives,* p. 475.

ACEBUTOLOL   (ah-seh-**BYOU**-toe-lohl)
Sectral (Rx)

See *Antihypertensives,* Chapter 26, p. 486.

ATENOLOL   (ah-**TEN**-oh-lohl)
Tenormin (Rx)

45

See *Antihypertensives,* Chapter 26, p. 487.

BETAXOLOL HYDROCHLORIDE   (beh-**TAX**-oh-lohl)
Kerlone (Rx)

See also *Beta-Adrenergic Blocking Agents, p. 483.*

Classification: Beta-adrenergic blocking agent.

Action/Kinetics: Inhibits beta$_1$- adrenergic receptors although beta$_2$- receptors will be inhibited at high doses. Has some membrane stabilizing activity but no intrinsic sympathomimetic activity. Low lipid solubility. **t^1/$_2$:** 14–22 hr. Metabolized in the liver with most excreted through the urine; about 15% is excreted unchanged.

Uses: Hypertension, alone or with other antihypertensive agents (especially diuretics).

Special Concerns: Pregnancy category: C. Use with caution during lactation. Safety and effectiveness have not been determined in children. Geriatric patients are at greater risk of developing bradycardia.

Dosage: Tablets. Initial: 10 mg once daily either alone or with a diuretic. If the desired effect is not reached, the dose can be increased to 20 mg although doses higher than 20 mg will not increase the therapeutic effect. In geriatric patients the initial dose should be 5 mg daily.

NURSING CONSIDERATIONS

See also *Nursing Considerations* for *Beta-Adrenergic Blocking Agents,* p. 485.

Administration/Storage

1. The full effect is usually observed within 7–14 days.
2. As the dose is increased, the heart rate decreases.
3. Drug therapy with betaxolol should be discontinued gradually over a 2-week period.

CARTEOLOL HYDROCHLORIDE   (KAR-tee-oh-lohl)
Cartrol (Rx)

See *Antihypertensives,* Chapter 26, p. 488.

DIHYDROERGOTAMINE MESYLATE   (dye-HY-droh-er-GOT-ah-meen)
D.H.E. 45, Dihydroergotamine-Sandoz (Rx)

Classification: Alpha-adrenergic blocking agent.

Action/Kinetics: Dihydroergotamine manifests alpha-adrenergic receptor blocking activity as well as a direct stimulatory action on vascular smooth muscle of peripheral and cranial blood vessels, resulting in vasoconstriction, thus preventing the onset of a migraine attack. Dihydroergotamine manifests greater adrenergic blocking activity, less pronounced vasoconstriction, less nausea and vomiting, and fewer oxytocic properties than does ergotamine. It is more effective when given early in the course of a migraine attack. **Onset: IM,** 15–30 min; **IV,** less than 5 min. **Duration: IM,** 3–4 hr. **t½: initial,** 1.4 hr; **final,** 18–22 hr. Metabolized in liver and excreted in feces with less than 10% excreted through the urine.

Uses: Migraine, migraine variant, histaminic cephalalgia, and cluster headaches. Especially useful when rapid effect is desired or when other routes of administration are not possible. *Investigational:* Adjunct in prophylaxis of deep venous and pulmonary thrombosis.

Contraindications: Lactation. Peripheral vascular disease, coronary heart disease, hypertension, impaired hepatic or renal function, sepsis, hypersensitivity, or malnutrition, severe pruritus, presence of infection. Not recommended for prophylaxis of migraine attack.

Special Concerns: Pregnancy category: X. Geriatric patients may be more affected by peripheral vasoconstriction which results in hypothermia.

Side Effects: *CV:* Precordial pain, transient tachycardia or bradycardia. Large doses may cause increased blood pressure, vasoconstriction of coronary arteries, and brandycardia. *GI:* Nausea, vomiting, diarrhea. *Other:* Numbness and tingling of fingers and toes, muscle pain in extremities, weakness in legs, localized edema, and itching. *Prolonged use:* Gangrene, ergotism.

Drug Interactions: Oral nitroglycerin ↑ bioavailability of hydroergotamine.

Dosage: IM. *Suppress vascular headache:* **initial,** 1 mg at first sign of headache; repeat every 1–2 hr to a total of 3 mg/attack or 6 mg/week. **IV.** *Suppress vascular headache:* Similar to IM but to a maximum of 2 mg/attack or 6 mg weekly. **SC.** *Prophylaxis of thrombosis:* **SC,** 0.5 mg 2 hr prior to surgery concurrently with heparin; **then,** repeat dose q 12 hr for 5–7 days.

NURSING CONSIDERATIONS

Administration/Storage

Adjust the dosage if the client complains of severe headaches. This dose should then be used when subsequent headaches begin.

Assessment

1. Obtain a thorough nursing, diet, and drug history.
2. Note any history of prior adverse reactions to ergotamine.
3. Determine if the client is taking nitroglycerin. Dihydroergotamine interacts with nitroglycerin and should be avoided.
4. Determine the severity of the client's headaches, how long they last and what, if any, medications have been effective in relieving them in the past.
5. If the client is of childbearing age and is sexually active, note the possibility of pregnancy. Ergotamine has an oxytoxic effect and therefore is contraindicated in this setting.

Client/Family Teaching

1. Advise the client to take the drug at the onset of a migraine headache. This drug is most effective when administered early in an attack.
2. Instruct the client on alternative methods for dealing with stress, such as relaxation techniques.
3. Advise the client to report any bothersome side effects. Any numbness or tingling of the extremities should be reported immediately to the physician.
4. Instruct the client to take the drug only as directed. Do not stop taking the drug abruptly or without the physician's knowledge.

ERGOTAMINE TARTRATE   (er-**GOT**-ah-meen)

Ergomar, Ergostat, Gynergen✿, Medihaler Ergotamine (Rx)

Classification: Alpha-adrenergic blocking agent.

Action/Kinetics: Ergot alkaloid with alpha-adrenergic blocking activity as well as direct stimulatory activity on vascular smooth muscle, causing vasoconstriction. The result is a decrease in pulsations responsible for migraine and other symptoms of vascular headaches. Ergotamine also has oxytocic and emetic effects. Absorption following inhalation is rapid and complete although absorption across the buccal membranes is poor. **Onset:** variable but usually between 1–2 hr. **Peak plasma levels:** 0.5–3 hr. **t½:** 2 hr. Metabolized by the liver and excreted in the bile. Trace amounts of unchanged drug are excreted through the feces and urine.

Uses: Drug of choice for acute attacks of migraine and cluster headaches.

Contraindications: Pregnancy (pregnancy category: X) and lactation. Peripheral vascular disease, coronary heart disease, hypertension, impaired hepatic or renal function, sepsis, hypersensitivity, or malnutrition, severe pruritus, presence of infection. Not recommended for prophylaxis of migraine attacks.

Special Concerns: Safety and efficacy have not been determined in children. Geriatric patients may be more affected by peripheral vasoconstriction which result in hypothermia.

Side Effects: *CV:* Precordial pain, transient tachycardia or bradycardia. Large doses may cause increased blood pressure, vasoconstriction of coronary arteries, and bradycardia. *GI:* Nausea, vomiting, diarrhea. *Other:* Numbness and tingling of fingers and toes, muscle pain in extremities, weakness in legs, localized edema, and itching. *Prolonged use:* Gangrene, ergotism.

Drug Interactions	
Caffeine	Caffeine ↑ rate of absorption of ergotamine
Troleandomycin	↑ Effect of ergotamine due to ↓ breakdown by liver
Vasoconstrictors	Significant hypertension

Dosage: Sublingual. Adults: 1 mg at start of migraine attack followed by 2 mg every 30 min if necessary, but not more than 5 mg in 24 hr and 10 mg in 1 week. **Pediatric, 10 years and older:** 1 mg repeated in 30 min if necessary.

   Inhalation Aerosol. Adults: 0.36 mg (one inhalation) at start of attack; may be repeated in 5-min intervals. Can take up to 6 doses (2.16 mg) in 24 hr or 15 doses (5.4 mg) per week. *Combination with caffeine:* 100 mg caffeine for every 1 mg ergotamine.

NURSING CONSIDERATIONS

See also *Nursing Considerations* for *Dihydroergotamine Mesylate,* p. 915.

Client/Family Teaching

1. Instruct clients to check for coldness of extremities or tingling of fingers when on long-term therapy and report. These symptoms appear before the onset of gangrene.
2. Remind female clients of childbearing age that they should not take ergotamine when pregnancy is suspected. Birth control should be practiced during therapy as drug has an oxytocic effect.
3. Instruct client to take the drug only as directed and not to stop abruptly without the physician's knowledge.
4. Review and demonstrate the appropriate method for use and care of inhalers.

LEVOBUNOLOL HYDROCHLORIDE   (lee-voh-**BYOU**-no-lohl)

Betagan ✿, Betagan C Cap Q.D., Betagan C Cap B.I.D. (Rx)

See also *Beta-Adrenergic Blocking Agents,* p. 483.

Classification: Beta-adrenergic blocking agent for glaucoma.

Action/Kinetics: Levobunolol acts on both $beta_1$- and $beta_2$-adrenergic receptors. The drug may act by decreasing the formation of aqueous humor. **Onset:** Less than 60 min. **Peak effect:** 2–6 hr. **Duration:** 24 hr.

Uses: To decrease intraocular pressure in chronic open-angle glaucoma or ocular hypertension.

Special Concerns: Use with caution during pregnancy (pregnancy category: C). Safety and effectiveness have not been determined in children. Significant absorption in geriatric patients may result in myocardial depression. Also, use with caution in angle-closure glaucoma (use with a miotic), in patients with muscle weaknesses, and in patients with decreased pulmonary function.

Additional Side Effects: *Ophthalmic:* Stinging and burning (transient), decreased corneal sensitivity, blepharoconjunctivitis. *Dermatologic:* Urticaria, pruritis.

Dosage: Ophthalmic Solution. Adults: usual, 1 gtt of 0.5% solution in affected eye(s) 1–2 times/day (depending on variations in diurnal intraocular pressure).

NURSING CONSIDERATIONS

See also *Nursing Considerations* for *Beta-Adrenergic Blocking Agents,* p. 485.

Administration/Storage

1. Instruct the client not to close the eyes tightly or blink more frequently than usual after instillation of the drug.
2. If other eye drops are to be administered, wait at least five minutes before instillation of other eye drops.
3. Apply gentle pressure to the inside corner of the eye for approximately 60 seconds following instillation.
4. If intraocular pressure is not decreased sufficiently, pilocarpine, epinephrine, or systemic carbonic anhydrase inhibitors may be used.

Client/Family Teaching

1. Review and demonstrate the appropriate method for instilling eye drops.
2. Explain the reasons for the medication and the side effects that should be reported to the physician, should they occur.
3. Stress the importance of return visits to evaluate intraocular pressure and the effectiveness of the medication.

METHYSERGIDE MALEATE (meth-ih-**SER**-jyd)

Sansert (Rx)

Classification: Prophylactic for vascular headaches.

Action/Kinetics: Methysergide is an ergot alkaloid derivative structurally related to LSD. It is thought to act by directly stimulating smooth muscle leading to vasoconstriction. The drug blocks the effects of serotonin, a powerful vasodilator believed to play a role in vascular headaches; it also inhibits the release of histamine from mast cells and prevents the release of serotonin from platelets. It has weak emetic and oxytocic activity. **Onset:** 1–2 days. **Peak plasma levels:** 60 ng/mL. **Duration:** 1–2 days. Excreted through the urine as unchanged drugs and metabolites.

Uses: Prophylaxis of migraine or other vascular headaches, such as cluster headaches. Use should be limited to 6 months or less and for patients with severe headaches or those who are refractory to other therapy. Patients should remain under supervision.

Contraindications: Severe renal or hepatic disease, severe hypertension, coronary artery disease, peripheral vascular disease, or tendency toward thromboembolic disease, cachexia (profound ill health or malnutrition), infectious disease, or peptic ulcer. Pregnancy, lactation, use in children.

Special Concerns: Geriatric patients may be more affected by peripheral vasoconstriction leading to the possibility of hypothermia.

Side Effects: The drug is associated with a high incidence of side effects. *Fibrosis:* Retroperitoneal fibrosis, cardiac fibrosis, pleuropulmonary fibrosis, Peyronies-like disease. The fibrotic condition may result in vascular insufficiency in the lower legs. *CV:* Vasoconstriction of arteries leading to paresthesia, chest pain, abdominal pain, or extremities that are cold, numb, or painful. Tachycardia, postural hypotension. *CNS:* Dizziness, ataxia, drowsiness, vertigo, insomnia, euphoria, lightheadedness, and psychic reactions such as depersonalization, depression, and hallucinations. *GI:* Nausea, vomiting, diarrhea, heartburn, abdominal pain. *Hematologic:* Eosinophilia, neutropenia. *Other:* Peripheral edema, flushing of face, skin rashes, transient alopecia, myalgia, arthralgia, weakness, weight gain.

Drug Interactions: Narcotic analgesics are inhibited by methysergide.

Dosage: Tablets. Administer 4–8 mg daily in divided doses. Continuous administration should not exceed 6 months. Drug may be readministered after a 3- to 4-week rest period.

NURSING CONSIDERATIONS

Administration/Storage
1. Administer the drug with meals or milk to minimize irritation due to increased hydrochloric acid production.
2. The drug must be discontinued gradually to avoid migraine headache rebound.

Assessment
1. Note any history of renal or hepatic disease. Obtain baseline liver and renal function studies prior to initiating therapy.
2. Obtain baseline eosinophil and neutrophil count prior to beginning therapy.
3. Note the frequency and severity of the client's headaches and efforts made in the past to control them.
4. Assess the client's behavior prior to initiating therapy.

Interventions
1. Compare behavior after the client has been taking methysergide maleate to ascertain changes, such as hallucinations, that would indicate an adverse response to the drug.
2. Closely observe the client for the presence of vascular headaches, lightheadedness, nervousness or insomnia and report these symptoms to the physician.
3. A client who develops general malaise, fatigue, weight loss, low grade fever, or urinary tract problems may be developing fibrosis (cardiac or pleuropulmonary fibrosis), and the drug should be discontinued.
4. If the client has no effect from the drug within 3 weeks, there is likely to be no response and the drug should be discontinued.

Client/Family Teaching
1. Advise the client to report nervousness, weakness, rashes, alopecia and peripheral edema to the physician.
2. Instruct client to weigh herself daily, record and report any unusual weight gain.
3. If the weight gain becomes excessive, instruct the client on how to adjust the caloric intake.
4. Instruct the client on how to check the extremities for edema.
5. Advise the client that administration of methysergide should not be continued on a regular basis for longer than 6 months.

6. Instruct the client on how to maintain a low-salt diet, if prescribed.

7. Remind the client to remain under medical supervision. Stress that blood tests must be done at periodic intervals to detect complications of drug therapy.

8. Advise client to report to the physician immediately any chest or flank pain and dyspnea as the drug should be discontinued.

9. Do not drive a car or engage in other hazardous tasks, until drug effects are realized because drug may cause drowsiness.

10. Discuss with the family psychological changes that may occur and advise them to report these to the physician.

11. Advise the client to be alert to signs of circulatory disturbances that should be reported to the physician.

12. If dizziness or lightheadedness occurs upon arising, instruct client to rise slowly from a supine position and dangle the legs for a few minutes before standing erect.

13. If feeling faint, lie down with the legs elevated.

14. Do not discontinue medication abruptly. Rebound migraine headaches may occur. Medication must be discontinued gradually.

METOPROLOL TARTRATE   (meh-toe-**PROH**-lohl)

Lopressor (Rx)

See *Antihypertensives,* Chapter 26, p. 490.

NADOLOL   (**NAY**-doh-lohl)

Corgard (Rx)

See *Antihypertensives,* Chapter 26, p. 491.

PENBUTOLOL SULFATE   (pen-**BYOU**-toe-lohl)

Levatol (Rx)

See also *Beta-Adrenergic Blocking Agents,* p. 492.

Action/Kinetics: Penbutolol has both beta$_1$- and beta$_2$- receptor blocking activity. It has no membrane-stabilizing activity but does possess minimal intrinsic sympathomimetic activity. High lipid solubility. **t½:** 5 hr. 80%–98% protein bound. Penbutolol is metabolized in the liver and excreted through the urine.

Uses: Mild to moderate arterial hypertension.

Special Concerns: Pregnancy category: C. Dosage has not been established in children. Geriatric patients may manifest increased or decreased sensitivity to the usual adult dose.

Dosage: Tablets. *Hypertension:* **initial,** 20 mg once daily either alone or with other antihypertensive agents. **Maintenance:** Same as initial dose. Doses greater than 40 mg daily do not result in a greater antihypertensive effect.

NURSING CONSIDERATIONS

See also *Nursing Considerations* for *Beta-Adrenergic Blocking Agents,* p. 485.

Administration/Storage

1. The full effect of a 20–40 mg dose may not be observed for 2 weeks.
2. Doses of 10 mg daily are effective but full effects are not seen for 4–6 weeks.

Client/Family Teaching

1. Review the signs and symptoms associated with postural hypotension and instruct client to rise slowly from a sitting or lying position.
2. Take medication only as prescribed since full effects may not be realized for a month or more.

PHENOXYBENZAMINE HYDROCHLORIDE   (feh-NOX-ee-BENS-ah-meen)

Dibenzyline (Rx)

Classification: Alpha-adrenergic blocking agent.

Action/Kinetics: Phenoxybenzamine is an irreversible alpha-adrenergic blocking agent. The drug increases blood flow to the skin, mucosa, and abdominal viscera as well as lowers blood pressure. Beneficial effects may not be noted for 2–4 weeks. **Onset:** gradual. **Peak effect:** 4–6 hr. **Duration:** 3–4 days after one dose. **t½:** 24 hr. Metabolized slowly and excreted in urine and feces.

Uses: To control hypertension and sweating in pheochromocytoma prior to surgery, when surgery is contraindicated, or in malignant pheochromocytoma.

Contraindications: Conditions in which a decrease in blood pressure is not desired. Essential hypertension.

Special Concerns: Geriatric patients may be more sensitive to the hypotensive hypothermic effects. Use with caution in coronary or cerebral arteriosclerosis, respiratory infections, and renal disease.

Side Effects: Due to adrenergic blockade and include: miosis, postural hypotension, tachycardia, nasal congestion, and inhibition of ejaculation. Also, drowsiness, fatigue, GI upset.

Dosage: Capsules. Adults: initial, 10 mg b.i.d.; may be increased every other day until desired effect is obtained. **Maintenance:** 20–40 mg b.i.d.–t.id. **Pediatric, initial:** 0.2 mg/kg (6 mg/m²) up to a maximum of 10 mg once daily; dose may be increased q 4 days until desired effect is reached. **Maintenance:** 0.4 mg (1.2 mg/m²) daily in 3–4 divided doses.

NURSING CONSIDERATIONS

Administration/Storage

1. Observe the client closely before increasing the dosage of drug.
2. Since the effects of phenoxybenzamine are irreversible, the drug is usually started in low doses and gradually increased.
3. It may take 2 weeks to titrate the medication to the optimum dosage.
4. Have levarterenol available to treat overdosage.

Assessment

1. Obtain baseline renal function studies prior to beginning therapy.

2. Note and report any evidence of hypotension.

3. Obtain blood pressure and pulse measurements to serve as baseline data against which to measure drug effects.

Interventions

1. Take BP every 4 hours with the client in both supine and erect positions to check for excessive hypotension.

2. Note the blood pressure, pulse, the quality of peripheral pulses. Assess the extremities for increased warmth for 4 days after a change in drug dosage. The results may help determine whether the client needs an adjustment in dosage.

3. If the client has a preexisting respiratory infection, it may be aggravated by the drug. Increased respiratory supportive care may be required.

4. Have levarterenol available to treat overdosage. Epinephrine is ineffective and may increase heart rate as well as cause further peripheral dilatation.

5. Keep the client in a supine position for 24 hours after overdosage. Wrap the legs in Ace bandages, and apply an abdominal binder, unless contraindicated.

Client/Family Teaching

1. Instruct client to rise slowly from a supine position and to dangle feet for a few minutes before standing erect.

2. If the client feels faint, have him lie down immediately and elevate the legs.

3. Instruct the client how to take a radial pulse and to report any evidence of tachycardia to the physician. This may be a sign of autonomic blockade.

4. It may take up to a month before the desired effects are obtained. Therefore, it is important to take medications as prescribed. If there are no changes after that time, report to the physician.

5. The drug affects mental alertness. Therefore, tasks that require concentration should be avoided until the drug effects are evident.

PHENTOLAMINE MESYLATE   (fen-TOE-lah-meen)

Regitine, Rogitine ✳ (Rx)

Classification: Alpha-adrenergic blocking agent.

Action/Kinetics: Phentolamine competitively blocks both presynaptic (alpha$_2$-) and postsynaptic (alpha$_1$-) adrenergic receptors producing vasodilation and a decrease in peripheral resistance. The drug has little effect on blood pressure. In congestive heart failure, phentolamine reduces afterload and pulmonary arterial pressure as well as increases cardiac output. **Onset** (parenteral): Immediate. **Duration:** Short. Poorly absorbed from the GI tract. About 10% excreted unchanged in the urine after parenteral use.

Uses: Treatment of hypertension caused by pheochromocytoma prior to or during surgery. Dermal necrosis and sloughing following IV use or extravasation of norepinephrine. *Investigational:* Treatment of congestive heart failure. In combination with papaverine as an intracavernous injection for impotence.

Contraindications: Coronary artery disease including angina, myocardial infarction, or coronary insufficiency.

Special Concerns: Use during pregnancy and lactation only if benefits clearly outweigh risks. Geriatric patients may have a greater risk of developing hypothermia. Use with great caution in the presence of gastritis, ulcers, and in patients with a history thereof.

Side Effects: *CV:* Acute and prolonged hypotension, tachycardia, and arrhythmias, especially after parenteral administration. Orthostatic hypotension, flushing. *GI:* Nausea, vomiting, diarrhea. *Other:* Dizziness, weakness, nasal stuffiness.

Drug Interactions	
Ephedrine	Phentolamine antagonizes vasoconstrictor and hypertensive effect
Epinephrine	Phentolamine antagonizes vasoconstrictor and hypertensive effect
Norepinephrine	Suitable antagonist to treat overdosage induced by phentolamine
Propranolol	Concomitant use during surgery for pheochromocytoma is indicated

Dosage: *Prevent hypertension in pheochromocytoma, preoperative:* **Adults, IV:** 5 mg 1–2 hr before surgery; dose may be repeated if needed. **Pediatric, IV, IM:** 1 mg (or 0.1 mg/kg) 1–2 hr before surgery; dose may be repeated if needed. *Prevent or control hypertension during surgery:* **Adults, IV:** 5 mg. **IV infusion:** 0.5–1 mg/min. **Pediatric, IV:** 0.1 mg/kg (3 mg/m^2). May be repeated, if necessary. During surgery 5 mg for adults and 1 mg for children may be given to prevent or control symptoms of epinephrine intoxication (e.g., paroxysms of hypertension, respiratory depression, seizures, tachycardia). *Dermal necrosis/sloughing following IV or extravasation of norepinephrine: Prevention,* 10 mg/1,000 mL norepinephrine solution; *treatment:* 5–10 mg/10 mL saline injected into area of extravasation within 12 hr. **Pediatric:** 0.1–0.2 mg/kg to a maximum of 10 mg. *Congestive heart failure:* **Adults, IV infusion:** 0.17–0.4 mg/min. *Impotence:* **Adults, intracavernosal:** papaverine, 30 mg and 0.5–1 mg phentolamine; adjust dose according to response.

NURSING CONSIDERATIONS

Interventions

1. Monitor the blood pressure and pulse before and after parenteral administration, until stabilized.
2. To avoid postural hypotension after parenteral administration, keep the client in a supine position for at least 30 min after injection. Then have the client dangle his legs over the side of the bed and rise slowly to avoid the effects of orthostatic hypotension.
3. If the client shows signs of drug overdose, place in the Trendelenburg position. Assist with the administration of parenteral fluids. Have levarterenol available to minimize hypotension. *Do not use epinephrine.*
4. If the IV administration of norepinephrine or dopamine results in infiltration, administer subcutaneous solutions of phentolamine at the site, within 12 hours for beneficial effects.

(For the Diagnosis of pheochromocytoma):

1. The test for pheochromocytoma should not be undertaken on normotensive clients.
2. Sedatives, analgesics, and other nonessential medication should be withheld for 24 hr (and preferably 72 hr) prior to the test.

3. When testing for pheochromocytoma, the client should be kept in a supine position, preferably in a dark, quiet room.

4. A positive response for pheochromocytoma is a drop in blood pressure of more than 35 mm Hg systolic and 25 mm Hg diastolic pressure. Maximal decreases in blood pressure usually occur within 2 min after injection of phentolamine and return to preinjection pressure within 15–30 min. A negative response is indicated when the blood pressure is unchanged, elevated, or reduced less than 35 mm Hg systolic and 25 mm Hg diastolic pressure.

5. The pheochromocytoma test is most reliable in clients with sustained hypertension and least reliable in clients with paroxysmal hypertension.

PINDOLOL   (PIN-doh-lohl)
Visken (Rx)

See *Antihypertensives,* Chapter 26, p. 493.

PROPRANOLOL HYDROCHLORIDE   (proh-PRAN-oh-lohl)
Inderal (Rx)

See *Antihypertensives,* Chapter 26, p. 493.

TIMOLOL MALEATE   (TIH-moh-lohl)
Blocadren, Timoptic (Rx)

See *Antihypertensives,* Chapter 26, p. 495.

TOLAZOLINE HYDROCHLORIDE   (toe-LAZ-oh-leen)
Priscoline (Rx)

Classification: Alpha-adrenergic blocking agent.

Action/Kinetics: Tolazoline is a peripheral vasodilator but with incomplete and transient effects as an alpha-adrenergic blocking agent. The vasodilation is due to a direct histamine-like effect on the smooth muscle of blood vessels. Other effects produced include cardiac and GI stimulation, increased cutaneous blood flow, and histamine-like effects. **Onset:** 30 min after first dose. **t½, in neonates:** 3–10 hr. Excreted unchanged in the urine.

Uses: Persistent pulmonary hypertension of the newborn when systemic arterial oxygenation cannot be maintained by mechanical ventilation or supplementary oxygen.

Special Concerns: Use with caution in mitral stenosis.

Side Effects: *CV:* Increase or decrease in blood pressure, tachycardia, arrhythmias, pulmonary hemorrhage. *GI:* Nausea, vomiting, diarrhea, aggravation of peptic ulcer, abdominal discomfort, GI hemorrhage. *Hematologic:* Thrombocytopenia, leukopenia. *Renal:* Oliguria, hematuria, edema. *Other:* Flushing, hepatitis, rashes, tingling or chilliness, increased pilomotor activity, rashes.

Drug Interactions	
Alcohol	Antabuse reaction when alcohol is ingested with tolazoline
Clonidine	Tolazoline ↓ effect of clonidine
Epinephrine	↓ Blood pressure with rebound (epinephrine reversal)

Dosage: IV. Initial: 1–2 mg/kg by a scalp vein over 5–10 min; **then,** administer 1–2 mg/kg hourly by IV infusion. Dose may be increased in increments of 1–2 mg/kg, up to 6–8 mg/kg/hr.

NURSING CONSIDERATIONS

Administration/Storage

1. If effective, the drug will cause a response within 30 min after the initial dose.
2. There has been little experience with infusions lasting longer than 36–48 hr. Withdraw drug when arterial blood gases become stable.
3. Pretreatment of the infant with an antacid may prevent GI bleeding.

Assessment

Obtain baseline blood pressure prior to administering the medication.

Interventions

1. Monitor the BP and pulse carefully. Clients are subject to either hypertension or hypotension. Document and report to the physician.
2. Routinely check the client's affected extremity for warmth. Note if there is a feeling of increased cold as this may result from a paradoxical reaction to the drug.
3. Observe the affected extremity for flushing and piloerection after the drug is administered. These are signs indicating that optimal dosage has been achieved.
4. To increase the effectiveness of the drug, keep the client warm.
5. To avoid postural hypotension after the drug has been administered, keep the client in a supine position for at least 30 min after administration. Have clients rise slowly and dangle their legs before standing.
6. If the client suffers from an overdosage of medication, place the client in Trendelenburg position. Assist with the administration of parenteral fluids and have ephedrine available for administration to minimize hypotension. (*Do not use epinephrine or norepinephrine.*)

Client/Family Teaching

1. Warn the client not to ingest alcohol before or after administration of this drug. A disulfiram-like reaction may occur.
2. Drug may aggravate stress ulcers as it stimulates gastric secretion. Report to physician so antacid therapy may be added.

CHAPTER FORTY-SIX

Parasympathomimetic (Cholinergic) Drugs

PARASYMPATHOMIMETICS

46

The neurohormone acetylcholine is necessary for nerve impulse transmission in the parasympathetic (cholinergic) portion of the autonomic nervous system (ANS).

Acetylcholine is stored at the neurojunction; after appropriate stimulation, the neurohormone is released, crosses the synapse, and interacts with receptors located on the postsynaptic membrane.

Although all postjunctional cholinergic receptors of the parasympathetic ANS share certain characteristics, they vary with respect to the intensity with which they respond to stimulation by acetylcholine and drugs that either mimic the effects of acetylcholine or block its action. This difference in response was first identified in studies on receptors involving the alkaloids muscarine and nicotine. The receptors were classified into a muscarinic type and a nicotinic type, some of which were recently further subdivided.

Cholinergic drugs can be divided into two classes: directly acting drugs that mimic the action of acetylcholine and indirectly acting drugs that increase the concentration of acetylcholine, usually by inhibiting acetylcholinesterase, the enzyme that degrades acetylcholine. The direct-acting drugs include bethanecol and guanidine while the indirect-acting drugs include ambenonium, edrophonium, neostigmine, physostigmine, and pyridostigmine.

Cholinergic drugs have the following pharmacologic effects on various structures:

GI Tract

Enhance secretion by gastric and other glands (may cause belching, heartburn, nausea, and vomiting). Increase smooth muscle tone and stimulate bowel movement.

Genitourinary System

Stimulation of ureter and relaxation of urinary bladder, resulting in micturition.

Cardiac Muscle

Slowing of heart rate (bradycardia), decrease in atrial contractility, impulse formation, and conductivity.

Blood Vessels

Vasodilation, resulting in increased skin temperature and local flushing.

Respiration

Increased mucus secretion and bronchial constriction, which causes coughing, choking, and wheezing, especially in patients with history of asthma.

Eyes

Contraction of radial and sphincter muscles of iris (pupillary constriction or miosis). Contraction of the ciliary body producing spasm of accommodation of the lens, which then no longer adjusts to see at various distances. Reduction of intraocular pressure.

Skin

Sweat and salivary glands: Activation, increased pilomotor response.

Note that some of these effects are more pronounced with some drugs than with others. Also, the cholinergic drugs are rather nonspecific because they affect so many different parts of the body and thus have many side effects.

Directly Acting Cholinergic Drugs

BETHANECHOL CHLORIDE   (beh-THAN-eh-kohl)

Duvoid, Urabeth, Urecholine (Rx)

Classification: Cholinergic (parasympathomimetic), direct-acting.

Action/Kinetics: Directly stimulates cholinergic receptors, primarily muscarinic type. This results in stimulation of gastric motility, increases gastric tone, and stimulates the detrusor muscle of the urinary bladder. Bethanechol produces a slight transient fall of diastolic BP, accompanied by minor reflex tachycardia. The drug is resistant to hydrolysis by acetylcholinesterase, which increases its duration of action. **PO: Onset,** 30–90 min; **maximum:** 60–90 min; **duration:** up to 6 hr. **SC: Onset,** 5–15 min; **maximum:** 15–30 min.; **duration:** 2 hr.

Uses: Postpartum or postoperative urinary retention, atony of the bladder with urinary retention. *Investigational:* Reflux esophagitis, congenital megacolon, postoperative gastric atony.

Contraindications: Hypotension, coronary artery disease, coronary occlusion, AV conduction defects, bradycardia. Also, peptic ulcer, asthma, hyperthyroidism, parkinsonism, epilepsy, obstruction of the bladder; if the strength or integrity of the GI or bladder wall is questionable, peritonitis, GI spastic disease, inflammatory lesions of the GI tract, vagotonia. Not to be used IM or IV.

Special Concerns: Pregnancy category: C. Use with caution during lactation. Safety and effectiveness have not been determined in children less than 8 years of age.

Side Effects: Serious side effects are uncommon with oral dosage; symptoms observed are those of overdosage. *GI:* Nausea, vomiting, diarrhea, salivation, GI upset, involuntary defecation, cramps, colic, belching. *CV:* Heart block, orthostatic hypotension, syncope with cardiac arrest, atrial fibrillation (in hyperthyroid patients). *CNS:* Headache, malaise. *Other:* Flushing, sweating, urinary urgency, attacks of asthma, dyspnea, chest pain or pressure.

Drug Interactions

Cholinergic inhibitors	Additive cholinergic effects
Ganglionic blocking agents	Critical hypotensive response
Procainamide	Antagonism of cholinergic effects
Quinidine	Antagonism of cholinergic effects

Dosage: Tablets: **Adults, usual,** 10–50 mg t.i.d.–q.i.d. to a maximum of 120 mg/day. The minimum effective dose can be determined by giving 5–10 mg initially and repeating this dose q 1–2 hr until a satisfactory response is observed or a maximum of 50 mg has been given. **Pediatric:** 0.2 mg/kg (6.7 mg/m^2) t.i.d. **SC: usual,** 5 mg t.i.d.–q.i.d. The minimum effective dose is determined by giving 2.5 mg initially and repeating this dose at 15–30-min intervals to a maximum of 4 doses or until a satisfactory response is obtained. **Pediatric:** 0.15–0.2 mg/kg (5–6.7 mg/m^2) t.i.d. Never give IM or IV.

NURSING CONSIDERATIONS

Administration/Storage

1. To avoid nausea and vomiting, bethanechol tablets should be taken on an empty stomach. Usually, 1 hr before or 2 hr after meals.
2. Administer orally or subcutaneously only.
3. The client should be observed closely for 30–60 min after drug administration for possible severe side effects. A syringe containing atropine should be available to reverse the effects of bethanechol.

Assessment

1. Take a complete nursing history.
2. Note the drugs the client is currently taking to determine if there are any that are likely to interact with bethanechol.
3. Obtain baseline data concerning the client's intake and output when the drug is to be used to treat urinary tract problems.
4. If the drug is to be used to treat GI atony, obtain baseline data concerning bowel sounds and habits.
5. If the client is taking antacids, investigate the reasons to determine if the client has a history of peptic ulcers.

Interventions

1. Monitor the client's vital signs, intake and output until it can be determined what the effects of the drug will be.
2. If the drug is to be administered SC, administer 2 hr before eating to reduce the potential for nausea.

3. Have atropine available during SC therapy to counteract manifestations of acute toxicity.

4. If the drug is being administered for GI atony, monitor for bowel sounds.

5. If the client complains of gnawing, aching, burning or epigastric pain in the left epigastric area, document and report to the physician for further investigation of the problem.

6. If the client complains of tightness in the region of the urinary bladder, monitor client intake and output closely. If the output is inadequate for the amount of intake, record and report to the physician immediately because the drug should be discontinued.

Client/Family Teaching

1. Advise clients to take oral medication when the stomach is empty to avoid nausea and vomiting.

2. Discuss with the client and family the expected results of the therapy.

3. Instruct the client to report any adverse side effects to the physician.

GUANIDINE HYDROCHLORIDE   (GWAH-nih-deen)

(Rx)

Classification: Cholinergic muscle stimulant.

Action/Kinetics: Guanidine hydrochloride increases the release of acetylcholine at the synapses following nerve impulse transmission; it slows the rate of depolarization and repolarization of the muscle cell membrane, therefore acting as a cholinergic muscle stimulant. It is ineffective in the treatment of myasthenia gravis.

Uses: Reduction of muscle weakness and relief of fatigue associated with Eaton-Lambert syndrome.

Contraindications: Hypersensitivity to and intolerance of drug. Lactation. Use in myasthenia gravis.

Special Concerns: Use during pregnancy only if benefits clearly outweigh risks. Safety for use in children not established.

Side Effects: *CNS:* Nervousness, tremors, irritability, lightheadedness, ataxia, jitteriness, psychoses, confusion, changes in mood and emotions, hallucinations. *Neurologic:* Paresthesia of face, feet, hands, and lips; hands and feet feel cold. *GI:* Nausea, cramps, diarrhea, anorexia, dry mouth, gastric irritation. *Dermatologic:* Rashes, petechiae, ecchymoses, sweating, dry skin, scaling of skin, folliculitis, purpura, flushing. *CV:* Hypotension, atrial fibrillation, tachycardia, palpitations. *Hematologic:* Anemia, leukopenia, thrombocytopenia. *Renal:* Uremia, renal tubular necrosis, chronic interstitial nephritis. *Other:* Sore throat, fever.

Laboratory Test Interferences: Increase in blood creatinine, uremia, abnormal liver function tests.

Dosage: Tablets. *Individualized,* **Adults: initial,** 10–15 mg/kg/day in 3–4 divided doses; **then,** increase dose gradually to 35 mg/kg/day or up to the development of side effects.

NURSING CONSIDERATIONS

Assessment

1. Take a complete nursing history.

2. Note any history of myasthenia gravis as the drug is contraindicated.

3. Obtain baseline CBC, liver and renal function studies prior to initiating therapy.

Interventions

1. Monitor CBC, liver and renal function tests periodically while client is receiving the drug because damage may be dose-related.
2. If client experiences anorexia, increased peristalsis, or diarrhea, notify the physician. These are early warnings that suggest the drug should be discontinued.
3. Symptoms of hyperirritability, tremors, convulsive contractions of muscles, increased salivation, vomiting, diarrhea, and hypoglycemia are usually toxic manifestations of drug therapy.
4. The drug is highly toxic and treatment should continue only as long as necessary.
5. Have calcium gluconate available to control neuromuscular and convulsive symptoms.
6. Have atropine available to reduce GI symptoms, circulatory disturbances, and changes in blood glucose levels.

Evaluation

1. Observe for freedom from complications of drug therapy.
2. Determine if client complaints of fatigue are decreased.

Indirectly Acting Cholinergic Drugs (Cholinesterase Inhibitors)

AMBENONIUM CHLORIDE   (am-beh-**NO**-nee-um)

Mytelase (Rx)

For additional information, see *Neostigmine*, p. 931.

Classification: Indirectly acting cholinergic-acetylcholinesterase inhibitor.

Action/Kinetics: Onset: 20–30 min. **Duration:** 3–8 hr. Has a longer duration of action than neostigmine or pyridostigmine.

Uses: Myasthenia gravis.

Additional Contraindications: Use with other cholinergics.

Special Concerns: Safe use during pregnancy and lactation has not been established.

Dosage: Tablets. *Individualized.* **Adults: initial,** 5 mg t.i.d.; **then,** dosage can be adjusted at 1–2-day intervals as needed to prevent toxicity. Doses as high as 200 mg/day have been used, but the patient must be carefully observed for toxicity. **Pediatric:** 0.3 mg/kg (10 mg/m^2) daily in 3–4 divided doses; dose can be increased to 1.5 mg/kg daily given in 3–4 divided doses.

NURSING CONSIDERATIONS

See also *Nursing Considerations* for *Neostigmine*, p. 932.

Administration/Storage

1. There is a narrow margin between the first appearance of side effects and subsequent serious toxic symptoms.
2. Have 0.5–1 mg of atropine sulfate available as an antidote to be administered slowly IV, in the event of drug overdose.
3. Oxygen and mechanical ventilation equipment should also be available for emergency treatment.

Interventions

1. Monitor vital signs and intake and output.
2. Observe client closely for side effects of drug therapy. These are indications of drug overdose and require immediate treatment.
3. Note client reactions peculiar to this cholinergic drug. These may include nervousness, dizziness, headache, and mental confusion. Document and report these incidents to the physician.
4. The response of the client to the drug is highly individualized. Therefore, careful monitoring of the client is essential. Any prior experience with the drug needs to be noted.

Client/Family Teaching

1. Remind clients to take their medication only as directed and to report for follow-up visits as scheduled. Resistance may develop to the drug and close follow-up is important to assure this has not occurred.
2. Explain that drug requirements are higher during times of greatest fatigue.
3. Provide the client with a printed list of adverse muscarinic effects and provide written guidelines concerning how to adjust the dosage during these events.
4. Take the medication with food or milk to minimize GI upset.
5. Provide the names and address of local support groups that may assist client to understand and cope with the disease.

EDROPHONIUM CHLORIDE   (ed-roh-**FOH**-nee-um)

Enlon, Reversol, Tensilon (Rx)

For additional information, see *Neostigmine*. p. 931.

Classification: Indirectly acting cholinergic-acetylcholinesterase inhibitor.

Action/Kinetics: Edrophonium is a short-acting agent mostly used for diagnosis and not for maintenance therapy. By increasing the duration of action at the motor end plate, edrophonium causes a transient increase in muscle strength in myasthenia gravis patients and either no change or a slight weakness in muscle strength in patients with other disorders. **Onset: IM,** 2–10 min; **IV,** less than 1 min. **Duration: IM,** 5–30 min; **IV,** 10 min. Eliminated through the kidneys.

Uses: Diagnosis of myasthenia gravis, adjunct to treat respiratory depression due to curare and similar nondepolarizing agents such as gallamine, pancuronium, and tubocurarine. *Investigational:* Treatment of supraventricular tachycardia.

Special Concerns: Pregnancy category: C.

Dosage: IM, IV. *Diagnosis of myasthenia gravis.* **IV: Adults,** 2 mg initially over 15–30 sec; with needle in place, wait 45 sec; if no response occurs after 45 seconds inject an additional 8 mg. If a reaction is obtained following 2 mg, test is discontinued and atropine, 0.4–0.5 mg, is given IV. The test may be repeated in 30 min. **Pediatric, up to 34 kg: IV,** 1 mg; if no response after 45 sec, can give up to 5 mg. **Pediatric, over 34 kg: IV,** 2 mg; if no response after 45 sec, can give up to 10 mg in 1 mg increments q 30–45 sec. **Infants:** 0.5 mg. If IV injection is not feasible, IM can be used. **IM: Adults,** 10 mg; if hyperreactivity occurs, retest after 30 min with 2 mg IM to rule out false negatives. **Pediatric, up to 34 kg:** 2 mg; **more than 34 kg:** 5 mg. (There is a 2–10-min delay in reaction with IM route.)

To evaluate treatment needs in myasthenic patients: 1 hr after PO administration of drug used to treat myasthenia, give edrophonium **IV,** 1–2 mg. (Note: Response will be myasthenic in undertreated patients, adequate in controlled patients, and cholinergic in overtreated patients.)

Curare antagonist: **Slow IV,** 10 mg over 30–45 seconds; repeat if necessary to maximum of 40 mg. *Treat supraventricular tachycardia:* **Adults, IV, initial** 5–10 mg repeated in 10 min if necessary. **Pediatric, IV:** 2 mg given slowly.

NURSING CONSIDERATIONS

See also *Nursing Considerations* for *Neostigmine* below.

Administration/Storage

1. Edrophonium should not be given before curare or curare-like drugs.
2. Have IV atropine sulfate available to use as an antagonist.

Interventions

1. Observe the client closely in a monitored environment during drug administration.
2. Monitor vital signs, intake and output at least every 4 hours.
3. Observe the client for side effects such as increased salivation, bronchial spasm, bradycardia, and cardiac dysrhythmia. This is particularly important when working with elderly clients. Document and report these symptoms to the physician immediately.
4. When the drug is being administered as an antidote for curare, assess the client for the effects of each dose of drug. Do not administer the next dose of drug unless the prior effects have been observed and recorded. Larger doses of medication may potentiate effects.
5. Evaluate the client's respiratory effort and provide assisted ventilation as needed.
6. Clients in cholinergic crisis should have their state of consciousness monitored closely.

NEOSTIGMINE BROMIDE   (nee-oh-**STIG**-meen)

Prostigmin Bromide (Rx)

NEOSTIGMINE METHYLSULFATE   (nee-oh-**STIG**-meen)

Prostigmin Methylsulfate (Rx)

Classification: Indirectly acting cholinergic-acetylcholinesterase inhibitor.

Action/Kinetics: By inhibiting the enzyme acetylcholinesterase, these drugs cause an increase in the concentration of acetylcholine at the myoneural junction, thus facilitating transmission of impulses across the myoneural junction. In myasthenia gravis, muscle strength is increased. The drug may also act on the autonomic ganglia of the CNS. Neostigmine also prevents or relieves postoperative distention by increasing gastric motility and tone and prevents or relieves urinary retention by increasing the tone of the detrusor muscle of the bladder. Shorter acting than ambenonium chloride and pyridostigmine. Atropine is often given concomitantly to control side effects. **Onset: PO,** 45–75 min; **IM,** 20–30 min; **IV,** 4–8 min. **Time to peak effect, parenteral:** 20–30 min. **Duration:** All routes, 2–4 hr. **t½, PO:** 42–60 min; **IM:** 51–90 min; **IV:** 47–60 min. Eliminated through the urine (about 40% unchanged).

Uses: Diagnosis and treatment of myasthenia gravis. Prophylaxis and treatment of postoperative GI ileus or urinary retention. Antidote for tubocurarine and other nondepolarizing drugs.

Contraindications: Hypersensitivity, mechanical obstruction of GI or urinary tract, peritonitis, history of bromide sensitivity, bradycardia, hypotension, vagotonia, peptic ulcer, asthma, hyperthyroidism, coronary occlusion, vesical neck obstruction of urinary bladder.

Special Concerns: Safe use during pregnancy (pregnancy category: C) and lactation not established. May cause uterine irritability and premature labor if given IV to pregnant women near term. In geriatric patients, the duration of action may be increased.

Side Effects: *GI:* Nausea, vomiting, diarrhea, abdominal cramps, involuntary defecation, salivation, dysphagia, flatulence, increased gastric and intestinal secretions. *CV:* Bradycardia, hypotension, ECG changes, nodal rhythm, cardiac arrest, syncope, AV block, substernal pain, thrombophlebitis after IV use. *CNS:* Headache, seizures, malaise, dysphonia, dysarthria, dizziness, drowsiness, loss of consciousness. *Respiratory:* Increased secretions, bronchoconstriction, skeletal muscle paralysis, laryngospasm, central respiratory paralysis, respiratory depression or arrest, bronchospasm, dyspnea. *Ophthalmologic:* Miosis, double vision, lacrimation, accommodation difficulties, hyperemia of conjunctiva, visual changes. *Musculoskeletal:* Muscle fasciculations or weakness, muscle cramps or spasms, arthralgia. *Other:* Skin rashes, urinary frequency and incontinence, sweating, flushing, allergic reactions, anaphylaxis, urticaria. These effects can usually be reversed by parenteral administration of 0.6 mg of atropine sulfate, which should be readily available.

Cholinergic crisis, due to overdosage, must be distinguished from myasthenic crisis (worsening of the disease), since cholinergic crisis involves removal of drug therapy, while myasthenic crisis involves an increase in anticholinesterase therapy.

Drug Interactions	
Aminoglycosides	↑ Neuromuscular blockade
Atropine	Atropine suppresses symptoms of excess GI stimulation caused by cholinergic drugs
Corticosteroids	↓ Effect of neostigmine
Magnesium salts	Antagonize the effects of anticholinesterases
Mecamylamine	Intense hypotensive response
Organophosphate-type insecticides/pesticides	Added systemic effects with cholinesterase inhibitors
Succinylcholine	↑ Neuromuscular blocking effects

Dosage: Tablets: Neostigmine bromide. *Treat myasthenia gravis:* **Adults,** 15 mg q 3–4 hr; adjust dose and frequency as needed. **Usual maintenance,** 150 mg/day with dosing intervals determined by patient response. **Pediatric,** 2 mg/kg (60 mg/m²) daily in 6–8 divided doses. **IM, IV, SC: Neostigmine methylsulfate.** *Treat myasthenia gravis:* **Adults: IM, SC,** 0.5 mg. **Pediatric: IM, SC,** 0.01–0.04 mg/kg q 2–3 hr. *Diagnosis of myasthenia gravis:* **Adults: IM, SC,** 1.5 mg given with 0.6 mg atropine; **pediatric, IM:** 0.04 mg/kg (1 mg/m²); or, **IV:** 0.02 mg/kg (0.5 mg/m²). *Antidote for tubocurarine,* **Adults: IV,** 0.5–2 mg slowly with 0.6–1.2 mg atropine sulfate. Can repeat if necessary up to total dose of 5 mg. **Pediatric: IV,** 0.04 mg/kg with 0.02 mg/kg atropine sulfate. *Prevention of postoperative GI distention or urinary retention:* **Adults: IM, SC,** 0.25 mg immediately after surgery repeated q 4–6 hr for 2–3 days. *Treatment of postoperative GI distention:* **Adults: IM, SC,** 0.5 mg as required. *Treatment of urinary retention:* **Adults: IM, SC,** 0.5 mg repeated q 3 hr for 5 doses after bladder has been emptied or patient has voided. If urination does not occur within 1 hr after 0.5 mg, the patient should be catheterized.

NURSING CONSIDERATIONS

Administration/Storage

1. The interval between doses must be individually determined in order to achieve optimum effects.

2. If greater fatigue occurs at certain times of the day, a larger part of the daily dose can be administered at these times.

3. Neostigmine should not be given if high concentrations of halothane or cyclopropane are present.

4. Have atropine available to treat overdose or toxicity.

5. If bradycardia is present, atropine should be administered first to get the heart rate to approximately 80 beats/min.

Assessment

1. Note any history of hypersensitivity to drugs in this category.

2. Identify any drugs the client is taking to determine if they are interactant with neostigmine.

3. Note any history of bromide sensitivity. The drug is contraindicated in these instances.

4. Take the client's pulse prior to administering the drug. If the client's pulse is less than 80, the drug should be withheld and the physician notified.

Interventions

1. Observe the client for generalized cholinergic stimulation. This is evidence of a toxic reaction and the physician should be notified immediately.

2. Assess clients for stability and vision. If the client has difficulty with coordination or vision caution them to avoid use of heavy machinery until the effects of the medication wear off. If the effects become severe, notify the physician.

3. Monitor the pulse and blood pressure for the first hour after drug administration. If hypotension occurs, have the client remain recumbent until the blood pressure stabilizes.

4. When the medication is used as an antidote for tubocurarine, assist in the ventilation of the client and maintain a patent airway.

5. If the client is taking the medication for treatment of myasthenia gravis, any onset of weakness 1 hr after administration usually indicates overdosage of drug. Notify the physician immediately. The onset of weakness 3 hr or more after administration usually indicates underdosage and/or resistance and should also be documented and reported to the physician. Also note any associated difficulty with respirations or increase in muscle weakness.

PHYSOSTIGMINE SALICYLATE   (fye-zoh-STIG-meen)

Antilirium, Eserine Salicylate, Isopto Eserine (Rx)

PHYSOSTIGMINE SULFATE   (fye-zoh-STIG-meen)

Eserine Sulfate (Rx)

See also *Neostigmine,* p. 931, and *Ophthalmic Cholinergic Agents,* p. 936.

Classification: Indirectly acting cholinergic-acetylcholinesterase inhibitor.

Action/Kinetics: Physostigmine is a reversible acetylcholinesterase inhibitor resulting in an increased concentration of acetylcholine at nerve endings which can antagonize anticholinergic drugs. It produces miosis, increased accommodation, and a decrease in intraocular pressure with decreased resistance to outflow of aqueous humor. When used for chronic open-angle glaucoma, ciliary muscle contraction may open the intertrabecular spaces facilitating aqueous humor outflow.

Onset, IV: 3–5 min. **Duration, IV:** 1–2 hr. **t½:** 1–2 hr. No dosage alteration is necessary in patients with renal impairment. **Onset, miosis:** 10–30 min; **duration, miosis:** 12–48 hr.

Uses: Overdosage due to cholinergic blocking drugs (e.g., atropine) and tricyclic antidepressant overdosage. Reduce intraocular pressure in open-angle glaucoma. Freidreich's and other inherited ataxias (FDA has granted orphan status for this use). *Investigational:* Angle-closure glaucoma during or after iridectomy, secondary glaucoma if no inflammation present.

Special Concerns: Use during pregnancy (pregnancy category: C) only when benefits clearly outweigh risks.

Additional Side Effects: If IV administration is too rapid, bradycardia, hypersalivation, breathing difficulties, and seizures may occur. Conjunctivitis when used for glaucoma.

Dosage: IM, IV. *Anticholinergic drug overdosage:* **Adults, IM, IV,** 0.5–2 mg at a rate of 1 mg/min; may be repeated if necessary. **Pediatric, IV:** 0.5 mg given over a period of at least 1 min. Dose may be repeated at 5–10 min if needed to a maximum of 2 mg if no toxic effects are manifested.
   Ophthalmic Solution. Adults and children: 1 gtt of the 0.25% or 0.5% salicylate solution in the eye b.i.d.–t.i.d. **Ophthalmic Ointment. Adults and children:** 1 cm of the 0.25% sulfate ointment in the conjunctiva 1–3 times daily.

NURSING CONSIDERATIONS

See also *Nursing Considerations* for *Neostigmine,* p. 932, *Cholinergic Blocking Agents,* p. 949, and *Ophthalmic Cholinergic Agents,* p. 937.

Administration/Storage

1. Following use of the ophthalmic solution, the lacrimal sac should be pressed for 1–2 min to avoid excessive systemic absorption.
2. The ophthalmic ointment may be used at night for prolonged effect of the medication.
3. Due to the possibility of allergic reactions, atropine should always be available as an antidote.

Interventions

1. Wipe away any excess solution from around the eyes.
2. Wash hands after administration to prevent systemic absorption.
3. When specifically ordered, monitor and record the heart rate and consult with the physician if not within normal limits.
4. Have the client void prior to administering the medication. If the client develops incontinence, it may be caused by too high a dose. Document and notify the physician.

Client/Family Teaching

1. Instruct the client to notify the physician immediately if any respiratory difficulty occurs.
2. Advise the client that nausea and vomiting may occur. If the symptoms are severe, the physician should be notified.
3. Some stinging and burning of the eyes may occur with the ophthalmic medication. Reassure the client that these symptoms should disappear as the use of the drug continues. If clients experiences painful spasms, instruct them to apply cold compresses. If itching, pain or tearing persists, do not continue using the medication until the physician has been consulted.

PYRIDOSTIGMINE BROMIDE   (pih-rid-oh-**STIG**-meen)

Mestinon, Regonol (Rx)

For all information, see also *Neostigmine,* p. 931.

Classification: Indirectly acting cholinergic-acetylcholinesterase inhibitor.

Action/Kinetics: Has a slower onset, longer duration of action, and fewer side effects than neostigmine. **Onset, PO:** 30–45 min for syrup and tablets and 30–60 min for extended-release tablets; **IM:** 15 min; **IV:** 2–5 min. **Duration, PO:** 3–6 hr for syrup and tablets and 6–12 hr for extended-release tablets; **IM, IV:** 2–4 hr. Poorly absorbed from the GI tract; excreted in urine up to 72 hr after administration.

Uses: Myasthenia gravis. Antidote for nondepolarizing muscle relaxants (e.g., tubocurarine).

Additional Contraindications: Sensitivity to bromides.

Special Concerns: Safe use during pregnancy and during lactation has not been established. May cause uterine irritability and premature labor if given IV to pregnant women near term. In geriatric patients, the duration of action may be increased.

Additional Side Effects: Skin rash. Thrombophlebitis after IV use.

Dosage: Syrup, Tablets. *Myasthenia gravis:* **Adults:** 60–120 mg q 3–4 hr with dosage adjusted to patient response. **Maintenance:** 600 mg daily (range: 60 mg–1.5 g). **Pediatric:** 7 mg/kg (200 mg/m²) daily in 5–6 divided doses. **Sustained-release Tablets. Adults:** 180–540 mg 1–2 times daily with at least 6 hr between doses. Extended-release tablets not recommended for use in children.

    IM, IV. *Myasthenia gravis:* **Adults, IM, IV,** 2 mg (about ¹/₃₀ the adult dose) q 2–3 hr. *Antidote for nondepolarizing drugs:* **Adults, IV,** 10–20 mg with 0.6–1.2 mg atropine sulfate given IV. *Myasthenia gravis:* **Neonates of myasthenic mothers, IM,** 0.05–0.15 mg/kg q 4–6 hr.

NURSING CONSIDERATIONS

See also *Nursing Considerations* for *Neostigmine,* p. 932.

Administration

1. During dosage adjustment, administer the drug to the client in a closely monitored environment.
2. Parenteral medication dosage is ¹/₃₀ of the oral dose.
3. After oral administration, onset of action occurs in 30–45 minutes and lasts for 3–6 hours. When administered IM, the onset of action occurs within 15 minutes. When administered IV, the onset of action occurs within 2–5 minutes.
4. Have atropine sulfate available to administer as an antidote.

Interventions

1. Observe the client for toxic reactions demonstrated by generalized cholinergic stimulation.
2. Assess the client for muscular weakness. This may be a sign of impending myasthenic crisis and cholinergic overdose.
3. Work with the client to determine the best individualized medication administration schedule.

Client/Family Teaching

1. Explain how extended-release tablets work. Caution clients not to crush them, and not to take these tablets more often than every 6 hours.

2. If ordered by the physician, extended-release tablets may be taken with conventional tablets.

3. Provide the client and family with printed instructions and a list of toxic side effects that should be reported to the physician.

4. Explain how to recognize symptoms of toxic reaction and myasthenic crisis.

5. Clients may develop resistance to the drug. Explain the importance of close medical supervision as well as the prompt reporting of all side effects so that drug therapy can be evaluated.

6. Provide the names and addresses of local support groups that may assist the client and family to understand and cope with the disease.

OPHTHALMIC CHOLINERGIC (MIOTIC) AGENTS

General Statement: Cholinergic agents are commonly used for the treatment of glaucoma and less frequently for the correction of accommodative esotropia.

Action/Kinetics: The ophthalmic cholinergic drugs fall into two classes: direct-acting (carbachol, pilocarpine) and indirect-acting (demecarium, echothiophate, isoflurophate, neostigmine, physostigmine), which inhibit the enzyme acetylcholinesterase. In the treatment of glaucoma, the drugs lead to an accumulation of acetylcholine, which stimulates the ciliary muscles and increases contraction of the iris sphincter muscle. This opens the angle of the eye and results in increased outflow of aqueous humor and consequently in a decrease of intraocular pressure. This effect is of particular importance in narrow-angle glaucoma. Hourly tonometric measurements are recommended during initiation of therapy. The drugs also cause spasms of accommodation.

Uses: Glaucoma: Primary acute narrow-angle glaucoma (acute therapy) and primary chronic wide-angle glaucoma (chronic therapy). Selected cases of secondary glaucoma. Diagnosis and treatment of accommodative esotropia. Antidote against harmful effects of atropine-like drugs in patients suffering from glaucoma. Alternately with a mydriatic drug to break adhesions between lens and iris. See also Table 17.

Contraindications: *Direct-acting drugs:* Inflammatory eye disease (iritis), asthma, hypertension. *Indirect-acting drugs:* Same as for direct-acting drugs, as well as acute-angle glaucoma, history of retinal detachment, ocular hypotension accompanied by intraocular inflammatory processes, intestinal or urinary obstruction, peptic ulcer, epilepsy, parkinsonism, spastic GI conditions, vasomotor instability, severe bradycardia or hypotension, and recent myocardial infarctions. During lactation.

Special Concerns: Pregnancy category: X for demecarium, echothiophate, and isoflurophate. Geriatric patients must be carefully monitored.

Side Effects: *Local:* Painful contraction of ciliary muscle, pain in eye, blurred vision, spasms of accommodation, darkened vision, failure to accommodate to darkness, twitching, headaches, painful brow. Most of these symptoms lessen with prolonged usage. Iris cysts and retinal detachment (indirect-acting drugs only).

Systemic: Systemic absorption of drug may cause nausea, GI discomfort, diarrhea, hypotension, bronchial constriction, and increased salivation.

Dosage: See Table 17.

NURSING CONSIDERATIONS

Administration

1. To prevent the overflow of solution into the nasopharynx after topical instillation of drops, exert pressure on the nasolacrimal duct for 1–2 min before the client closes the eyelids.
2. Have epinephrine and atropine available for emergency treatment of increased intraocular pressure.

Interventions

Report redness around the cornea. Epinephrine or phenylephrine hydrochloride (10%) may be ordered with demecarium bromide, echothiophate iodide or isoflurophate to minimize this kind of reaction.

Client/Family Teaching

1. Stress the importance of taking the eye drops exactly as prescribed.
2. Side effects can be minimized by taking at least one dose of medication at bedtime.
3. Review and demonstrate the appropriate method for instilling eye drops.
4. Advise the client not to drive for 1–2 hr after administering eye drops.
5. Pain and blurred vision may occur. This problem usually diminishes with prolonged use of the drug. However, if these symptoms persist, call the physician.
6. If bothersome side effects persist, notify the physician. The dosage of medication may need to be changed.
7. Explain that painful eye spasms may be relieved by applying cold compresses.
8. Provide the client with a schedule for eye examinations. Stress the importance of adhering to the schedule and refilling the prescriptions as needed.

Table 17 Ophthalmic Cholinergic Drugs (Miotics)

Drug	Uses	Dosage	Remarks
Acetylcholine chloride, intraocular (Miochol Intraocular) (Rx)	Rapid intense miosis during cataract surgery; for rapid miosis in iridectomy, keratoplasty, anterior segment surgery	**Solution, 1%:** 0.5–2 mL.	Irrigate slowly to avoid atrophy of iris. Rapid acting, short duration (10–20 min). Since aqueous solutions of acetylcholine are unstable, prepare immediately before use. Pilocarpine may be used before the dressing is applied in order to maintain miosisis.
Carbachol, intraocular (Miostat Intraocular) (Rx)	Miosis during surgery	**Solution:** 0.5 mL of 0.01% solution placed in anterior chamber.	Administered together with wetting agent. **Maximum effects:** Within 2–5 min. **Duration, miosis:** 8 hr. **Decrease in intraocular pressure:** 8 hr.
Carbachol, ophthalmic (Isopto Carbachol) (Rx)	Glaucoma, open-angle. *Investigational:* Angle-closure glaucoma (including during or after iridectomy), secondary glaucoma.	**Solution:** 1 gtt of the solution in the conjunctiva 1–3 times daily.	Available as a 0.75%, 1.5%, 2.25%, and 3% solution. *Side Effects:* Slight hyperemia during first few days, aching of eyes and head which usually passes after third day of treatment. *Nursing Considerations:* After instillation of gtt, absorption may be improved by gentle massage of the lids, unless contraindicated.
Demecarium bromide (Humorsol Ophthalmic) (Rx) Pregnancy category: X.	Open-angle glaucoma, accommodative esotropia, angle-closure glaucoma after iridectomy	**Solution.** *Glaucoma:* **Adults, children,** 1 gtt of the 0.125 or 0.25% solution 1–2 times daily. *Esotropia:* **Adults, children,** 1 gtt of the 0.125 or 0.25% solution once daily for 2–4 weeks; **then,** 1 gtt q 2 days for 3–4 weeks after which the patient is re-evaluated. Then, 1 gtt once every 2 days. *Diagnosis of accommodative esotropia:* 1 gtt of the 0.125 or 0.25% solution once daily for 2 weeks; **then,** 1 gtt q 2 days for 2–3 weeks.	1. *Kinetics:* **Onset,** 15–60 min. **Duration:** 3–10 days. **Peak effect, miosis:** 2–4 hr. 2. Available as a 0.125% and a 0.25% solution. 3. To prevent overdosage, use the lowest possible dose to achieve adequate control. 4. Observe patient closely during first 24 hr of therapy; if response is not adequate, other therapy should be undertaken.

Drug	Indications	Route/Dosage	Nursing Considerations
Echothiophate iodide (Phospholine Iodide) (Rx) Pregnancy category: C.	Open-angle glaucoma; angle-closure glaucoma after iridectomy; secondary glaucoma. Diagnosis and treatment of accommodative esotropia.	**Solution.** *Antiglaucoma agent:* **Adults and children,** 1 gtt of the 0.03–0.25% solution 1–2 times daily. *Accommodative esotropia:* 1 gtt of the 0.03–0.25% solution once daily or every 2 days. *Diagnosis of accommodative esotropia:* 1 gtt of the 0.125% solution once daily at bedtime for 2–3 weeks.	1. *Kinetics:* **Onset:** 10–30 min. **Duration:** 1–4 weeks. **Time to peak, miosis:** 30 min. 2. Available as powder for reconstitution to 0.03%, 0.06%, 0.125%, and 0.25% solutions. 3. To prevent toxic effects, use the lowest possible dose. 4. If tolerance develops after long-term use, a rest period may restore response. 5. May be used together with epinephrine, a carbonic anhydrase inhibitor, or both.
Isoflurophate (Floropryl) (Rx) Pregnancy category: X.	Open-angle glaucoma. Angle-closure glaucoma after iridectomy; secondary glaucoma. Diagnosis and treatment of accommodative esotropia.	**Ointment.** *Antiglaucoma drug:* **Adults and children:** thin strip (0.5 cm) of 0.025% ointment once q 3 days to three times daily. *Accommodative esotropia:* **Adults, children,** thin strip (0.5 cm) of the 0.025% ointment once daily at bedtime for 2 weeks; **then,** once a week to once q 2 days for 2 months. *Diagnosis of accommodative esotropia:* thin strip (0.5 cm) of the 0.025% ointment once daily at bedtime for 2 weeks.	1. *Kinetics:* **Onset:** 5–10 min. **Duration:** 1–4 weeks. **Time to peak, miosis:** 15–20 min. 2. The ointment tube should be kept closed tightly to prevent loss of potency and absorption of moisture. 3. Apply before bedtime to lessen blurring of vision. 4. Hands should be washed immediately after administration. 5. A rest period may restore response if tolerance develops.
Physostigmine salicylate (Eserine Salicylate, Isopto Eserine) (Rx) Pregnancy category: C. Physostigmine sulfate (Eserine Sulfate) (Rx) Pregnancy category: C.	Open-angle glaucoma. *Investigational:* Angle-closure glaucoma during or after iridectomy. Secondary glaucoma.	**Salicylate Solution. Adults and children:** 1 gtt of the 0.25 or 0.5% solution b.i.d.–t.i.d. **Sulfate Ointment. Adults and children:** 1 cm of the 0.25% ointment 1–3 times daily.	1. *Kinetics:* **Onset:** 10–30 min. **Duration:** 12–48 hr. 2. Chronic use may cause conjunctivitis. 3. Solution should not be used if it is cloudy or dark brown.
Pilocarpine hydrochloride (Adsorbocarbine,	Open-angle glaucoma, angle-closure glaucoma	**Gel. Adults and children:** ½-inch strip of 4% gel once	1. *Kinetics:* **Onset:** 10–30 min. **Duration:** 4–8 hr.

Table 17 *(Continued)*

Drug	Uses	Dosage	Remarks
Akarpine, Almocarpine, I-Pilopine, Isopto Carpine, Miocarpine ✦, Ocu-Carpine, Pilocar, Pilokair, Piloptic-1, -2, and -4) (Rx) Pregnancy category: C.	including during or after iridectomy, secondary glaucoma. To produce miosis thus reversing the effects of cycloplegic and mydriatic drugs.	daily at bedtime. **Solution.** All doses are for both adults and children. *Chronic glaucoma:* 1 gtt of a 0.5–4% solution q.i.d. *Acute angle-closure glaucoma:* 1 gtt of a 1 or 2% solution q 5–10 min for 3–6 doses; **then,** 1 gtt q 1–3 hr until pressure is decreased. *Miotic, to counteract sympabomimetics:* 1 gtt of a 1% solution. *Miosis, prior to surgery:* 1 gtt of 2% solution q 4–6 hr for 1 or 2 doses before surgery. *Miosis before iridectomy:* 1 gtt of a 2% solution for 4 doses before surgery.	2. Available as a 0.25%, 0.5%, 1%, 2%, 3%, 4%, 5%, 6%, 8%, and 10% solutions and as a 4% gel. 3. Since pilocarpine is absorbed by melanin, patients with dark pigmented eyes may respond better to solutions greater than 4%. 4. To prevent an attack of angle-closure glaucoma, instill pilocarpine into the unaffected eye during acute, narrow-angle glaucoma.
Pilocarpine nitrate (Minims Pilocarpine ✦, PV. Carpine Liquifilm, Spectro-Pilo) (Rx) Pregnancy category: C.	See Pilocarpine HCl. Also used for emergency miosis.	**Solution.** All doses are for both adults and children. *Chronic glaucoma:* 1 gtt of a 1–4% solution q.i.d. *Acute angle-closure glaucoma:* 1 gtt of a 1 or 2% solution q 5–10 min for 3–6 doses; **then,** 1 gtt q 1–3 hr until pressure is decreased. *Miosis:* 1 gtt of a 1% solution (to counter sympathomimetics), 1 gtt of a 2% solution q 4–6 hr before surgery for glaucoma, 1 gtt of a 2% solution for 4 doses just before surgery for iridectomy.	1. Available as a 1%, 2%, or 4% solution. 2. The dose needed to reverse mydriasis will depend on the dose and strength of cycloplegic used.
Pilocarpine ocular therapeutic system (Ocusert Pilo-20 and -40) (Rx) Pregnancy category: C.	See Pilocarpine HCl.	A unit designed to be placed in the cul-de-sac of the eye for slow release of pilocarpine at a rate of 20 or 40 mcg/hr for 1 week. Ocuset Pilo-20 is equivalent to the 0.5% or 1% drops; Ocusert Pilo-40 is equivalent to the 2% or 3% solution.	1. *Kinetics:* Releases the drug three times faster during the first few hours and then decreases to the rated value (*see Dosage*) within 6 hr. 2. Myopia may be observed during the first several hours of therapy. 3. The system allows a reduction of intraocular pressure around the clock.

| Pilocarpine and Epinephrine (E-Pilo-1, E-Pilo-2, E-Pilo-3, E-Pilo-4, E-Pilo-6, P_1E_1, P_2E_1, P_3E_1, P_4E_1, P_6E_1) (Rx) | Glaucoma | **Solution.** 1–2 gtt into the eye(s) 1–4 times daily. | 1. Pilocarpine and epinephrine exert an additive effect to reduce intraocular pressure; the combination exerts opposite effects on the pupil, which prevents significant mydriasis or miosis.
2. The solutions all contain epinephrine, 1% with varying concentrations of pilocarpine, indicated by the number in the name (e.g., E-Pilo-1 contains 1% pilocarpine and P_2E_1 contains 2% pilocarpine). |
| Pilocarpine and Physostigmine (Isopto P-ES) (Rx) | Glaucoma | **Solution.** 2 gtt into the eye(s) up to q.i.d. | 1. This product contains pilocarpine HCl, 2%, and physostigmine salicylate, 0.25%.
2. There is no evidence to suggest that this combination exerts greater effects to lower intraocular pressure than either drug alone. |

CHAPTER FORTY-SEVEN

Cholinergic Blocking (Parasympatholytic) Drugs

CHOLINERGIC BLOCKING AGENTS

Action/Kinetics: The cholinergic blocking agents prevent the neurotransmitter acetylcholine from combining with receptors on the postganglionic parasympathetic nerve terminal (muscarinic site). In therapeutic doses, these drugs have little effect on transmission of nerve impulses across ganglia (nicotinic sites) or at the neuromuscular junction.

The main effects of cholinergic blocking agents are:

1. to reduce spasms of smooth muscles like those controlling the urinary bladder or spasms of bronchial and intestinal smooth muscle.
2. to block vagal impulses to the heart, resulting in an increase in the rate and speed of impulse conduction through the atrioventricular conducting system.
3. to suppress or decrease gastric secretions, perspiration, salivation, and secretion of bronchial mucus.
4. to relax the sphincter muscles of the iris and cause pupillary dilation (mydriasis) and loss of accommodation for near vision (cycloplegia).
5. to act in diverse ways on the CNS, producing such reactions as depression (scopolamine) or stimulation (toxic doses of atropine). Many of the anticholinergic drugs also have antiparkinson-

ism effects. They abolish or reduce the signs and symptoms of Parkinson's disease, such as tremors and rigidity, and result in some improvement in mobility, muscular coordination, and motor performance. These effects may be due to blockade of the effects of acetylcholine in the CNS. This section also discusses miscellaneous synthetic antispasmodics related to anticholinergic drugs.

The anticholinergics that are related to atropine are quickly absorbed following oral ingestion. These agents cross the blood-brain barrier and may exert significant CNS effects. Examples of these drugs are scopolamine, *l*-hyoscyamine, and belladonna alkaloids. The drugs classified as quaternary ammonium anticholinergic drugs are erratically absorbed from the GI tract and exert minimal CNS effects, since they do not cross the blood-brain barrier. Examples of these drugs are glycopyrrolate, methantheline, propantheline, tridihexethyl chloride, clidinium bromide, isopropamide, and others.

Uses: See individual drugs.

Contraindications: Glaucoma, adhesions between iris and lens of the eye, tachycardia, myocardial ischemia, unstable cardiovascular state in acute hemorrhage, partial obstruction of the GI and biliary tracts, prostatic hypertrophy, renal disease, myasthenia gravis, hepatic disease, paralytic ileus, pyloroduodenal stenosis, pyloric obstruction, intestinal atony, ulcerative colitis, obstructive uropathy. Cardiac patients, especially when there is danger of tachycardia; older persons suffering from atherosclerosis or mental impairment. Lactation.

Special Concerns: Use with caution in pregnancy. Infants and young children are more susceptible to the toxic side effects of anticholinergic drugs. Of particular importance is use of such drugs in children when the ambient temperature is high; due to suppression of sweat glands, the body temperature may increase rapidly. Geriatric patients are particularly likely to manifest anticholinergic side effects such as dry mouth, constipation, and urinary retention (especially in males). Geriatric patients are also more likely to experience agitation, confusion, drowsiness, excitement, glaucoma, and impaired memory. Use with caution in hyperthyroidism, congestive heart failure, cardiac arrhythmias, hypertension, Down's syndrome, asthma, spastic paralysis, blonde individuals, allergies, and chronic lung disease.

Side Effects: These are desirable in some conditions and undesirable in others. Thus, the anticholinergics have an antisalivary effect that is useful in parkinsonism. This same effect is unpleasant when the drug is used for spastic conditions of the GI tract.

Most untoward reactions are dose-related and decrease when dosage decreases. Sometimes it helps to discontinue the medication for several days. With this in mind, anticholinergic drugs have the following untoward reactions. *GI:* Nausea, vomiting, dry mouth, dysphagia, constipation, heartburn, change in taste perception, bloated feeling, paralytic ileus. *CNS:* Dizziness, drowsiness, nervousness, disorientation, headache, weakness, insomnia, fever (especially in children). Large doses may produce CNS stimulation including tremor and restlessness. Anticholinergic psychoses: ataxia, euphoria, confusion, disorientation, loss of short-term memory, decreased anxiety, fatigue, insomnia, hallucinations, dysarthria, agitation. *CV:* Palpitations. *GU:* Urinary retention or hesitancy, impotence. *Ophthalmologic:* Blurred vision, dilated pupils, photophobia, cycloplegia, precipitation of acute glaucoma. *Allergic:* Urticaria, skin rashes, anaphylaxis. *Other:* Flushing, decreased sweating, nasal congestion, suppression of glandular secretions including lactation. Heat prostration (fever and heat stroke) in presence of high environmental temperatures due to decreased sweating.

Note: Even small doses of anticholinergic drugs in geriatric patients may cause agitation, drowsiness, excitement, and other untoward reactions.

Belladonna Poisoning: Infants and children are especially susceptible to the toxic effects of atropine and scopolamine. Poisoning (dose-dependent) is characterized by the following symptoms: dry mouth, burning sensation of the mouth, difficulty in swallowing and speaking, blurred vision, photophobia, rash, tachycardia, increased respiration, increased body temperature (up to 109°F,

42.7°C), restlessness, irritability, confusion, muscle incoordination, dilated pupils, hot dry skin, respiratory depression and paralysis, tremors, seizures, hallucinations, and death.

Treatment of Belladonna Poisoning: *After PO intake:* gastric lavage or induction of vomiting followed by activated charcoal.

Systemic antidote: physostigmine (Eserine), 1–3 mg IV (effectiveness uncertain; thus use other agents if possible). Neostigmine methylsulfate, 0.5–2 mg IV, repeated as necessary. If there is excitation, diazepam or a short-acting barbiturate may be given. For fever, cool baths may be used. Keep patient in a darkened room if photophobia is manifested.

Drug Interactions

Amantadine	Additive anticholinergic side effects
Antacids	↓ Absorption of anticholinergics from GI tract
Antidepressants, tricyclic	Additive anticholinergic side effects
Antihistamines	Additive anticholinergic side effects
Atenolol	Anticholinergics ↑ effects of atenolol
Benzodiazepines	Additive anticholinergic side effects
Corticosteroids	Additive increase in intraocular pressure
Cyclopropane	↑ Chance of ventricular arrhythmias
Digoxin	↑ Effect of digoxin due to ↑ absorption from GI tract
Disopyramide	Potentiation of anticholinergic side effects
Guanethidine	Reversal of inhibition of gastric acid secretion caused by anticholinergics
Haloperidol	Additive increase in intraocular pressure
Histamine	Reversal of inhibition of gastric acid secretion caused by anticholinergics
Levodopa	Possible ↓ effect of levodopa due to ↑ breakdown of levodopa in stomach (due to delayed gastric emptying time)
Meperidine	Additive anticholinergic side effects
Methylphenidate	Potentiation of anticholinergic side effects
Metoclopramide	Anticholinergics block action of metoclopramide
Monoamine oxidase inhibitors	↑ Effect of anticholinergics due to ↓ breakdown by liver
Nitrates, nitrites	Potentiation of anticholinergic side effects
Nitrofurantoin	↑ Bioavailability of nitrofurantoin
Orphenadrine	Additive anticholinergic side effects
Phenothiazines	Additive anticholinergic side effects; also, effects of phenothiazines may be ↓
Primidone	Potentiation of anticholinergic side effects
Procainamide	Additive anticholinergic side effects
Quinidine	Additive anticholinergic side effects
Reserpine	Reversal of inhibition of gastric acid secretion caused by anticholinergics
Sympathomimetics	↑ Bronchial relaxation
Thiazide diuretics	↑ Bioavailability of thiazide diuretics
Thioxanthines	Potentiation of anticholinergic side effects

Dosage: See individual drugs and Table 18, p. 945.

Table 18 Cholinergic Blocking Agents

Drug	Use	Dosage	Remarks*
Anisotropine methyl-bromide (Valpin 50) (Rx) Pregnancy category: C.	Adjunct in peptic ulcer therapy before meals.	**Tablets. Adults:** 50 mg t.i.d.	Quaternary ammonium compound. **Onset:** 1 hr; **duration:** 4–6 hr. Geriatric patients may be more sensitive to the usual adult dose.
Belladonna Extract (Rx) Pregnancy category: C. Belladonna Tincture (Rx) Pregnancy category: C.	**GI:** Adjunct to treat peptic ulcer; spastic colon, mucous and ulcerative colitis; pancreatitis; diarrhea; diverticulitis. **CNS:** Idiopathic or postencephalitic parkinsonism, motion sickness. **GU:** Dysmenorrhea, nocturnal enuresis. **Dentistry:** Antisialagogue.	**PO: Tablets (Extract):** 15 mg t.i.d.–q.i.d. 30–60 min before meals and at bedtime. **Tincture. Adults:** 0.18–0.3 mg t.i.d.–q.i.d. 30–60 before meals and at bedtime. **Pediatric:** 0.009 mg/kg daily in 3–4 divided doses.	1. Belladonna contains hyoscyamine, scopolamine (hyoscine), and other alkaloids. 2. Extract contains 1.25 mg alkaloids/g while tincture contains 0.3 mg alkaloids/mL. 3. **Onset:** 1–2 hr; **Duration:** 4 hr.
Clidinium bromide (Quarzan) (Rx) Pregnancy category: C.	Adjunct in peptic ulcer therapy	**Capsules. Adults,** 2.5–5.0 mg t.i.d.–q.i.d. before meals and at bedtime. **Geriatric or debilitated patients:** 2.5 mg t.i.d before meals.	1. Clidinium is a synthetic quaternary ammonium compound. 2. Also found in Librax (see Chapter 53, p. 1039). 3. **Onset:** 1 hr; **duration:** Up to 3 hr.
Hexocyclium methylsulfate (Tral Filmtabs) (Rx) Pregnancy category: C.	Adjunct in peptic ulcer therapy	**Tablets. Adults:** 25 mg q.i.d. before meals and at bedtime.	1. Synthetic, quaternary ammonium compound. 2. **Onset:** 1 hr; **duration:** 3–4 hr. 3. Not for use in children.
Hyoscyamine sulfate (Anaspaz, Cystospaz, Cystospaz-M, Levsin, Levsinex Timecaps, Neoquess) (Rx) Pregnancy category: C.	**GI:** Adjunct in peptic ulcer therapy; spastic colon; mucous colitis, acute enterocolitis; mild dysenteries and diverticulitis; biliary and infant colic; neurogenic bowel disturbances. **Respiratory:** Preanesthetic to dry secretions. **CNS:** Poisoning by anticholinesterase agents. Parkinsonism. **GU:** Cystitis, renal colic.	**Elixir, Oral Solution, Tablets. Adults:** 0.125–0.5 mg t.i.d.–q.i.d. 30–60 min before meals and at bedtime. **Elixir, Pediatric, weight in kg: 2.3–3.3 kg:** 0.0125 mg q 4 hr; **3.4–4.4 kg:** 0.0156 mg q 4 hr; **4.5–6.7 kg:** 0.0188 mg q 4 hr; **6.8–9 kg:** 0.025 mg q 4 hr; **9.1–13.5 kg:** 0.0313 mg q 4 hr; **13.6–22.6 kg:** 0.063 mg q 4 hr; **22.7–33 kg:** 0.125–0.187 mg q 4 hr; **34–36 kg:** 0.125–0.187 mg q 4 hr. **Extended-release Capsules. Adults:** 0.375 mg b.i.d. in the morning and at bedtime.	1. Also found in Donnagel, Donnagel PG, and Donnatal. 2. **Onset:** 20–30 min after PO and 2–3 min parenterally. **Duration:** 4–6 hr. 3. If used during pregnancy, may produce tachycardia in the fetus. 4. Geriatric patients may be more sensitive to the usual adult dose.

945

Table 18 (*continued*)

Drug	Use	Dosage	Remarks*
		IM, IV, SC. *Anticholinergic:* **Adults,** 0.25–0.5 mg q 4–6 hr. *GI radiography:* **Adults,** 0.25–0.5 mg 5–10 min before procedure. *Antisialagogue:* **Adults,** 0.5 mg 30–60 min before anesthesia; **pediatric:** 0.005 mg/kg 30–60 min before surgery.	
Isopropamide iodide (Darbid) (Rx) Pregnancy category: C.	Adjunct in peptic ulcer therapy	**Tablets. Adults:** 5 mg q 12 hr up to 10 mg q 12 hr. Not for use in children under 12 years.	1. Synthetic quaternary ammonium compound. 2. **Duration:** 12 hr. 3. Sedatives and antacids can be given concomitantly. 4. Also found in Combid, Ornade, and Tuss-Ornade (see Chapter 50, p. 991 and p. 999). 5. The drug may interfere with thyroid function tests. Should be discontinued 1 wk before tests.
Mepenzolate bromide (Cantil) (Rx) Pregnancy category: C.	Adjunct in peptic ulcer therapy	**Tablets. Initial:** 25–50 mg q.i.d. before meals and at bedtime. Increase gradually to 50 mg q.i.d. until therapeutic response is attained or side effects appear.	1. Synthetic quaternary ammonium compound. 2. Safety and efficacy have not been established in children. *Additional Nursing Considerations:* Observe carefully for onset of therapeutic response and any side effects so maintenance dose may be determined.
Methscopolamine bromide (Pamine) (Rx) Pregnancy category: C.	Adjunct in peptic ulcer therapy	**Tablets. Adults:** 2.5 mg 1/2 hr before meals and 2.5–5 mg at bedtime. *Severe symptoms:* **Initial,** 5 mg q.i.d. 30 min before meals and at bedtime. **Pediatric:** 0.2 mg/kg daily in 4 divided doses before meals and at bedtime.	1. Quaternary ammonium derivative of belladonna. 2. **Onset:** 1 hr; **duration:** 4–6 hr. 3. Dose-related side effects may be relieved by decreasing dose for 5–7 days. 4. Geriatric patients may be more sensitive to the usual adult dose.

Drug	Uses	Dosage	Nursing Implications
Oxyphencyclimine HCl (Daricon) (Rx) Pregnancy category: C.	Adjunct in peptic ulcer therapy. Antispasmodic.	**Tablets. Adults,** 5–10 mg b.i.d.–t.i.d. (in the morning and at bedtime). Not recommended for children under 12 years.	1. Tertiary amine anticholinergic. 2. Can be given with antacids and sedatives. 3. High doses may cause CNS stimulation; use neostigmine to treat overdose. 4. **Onset:** 1–2 hr; **duration:** > 2 hr. 5. Geriatric patients may be more sensitive to the usual adult dose.
Oxyphenonium bromide (Antrenyl) (Rx) Pregnancy category: C.	Adjunct in peptic ulcer therapy	**PO. Adults:** 10 mg q.i.d. before meals and at bedtime for several days; **then,** adjust dosage according to response. Not for use in children.	1. Tertiary amine anticholinergic. 2. **Onset:** 30 min; **duration:** 6 hr; **t½:** 3.2 hr. 3. High incidence of side effects; treat overdosage with neostigmine.
Scopolamine hydrobromide (Hyoscine Hydrobromide) (Rx) Pregnancy category: C.	**PO:** Motion sickness. **Parenteral:** Preanesthetic sedation and antisialagogue, obstetrical amnesia, antiarrhythmic during anesthesia and surgery. Mydriatic and cycloplegic (See Table 19, p. 955)	**IM, IV, SC.** *Anticholinergic:* **Adults,** 0.3–0.6 mg as a single dose. **Pediatric:** 0.006 mg/kg as a single dose. *Antiemetic:* **Adults,** 0.3–0.6 mg as a single dose. **Pediatric:** 0.006 mg/kg as a single dose. *Antisialagogue, in anesthesia:* **Adults, IM,** 0.2–0.6 mg 30–60 min before induction of anesthesia. **Pediatric, IM, 8–12 years:** 0.3 mg; **3–8 years:** 0.2 mg; **7 months–3 years:** 0.15 mg; **4–7 months:** 0.1 mg. For children dose should be given 45–60 min before induction of anesthesia. Should not be used in infants less than 4 months of age. *Adjunct to anesthesia, sedation/hypnosis:* **Adults, IM, SC, IV,** 0.6 mg t.i.d.–q.i.d. *Adjunct to anesthesia, amnesia:* **Adults, IM, IV, SC,** 0.32–0.65 mg.	1. Produces amnesia when given with morphine or meperidine. 2. In the presence of pain, may produce delirium. 3. Also present in Donnagel, Donnagel PG, and Donnatal. 4. May cause disorientation, delirium, increased heart rate, decreased respiratory rate. 5. **Onset, PO:** 30–60 min; **parenteral:** 30 min. **Duration, PO:** 4–6 hr; **parenteral:** 4 hr. 6. If given parenterally before onset of labor, may cause CNS depression and hemorrhage in the infant. 7. May cause additive sedation with other CNS depressants. *Additional Nursing Implications:* 1. Assess a. for additional side effects. b. for tolerance after a long course of therapy. 2. Do not administer drug alone for pain, as it is likely to cause delirium. 3. Orient and reassure patient who experiences amnesia after receiving drug.

Table 18 (*Continued*)

Drug	Use	Dosage	Remarks*
Scopolamine trans-dermal therapeutic system (Transderm-Scop, Transderm-V✿) (Rx) Pregnancy category: C.	Prophylaxis of nausea and vomiting associated with motion sickness. Treatment of vertigo.	One system is applied to post-auricular skin several hours before effect needed. System should be replaced q 3 days if continuous therapy required. Apply system 4 hr before antiemetic effect is desired.	1. *Kinetics*: The system contains 1.5 mg scopolamine in a mineral oil/polyisobutylene matrix. The system will deliver a total of 0.5 mg scopolamine over 3 days. 2. Contraindicated in children and during lactation. 3. Drug may cause drowsiness, confusion, and disorientation. 4. Geriatric patients may be more sensitive to the usual adult dose.
Tridihexethyl (Pathilon) (Rx)	Adjunct in peptic ulcer therapy	**Tablets. Adults:** 25–50 mg t.i.d.–q.i.d. before meals and at bedtime. Usual bedtime dose is 50 mg. Adjust dosage as needed.	1. Synthetic quaternary ammonium compound. 2. Dosage not established in children. 3. Geriatric patients may be more sensitive to the usual adult dose.

*For General Nursing Considerations for these agents, see *Nursing Considerations* for *Parasympatholytics*, p. 949

NURSING CONSIDERATIONS

Administration/Storage

1. Check dosage and measure the drug exactly. Some drugs in this category are given in small amounts. As a consequence, overdosage is quickly achieved and can lead to toxicity.
2. Review the list of medications with which drugs in this category interact.

Assessment

1. Assess for a history of asthma, glaucoma, or duodenal ulcer, all of which contraindicate the use of these drugs.
2. Note client history of renal disease, cardiac problems or hepatic disease.
3. Determine the age of the client. Elderly clients, especially those with mental impairment or atherosclerosis, should not receive these drugs.

Interventions

1. If the client complains of a dry mouth, provide frequent mouth care and cold drinks, especially postoperatively. Sugarless hard candies and chewing gum may also be of some benefit.
2. Observe the client for evidence of drug interactions that may occur. A reduction in dosage of one of the medications may be necessary.

Client/Family Teaching

1. Explain that certain side effects are to be expected and describe these. Advise the client to report these to the physician, who may alleviate symptoms by reducing the dose of drug or by temporarily stopping the drug. Sometimes the client may be expected to tolerate certain side effects such as dry mouth or blurred vision because of the overall beneficial effects of drug therapy.
2. Stress the importance of maintaining the dietary regimen prescribed by the physician. Assist the client to understand and plan diet. Consult with the dietitian as necessary for instruction in meal planning.
3. Remind the client that antiparkinsonism drugs are not to be withdrawn abruptly. If the medication is changed, one drug should be withdrawn slowly and the other started in small doses.

ADDITIONAL NURSING CONSIDERATIONS RELATED TO PATHOLOGIC CONDITIONS FOR WHICH THE DRUG IS ADMINISTERED

Cardiovascular

Interventions

1. Assess the client for changes in pulse rate.
2. Note any client complaints of palpitations, document and report to the physician.

Ocular

Interventions

Note any client complaint of dizziness or blurred vision. Provide assistance with ambulation and institute safety measures.

Client/Family Teaching

1. Explain to the client and family how long vision will be affected by the medication and assist the client in planning activities for safety.
2. Explain that photophobia, which may occur, can be relieved by wearing dark glasses.
3. Advise client to report any marked changes in vision.

Gastrointestinal

Client/Family Teaching

1. Advise clients receiving medication for treatment of GI pathology to take the medication early enough before a meal (at least 20 min) so that the medication will be effective when needed.
2. Clients with GI pathology should be instructed on how to maintain the prescribed diet. Provide printed information related to the diet and refer to the dietitian as needed.
3. Instruct the client to continue taking the medication as ordered and to notify the physician of any adverse side effects.

Genitourinary

Interventions

1. Assess middle-aged male clients in particular for infrequent voiding. This is evidence of urinary retention and should be documented and reported to the physician.
2. If impotence occurs, it may be drug-related. The client should be encouraged to consult with the physician.

ATROPINE SULFATE   (AH-troh-peen)

Atropair, Atropine Sulfate S.O.P., Atropine-Care Ophthalmic, Atropisol Ophthalmic, Isopto Atropine Ophthalmic, I-Tropine, Minims Atropine✸, Ocu-Tropine, S.M.P. Atropine✸ (Rx)

See also *Cholinergic Blocking Agents,* p. 942.

Classification: Cholinergic blocking agent.

Action/Kinetics: Atropine blocks the action of acetylcholine on postganglionic cholinergic receptors in smooth muscle, cardiac muscle, exocrine glands, urinary bladder, and the AV and SA nodes in the heart. Ophthalmologically, atropine blocks the effect of acetylcholine on the sphincter muscle of the iris and the accommodative muscle of the ciliary body. This results in dilation of the pupil (mydriasis) and paralysis of the muscles required to accommodate for close vision (cycloplegia). This enables the physician to examine the inner structure of the eye, including the retina. It also permits examination of refractive errors of the lens without the patient automatically accommodating. **Peak effect:** *Mydriasis,* 30–40 min; *cycloplegia,* 1–3 hr. **Recovery:** Up to 12 days. **Duration, oral:** 4–6 hr. t½: 2.5 hr. Metabolized by the liver although 30–50% is excreted through the kidneys unchanged.

Uses: Oral: Adjunct in peptic ulcer treatment. Irritable bowel syndrome. Adjunct in treatment of spastic disorders of the biliary tract. Urologic disorders, urinary incontinence. During anesthesia to control salivation and bronchial secretions. Has been used for parkinsonism but more effective drugs are available.

   Parenteral: Antiarrhythmic, adjunct in GI radiography. Prophylaxis of arrhythymias induced by succinylcholine or surgical procedures. Reduce sinus bradycardia (severe) and syncope in hyperactive carotid sinus reflex. Prophylaxis and treatment of toxicity due to cholinesterase inhibitors, including organophosphate pesticides. Treatment of curariform block. As a preanesthetic or in dentistry to decrease secretions.

Ophthalmologic: Cycloplegic refraction, treatment of uveitis. *Investigational:* Treatment and prophylaxis of posterior synechiae; pre-and postoperative mydriasis; treatment of malignant glaucoma.

Additional Contraindications: Ophthalmic use: Infants less than 3 months of age.

Special Considerations: Pregnancy category: C. Use with caution in infants, children, geriatric patients, diabetes, hypo- or hyperthyroidism, narrow anterior chamber angle.

Additional Side Effects: *Ophthalmologic:* Blurred vision, stinging, increased intraocular pressure, contact dermatitis. Long-term use may cause irritation, photophobia, ecxzematoid dermatitis, conjunctivitis, hyperemia, or edema.

Dosage: Tablets, Soluble Tablets. *Anticholinergic or antispasmodic.* **Adults:** 0.3–1.2 mg q 4–6 hr. **Pediatric, over 41 kg:** same as adult; **29.5–41 kg:** 0.4 mg q 4–6 hr; **18–29.5 kg:** 0.3 mg q 4–6 hr; **11–18 kg:** 0.2 mg q 4–6 hr; **7–11 kg:** 0.15 mg q 4–6 hr; **3–7 kg:** 0.1 mg q 4–6 hr. *Prophylaxis of respiratory tract secretions and excess salivation during anesthesia:* **Adults,** 2 mg. *Parkinsonism:* **Adults:** 0.1–0.25 mg q.i.d.

IM, IV, SC. *Anticholinergic:* **Adults, IM, IV, SC,** 0.4–0.6 mg q 4–6 hr. **Pediatric, SC,** 0.01 mg/kg, not to exceed 0.4 mg (or 0.3 mg/m²). *Reverse curariform block:* **Adults, IV** 0.6–1.2 mg given at the same time or a few minutes before 0.5–2 mg neostigmine methylsulfate (use separate syringes). *Treatment of toxicity from cholinesterase inhibitors:* **Adults, IV, initial,** 2–4 mg; **then,** 2 mg repeated q 5–10 min until muscarinic symptoms disappear and signs of atropine toxicity begin to appear. **Pediatric, IM, IV, initial:** 1 mg; **then,** 0.5–1 mg q 5–10 min until muscarinic symptoms disappear and signs of atropine toxicity appear. *Treatment of mushroom poisoning due to muscarine:* **Adults, IM, IV,** 1–2 mg q hr until respiratory effects decrease. *Treatment of organophosphate poisoning:* **Adults, IM, IV, initial,** 1–2 mg; **then,** repeat in 20–30 min (as soon as cyanosis has disappeared). Dosage may be continued for up to 2 days until symptoms improve. *Arrhythmias:* **Pediatric, IV,** 0.01–0.03 mg/kg. *Prophylaxis of respiratory tract secretions, excessive salivation, succinylcholine- or surgical procedure-induced arrhythmias:* **Pediatric, SC: up to 3 kg,** 0.1 mg; **7–9 kg:** 0.2 mg; **12–16 kg:** 0.3 mg; **20–27 kg:** 0.4 mg; **32 kg:** 0.5 mg; **41 kg:** 0.6 mg.

NURSING CONSIDERATIONS

See also *Nursing Considerations* for *Cholinergic Blocking Agents,* p. 949.

Administration/Storage

For ophthalmologic use, atropine sulfate is available in 0.5–3% solutions or 1.0% ointment.

Assessment

Check for a history of angle-closure glaucoma, before administering the drug in the eye. Atropine may precipitate an acute crisis.

Client/Family Teaching

Warn the client that when atropine is used in the eye, vision will be temporarily impaired. Therefore, close work, operating machinery, or driving a car should be avoided until the effects of the medication have worn off.

DICYCLOMINE HYDROCHLORIDE   (dye-**SYE**-kloh-meen)

Antispas, A-Spas, Bentyl, Bentylol✿, Byclomine, Dibent, Di-Cyclonex, Dilomine, Di-Spaz, Formulex✿, Lomine✿, Neoquess, Or-Tyl, Protylol✿, Spasmoban✿, Spasmoject, Viscerol✿ (Rx)

See also *Cholinergic Blocking Agents,* p. 942.

Classification: Cholinergic blocking agent.

Action/Kinetics: t$^{1}/_{2}$, initial: 1.8 hr; **secondary:** 9–10 hr.

Uses: Hypermotility and spasms of GI tract associated with irritable colon and spastic colitis, mucous colitis.

Additional Contraindications: Use for peptic ulcer.

Special Concerns: Pregnancy category: C. Pediatric dosage of the injectable form has not been established. Use of capsules and tablets in children less than 6 years of age not recommended; use of the syrup in children less than 6 months of age not recommended.

Additional Side Effects: Brief euphoria, slight dizziness, feeling of abdominal distention. **Use of the syrup in infants less than 3 months of age:** Seizures, syncope, respiratory symptoms, fluctuations in pulse rate, asphyxia, muscular hypotonia, coma.

Dosage: Capsules, Syrup, Tablets. Adults: 10–20 mg t.i.d.–q.i.d.; **then,** may increase to total daily dose of 160 mg (only oral dose shown to be effective) if side effects do not limit this dosage. **Pediatric, 6 years and older, capsules or tablets:** 10 mg t.i.d.–q.i.d.; adjust dosage to need and incidence of side effects. **Pediatric, 6 months–2 years, syrup:** 5–10 mg t.i.d.–q.i.d.; **2 years and older:** 10 mg t.i.d.–q.i.d. The dose should be adjusted to need and incidence of side effects.

   IM. Adults: 20 mg q 4–6 hr. **Not for IV use.**

NURSING CONSIDERATIONS

See *Nursing Considerations* for *Cholinergic Blocking Agents,* p. 949.

Administration/Storage

Drug can be administered to clients with glaucoma.

GLYCOPYRROLATE   (glye-koh-**PIER**-roh-layt)

Robinul, Robinul Forte (Rx)

See also *Cholinergic Blocking Agents,* p. 942.

Classification: Cholinergic blocking agent.

Action/Kinetics: Onset: PO, 1 hr; **IV,** 1 min; **IM, SC:** 15–30 min. **Duration: decrease salivation,** Up to 7 hr; **block vagal activity:** 2–3 hr. **t$^{1}/_{2}$:** 0.6–4.6 hr.

Uses: PO. Adjunct in treatment of peptic ulcer. Antidiarrheal. **IM, IV.** To reduce salivation, tracheobronchial and pharyngeal secretions during surgery. To decrease acidity and volume of gastric secretions; to block cardiac vagal inhibitory reflexes during induction of anesthesia and intubation. Prophylaxis of aspiration of gastric contents during anesthesia. Adjunct with neostigmine or pyridostigmine to reverse neuromuscular blockade due to nondepolarizing muscle relaxants.

Additional Contraindication: Peptic ulcer in children under 12 years of age.

Special Concerns: Pregnancy category: B. Dosage has not been determined for the injection in children with peptic ulcer.

Laboratory Test Interferences: ↓ Serum uric acid in patients with gout or hyperuricemia.

Dosage: Tablets. *Peptic ulcer:* **Adults, initial** 1–2 mg t.i.d. or 2 mg b.i.d.–t.i.d. (may also give 2 mg at bedtime); **maintenance:** 1 mg b.i.d. with dose adjusted as needed up to a maximum of 8 mg.
  IM, IV. *Peptic ulcer:* **Adults, IM, IV,** 0.1–0.2 mg t.i.d.–q.i.d. *Prophylaxis of excessive salivation, respiratory tract secretions, gastric hypersecretion during anesthesia:* **Adults, IM,:** 0.0044 mg/kg 30–60 min prior to anesthesia or at the time the preanesthetic sedative and/or narcotic are given; **pediatric, less than 12 years:** 0.0044–0.0088 mg/kg 30–60 min before anesthetic or at the time preanesthetic medication is given. *Prophylaxis of arrhythmias during anesthesia and surgery:* **Adults, IV,** 0.1 mg repeated, as needed, q 2–3 min; **pediatric, IV,** 0.0044 mg/kg not to exceed 0.1 mg per dose, repeated, as needed, q 2–3 min. *Reversal of neuromuscular blockade.* **IV: Adults and children:** 0.2 mg for each 1 mg neostigmine or 5 mg pyridostigmine. Give IV at the same time and in the same syringe.

NURSING CONSIDERATIONS

See *Nursing Considerations* for *Cholinergic Blocking Agents,* p. 949.

Administration/Storage

1. Do not add to IV solution containing sodium chloride or bicarbonate.
2. Parenteral use may slow stomach emptying and cause pain at the injection site.

Assessment

Note the age of the client. Elderly clients are more sensitive to the side effects of drug therapy than younger clients.

METHANTHELINE BROMIDE   (meth-**ANTH**-eh-leen)

Banthine (Rx)

See also *Cholinergic Blocking Agents,* p. 942.

Classification: Synthetic anticholinergic, antispasmodic (quaternary ammonium compound).

Action/Kinetics: PO: Onset, 30 min; **duration:** 6 hr. **IM: Duration,** 2–4 hr. Drug has some ganglionic blocking activity.

Uses: Adjunct in peptic ulcer therapy. Urinary incontinence.

Special Concerns: Pregnancy category: C.

Additional Side Effects: Postural hypotension, impotence. Respiratory paralysis and tachycardia (overdosage).

Dosage: Tablets. Adults: 50–100 mg q.i.d. **Pediatric, over 1 year:** 12.5–50 mg q.i.d. **Infants, 1–12 months:** 12.5 up to 25 mg q.i.d. **Newborns:** 12.5 mg b.i.d.; **then,** 12.5 mg t.i.d.

NURSING CONSIDERATIONS

See also *Nursing Considerations* for *Cholinergic Blocking Agents,* p. 949.

Interventions

1. Initiate therapy for clients with duodenal ulcer while the client is on a liquid diet.

2. If the client is taking potassium chloride, anticholinergic agents may delay absorption of the potassium. Special attention should be given to client complaints that could indicate lesions in the GI mucosa. These should be reported to the physician.

3. Auscultate for bowel sounds and assess the client for abdominal distention, epigastric distress, and vomiting. The drug reduces gastric motility.

Client/Family Teaching

1. Advise clients to rise slowly from a supine position to prevent hypotension.
2. Remind male clients that drug-induced impotence may occur. This should be reported to the physician.

PROPANTHELINE BROMIDE   (proh-**PANTH**-eh-leen)

Norpanth, Pro-Banthine, Propanthel ✸ (Rx)

See also *Cholinergic Blocking Agents,* p. 942.

Classification: Anticholinergic, antispasmodic (quaternary ammonium compound).

Action/Kinetics: Duration: 6 hr. Metabolized in the liver and excreted through the urine.

Uses: Adjunct in peptic ulcer therapy. Spastic and inflammatory disease of GI and urinary tracts. Control of salivation and enuresis. Duodenography. Urinary incontinence.

Special Concerns: Pregnancy category: C. Safety and effectiveness for use in children with peptic ulcer have not been established.

Dosage: Tablets. Adults: 15 mg 30 min before meals and 30 mg at bedtime. Reduce dose to 7.5 mg t.i.d. for mild symptoms, geriatric patients, or patients of small stature. **Pediatric:** 0.375 mg/kg (10 mg/m²) q.i.d. with dose being adjusted as needed.

NURSING CONSIDERATIONS

See also *Nursing Considerations* for *Cholinergic Blocking Agents,* p. 949.

Interventions

A liquid diet is recommended during initiation of therapy in clients with edematous duodenal ulcer.

MYDRIATICS AND CYCLOPLEGICS

Action/Kinetics: These agents block the effect of acetylcholine on the sphincter muscle of the iris and the accommodative muscle of the ciliary body. This results in dilation of the pupil (mydriasis) and paralysis of the muscles required to accommodate for close vision (cycloplegia). This enables the physician to examine the inner structure of the eye, including the retina. It also permits examination of refractive errors of the lens without the patient automatically accommodating.

Uses: Diagnostic ophthalmoscopic examination, refraction in children, dilation of pupil in inflammation of the iris and uveal tract.

Contraindications: Glaucoma, infants less than three months of age.

Special Concerns: Use during pregnancy and during lactation only if the benefits clearly outweigh the risks. Use with caution in infants, children, geriatric patients, diabetes, hypo- or hyperthyroidism, narrow anterior chamber angle.

Side Effects: *Ophthalmologic:* Blurred vision, stinging, increased intraocular pressure. Long-term use may cause irritation, photophobia, conjunctivitis, hyperemia, edema, vascular congestion, and eczematoid dermatitis. For systemic side effects, see *Side Effects* for *Parasympatholytics,* p. 943.

Dosage: See individual agents, Table 19.

Table 19   Mydriatics and Cycloplegics

Drug	Dosage	Remarks
Atropine sulfate (Atropair, Atropine Sulfate Ophthalmic, Atropine Sulfate S.O.P., Atropine-Care Ophthalmic, Atropisol Ophthalmic, Isopto Atropine, I-Tropine, Minims Atropine✿, Ocu-Tropine, S.M.P. Atropine✿) (Rx) Pregnancy category: C.	*Refraction,* **adults and children:** 1 gtt in eyes b.i.d. for 1–3 days before examination using the following concentrations: **Ointment: Children, up to 2 years:** 0.5% for blue irides and 1% for dark irides; **Over 2 years:** 1%. **Solution: Infants up to 1 year:** 0.125%; **1–5 years:** 0.25%; **5 years or over:** 0.25% for blue irides and 0.5 or 1% for dark irides. *Uveitis or postoperative mydriasis:* **Pediatric:** 0.3–0.5 cm of 0.5% or 1% ointment 1–3 times daily or 1 gtt of 0.1–1% solution 1–2 times daily.	1. **Peak effect:** *Mydriasis,* 30–40 min; *cycloplegia,* 1–3 hr. **Recovery:** Up to 12 days. 2. Drug particularly prone to have systemic effects such as contact dermatitis, allergic conjunctivitis. 3. Strengths of 0.125% and 0.25% must be compounded as they are not available commercially. Available in 0.5%, 1%, 2%, and 3% solutions and 0.5% and 1% ointments. 4. Infants, young children, children with blond hair, blue eyes, Down's syndrome or brain damage are particularly susceptible to atropine.
Cylcopentolate HCl (AK-Pentolate, Cyclogyl, I-Pentolate, Minims Pentolate✿, Ocu-Pentolate, Pentolair, Spectro-Pentolate) (Rx)	*Mydriasis and cyclopegia:* **Adults,** 1 gtt of 0.5–2% solution followed in 5–10 min by a second drop. **Children:** 1 gtt of 0.5%, 1%, or 2% solution followed in 5 min by a second drop of 0.5% or 1% solution. **Infants:** 1 gtt of 0.5% solution in each eye. *Uveitis:* **Adults and children:** 1 gtt of 0.5% or 1% solution t.i.d.–q.i.d.	1. **Peak effect,** *mydriasis:* 30–60 min; *cycloplegia:* 25–75 min. **Recovery,** *mydriasis:* 24 hr; *cylcoplegia,* 6–24 hr. 2. In adults, recovery time can be reduced by instilling 1–2 gtt of 1% or 2% pilocarpine. 3. To reduce absorption in children, pressure should be applied over the nasolacrimal sac for 2–3 min. 4. Larger doses may be needed for patients with heavily pigmented irides. 5. Concentrations above 0.5% are not to be used in small infants. Infants should be observed closely for 30 min for toxic side effects.

Table 19   *(Continued)*

Drug	Dosage	Remarks
Homatropine HBr (AK-Homatropine, Homatrine, I-Homatropine, Isopto Homatropine, Minims Homatropine✤) (Rx) Pregnancy category: C.	*Refraction:* **Adults,** 1 gtt of the 2% or 5% solution; may be repeated q 5–10 min for 2–3 doses just before refraction. **Pediatric:** 1 gtt of a 1% or 2% solution q 10 min for 2–3 doses just before refraction. *Uveitis:* **Adults,** 1 gtt of a 2% or 5% solution b.i.d.–t.i.d. (Doses up to q 3–4 hr may be needed). **Pediatric:** 1 gtt of 1% or 2% solution b.i.d.–t.i.d.	1. **Peak effect,** *mydriasis:* 40–60 min; *cycloplegia:* 30–60 min. **Recovery,** *mydriasis or cycloplegia:* 1–3 days. 2. Larger doses may be needed for patients with heavily pigmented irides. 3. Available as a 2% or 5% solution. 4. See also *Atropine Sulfate,* under *Remarks*.
Scopolamine HBr (Isopto Hyoscine Ophthalmic) (Rx)	**Solution.** *Refraction:* **Adults,** 1 gtt of the 0.25% solution 1 hr before refraction. **Pediatric:** 1 gtt of the 0.25% solution b.i.d. for 2 days before refraction. *Uveitis:* **Adults,** 1 gtt of solution 1–3 times daily; **Pediatric:** 1 gtt of solution 1–3 times daily. *Posterior synechiae:* **Adults, children,** 1 gtt of solution q min for 5 min. *Postoperative mydriasis:* **Adults,** 1 gtt of solution once daily. *Postoperative or preoperative iridocyclitis:* **Adults and children,** 1 gtt of solution 1–4 times daily to maintain mydriasis; decrease dose as inflammation decreases.	**Peak effects** *mydriasis:* 20–30 min; *cycloplegia:* 30–60 min. **Recovery,** *mydriasis or cycloplegia:* 3–7 days.
Tropicamide (I-Picamide, Minims Tropicamide✤, Mydriacyl, Mydriafair, Ocu-Tropic, Spectro-Cyl, Tropicacyl) (Rx)	*Refraction:* **Adults,** 1 gtt of the 1% solution repeated in 5 min. An additional drop should be instilled if the patient is not seen within 20–30 min. **Pediatric:** 1 gtt of the 0.5% or 1% solution repeated once after 5 min. *Examination of fundus of eye:* **Adults and children:** 1 gtt of the 0.5% or 1% solution repeated once after 5 min.	**Peak effect** *mydriasis:* 20–40 min; *cycloplegia:* 20–35 min; **Recovery,** *mydriasis and cycloplegia:* 6 hr. Also used pre- or postoperatively if a short-acting mydriatic is needed.

NURSING CONSIDERATIONS

Administration/Storage

Drops are instilled in the conjunctival sac.

Assessment

Check the client's history, before administration, to determine if they have angle-closure glaucoma. The drug could precipitate an acute crisis in these clients.

Interventions

1. Apply finger pressure to the lacrimal sac during and for several minutes following instillation. This to prevent systemic absorption and associated effects from drug therapy.
2. These drugs will temporarily impair vision. The client should be advised not to perform close work, operate machinery, or drive a car when the eyes are dilated. Activities may be resumed once the drug effects have worn off.

CHAPTER FORTY-EIGHT

Neuromuscular Blocking Agents

48

General Statement: The drugs considered in this section interfere with nerve impulse transmission between the motor end plate and the receptors of skeletal muscle (i.e., peripheral action). Upon stimulation, these muscles normally contract when acetylcholine is released from storage sites embedded in the motor end plate.

The drugs fall into two groups: competitive (nondepolarizing) agents and depolarizing agents. Competitive agents—atracurium, gallamine, metocurine, pancuronium, tubocurarine, vecuronium—compete with acetylcholine for the receptor site in the muscle cells. These agents are also called *curariform* because their mode of action is similar to that of the poison curare. The depolarizing agent—succinylcholine—initially excites skeletal muscle and then prevents the muscle from contracting by prolonging the time during which the receptors at the end plate cannot respond to acetylcholine (depolarization during refractory time).

The muscle paralysis caused by the neuromuscular blocking agents is sequential. Therapeutic doses produce muscle depression in the following order: heaviness of eyelids, difficulty in swallowing and talking, diplopia, progressive weakening of the extremities and neck, followed by relaxation of the trunk and spine. The diaphragm (respiratory paralysis) is affected last. The drugs do not affect consciousness, and their use, in the absence of adequate levels of general anesthesia, may be frightening to the patient.

There is a narrow margin of safety between a therapeutically effective dose causing muscle relaxation and a toxic dose causing respiratory paralysis. **The neuromuscular blocking agents are always administered by a physician.** However, the nurse must be prepared to maintain and monitor a patient's respiration until the effect of the drug subsides.

Uses: See individual agents.

Special Concerns: The neuromuscular blocking agents should be used with caution in patients with myasthenia gravis; renal, hepatic, or pulmonary impairment; respiratory depression; and in elderly or debilitated patients.

Depolarizing agents should be used with caution for patients with electrolyte imbalance, especially hyperkalemia, and in patients on digitalis.

Side Effects: Respiratory paralysis. Severe and prolonged muscle relaxation. Some neuromuscular blocking agents cause hypotension, bronchospasms, cardiac disturbances, hyperthermia. See also individual agents.

Drug Interactions: The following drug interactions are for nondepolarizing skeletal muscle relaxants. For succinylcholine, see p. 965.

Drug Interactions	
Aminoglycoside antibiotics	Additive muscle relaxation
Amphotericin B	↑ Muscle relaxation
Anesthetics, inhalation	Additive muscle relaxation
Clindamycin	Additive muscle relaxation
Colistin	↑ Muscle relaxation
Furosemide	Furosemide ↑ effect of skeletal muscle relaxants
Lincomycin	↑ Muscle relaxation
Magnesium salts	↑ Muscle relaxation
Methotrimeprazine	↑ Muscle relaxation
Narcotic analgesics	↑ Respiratory depression and ↑ muscle relaxation
Phenothiazines	↑ Muscle relaxation
Polymyxin B	↑ Muscle relaxation
Procainamide	↑ Muscle relaxation
Procaine	↑ Muscle relaxation by ↓ plasma protein binding
Quinidine	↑ Muscle relaxation
Thiazide diuretics	↑ Muscle relaxation due to hypokalemia

NURSING CONSIDERATIONS

Administration

1. When the drug is to be administered by a constant infusion, use a microdrip tubing administration set and an infusion control device.
2. During drug administration, have a suction machine, oxygen, and resuscitation equipment immediately available for emergency use.
3. Have anticholinesterase drugs, such as neostigmine, available to counteract respiratory depression should it occur. Neostigmine increases the body's production of acetylcholine.
4. The antidote for depolarizing drugs in this class, is oxygen under pressure, followed by whole blood or plasma if apnea is prolonged.
5. Use a peripheral nerve stimulator to monitor the client's response to the neuromuscular blocking medication.

Assessment

1. If the client has any history of renal disease, obtain renal function studies prior to beginning therapy.
2. Note age and condition of the client. Elderly and debilitated clients should not receive drugs in this category.
3. Note all other drugs the client is receiving. Often clients requiring neuromuscular blocking agents are also receiving other drugs which may have the effect of prolonging client response to the neuromuscular blocking agent being used.

Interventions

1. Drugs should be administered in a closely monitored environment.
2. Monitor the client's blood pressure, pulse, respirations and pulmonary status at frequent intervals. Report any signs of respiratory distress, such as apnea.
3. Observe for excessive bronchial secretions or respiratory wheezing. If evident, report these immediately to the physician.
4. Question the client concerning changes in vision, ability to chew or to move the fingers and document findings.
5. Observe the client closely for drug interactions. These can potentiate muscular relaxation and prove fatal. If interactions occur, consult the physician immediately to obtain orders for the appropriate medication to counteract the observed effects.
6. Most clients can still hear, feel and see while they are receiving blocking agents. Therefore, inappropriate talking should be avoided.

ATRACURIUM BESYLATE   (ah-trah-**KYOU**-ree-um)

Tracrium Injection (Rx)

See also *Neuromuscular Blocking Agents,* p. 957.

Classification: Nondepolarizing skeletal muscle relaxant.

Action/Kinetics: Atracurium prevents the action of acetylcholine by competing for the cholinergic receptor at the neuromuscular junction. It may also release histamine, leading to hypotension. **Onset:** Within 2 min. **Peak effect:** 1–2 min. **Duration:** 20–40 min with balanced anesthesia. Recovery occurs more quickly than with other nondepolarizing agents (e.g., *d*-tubocurarine). **t½:** 20 min. Drug is metabolized in the plasma.

Uses: Skeletal muscle relaxant during surgery; adjunct to general anesthesia; assist in endotracheal intubation. *Investigational:* Treat seizures due to drugs or electrically induced.

Contraindications: In patients with myasthenia gravis, Eaton-Lambert syndrome, electrolyte disorders, bronchial asthma.

Special Concerns: Use with caution in pregnancy (category: C) and during labor and delivery. Safety and efficacy have not been determined during lactation. Children up to 1 month of age may be more sensitive to the effects of atracurium.

Additional Side Effects: *CV:* Bradycardia. Other untoward reactions may be due to histamine release and include flushing, erythema, wheezing, urticaria, bronchial secretions, blood pressure and heart rate changes.

Additional Drug Interactions

Enflurane	↑ Muscle relaxation
Halothane	↑ Muscle relaxation
Isoflurane	↑ Muscle relaxation
Lithium	↑ Muscle relaxation
Phenytoin	↓ Effect of atracurium
Succinylcholine	↑ Onset and depth of muscle relaxation
Theophylline	↓ Effect of atracurium
Trimethaphan	↑ Muscle relaxation
Verapamil	↑ Muscle relaxation

Dosage: IV only. Adults and children over 2 years, initial: 0.4–0.5 mg/kg as IV bolus; **maintenance:** 0.08–0.1 mg/kg. *Following use of succinylcholine for intubation under balanced anesthesia:* **initial,** 0.3–0.4 mg/kg; if using potent inhalation anesthetics, further reductions may be required. *Use in cardiovascular disease or patients with history of asthma or anaphylaxis:* **initial,** 0.3–0.4 mg/kg, given slowly over 1 min. *Use after steady-state enflurane or isoflurane anesthesia established:* 0.25–0.35/kg (about ⅓ less than the usual initial dose). *Use in infants 1 month to 2 years of age under halothane anesthesia:* 0.3–0.4 mg/kg.

Supplemental use: **IV,** 0.08–0.1 mg/kg 20–45 min after the initial dose; then q 15–25 min or as needed. *IV Infusion, balanced anesthesia:* **IV infusion,** 0.009–0.01 mg/kg until the level of neuromuscular blockade is re-established; **then,** rate of infusion is adjusted according to patient needs (usually 0.005–0.009 mg/kg/min although some patients may require as little as 0.002 mg/kg/min and others as much as 0.015 mg/kg/min). *For cardiopulmonary bypass surgery in which hypothermia is induced:* **IV infusion,** Reduce rate of infusion by 50%.

NURSING CONSIDERATIONS

See also *Nursing Considerations* for *Neuromuscular Blocking Agents,* p. 959.

Administration/Storage

1. Initial dosage should be reduced to 0.25–0.35 mg/kg if drug is being used with steady-state enflurane or isoflurane (smaller reductions if halothane is being used).
2. Dosage should be reduced in clients with myasthenia gravis or other neuromuscular diseases, electrolyte disorders, or carcinomatosis.

3. Atracurium should not be mixed with alkaline solutions.
4. Maintenance doses can be given by continuous infusion of a diluted solution to clients 2 years of age to adulthood.
5. Solutions for infusion should be used within 24 hr.
6. To preserve potency, the drug should be refrigerated at 2°–8° C (36°–46°F).
7. IM administration may cause tissue irritation.
8. IV atropine may be used to treat bradycardia due to atracurium.

GALLAMINE TRIETHIODIDE (GAL-ah-meen)

Flaxedil (Rx)

See also *Neuromuscular blocking Agents,* p. 957.

Classification: Nondepolarizing neuromuscular blocking agent.

Action/Kinetics: Similar to tubocurarine. Does not release histamine or produce bronchospasms. Has no effect on GI tract or autonomic ganglia although it does manifest vagolytic activity. Effects can be antagonized by anticholinesterase agents. In usual doses, the duration is shorter than that for tubocurarine. **Onset, IV:** 1–2 min. **Time to peak effect:** 3–5 min. **Duration:** 15–30 min after a single dose (duration increased with repeated dosing). Excreted unchanged by kidney.

Uses: Muscle relaxant during surgery; adjunct to manage patients requiring mechanical ventilation. *Investigational:* Treat seizures electrically induced or induced by drugs.

Additional Contraindications: Myasthenia gravis. Cardiac disease, especially for patients in whom tachycardia may be dangerous. Also in presence of hypertension, hyperthyroidism, impaired renal function or respiratory depression, and hypersensitivity to iodine.

Special Concerns: Use with caution during pregnancy. Use with caution in patients weighing less than 5 kg. Children up to 1 month of age may be more sensitive to the effects of atracurium.

Additional Side Effects: Anaphylaxis.

Drug Interactions

Aminoglycosides	↑ Effect of gallamine
Azathioprine	↓ Or reverse the effect of gallamine
Methoxyflurane	↑ Effect of gallamine
Polymyxins	↑ Effect of gallamine

Dosage: IV. Adults and children: *After general anesthesia has been introduced: highly individualized.* **Initial,** 1 mg/kg body weight up to maximum of 100 mg; an additional dose of 0.5–1 mg/kg body weight may be given at 30–40 min intervals.

NURSING CONSIDERATIONS

See also *Nursing Considerations* for *Neuromuscular Blocking Agents,* p. 959.

Administration/Storage

1. Dose should be reduced if used with cyclopropane, ether, halothane, or methoxyflurane.
2. A precipitate will form if gallamine is mixed with anesthetic agents.
3. Gallamine can be used with preanesthetic medications (e.g., atropine) and anesthetic agents.

4. A dose of 1 mg/kg produces a 50% decrease in respiratory minute volume. A dose of 1.5 mg/kg produces a 75 % decrease in respiratory minute volume.

5. Anticipate the peak effect to occur in 3 minutes and to last approximately 15–20 minutes.

Assessment

1. Obtain baseline electrolyte levels before administering a neuroblocking agent.

2. Obtain liver and renal function studies prior to initiating therapy.

Interventions

Administer only in a closely monitored environment. Assess vital signs and intake and output and report any abnormal findings.

METOCURINE IODIDE   (met-oh-**KYOU**-reen)

Metubine Iodide Injection (Rx)

See also *Neuromuscular Blocking Agents,* p. 957.

Classification: Nondepolarizing neuromuscular blocking agent.

Action/Kinetics: Metocurine is two times as potent as tubocurarine and does not cause ganglionic blockade. Histamine may be released. Effects are cumulative. The effects may be reversed by anticholinesterase agent. **Onset:** few minutes; maximal effects persist for 35–60 min; **Duration:** 25–90 min. **t½:** 3.6 hr. About 50% excreted unchanged in urine.

Uses: Muscle relaxation during surgery; to decrease muscle contractions during seizures; as adjunct in patients requiring mechanical ventilation; adjunct in electroshock therapy.

Contraindications: Patients sensitive to iodide.

Special Concerns: Pregnancy category: C. Dosage has not been established in children. Children up to 1 month of age may be more sensitive to the effects of atracurium.

Additional Side Effects: Allergic reactions to drug or iodine. *Symptoms due to histamine release: CV:* Hypotension, erythema, tachycardia, flushing, circulatory collapse. *Other:* Edema, bronchospasm, skin rash.

Additional Drug Interactions: Succinylcholine chloride ↑ relaxant effect of both drugs.

Dosage: IV only. Adults, initial: 0.15–0.4 mg/kg given over 30–60 seconds; **then,** supplemental doses of 0.5–1 mg (total dose) may be given q 30–90 min as needed. *When used with enflurane or isoflurane anesthesia:* Reduce dose by 33%–50%. (The dose may also need to be reduced during halothane anesthesia.) *During electroshock therapy:* 2–3 mg (range: 1.75–5.5 mg).

NURSING CONSIDERATIONS

See also *Nursing Considerations* for *Neuromuscular Blocking Agents,* p. 959.

Administration/Storage

1. For use in electroshock therapy, give IV slowly until head-drop occurs. Subsequent injections should be given within 15–50 sec.

2. Metocurine is incompatible with alkaline solutions.

3. IM use is not recommended.

4. Have neostigmine methylsulfate on hand during IV administration to combat respiratory depression.

Interventions

Monitor the client's blood pressure. If the client has a fall in blood pressure associated with respiratory depression, do not give neostigmine, as it may aggravate shock.

PANCURONIUM BROMIDE (pan-kyou-**ROH**-nee-um)

Pavulon (Rx)

See also *Neuromuscular Blocking Agents,* p. 959.

Classification: Nondepolarizing neuromuscular blocking agent.

Action/Kinetics: Effects similar to *d*-tubocurarine although pancuronium is 5 times as potent. Drug effects can be reversed by anticholinesterase agents. Pancuronium possesses vagolytic activity although it is not likely to cause histamine release. **Onset:** Within 45 sec. **Time to peak effect:** 3–4.5 min (depending on the dose). **Duration:** 35–45 min (increased with multiple doses). **t½, elimination:** 114–116 min. Ninety percent of the total dose is excreted through the urine either unchanged or as metabolites; 10% is excreted through the bile. In patients with renal failure, the t½ is doubled. Significantly bound to plasma protein.

Uses: Muscle relaxation during anesthesia, endotracheal intubation, management of patients undergoing mechanical ventilation.

Special Concerns: Pregnancy category: C. Children up to 1 month of age may be more sensitive to the effects of atracurium.

Additional Side Effects: *Respiratory:* Apnea, respiratory insufficiency. *CV:* Increased heart rate and increased mean arterial pressure. *Miscellaneous:* Salivation, skin rashes, hypersensitivity reactions (e.g., bronchospasm, flushing, hypotension, redness, tachycardia).

Additional Drug Interactions	
Azathioprine	Reverses effects of pancuronium
Bacitracin	Additive muscle relaxation
Enflurane	↑ Muscle relaxation
Isoflurane	↑ Muscle relaxation
Quinine	↑ Effect of pancuronium
Succinylcholine	↑ Intensity and duration of action of pancuronium
Tetracyclines	Additive muscle relaxation
Theophyllines	↓ Effects of pancuronium; also, possible cardiac arrhythmias

Dosage: IV only. Adults and children over 1 month of age, initial: 0.04–0.1 mg/kg. Additional doses of 0.01 mg/kg may be administered as required (usually q 20–60 min). **Neonates:** A test dose of 0.02 mg/kg should be administered first to determine responsiveness. *Endotracheal intubation:* 0.06–0.1 mg/kg as a bolus dose. *When used with enflurane or isoflurane anesthesia and/or after succinylcholine-assisted endotracheal intubation:* 0.05 mg/kg initially; **then,** adjust to patient response.

NURSING CONSIDERATIONS

See also *Nursing Considerations* for *Neuromuscular Blocking Agents*, p. 959.

Administration/Storage

1. Additional doses of pancuronium significantly increase the duration of skeletal muscle relaxation.
2. The drug may be mixed with 5% dextrose, 5% dextrose and sodium chloride, lactated Ringer's injection, and 0.9% sodium chloride injection. When mixed with any of these solutions, the drug is stable for 2 days.
3. Anticipate the medication will act within 3 minutes upon administration and last 35–45 minutes.
4. Administer IV drug in a continuously monitored environment.

Interventions

1. Provide ventilatory support.
2. Monitor and record vital signs, input and output.
3. Position the client for comfort and so that the body is in proper alignment. Turn the client and perform mouth care and eye care frequently.
4. Assess the client's airway at frequent intervals. Have a suction machine at the bedside.
5. Check to be certain that the ventilator alarms are set and on at all times.

SUCCINYLCHOLINE CHLORIDE   (suk-sin-ill-**KOH**-leen)

Anectine, Anectine Flo-Pack, Quelicin, Succinylcholine Chloride Min-I-Mix, Sucostrin High Potency (Rx)

See also *Neuromuscular Blocking Agents*, p. 957.

Classification: Depolarizing neuromuscular blocking agent.

Action/Kinetics: Succinylcholine initially excites skeletal muscle by combining with cholinergic receptors preferentially to acetylcholine. Subsequently, it prevents the muscle from contracting by prolonging the time during which the receptors at the neuromuscular junction cannot respond to acetylcholine. Short-acting. It has no effect on pain threshold, cerebration, or consciousness; thus, it should be used with sufficient anesthesia. Effects are not blocked by anticholinesterase drugs and may even be enhanced by them. **IV: onset,** 1 min; **duration:** 4–6 min; **recovery:** 8–10 min. **IM: Onset,** 3 min; **duration:** 10–30 min. Metabolized by plasma pseudocholinesterase to succinyl-monocholine, which is a nondepolarizing muscle relaxant. About 10% succinylcholine is excreted unchanged in the urine.

Uses: Muscle relaxant during surgery, endotracheal intubation, endoscopy and short manipulative procedures. *Investigational:* Reduce intensity of electrically induced seizures or seizures due to drugs.

Special Concerns: Safe use during pregnancy (pregnancy category: C) not established. Use with caution during lactation. Pediatric patients may be especially prone to myoglobinemia, myoglobinuria, and cardiac effects. Use of IV infusion is not recommended in children due to the risk of malignant hyperpyrexia. Use with caution in patients with severe liver disease, severe anemia, malnutrition, impaired cholinesterase activity, genetic disorders of plasma pseudocholinesterase, myopathies associated with increased creatine phosphokinase, acute narrow-angle glaucoma, history of malignant hyperthermia, penetrating eye injuries, fractures. Also, in cardiovascular, pulmonary, renal, or metabolic diseases.

Side Effects: *Skeletal muscle:* May cause severe, persistent respiratory depression or apnea. Muscle fasciculations, postoperative muscle pain. *CV:* Bradycardia or tachycardia, blood pressure changes, arrhythmias, cardiac arrest. *Respiratory:* Apnea, respiratory depression. *Other:* Fever, malignant hyperthermia, salivation, hyperkalemia, postoperative muscle pain, anaphylaxis, myoglobinemia, myoglobinuria, skin rashes, increased intraocular pressure. Repeated doses may cause tachyphylaxis.

Drug Interactions	
Aminoglycoside antibiotics	Additive skeletal muscle blockade
Amphotericin B	↑ Effect of succinylcholine
Antibiotics, nonpenicillin	Additive skeletal muscle blockade
Anticholinesterases	Additive skeletal muscle blockade
Beta-adrenergic blocking agents	Additive skeletal muscle blockade
Chloroquine	Additive skeletal muscle blockade
Clindamycin	Additive skeletal muscle blockade
Cyclophosphamide	↑ Effect of succinylcholine by ↓ breakdown of drug in plasma by pseudocholinesterase
Diazepam	↓ Effect of succinylcholine
Digitalis glycosides	↑ Chance of cardiac arrhythmias
Echothiophate iodide	↑ Effect of succinylcholine by ↓ breakdown of drug in plasma by pseudocholinesterase
Furosemide	↑ Action of succinylcholine
Isoflurane	Additive skeletal muscle blockade
Lidocaine	Additive skeletal muscle blockade
Lincomycin	Additive skeletal muscle blockade
Lithium	↑ Effect of succinylcholine
Magnesium salts	Additive skeletal muscle blockade
Narcotics	↑ Risk of bradycardia and sinus arrest
Oxytocin	↑ Effect of succinylcholine
Phenelzine	↑ Effect of succinylcholine
Phenothiazines	↑ Effect of succinylcholine
Polymyxin	Additive skeletal muscle blockade
Procainamide	↑ Effect of succinylcholine
Procaine	↑ Effect of succinylcholine by inhibiting plasma pseudocholinesterase activity
Promazine	↑ Effect of succinylcholine
Quinidine	Additive skeletal muscle blockade
Quinine	Additive skeletal muscle blockade
Thiotepa	↑ Effect of succinylcholine by ↓ breakdown of drug in plasma by pseudocholinesterase
Trimethophan	↑ Effect of succinylcholine by inhibiting plasma pseudocholinesterase activity

Dosage: IM, IV. *Short or prolonged surgical procedures:* **Adults, IV: initially,** 0.3–1.1 mg/kg; **then,** repeated doses can be given based on patient response. **Adults, IM:** 3–4 mg/kg not to exceed a total dose of 150 mg. *Prolonged surgical procedures, IV infusion (preferred),* 0.1%–0.2% solution in 5% dextrose, sodium chloride injection, or other diluent given at a rate of 0.5–10 mg/min depending on patient response and degree of relaxation desired, for up to 1 hr.

Electroshock therapy: **Adults, IV:** 10–30 mg given 1 min prior to the shock (individualize dosage). **IM:** Up to 2.5 mg/kg, not to exceed a total dose of 150 mg. *Endotracheal intubation:* **Pediatric, IV:** 1–2 mg/kg; if necessary, dose can be repeated. **IM:** Up to 2.5 mg/kg, not to exceed a total dose of 150 mg.

NURSING CONSIDERATIONS

See also *Nursing Considerations* for *Neuromuscular Blocking Agents,* p. 959.

Administration/Storage

1. An initial test dose of 0.1 mg/kg should be given to assess sensitivity and recovery time.
2. Review the drugs with which succinylcholine interacts.
3. Do not mix with anesthetic.
4. For IV infusion, use 1 or 2 mg/mL solution of drug in 5% dextrose injection, 0.9% sodium chloride, or other suitable IV solution. Succinylcholine is not compatible with alkaline solutions.
5. Alter the degree of relaxation by altering the rate of flow.
6. To reduce salivation, premedication with atropine or scopolamine is recommended.
7. A low dose of a nondepolarizing agent may be given to reduce the severity of muscle fasciculations.
8. Store the drug in the refrigerator.

Assessment

1. Note if the client is taking digitalis products. These clients are sensitive to the release of intracellular potassium.
2. Assess clients with low plasma pseudocholinesterase levels. They are sensitive to the effects of succinylcholine and require lower doses.

Interventions

1. Monitor the client's blood pressure and pulse. Succinylcholine can cause vagal stimulation resulting in bradycardia, hypotension and cardiac arrhythmias.
2. Observe the client for excessive, transient increase in intraocular pressure. This can be dangerous to the eye. Document and report to the physician.
3. Muscle fasciculations may cause the client to be sore after recovery. Administer prescribed nondepolarizing agent and reassure the client that the soreness is likely caused by the drug.
4. Document the length of time the client is taking the drug. It should be used only on a short-term basis and in a continuously monitored environment.

TUBOCURARINE CHLORIDE (too-boh-kyour-**AR**-een)

Tubarine ✱ **(Rx)**

See also *Neuromuscular Blocking Agents,* p. 957.

Classification: Nondepolarizing neuromuscular blocking agent.

Action/Kinetics: Cumulative effects may occur. Most likely of the nondepolarizing drugs to cause histamine release. Narrow margin between therapeutic dose and toxic dose. Overdosage chiefly treated by artificial respiration, although neostigmine, atropine, and edrophonium chloride should also be on hand. **Onset, IV:** 1 min; **IM:** 15–25 min. **Time to peak effect, IV:** 2–5 min. **Duration, IV:** 20–40 min. **t½:** 1–3 hr. About 43% excreted unchanged in urine.

Uses: Muscle relaxant during surgery or setting of fractures and dislocations; spasticity caused by injury to or disease of CNS. Treat seizures electrically induced or induced by drugs. Diagnosis of myasthenia gravis.

Additional Contraindications: Drug may cause excessive secretion and circulatory collapse. Patients in whom release of histamine is hazardous.

Special Concerns: Use with caution during pregnancy (pregnancy category: C) and lactation and in children. If repeated doses are used before delivery, the newborn may manifest decreased skeletal muscle activity. Children up to 1 month of age may be more sensitive to the effects of tubocurarine. Use with extreme caution in patients with renal dysfunction, liver disease, or obstructive states.

Additional Side Effects: Allergic reactions.

Additional Drug Interactions

Acetylcholine	Acetylcholine antagonizes effect of tubocurarine
Anticholinesterases	Anticholinesterases antagonize effect of tubocurarine
Calcium salts	↑ Effect of tubocurarine
Diazepam	Diazepam may cause malignant hyperthermia with tubocurarine
Potassium	Antagonizes effect of tubocurarine
Propranolol	↑ Effect of tubocurarine
Quinine	↑ Effect of tubocurarine
Succinylcholine chloride	↑ Relaxant effect of both drugs
Trimethophan	↑ Effect of tubocurarine

Dosage: IV, IM: *Adjunct to surgical anesthesia:* **Adults, IM, IV, initial,** 6–9 mg/kg; **then,** 3–4.5 mg in 3–5 min if needed. Supplemental doses of 3 mg can be given for prolonged procedures. Dosage can be calculated on the basis of 0.165 mg/kg. **Pediatric, up to 4 weeks of age, IV, initial:** 0.25–0.5 mg/kg; **then,** give subsequent doses in increments of ⅕–⅙ the initial dose. **Infants and children, IV:** 0.5 mg/kg. *Aid to controlled respiration:* **Adults, IV, initial,** 0.0165 mg/kg with additional doses adjusted as required. *Electroshock therapy:* **Adults, IV,** 0.165 mg/kg given over 30–90 seconds. It is recommended that the initial dose be 3 mg less than the calculated total dose. *Diagnosis of myasthenia gravis:* **Adults, IV,** 0.004–0.033 mg/kg. A test dose should be given within 2–3 min with IV neostigmine, 1.5 mg, to minimize prolonged respiratory paralysis.

NURSING CONSIDERATIONS

See also *Nursing Considerations* for *Neuromuscular Blocking Agents,* p. 959.

Administration/Storage

1. Review the drugs with which tubocurarine interacts.
2. Tubocurarine is incompatible with alkaline solutions and may form a precipitate when mixed with them (e.g., methohexital sodium or thiopental sodium).
3. After IV administration, expect the peak action to occur in 2–5 minutes and the effect to last 25–90 minutes.
4. Have neostigmine methylsulfate available as an antidote.

VECURONIUM BROMIDE   (ve-kyour-OH-nee-um)

Norcuron (Rx)

See also *Neuromuscular Blocking Agents,* p. 957.

Classification: Nondepolarizing neuromuscular blocking agent.

Action/Kinetics: Less likely than other agents to cause histamine release. Effects can be antagonized by anticholinesterase drugs.

Onset: 2.5–3 min; **peak effect:** 3–5 min; **duration:** 25–30 min using balanced anesthesia. No cumulative effects noted after repeated administration. Metabolized in liver and excreted through the kidney and bile. Is bound to plasma protein.

Uses: To induce skeletal muscle relaxation during surgery or to assist in endotracheal intubation. As an adjunct to general anesthesia. *Investigational:* To treat electrically induced seizures or seizures induced by drugs.

Additional Contraindications: Use in neonates, obesity. Sensitivity to bromides.

Special Concerns: Pregnancy category: C. Pediatric patients from 7 weeks to 1 year of age are more sensitive to the effects of vecuronium leading to a recovery time up to 1½ times that for adults. The dose for children aged 1–10 years of age must be individualized and may, in fact, require a somewhat higher initial dose and a slightly more frequent supplemental dosing schedule than adults.

Additional Side Effects: Moderate to severe skeletal muscle weakness, which may require artificial respiration. Malignant hyperthermia.

Additional Drug Interaction: Succinylcholine ↑ effect of vecuronium.

Dosage: IV only. Adults and children over 10 years of age. *Intubation:* 0.08–0.1 mg/kg. *For use after succinylcholine-assisted endotracheal intubation:* 0.04–0.06 mg/kg for inhalation anesthesia and 0.05–0.06 mg/kg using balanced anesthesia. (**Note:** For halothane anesthesia, doses from 0.15–0.28 mg/kg may be given without adverse effects.) *For use during anesthesia with enflurane or isoflurane after steady-state established:* 0.06–0.085 mg/kg (about 15% less than the usual initial dose). *Supplemental use:* **IV:** 0.01–0.015 mg/kg given 25–40 min following the initial dose; **then,** given q 12–15 min as needed. **IV infusion:** Initiated after recovery from effects of initial IV dose of 0.08–0.1 mg/kg has started. Infusion rate: 0.0008–0.0012 mg/kg. After steady-state enflurane, isoflurane, and possibly halothane anesthesia has been established: IV infusion should be reduced by 25%–60%.

NURSING CONSIDERATIONS

See also *Nursing Considerations* for *Neuromuscular Blocking Agents,* p. 959.

Administration/Storage

1. Dosage must be individualized and depends on prior or concomitant use of anesthetics or succinylcholine.
2. Vecuronium may be mixed with saline, 5% dextrose alone or with saline, lactated Ringer's solution, and sterile water for injection.
3. Vecuronium should be used within 8 hr of reconstitution.
4. Anticipate the onset of action to occur within 1–5 minutes, and the effect to last 20–40 minutes.
5. The drug should be refrigerated after reconstitution.

PART EIGHT
Drugs Affecting the Respiratory System

CHAPTER FORTY-NINE
Antiasthmatic Drugs

General Statement: Asthma is a disease characterized by difficulty in breathing which may result from smooth muscle contraction of the bronchi and bronchioles, edema of the mucosa of the respiratory tract, or mucus secretions that adhere to the walls of the bronchi and bronchioles. The cause of asthma is not known with certainty but, in some patients allergy is the underlying reason.

The overall objectives of drug therapy for asthma are to open blocked airways and to alter the characteristics of respiratory tract fluid. The drugs and drug classes that are used to treat asthma are bronchodilators such as theophyllines and sympathomimetic amines (see Chapter 44, p. 883), mucolytics (see Chapter 50, p. 979), corticosteroids (see Chapter 61, p. 1148), and cromolyn sodium. Theophyllines and cromolyn sodium are discussed in this chapter.

THEOPHYLLINE DERIVATIVES

Action/Kinetics: The theophylline derivatives are plant alkaloids, which, like caffeine, belong to the xanthine family. They stimulate the CNS, relax the smooth muscles of the bronchi and pulmonary blood vessels (relieve bronchospasms), produce diuresis, stimulate gastric acid secretion, and increase the rate and force of contraction of the heart. The bronchodilator activity of theophyllines is due to direct relaxation of the bronchiolar smooth muscle and pulmonary blood vessels which relieves bronchospasm. The proposed mechanism (which is controversial) for this effect may be due to competitive inhibition of phosphodiesterase, which is the enzyme responsible for metabolizing cyclic AMP to 5-AMP. The resultant increase in cyclic AMP increases the release of endogenous epinephrine, which can cause bronchodilation. Theophyllines may also act by altering the calcium levels of smooth muscle, blocking adenosine receptors, inhibiting the effect of prostaglandins on smooth muscle, and inhibition of the release of slow-reacting substance of anaphylaxis (SRS-A) and histamine. Aminophylline, oxtriphylline, and theophylline sodium glycinate release free theophylline in vivo. Response to the drugs is highly individualized. *Theophylline salts:* **Onset:** 1–5 hr, depending on route and formulation. **Therapeutic plasma levels:** 10–20 mcg/mL. **t½:** 7–9 hr in nonsmoking adults, 4–5 hr in adult heavy smokers, and 3–5 hr in children. Because of great variations in the rate of absorption (due to dosage form, food, dose level) as well as its extremely narrow therapeutic range, theophylline therapy is best monitored by determination of the serum levels. If these determinations cannot be obtained, saliva (which contains 60% of corresponding theophylline serum levels) determinations can be used. Metabolized in liver to caffeine which may accumulate in neonates less than 3 months of age. Excretion is through the kidneys (about 10% unchanged in adults).

Uses: Prophylaxis and treatment of bronchial asthma. Reversible bronchospasms associated with chronic bronchitis, emphysema, and chronic obstructive pulmonary disease. *Investigational:* Treatment of neonatal apnea and Cheyne-Stokes respiration.

Contraindications: Hypersensitivity to drug, hypotension, coronary artery disease, angina pectoris.

Special Concerns: Safe use during pregnancy (pregnancy category: C) has not been established. Use during lactation may result in irritability, insomnia, and fretfulness in the infant. Use with caution in premature infants due to the possible accumulation of caffeine. Xanthines are not usually tolerated by small children because of excessive CNS stimulation. Geriatric patients may manifest an increased risk of toxicity. Use with caution in the presence of gastritis, peptic ulcer, alcoholism, acute cardiac diseases, hypoxemia, severe renal and hepatic disease, severe hypertension, severe myocardial damage, hyperthyroidism, glaucoma.

Side Effects: *GI:* Nausea, vomiting, diarrhea, anorexia, epigastric pain, hematemesis, dyspepsia, rectal irritation (following use of suppositories). *CNS:* Headache, insomnia, irritability, fever, dizziness, lightheadedness, vertigo, reflex hyperexcitability, seizures, depression, speech abnormalities, alternating periods of mutism and hyperactivity, brain damage, death. *CV:* Hypotension, arrhythmias, palpitations, tachycardia, peripheral vascular collapse, extrasystoles. *Renal:* Proteinuria, excretion of erythrocytes and renal tubular cells, dehydration due to diuresis, urinary retention (males with prostatic hypertrophy). *Other:* Tachypnea, respiratory arrest, fever, flushing, hyperglycemia, antidiuretic hormone syndrome, leukocytosis.

Note: Aminophylline given by rapid IV may produce hypotension, flushing, palpitations, precordial pain, headache, dizziness, or hyperventilation. Also, the ethylenediamine in aminophylline may cause allergic reactions, including urticaria and skin rashes.

Overdosage: Early signs of toxicity include anorexia, nausea, vomiting, wakefulness, restlessness, irritability. Later symptoms include agitation, manic behavior, frequent vomiting, extreme thirst, delirium, convulsions, hyperthermia, vasomotor collapse. Serious toxicity can develop without earlier signs of toxicity. Toxicity is usually associated with parenteral administration but can be observed after oral administration, especially in children.

Drug Interactions

Beta-adrenergic blocking agents	↓ Effect of theophylline
Cimetidine	↑ Theophylline toxicity due to ↓ breakdown by liver
Ciprofloxacin	↑ Plasma levels of theophylline with ↑ possibility of untoward reactions
Digitalis	Theophylline ↑ toxicity of digitalis
Ephedrine and other sympathomimetics	↑ CNS stimulation
Erythromycin	↑ Effect of theophylline due to ↓ breakdown by liver
Furosemide	↑ Effect of theophylline
Halothane	↑ Risk of cardiac arrhythmias
Lithium	↓ Effect of lithium due to ↑ rate of excretion
Muscle relaxants, nondepolarizing	Theophylline ↓ effect of these drugs
Oral contraceptives	↑ Effect of theophyllines due to ↓ breakdown by liver
Phenytoin	↓ Effect of both drugs due to ↑ breakdown by liver
Reserpine	Concomitant use → tachycardia
Tobacco smoking	↓ Effect of theophylline due to ↑ breakdown by liver
Troleandomycin	↑ Effect of theophylline due to ↓ breakdown by liver
Verapamil	↑ Effect of theophyllines

Laboratory Test Interferences: ↑ Plasma free fatty acids, bilirubin, urinary catecholamines, RBC sedimentation rate. Interference with uric acid tests and tests for furosemide, probenecid, theobromine, and phenylbutazone.

Dosage: Individualized. Initially, dosage should be adjusted according to plasma level of drug. Usual: 10–20 mcg theophylline/mL plasma. The dose of the various salts should be equivalent based on the content of anhydrous theophylline. See individual agents and Table 20.

Table 20   Theophylline Derivatives

Drug	Dosage	Remarks
Dyphylline (Dilor, Dilor-400, Dyflex, Dyflex 400, Lufyllin, Lufyllin-400, Neothylline, Protophylline, Thylline) (Rx) Pregnancy category: C.	**Elixir, Oral Solution, Tablets. Adults,** 15 mg/kg q 6 hr up to q.i.d. **IM. Adults, initial:** 250–500 mg q 2–6 hr. Pediatric oral and IM doses must be individualized by the physician.	**Peak plasma levels:** 1 hr. **t$^{1}/_{2}$:** 2–2.5 hr. **Minimum effective concentration:** 2 mg/mL. Excreted unchanged in the urine. Not to be used IV. Fewer side effects than theophylline salts. Equivalent to 70% theophylline although serum theophylline levels are not used to measure dyphylline. Use with caution in patients with impaired renal function.

Table 20 (*continued*)

Drug	Dosage	Remarks
Oxtriphylline (Apo-Oxtriphylline✦, Choledyl, Choledyl Delayed Release, Choledyl SA, Novotriphyl✦) (Rx) Pregnancy category: C.	**Syrup, Tablets.** *Acute attack:* **Adults,** not on any theophylline products, 5–6 mg/kg (as anhydrous theophylline). **Patients on theophylline:** Loading dose based on premise that 0.5 mg/kg theophylline increases serum levels by 0.5–1.6 mcg/mL. **Maintenance:** 3 mg/kg q 8 hr (nonsmokers) (2 mg/kg q 8 hr for geriatric patients and 4 mg/kg q 6 hr for smokers). **Pediatric, loading dose, up to 16 years:** 5–6 mg/kg (as anhydrous theophylline) for patients not on theophylline. See Adult dose for patients on theophylline. **Maintenance, 12–16 years:** 3 mg/kg q 6 hr; **9–12 years:** 4 mg/kg q 6 hr; **1–9 years:** 5 mg/kg q 6 hr; **6–12 months:** dose (mg/kg) q 6 hr = (0.05) (age in weeks) + 1.25; **up to 6 months:** dose (mg/kg) q 8 hr = (0.07) (age in weeks) + 1.7. Dose based on anhydrous theophylline. *Chronic use:* **Adults, initial,** Up to 400 mg daily in divided doses q 6–8 hr; dose can then be increased to a maximum of 900 mg daily. **Pediatric, initial:** 16 mg/kg (maximum of 400 mg) daily in 3–4 divided doses q 6–8 hr. Dose can be increased as follows: **Over 16 years:** 13 mg/kg or 900 mg daily (whichever is less); **12–16 years:** 18 mg/kg daily; **9–12 years:** 20 mg/kg daily; **1–9 years:** 24 mg/kg daily; **Up to 1 year:** daily dose (mg/kg) (0.3) (age in weeks) + 8.0. **Delayed-release Tablets.** *Chronic therapy:* **Adults,** See *Chronic therapy* for Syrup/Tablets. **Extended-release Tablets.** *Chronic therapy:* **Adults, initial,** 4 mg/kg q 8–12 hr; dose may be increased to a maximum of 13 mg/kg or 900 mg daily (whichever is less).	Choline salt of theophylline containing 64% theophylline. Less irritating than aminophylline. Preferably given after meals and at bedtime. **Note:** Dosage is based on the equivalent of anhydrous theophylline. Serum theophylline levels should be monitored to decrease risk of side effects and increase the chance of optimal response.

Table 20   (*continued*)

Drug	Dosage	Remarks
Theophylline sodium glycinate (Synophylate) (Rx) Pregnancy category: C.	**Elixir. Adults:** 330–600 mg q 6–8 hr after meals; **pediatric, 6–12 years:** 220–330 mg q 6–8 hr after meals; **pediatric, 3–6 years:** 110–165 mg q 6–8 hr after meals; **pediatric, 1–3 years:** 55–110 mg q 6–8 hr after meals.	Contains 44.5%–47.3% theophylline in an elixir.

NURSING CONSIDERATIONS

Administration/Storage
1. Review the list of agents with which theophylline derivatives interact.
2. Dilute drugs and maintain proper infusion rates to minimize problems of overdosage. Use an infusion pump to regulate infusion of IV solutions.
3. Wait to initiate oral therapy for at least 4–6 hr after switching from IV therapy.
4. Have ipecac syrup, gastric lavage equipment and cathartics available to treat overdose if the client is conscious and not having seizures. Otherwise a respirator, oxygen, diazepam, and IV fluids may be necessary for the treatment of overdosage.

Assessment
1. Assess the client for any history of hypersensitivity to xanthine compounds.
2. Note if the client has a history of hypotension, coronary artery disease or angina. These drugs generally should not be used in clients with these problems.
3. Determine if the client smokes or has a history of smoking marijuana. These habits induce hepatic metabolism of the drug. Smokers require an increase in the dosage of drug from 50–100%.
4. Assess diet habits as these can influence the excretion of theophylline. A client eating a high protein and/or low carbohydrate diet will have an increased excretion of the drug. Clients eating a low protein and/or high carbohydrate diet will have a decrease in the excretion of theophylline. Therefore, dietary intake is an important part of the premedication assessment.
5. Obtain baseline blood pressure and pulse prior to starting drug therapy.

Interventions
1. Monitor BP and pulse closely during therapy. Report any wide variations from normal to the physician.
2. Observe closely for signs of toxicity such as nausea, anorexia, insomnia, irritability, hyperexcitability, or cardiac arrhythmias. Document and report to the physician.
3. Observe small children in particular, for excessive CNS stimulation, because children often are unable to report side effects.

4. To avoid epigastric pain when the drug is administered orally, give the medication with a snack or with meals.

5. Monitor for serum levels of theophylline in the 10–20 mcg/mL range. Levels above 20 mcg/mL require an adjustment in the dosage of drug.

Client/Family Teaching

1. If nausea, vomiting, GI pain, or restlessness occurs, instruct the client to notify the physician.

2. Take the medication only as prescribed, because more is *not* better.

3. Do not smoke as smoking may aggravate underlying medical conditions as well as interfere with drug absorption.

4. Explain to clients how to protect themselves from acute exacerbations of illness by: avoiding crowds, dressing warmly in cold weather, covering their mouth and nose so that cold air is not directly inhaled, staying in air conditioning during excessively hot and humid weather, proper diet and nutrition and adequate fluid intake.

5. Provide printed material listing the early signs and symptoms of infections, adverse side effects of drug therapy and when to call the physician.

6. When secretions become thick and tacky, instruct the client to increase intake of fluids. This thins secretions and assists in their removal.

7. Avoid overexertion at all times.

AMINOPHYLLINE (am-in-**OFF**-ih-lin)

Aminophyllin, Corophyllin✼, Palaron✼, Phyllocontin, Phyllocontin-350✼, Somophyllin, Somophyllin-DF, Truphyllin (Rx)

See also *Theophylline Derivatives,* p. 976.

Action/Kinetics: Aminophylline contains 79–86% theophylline.

Additional Uses: Neonatal apnea, respiratory stimulant in Cheyne-Stokes respiration. Parenteral form has been used for biliary colic, as a cardiac stimulant, diuretic, and an adjunct in treating congestive heart failure although such uses have been replaced by more effective drugs.

Special Concerns: Pregnancy category: C. Use with caution when aminophylline and sodium chloride are used with adrenocorticosteroids or in patients with edema.

Additional Side Effects: The ethylenediamine in the product may cause exfoliative dermatitis or urticaria.

Dosage: Oral Solution, Tablets. *Bronchodilator, acute attacks, in patients not currently on theophylline therapy:* **Adults and children up to 16 years of age, loading dose:** equivalent of 5–6 mg of anhydrous theophylline/kg. *Bronchodilator, acute attacks, in patients currently receiving theophylline:* **Adults and children up to 16 years of age:** If possible, a serum theophylline level should be obtained first. Then, base loading dose on the premise that each 0.5 mg theophylline/kg of lean body weight will result in a 0.5–1.6 mcg/mL increase in serum theophylline levels. If immediate therapy is needed and a serum level cannot be obtained, a single dose of the equivalent of 2.5 mg/kg of anhydrous theophylline can be given. *Maintenance in acute attack, based on equivalent of anhydrous theophylline:* **Young adult smokers,** 4 mg/kg q 6 hr; **healthy, nonsmoking adults,** 3 mg/kg q 8 hr; **geriatric patients or patients with cor pulmonale,** 2 mg/kg q 8 hr; **patients with congestive heart failure or liver failure,** 2 mg/kg 8–12 hr. **Pediatric, 12–16 years,** 3 mg/kg q 6 hr; **9–12 years:** 4 mg/kg q 6 hr; **1–9 years:** 5 mg/kg q 6 hr; **6–12 months,** Use the formula: dose (mg/kg q 8 hr) = (0.05) (age in weeks) + 1.25; **Up to 6 months,** Use the formula: dose (mg/kg q 8 hr) = (0.07) (age in weeks) + 1.7. *Chronic therapy, based on equivalent of anhydrous theophylline:* **Adults, initial,** 6–8 mg/kg up to a maximum of 400 mg daily in 3–4 divided doses at 6–8 hr intervals; **then,** dose can be increased in 25% increments at 2–3 day intervals up to a maximum of 13 mg/kg or 900 mg daily, whichever is less. **Pediatric, initial,** 16 mg/kg up to a maximum of 400 mg daily in 3–4 divided doses at 6–8 hr intervals; **then,** dose may be increased in 25% increments at 2–3 day intervals up to the following maximum doses (without measuring serum theophylline): **16 years and older,** 13 mg/kg or 900 mg daily, whichever is less; **12–16 years:** 18 mg/kg daily; **9–12 years:** 20 mg/kg daily; **1–9 years:** 24 mg/kg daily; **Up to 12 months,** Use the following formula: dose (mg/kg daily) = (0.3) (age in weeks) + 8.0.

Enteric-coated Tablets. *Bronchodilator, chronic therapy, based on equivalent of anhydrous theophylline:* **Adults, initial,** 6–8 mg/kg up to a maximum of 400 mg daily in 3–4 divided doses q 6–8 hr; **then,** dose may be increased, if needed and tolerated, by increments of 25% at 2–3 day intervals up to a maximum of 13 mg/kg/day or 900 mg/day, whichever is less, without measuring serum theophylline. **Pediatric, over 12 years of age, initial,** 4 mg/kg q 8–12 hr; **then,** dose may be increased by 2–3 mg/kg/day at 3-day intervals up to the following maximum doses (without measuring serum levels): **16 years and older:** 13 mg/kg/day or 900 mg/day, whichever is less; **12–16 years:** 18 mg/kg daily.

Extended-release Tablets. *Bronchodilator, chronic therapy, based on equivalent of anhydrous theophylline:* **Adults, initial,** 4 mg/kg q 8–12 hr; **then,** dose may be increased by 2–3 mg/kg/day at 3-day intervals to a maximum of 13 mg/kg or 900 mg/day, whichever is less. **Pediatric, initial,** Same as adults; **then,** dose may be increased by 2–3 mg/kg/day at 3-day intervals up to the following maximum doses: **16 years and older:** 13 mg/kg/day or 900 mg/day, whichever is less. **12–16 years:** 18 mg/kg/day.

Enema. For use as a bronchodilator for loading doses and for maintenance in acute attacks, see doses for oral solution and tablets.

IV infusion. *Bronchodilator, acute attacks, for patients not currently on theophylline:* **Adults and children up to 16 years, loading dose based on anhydrous theophylline,** 5 mg/kg given over a period of 20 min. *Bronchodilator, acute attack, for patients currently on theophylline:* **Adults and children up to 16 years, loading dose based on anhydrous theophylline,** If possible, a serum theophylline level should be obtained first. Then, base loading dose on the premise that each 0.5 mg theophylline/kg of lean body weight will result in a 0.5–1.6 mcg/mL increase in serum theophylline levels. If immediate therapy is needed and a serum level can not be obtained, a single dose of the equivalent of 2.5 mg/kg of anhydrous theophylline can be given. *Maintenance for acute attacks, based on equivalent of anhydrous theophylline:* **Young adult smokers,** 0.7 mg/kg/hr; **nonsmoking, healthy adults,** 0.43 mg/kg/hr; **geriatric patients or cor pulmonale:** 0.26 mg/kg/hr; **patients with congestive heart failure or liver failure:** 0.2 mg/kg/hr. **Pediatric, 12–16 years, nonsmokers,** 0.5 mg/kg/hr; **9–12 years of age,** 0.7 mg/kg/hr; **1–9 years of age,** 0.8 mg/kg/hr; **up to 1 year,** Based on the following formula: dose (mg/kg/hr) = (0.008) (age in weeks) + 0.21.

NURSING CONSIDERATIONS

See also *Nursing Considerations* for *Theophylline Derivatives,* p. 977.

Administration/Storage

1. To avoid hypotension, administer IV doses of medication at a rate not to exceed 25 mg/min.

2. Only the 25 mg/mL injection (which should be further diluted) should be used for IV administration. Use an infusion pump to regulate infusion rates of IV solutions.

3. IM injection is not recommended due to severe, persistent pain at the site of injection.

4. A minimum of 4–6 hr should elapse when switching from IV infusion to the first dose of PO therapy.

5. Enteric-coated tablets may be incompletely and slowly absorbed.

6. Enteric-coated and extended-release tablets are not recommended for children less than 12 years of age.

7. Use of aminophylline suppositories is not recommended (dose not provided) due to the possibility of slow and unreliable absorption.

8. Serum levels of theophylline should be determined to monitor for side effects and client response.

Interventions

Monitor pulse and BP closely during IV administration. Aminophylline may cause a transitory lowering of the blood pressure. If this occurs, the dosage of drug and rate of flow should be adjusted immediately.

THEOPHYLLINE   (thee-OFF-ih-lin)

Immediate-release Capsules, Tablets, Liquid Products: Accurbron, Aerolate, Aquaphyllin, Asmalix, Bronkodyl, Elixicon, Elixomin, Elixophyllin, Lanophyllin, Lixolin, PMS Theophylline ✳, Pulmophylline ✳, Quibron-T ✳, Quibron-T Dividose, Slo-Phyllin, Solu-Phyllin, Somnophyllin-T, Theo, Theoclear-80, Theolair, Theomar, Theon, Theostat-80, Truxophyllin. Timed-release Capsules and Tablets: Aerolate III, Aerolate Jr., Aerolate Sr., Constant-T, Duraphyl, Elixophyllin SR, Quibron-T/SR Dividose, Respid, Slo-Bid Gyrocaps, Slo-Phyllin Gyrocaps, Somophyllin-12 ✳, Somophyllin-CRT, Sustaire, Theo-24, Theo 250, Theobid Duracaps, Theobid Jr Duracaps, Theoclear L.A.-130 Cenules, Theoclear L.A.-260 Cenules, Theocot, Theocron, Theo-Dur, Theo-Dur Sprinkle, Theo-SR ✳, Theolair-SR, Theospan-SR, Theo-Time, Theophylline SR, Theovent Long-Acting, Uniphyl (Rx)

See also *Theophylline Derivatives*, p. 976.

Classification: Antiasthmatic, bronchodilator.

Action/Kinetics: Time to peak serum levels, oral solution: 1 hr; **uncoated tablets:** 2 hr; **chewable tablets:** 1–1.5 hr; **enteric-coated tablets:** 5 hr; **extended-release capsules and tablets:** 4–7 hr. In healthy adults, about 60% is bound to plasma protein whereas in neonates 36% is bound to plasma protein.

Additional Uses: Oral liquid: Neonatal apnea as a respiratory stimulant. Theophylline and dextrose injection: Respiratory stimulant in neonatal apnea and Cheyne-Stokes respiration.

Dosage: Capsules, Elixir, Oral Solution, Oral Suspension, Syrup, Tablets. See *Dosage for Oral Solution, Tablets,* p. 974, under *Aminophylline.*

Extended-release Capsules, Extended-release Tablets. See *Dosage* for *Extended-release Tablets,* p. 974, under *Aminophylline. Bronchodilator, chronic therapy:* **9–12 years:** 20 mg/kg daily; **6–9 years:** 24 mg/kg daily.

Elixir, Oral Solution, Oral Suspension, Syrup. *Neonatal apnea,* **loading dose:** Using the equivalent of anhydrous theophylline administered by nasogastric tube, 5 mg/kg.

NURSING CONSIDERATIONS

See also *Nursing Considerations* for *Theophylline Derivatives*, p. 977.

Administration/Storage

1. Dosage is individualized to maintain serum levels of 10–20 mcg/mL.
2. Dosage should be calculated based on lean body weight (theophylline does not distribute to body fat).
3. Serum theophylline levels should be monitored in chronic therapy if the maximum maintenance doses are used or exceeded.
4. The extended-release tablets or capsules are not recommended for children less than 6 years of age. Dosage for once-a-day products has not been established in children less than 12 years of age.

Client/Family Teaching

1. Stress the importance of taking the drug only as prescribed by the physician.
2. Instruct the client not to crush or break slow-release forms of the drug.

MISCELLANEOUS ANTIASTHMATIC

CROMOLYN SODIUM   (CROW-mo-lin)

Fivent✵, Gastrocrom, Intal, Nasalcrom, Opticrom, Rynacrom✵, Vistacrom✵ (Rx)

Classification: Respiratory inhalant for bronchial asthma.

Action/Kinetics: Cromolyn sodium appears to act locally on the lung mucosa, preventing the release of histamine, leukotrienes, and other endogenous substances causing hypersensitivity reactions. The drug, when effective, reduces the number and intensity of asthmatic attacks. The drug has no antihistaminic, anti-inflammatory, or bronchodilator effects and has no role in terminating an acute attack of asthma. After inhalation some of the drug is absorbed systemically. It is excreted about equally in urine and bile (feces). $t\frac{1}{2}$: 81 min; from lungs: 60 min. About 50% excreted unchanged through the urine and 50% through the bile. When used in the eye, approximately 0.03% is absorbed. **Onset, ophthalmic:** Several days. **Onset, nasal:** Less than 1 week. **Time to peak effect, nasal:** Up to 4 weeks.

Uses: *Inhalation:* Prophylactic and adjunct in the management of severe bronchial asthma in selected patients. Prophylaxis of exercise-induced bronchospasms and bronchospasms due to allergens, cold dry air, or environmental pollutants. *Ophthalmologic:* Treat allergic ocular disorders, including allergic conjunctivitis and keratoconjunctivitis, giant papillary conjunctivitis, and vernal keratoconjunctivitis. *Nasal:* Prophylaxis and treatment of allergic rhinitis. *Oral:* Mastocytosis. *Investigational:* Orally to treat food allergies.

Contraindications: Hypersensitivity. Children under 4 years of age. Acute attacks and status asthmaticus. Soft contact lenses should not be worn if the drug is used in the eye.

Special Concerns: Safe use in pregnancy not established (pregnancy category: B). Dosage of the ophthalmic product has not been established in children less than 4 years of age while dosage of the nasal product has not been established in children less than 6 years of age. Use with caution for long periods of time or in the presence of renal or hepatic disease.

Side Effects: *Respiratory:* Bronchospasm, cough, laryngeal edema (rare), eosinophilic pneumonia. *CNS:* Dizziness, drowsiness, headache. *Allergic:* Urticaria, rash, angioedema, serum sickness, anaphylaxis. *Other:* Nausea, urinary frequency, dysuria, joint swelling and pain, lacrimation, swollen parotid gland.
Following nebulization: Sneezing, wheezing, itching, nose bleeds, burning, nasal congestion.
Following nasal solution: Burning, stinging, irritation of nose; sneezing, nose bleeds, headache, bad taste in mouth, postnasal drip. **Following ophthalmic use:** Stinging and burning after use.
Following oral use: *GI:* Diarrhea, taste perversion, spasm of esophagus, flatulence, dysphagia, burning of mouth and throat. *CNS:* Headache, dizziness, fatigue, migraine, paresthesia, anxiety, depression, psychosis, behavior changes, insomnia, hallucinations, lethargy, lightheadedness after eating. *Dermatologic:* Flushing, angioedema, urticaria, skin burning, skin erythema. *Musculoskeletal:* Arthralgia, stiffness and weakness in legs. *Miscellaneous:* Altered liver function test, dyspnea, dysuria, polycythemia, neutropenia.

Dosage: Capsules or Solution for Inhalation. *Prophylaxis of bronchial asthma:* **Adults:** 20 mg q.i.d. at regular intervals. Adjust dosage as required. *Prophylaxis of bronchospasm:* **Adults:** 20 mg as a single dose just prior to exposure to the precipitating factor. If used chronically, 20 mg q.i.d, up to a maximum of 160 mg daily.
Ophthalmic Solution. Adults and children over 4 years of age: 1 drop of the 2% or 4% solution 4–6 times daily at regular intervals.
Nasal Solution. Adults and children over 6 years of age: 2.6 mg in each nostril six times daily or 5.3 mg in each nostril 3–4 times daily at regular intervals.
Oral Capsules. Adults: 200 mg q.i.d. 30 min before meals and at bedtime. **Pediatric, term to 2 years:** 20 mg/kg daily in four divided doses; should be used in this age group only in severe incapacitating disease where benefits outweigh risks. **Pediatric, 2–12 years:** 100 mg q.i.d. 30 min before meals and at bedtime. If relief is not seen within 2–3 weeks, dose may be increased, but should not exceed 40 mg/kg daily for adults and children over 2 years of age and 30 mg/kg daily for children 6 months–2 years.

NURSING CONSIDERATIONS

Administration/Storage

1. Institute only after acute episode is over, when airway is clear and client can inhale adequately.
2. Corticosteroid dosage should be continued when initiating cromolyn therapy. However, if improvement occurs, the steroid dosage may be tapered slowly. Steroid therapy may have to be reinstituted if cromolyn inhalation is impaired, in times of stress, or in adrenocortical insufficiency.
3. One drop of the ophthalmic solution contains 1.6 mg cromolyn sodium.
4. The ophthalmic solution should be protected from sunlight and, once opened, should be discarded after 4 weeks.

Client/Family Teaching

1. When the medication is administered by inhaler, the following procedure should be used:
   - Demonstrate how to load the capsule into the inhaler.
   - Instruct clients to inhale and exhale fully and then to introduce the mouthpiece between their lips.

- Tilt their head back and inhale deeply and rapidly through the inhaler. This causes the propeller to turn rapidly and to supply more medication in one breath.
- Remove inhaler, hold breath a few seconds and exhale slowly.
- Repeat this procedure until the powder is completely administered.
- Do not wet powder with breath while exhaling.

2. When used orally, the following procedure should be used to prepare the solution in water:
   - Open the capsule (which is oversized to prevent spilling of powder when opened) and pour the powder into one-half glass of hot water.
   - Stir the mixture until the powder is completely dissolved and the solution is clear.
   - While stirring, add an equal quantity of cold water.
   - The drug should **not** be mixed with milk, foods, or fruit juice.
   - The entire glass of liquid should be consumed.

3. Provide the client and family with written guidelines concerning the prescribed method of medication administration.

4. Encourage the client to continue self-administration of medication as ordered. It may take up to 4 weeks for frequency of asthmatic attacks to decrease.

5. If the client wishes to discontinue medication, stress the importance of notifying the physician. Rapid withdrawal of the drug may precipitate an asthmatic attack, and concomitant corticosteroid therapy may require adjustment.

CHAPTER FIFTY

50

Antitussives, Expectorants, and Mucolytics

ANTITUSSIVES

General Statement: The cough is a useful protective reflex mechanism through which the body attempts to clear the respiratory tract of excess mucus or foreign particles. Coughing may accompany upper respiratory tract infections and as such will usually clear up by itself within a few days. It may also indicate an underlying organic disease whose cause should be ascertained.

There are two common types of cough: productive (cough accompanied by expectoration of mucus and phlegm) and nonproductive (dry cough). When a cough becomes excessive and interferes with normal activities or sleep, it should be treated symptomatically. An important treatment for cough is also proper humidification and/or intake of fluids.

Antitussive agents can be divided into narcotic (see *Codeine,* Chapter 37, p. 750) and nonnarcotic products. Such agents depress a cough either by depressing the activity of the cough center in the medulla or by a local action to decrease nerve impulses.

NARCOTIC ANTITUSSIVE

CODEINE   (KOH-deen)

See *Narcotic Analgesics,* Chapter 37, p. 750.

NONNARCOTIC ANTITUSSIVES

General Statement: The drugs belonging to this category depress the cough reflex by a variety of mechanisms, including depression of the cough reflex in the medulla and a local anesthetic effect. All of them are more effective in the treatment of nonproductive cough than in cough associated with copious sputum. Unlike narcotics, they do not produce physical dependence.

Contraindication: Antitussive medication should be avoided during the first trimester of pregnancy unless otherwise decided by a physician.

NURSING CONSIDERATIONS

Assessment

1. Note any client allergic response to drugs in this category.
2. Question the client concerning the amount of sputum that results from coughing. Drugs in this category are most effective with clients who have a dry, nonproductive cough.
3. Assess the amount of congestion the client has prior to administering the medication. Document baseline lung sounds.
4. If the client is of childbearing age and sexually active, determine if the client is pregnant. Antitussives are generally contraindicated in pregnancy.

Interventions

1. Routinely auscultate the client's chest. If the client continues to have congestion or is unable to bring up secretions, record on the chart and report to the physician.
2. Encourage the client to increase fluid intake.
3. Before instituting a procedure designed to encourage production of sputum, give the client warm, soothing liquids. This will reduce mucosal irritation.
4. When asking the client to cough, have the client sit upright. Place a pillow in front of the chest, and ask the client to put his/her arms around the pillow to support their abdomen and if applicable, splint their incision. Then encourage the client to cough.
5. Clap and vibrate the chest and position the client in the proper positions for postural drainage to assist in the removal of secretions.
6. Document and report to the physician the results of therapy.

Client/Family Teaching

1. Advise the client not to eat or drink fluids for at least 15 minutes after taking a cough syrup that has a demulcent effect.
2. Female clients of childbearing age, should be advised to use some form of birth control during therapy.
3. Advise the client to seek further medical assistance if the symptoms persist.

Evaluation

1. Review with the client and family the goals of therapy and determine the client's response.
2. Assess lung sounds and client for verbal reports of improvement in breathing as well as a decrease in the amount of chest congestion and production of secretions.

BENZONATATE   (ben-**ZOH**-nah-tayt)

Tessalon Perles (Rx)

Classification: Nonnarcotic antitussive.

Action/Kinetics: Antitussive action is due to local anesthetic effect on stretch receptors in respiratory tract, lungs, and pleura, thus depressing the cough reflex at its source. It is as effective as codeine. **Onset:** 15–20 min. **Duration:** 3–8 hr.

Uses: Nonproductive cough.

Contraindications: Sensitivity to benzonatate or related drugs such as tetracaine.

Special Concerns: Safety has not been established for use during pregnancy and during lactation.

Side Effects: *GI:* Nausea, gastric upset, constipation. *CNS:* Drowsiness, dizziness, headache. *Other:* Skin rash, pruritus, nasal congestion, chills, burning of the eyes, numbness of the chest, hypersensitivity.

Dosage: Capsules. Adults and children over 10: 100 mg t.i.d. up to maximum of 600 mg/day.

NURSING CONSIDERATIONS

See also *Nursing Considerations* for *Nonnarcotic Antitussives,* p. 981.

Administration/ Storage

Perles should be swallowed without chewing to avoid local anesthetic effect on the oral mucosa.

Assessment

1. Note the client's history for prior sensitivity to benzonatate or tetracaine.
2. If the client is of childbearing age, determine the possibility of pregnancy. The safety of the drug in pregnancy has not been established.

Interventions

1. Observe the client for nausea, gastric upset or constipation. If the problem persists notify the physician.
2. Observe for drowsiness and client complaints of dizziness. If these symptoms occur, have the client sit on the side of the bed a few seconds when arising from a recumbent position and then slowly stand up.

Client/Family Teaching

1. Advise the client to report any bothersome side effects.
2. Instruct the client not to perform tasks that require mental alertness until the drug effects have been realized.

DEXTROMETHORPHAN HYDROBROMIDE   (dex-troh-meth-**OR**-fan)

Balminil D.M. Syrup✹, Benylin DM, Broncho-Grippol-DM✹, Congespirin For Children, Cremacoat 1, Delsym, DM Cough, DM Syrup✹, Hold, Koffex✹, Mediquell, Neo-DM✹, Pedia Care 1, Pertussin Cough Suppressant, Pertussin 8 Hour Cough Formula, Robidex✹, St. Joseph For Children, Sedatuss✹, Sucrets Cough Control Formula (OTC)

Classification: Nonnarcotic antitussive.

Action/Kinetics: Dextromethorphan selectively depresses the cough center in the medulla, and its antitussive activity is about equal to that of codeine. It is a common ingredient of nonprescription cough medications; it does not produce physical dependence or respiratory depression. Well absorbed from GI tract. **Onset:** 15–30 min. **Duration:** 3–6 hr.

Use: Symptomatic relief of nonproductive cough due to colds or inhaled irritants.

Contraindications: Persistent or chronic cough. Use during first trimester of pregnancy unless directed otherwise by physician.

Special Concerns: Use is not recommended in children less than 2 years of age. Use with caution in patients with nausea, vomiting, high fever, rash, or persistent headache.

Side Effects: *CNS:* Dizziness, drowsiness. *GI:* Nausea, vomiting, stomach pain.

Drug Interaction: Contraindicated with monoamine oxidase inhibitors.

Dosage: Syrup, Lozenges, Chewable Tablets. Adults and children over 12: 10–20 mg q 4–8 hr or 30 mg q 6–8 hr, not to exceed 120 mg/day; **pediatric, 6–12 years:** either 5–10 mg q 4 hr or 15 mg q 6–8 hr, not to exceed 60 mg/day; **pediatric, 2–6 years:** either 2.5–5 mg q 4 hr or 7.5 mg q 6–8 hr, not to exceed 30 mg/day. **Controlled-release Oral Suspension. Adults:** 60 mg q 12 hr; **pediatric, 6–12 years:** 30 mg q 12 hr, not to exceed 60 mg daily; **pediatric, 2–6 years:** 15 mg q 12 hr, not to exceed 30 mg daily.

NURSING CONSIDERATIONS

See *Nursing considerations for Nonnarcotic antitussives,* p. 981.

Administration/Storage

1. Increasing the dose of dextromethorphan will not increase its effectiveness but will increase the duration of action.
2. The lozenges should not be given to children under 6 years of age.

Assessment

1. Note the length of time the client has had the cough. If the cough is persistent, dextromethorphan should not be given.
2. In taking the client's history, note if the client has had nausea, vomiting, persistent headache or a high fever.
3. If the client is pregnant, determine if she is in the first trimester of pregnancy. The drug is contraindicated in this instance.

DIPHENHYDRAMINE HYDROCHLORIDE   (dye-fen-**HY**-drah-meen)

Allerdryl✱, AllerMax, Beldin Cough, Belix, Bena-D, Bena-D 50, Benadryl, Benadryl Complete Allergy, Benahist 10 and 50, Ben-Allergin-50, Benoject-10 and -50, Benylin Cough, Benaphen, Bydramine Cough, Diahist, Dihydrex, Diphenacen-10 and -50, Diphenadryl, Diphen Cough, Fenylhist, Fynex, Hydramine, Hydramine Cough, Hydril, Hyrexin-50, Noradryl, Nordryl, Nordryl Cough, Tusstat, Valdrene, Wehdryl (OTC and Rx).

Sleep-Aids: Compoz, Dormarex 2, Insomnal✱, Nervine Nighttime Sleep-Aid, Nytol with DPH, Sleep-Eze 3, Sominex 2, Twilite (OTC)

See also *Antihistamines,* p. 1003, *Antiemetics,* p. 1076, and *Antiparkinson Agents,* p. 681.

Classification: Antihistamine, antiemetic (ethanolamine-type).

Additional Uses: Treatment of parkinsonism in geriatric patients unable to tolerate more potent drugs. Also for mild parkinsonism in other age groups. Drug-induced extrapyramidal symptoms. Motion sickness, antiemetic, as a sleep-aid. Coughs, including those due to allergy.

Special Concerns: Pregnancy category: B.

Dosage: Capsules, Elixir, Syrup, Tablets. *Antihistamine, antiemetic, antimotion sickness, parkinsonism:* **Adults,** 25–50 mg t.i.d.–q.i.d.; **pediatric, over 44 kg:** 12.5–25 mg t.i.d.–q.i.d. (or 5 mg/kg/day not to exceed 300 mg daily). *Sleep aid:* **Adults,** 50 mg at bedtime. *Antitussive:* **Adults,** 25 mg q 4 hr, not to exceed 150 mg daily; **pediatric, 6–12 years:** 12.5 mg q 4 hr, not to exceed 75 mg daily; **pediatric, 2–6 years:** 6.25 mg q 4 hr, not to exceed 25 mg daily.

   IV, deep IM: Adults 10–50 mg up to 100 mg, not to exceed 400 mg daily; **pediatric:** 5 mg/kg/day, not to exceed 300 mg daily.

NURSING CONSIDERATIONS

See also *Nursing Considerations* for *Antihistamines,* p. 1007, *Antiemetics,* p. 1076, and *Antiparkinson Agents,* p. 681.

Administration/Storage

1. For motion sickness, the full prophylactic dose should be given 30 min prior to travel with similar doses with meals and at bedtime.
2. Note if the products contain ammonium chloride or sodium citrate. These ingredients no longer claim to have any effect as an expectorant and are present only as inactive ingredients.

Assessment

1. Note if the client has any allergies to ammonium compounds or sodium citrate. Medications containing these ingredients should be avoided.
2. Determine if the client is on any sodium restrictions. These clients should avoid diphenhydramine if the preparation contains sodium.

EXPECTORANTS

GUAIFENESIN (GLYCERYL GUAIACOLATE)   (gwye-FEN-eh-sin)

Amonidrin, Anti-Tuss, Balminil Expectorant✹, Breonesin, Colrex Expectorant, Cremacoat 2, Gee-Gee, Genatuss, GG-Cen, Glyate, Glycotuss, Glytuss, Guiatuss, Halotussin, Humibid L.A., Humibid Sprinkle, Hytuss, Hytuss-2X, Malotuss, Mytussin, Naldecon Senior EX, Nortussin, Resyl✹, Robafen, Robitussin, Scottussin (OTC)

Classification: Expectorant.

Action/Kinetics: Guaifenesin increases the output of fluid of the respiratory tract by reducing the viscosity and surface tension of respiratory secretions, thereby facilitating their expectoration. Data on efficacy are lacking; however, guaifenesin is an ingredient of many nonprescription cough preparations.

Uses: Dry, nonproductive cough due to colds and minor upper respiratory tract infections.

Contraindications: Chronic cough, cough accompanied by excess secretions.

Side Effects: *GI:* Nausea, vomiting, GI upset. *CNS:* Drowsiness.

Drug Interaction: Inhibition of platelet adhesiveness by guaifenesin may result in bleeding tendencies.

Laboratory Test Interferences: False + urinary 5-hydroxyindoleacetic acid. Color interference with determination of urinary vanillylmandelic acid.

Dosage: Capsules, Oral Solution, Syrup, Tablets. Adults and children over 12 years: 200–400 mg q 4 hr, not to exceed 2.4 g/day; **pediatric, 6–12 years:** 100–200 mg q 4 hr, not to exceed 600 mg/day; **pediatric, 2–6 years:** 50–100 mg q 4 hr, not to exceed 300 mg/day. If less than 2 years of age, the dosage must be individualized by the physician.
  Extended-release Capsules, Extended-release Tablets. Adults and children over 12 years: 600–1,200 mg q 12 hr, not to exceed 2.4 g/day; **pediatric, 6–12 years:** 600 mg q 12 hr, not to exceed 1.2 g/day; **pediatric, 2–6 years:** 300 mg q 12 hr, not to exceed 600 mg/day. *Note:* The liquid dosage forms may be more suitable for children less than 6 years of age.

TERPIN HYDRATE ELIXIR   (TER-pin)
(OTC)

TERPIN HYDRATE AND CODEINE ELIXIR   (TER-pin, KOH-deen)
(C-V, Rx or OTC)

See also *Codeine,* p. 760.

Classification: Antitussive and expectorant.

General Statement: Terpin hydrate is alleged to increase respiratory tract fluid secretion, liquefy sputum, and facilitate expectoration; however, the recommended doses probably do not cause this effect and the FDA does not recommend its use as an expectorant. Terpin hydrate is combined with codeine, a narcotic, which specifically depresses the cough reflex. Terpin hydrate and codeine elixir contains 40% alcohol, 85 mg terpin hydrate, and 10 mg codeine per 5 mL and is subject to federal narcotic regulations.

Use: Symptomatic treatment of cough.

Contraindications: Peptic ulcer and severe diabetes mellitus. Use in children less than 12 years of age due to the high alcohol content of the elixir.

Special Concerns: Use during pregnancy and during lactation only if benefits outweigh risks.

Side Effects: *CNS:* Drowsiness (due to alcohol). *GI:* Epigastric pain if taken on an empty stomach. Also, see *Codeine,* p. 760.

Dosage: Adults.. *Terpin hydrate and codeine elixir,* **PO:** 5 mL q 3–4 hr.

NURSING CONSIDERATIONS

Administration/Storage

Administer with a full glass of water in order to facilitate the loosening of mucus.

Assessment

1. Note any evidence the client may present that would suggest an addiction to any medication, particularly opiates.
2. In taking the client's history, note if the client has complaints that would suggest the presence of a peptic ulcer. This drug should not be given to these clients.
3. If the client has diabetes mellitus, note the severity of his illness. Clients with severe diabetes should not be given this compound.
4. Note any history of alcohol addiction. Terpin hydrate and terpin hydrate and codeine elixir have a high alcohol content.

Interventions

1. Observe the client for undue drowsiness. Document and report. Discuss the amount of drug the client is taking and the frequency since excessive use may lead to oversedation and possibly drug dependence.
2. If the client is hospitalized, do not leave the medication at the bedside. Those on the unit who are alcoholic or drug-dependent would have access to a medication that is contraindicated for them.

Client/Family Teaching

1. Warn the client that excessive use of this medication may lead to oversedation and prolonged use may lead to dependence.
2. Instruct the client to report any epigastric pain to the physician.
3. If purchasing any OTC preparations, check first with the physician, pharmacist or nurse. Avoid drugs that have alcohol as a base.

COMBINATION DRUGS COMMONLY USED FOR COUGHS, COLDS, AND CONGESTION

ACTIFED   (AK-tih-fed)

(OTC)

Classification/Contents: Each capsule or tablet contains: *Antihistamine:* Triprolidine HCl, 2.5 mg. *Decongestant:* Pseudoephedrine HCl, 60 mg. Each 5 mL of the syrup contains one-half the amount of the above drugs, while the 12-Hour Capsule contains twice the amount of the above drugs. Also see information on individual components.

Uses: Treatment of nasal congestion, runny nose, itching of nose or throat, itchy or watery eyes due to the common cold, allergic rhinitis (i.e., hay fever), or other upper respiratory problems.

Dosage: Capsules: One q 4–6, hr not to exceed four capsules daily. Consult physician if capsules are indicated for children under 12 years of age. **Tablets: Adults and children over 12 years of age:** One q 4–6 hr; **pediatric, 6–12 years of age:** ½ tablet q 4–6 hr. Consult physician if tablets are indicated for children under 6 years of age. No more than four doses of the tablets should be given daily. **Syrup: Adults and children over 12 years of age:** 10 mL q 4–6 hr; **pediatric, 6–12 years of age:** 5 mL q 4–6 hr. Consult physician if syrup is indicated for children under 6 years of age. No more than four doses of the syrup should be given daily. **12-Hour Capsules: Adults and children over 12 years of age:** One q 12 hr, not to exceed two capsules daily.

NURSING CONSIDERATIONS

See *Nursing Considerations* for *Antihistamines,* p. 1007, and *Sympathomimetics,* p. 887.

COADVIL   (koh-**AD**-vil)
(OTC)

Classification/Content: Each tablet contains: *Nonsteroidal anti-inflammatory agent:* Ibuprofen, 200 mg. *Decongestant:* Pseudoephedrine HCl, 30 mg. See also information on individual components.

Uses: Temporary relief of symptoms associated with the common cold, flu, or sinusitis including fever, headache, nasal congestion, body aches, and pains.

Contraindications: Patients sensitive to aspirin. Hypertension, heart disease, diabetes, thyroid disease, difficulty in urination due to enlarged prostate. During the last three months of pregnancy. Should not be taken for more than seven days for a cold or for more than three days for fever.

Special Concerns: Use with caution during lactation. Use in children under 12 years of age only on the advice of a physician.

Side Effects: *Higher doses:* Nervousness, dizziness, or sleeplessness. See also individual drugs.

Dosage: Tablets. 1 caplet q 4–6 hr while symptoms persist. If no response, dose can be increased to 2 caplets but the total dose should not exceed 6 caplets in 24 hr, unless directed otherwise by a physician.

NURSING CONSIDERATIONS

See *Nursing Considerations* for *Nonsteroidal Anti-Inflammatory Agents* p. 803, and *Sympathomimetics,* p. 887.

Administration/Storage

The drug can be taken with food or milk if mild heartburn, stomach upset, or stomach pain occurs.

DECONAMINE SYRUP AND TABLETS   (de-**KON**-ah-meen)
(Rx)

DECONAMINE SR CAPSULES   (de-**KON**-ah-meen)
(Rx)

Classification/Content: Syrup. *Antihistamine:* Chlorpheniramine maleate, 2 mg/5 mL and *Decongestant:* Pseudoephedrine sulfate, 30 mg/5 mL. **Tablets.** *Antihistamine:* Chlorpheniramine

maleate, 4 mg and *Decongestant:* Pseudoephedrine sulfate, 60 mg. The SR Capsules contain twice the amount of each drug in each capsule.
See also information on individual components.

Uses: Nasal congestion due to hay fever and other allergies, the common cold, sinusitis, allergic and vasomotor rhinitis, blockage of eustachian tubes.

Special Concerns: Pregnancy category: C.

Dosage: Extended-release Capsules, Syrup, Tablets. Adults and children over 12 years of age: 1 tablet t.i.d.–q.i.d. or 1 SR capsule q 12 hr, or 5–10 mL syrup t.i.d.–q.i.d. **Pediatric, 6–12 years of age:** 2.5–5 mL t.i.d.–q.i.d., not to exceed 20 mL daily; **pediatric, 2–6 years of age:** 2.5 mL t.i.d.–q.i.d., not to exceed 10 mL daily.

NURSING CONSIDERATIONS

See *Nursing Considerations* for *Antihistamines,* p. 1007, and *Sympathomimetics,* p. 887.

DIMETANE DECONGESTANT   (DYE-meh-tayn)
(OTC)

Classification/Content: *Antihistamine:* Brompheniramine maleate, 4 mg/tablet or 2 mg/5 mL elixir. *Decongestant:* Phenylephrine HCl, 10 mg/tablet or 5 mg/5 mL elixir.
Also see information on individual components.

Uses: Relief of symptoms due to the common cold, hay fever, sinusitis or other upper respiratory tract allergies including sneezing, itchy nose or throat, runny nose, itchy and watery eyes.

Dosage: Tablets. Adults and children over 12 years: One tablet q 4 hr not to exceed 6 tablets daily; **pediatric, 6–12 years:** ½ tablet q 4 hr, not to exceed three whole tablets daily. **Elixir. Adults and children over 12 years:** 10 mL q 4 hr, not to exceed 60 mL daily; **pediatric, 6–12 years of age:** 5 mL q 4 hr, not to exceed 30 mL daily.

NURSING CONSIDERATIONS

See *Nursing Considerations* for *Antihistamines,* p. 1003, and *Sympathomimetics,* p. 887.

DIMETAPP ELIXIR AND TABLETS   (DYE-meh-tap)
(OTC)

Classification/Content: Each tablet contains: *Antihistamine:* Brompheniramine maleate, 4 mg. *Decongestant:* Phenylpropanolamine HCl, 25 mg. The long-acting tablets contain three times the amount of the drugs while 5 mL of the elixir contains one-half the amount of the drugs.
See also information on individual components.

Uses: Relief of symptoms due to the common cold, hay fever, sinusitis, or other upper respiratory tract allergies including sneezing, itchy nose or throat, runny nose, or itchy and watery eyes.

Dosage: Tablets. Adults and children over 12 years: One tablet q 4 hr; **pediatric, 6–12 years:** ½ tablet q 4 hr. Dosage should not exceed six tablets daily. **Long-acting tablets. Adults and**

children over 12 years: One tablet q 12 hr, not to exceed two tablets in a 24-hr period. **Elixir. Adults and children over 12 years:** 10 mL q 4 hr, not to exceed 60 mL daily; **pediatric, 6–12 years:** 5 mL q 4 hr, not to exceed 30 mL daily. Consult physician if elixir is indicated in children less than 6 years of age.

NURSING CONSIDERATIONS
See *Nursing Considerations* for *Antihistamines,* p. 1007, and *Sympathomimetics,* p. 887.

DRIXORAL   (drix-**OR**-al)
(OTC)

Classification/Content: *Antihistamine:* Brompheniramine maleate, 2 mg/5 mL elixir or 6 mg/ sustained-release tablet. *Decongestant:* Pseudoephedrine sulfate, 30 mg/5 mL elixir or 120 mg/ sustained-release tablet.
See also information on individual components.

Uses: Symptoms of the common cold, allergic rhinitis (i.e., hay fever), or other upper respiratory allergies with symptoms of nasal congestion, runny nose, sneezing, itchy nose or throat, itchy and watery eyes.

Dosage: Sustained-release Tablets. Adults and children over 12 years: One tablet q 12 hr, not to exceed 2 tablets in 24 hr. **Syrup. Adults and children over 12 years:** 10 mL q 4–6 hr; **pediatric, 6–12 years:** 5 mL q 4–6 hr. No more than four doses should be given in 24 hr.

NURSING CONSIDERATIONS
See *Nursing Considerations* for *Antihistamines,* p. 1007, and *Sympathomimetic Drugs,* p. 887.

ENTEX LA   (EN-tex)
(Rx)

Classification/Content: *Expectorant:* Guaifenesin, 400 mg. *Decongestant:* Phenylpropanolamine HCl, 75 mg.
See also information on individual components.

Uses: Nasal congestion and viscous mucus in the lower respiratory tract accompanying bronchitis, sinusitis, pharyngitis, coryza.

Special Concerns: Pregnancy category: C.

Dosage: Tablets. Adults and children over 12 years: 1 tablet q 12 hr; **children, 6–12 years:** one-half tablet q 12 hr. Not recommended for children under 6 years of age.

NURSING CONSIDERATIONS
See *Nursing Considerations* for *Sympathomimetics,* p. 887.

Administration/Storage
Tablets should not be crushed or chewed before swallowing.

HYCODAN SYRUP AND TABLETS   (HI-koh-dan)

(Rx) (C-III)

Classification/Content: Each tablet or 5 mL contains: *Antitussive, narcotic:* hydrocodone bitartrate, 5 mg; *anticholinergic:* homatropine methylbromide, 1.5 mg.

See also information on narcotic analgesics, p. 750, and cholinergic blocking drugs, p. 942.

Uses: Relief of symptoms of cough.

Dosage: Syrup, Tablets. Adults and children over 12 years: 1 tablet or 5 mL after meals and at bedtime. **Pediatric, 2–12 years:** ½ tablet or 2.5 mL after meals and at bedtime; **pediatric, less than 2 years:** ¼ tablet or 1.25 mL after meals and at bedtime.

NURSING CONSIDERATIONS

See also *Nursing Considerations* for *Cholinergic Blocking Agents*, p. 949, and *Narcotic Analgesics*, p. 753.

Administration/Storage

1. The single maximum dose of medication for adults is 3 tablets or 15 mL of syrup after meals and at bedtime.
2. For children over 12 years of age, the maximum dosage is 2 tablets or 10 mL of syrup after meals and at bedtime.
3. For children 2–12 years of age, the maximum dosage is 1 tablet or 5 mL of syrup after meals and at bedtime.
4. For children less than 2 years old, the maximum dosage is ¼ tablet or 1.25 mL of syrup after meals and at bedtime.
5. Doses should be taken at least 4 hr apart.

Client/Family Teaching

1. Caution that the drug may cause drowsiness and/or dizziness. Advise client to avoid tasks that require mental alertness, such as operating machinery or driving a car.
2. Instruct the client to notify the physician if symptoms persist or intensify.
3. Explain that the drug may be habit-forming if used over a prolonged period of time.

NALDECON SYRUP AND TABLETS   (NAL-dek-on)

(Rx)

Classification/Content: Each sustained action tablet contains the following (one-half for immediate release and one-half for delayed action):
Antihistamine: Chlorpheniramine maleate, 5 mg.
Decongestant: Phenylpropanolamine HCl, 40 mg.
Decongestant: Phenylephrine HCl, 10 mg.
Antihistamine: Phenyltoloxamine citrate, 15 mg.
Note: The syrup contains one-half the amount of the above components in each 5 mL, whereas the pediatric syrup (in each 5 mL) and pediatric drops (in each 1 mL) contain chlorpheniramine

maleate, 0.5 mg; phenylpropanolamine HCl, 5 mg; phenylephrine HCl, 1.25 mg; and phenyltoloxamine citrate, 2 mg.

Uses: Nasal congestion and eustachian tube congestion observed with the common cold, acute upper respiratory tract infections, or sinusitis. Also, seasonal allergic rhinitis or vasomotor rhinitis. Also used to relieve eustachian tube congestion associated with serous otitis media, acute eustachian salpingitis, or aerotitis.

Special Concerns: Pregnancy category: C.

Dosage: Pediatric Drops and Syrup, Syrup, Tablets. Adults and children over 12 years: 1 tablet on arising, in midafternoon, and at bedtime; or 5 mL syrup q 3–4 hr not to exceed 4 doses daily. **Pediatric, 6–12 years:** 10 mL pediatric syrup q 3–4 hr, not to exceed 4 doses daily; **1–6 years:** 5 mL pediatric syrup or 1 mL pediatric drops q 3–4 hr, not to exceed 4 doses daily; **6–12 months:** 2.5 mL pediatric syrup or 0.5 mL pediatric drops q 3–4 hr, not to exceed 4 doses daily; **3–6 months:** 0.25 mL pediatric drops q 3–4 hr, not to exceed 4 doses daily.

NURSING CONSIDERATIONS

See *Nursing Considerations* for *Antihistamines,* p. 1007, and *Sympathomimetics,* p. 887.

NOVAHISTINE ELIXIR   (no-vah-**HISS**-teen)
(OTC)

Classification/Content: *Antihistamine:* Chlorpheniramine maleate, 2 mg/5 mL. *Decongestant:* Phenylephrine HCl, 5 mg/5 mL.
   See also information on individual components.

Uses: To treat congestion of the nose and eustachian tubes manifested by hay fever, the common cold, and sinusitis. Also useful for relief of other symptoms (e.g., runny nose, sneezing, itchy nose and throat, water eyes) due to hay fever or the common cold.

Dosage: Elixir. Adults: 10 mL q 4 hr; **pediatric, 6–12 years:** 5 mL q 4 hr; **pediatric, 2–6 years:** 2.5 mL q 4 hr. Use only on advice of physician if child is less than 2 years of age.

NURSING CONSIDERATIONS

See *Nursing Considerations* for *Antihistamines,* p. 1007, and *Sympathomimetics,* p. 887.

ORNADE   (OR-nayd)
(Rx)

Classification/Content: *Antihistamine:* Chlorpheniramine maleate, 12 mg. *Decongestant:* Phenylpropanolamine HCl, 75 mg.
   See also information on individual components.

Uses: Symptoms of allergic rhinitis or the common cold including runny nose, nasal congestion, sneezing, itching throat or nose, itchy and watery eyes.

Special Concerns: Pregnancy category: B.

Dosage: Capsules. Adults and children over 12 years: One capsule q 12 hr. Not to be used in children under 12 years of age.

NURSING CONSIDERATIONS

See *Nursing Considerations* for *Antihistamines,* p. 1007, and *Synpathomimetics,* p. 887.

PHENERGAN WITH CODEINE SYRUP   (FEN-er-gan, KOH-deen)
(Rx) (C-V)

Classification/Content: *Antihistamine:* Promethazine HCl, 6.25 mg/5 mL. *Antitussive, narcotic:* Codeine phosphate, 10 mg/5 mL.
   See also information on individual components.

Uses: Relief of coughs and other upper respiratory tract problems associated with the common cold or with allergy.

Special Concerns: Pregnancy category: C.

Dosage: Syrup. Adults: 5 mL q 4–6 hr, not to exceed 30 mL daily; **pediatric, 6–12 years:** 2.5–5 mL q 4–6 hr, not to exceed 30 mL daily; **pediatric, less than 6 years:** 0.25–0.5 mL q 4–6 hr. Not recommended for children under 2 years of age.

NURSING CONSIDERATIONS

See *Nursing Considerations* for *Antihistamines,* p. 1007, and *Codeine,* p. 887.

Administration/Storage

The maximum daily dose of medication for children between 2 and 6 years of age depends on body weight. The amount of drug administered should not exceed:
- 9 mL for 18 kg of body weight, or
- 8 mL for 16 kg of body weight, or
- 7 mL for 14 kg of body weight, or
- 6 mL for 12 kg of body weight.

Assessment

Take a thorough nursing history to determine how long the client has had the symptoms and whether or not the problem may be related to an allergy.

Client/Family Teaching
1. Instruct the client to notify the physician if the symptoms persist or intensify.
2. Advise that constipation may be a side effect of the medication therapy. To avoid the problem, instruct the client to drink approximately 2,500 cc of fluid per day and to include additional roughage in the diet.
3. Explain that the drug may be habit-forming and is not for long-term indiscriminate use.

PHENERGAN WITH DEXTROMETHORPHAN SYRUP   (FEN-er-gan, dex-troh-meth-OR-fan)
(Rx)

Classification/Content: *Antihistamine:* Promethazine HCl, 6.25 mg/5 mL. *Nonnarcotic antitussive:*

Dextromethorphan HCl, 15 mg/5 mL.

Uses: To treat symptoms of cough and upper respiratory problems observed with the common cold and allergies.

Special Concerns: Pregnancy category: C.

Dosage: Syrup. Adults: 5 mL q 4–6 hr, not to exceed 30 mL daily. **Pediatric, 6–12 years:** 2.5–5 mL q 4–6 hr, not to exceed 20 mL daily; **2–6 years:** 1.25–2.5 mL q 4–6 hr, not to exceed 10 mL daily. This product is not recommended for children under 2 years of age.

NURSING CONSIDERATIONS

See *Nursing Considerations* for *Antihistamines* p. 1007, and *Dextromethorphan,* p. 983.

PHENERGAN VC SYRUP   (FEN-er-gan)

PHENERGAN VC WITH CODEINE SYRUP   (FEN-er-gan, KOH-deen)
(C-V) (Rx)

Classification/Content: Phenergan VC contains the following: *Antihistamine:* Promethazine HCl, 6.25 mg/5 mL. *Decongestant:* Phenylephrine HCl, 5 mg/5 mL. Phenergan VC with Codeine contains the above plus: *Narcotic antitussive:* Codeine phosphate, 10 mg/5 mL.

Uses: Phenergan VC: Nasal congestion accompanying allergy or the common cold. Phenergan VC with Codeine: Cough and nasal congestion accompanying allergy or the common cold.

Special Concerns: Pregnancy category: C.

Dosage: *Phenergan VC Syrup, Phenergan VC with Codeine Syrup.* **PO. Adults:** 5 mL q 4–6 hr, not to exceed 30 mL daily. **Pediatric, 6–12 years:** 2.5–5 mL q 4–6 hr not to exceed 30 mL daily; **2–6 years:** 1.25–2.5 mL q 4–6 hr (the maximum daily dose of Phenergan VC with Codeine ranges from 6 to 9 mL depending on the body weight). These products are not recommended for children under 2 years of age.

NURSING CONSIDERATIONS

See *Nursing Considerations* for *Antihistamines,* p. 1007, and *Phenergan with Codeine syrup,* p. 992, and *Codeine,* p. 761.

ROBITUSSIN-AC   (roh-bih-TUSS-in)
(C-V) (Rx)

Classification/Content: *Expectorant:* Guaifenesin, 100 mg/5 mL. *Antitussive:* Codeine phosphate, 10 mg/5 mL.
See also information on individual components.

Uses: Coughs associated with bronchitis, the common cold, laryngitis, pharyngitis, pertussis, tracheitis, flu, and measles.

Contraindications: Use with caution in patients with chronic coughs.

Laboratory Test Interferences: Guaifenesin may interfere with determination of 5-hydroxyin-doleacetic acid (5-HIAA) or vanillylmandelic acid (VMA).

Dosage: Syrup. Adults and children over 12 years: 10 mL q 4 hr, not to exceed 60 mL daily; **pediatric, 6–12 years:** 5 mL q 4 hr, not to exceed 30 mL daily; **pediatric, 2–6 years:** 2.5 mL q 4 hr, not to exceed 15 mL daily. Should not be used in children less than 2 years of age.

NURSING CONSIDERATIONS

See also *Nursing Considerations* for *Narcotic Analgesics,* p. 753.

Assessment

Review the client history. If the cough is chronic, the drug is contraindicated.

Client/Family Teaching

1. Instruct the client to take only as directed and to notify the physician if symptoms persist or intensify.
2. Constipation may occur with drug therapy. Advise the client to drink between 2,500 and 3,000 cc of fluid per day and to increase intake of fruits, grains, and other high-fiber foods. If the problem persists a stool softener may be recommended. If the stool softener is not effective, report to the physician. Other reasons for the constipation may then need to be ruled out.
3. Advise the client that the drug may be habit-forming.

ROBITUSSIN-CF   (roh-bih-**TUSS**-in)
(OTC)

ROBITUSSIN-DM   (roh-bih-**TUSS**-in)
(OTC)

ROBITUSSIN-PE   (roh-bih-**TUSS**-in)
(OTC)

Classification/Content: Robitussin-CF. *Expectorant:* Guaifenesin, 100 mg/5 mL; *Decongestant:* Phenylpropanolamine HCl, 12.5 mg/5 mL; and, *Antitussive:* Dextromethorphan HBr, 10 mg/5 mL.
Robitussin-DM. *Expectorant:* Guaifenesin, 100 mg/5 mL and *Antitussive:* Dextromethorphan HBr, 15 mg/5 mL.
Robitussin-PE. *Expectorant:* Guaifenesin, 100 mg/5 mL and *Decongestant:* Pseudoephedrine HCl, 30 mg/5 mL.
See also information on individual components.

Uses: Coughs associated with bronchitis, laryngitis, pharyngitis, the common cold, flu, pertussis, tracheitis, and measles. Robitussin-CF is indicated for coughs with congestion and irritating cough; Robitussin-DM is indicated for irritating coughs; and Robitussin-PE is indicated for coughs with congestion.

Contraindications: Products containing sympathomimetic decongestants should be used with caution in patients with hypertension, diabetes, cardiac disorders, peripheral vascular disease, glaucoma, prostatic hypertrophy.

Laboratory Test Interferences: Guaifenesin may interfere with determination of 5-hydroxyindoleacetic acid (5-HIAA) and vanillylmandelic acid (VMA).

Dosage: Robitussin-CF Syrup. Adults and children over 12 years: 10 mL q 4 hr, not to exceed 60 mL daily; **pediatric, 6–12 years:** 5 mL q 4 hr, not to exceed 30 mL daily; **pediatric, 2–6 years:** 2.5 mL q 4 hr, not to exceed 15 mL daily.
   Robitussin-DM Syrup. Adults and children over 12 years: 10 mL q 6–8 hr, not to exceed 40 mL daily; **pediatric, 6–12 years:** 5 mL q 6–8 hr, not to exceed 20 mL daily; **pediatric, 2–6 years:** 2.5 mL q 6–8 hr, not to exceed 10 mL daily.
   Robitussin-PE Syrup. Adults and children over 12 years: 10 mL q 4 hr, not to exceed 40 mL daily; **pediatric, 6–12 years:** 5 mL q 4 hr, not to exceed 20 mL daily; **pediatric, 2–6 years:** 2.5 mL q 4 hr, not to exceed 10 mL daily.
   None of these products should be used in children under 2 years of age.

NURSING CONSIDERATIONS

See also *Nursing Considerations* for *Sympathomimetics,* p. 887, and *Dextromethophan*, p. 983.

Assessment

1. Note if the client has a history of hypertension, cardiac disease or peripheral vascular disorders. The drug is contraindicated in these conditions.
2. Determine if the client has diabetes mellitus and document. Syrups and other drugs in this class may upset blood sugar levels and alter the amount of hypoglycemic agent required for adequate control.
3. When working with elderly male clients, discuss any possible problems they may have with urinary output or knowledge the client may have of prostatic hypertrophy and document.

RONDEC-DM ORAL DROPS   (RON-dec)
(Rx)

RONDEC-DM SYRUP   (RON-dec)
(Rx)

Classification/Content: *Antitussive:* Dextromethorphan HBr, 4 mg/mL Oral Drops or 15 mg/5 mL Syrup. *Decongestant:* Pseudoephedrine HCl, 25 mg/mL Oral Drops or 60 mg/5 mL Syrup. *Antihistamine:* Carbinoxamine maleate, 2 mg/mL Oral Drops or 4 mg/5 mL Syrup.
   See also information on individual components.

Uses: Treatment of coughs, nasal congestion, and other upper respiratory tract symptoms due to the common cold or allergy.

Contraindications: Safe use during pregnancy has not been established.

Dosage: Syrup. Adults and children over 6 years: 5 mL q.i.d.; **children 18 months–6 years:** 2.5 mL q.i.d. **Oral Drops. Pediatric, 9–18 months:** 1 mL q.i.d.; **6–9 months:** 0.75 mL q.i.d.; **3–6 months:** 0.5 mL q.i.d.; **1–3 months:** 0.25 mL q.i.d.

NURSING CONSIDERATIONS

See also *Nursing Considerations* for *Antihistamines* p. 1007, *Dextromethorphan,* p. 983, and *Sympathominetics*, p. 887.

Assessment

If female is sexually active and of childbearing age, determine if she is pregnant. Safe use of drug during pregnancy has not been established.

RYNATAN   (RYE-nat-an)
(Rx)

Classification/Content: *Antihistamine:* Chlorpheniramine tannate, 8 mg (tablet) or 2 mg (per 5 mL suspension). *Antihistamine:* Pyrilamine tannate, 25 mg (tablet) or 12.5 mg (per 5 mL suspension). *Decongestant:* Phenylephrine tannate, 25 mg (tablet) or 5 mg (per 5 mL suspension).
See also information on individual components.

Uses: Nasal congestion and runny nose due to upper respiratory tract conditions including the common cold, allergic rhinitis, and sinusitis.

Special Concerns: Pregnancy category: C.

Dosage: Oral Suspension Tablets. Adults: 1–2 tablets q 12 hr. **Pediatric, over 6 years:** 5–10 mL of the suspension q 12 hr; **pediatric, 2–6 years:** 2.5–5 mL of the suspension q 12 hr. The dose should be carefully individualized in children under 2 years of age.

NURSING CONSIDERATIONS

See *Nursing Considerations* for *Antihistamines,* p. 1007, and *Sympathominetics,* p. 887.

TAVIST-D   (TAV-ist)
(Rx)

Classification/Content: *Antihistamine:* Clemastine fumarate, 1.34 mg. *Decongestant:* Phenylpropanolamine HCl, 75 mg.
The clemastine is formulated in the outer shell of the tablet and is released immediately. The phenylpropanolamine component is incorporated into a sustained-release matrix, which releases the drug over a period of 12 hr; the slow release achieves blood levels equivalent to those achieved by giving 25 mg phenylpropanolamine q 4 hr for 3 doses.
See also information on individual components.

Uses: To treat symptoms of allergic rhinitis (i.e., hay fever) including nasal congestion; sneezing; itchy eyes, nose, or throat; runny nose or eyes.

Special Concerns: Pregnancy category: B.

Dosage: Tablets. Adults and children over 12 years: One tablet (taken whole) q 12 hr.

NURSING CONSIDERATIONS

See *Nursing Considerations* for *Antihistamines,* p. 1007, and *Sympathominetics,* p. 887.

Client/Family Teaching

Instruct the client not to break tablets or crush them, but to take tablets whole. This permits the specially designed release system to remain intact.

TEDRAL ELIXIR, SUSPENSION, AND TABLETS   (TED-ral)

(OTC)

TEDRAL SA TABLETS   (TED-ral)

(Rx)

Classification/Content: *Sympathomimetic bronchodilator:* Theophylline anhydrous, 29.5 mg/5 mL (Elixir), 59.1 mg/5 mL (Suspension), 118 mg (Tablets) or 180 mg (SA Tablets). *Sympathomimetic bronchodilator:* Ephedrine HCl, 6 mg/5 mL (Elixir), 12 mg/5 mL (Suspension), 24 mg (Tablets) or 48 mg (SA Tablets). *Sedative:* Phenobarbital, 2 mg/5 mL (Elixir), 4 mg/5 mL (Suspension), 8 mg (Tablets) or 25 mg (SA Tablets).

See also information on individual components.

Uses: Adjunct in the treatment of bronchial asthma, asthmatic bronchitis, or other bronchial disorders. Prophylactically to prevent or minimize incidence of asthmatic attacks. Treatment of occasional, seasonal, or perennial asthma.

Dosage: Elixir. Adults, 15–30 mL q 4 hr; **pediatric:** 5 mL/30 lb body weight q 4–6 hr. **Suspension. Adults,** 10–20 mL q 4 hr; **pediatric:** 5 mL/60 lb body weight q 4–6 hr. **Tablets. Adults:** 1–2 tablets q 4 hr; **children (6–12 years:)** ½–1 tablet q 4 hr. **SA Tablets. Adults,** One tablet on arising and one 12 hr later.

NURSING CONSIDERATIONS

See *Special Nursing Considerations For Adrenergic Bronchodilators* under *Sympathomimetic Drugs,* p. 887, *Theophylline,* p. 973, and *Barbiturates,* p. 585.

Administration/Storage

1. The Elixir and Suspension should be administered to children under 2 years of age with extreme caution.
2. SA Tablets are not indicated for children under 12 years of age.
3. Tablets should not be chewed.
4. If the medication is in suspension form, the container should be shaken well before administering.

Assessment

If the client is receiving the drug to treat asthma, note the extent and severity of asthma attacks. Also, document the compounds that have been used with positive clinical results prior to this drug therapy.

TRINALIN   (TRIN-al-in)

Classification/Content: *Antihistamine:* Azatadine maleate, 1 mg. *Decongestant:* Pseudoephedrine sulfate, 120 mg.

See also information on individual components.

Action/Kinetics: The tablet is formulated so that the azatadine and one-half of the pseudo-ephedrine are released immediately; the remaining one-half of the pseudoephedrine is released after several hours.

Uses: Symptoms of allergic rhinitis and perennial rhinitis, including nasal and eustachian tube congestion.

Additional Contraindications: Children under 12 years of age.

Special Concerns: Pregnancy category: C.

Dosage: Tablets. Adults: One tablet b.i.d.

NURSING CONSIDERATIONS

See also *Nursing Considerations* for *Antihistamines,* p. 1007, and *Sympathomimetics,* p. 887.

Administration/Storage

1. Trinalin may be used in conjunction with other analgesics and/or antibiotics.
2. Do not administer to children under 12 years of age.

TUSSIONEX CAPSULES, SUSPENSION, AND TABLETS   (TUSS-ee-oh-nex)

(Rx) (C-III)

Classification/Content: Each capsule, tablet, or 5 mL of suspension contains: *Narcotic antitussive:* Hydrocodone, 5 mg. *Nonnarcotic antitussive:* Phenyltoloxamine, 10 mg.
   See also *Narcotic Analgesics,* p. 750.

Uses: Antitussive.

Dosage: Capsules, Suspension, Tablets. Adults: 1 capsule, tablet, or 5 mL of suspension q 8–2 hr. **Pediatric, over 5 years:** 5 mL q 12 hr; **pediatric, 1–5 years:** 2.5 mL of the suspension q 12 hr; **infants, less than 1 year:** 1.25 mL of the suspension q 12 hr.

NURSING CONSIDERATIONS

See also *Nursing Considerations* for *Narcotic Analgesics,* p. 753.

Client/Family Teaching

1. Advise the client to notify the physician if the symptoms persist or intensify.
2. Explain that the drug may be habit-forming if it is used for long periods of time.

TUSSI-ORGANIDIN   (TUSS-ee-or-GAN-ih-din)

(C-V) (Rx)

TUSSI-ORGANIDIN DM   (TUSS-ee-or-GAN-ih-din)

(Rx)

Classification/Content: Each 5 mL of Tussi-Organidin contains: *Mucolytic/expectorant:* Iodinated glycerol, 30 mg. *Narcotic antitussive:* Codeine phosphate, 10 mg. Each 5 mL of Tussi-Organidin DM contains: *Mucolytic/expectorant:* Iodinated glycerol, 30 mg. *Nonnarcotic antitussive:* Dextromethorphan, 10 mg.

See also information on *Narcotic Analgesics,* p. 750, and *Dextromethorphan,* p. 982.

Uses: Relief of irritating, nonproductive cough due to a variety of respiratory tract problems including the common cold, chronic bronchitis, bronchial asthma, tracheobronchitis, laryngitis, pharyngitis, pertussis, emphysema, and croup.

Special Concerns: Pregnancy category: X.

Dosage: Liquid. Adults: 5–10 mL q 4 hr; **pediatric:** 2.5–5 mL q 4 hr.

NURSING CONSIDERATIONS

See also *Nursing Considerations* for *Narcotic Analgesics,* p. 753, and *Dextromethorphan,* p. 983.

Assessment

1. Tussi-Organidin contains codeine. Therefore, assess the client for any history of drug addiction.
2. Determine how long the client has had the cough, the length of time he has had an infection of the upper respiratory tract and what the client has done to correct the problems.

Client/Family Teaching

1. Instruct the client to notify the physician if the symptoms persist beyond a week or 10 days and/or intensify.
2. Explain that the drug may be habit-forming and is not for long-term indiscriminate use.
3. Constipation may develop as a side effect of therapy. Advise the client to drink 2,500–3,000 cc of fluid per day and to increase the intake of fruits, fruit juices and grains as a preventive action.

TUSS-ORNADE CAPSULES AND LIQUID   (TUSS-OR-nayd)

(Rx)

Classification/Content: *Antihistamine:* Caramiphen edisylate, 40 mg (Capsule) or 6.7 mg/5 mL (Liquid). *Decongestant:* Phenylpropanolamine HCl, 75 mg (Capsule) or 12.5 mg/5 mL (Liquid).
See also information on individual components.

Uses: Nasal congestion and cough due to the common cold.

Contraindications: Use during pregnancy only if benefits outweigh risks.

Dosage: Capsules. Adults and children over 12 years, One capsule q 12 hr. **Liquid. Adults and children over 12 years of age:** 10 mL q 4 hr; **pediatric, 6–12 years:** 5 mL q 4 hr, not to exceed 30 mL daily; **pediatric, 2–6 years:** 2.5 mL q 4 hr, not to exceed 15 mL daily.

NURSING CONSIDERATIONS

See also *Nursing Considerations* for *Antihistamines,* p. 1007, and *Sympathomimetics,* p. 887.

Administration/Storage

1. The capsules should not be used in children who are under 12 years of age.

2. The liquid should not be used for children who are under 6 months of age or who weigh less than 15 lb.

3. Pregnant women should avoid using the drug.

MUCOLYTIC

ACETYLCYSTEINE (ah-see-till-SISS-teen)

Airbron✿, Mucomyst, Mucosol (Rx)

Classification: Mucolytic.

General Statement: Acetylcysteine reduces the viscosity of purulent and nonprurulent pulmonary secretions and facilitates their removal by splitting disulfide bonds. Action increases with increasing pH (peak: pH 7–9). **Onset, inhalation:** Within 1 min; **by direct instillation:** immediate. **Time to peak effect:** 5–10 min.

Uses: Adjunct in the treatment of acute and chronic bronchitis, emphysema, tuberculosis, pneumonia, bronchiectasis, atelectasis. Routine care of patients with tracheostomy, pulmonary complications after thoracic or cardiovascular surgery, or in posttraumatic chest conditions. Pulmonary complications of cystic fibrosis. Diagnostic bronchial asthma. Antidote in acetaminophen poisoning to reduce hepatotoxicity. *Investigational:* As an ophthalmic solution for dry eye.

Contraindications: Sensitivity to drug.

Special Concerns: Pregnancy category: B. Use with caution during lactation, in the elderly, and in patients with asthma.

Side Effects: *Respiratory:* Acetylcysteine increases the incidence of bronchospasm in patients with asthma. The drug may also increase the amount of liquefied bronchial secretions, which must be removed by suction if cough is inadequate. Bronchial and tracheal irritation, tightness in chest, bronchoconstriction. *GI:* Nausea, vomiting, stomatitis. *Other:* Rashes, fever, drowsiness, rhinorrhea.

Drug Interactions: Acetylcysteine is incompatible with antibiotics and should be administered separately.

Dosage: Nebulization, direct application, or direct intratracheal instillation using 10% or 20% solution. *Nebulization into face mask, tracheostomy, mouth piece:* 1–10 mL of 20% solution or 2–10 mL of 10% solution 3 to 4 times daily. *Closed tent or croupette:* 300 mL of 10% or 20% solution per treatment. *Direct instillation into tracheostomy:* 1–2 mL of 10–20% solution every 1 to 4 hr. *Percutaneous intratracheal catheter:* 1–2 mL of 20% solution or 2–4 mL of 10% solution q 1–4 hr by syringe attached to catheter. *Instillation to particular portion of bronchopulmonary tree using small plastic catheter into the trachea:* 2–5 mL of 20% solution instilled into the trachea by means of a syringe connected to a catheter. *Diagnostic procedures:* 2 to 3 doses of 1–2 mL of 20% or 2–4 mL of 10% solution by nebulization or intratracheal instillation before the procedure. *Acetaminophen overdosage:* **PO, initial,** 140 mg/kg; **then,** 70 mg/kg q 4 hr for a total of 17 doses.

NURSING CONSIDERATIONS

Administration/ Storage

1. Use nonreactive plastic, glass, or stainless steel equipment for administration.
2. The 10% solution may be used undiluted.
3. Use either water for injection or saline to dilute the 20% solution.
4. Administer the medication via face mask, face tent, oxygen tent, head tent, or by positive pressure breathing machine as indicated.
5. Administer with compressed air for nebulization. Hand nebulizers are contraindicated.
6. After prolonged nebulization, dilute the last fourth of the medication with sterile water for injection to prevent concentration of the medication.
7. The solution may develop a light purple color. This does not affect the action of the medication.
8. Closed bottles of solution remain stable for 2 years when stored at 20°C. Open bottles should be stored at 2°C–8°C and should be used within 96 hr. Once a bottle has been opened, record the time and date of opening so that the drug will not be used beyond the 96-hr period.
9. Acetylcysteine is incompatible with antibiotics and must be administered separately.
10. Have a suction machine at the bedside and an endotracheal tube available.

Assessment

1. Determine from the client and history when bronchial spasms occur.
2. Discuss the conditions that are likely to cause congestion and wheezing and document.
3. Identify the treatments that have been successful in treating these conditions in the past and those that have failed.
4. Determine if the client is currently taking any antibiotic medications.

Interventions

1. If bronchospasm occurs, have a bronchodilator such as isoproterenol for aerosol inhalation available for use.
2. Position the client to facilitate the removal of secretions.
3. If the client is unable to cough up secretions, provide mechanical suction for their removal.
4. Advise the client that the nauseous odor that is present when the treatment begins will likely become less noticeable.
5. Monitor vital signs, intake and output.
6. Wash the client's face following nebulization treatment. The medication may cause the face to be sticky.

CHAPTER FIFTY-ONE
Histamine and Antihistamines

Histamine

Antihistamines (H₁ Blockers)

HISTAMINE

General Statement: Histamine is stored in almost every type of tissue in the body; to date, however, the pharmacologic importance of histamine rests primarily on the suppression of its action by various histamine receptor blockers (antihistamines). Appropriate stimuli, including tissue injury, antigen-antibody (allergic) reactions, and extreme cold trigger the release of histamine from its storage sites into the vascular system, where it induces the following responses.

1. Dilation and increased permeability of the small arterioles, capillaries, and precapillaries, which result in increased permeability to fluid. This causes a fall of blood pressure in humans. The outflow of fluid into the subcutaneous spaces results in edema. The local edema in the nasal mucosa caused by histamine is responsible for the nasal congestion associated with allergies. It may also cause laryngeal edema.
2. Contraction of some smooth muscles such as those in the bronchioles; the resulting broncho-constriction is believed to account for the role histamine plays in bronchial asthma. Histamine also causes the uterus to contract.
3. Stimulation of acid secretion in the stomach. It is used diagnostically to stimulate the gastric glands to test gastric function. It also increases bronchial, intestinal, and mild salivary secretions.
4. Dilation of cerebral vessels and small doses can cause an intense headache.
5. Pain and itch, because it stimulates the sensory nerve endings.

Action/Kinetics: Upon release, histamine interacts with specific histamine receptors currently subdivided into H_1 receptors and H_2 receptors. Bronchoconstriction and intestinal motility are controlled by H_1 receptors, whereas gastric secretion involves H_2 receptors. Other processes in which histamine has a role, such as hypotension resulting from vascular dilation, involve both H_1 and H_2 receptors. When administered, onset is rapid and duration is transient.

Uses: Diagnostic aid for assessment of gastric acid secretory function.

Contraindications: Severe cardiac disease, hypotension, hypertension, impaired renal function, bronchial disease, history of urticaria, vasomotor instability, pheochromocytoma.

Special Concerns: Pregnancy category: C.

Side Effects: *CV:* Hypotension, hypertension, tachycardia, flushing or redness of face. *Respiratory:* Difficulty in breathing, chest discomfort or pain. *GI:* Severe vomiting, severe diarrhea, abdominal cramps or spasms, nausea, metallic taste. *CNS:* Nervousness, seizures. *Miscellaneous:* Headache (due to dilation of cerebral vessels), hives, skin rash, bluish coloration of face, blurred vision.

Dosage: SC. *Diagnosis of gastric acid function:* **Adults,** 0.0275 mg/kg given after collection of basal gastric secretion.

NURSING CONSIDERATIONS

Interventions

1. Advise client that no food should be ingested for 12 hr before the histamine test is given.
2. Remind client that saliva should not be swallowed during the histamine test.
3. In the event of a severe hypotensive response, have epinephrine available.
4. Pulse rate and blood pressure should be determined immediately following injection of histamine and monitored until stabilized.

ANTIHISTAMINES (H_1 BLOCKERS)

51

Action/Kinetics: The effects of histamine may be reversed either by drugs that block histamine receptors (antihistamines) or by drugs that have effects opposite to those of histamine (e.g., epinephrine). Antihistamines used for the treatment of allergic conditions are referred to as *H_1-receptor blockers* while antihistamines used for the treatment of GI disorders (e.g., peptic ulcer) are referred to as *H_2-receptor blockers* (see *Cimetidine, Famotidine, Nizatidine,* and *Ranitidine,* Chapter 53, p. 1044).

Antihistamines do not prevent the release of histamine; rather, they compete with histamine for histamine receptors (competitive inhibition), thus preventing or reversing the effects of histamine. Antihistamines prevent or reduce increased capillary permeability (i.e., decrease edema, itching) and bronchospasms. Allergic reactions unrelated to histamine release are not affected by antihistamines.

The H_1-blockers manifest varying degrees of CNS depression, as well as anticholinergic, antiemetic, and antiserotonin effects.

From a chemical point of view, the antihistamines can be divided into the following classes.

1. **Ethylenediamine Derivatives.** This group manifests low to moderate sedative effects and almost no anticholinergic or antiemetic activity. They frequently cause GI distress. Available agents: pyrilamine, tripelennamine.
2. **Ethanolamine Derivatives.** This group is most likely to cause CNS depression (drowsiness).

There is a low incidence of GI side effects. There are significant anticholinergic and antiemetic effects. Available agents: carbinoxamine, clemastine, diphenhydramine.

3. **Alkylamines.** Members of this group are among the most potent antihistamines. They are effective at relatively low dosage and are most suitable agents for daytime use. This group manifests minimal sedation, moderate anticholinergic effects, and no antiemetic effects. Paradoxical excitation may also occur. Individual response to agents is variable. Available agents: brompheniramine, chlorpheniramine, dexchlorpheniramine, triprolidine.

4. **Phenothiazines.** These agents possess significant antihistaminic action, varying degrees of sedation, and a high degree of both anticholinergic and antiemetic effects. Available agents: methdilazine, promethazine, trimeprazine.

5. **Piperidines.** Members of this group have prolonged antihistaminic activity, with a comparatively low incidence of drowsiness, moderate anticholinergic activity, and no antiemetic effects. Available agents: azatadine, cyproheptadine, diphenylpyraline, phenindamine.

6. **Miscellaneous.** The two drugs in this group are specific in that they bind to peripheral rather than central H_1 histamine receptors. They have no sedative, anticholinergic, or antiemetic effects. Available agents: astemizole, terfenadine.

The kinetics of most antihistamines are similar. **Onset:** 15–30 min; **peak:** 1–2 hr; **duration:** 4–6 hr (piperidines have a longer duration). Many antihistamines are available as timed-release preparations. Most antihistamines are metabolized by the liver and excreted in the urine.

Uses: Treatment of vasomotor, perennial, or seasonal allergic rhinitis and allergic conjunctivitis. Treatment of angioedema, urticarial transfusion reactions, urticaria, pruritus. Atopic dermatitis, contact dermatitis, pruritus ani, pruritus vulvae, insect bites. Sneezing and rhinorrhea due to the common cold. Treatment of anaphylaxis, parkinsonism, drug-induced extrapyramidal reactions, vertigo. Prophylaxis and treatment of motion sickness, including nausea and vomiting. Night-time sleep aid.

Contraindications: Hypersensitivity to the drug, narrow-angle glaucoma, prostatic hypertrophy, stenosing peptic ulcer, and pyloroduodenal or bladder neck obstruction. Pregnancy or possibility thereof (some agents), lactation, premature and newborn infants. The phenothiazine-type antihistamines are contraindicated in CNS depression from any cause, bone marrow depression, jaundice, dehydrated or acutely ill children, and in comatose patients.

Special Concerns: Administer with caution to patients with convulsive disorders, to geriatric patients, in respiratory disease, and to infants and children (may cause hallucinations, convulsions, and death).

Side Effects: *CNS:* Sedation ranging from mild drowsiness to deep sleep. Dizziness, lassitude, headache, confusion, disturbed coordination, muscular weakness. Paradoxical excitation (especially in children and the elderly) including restlessness, irritability, insomnia, hysteria, tremors, euphoria, nervousness, delirium, palpitations, and even convulsions. Also, hallucinations, disorientation, disturbing dreams or nightmares, catatonia, pseudoschizophrenia, extrapyramidal reactions. Antihistamines can precipitate epileptiform seizures in patients with focal lesions. *GI:* Epigastric distress, dryness of mouth, anorexia or increased appetite, weight gain, nausea, vomiting, and diarrhea or constipation. *CV:* Palpitations, increased heart rate, postural hypotension, extrasystoles, bradycardia, reflex tachycardia, ECG changes, cardiac arrest. *GU:* Urinary frequency, retention, or difficulty. Impotence, decreased libido, menstrual irregularities, induced lactation, gynecomastia, inhibition of ejaculation. *Respiratory:* Dryness of nose, mouth, throat; nasal stuffiness, respiratory depression, wheezing and tightness of chest. *Hematologic:* Anemias (hemolytic, hypoplastic, aplastic), leukopenia, pancytopenia, thrombocytopenic purpura, agranulocytosis, thrombocytopenia. *Allergic:* Edema (peripheral, angioneurotic, laryngeal), anaphylaxis, rash, photosensitivity, urticaria, dermatitis, lupus-like syndrome, asthma. *Miscellaneous:* Hands become heavy and weak, tingling, excess sweating, chills, erythema, stomatitis, glycosuria, double vision, vertigo, tinnitus, acute labyrinthitis, neuritis, blurred vision, oculogyric crisis, torticollis.

Topical use: Prolonged use may result in local irritation and allergic contact dermatitis.

Acute Toxicity: Antihistamines have a wide therapeutic range. Overdosage can nevertheless be fatal. Children are particularly susceptible. Overdosage can cause both CNS overstimulation and depression. The overstimulation is characterized by hallucinations, incoordination, and tonic-clonic convulsions. Fixed, dilated pupils, flushing, and fever are common in children. Cerebral edema, deepening coma, and respiratory collapse occur usually within 2 to 18 hr.

Overdosage in adults usually starts with severe CNS depression. Treatment of overdosage is symptomatic and supportive. Vomiting is induced with syrup of ipecac (do not use for phenothiazine overdosage) followed by activated charcoal and a cathartic. If vomiting has not been induced within 3 hr of ingestion, gastric lavage can be undertaken. Hypotension can be treated with a vasopressor such as norepinephrine, dopamine, or phenylephrine (do not use epinephrine). For convulsions, IV phenytoin is indicated; **do not use CNS depressants, including diazepam.**

Drug Interactions	
Alcohol, ethyl	See *CNS depressants*
Anticoagulants	Antihistamines may ↓ the anticoagulant effects
Antidepressants, tricyclic	Additive anticholinergic side effects
CNS depressants, antianxiety agents, barbiturates, narcotics, phenothiazines, procarbazine, sedative-hypnotics	Potentiation or addition of CNS depressant effects. Concomitant use may lead to drowsiness, lethargy, stupor, respiratory depression, coma, and possibly death
Heparin	Antihistamines may ↓ the anticoagulant effects
MAO inhibitors	Intensification and prolongation of anticholinergic side effects

Note: Also see *Drug Interactions* for *Phenothiazines,* p. 629.

Laboratory Test Interference: Discontinue antihistamines 4 days before skin testing to avoid false-negatives.

Dosage: Usually PO. Parenteral administration is seldom used because of irritating nature of drugs. Topical usage is also limited because antihistamines often cause hypersensitivity reactions. When given for motion sickness, antihistamines are usually given 30 to 60 minutes before anticipated travel. See individual drugs.

NURSING CONSIDERATIONS

Administration/Storage

1. Inject IM preparations deep into the muscle. Preparations tend to be irritating to the tissues.
2. Sustained release preparations should be swallowed whole. Scored tablets may be broken before swallowing. If the client has difficulty swallowing capsules, they can be opened and the contents put into soft food for ingestion.
3. Topical preparations should not be applied to raw, blistered, or oozing areas of the skin.
4. Do not apply to the eyes, around the genitalia, or to mucous membranes.
5. Oral preparations may cause gastric irritation. Therefore, administer the medication with meals, milk or a snack.

Table 21 Antihistamines

Drug	Type*	Dosage	Remarks
Azatadine maleate (Optimine) (Rx) Pregnancy Category: B	5	**Tablets. Adults:** 1–2 mg q 8–12 hr. **Pediatric, 12 years and older:** 0.5–1 mg b.i.d. Geriatric patients are more sensitive to the usual adult dose.	Has prolonged action. Used for allergic rhinitis and chronic urticaria. Should not be used in children under 12 years of age. **t½:** 12 hr. **Duration:** 12 hr.
Carbinoxamine maleate (Clistin) (Rx) Pregnancy Category: C	2	**Tablets. Adults:** 4–8 mg t.i.d.–q.i.d. **Pediatric 1–3 years,** 2 mg t.i.d.–q.i.d.; **3–6 years:** 2–4 mg t.i.d.–q.i.d.; **over 6 years:** 4–6 mg t.i.d.–q.i.d.	Some patients respond to doses as small as 4 mg/day while others can tolerate up to 24 mg daily. **t½:** 10–20 hr. **Duration:** 6–8 hr.
Clemastine fumarate (Tavist, Tavist 1) (Rx) Pregnancy Category: B	2	**Syrup/Tablets. Adults and children over 12 years:** 1.34 mg b.i.d. to 2.68 mg t.i.d. not to exceed 8.04 mg daily. **Pediatric, 6–12 years:** 0.67–1.34 mg b.i.d. not to exceed 4.02 mg daily. *Dermatoses:* Use 2.68 mg tablet only.	Do not use in children under 12 years of age. Frequently causes drowsiness. **Duration:** 12 hr.
Diphenylpyraline hydrochloride (Hispril) (Rx)	5	**Capsules. Adults,** 5 mg q 12 hr. **Pediatric, 6–12 years:** 5 mg/day. **Not for children under 6 years.** Geriatric patients may be more sensitive to the usual adult dose.	Low incidence of side effects: drowsiness, headaches, dizziness, dry mouth. Safe use during pregnancy has not been determined.
Methdilazine hydrochloride (Dilosyn✦, Tacaryl) (Rx)	4	**Syrup, Tablets, Chewable Tablets. Adults:** 8 mg b.i.d.–q.i.d.; **pediatric, over 3 years:** 4 mg b.i.d.–q.i.d.	Indicated for allergic and nonallergic pruritus. Tablet must be chewed properly. May cause drowsiness. See also *Phenothiazines*, p. 627. Safe use during pregnancy has not been determined.

Drug	Type*	Dosage	Remarks
Phenindamine tartrate (Nolahist) (OTC)	5	**Tablets. Adults:** 25 mg q 4–6 hr not to exceed 150 mg/day. **Pediatric, 6–12 years;** 12.5 mg q 4–6 hr not to exceed 75 mg/day.	For children under 6 years, physician should be consulted. **Duration:** 4–6 hr.
Pyrilamine maleate (OTC)	1	**PO. Adults:** 25–50 mg t.i.d. up to a maximum of 200 mg daily. **Pediatric, 6 years and older:** 12.5–25 mg q 8 hr. Use not recommended for children less than 6 years of age.	Geriatric patients may be more sensitive to the usual adult dose. **Duration:** 8 hr.
Trimeprazine tartrate (Panectyl ✿, Temaril) (Rx)	4	**Extended-release Capsules, Syrup, Tablets. Adults:** 2.5 mg q.i.d. or 5 mg sustained-release q 12 hr. **Pediatric, 6 months to 3 years:** 1.25 mg t.i.d., or at bedtime (use syrup); **over 3 years:** 2.5 mg t.i.d. or at bedtime; **over 6 years:** 5 mg/day of sustained-release.	Symptomatic relief of acute and chronic pruritus. Also see *Phenothiazines*, p. 627. May cause drowsiness (decreasing with usage), dizziness, dry mouth. Safe use during pregnancy has not been established.

*Type 1: Ethylenediamine derivatives. Type 2: Ethanolamine derivatives. Type 3: Alkylamines. Type 4: Phenothiazines. Type 5: Piperidines.

6. Have syrup of ipecac available to induce vomiting in the event of overdosage.

Assessment

1. Determine if the client is to have skin testing conducted. Antihistamines should be discontinued 4 days prior to testing to avoid false negative results.
2. Note any history of drug sensitivity to antihistamines and record.
3. Note if the client has any medical history of ulcers, glaucoma or if the client is pregnant. Antihistamines are contraindicated under these circumstances.
4. Assess the extent of the allergic response for which the antihistamine is being ordered.
5. Review the medications the client is currently taking, noting those with which there may be an interaction.
6. Obtain a baseline blood pressure, pulse and respirations and document.

Interventions

1. Note client complaints of severe CNS depression. This is a symptom of overdosage and may require the administration of syrup of ipecac.
2. Monitor the blood pressure, pulse and respirations. If the client develops hypotension or palpitations, document and report to the physician.
3. If the client experiences difficulty in voiding, have them void prior to receiving the medication.
4. If the client complains of constipation, encourage the client to take at least 3000 cc of fluids per day, unless the client's condition requires restriction of fluids. Instruct them to increase the amount of exercise performed and increase their intake of fruits, fruit juices, and fiber. A stool softener may also be indicated if these measures are not successful.
5. If the client is hospitalized and sedated with antihistamines, put up the side rails and incorporate safety precautions.
6. If the client complains of dizziness, weakness, or lassitude, assist with ambulation and report these symptoms.
7. If the client complains of local irritation, he/she may have developed an adverse reaction to the drug. Document and report to the physician.

Client/Family Teaching

1. Advise the client to report side effects to the physician immediately. Instruct the client to include onset of the side effects and duration, describing exactly what occurred. The physician may order a drug with fewer side effects. However, the client should not discontinue taking the medication without consulting the physician.
2. Provide the client with a list of drugs to avoid. Advise the client to consult with the physician concerning any depressants that may be ordered since antihistamines tend to potentiate the effects of other CNS depressants.
3. Instruct the client to report the development of sore throat, fever, unexplained bruising, bleeding or petechiae. A CBC and platelets may be indicated to rule out a blood dyscrasia.
4. Advise the client that there is potential for developing a sensitivity to sun or ultraviolet light. Instruct them to avoid undue exposure to the sun, use a sunscreen, and to wear a hat and long sleeves when in the sun.
5. If the drug is being used for motion sickness, it should be taken 30 minutes before it is time to use the vehicle or board a plane.
6. Instruct the client to avoid using OTC products unless ordered by the physician.
7. Caution the client not to drive a car or operate other machinery until response to the

medication (drowsiness) has worn off. Sedative effect may disappear spontaneously after several days of therapy.

Evaluation

Determine the effectiveness of the treatment by interviewing the client and family concerning the client's response. There should be a reduction in the original complaints.

ASTEMIZOLE   (ah-**STEM**-ih-zohl)

Hismanil (Rx)

See also *Antihistamines,* p. 1003.

Classification: Antihistamine, miscellaneous.

Action/Kinetics: Low to no sedative effect, antiemetic effect, or anticholinergic activity. The drug is metabolized in the liver to both active and inactive metabolites and is excreted through the feces. $t^{1}/_{2}$: About 1.6 days. **Onset:** 2–3 days. **Duration:** Up to several weeks. Over 95% is bound to plasma protein. Mainly excreted through the feces.

Special Concerns: Pregnancy category: C. Safety and efficacy have not been established in children less than 12 years of age.

Dosage: Tablets. Adults and children over 12 years of age, maintenance: 10 mg once daily; **pediatric, 6–12 years:** 5 mg once daily. The pharmacokinetics of the drug are proportional following single doses of 10–30 mg. Thus, to reduce the time required to reach steady state concentration, a single dose of 30 mg may be given on Day 1, followed by 20 mg on Day 2 and then on Day 3, the recommended 10 mg daily dose may be given.

NURSING CONSIDERATIONS

See also *Nursing Considerations* for *Antihistamines,* p. 1007.

Client/Family Teaching

1. Take medication on an empty stomach.
2. Do not eat until at least one hour after medication administration as food interferes with the drug absorption.
3. Take medication only as directed since desired effects may not be noticeable immediately.
4. Report any persistent side effects, including depression, to the physician.

BROMPHENIRAMINE MALEATE   (brohm-feh-**NEER**-ah-meen)

Brombay, Bromphen, Chlorphed, Codimal-A, Conjec-B, Cophene-B, Dehist, Diamine T.D., Dimetane, Dimetane Extentabs, Dimetane-Ten, Histaject Modified, Nasahist B, ND Stat Revised, Oraminic II, Sinusol-B, Veltane (Rx; Dimetane and Dimetane Extentabs are OTC)

See also *Antihistamines,* p. 1003.

Classification: Antihistamine, alkylamine type.

Action/Kinetics: Fewer sedative effects. $t^{1}/_{2}$: 25 hr. **Time to peak effect:** 3–9 hr. **Duration:** 4–25 hr.

Special Concerns: Pregnancy category: B. Use is not recommended for neonates. Geriatric patients may be more sensitive to the usual adult dose.

Dosage: Elixir, Tablets. Adults and children over 12: 4 mg q 4–6 hr, or 8–12 mg sustained-release b.i.d.–t.i.d., not to exceed 24 mg/day. **Pediatric, 6–12 years:** 2 mg q 4–6 hr, not to exceed 12 mg daily; **2–6 years:** 1 mg q 4–6 hr, not to exceed 6 mg daily. **Extended-release Tablets. Adults and children over 12:** 8 mg q 8–12 hr or 12 mg q 12 hr; **pediatric, 6–12 years:** 8–12 mg q 12 hr.

    IM, IV, SC. Adults: usual, 10 mg (range: 5–20 mg) q 8–12 hr (maximum daily dose: 40 mg); **pediatric, under 12 years:** 0.125 mg/kg (3.75 mg/m^2) 3–4 times daily.

NURSING CONSIDERATIONS

See *Nursing Considerations* for *Antihistamines,* p. 1007.

Administration/Storage

1. Do not use solutions containing preservatives for IV injection.
2. Sustained-release preparations for children aged 6–12 years old require the supervision of a physician.
3. For IV administration, the 10 mg/mL preparations may be used undiluted or diluted 1:10 with sterile saline for injection.
4. The 10 mg/mL preparations may also be added to 5% glucose, normal saline, or whole blood.
5. The 100 mg/mL preparation is not recommended for IV use.
6. For IM or SC use, the drug may be used undiluted or diluted 1:10 with saline.

BUCLIZINE HYDROCHLORIDE   (BYOU-klih-zeen)

Bucladin-S Softabs (Rx)

See also *Antiemetics,* p. 1076, and *Antihistamines,* p. 1003.

Classification: Antiemetic, antihistamine, piperazine type.

Action/Kinetics: Buclizine suppresses nausea and vomiting through an action on the CNS to decrease vestibular stimulation and depress labyrinthine function. The drug may also act on the chemoreceptor trigger zone to decrease vomiting. **Duration:** 4–6 hr.

Uses: Nausea, vomiting, dizziness of motion sickness.

Additional Contraindications: Hypersensitivity to drug, pregnancy, lactation.

Special Concerns: Pregnancy category: B. Safe use in children not established. Geriatric patients may be more susceptible to the usual adult dose.

Side Effects: Drowsiness, dry mouth, headache, nervousness.

Dosage: Chewable Tablets. Adults: 50 mg 30 min before travel; dosage may be repeated after 4–6 hr. *Severe nausea:* up to 150 mg daily.

NURSING CONSIDERATIONS

See *Nursing Considerations* for *Antiemetics,* p. 1076, and *Antihistamines,* p. 1007.

Administration/Storage

1. To prevent motion sickness, take medication 30 min before departure.
2. Tablets can be chewed, swallowed whole, or dissolved in the mouth.

CHLORPHENIRAMINE MALEATE   (klor-feh-**NEER**-ah-meen)

Syrup, Tablets, Chewable Tablets: Aller-Chlor, Chlo-Amine, Chlorate, Chlor-Niramine, Chlortab 4, Chlor-Trimeton, Chlor-Tripolon✱, Genallerate, Novopheniram✱, Pfeiffer's Allergy, Phenetron, Trymegen. Extended-release Capsules, Extended-release Tablets: Chlorspan-12, Chlortab 8, Chlor-Trimeton Repetabs, Chlor-Tripolon✱, Phenetron Telachlor, Teldrin. Injectables: Chlor-100, Chlor-Pro, Chlor-Pro 10, Chlor-Trimeton. (OTC and Rx)

See also *Antihistamines,* p. 1003.

Classification: Antihistamine, alkylamine type.

Action/Kinetics: Sedation less pronounced. **t½:** 21–27 hr. **Time to peak effect:** 6 hr. **Duration:** 4–8 hr.

Additional Contraindication: Not recommended for children under 6 years of age.

Special Concerns: Pregnancy category: B. Geriatric patients may be more sensitive to the adult dose. The parenteral route is not recommended for neonates.

Dosage: Syrup, Tablets, Chewable Tablets. Adults: 4 mg q 6 hr as needed; **pediatric, 6–12 years:** 2 mg t.i.d.–q.i.d., not to exceed 12 mg daily. **Extended-release Capsules, Extended-release Tablets. Adults:** 8–12 mg q 8–12 hr as needed; **pediatric, 12 years and older:** 8 mg q 12 hr as needed.
   IM, IV, SC. Adults: 5–40 mg as a single dose as needed, up to 40 mg daily; **pediatric, SC:** 0.0875 mg/kg (2.5 mg/m²) q 6 hr as needed.

NURSING CONSIDERATIONS

See *Nursing Considerations* for *Antihistamines,* p. 1007.

Administration/Storage

1. If administered with food, the absorption of drug is delayed.
2. The injection containing 10 mg/mL may be administered IV, IM, or SC.
3. The injection containing 100 mg/mL should only be administered IM or SC.
4. Expect the onset of action to occur within 15–30 min and to last 3–6 hr.

CYCLIZINE HYDROCHLORIDE   (SYE-klih-zeen)

Marezine (OTC)

CYCLIZINE LACTATE   (SYE-klih-zeen)

Marezine (Rx)

See also *Antihistamines,* p. 1003.

Classification: Antihistamine, antiemetic.

Action/Kinetics: The mechanism for the antiemetic effect is not known with certainty but may be due to central anticholinergic effects to cause reduced labyrinthine function and decreased vestibular stimulation. This action is thought to be mediated through pathways to the vomiting center from the chemoreceptor trigger zone or peripheral nerve pathways. **Onset:** 30–60 min; **Duration:** 4–6 hr.

Uses: Nausea, vomiting, dizziness of motion sickness. *Investigational:* Postoperative vomiting.

Contraindications: Pregnancy and lactation.

Special Concerns: Safety for use in children less than 12 years of age has not been determined; children may be more sensitive to the anticholinergic effects of the drug. Geriatric patients may experience a greater incidence of constipation, dry mouth, and urinary retention (i.e., due to the anticholinergic effects).

Side Effects: *CNS:* Drowsiness, excitation, nervousness, restlessness, insomnia, euphoria, vertigo, hallucinations (auditory or visual). *GI:* Nausea, vomiting, diarrhea, constipation, anorexia). *GU:* Urinary frequency or retention; difficulty in urination. *CV:* Hypotension, tachycardia, palpitations. *Miscellaneous:* Dry nose and throat, blurred or double vision, tinnitus, rash, urticaria.

Dosage: Tablets, Injection (IM). *Motion sickness:* **Adults,** 50 mg 30 min before leaving and q 4–6 hr thereafter, not to exceed 200 mg/day; **pediatric, 6–12 years:** 1 mg/kg (33 mg/m²) t.i.d. or 25 mg 30 min before travel and repeated in 6–8 hr if needed, not to exceed 75 mg daily. *Postoperative vomiting:* **Adults, IM:** 50 mg 30 min before end of surgery; may be repeated t.i.d. during first few postoperative days. **Pediatric, 6–12 years:** 25 mg 30 min before end of surgery and repeated t.i.d. during first few postoperative days; **Less than 6 years:** 12.5 mg given same as for older children.

NURSING CONSIDERATIONS

See *Nursing Considerations* for *Antihistamines,* p. 1007

CYPROHEPTADINE HYDROCHLORIDE   (sye-proh-**HEP**-tah-deen)

Periactin (Rx)

See also *Antihistamines,* p. 1003.

Classification: Antihistamine, piperidine-type.

Action/Kinetics: Cyproheptadine also possesses antiserotonin activity. **Duration:** 8 hr.

Additional Uses: Cold urticaria. *Investigational:* Cluster headaches, appetite stimulant in underweight patients and those with anorexia nervosa.

Additional Contraindications: Glaucoma, urinary retention.

Special Concerns: Pregnancy category: B. Geriatric patients may be more sensitive to the usual adult dose.

Additional Side Effect: Increased appetite.

Laboratory Test Interferences: ↑ Serum amylase and prolactin if given with thyroid-releasing hormone.

Dosage: Syrup, Tablets. *Antihistaminic:* **Adults, initial:** 4 mg q 8 hr; **then,** 4–20 mg daily, not to exceed 0.5 mg/kg daily. **Pediatric, 2–6 years:** 2 mg q 8–12 hr, not to exceed 12 mg daily; **6–14 years:** 4 mg q 8–12 hr, not to exceed 16 mg daily. *Appetite stimulant:* **Adults,** 4 mg t.i.d. with meals. **Pediatric, 6–14 years, initial:** 2 mg t.i.d.–q.i.d. with meals; **then,** reduce dose to 4 mg t.i.d. **Pediatric, 2–6 years, initial:** 2 mg t.i.d. with meals; **then,** dose may be increased to a total of 8 mg daily.

NURSING CONSIDERATIONS

See *Nursing Considerations* for *Antihistamines,* p. 1007.

Administration/Storage

1. Drug should not be given more than 6 months to adults and 3 months to children for appetite stimulation.
2. Anticipate the onset of action to occur within 15–30 min and to last from 3–6 hr.

DEXCHLORPHENIRAMINE MALEATE (dex-klor-feh-**NEER**-ah-meen)

Dexchlor, Poladex T.D., Polaramine, Polargen (Rx)

See also *Antihistamines,* p. 1003.

Classification: Antihistamine, alkylamine type.

Action/Kinetics: Less severe sedative effects. **Duration:** 8 hr.

Special Concerns: Pregnancy category: B. Extended-release tablets should not be used in children. Geriatric patients may be more sensitive to the usual adult dose.

Dosage: Syrup, Tablets. Adults: 2 mg q 4–6 hr as needed. **Pediatric, 5–12 years:** 1 mg q 4–6 hr as needed; **2–5 years:** 0.5 mg q 4–6 hr as needed. **Extended-release Tablets. Adults:** 4–6 mg q 8–12 hr as needed.

NURSING CONSIDERATIONS

See *Nursing Considerations* for *Antihistamines,* p. 1007.

DIMENHYDRINATE (dye-men-**HY**-drih-nayt)

Elixir, Syrup, Tablets, Chewable Tablets: Apo-Dimenhydrinate✴, Calm-X, Dimentabs, Dramamine, Gravol✴, Marmine, Motion-Aid, Nauseatol✴, Novodimenate✴, PMS-Dimenhydrinate✴, Travamine, Triptone (OTC). Injection: Dinate, Dommanate, Dramamine, Dramanate, Dramilin, Dramocen, Dramoject, Dymenate, Gravol✴, Hydrate, Marmine, Reidamine, Wehamine (Rx)

See also *Antihistamines,* p. 1003, and *Antiemetics,* p. 1076.

Classification: Antiemetic/antihistamine.

Action/Kinetics: Dimenhydrinate contains both diphenhydramine and chlorotheophylline. The precise mechanism for the antiemetic effect is not known but the drug does depress labyrinthine and vestibular function. The drug may mask ototoxicity due to aminoglycosides. Possesses anticholinergic activity. **Duration:** 3–6 hr.

Uses: Motion sickness, especially to relieve nausea, vomiting, or dizziness. Treat vertigo.

Special Concerns: Pregnancy category: B. Use of the injectable form is not recommended in neonates. Geriatric patients may be more sensitive to the usual adult dose.

Dosage: Elixir, Syrup, Tablets, Chewable Tablets. Adults: 50–100 mg q 4 hr not to exceed 400 mg/day. **Pediatric, 6–12 years:** 25–50 mg q 6–8 hr, not to exceed 150 mg/day; **2–6 years:**

12.5–25 mg q 6–8 hr, not to exceed 75 mg/day. **Extended-release Capsules. Adults:** 1 capsule q 12 hr. Use is not recommended in children. **IM, IV. Adults:** 50 mg as required. **Pediatric, over 2 years:** 1.25 mg/kg (37.5 mg/m^2) q.i.d., not to exceed 300 mg/day. **IV. Adults:** 50 mg in 10 mL sodium chloride injection given over 2 min; may be repeated q 4 hr as needed. **Pediatric:** 1.25 mg/kg (37.6 mg/m^2) in 10 mL of 0.9% sodium chloride injection given slowly over 2 min; may be repeated q 6 hr, not to exceed 300 mg daily. **Suppositories. Adults:** 50–100 mg q 6–8 hr. **Pediatric, 12 years and older:** 50 mg q 8–12 hr; **8–12 years:** 25–50 mg q 8–12 hr; **6–8 years:** 12.5–25 mg q 8–12 hr. Dosage not established in children less than 6 years of age.

NURSING CONSIDERATIONS

See *Nursing Considerations* for *Antihistamines,* p. 1007, and *Antiemetics,* p. 1076.

DIPHENHYDRAMINE HYDROCHLORIDE   (dye-fen-**HY**-drah-meen)

Allerdryl✽, AllerMax, Beldin Cough, Belix, Bena-D, Bena-D 50, Benadryl, Benadryl Complete Allergy, Benahist 10 and 50, Ben-Allergin-50, Benoject-10 and -50, Benylin Cough, Benaphen, Bydramine Cough, Diahist, Dihydrex, Diphenacen-10 and -50, Diphenadryl, Diphen Cough, Fenylhist, Fynex, Hydramine, Hydramine Cough, Hydril, Hyrexin-50, Noradryl, Nordryl, Nordryl Cough, Tusstat, Valdrene, Wehdryl (OTC and Rx).

Sleep-Aids: Compoz, Dormarex 2, Insomnal✽, Nervine Nighttime Sleep-Aid, Nytol with DPH, Sleep-Eze 3, Sominex 2, Twilite (OTC)

See also *Antihistamines,* p. 1003, *Antiemetics,* p. 1076, and *Antiparkinson Agents,* p. 681.

Classification: Antihistamine, antiemetic (ethanolamine-type).

Additional Uses: Treatment of parkinsonism in geriatric patients unable to tolerate more potent drugs. Also for mild parkinsonism in other age groups. Drug-induced extrapyramidal symptoms. Motion sickness, antiemetic, as a sleep-aid. Coughs, including those due to allergy.

Special Concerns: Pregnancy category: B.

Dosage: Capsules, Elixir, Syrup, Tablets. *Antihistamine, antiemetic, antimotion sickness, parkinsonism:* **Adults,** 25–50 mg t.i.d.–q.i.d.; **pediatric, over 20 lb:** 12.5–25 mg t.i.d.–q.i.d. (or 5 mg/kg/day not to exceed 300 mg daily). *Sleep aid:* **Adults,** 50 mg at bedtime. *Antitussive:* **Adults,** 25 mg q 4 hr, not to exceed 150 mg daily; **pediatric, 6–12 years:** 12.5 mg q 4 hr, not to exceed 75 mg daily; **pediatric, 2–6 years:** 6.25 mg q 4 hr, not to exceed 25 mg daily.

IV, deep IM: Adults 10–50 mg up to 100 mg, not to exceed 400 mg daily; **pediatric:** 5 mg/kg/day, not to exceed 300 mg daily.

NURSING CONSIDERATIONS

See also *Nursing Considerations* for *Antihistamines,* p. 1007, *Antiemetics,* p. 1076, and *Antiparkinson Agents,* p. 681.

Administration/Storage

1. When using for motion sickness, the full prophylactic dose should be administered 30 min prior to travel.
2. Similar doses should also be taken with meals and at bedtime.

MECLIZINE HYDROCHLORIDE   (MEK-lih-zeen)

Antivert, Antivert/25 and /50, Antivert/25 Chewable, Antrizine, Bonamine✽, Bonine, Dizmiss, Meni-D, Ru-Vert-M (OTC and Rx)

See also *Antihistamines,* p. 1003, and *Antiemetics,* p. 1076.

Classification: Antihistamine (piperidine-type), antiemetic, antimotion sickness.

Action/Kinetics: The mechanism for the antiemetic effect is not known but may be due to a central anticholinergic effect to decrease vestibular stimulation and depress labyrinthine activity. The drug may also act on the chemoreceptor trigger zone to decrease vomiting.
   Onset: 30–60 min. **Duration:** 8–24 hr. **t½:** 6 hr.

Uses: Nausea, vomiting, dizziness of motion sickness, vertigo associated with diseases of the vestibular system.

Special Concerns: Pregnancy category: B. Safety for use during lactation and in children less than 12 years of age has not been determined. Pediatric and geriatric patients may be more sensitive to the anticholinergic effects of meclizine.

Side Effects: *CNS:* Drowsiness, excitation, nervousness, restlessness, insomnia, euphoria, vertigo, hallucinations (auditory or visual). *GI:* Nausea, vomiting, diarrhea, constipation, anorexia. *GU:* Urinary frequency or retention; difficulty in urination. *CV:* Hypotension, tachycardia, palpitations. *Miscellaneous:* Dry nose and throat, blurred or double vision, tinnitus, rash, urticaria.

Dosage: Capsules, Tablets, Chewable Tablets. *Motion sickness:* **Adults,** 25–50 mg 1 hr before travel; may be repeated q 24 hr during travel. *Vertigo:* **Adults:** 25–100 mg daily in divided doses.

NURSING CONSIDERATIONS

See also *Nursing Considerations* for *Antihistamines,* p. 1003, and *Antiemetics,* p. 1076.

Interventions

1. Assess the client for other adverse symptoms in addition to nausea. An antiemetic drug may mask signs of drug overdose as well as signs of pathology such as increased intracranial pressure or intestinal obstruction.
2. Antiemetics tend to cause drowsiness and dizziness. Therefore, caution clients against driving or performing other hazardous tasks until individual response to the drug has been evaluated.

PROMETHAZINE HYDROCHLORIDE   (proh-METH-ah-zeen)

Syrup, Tablets: Phenergan Fortis, Phenergan Plain, PMS Promethazine✽, Prothazine Plain. Parenteral: Anergan 25 and 50, K-Phen, Mallergan, Pentazine, Phenazine 25 and 50, Phencen-50, Phenergan, Phenoject-50, Pro-50, Prometh-25 and -50, Prorex-25 and -50, Prothazine, V-Gan-25 and -50. Rectal: Phenergan, Promethagan (Rx)

See also *Antihistamines,* p. 1003, and *Antiemetics,* p. 1076.

Classification: Antihistamine, phenothiazine-type.

Action/Kinetics: Promethazine is a potent antihistamine with prolonged action. It may cause severe drowsiness. The antiemetic effects are likely due to inhibition of the chemoreceptor trigger zone. The drug is effective in vertigo by its central anticholinergic effect which inhibits the vestibular apparatus and the integrative vomiting center as well as the chemoreceptor trigger zone. **Onset,**

PO, IM, rectal: 20 min; **IV:** 3–5 min. **Duration, antihistaminic:** 6–12 hr; **sedative:** 2–8 hr. Slowly eliminated through urine and feces.

Uses: Treatment and prophylaxis of motion sickness. Nausea and vomiting due to anesthesia or surgery. Pre- or postoperative sedative, obstetrical sedative. Treatment of pruritus, urticaria, angioedema, dermographism, nasal and ophthalmic allergies. Adjunct in the treatment of anaphylaxis or anaphylactoid reactions. Adjunct to analgesics for postoperative pain. IV with meperidine or other narcotics in special surgical procedures as bronchoscopy, ophthalmic surgery, or in poor-risk patients.

Contraindications: Lactation. Children up to 2 years of age.

Special Concerns: Safe use during pregnancy has not been established. Use in children may cause paradoxical hyperexcitability and nightmares. Injection not recommended for children less than 2 years of age. Geriatric patients are more likely to experience confusion, dizziness, hypotension, and sedation.

Additional Side Effects: Leukopenia and agranulocytosis (especially if used with cytotoxic agents).

Dosage: Syrup, Tablets. *Antihistaminic:* **Adults,** 12.5 mg q.i.d. before meals and at bedtime (or 25 mg at bedtime if needed). **Pediatric,** 0.125 mg/kg (3.75 mg/m^2) q 4–6 hr; 0.5 mg/kg (15 mg/m^2) at bedtime if needed; or, 6.26–12.6 mg t.i.d. (or 25 mg at bedtime if needed). *Anivertigo:* **Adults,** 25 mg b.i.d.; **pediatric,** 0.5 mg/kg (15 mg/m^2) q 12 hr or 12.5–25 mg b.i.d. *Antiemetic:* **Adults,** 25 mg b.i.d. as needed; **pediatric,** 0.25–0.5 mg/kg (7.5–15 mg/m^2) q 4–6 hr as needed (or 12.5–25 mg 4–6 hr). *Sedative-Hypnotic:* **Adults,** 25–50 mg; **pediatric,** 0.5–1 mg/kg (15–30 mg/m^2) or 12.5–25 mg as needed.

    Injectable, Suppositories. *Antihistaminic:* **Adults, IM, IV, Rectal,** 25 mg repeated in 2 hr if needed; **pediatric, IM, Rectal,** 0.125 mg/kg q 4–6 hr (or 0.5 mg/kg at bedtime). *Antiemetic:* **Adults, IM, IV, Rectal,** 12.5–25 mg q 4 hr; **pediatric, IM, Rectal,** 0.25–0.5 mg/kg q 4–6 hr (or 12.5–25 mg q 4–6 hr). *Sedative-Hypnotic:* **Adults, IM, IV, Rectal,** 25–50 mg; **pediatric, IM, Rectal,** 0.5–1 mg/kg (or 12.5–25 mg). *Antivertigo:* **Adults, Rectal,** 25 mg b.i.d.; **pediatric, Rectal,** 0.5 mg/kg q 12 hr (or 12.5–25 mg b.i.d.)

NURSING CONSIDERATIONS

See *Nursing Considerations* for *Antihistamines,* p. 1007, and *Antiemetics,* p. 1076.

Administration/Storage

1. Drug may be taken with food or milk to lessen GI irritation.
2. Dosage should be decreased in dehydrated clients or those with oliguria.
3. When used to prevent motion sickness, the medication should be taken 30 min, and preferably 1–2 hr, before travel.

TERFENADINE   (ter-**FEN**-ah-deen)

Seldane (Rx)

See also *Antihistamines,* p. 1003.

Classification: Antihistamine, piperidine type.

Action/Kinetics: Is said to manifest significantly less drowsiness and anticholinergic effects than other antihistamines. **Onset:** 1–2 hr; **peak effect:** 3–4 hr; **peak plasma levels:** 2 hr. **t½:** About 20 hr. **Duration:** Over 12 hr. Metabolized in the liver and excreted in the urine and feces.

Additional Uses: *Investigational:* Histamine-induced bronchoconstriction in asthmatics; exercise and hyperventilation-induced bronchospasm.

Special Concerns: Pregnancy category: C. Safety and efficacy in children less than 12 years of age have not been established.

Dosage: Tablets. Adults and children over 12 years: 60 mg q 8–12 hr as needed.

NURSING CONSIDERATIONS
See *Nursing Considerations* for *Antihistamines,* p. 1007.

TRIPELENNAMINE HYDROCHLORIDE   (trih-pell-**ENN**-ah-meen)
PBZ, PBZ-SR, Pelamine (Rx)

See also *Antihistamines,* p. 1003.

Classification: Antihistamine, ethylenediamine derivative.

Action/Kinetics: GI effects more pronounced than other antihistamines. **Duration:** 4–6 hr.

Special Concerns: Safe use during pregnancy has not been established. Use is not recommended in neonates. Geriatric patients may be more sensitive to the usual adult dose.

Side Effects: Low incidence. Moderate sedation, mild GI distress, paradoxical excitation, hyperirritability.

Dosage: Elixir, Tablets. Adults: usual, 25–50 mg q 4–6 hr; **pediatric:** 1.25 mg/kg (37.5 mg/m^2) q 6 hr as needed, not to exceed 300 mg daily. **Extended-release Tablets. Adults:** 100 mg q 8–12 hr as needed, up to a maximum of 600 mg daily. Do not use sustained-release form in children.

NURSING CONSIDERATIONS
See *Nursing Considerations* for *Antihistamines,* p. 1007.

TRIPROLIDINE HYDROCHLORIDE   (try-**PROH**-lih-deen)
Actidil, Alleract, Myidyl (OTC and Rx)

See also *Antihistamines,* p. 1003.

Classification: Antihistamine, alkylamine-type.

Action/Kinetics: Sedative effects less pronounced. **Time to peak effect:** 2–3 hr. **t½:** 3–3.3 hr. **Duration:** 4–25 hr. Also found in Actifed and Actifed-C.

Special Concerns: Pregnancy category: B. Geriatric patients may be more susceptible to the usual adult dose.

Additional Side Effects: Low incidence of side effects. *CNS:* Drowsiness, dizziness, paradoxical excitement, hyperirritability. *GI:* GI distress.

Dosage: Syrup, Tablets. Adults: 2.5 mg q 4–6 hr. **Pediatric 6–12 years:** 1.25 mg q 6–8 hr; **4–6 years:** 0.937 mg q 6–8 hr; **2–4 years:** 0.625 mg q 6–8 hr; **4 months–2 years:** 0.312 mg q 6–8 hr.

NURSING CONSIDERATIONS
See *Nursing Considerations* for *Antihistamines,* p. 1007.

PART NINE

Drugs Affecting the Gastrointestinal System

CHAPTER FIFTY-TWO

Antacids

General Statement: Hydrochloric acid maintains the stomach at a pH (1–2) necessary for optimum activity of the digestive enzyme pepsin and to stimulate the release of secretin when the acid contents of the stomach pass into the duodenum. Under certain circumstances, however, people suffer adverse reactions due to gastric acidity ranging from heartburn to life-threatening peptic or duodenal ulcers. Although production of acid plays an important role in the development of gastric and duodenal ulcers, other factors are also believed to play a role. These include endogenous histamine (which can stimulate gastric acid secretion), antigen-antibody reactions, and the psychological makeup of the patient. Acute and chronic GI disturbances are among the most common medical conditions requiring treatment. Various drugs and dietary measures are used for the treatment of hyperacidity states and ulcers, and the use of antacids is an important part of such regimens.

Action/Kinetics: Antacids act by neutralizing or reducing gastric acidity, thus increasing the pH of the stomach and relieving hyperacidity. If the pH is increased to 4, the activity of pepsin is inhibited. The ability of a specific antacid to neutralize acid is termed *acid-neutralizing capacity,* and antacids are selected on this basis. Acid-neutralizing capacity is expressed as mEq/mL and is defined as the HCl required to maintain an antacid suspension at pH 3 for 2 hr in vitro. Ideally, antacids should not be absorbed systemically, although substances such as sodium bicarbonate or calcium carbonate may produce significant systemic effects. The most effective dosage form for antacids is suspensions. Antacids also promote healing of peptic ulcers.

Antacids containing magnesium have a laxative effect, while those containing aluminum or calcium have a constipating effect. This is why patients are often given alternating doses of laxative and constipating antacids. Antacids containing aluminum bind with phosphate ions in the intestine forming the insoluble aluminum phosphate which is excreted in the feces. This is of value in treating hyperphosphatemia of chronic renal failure. **Onset:** Depends on ability of the antacid to solubilize in the stomach and react with hydrochloric acid. The poorly soluble antacids (e.g., magnesium trisilicate) react slower with hydrochloric acid than do the more soluble compounds. **Duration of antacids:** 30 min if fasting; up to 3 hr if taken after meals.

Uses: Treatment of hyperacidity (heartburn, acid indigestion, sour stomach), gastric ulcer, duodenal ulcer, gastroesophageal reflux. Adjunct (with histamine H_2-receptor antagonists) in the treatment of hypersecretory conditions (e.g., Zollinger-Ellison syndrome), systemic mastocytosis, and multiple endocrine adenoma. Treatment of hypocalcemia, hypophosphatemia. Prophylaxis of renal calculi.

Contraindications: Sodium-containing products are contraindicated in congestive heart failure, hypertension, or conditions requiring a low sodium diet. Pregnant or lactating women should not use antacids without physician approval. Children less than six years of age.

Special Concerns: Chronic use of aluminum-containing antacids may aggravate metabolic bone disease seen in geriatric patients; also, chronic use of aluminum-containing antacids may contribute to development of Alzheimer's disease.

Drug Interactions:

1. *Aluminum-containing antacids:* ↑ Effect of benzodiazepines. ↓ Effect of allopurinol, corticosteroids, diflunisal, digoxin, iron products, isoniazid, penicillamines, phenothiazines, ranitidine, and tetracyclines by ↓ absorption from GI tract.
2. *Aluminum and magnesium-containing antacids:* ↑ Effect of levodopa, quinidine, and valproic acid probably by ↓ excretion. ↓ Effect of benzodiazepines, captopril, cimetidine, corticosteroids, iron products, ketoconazole, penicillamine, phenothiazines, phenytoin, quinolones, ranitidine, salicylates, tetracyclines either by ↓ absorption from GI tract or ↑ excretion.
3. *Calcium-containing antacids:* ↑ Effect of quinidine by ↓ excretion. ↓ Effect of iron products, phenytoin, salicylates, and tetracyclines either by ↓ absorption from GI tract or ↑ excretion.
4. *Magnesium-containing antacids:* ↑ Effect of dicumarol and quinidine probably by ↓ excretion. ↓ Effect of benzodiazepines, corticosteroids, digoxin, iron products, nitrofurantoin, penicillamine, phenothiazines, and tetracyclines either by ↓ absorption from GI tract or ↑ excretion. Also, systemic antacids ↓ excretion of amphetamines leading to ↑ effect and the effect of anticholinergics is ↓ due to ↓ absorption.

Dosage: See individual drugs.

NURSING CONSIDERATIONS

Administration/Storage

1. Clients who have an active peptic ulcer should take antacids every hour during waking hours for the first 2 weeks.

2. For peptic ulcer disease, it is recommended that most antacids be taken 1 and 3 hr after meals and at bedtime.

3. Tablets should be thoroughly chewed before swallowing and followed by a glass of milk or water.

4. Liquid preparations have a more rapid action time and greater activity than tablets.

5. Shake liquid suspensions thoroughly before pouring the medication.

6. The absorption rate of many drugs may be affected by antacids. Therefore, if other oral drugs are to be taken, it should be done at least two hours after ingestion of the antacid.

7. Administer laxative or cathartic dose at bedtime, as medication takes about 8 hr to be effective and the effect should not interfere with the client's rest.

Assessment

1. Determine if the client has a history of cardiac disease or hypertension. These clients often are on low sodium diets, so prescribed antacids should also be low in sodium.

2. Note if the client has problems with diarrhea. Antacids containing magnesium may have a laxative effect, worsening this problem.

3. List other drugs the client may be taking to ascertain if any have an unfavorable interaction with the antacid ordered.

Interventions

1. Clients taking antacid preparations that contain calcium or aluminum are prone to constipation. Encourage them to drink 2500–3000 cc of fluid, unless contraindicated and also to increase consumption of foods high in bulk.

2. If constipation persists, consult with the physician concerning either changing the antacid or using laxatives and/or enemas.

3. If the client has renal failure, increasing fluid intake to avoid constipation is not an option. Stool softeners may be necessary.

4. Clients taking antacids that contain magnesium may report having diarrhea. Document and report this to the physician. A change in antacid or alternating a magnesium-based antacid with an aluminum- or calcium-based antacid may be indicated.

Client/Family Teaching

1. Instruct client to take the medication with water or milk. The liquid acts as a vehicle, transporting the medication to the stomach, where the desired drug action occurs.

2. Encourage the client to take the drug at the prescribed times. Some may need to be taken on an empty stomach, while others, such as those used to bind phosphate, may need to be taken with meals.

3. Advise the client to report persistent constipation or diarrhea to the physician.

4. Encourage the client to avoid taking OTC preparations unless specifically ordered by the physician.

5. Encourage the client to avoid smoking or using alcoholic beverages.

6. Discuss the importance of following the specific dietary regime established as well as adhering to the medication protocol. Explain that antacids should be taken for 4–6 weeks after symptoms have disappeared as healing of the ulcer is not correlated with the disappearance of symptoms.

7. Instruct client to report to the physician if the symptoms for which they are being treated show little or no improvement.

ALUMINUM HYDROXIDE GEL (ah-LOO-mih-num)

Alternagel, Amphojel, Concentrated Aluminum Hydroxide, Gaviscon✿, Nephrox (OTC)

ALUMINUM HYDROXIDE GEL, DRIED (ah-LOO-mih-num)

Alu-Cap, Alu-Tab, Amphojel Tablets, Basaljel✿, Dialume (OTC)

See also *Antacids,* p. 1019.

Classification: Antacid.

Action/Kinetics: Aluminum hydroxide is nonsystemic, has demulcent activity, and is constipating. Aluminum hydroxide and phosphorus form insoluble phosphates that are eliminated in the feces. This yields a relatively phosphorus-free urine and prevents phosphate stone formation in susceptible patients. Acid-neutralizing capacity: 6.5–18 mEq/tablet, capsule, or 5 mL. Aluminum-containing antacids are believed to have a cytoprotective effect on the gastric mucosa (perhaps by stimulating prostaglandin synthesis), which protects against mucosal damage by aspirin and ethanol. Small amounts are absorbed from the intestine.

Additional Uses: Hyperphosphatemia, chronic renal failure.

Contraindications: Sensitivity to aluminum. Peptic ulcer associated with pancreatic deficiency, diarrhea, or low-phosphorus diet. Aluminum hydroxide preparations contain sodium and thus should not be administered to patients on a low-sodium diet.

Side Effects: Chronic use may lead to bone pain, muscle weakness, or malaise due to chronic phosphate deficiency and osteomalacia. Constipation, intestinal obstruction. Decreased absorption of fluoride. Accumulation of aluminum in bone, CNS, and serum which may be neurotoxic (e.g., encephalopathy has been reported).

Additional Drug Interactions: Aluminum hydroxide gel inhibits the absorption of barbiturates, digoxin, phenytoin, corticosteroids, quinidine, warfarin, and isoniazid, thereby decreasing their effect.

Dosage: Capsules, Suspension, Tablets. *Antacid:* **Adults, usual:** 500–1,800 mg 3–6 times/day after meals, between meals, and at bedtime. *Hyperphosphatemia:* **Children:** 50–150 mg/kg/day in divided doses q 4–6 hr; adjust dosage until normal serum phosphate levels achieved.

NURSING CONSIDERATIONS

See also *Nursing Considerations* for *Antacids,* p. 1020.

Administration/Storage

1. Administer the gel in a half glass of water.
2. If administering the medication via stomach tube, dilute commercial solution 2 or 3 times with water. Administer this solution at a rate of 15–20 mL/min. The total daily dose should be approximately 1.5 L of the diluted suspension.

Assessment

1. Note any client history of hypersensitivity to aluminum products.
2. Determine if the client is, for any reason, on a prescribed low-sodium diet. Aluminum preparations may then be contraindicated.
3. Discuss with the client the kind of epigastric discomfort being experienced. Determine if the pain is localized, burning and gnawing, if it occurs 2–3 hr after a meal, and/or if it occurs during the early morning.
4. Obtain baseline data concerning the presence of occult blood in the stools.

5. Obtain laboratory tests such as complete blood cell counts, liver and renal function studies.
6. Assess the client's bowel sounds, skin integrity and neurological status and document findings.
7. List any other drugs the client may be taking, either prescribed or OTC preparations.

Interventions

1. Monitor the client for relief of epigastric pain and report any incidence of continued distress.
2. Monitor for additive effects the drug may have on GI motility. Palpate the abdomen and listen to bowel sounds for evidence of any problems.
3. Observe the client for acid rebound effects, evidenced by client complaint of nocturnal pain. Document and report to the physician.
4. Determine the urinary phosphate level monthly when the drug is used in the management of phosphatic urinary calculi.
5. If clients are being treated for phosphatic urinary calculi, refer them to a dietitian for a low-phosphate diet. The diet generally should consist of 1.3 g phosphorus, 700 mg calcium, 13 g nitrogen, and 2,500 cal/day for the duration of the therapy.

Client/Family Teaching

1. If clients are given tablets, instruct them to chew the tablets before swallowing and to take them with a glass of milk or water.
2. Advise the client to report any changes in bowel elimination to the physician.
3. Remind the client that these products are not indicated for prolonged, continual use except under the supervision of a physician. If the symptoms persist, report them to the physician so that further evaluation and therapy may be prescribed.

BASIC ALUMINUM CARBONATE GEL   (ah-**LOO**-mih-num)

Basaljel (OTC)

Classification: Antacid.

Action/Kinetics: The acid neutralizing capacity of the capsules, suspension, or tablets is 12–13 mEq/capsule, tablet, or 5 mL. The acid neutralizing capacity of the extra-strength suspension is 22 mEq/5 mL.

Uses: Hyperacidity. With low-phosphorus diet to prevent phosphate urinary stones by reducing urinary phosphate levels.
   Note: See *Aluminum Hydroxide Gel,* p. 1022, for Contraindications, Side Effects, and Additional Drug Interactions.

Dosage: *Antacid:* 2 tablets or capsules, 2 teaspoons of regular strength suspension, or 1 teaspoon of extra-strength suspension q 2 hr, if necessary, up to 12 times each day. *Hyperphosphatemia:* 2 capsules or tablets, 12 mL suspension, or 5 mL extra-strength suspension t.i.d.–q.i.d. after meals.

NURSING CONSIDERATIONS
See also *Nursing Considerations* for *Antacids,* p. 1022.

Administration/Storage

1. Dilute the liquid form in water or fruit juice.
2. Administer medication after meals and at bedtime.

Interventions

Monitor appropriate laboratory data. Prolonged use may lead to hypophosphatemia, reabsorption of calcium, and bone demineralization.

CALCIUM CARBONATE PRECIPITATED   (KAL-see-um)

Alka-Mints, Amitone, Calcilac, Calglycine, Chooz, Dicarbosil, Equilet, Genalac, Glycate, Gustalac, Mallamint, Pama No. 1, Rolaids Calcium Rich, Titralac, Tums, Tums E-X Extra Strength, Tums Liquid Extra Strength (OTC)

See also *Antacids,* p. 1019.

Classification: Antacid.

Action/Kinetics: Nonsystemic antacid regarded by some as the antacid of choice. Since calcium carbonate is constipating, it is often alternated or even mixed with magnesium salts. Acid-neutralizing capacity: 8.25–10 mEq/tablet. Contains 40% calcium. Chronic use may lead to systemic effects. Rapid onset of action and relatively prolonged activity.

Uses: Antacid; adjunct in peptic ulcer therapy. Calcium deficiency.

Side Effects: *GI:* Constipation, rebound hyperacidity, flatulence, eructation, intestinal obstruction. *Milk-alkali syndrome:* Hypercalcemia, metabolic alkalosis, renal dysfunction.

Dosage: Chewing Gum, Oral Suspension, Tablets, Chewable Tablets. Adults, individualize, usual: 0.5–1 g as necessary (or 0.5–1.5 g q 2–4 hr).

NURSING CONSIDERATIONS

See also *Nursing Considerations* for *Antacids,* p. 1020.

Administration/Storage

Tablets should be chewed before being swallowed.

DIHYDROXYALUMINUM SODIUM CARBONATE   (dye-hi-DROK-see-ah-LOO-mih-num)

Rolaids Antacid (OTC)

See also *Antacids,* p. 1019.

Classification: Antacid.

Action/Kinetics: Nonsystemic antacid with adsorbent and protective properties similar to those of aluminum hydroxide but reported to act more rapidly. Acid-neutralizing capacity: 7 mEq/tablet.
   Note: See *Aluminum Hydroxide Gel,* p. 1022, for Uses, Contraindications, Side Effects, and Drug Interactions.

Dosage: Chewable Tablets. Adults: 1–2 tablets chewed after meals and at bedtime; 1–2 tablets chewed q 2–4 hr may be required to alleviate severe discomfort.

NURSING CONSIDERATIONS

See *Nursing Considerations* for *Antacids* p. 1020.

GELUSIL AND GELUSIL-II   (JELL-you-sill)

See also *Antacids,* p. 1019.

Classification/Content: Gelusil contains the following in each tablet or 5 mL:
Antacid: Aluminum hydroxide, 200 mg.
Antacid: Magnesium hydroxide, 200 mg.
Antiflatulent: Simethicone, 25 mg.
Gelusil-II contains aluminum hydroxide and magnesium hydroxide, each 400 mg and simethicone, 30 mg. See also information on individual components.

Action/Kinetics: Gelusil has a high capacity to neutralize acid and has a low sodium content.

Uses: To treat acid indigestion, heartburn, sour stomach; relieve symptoms of gas. Also as an adjunct in the treatment of peptic ulcer.

Additional Contraindication: Kidney disease.

Dosage: Oral Suspension, Chewable Tablets. *Gelusil, Gelusil-II:* Two or more tablets or teaspoonsful 1 hr after meals and at bedtime.

NURSING CONSIDERATIONS

See also *Nursing Considerations* for *Antacids,* p. 1020.

Administration/Storage

1. Tablets should be chewed before being swallowed.
2. The maximum daily dosage of Gelusil should be 12 tablets or teaspoons, and the maximum daily dosage for Gelusil-II should be 8 tablets or teaspoonsful. Maximum dosage should not be taken for more than 2 weeks.

MAALOX NO. 1 TABLETS, ORAL SUSPENSION, DOUBLE STRENGTH TABLETS   (MAY-lox)

See also *Antacids,* p. 1019.

Classification/Content: Maalox No. 1 Tablets. *Antacids:* Aluminum hydroxide, 200 mg, and magnesium hydroxide, 200 mg. **Note:** The Double Strength Tablets contain twice the amount of each antacid per tablet. **Maalox Suspension.** *Antacids:* Aluminum hydroxide, 225 mg/5 mL, and magnesium hydroxide, 200 mg/5 mL.

Uses: Relief of hyperacidity due to peptic ulcer, gastritis, gastric hyperacidity, peptic esophagitis, hiatal hernia, or heartburn.

Dosage: No. 1 Tablets: 2–4 tablets 20–60 min after meals and at bedtime. **Double Strength Tablets:** 1–2 tablets q.i.d. 20–60 min after meals and at bedtime. **Suspension:** 10–20 mL q.i.d. 20–60 min after meals and at bedtime.

NURSING CONSIDERATIONS

See also *Nursing Considerations* for *Antacids*, p. 1022.

Client/Family Teaching

1. Advise client to chew tablets well before swallowing.

2. If a suspension is to be used, shake the container well before pouring the medication.

3. Advise the client not to take more than 80 mL of the Oral Suspension in a 24 hour period.

4. If the client is taking No. 1 Tablets, advise the client to take no more than 16 tablets per day. If there is no relief, notify the physician.

5. If the client is to take Double Strength Tablets, advise him/her to take no more than 8 tablets in a 24 hour period.

6. If the client is taking tetracycline advise the physician so that antacid therapy can be avoided.

MAALOX PLUS ORAL SUSPENSION AND TABLETS (MAY-lox)
(OTC)

See also *Antacids,* p. 1019.

Classification/Content: *Antacid:* Magnesium hydroxide, 200 mg (tablet or 5-mL suspension). *Antacid:* Aluminum hydroxide, 200 mg (tablet) or 225 mg (5-mL suspension). *Antiflatulent:* Simethicone, 25 mg (tablet or 5 mL suspension).
   See also information on individual components.

Uses: Relief of hyperacidity due to peptic ulcer, peptic esophagitis, gastric hyperacidity, gastritis, hiatal hernia, or heartburn. Also, to relieve symptoms of gas, including postoperative gas pain.

Dosage: Suspension: 10–20 mL q.i.d. 20–60 min after meals and at bedtime. **Tablets:** 1–4 tablets q.i.d. 20–60 min after meals and at bedtime.

NURSING CONSIDERATIONS

See also *Nursing Considerations* for *Maalox No. 1 Tablets, Oral Suspension, Double Strength Tablets,* p. 1025, and *Antacids,* p. 1020.

MAALOX TC SUSPENSION AND TABLETS (MAY-lox)
(OTC)

Classification/Content: Maalox TC (therapeutic concentrate) is a high-potency antacid preparation. *Antacid:* Magnesium hydroxide, 300 mg (tablet or 5-mL suspension). *Antacid:* Aluminum hydroxide, 600 mg (tablet or 5-mL suspension). See also information on individual components.

Uses: Relief of hyperacidity due to peptic ulcer, gastritis, gastric hyperacidity, peptic esophagitis, hiatal hernia, or heartburn.

Dosage: Suspension: 5–10 mL q.i.d. 20–60 min after meals and at bedtime. **Tablets:** 1–2 tablets between meals and at bedtime.

NURSING CONSIDERATIONS

See *Nursing Considerations* for *Maalox No. 1 Tablets, Oral Suspension, Double Strength Tablets,* p. 1025, and *Antacids,* p. 1020.

MAGALDRATE (HYDROXYMAGNESIUM ALUMINATE)   (MAG-al-drayt)

Antiflux❁, Lowsium, Riopan, Riopan Extra Strength❁ (OTC)

Classification: Antacid.

Action/Kinetics: Chemical combination of aluminum hydroxide and magnesium hydroxide. This compound is an effective nonsystemic antacid. It buffers (pH 3.0–5.5) without causing alkalosis. Acid-neutralizing capacity: 13.5 mEq/tablet or 15 mEq/5 mL suspension.

Use: Antacid.

Contraindication: Sensitivity to aluminum. Use with caution in patients with impaired renal function.

Side Effects: Mild constipation and hypermagnesemia. Rebound hyperacidity, milk-alkali syndrome.

Dosage: Oral Suspension, Tablets, Chewable Tablets. Adults: 480–1,080 mg q.i.d. between meals and at bedtime. Frequency of administration may have to be increased initially to every hour to control severe symptoms. The suspension contains 540 mg/5 mL.

NURSING CONSIDERATIONS

See also *Nursing Considerations* for *Antacids*, p. 1020.

Assessment

Baseline renal function studies may be indicated prior to administering drug therapy.

MAGNESIUM HYDROXIDE (MAGNESIA)   (mag-NEE-see-um)

Phillips' Milk of Magnesia, M.O.M (OTC)

See also *Antacids*, p. 1019, and *Laxatives*, p. 1048.

Classification: Antacid, laxative.

Action/Kinetics: Depending on dosage, drug acts as an antacid or as a laxative. Neutralizes hydrochloric acid. Does not produce alkalosis and has a demulcent effect. A dose of 1 mL neutralizes 2.7 mEq of acid. As an antacid, often alternated with aluminum hydroxide to counteract laxative effect.

As a laxative, magnesium hydroxide increases the bulk of the stools by attracting and holding large amounts of fluids. The increased bulk results in the mechanical stimulation of peristalsis. **Onset:** 2–6 hr.

Uses: Antacid. As a laxative to empty the bowl prior to diagnostic or surgical procedures, to eliminate parasites following anthelmintic therapy, to remove toxic materials following poisoning, and to collect a stool specimen for parasite examination.

Contraindications: Poor renal function.

Side Effects: Diarrhea, abdominal pain, nausea, vomiting. Hypermagnesemia and CNS depression (especially in patients with renal failure). Magnesium intoxication is manifested by drowsiness, dizziness, other signs of CNS depression, and thirst.

Additional Drug Interactions

Procainamide	Procainamide ↑ muscle relaxation produced by Mg salts
Skeletal muscle relaxants (surgical), succinylcholine, tubocurarine	↑ Muscle relaxation

---

Dosage: Oral Suspension, Tablets, Chewable Tablets. Adults and children over 12 years: *Antacid,* 5–15 mL liquid or 650–1,300 mg tablets q.i.d. *Laxative:* 15–40 mL liquid once daily with water. **Children 6–12 years:** *Antacid,* 2.5–5 mL liquid with water; *laxative,* 15–30 mL (depending on age) once daily with water. **Children 2–6 years:** *laxative,* 5–15 mL liquid once daily with water.

NURSING CONSIDERATIONS

See *Nursing Considerations* for *Antacids,* p. 1020, and *Laxatives,* p. 1049.

Administration/Storage

1. Suspensions should be administered with water.
2. Administer combined magnesia magma and aluminum hydroxide gel with one-half glass of water.
3. Provide a slice of orange or glass of orange juice after administration as a laxative, to minimize the unpleasant aftertaste.
4. Administer laxative dose at bedtime, as medication takes about 8 hr to be effective and therefore will not interfere with client's rest.

MAGNESIUM OXIDE   (mag-NEE-see-um)

Mag-Ox 400, Maox, Par-Mag, Uro-Mag (OTC)

See also *Antacids,* p. 1019, and *Laxatives,* p. 1048.

Classification: Antacid, laxative.

Action/Kinetics: Magnesium oxide is a nonsystemic antacid with a laxative effect. The compound has a rather high neutralizing capacity (1.0 g neutralizes 50 mEq acid). Magnesium oxide is slower acting than sodium bicarbonate but has a more prolonged activity.

Uses: Antacid.

Contraindication: Poor renal function.

Side Effects: Abdominal pain, nausea, diarrhea. Hypermagnesemia and CNS depression in patients with poor renal function. Symptoms of magnesium intoxication include drowsiness, dizziness, other signs of CNS depression, and thirst. Rebound hyperacidity, milk-alkali syndrome.

Drug Interactions: See *Magnesium Hydroxide,* p. 1027.

Dosage: Capsules, Tablets. *Antacid:* **Capsules,** 140 mg with water or milk t.i.d.–q.i.d. **Tablets:** 400–840 mg daily.

NURSING CONSIDERATIONS

See *Nursing Considerations* for *Antacids,* p. 1019, and *Laxatives,* p. 1049.

MYLANTA LIQUID AND TABLETS   (my-LAN-tah)
(OTC)

MYLANTA-II LIQUID AND TABLETS   (my-LAN-tah)
(OTC)

See also *Antacids,* p. 1019.

Classification/Content: Mylanta. Each tablet or 5 mL contains: *Antacid:* Aluminum hydroxide, 200 mg; *Antacid:* Magnesium hydroxide, 200 mg; and, *Antiflatulent:* Simethicone, 20 mg.

Mylanta-II. Each tablet or 5 mL contains: *Antacid:* Aluminum hydroxide, 400 mg; *Antacid:* Magnesium hydroxide, 400 mg; and, *Antiflatulent:* Simethicone, 40 mg.

See also information on individual components.

Uses: Symptoms due to heartburn, gastritis, peptic ulcer, hiatal hernia, and peptic esophagitis. The product also relieves accompanying distress due to gas and swallowed air.

Dosage: Oral Suspension, Chewable Tablets. *Mylanta or Mylanta-II.* **Adults:** 10–20 mL of the liquid or 2–4 tablets between meals and at bedtime.

NURSING CONSIDERATIONS

Administration/Storage

The gastric acid output and gastric emptying time vary greatly; thus, the dosage schedule should be individualized.

Client/Family Teaching

1. Advise client to chew tablets well before swallowing.
2. If a suspension is to be used, shake the container well before pouring the medication.
3. Advise the client not to take more than 120 mL of the Oral Mylanta Suspension or 60 mL of the Oral Mylanta II suspension in a 24-hour period.
4. If the client is taking Mylanta Tablets, advise the client to take no more than 24 Mylanta tablets or 12 Mylanta II tablets per day. If there is no relief, notify the physician.
5. If the client is taking tetracycline advise the physician so that therapy with these products can be avoided.

SODIUM BICARBONATE
Arm and Hammer Pure Baking Soda, Bell/ans, Citrocarbonate, Neut, Soda Mint (Rx and OTC)

Classification: Alkalinizing agent, antacid, electrolyte.

Action/Kinetics: The antacid action is due to neutralization of hydrochloric acid by forming sodium chloride and carbon dioxide (1 g of sodium bicarbonate neutralizes 12 mEq of acid). Provides temporary relief of peptic ulcer pain and of discomfort associated with indigestion. Although widely used by the public, sodium bicarbonate is rarely prescribed as an antacid because of its high sodium content, short duration of action, and ability to cause alkalosis (sometimes desired). Sodium bicarbonate is also a systemic and urinary alkalinizer by increasing plasma and urinary bicarbonate, respectively.

Uses: Treatment of hyperacidity, severe diarrhea (where there is loss of bicarbonate), nonspecific treatment of drug toxicity (e.g., barbiturates, salicylates, methanol). Treatment of acute mild to moderate metabolic acidosis due to shock, severe dehydration, renal disease, cardiac arrest, severe primary lactic acidosis. Prophylaxis of renal calculi in gout. During sulfonamide therapy to prevent renal calculi and nephrotoxicity. *Investigational:* Sickle-cell anemia.

Contraindications: Renal impairment, congestive heart failure, pyloric obstruction, patients on restricted-sodium diet, edema, cirrhosis of the liver, metabolic or respiratory alkalosis, toxemia of pregnancy. Do not use as an antidote for strong mineral acids because carbon dioxide is formed, which may cause discomfort and even perforation. Children less than 6 years of age.

Special Concerns: Pregnancy category: C. Use with extreme caution in patients losing chloride through vomiting or continuous GI suction and in those in whom diuretics produce hypochloremic alkalosis. Use with caution in patients with edema and cirrhosis.

Side Effects: *GI:* Acid rebound, gastric distention. *Milk-alkali syndrome:* Hypercalcemia, metabolic alkalosis (dizziness, cramps, thirst, anorexia, nausea, vomiting, hyperexcitability, tetany, diminished breathing, seizures), renal dysfunction. Extravasation following IV use may manifest ulceration, sloughing, cellulitis, or tissue necrosis at the site of injection.

Drug Interactions	
Amphetamines	↑ Effect of amphetamines by ↑ renal tubular reabsorption
Antidepressants, tricyclic	↑ Effect of tricyclics by ↑ renal tubular reabsorption
Benzodiazepines	↓ Effect due to ↑ alkalinity of urine
Ephedrine	↑ Effect of ephedrine by ↑ renal tubular reabsorption
Erythromycin	↑ Effect of erythromycin in urine due to ↑ alkalinity of urine
Flecainide	↑ Effect due to ↑ alkalinity of urine
Iron products	↓ Effect due to ↑ alkalinity of urine
Ketoconazole	↓ Effect due to ↑ alkalinity of urine
Lithium carbonate	Excretion of lithium is proportional to amount of sodium ingested. If patient on sodium-free diet, may develop lithium toxicity, since less lithium is excreted
Methenamine compounds	↓ Effect of methenamine due to ↑ alkalinity of urine
Nitrofurantoin	↓ Effect of nitrofurantoin due to ↑ alkalinity of urine
Procainamide	↑ Effect of procainamide due to ↓ excretion by kidney
Pseudoephedrine	↑ Effect of pseudoephedrine due to ↑ tubular reabsorption
Quinidine	↑ Effect of quinidine by ↑ renal tubular reabsorption
Salicylates	↓ Effect due to ↑ alkalinity of urine
Sulfonylureas	↓ Effect due to ↑ alkalinity of urine
Tetracyclines	↓ Effect of tetracyclines due to ↑ excretion by kidney

Dosage: Effervescent Powder. *Antacid:* **Adults,** 3.9–10 g in a glass of cold water after meals. **Geriatric and pediatric, 6–12 years:** 1.9–3.9 g after meals.

Oral Powder. *Antacid:* **Adults,** ½ teaspoonful in a glass of water q 2 hr; adjust dosage as required. *Urinary alkalinizer:* **Adults,** 1 teaspoonful in a glass of water q 4 hr; adjust dosage as required. Dosage not established for this form for children.

Tablets. *Antacid:* **Adults,** 0.325–2 g 1–4 times daily; **pediatric, 6–12 years:** 520 mg; may be repeated once after 30 min. *Urinary alkalinizer:* **Adults, initial,** 4 g; **then,** 1–2 g q 4 hr. **Pediatric,** 23–230 mg/kg daily; adjust dosage as needed.

Injection. *Systemic alkalizer, cardiac arrest:* **Adults, IV, initial,** 1 mEq/kg; **then,** 0.5 mEq/kg which may be repeated q 10 min of continued arrest. **Pediatric, IV, initial:** 1 mEq/kg; **then,** 0.5 mEq/kg q 10 min of continued arrest. *Systemic alkalinizer, less severe metabolic acidosis:* **Adults and older children, IV infusion,** 2–5 mEq/kg given over 4–8 hr. *Urinary alkalinizer:* **Adults and children, IV,** 2–5 mEq/kg over 4–8 hr.

NURSING CONSIDERATIONS

Administration/Storage

1. Hypertonic solutions must be administered by trained personnel.
2. IV dose should be determined by arterial blood pH, pCO_2, and base deficit.
3. Isotonic solutions should be administered slowly as ordered. Too-rapid administration may result in death due to cellular acidity. Therefore, check rate of flow frequently.
4. If only the 7.5% or 8.4% solutions are available, they should be diluted 1:1 with 5% dextrose in water when used in infants for cardiac arrest.
5. Have available a parenteral solution of calcium gluconate and 2.14% solution of ammonium chloride in the event of severe alkalosis or tetany.

Assessment

1. Note any client history of renal impairment, congestive heart failure or if the client is on a sodium-restricted diet.
2. Assess the client for evidences of edema that may indicate the inability to use sodium bicarbonate.
3. If the client is on low continuous or intermittent NG suctioning, or is vomiting, assess for evidence of excessive loss of chloride.
4. Note if the client is taking other medications. List the names and what their potential interactive effect may be.
5. If the client is to receive sodium bicarbonate to counteract metabolic acidosis, obtain arterial blood for pH, pCO_2, and HCO_3, and other designated electrolytes, as baseline data.

Interventions

1. Observe the client for dry skin and mucous membranes, polydipsia, polyuria and air hunger. These are indications of a reversal of symptoms of metabolic acidosis and need to be documented and reported to the physician.
2. Compare the pH and electrolytes with the values taken prior to administering sodium bicarbonate to assure that the client is not developing an alkalosis. If there is evidence of alkalosis, notify the physician and be prepared to have the client breathe in and out of a paper bag.

3. Periodically assess the client's serum pH during the therapy.

4. Assess the client with acidosis who is being treated with sodium bicarbonate for the relief of dyspnea and hyperpnea. Relief of these symptoms indicates that the drug may be discontinued.

5. Observe if the client being treated for acidosis develops edema. Report to the physician and anticipate the order will be changed to potassium bicarbonate.

6. At intervals during the day, test the client's urine with nitrazine paper to determine if the urine is becoming alkaline. Adjust the dosage of sodium bicarbonate accordingly.

Client/Family Teaching

1. Warn clients taking excessive oral preparations of sodium bicarbonate routinely to relieve gastric distress that there may be a rebound reaction resulting either in an increased acid secretion or systemic alkalosis. Remind them to consult a physician with persistent symptoms of gastric distress.

2. Also, advise the client taking sodium bicarbonate on a routine basis of the danger of forming phosphate crystals in the kidney.

3. Explain to clients that if they take sodium bicarbonate with milk or calcium, a milk-alkali syndrome may result. Clients may develop anorexia, nausea and vomiting when this occurs. They may also become mentally confused. The physician should be notified immediately if these symptoms occur.

4. Explain to the client the need to avoid OTC preparations such as Alka-Seltzer, or Fizrin that contain sodium bicarbonate.

CHAPTER FIFTY-THREE
Antiulcer and other GI Drugs

CIMETIDINE (sye-**MEH**-tih-deen)

Apo-Cimetidine✿, Novocimetidine✿, Peptol✿, Tagamet (Rx)

Classification: Histamine H_2-receptor blocking agent.

Action/Kinetics: Cimetidine decreases the acidity of the stomach by blocking the action of histamine, a substance involved in triggering gastric acid secretion. Cimetidine blocks the action of histamine by competitively occupying the histamine H_2-receptors in the gastric mucosa. This, in turn, inhibits the release of gastric (hydrochloric) acid. Cimetidine reduces postprandial daytime and nighttime gastric acid secretion by about 50–80%. It is well absorbed from GI tract. The drug may increase gastromucosal defense and healing in acid-related disorders (e.g., stress-induced ulcers) by increasing production of gastric mucus, increasing mucosal secretion of bicarbonate and gastric mucosal blood flow as well as increasing endogenous mucosal synthesis of prostaglandins. It also inhibits cytochrome P-450 and P-448 which will affect metabolism of drugs. Cimetidine also possesses antiandrogenic activity and will increase prolactin levels following an IV bolus injection. **Peak plasma level, PO:** 45–90 min. **Time to peak effect, after PO:** 1–2 hr. **Duration, nocturnal:** 6–8 hr; **basal:** 4–5 hr. **t½:** 2 hr, longer in presence of renal impairment. After PO use, most metabolized in liver; after parenteral use, about 75% of drug excreted unchanged in the urine.

Uses: Short-term (up to 8 weeks) and maintenance treatment of active duodenal ulcers; short-term treatment of benign gastric ulcers. Management of gastric acid hypersecretory states (Zollinger-Ellison syndrome, systemic mastocytosis). *Investigational:* Prior to surgery to prevent aspiration pneumonitis, secondary hyperparathyroidism in chronic hemodialysis patients, prophylaxis of stress-induced ulcers, upper GI bleeding, hyperparathyroidism, herpes virus infections, tinea capitis, prevent gastric damage due to nonsteroidal anti-inflammatory agents, hirsute women, chronic idiopathic urticaria, dermatological anaphylaxis, acetaminophen overdosage.

Contraindications: Children under 16, nursing mothers. Cirrhosis, impaired liver and renal function.

Special Concerns: Pregnancy category: B. In geriatric patients with impaired renal or hepatic function, confusion is more likely to occur.

Side Effects: *GI:* Diarrhea, pancreatitis, hepatitis, hepatic fibrosis. *CNS:* Dizziness, sleepiness, headache, confusion, delirium, hallucinations, double vision, dysarthria, ataxia. *CV:* Hypotension and arrhythmias following rapid IV administration. *Hematologic:* Agranulocytosis, thrombocytopenia, hemolytic or aplastic anemia, granulocytopenia. *GU:* Impotence (high doses for prolonged periods of time), gynecomastia (long-term treatment). *Other:* Arthralgia, myalgia, rash, vasculitis, galactorrhea, alopecia, bronchoconstriction.

Drug Interactions

Antacids	↓ Effect of cimetidine due to ↓ absorption from GI tract
Anticholinergics	↓ Effect of cimetidine due to ↓ absorption from GI tract
Anticoagulants, oral	↑ Effect of anticoagulant due to ↓ breakdown by liver
Barbiturates	↓ Effect of cimetidine due to ↓ absorption from GI tract and ↑ breakdown by liver
Benzodiazepines	↑ Effect of benzodiazepines due to ↓ breakdown by liver
Beta-adrenergic blocking drugs	↑ Effect of beta blockers due to ↓ breakdown by liver
Caffeine	↑ Effect of caffeine due to ↓ breakdown by liver
Carbamazepine	Cimetidine ↑ effect of carbamazepine
Carmustine	Additive bone marrow depression
Chlorpromazine	↓ Effect of chlorpromazine due to ↓ absorption from GI tract
Iron salts	↓ Effect of iron due to ↓ absorption from GI tract
Ketoconazole	↓ Effect of ketoconazole due to ↓ absorption from GI tract
Lidocaine	↑ Effect of lidocaine due to ↓ breakdown by liver
Metoclopramide	↓ Effect of cimetidine due to ↓ absorption from GI tract
Metronidazole	↑ Effect of metronidazole due to ↓ breakdown by liver
Narcotics	Possible ↑ toxic effects of narcotics
Phenytoin	↑ Effect of phenytoin due to ↓ breakdown by liver
Procainamide	↑ Effect of procainamide due to ↓ excretion by kidney
Quinidine	↑ Effect of quinidine due to ↓ breakdown by liver
Tetracyclines	↓ Effect of tetracyclines due to ↓ absorption from GI tract
Theophylline	↑ Effect of theophyllines due to ↓ breakdown by liver

Dosage: Tablets, Oral Solution. Adults: *Duodenal ulcers:* 300 mg q.i.d. with meals and at bedtime for 4–6 weeks (administer with antacids). Alternate dosage: 800 mg at bedtime or 400–600 mg b.i.d. (in the morning and evening). *Prophylaxis of recurrent duodenal ulcers:* 400 mg at bedtime or 300 mg b.i.d. in the morning and evening. *Active benign peptic ulcers:* 300 mg q.i.d. with meals and at bedtime for no more than 8 weeks. Alternative dosage: 600 mg b.i.d. in the morning and at bedtime or 800 mg at bedtime. *Hypersecretory conditions:* 300 mg q.i.d. with meals and at bedtime up to a maximum of 2,400 mg daily. *Gastroesophageal reflux:* 300 mg q.i.d. with meals and at bedtime. Alternative dosage: 600 mg b.i.d. in the morning and at bedtime or 800 mg at bedtime. *Upper GI bleeding:* 300 mg q 6 hr or 600 mg b.i.d. in the morning and at bedtime. In impaired renal function, a dose of 300 mg q 8–12 hr may be necessary. **Pediatric, all uses:** 20–40 mg/kg daily in divided doses q.i.d. with meals and at bedtime.

IM, IV, IV infusion. *Duodenal ulcer, gastric ulcer, hypersecretory conditions, upper GI bleeding:* **Adults:** 300 mg (as the base) q 6–8 hr. *Prophylaxis of stress ulcers:* **Adults:** 300 mg (base) q 6 hr (or more frequently to maintain the gastric pH above 4). *Prophylaxis of aspiration pneumonitis:* **Adults, IM:** 300 mg (base) 1 hr before induction of anesthesia and 300 mg (base) IM or IV q 4 hr until patient is conscious. **Pediatric, all uses:** 5–10 mg/kg q 6–8 hr.

NURSING CONSIDERATIONS

Administration/Storage

1. For IV injections or infusions, dilute as specified by the manufacturer and inject over a period of 1–2 min, or infuse intermittently.
2. Administer oral medication with meals and a snack at bedtime.
3. If antacids are to be used, stagger the dose with that of cimetidine.

Assessment

1. Note the general over all condition of the client. Clients receiving radiation therapy or myelosuppressive drugs may have their action potentiated by cimetidine.
2. Review the list of drug interactions prior to administering the drug. Determine if any of the drugs the client is taking may interact unfavorably with cimetidine.

Interventions

1. Be alert to mood swings that may occur. These are more common among the elderly than among people in other age groups.
2. Note if the client appears to have an increased susceptibility to infections. Clients taking cimetidine may develop agranulocytosis, thrombocytopenia, or anemia and should have periodic hematologic evaluations.
3. For the elderly, severely ill client or one who has renal impairment, monitor renal function, fluid intake and output for the duration of the therapy.
4. Some clients develop diarrhea. Monitor the frequency of the episodes, their severity and persistence. Help the client to maintain adequate hydration, monitor the electrolytes and if the problem persists, notify the physician.
5. Inspect the skin routinely for rashes or other skin changes. Document and report any abnormalities to the physician.

Client/Family Teaching

1. Review with the client and family the goals of the prescribed therapy.

2. Discuss with clients other drugs that have been ordered and assist them to establish an appropriate schedule to assure compliance with drug therapy.

3. Discuss dietary modifications that may be required while taking the drug, especially if the client is being treated for GI problems. Evaluate carefully, as it may be necessary to have a dietitian work with the client.

4. Instruct clients about the symptoms of gynecomastia or galactorrhea and advise them to report these side effects to the physician should they occur.

5. Advise clients to report immediately if they have abdominal pain, bloody stools or other indications that the ulcer has been reactivated.

6. Explain the need for the client to continue taking the drug even though the symptoms may have disappeared.

DEXPANTHENOL   (dex-PAN-the-nohl)

Ilopan, Panthoderm (Rx)

Classification: Gastrointestinal stimulant.

Action/Kinetics: Dexpanthenol (*d*-pentothenyl alcohol), a precursor of coenzyme A, stimulates the smooth muscles of the GI tract, probably by increasing the synthesis of acetylcholine. Satisfactory response is unlikely in the presence of hypokalemia. Topically, the drug relieves itching and facilitates healing of skin lesions by stimulating epithelialization and granulation.

Uses: Prophylactic after major abdominal surgery to minimize development of paralytic ileus or abdominal distention. To treat retention of flatus or delay in resumption of normal intestinal motility after surgery or parturition. Paralytic ileus. **Topical:** Treat minor wounds, poison ivy, insect bites, poison oak, minor skin irritations, diaper rash.

Contraindications: Hemophilia. Ileus due to mechanical obstruction. Within one hour of succinylcholine.

Special Concerns: Safety and effectiveness in pregnancy, lactation, and in children have not been established.

Side Effects: *GI:* Intestinal colic, vomiting, diarrhea. *Allergic:* Pruritus, dermatitis, urticaria, tingling, itching, breathing difficulties. *Other:* Hypotension.

Drug Interactions	
Antibiotics Barbiturates Narcotics	Allergic reactions of unknown cause
Succinylcholine	↑ Effect of succinylcholine with respiratory difficulties

Dosage: IM. *Prophylaxis or postoperative abdominal distention:* 250–500 mg. Repeat once after 2 hr; **then** q 6 hr until danger of distention has passed. *Paralytic ileus:* 500 mg; repeat after 2 hr, **then** q 4–6 hr. Continue above regimens until all danger of distention has passed (usually for a period of 48 to 72 hr or longer).

Topical Cream. Apply 1–2 times daily to affected areas.

NURSING CONSIDERATIONS

Administration/Storage

1. Dexpanthenol can be administered by IV drip when mixed with 5% dextrose or lactated Ringer's solution.
2. Delay administration of dexpanthenol for 12 hours after administration of neostigmine or similar drug, or for 1 hour after administration of succinylcholine.
3. Do not administer full strength solution into vein.

Assessment

1. If the client is female, note a history of pregnancy. If the client is nursing it may not be advisable to use this medication since it is not known if the drug is excreted in breast milk.
2. Review other drugs the client is taking for potential unfavorable interactions.

Interventions

1. Observe for reactions such as vomiting, or diarrhea which could indicate an adverse reaction to the drug. Record the events, monitor closely and report them to the physician.
2. Monitor and record vital signs and intake and output.
3. Auscultate for the presence of bowel sounds to evaluate the effectiveness of dexpanthenol.
4. Check the abdomen for continued distention and whether or not the client is passing flatus.
5. If the client appears apathetic, complains of muscle weakness, has impaired respirations or experiences cardiac arrhythmias, check the serum potassium levels. These are symptoms of hypokalemia and dexpanthenol is not effective if the client is in a hypokalemic state. Notify the physician and anticipate discontinuation of the medication.

DONNATAL CAPSULES, ELIXIR, TABLETS

(Rx)

Classification/Content: Each tablet, capsule, or 5-mL elixir contains:
Anticholinergic: Atropine sulfate, 0.0194 mg.
Anticholinergic: Hyoscyamine sulfate, 0.1037 mg.
Anticholinergic: Scopolamine hydrobromide, 0.0065 mg.
Sedative: Phenobarbital, 16.2 mg.
Note: The Extentabs contain three times the amount of drugs found in tablets.

Uses: Adjunct in the treatment of irritable colon, spastic colon, mucous colitis, and acute enterocolitis. Has also been used in the treatment of duodenal ulcer.

Special Concerns: Pregnancy category: C.

Dosage: Capsules, Elixir, Tablets. Adults, usual: 1–2 tablets or capsules t.i.d.–q.i.d. (or one Extentab q 12 hr). If the elixir is used, **adult, usual:** 5–10 mL t.i.d.–q.i.d. **Pediatric:** Use elixir as follows: **4.5–8.6 kg:** 0.5 mL q 4 hr or 0.75 mL q 6 hr; **9–13.2 kg:** 1.0 mL q 4 hr or 1.5 mL q 6 hr; **13.6–22.3 kg:** 1.5 mL q 4 hr or 2.0 mL q 6 hr; **22.7–33.6 kg:** 2.5 mL q 4 hr or 3.75 mL q 6 hr. **34–45 kg:** 3.75 mL q 4 hr or 5 mL q 6 hr; **44.5 kg:** 5 mL q 4 hr or 7.5 mL q 6 hr.

NURSING CONSIDERATIONS

See *Nursing Considerations* for *Cholinergic Blocking Agents,* p. 949, and *Barbiturates,* p. 585.

FAMOTIDINE   (fah-**MOH**-tih-deen)

Pepcid (Rx)

Classification: Histamine H_2-receptor antagonist

Action/Kinetics: Famotidine is a competitive inhibitor of histamine H_2-receptors, thus leading to inhibition of gastric acid secretion. Both basal and nocturnal gastric acid secretion, as well as secretion stimulated by food or pentagastrin, are inhibited. **Peak plasma levels:** 1–3 hr. **t½:** 2.5–3.5 hr. **Onset:** 1 hr. **Duration:** 10–12 hr. From 25%–30% of an oral dose is eliminated through the kidney unchanged.

Uses: Short-term treatment of active duodenal ulcer (up to 8 weeks). Maintenance therapy for duodenal ulcer, at reduced dosage, after active ulcer has healed. Pathological hypersecretory conditions such as Zollinger-Ellison syndrome or multiple endocrine adenomas. Benign gastric ulcer. *Investigational:* Gastroesophageal reflux disease.

Contraindications: Cirrhosis of the liver, impaired renal or hepatic function.

Special Concerns: Pregnancy category: B. Assess benefits versus risks during lactation. Safety and efficacy in children have not been established.

Side Effects: *GI:* Constipation, diarrhea, nausea, vomiting, anorexia, dry mouth, abdominal discomfort. *CNS:* Dizziness, headache, paresthesias, depression, anxiety, decreased libido, insomnia, sleepiness. *Skin:* Rash, acne, pruritus, alopecia, dry skin, flushing. *CV:* Palpitations. *Other:* Fever, asthenia, fatigue, liver enzyme abnormalities, thrombocytopenia, musculoskeletal pain, arthralgia, orbital edema, conjunctival injection, bronchospasm, tinnitus, taste disorders.

Dosage: Oral Suspension, Tablets. *Duodenal ulcer, acute therapy:* 40 mg once daily at bedtime or 20 mg b.i.d. for up to 8 weeks. *Duodenal ulcer, maintenance therapy:* 20 mg once daily at bedtime. *Benign gastric ulcers:* 40 mg at bedtime. *Hypersecretory conditions:* **Individualized. Initial, adults:** 20 mg q 6 hr; **then,** adjust dose to response, although doses of up to 160 mg q 6 hr may be required for severe cases.

IV, IV infusion. *Hospitalized patients with hypersecretory conditions, duodenal ulcers, gastric ulcers, patients unable to take PO medication:* 20 mg q 12 hr.

In severe renal insufficiency, dosage should be reduced to 20 mg at bedtime, or the dosing interval may be increased to 36–48 hr.

NURSING CONSIDERATIONS

Administration/Storage

Antacids may be used concomitantly if required.

Assessment

1. If the client is pregnant, discuss with the physician the advisability of using the drug.
2. Prior to administering the drug, determine if the client has a history of seizures, document and report to the physician.
3. Perform a baseline exam of the client's mental status.

Interventions

1. Observe the client for CNS effects such as dizziness, headaches, and anxiety.
2. Periodically assess the client for signs of depression. Report any changes in client attitude such as increasing lack of concern for personal appearance or sleeplessness.

3. Check the client's eyes routinely and report any complaints of eye problems.

4. Monitor for GI effects, such as diarrhea, constipation, or loss of appetite, document and report.

5. Check urinary output. If there is evidence of renal insufficiency, order a urinalysis, BUN, and serum creatinine and report the results to the physician as a reduction in dosage may be indicated.

LIBRAX   (LIB-rax)
(Rx)

Classification/Content: *Antianxiety agent:* Chlordiazepoxide, 5 mg. *Anticholinergic agent:* Clidinium bromide, 2.5 mg.
 See also information on individual components.

Uses: Treatment of peptic ulcer, irritable colon, spastic colon, mucous colitis, enterocolitis.

Contraindications: Pregnancy.

Dosage: Capsules. Individualized. Adults, usual: 1–2 capsules t.i.d.–q.i.d. before meals and at bedtime.

NURSING CONSIDERATIONS

See *Nursing Considerations* for *Benzodiazepines,* p. 596, and *Cholinergic Blocking Agents,* p. 949.

METOCLOPRAMIDE   (meh-toe-KLOH-prah-myd)
Clopra, Emex✿, Maxeran✿, Maxolon, Octamide, Reclomide, Reglan (Rx)

Classification: Gastrointestinal stimulant.

Action/Kinetics: Metoclopramide, by increasing sensitivity to acetylcholine, increases motility of the upper GI tract and relaxes the pyloric sphincter and duodenal bulb. This results in shortened gastric emptying and GI transit time. Metoclopramide is considered a dopamine antagonist. The drug facilitates intubation of the small bowel and speeds transit of a barium meal. **Onset, IV:** 1–3 min; **IM,** 10–15 min; **PO,** 30–60 min. **Duration:** 1–2 hr. **t½:** 4–6 hr. Significant first-pass effect following PO use; unchanged drug and metabolites excreted in urine.

Uses: PO: Acute and recurrent diabetic gastroparesis, gastroesophageal reflux. **Parenteral:** Facilitate small bowel intubation, stimulate gastric emptying, and increase intestinal transit of barium to aid in radiologic examination of stomach and small intestine, prophylaxis of nausea and vomiting in cancer chemotherapy. *Investigational:* Postoperative drug-related nausea and vomiting, treatment of slow gastric emptying time, gastric stasis in premature infants, prophylaxis of aspiration pneumonitis, vascular headaches, increase milk secretion.

Contraindications: Gastrointestinal hemorrhage, obstruction, or perforation; epilepsy, patients taking drugs likely to cause extrapyramidal symptoms, such as phenothiazines. Pheochromocytoma.

Special Concerns: Safe use during pregnancy (pregnancy category: B) and lactation not established. Extrapyramidal effects are more likely to occur in children and geriatric patients.

Side Effects: *CNS:* Restlessness, drowsiness, fatigue, lassitude, insomnia. Headaches, dizziness, extrapyramidal symptoms, Parkinsonlike symptoms, dystonia, myoclonus, depression, dyskinesia. *GI:* Nausea, bowel disturbances. *CV:* Hypertension (transient).

Drug Interactions

Acetaminophen	↑ GI absorption of acetaminophen
Anticholinergics	↓ Effect of metoclopramide
Cimetidine	↓ Effect of cimetidine due to ↓ absorption from GI tract
CNS depressants	Additive sedative effects
Digoxin	↓ Effect of digoxin due to ↓ absorption from GI tract
Ethanol	↑ GI absorption of ethanol
Levodopa	↑ GI absorption of levodopa
Narcotic analgesics	↓ Effect of metoclopramide
Tetracyclines	↑ GI absorption of tetracyclines

Dosage: Tablets, Syrup. *Diabetic gastroparesis:* **Adults,** 10 mg 30 min before meals and at bedtime for 2–8 weeks (therapy should be reinstituted if symptoms recur). *Gastroesophageal reflux:* 10–15 mg q.i.d. 30 min before meals and at bedtime.

Delayed GI emptying, peristaltic stimulant: **Pediatric, 5–14 years of age:** 2.5–5 mg t.i.d. 30 min before meals.

IV. *Prophylaxis of vomiting due to chemotherapy:* **initial,** 1–2 mg/kg for 2 doses, with the first dose 30 min before chemotherapy; **then,** 10 mg or more q 3 hr for 3 doses. Inject slowly IV over 15 min. *Facilitate small bowel intubation:* **Adults,** 10 mg given over 1–2 min; **pediatric, 6–14 years:** 2.5–5 mg; **pediatric, less than 6 years:** 0.1 mg/kg. *Radiologic examinations to increase intestinal transit time:* 10 mg as a single dose given over 1–2 min. *Delayed GI emptying, peristaltic stimulant:* **Pediatric, up to 6 years:** 0.1 mg/kg; **pediatric, 6–14 years:** 2.5–5 mg as a single dose. Pediatric dosage should not exceed 0.5 mg/kg.

NURSING CONSIDERATIONS

Administration/Storage

1. Inject slowly over 1–2 min to prevent transient feelings of anxiety and restlessness.
2. After oral use, absorption of certain drugs from the GI tract may be affected (see *Drug Interactions*).
3. Metoclopramide is physically and/or chemically incompatible with a number of drugs; check package insert if drug is to be admixed.
4. For IV use, doses greater than 10 mg should be diluted in 50 mL of either dextrose 5% in water, dextrose 5% in 0.45% sodium chloride, lactated Ringer's injection, Ringer's injection, or sodium chloride injection.

Client/Family Teaching

1. Advise the client that metoclopramide will have an added sedative effect if she is taking any other CNS depressants such as tranquilizers or sleeping pills.
2. Instruct client that operating a car or hazardous machinery should not be attempted, as medication has a sedative effect.

3. Discuss the side effects related to this drug. Instruct the client to keep a record of events to share with the physician so the adverse side effects can be properly evaluated and counteracted.

MISOPROSTOL   (my-soh-PROS-tohl)

Cytotec (Rx)

Classification: Prostaglandin.

Action/Kinetics: Misoprostol is a synthetic prostaglandin E↑1 analog which inhibits gastric acid secretion, protects the gastric mucosa by increasing bicarbonate and mucus production, and decreases pepsin levels during basal conditions. The drug may also stimulate uterine contractions that may endanger pregnancy. Misoprostol is rapidly converted to the active misoprostol acid. **Time for peak levels of misoprostol acid:** 12 min. **t½, misoprostol acid:** 20–40 min. Misoprostol acid is less than 90% bound to plasma protein. *Note:* Misoprostol does not prevent development of duodenal ulcers in patients on nonsteroidal anti-inflammatory drugs.

Uses: Prevention of aspirin and other nonsteroidal anti-inflammatory-induced gastric ulcers in patients with a high risk of gastric ulcer complications (e.g., geriatric patients with debilitating disease) or in patients with a history of ulcer.

Contraindications: Allergy to prostaglandins, pregnancy (pregnancy category: X), during lactation (may cause diarrhea in nursing infants).

Special Concerns: Use with caution in patients with renal impairment and in patients older than 64 years of age. Safety and efficacy have not been established in children less than 18 years of age.

Side Effects: *GI:* Diarrhea, abdominal pain, nausea, dyspepsia, flatulence, vomiting, constipation. *Gynecological:* Cramps, dysmenorrhea, hypermenorrhea, menstrual disorders, postmenopausal vaginal bleeding. *Miscellaneous:* Headache.

Dosage: Tablets. Adults: 200 mcg q.i.d. with food. Dose can be reduced to 100 mcg if the larger dose can not be tolerated. In renal impairment, the 200 mcg dose can be reduced if necessary.

NURSING CONSIDERATIONS

Administration/Storage

1. The incidence of diarrhea can be reduced by giving the drug after meals and at bedtime as well as by avoiding magnesium-containing antacids. Diarrhea is usually self-limiting, however.
2. Maximum plasma levels of misoprostol are decreased if the drug is taken with food.
3. Misoprostol should be taken for the duration of nonsteroidal anti-inflammatory therapy.
4. Drug may increase gastric bicarbonate and mucus production.

Assessment

Obtain a negative pregnancy test on females of childbearing age prior to initiating drug therapy.

Client/Family Teaching

1. Provide client with both oral and written warnings of adverse drug effects. Instruct her to keep a record of events to share with the physician so that side effects and drug therapy can be evaluated.

2. Remind clients not to share medications with anyone.

3. Instruct client to take misoprostol exactly as prescribed for the duration of aspirin or nonsteroidal anti-inflammatory drug therapy.

4. Stress that all women of childbearing age must practice effective contraceptive measures as drug has abortifacient properties.

5. Clients may experience abdominal discomfort and/or diarrhea. Instruct them to take misoprostol after meals and at bedtime to minimize these side effects.

NIZATIDINE   (nye-ZAY-tih-deen)

Axid (Rx)

Classification: Histamine H$_2$-receptor antagonist.

Action/Kinetics: Nizatidine decreases gastric acid secretion by blocking the effect of histamine on histamine H$_2$-receptors. Does not affect the P-450 and P-448 drug metabolizing enzymes. **Peak plasma levels:** 0.5–3 hr after an oral dose. **Time to peak effect:** 0.5–3 hr. **Duration, nocturnal:** Up to 12 hr; **basal:** Up to 8 hr. **t½:** 1–2 hr. Approximately 60% of an oral dose is excreted unchanged in the urine. Patients with moderate to severe renal impairment manifest a significant prolongation of t½ with decreased clearance.

Uses: Acute duodenal ulcer. Prophylaxis of duodenal ulcer following healing of an active ulcer. *Investigational:* Benign gastric ulcer, gastroesophageal reflux disease.

Contraindications: Hypersensitivity to H$_2$-receptor antagonists. Cirrhosis of the liver, impaired renal or hepatic function.

Special Concerns: Pregnancy category: C. Use with caution during lactation. Safety and efficacy have not been determined in children.

Side Effects: *Hepatic:* Hepatocellular damage manifested by ↑ SGOT (AST), SGPT (ALT), or alkaline phosphatase. *Miscellaneous:* Somnolence, urticaria, sweating, rash, exfoliative dermatitis, hyperuricemia.

Drug Interactions: Following high doses of aspirin, nizatidine → ↑ salicylate serum levels.

Laboratory Test Interference: False + test for urobilinogen.

Dosage: Capsules. *Active duodenal ulcer:* Either 300 mg once daily at bedtime or 150 mg b.i.d. *Prophylaxis following healing of duodenal ulcer:* 150 mg once daily at bedtime. Dosage must be decreased for patients with moderate to severe renal insufficiency.

NURSING CONSIDERATIONS

Administration/Storage

1. Treatment for active duodenal ulcer should be maintained for up to 8 weeks.

2. Gastric malignancy may be present even though there has been a clinical response to nizatidine.

Assessment

1. Take a drug history to determine if the client has any allergies to H$_2$-receptor antagonists.

2. Obtain baseline laboratory studies including hepatic and renal function studies prior to initiating therapy.

Interventions

1. Assess the client for evidence of renal insufficiency. Document and report to the physician. Anticipate reduced dosage in clients with renal insufficiency.

2. Drug may cause a false-positive test for urobilinogen. If this test has been ordered, notify the lab that the client is taking nizatidine.

Client/Family Teaching

1. Instruct the client to notify the physician of any side effects, such as rashes, flaking of skin, or extreme sleepiness.

2. Take the medication at bedtime due to potential sedative effects.

3. Use caution when performing tasks that require mental alertness.

4. Continue to take the medication as ordered even if symptoms subside.

OMEPRAZOLE   (oh-MEP-rah-zohl)

Prilosec (formerly Losec)(Rx)

Classification: Agent to suppress gastric acid secretion.

Action/Kinetics: Omeprazole does not possess either anticholinergic or histamine H_2-receptor antagonist effects. Rather, the drug is thought to be a gastric pump inhibitor in that it blocks the final step of acid production by inhibiting the H^+-K^+ ATPase system at the secretory surface of the gastric parietal cell. Both basal and stimulated acid secretion is inhibited. Serum gastrin levels are increased during the first one or two weeks of therapy and are maintained at such levels during the course of therapy. Because omeprazole is acid-labile, the product contains an enteric-coated granule formulation; however, absorption is rapid. **Peak plasma levels:** 0.5–3.5 hr. **Onset:** Within 1 hr. **t½:** 0.5–1 hr. **Duration:** Up to 72 hr (due to prolonged binding of the drug to the parietal H^+-K^+ ATPase enzyme). The drug is significantly bound (95%) to plasma protein. Omeprazole is metabolized in the liver and inactive metabolites are excreted through the urine. Although plasma levels of omeprazole are increased in patients with chronic hepatic disease and in the elderly, dosage adjustment is not necessary.

Uses: Short-term (4–8 weeks) treatment of severe erosive esophagitis and poorly responsive gastroesophageal reflux disease. Long-term treatment of pathological hypersecretory conditions such as Zollinger-Ellison syndrome, multiple endocrine adenomas, and systemic mastocytosis. *Investigational:* Duodenal ulcers.

Contraindications: Long-term treatment of gastroesophageal reflux disease and esophagitis. Lactation.

Special Concerns: Use during pregnancy (pregnancy category: C) only if potential benefits outweigh potential risks. Safety and effectiveness have not been determined in children.

Side Effects: *CNS:* Headache, dizziness. Possibly, anxiety disorders, abnormal dreams, vertigo, insomnia, nervousness, apathy, somnolence, hemifacial dysesthesia. *GI:* Diarrhea, nausea, abdominal pain, vomiting, constipation, flatulence, acid regurgitation, abdominal swelling. Possibly, anorexia, fecal discoloration, esophageal candidiasis, mucosal atrophy of the tongue, dry mouth, irritable colon. *CV:* Angina, chest pain, tachycardia, bradycardia, palpitation, peripheral edema. *Respiratory:* Upper respiratory infection, pharyngeal pain. *Skin:* Inflammation, alopecia, urticaria, pruritus, dry skin, hyperhidrosis. *GU:* Urinary tract infection, urinary frequency, hematuria, proteinuria, glycosuria, testicular pain, microscopic pyuria. *Hematologic:* Pancytopenia, thrombocytopenia, anemia, leukocytosis, neutropenia. *Miscellaneous:* Rash, asthenia, cough, back pain, fever, pain, fatigue, malaise, hypoglycemia, weight gain, epistaxis, tinnitus, alteration in taste.

Note: Data are lacking on the effect of long-term hypochlorhydria and hypergastrinemia on the risk of developing tumors.

Drug Interactions	
Ampicillin (esters)	Possible ↓ absorption of ampicillin esters due to ↑ pH of stomach
Diazepam	↑ Plasma levels of diazepam due to ↓ rate of metabolism by the liver
Iron salts	Possible ↓ absorption of iron salts due to ↑ pH of stomach
Ketoconazole	Possible ↓ absorption of ketoconazole due to ↑ pH of stomach
Phenytoin	↑ Plasma levels of phenytoin due to ↓ rate of metabolism of the liver
Warfarin	Prolonged rate of elimination of warfarin due to ↓ rate of metabolism by the liver

Dosage: Capsules. *Severe erosive esophagitis, poorly responsive gastroesophageal reflux disease:* **Adults,** 20 mg daily for 4–8 wk. *Pathological hypersecretory conditions:* **Adults, initial,** 60 mg once daily; **then,** dose individualized although doses up to 120 mg t.i.d. have been used. Daily doses greater than 80 mg should be divided. *Duodenal ulcer:* 10–60 mg daily.

NURSING CONSIDERATIONS

Administration/Storage

1. Antacids can be administered with omeprazole.
2. The capsule should be swallowed whole and should not be opened, chewed, or crushed.

Assessment

1. If female of childbearing age, determine if pregnant.
2. Obtain baseline CBC, prior to initiating therapy.

Client/Family Teaching

1. Review the list of side effects associated with drug therapy. Instruct client to report any adverse effects to the physician.
2. Take drug as prescribed and before meals.
3. Report any changes in urinary elimination or pain and discomfort associated with voiding.

RANITIDINE HYDROCHLORIDE (rah-**NIT**-ih-deen)

Zantac (Rx)

Classification: H₂-receptor antagonist.

Action/Kinetics: Ranitidine competitively inhibits gastric acid secretion by blocking the effect of histamine on histamine H_2-receptors. Both daytime and nocturnal basal gastric acid secretion, as well as food- and pentagastrin-stimulated gastric acid are inhibited. It is a weak inhibitor of cytochrome P-450 (drug-metabolizing enzymes). **Peak effect: PO,** 1–3 hr; **IM, IV,** 15 min. **t¹/₂:** 2.5–3 hr. **Duration, nocturnal:** 13 hr; **basal:** 4 hr. **Serum level to inhibit 50% stimulated gastric acid secretion:** 36–94 ng/mL. Excreted in urine.

Uses: Short-term (4–8 weeks) and maintenance treatment of duodenal ulcer. Pathologic hyper-secretory conditions such as Zollinger-Ellison syndrome and systemic mastocytosis. Active, benign gastric ulcers, reflux esophagitis, *Investigational:* Prophylaxis of pulmonary aspiration of acid during anesthesia, prevent gastric damage from nonsteroidal anti-inflammatory drugs.

Contraindications: Cirrhosis of the liver, impaired renal or hepatic function.

Special Concerns: Use with caution during pregnancy (pregnancy category: B) and lactation and in patients with decreased hepatic or renal function. Safety and efficacy not established in children.

Side Effects: *GI:* Constipation, nausea, vomiting, diarrhea, abdominal pain. *CNS:* Headache, dizziness, malaise, insomnia, vertigo. *CV:* Bradycardia or tachycardia, premature ventricular beats. *Hematologic:* Thrombocytopenia, granulocytopenia, leukopenia, pancytopenia. *Hepatic:* Hepato-toxicity, jaundice, hepatitis, increase in SGPT. *Allergic:* Bronchospasm, rashes, fever, eosinophilia. *Other:* Arthralgia, alopecia.

Drug Interactions

Antacids	Antacids may ↓ the absorption of ranitidine
Glipizide	Ranitidine ↑ effect of glipizide
Warfarin	Ranitidine may ↑ hypoprothrombinemic effects of warfarin

---

Dosage: Syrup, Tablets. Adults: *Duodenal ulcer:* 150 mg b.i.d. or 300 mg at bedtime to heal ulcer, although 100 mg b.i.d. will inhibit acid secretion. **Maintenance:** 150 mg at bedtime. *Hypersecretory conditions:* 150 mg b.i.d. (up to 6 g/day has been used in severe cases). *Gastroesophageal reflux, benign gastric ulcer:* 150 mg b.i.d. In impaired renal function (creatinine clearance less than 50 mL/min): **PO,** 150 mg/day; **IM, IV.** *All uses:* **Adults, IM,** 50 mg q 6–8 hr. **IV injection or infusion:** 50 mg q 6–8 hr, not to exceed 400 mg daily.

NURSING CONSIDERATIONS

Administration/Storage

1. Antacids should be given concomitantly for pain, although they may interfere with absorption of ranitidine.
2. About one-half of clients may heal completely within 2 weeks; thus, endoscopy may show no need for further treatment.
3. No dilution is required for IM use. For IV injection, 50 mg should be diluted with 0.9% sodium chloride injection to a total volume of 20 mL. The diluted solution should be given over 5 min or more. For intermittent IV infusion, dilute 50 mg in 100 mL 5% dextrose injection and give over 15–20 min.

Assessment

1. Note any evidence of renal or liver disease.
2. Obtain baseline liver and renal function studies.
3. When working with sexually active female clients, determine the potential of an existing pregnancy. The drug should be used cautiously in these instances.

> **Interventions**
>
> 1. Monitor for any increase in the incidence of infections. Have a CBC with differential conducted routinely to detect any potential increased risk of infection.
> 2. If the client complains of diarrhea, notify the physician. Encourage the client to maintain adequate hydration and monitor serum electrolytes.
>
> **Client/Family Teaching**
>
> 1. Follow the scheduled visits to the physician so they can determine the extent of healing and when the drug can be safely discontinued.
> 2. Encourage the client not to smoke, because smoking may interfere with the healing of duodenal ulcers.
> 3. Explain to the client with symptoms that breast tenderness will usually disappear after several weeks. If it persists, the physician should be notified as the drug therapy may need to be discontinued.

SIMETHICONE   (sye-**METH**-ih-kohn)

Extra-Strength Gas-X, Gas-X, Mylicon, Mylicon-80, Mylicon-125, Ovol✽, Ovol-40 and -80✽, Phazyme, Phazyme 55✽, Phazyme 95 and 125, Silain (OTC)

Classification: Antiflatulent.

Action/Kinetics: Simethicone acts as a defoamant, which decreases surface tension of gas bubbles, thus facilitating their coalescence and expulsion as flatus or belching. It also prevents the accumulation of mucus-enclosed pockets of gas. Excreted in feces unchanged.

Uses: Relief of pain caused by excess gas in digestive tract. Adjunct in the treatment of postoperative gaseous distention, air swallowing, functional dyspepsia, peptic ulcer, spastic irritable colon, or diverticulitis. *Investigational:* Adjunct during gastroscopy to increase visualization and prior to radiography to reduce gas shadows in the bowel.

Dosage: Tablets: 50–100 mg after each meal and at bedtime (up to a maximum of 500 mg daily if used OTC). **Chewable Tablets:** 40–125 mg q.i.d. after each meal and at bedtime (up to 480 mg daily if used OTC). **Capsules:** 125 mg after each meal and at bedtime. **Oral Suspension:** 40 mg q.i.d. after meals and at bedtime. Also, for *gastroscopy, radiography of the bowel:* 67 mg in 2.5 mL water as a single dose.

NURSING CONSIDERATIONS

Administration/Storage

1. Tablets should be chewed thoroughly or dissolved in mouth.
2. Use calibrated dropper to administer medication.
3. Suspension should be shaken well before using.

Interventions

1. Assess bowel sounds periodically during therapy.
2. Question client concerning the effectiveness of prescribed therapy as dosage may need to be adjusted.

SUCRALFATE (sue-KRAL-fayt)

Carafate, Sulcrate ✳ (Rx)

Action/Kinetics: Sucralfate is the aluminum salt of a sulfurated disaccharide. It is thought to form an ulcer-adherent complex with albumin and fibrinogen at the site of the ulcer protecting it from further damage by gastric acid. It may also form a viscous, adhesive barrier on the surface of the gastric mucosa and duodenum. The drug adsorbs pepsin, thus inhibiting its activity. May be used in conjunction with antacids. Approximately 90% excreted in the feces. **Duration:** 5 hr.

Use: Short-term treatment (up to 8 weeks) of duodenal ulcers. *Investigational:* Hasten healing of gastric ulcers, chronic treatment of gastric or duodenal ulcers. Treatment of oral and esophageal ulcers due to chemotherapy, radiation, or sclerotherapy (suspension used). Treatment of aspirin- and NSAID-induced GI symptoms; prevention of stress ulcers and GI bleeding in critically ill patients.

Special Concerns: Safety for use in children and during pregnancy (pregnancy category: B) and lactation has not been fully established.

Side Effects: *GI:* Constipation (most common); also, nausea, diarrhea, indigestion, dry mouth, gastric discomfort. *Miscellaneous:* Back pain, dizziness, drowsiness, vertigo, rash, pruritus.

Drug Interactions: Sucralfate may prevent the absorption of cimetidine, phenytoin, or tetracyclines from the GI tract.

Dosage: Tablets. Adults: usual: 1 g q.i.d. 1 hr before meals and at bedtime (it may also be taken 2 hr after meals). The drug should be taken for 4–8 weeks unless x-ray films or endoscopy have indicated significant healing.

NURSING CONSIDERATIONS

Administration/Storage

1. If antacids are used, they should be taken 30 min before or after sucralfate.
2. Even though healing of ulcers may result, the frequency or severity of subsequent attacks is not altered.

Interventions

Assess for effectiveness of sucralfate therapy by examining for reduction in signs and symptoms of ulcer.

Client/Family Teaching

1. Stress the importance of taking the medication exactly as prescribed.
2. Instruct the client to report any bothersome side effects to the physician.

CHAPTER FIFTY-FOUR

Laxatives

General Statement: Difficult or infrequent passage of stools (constipation) is a symptom of many conditions ranging from purely organic causes (obstruction, megacolon) to common functional disorders. Patients confined to bed may often develop constipation. Constipation may also be of psychologic origin. The underlying cause of constipation should be elucidated by a physician, especially since a marked change in bowel habits may be a symptom of a pathologic condition.

Laxatives are effective because they act locally, either by specifically stimulating the smooth muscles of the bowel or by changing the bulk or consistency of the stools. The laxatives can be divided into four categories:

1. *Stimulant laxatives:* Substances that chemically stimulate the smooth muscles of the bowel so as to increase contractions. Drugs include bisacodyl, cascara, castor oil, phenolphthalein, and senna.
2. *Saline laxatives:* Substances that increase the bulk of the stools by retaining water. Includes magnesium salts and sodium phosphate.
3. *Bulk-forming laxatives:* Nondigestible substances that pass through the stomach and then increase the bulk of the stools. Examples are methylcellulose and psyllium.
4. *Emollient and lubricant laxatives:* Agents that soften hardened feces and facilitate their passage through the lower intestine. Examples include docusate and mineral oil.

There are many laxative products which contain two or more drugs with laxative properties. Today laxatives are prescribed less frequently for chronic constipation than in the past. In fact, continued use of laxatives has been held responsible for some cases of chronic constipation and other intestinal disorders because the patient may start to depend on the psychological effect and physical stimulus of the drug rather than on the body's own natural reflexes. Prevention of constipation should include adequate fluid intake and diet, as well as daily exercise.

Uses: Laxatives are indicated for the following conditions: anorectal lesions like hemorrhoids; for diagnostic procedures and in conjunction with surgery or anthelmintic therapy; and in cases of chemical poisoning. Short-term treatment of constipation.

Contraindications: Severe abdominal pain that *might* be caused by appendicitis, enteritis, ulcerative colitis, diverticulitis, intestinal obstruction. The administration of laxatives in such cases might cause rupture of the abdomen or intestinal hemorrhage. Children under the age of 2.

Side Effects: Excess activity of the colon resulting in nausea, diarrhea, or vomiting. Dehydration, disturbance of the electrolyte balance. Dependency occurs if used chronically.
   Bulk laxatives: Obstruction in the esophagus, stomach, small intestine, or rectum. *Stimulant laxatives:* Chronic abuse may lead to malfunctioning colon.

Drug Interactions	
Anticoagulants, oral	↓ Absorption of vitamin K from GI tract induced by laxatives may ↑ effects of anticoagulants and result in bleeding
Digitalis	Cathartics may ↓ absorption of digitalis
Tetracyclines	↓ Effect of tetracyclines due to ↓ absorption from GI tract

NURSING CONSIDERATIONS

Administration/Storage

1. When administering a laxative, note the length of time it takes for the laxative to take effect and give it so that the result of the laxative will not interfere with the client's rest.
2. Administer laxatives at a temperature that makes them more agreeable to the client.
3. If the laxative is to be administered in a liquid, try to select one that the client finds palatable.
4. Administer laxatives at a time that will not interfere with the client's digestion and absorption of nutrients.
5. If the laxative is ordered to prepare the client for a diagnostic study, check the directions carefully to ensure accurate administration in preparation for the study.

Assessment

1. Determine the extent of the client's problem with constipation. Note how long the client has had to rely on laxatives.
2. Note if the client has abdominal pain and discomfort, its exact location and the type of discomfort. The symptoms may indicate appendicitis or some other intestinal disorder and laxatives would be contraindicated.
3. Note the age of the client, their state of health and the client's nutritional status.
4. List other medications the client is taking that may contribute to a constipation problem.
5. Identify if the client has had any recent changes in lifestyle that may contribute to the current problem.

54

6. Determine the character of the client's stool and the frequency of bowel movements expected by the client. The client's definition of constipation may determine if, in fact, constipation exists.

7. Note the type of laxative the client has been taking and the relative effectiveness associated with this laxative.

Interventions

1. If the client is in a hospital or is ill at home, provide a commode at the bedside. This will promote better bowel function by encouraging the client to move about and ensure privacy.

2. Encourage the client to alter dietary habits to include bulk foods and sufficient fluid in the daily diet to enhance elimination.

3. Discuss with the client the need for exercise and reduction of a dependence on laxatives.

Client/Family Teaching

1. Discuss with the client the need to have a regular schedule for defecation.

2. Instruct the client in keeping a record of bowel function and response to laxatives taken.

3. If the laxative is to be taken in preparation for a diagnostic study, review the directions with the client and provide a printed set of instructions to follow. If the client is unable to read, try to assure that someone in the family or a friend can review the directions with the client so that an accurate result of the test can be obtained.

4. Instruct the client in techniques that facilitate elimination. Sitting with the legs slightly elevated and leaning forward to increase abdominal pressure often encourages elimination.

5. Discuss with the client the dangers of relying on laxatives for bowel movements and the use of diet to achieve the same purpose. Two or three prunes a day are preferable to laxatives.

6. Advise the client to consult the physician if constipation persists. There could be a physiological problem that requires attention.

7. If the client is pregnant, advise the client to consult with the physician before taking any laxatives to treat constipation.

8. Advise nursing mothers to avoid using laxatives unless approved by the physician. Many are excreted in breast milk and can cause the infant to develop diarrhea.

Evaluation

1. The client regularly passes stools with minimum difficulty.

2. The client reports that bowel movements occur without having to resort to the use of laxatives, enemas, or suppositories.

STIMULANT LAXATIVES

BISACODYL (bis-ah-KOH-dill)

Bisac-Evac, Bisacolax✿, Carter's Little Pills, Dacodyl, Deficol, Dulcolax, Fleet Bisacodyl, Fleet Bisacodyl Prep, Laxit✿, Theralax (OTC)

BISACODYL TANNEX (bis-ah-KOH-dill)

Clysodrast (Rx)

See also *Laxatives,* p. 1048.

Classification: Laxative, stimulant.

Action/Kinetics: Bisacodyl is a local chemical stimulant that acts by increasing the contraction of the muscles of the colon by stimulating the intramural nerve plexi. Bisacodyl is not absorbed systemically and can be administered orally or as a rectal suppository or solution. It produces a gentle bowel movement with soft, formed stools. It usually acts within 6 to 8 hr after PO administration and 15 to 60 minutes after rectal administration.

Uses: Cleansing of colon preoperatively and postoperatively and for diagnostic procedures (radiology, barium enemas, proctoscopy), colostomies. Short-term treatment of constipation.

May be used during pregnancy or in the presence of cardiovascular, renal, or hepatic disease.

Contraindications: Acute surgical abdomen or acute abdominal pain. Children less than 6 years of age.

Additional Side Effects: Suppositories may cause burning sensation.

Drug Interaction: Use of bisacodyl with antacids, milk, or cimetidine may result in premature dissolution of the enteric coating, leading to cramping and vomiting.

Dosage: Tablets. Adults: 10–15 mg at bedtime or before breakfast. *Preparation of lower GI tract:* Up to 30 mg; **Pediatric, over 6 years:** 5–10 mg at bedtime or before breakfast. **Rectal suppository, adults and children over 2 years:** 10 mg; **under 2 years:** 5 mg.

Bisacodyl Tannex. **Cleansing enema:** 2.5 g in 1 L warm water. *Barium enema:* 2.5 or 5 g in 1 L barium suspension. *Note:* No more than 10 g should be given within a 3-day period. Also, the total dose for one examination of the colon should not exceed 7.5 g.

NURSING CONSIDERATIONS

See also *Nursing Considerations* for *Laxatives,* p. 1049.

Administration/Storage

1. Bisacodyl tablets should be taken either at bedtime for effectiveness in the morning, or before breakfast so as not to interfere with the client's rest at night. The tablets should be effective within 6 hr.
2. If the tablets are being given to prepare the client for surgery, radiography, or sigmoidoscopy, the drug should be taken orally the night before the procedure and by rectal suppository early that morning.
3. Bisacodyl tablets should be refrigerated at temperatures not to exceed 30°C (86°F).
4. Lubricate suppositories with warm water prior to administration.

Client/Family Teaching

1. Instruct the client to swallow the tablet whole. Do not crush or chew the tablets.
2. Children who cannot swallow tablets will be unable to take the laxative by mouth.
3. Advise the client not to take the laxative within 1 hr of ingesting milk or an antacid.

CASCARA SAGRADA (kas-KAR-ah sah-GRAD-ah)

Cascara Sagrada Fluid Extract, Cascara Sagrada Aromatic Fluid Extract, Cascara Tablets (OTC)

See also *Laxatives,* p. 1048.

Classification: Stimulant laxative.

Action/Kinetics: Cascara sagrada directly stimulates the intestinal mucosa and the myenteric plexus. The drug alters secretion of water and electrolytes. It produces stools within 6–10 hr. The drug is available in tablet form as well as an aromatic fluid extract.

Uses: Short-term treatment of constipation.

Additional Contraindication: The drug gets into breast milk and may cause diarrhea in the infant.

Additional Side Effects: Dark pigmentation of the mucosa of the colon (called melanosis coli), which is slowly reversed after the drug is discontinued. Acid urine may be colored yellowish-brown while an alkaline urine may be colored pink, red, or violet.

Dosage: Aromatic fluid extract. Adults: 5 mL at bedtime; **pediatric, over 2 years of age:** 1–3 mL. **Fluid extract. Adults:** 1 mL at bedtime. **Tablets:** 1 tablet at bedtime.

NURSING CONSIDERATIONS

See also *Nursing Considerations* for *Laxatives,* p. 1049.

Assessment

Determine how long and how often the client has been using cascara.

Interventions

If the client has taken cascara over an extended period of time, monitor electrolyte levels.

Client/Family Teaching

1. Advise client that cascara sagrada may cause the urine to appear yellow-brown or reddish. This should not cause alarm.
2. Remind client to read the bottle carefully to distinguish between the Aromatic Fluid Extract and the Fluid Extract as the dosage is different.
3. If working with a pregnant client, advise the client to consult with the physician prior to taking cascara.
4. Advise clients to use cascara for a short time only. Cascara sagrada can cause electrolyte imbalance, especially hypokalemia. This can be particularly dangerous for elderly clients.

CASTOR OIL   (CAS-tor)

Kellogg's Castor Oil, Purge (OTC)

CASTOR OIL, EMULSIFIED   (CAS-tor)

Alphamul, Emulsoil, Fleet Flavored Castor Oil, Neoloid (OTC)

See also *Laxatives,* p. 1048.

Classification: Laxative, stimulant.

Action/Kinetics: The active ingredient is ricinoleic acid, which is liberated in the small intestine. This substance inhibits water and electrolyte absorption, leading to fluid accumulation and increased peristalsis. Prompt (within 2–6 hr) and complete evacuation of the bowel occurs, often with a watery stool.

Use: Short-term relief of constipation.

Contraindications: Pregnancy, menstruation, abdominal pain, and intestinal obstruction. Common constipation. Concomitantly with fat-soluble anthelmintics.

Side Effects: Severe diarrhea, abdominal pain and colic, altered mucosal permeability in the small intestine, dehydration, and changes in electrolyte balance, including hyperkalemia, acidosis, or alkalosis.

Dosage: *Castor oil:* 15–60 mL before diagnostic procedures; **infants:** 1–5 mL; **children over 2 years:** 5–15 mL. *Castor oil emulsified,* **PO:** 15–60 mL; **infants less than 2 years:** 1.25–7.5 mL; **children over 2 years:** 5–30 mL. Dose depends on strength of preparation.

NURSING CONSIDERATIONS
See also *Nursing Considerations* for *Laxatives,* p. 1049.

Administration/Storage
1. Shake emulsions well prior to administering. They may be further diluted in water, juice or cola before administering unless otherwise indicated.
2. Regular castor oil does not mix well with water-based materials. Adding a small amount of sodium bicarbonate to castor oil immediately before administering it will cause the mixture to fizz, particularly suspending the castor oil for a few minutes in the diluent. Discuss this with the physician prior to administering the laxative, unless the client's condition does not permit.

Client/Family Teaching
1. Clients usually prefer the more palatable oil-in-water emulsions that have been aromatized with flavoring agents.
2. Disguise the taste of plain castor oil by mixing with a glass of orange juice.

PHENOLPHTHALEIN   (fee-nohl-**THAY**-leen)

Alophen, Espotabs, Evac-U-Gen, Evac-U-Lax, Ex-Lax, Ex-Lax Pills, Feen-A-Mint Gum, Modane, Phenolax (OTC)

See also *Laxatives,* p. 1048.

Classification: Laxative, stimulant.

Action/Kinetics: The drug acts primarily on the large intestine to produce a semifluid stool with little or no accompanying colic. **Onset:** 4–8 hr. **Duration:** May be 3–4 days due to residual effect.

Use: Short-term use for constipation.

Additional Side Effects: Hypersensitivity reactions: Dermatitis, pruritus; rarely, nonthrombocytopenic purpura or anaphylaxis. Phenolphthalein may color alkaline urine pink-red and acidic urine yellow-brown.

Dosage: Gum, Tablets, Chewable Tablets, Wafers. Adults: 60–194 mg/day; **pediatric, over 6 years:** 30–60 mg/day; **2–5 years:** 15–20 mg/day. Usually taken at bedtime.

NURSING CONSIDERATIONS
See also *Nursing Considerations* for *Laxatives,* p. 1049.

Administration/Storage
1. Oral doses take 6–8 hours to be effective.
2. Suppositories are usually effective in 15–60 minutes.

Client/Family Teaching

1. Advise client that phenolphthalein colors alkaline stools and urine red.
2. Store medication out of the reach of children. This is particularly important when the laxative looks like chocolate and may be accidentally ingested as candy.
3. Remind clients that Ex-Lax is a medication, and to use only as directed.

SENNA   (SEN-nah)

Black-Draught Lax–Senna, Dr. Caldwell Senna Laxative, Fletcher's Castoria for Children, Senexon, Senokot, Senolax, X-Prep Liquid (OTC)

SENNOSIDES A AND B, CALCIUM SALTS   (SEN-noh-syds)

Gentle Nature, Glysennid ✹, Nytilax (OTC)

Classification: Stimulant laxative.

Action/Kinetics: Senna is prepared from the dried leaf or fruit of the *Cassia acutifolia* or *Cassia angustifolia* tree. Senna is similar to cascara although it is more potent. It increases peristalsis of the colon by stimulating the intestinal mucosa and the myenteric plexus; it also alters electrolyte secretion. **Onset:** 6–10 hr.

Uses: Constipation, preoperative and prediagnostic procedures involving the GI tract.

Contraindications: Irritable colon, nausea, vomiting, abdominal pain, and appendicitis or possibility thereof.

Special Concerns: Administer with caution to nursing mothers.

Side Effects: Abdominal pain, colic, and diarrhea. Senna colors alkaline urine pink, red, or violet and acid urine yellow-brown.

Dosage: *Senna.* **Tablets: Adults,** 2 at bedtime; **pediatric, over 60 lb:** 1 tablet at bedtime. **Suppositories: Adults,** 1 at bedtime; **pediatric, over 60 lb:** ½ suppository at bedtime. **Black-Draught Granules: Adults,** ¼–½ level teaspoon with water (not recommended for children). **Senokot Granules: Adults,** 1 teaspoon; **pediatric, over 60 lb:** ½ teaspoon. Taken at bedtime. **Senokot Syrup: Adults,** 10–15 mL at bedtime; **pediatric, 1–12 months:** 1.25–2.5 mL at bedtime; **pediatric, 1–5 years:** 2.5–5 mL; **5–15 years:** 5–10 mL. **Dr. Caldwell Senna Laxative: Adults,** 15–30 mL with or after meals or at bedtime; **pediatric, 6–15 years:** 10–15 mL at bedtime; **1–5 years:** 5–10 mL at bedtime. **Fletcher's Castoria for Children, 6–12 years:** 10–15 mL; **1–5 years:** 5–10 mL; **7–12 months:** 2.5–5 mL; **1–6 months:** 1.25–2.5 mL.
Sennosides A and B. **Gentle Nature, Adults,** 1–2 tablets at bedtime taken with water; **children 6 years and older:** 1 tablet at bedtime. **Nytilax, Adults:** 12–36 mg (1–3 tablets) at bedtime.

NURSING CONSIDERATIONS

See also *Nursing Considerations* for *Laxatives,* p. 1048.

Client/Family Teaching

1. Advise the client that gripping pain may be a symptom of overdosage. Omit drug when this occurs and notify physician.
2. Explain to the client that the drug causes acid urine to have a yellowish-brown color. Alkaline urine will develop a reddish color.

SALINE LAXATIVES

Action/Kinetics: Saline laxatives increase the bulk of the stools by attracting and holding large amounts of fluids. The increased bulk results in the mechanical stimulation of peristalsis. The saline cathartics should be administered with sufficient fluid so as not to cause dehydration of the patient. **Onset:** 0.5–3 hr.

The saline cathartics, which include magnesium sulfate, milk of magnesia (see *Antacids*), magnesium citrate, sodium phosphate, and sodium biphosphate are similar in activity, differing mostly with respect to palatability, cost, and efficiency.

There is always some systemic absorption of the saline cathartics. This presents a problem in the case of magnesium ions, which may cause magnesium intoxication when given to patients with poor renal function. Magnesium intoxication is characterized by drowsiness, dizziness, and other signs of CNS depression. Thirst may be an early sign of magnesium intoxication.

See Table 22 for individual agents.

Use: To empty the bowel prior to diagnostic or surgical procedures; to eliminate parasites following anthelmintic therapy; to remove toxic material following poisoning; to collect of stool specimen for parasite examination.

BULK-FORMING LAXATIVES

Action/Kinetics: Bulk-forming laxatives increase the bulk of the feces and stimulate peristalsis by mechanical means. These are the safest of the available laxatives. **Onset:** 12–24 hr. Stool is soft and formed.

Side Effects: Obstruction of the esophagus, stomach, small intestine, and rectum.

NURSING CONSIDERATIONS

Client/Family Teaching

1. Advise clients that good fluid intake is necessary to prevent intestinal obstruction.
2. Instruct client that they can anticipate results in 12–24 hours after taking the laxative.

METHYLCELLULOSE   (meth-ill-**SELL**-you-lohs)

Citrucel, Cologel (OTC)

Classification: Bulk-forming laxative.

Action/Kinetics: Methylcellulose is composed of indigestible fibers that form a colloidal, bulky gelatinous mass on contact with water. The fibers pass through the stomach and increase the bulk of the feces, stimulating peristalsis. The drug is usually effective within 12–24 hours.

Uses: Prophylaxis of constipation in patients who should not strain during defecation. Short-term treatment of constipation; useful in geriatric patients with diminished colonic motor response and during pregnancy and postpartum to reestablish normal bowel function. To soften feces during fecal impaction.

Contraindications: Intestinal obstruction, ulceration, and severe abdominal pain.

Table 22   Saline Laxatives

Drug	Dosage	Remarks
Magnesium citrate (Citrate of Magnesia, Citroma, Citro-Mag✱, Citro-Nesia) (OTC)	**Oral Solution. Adults:** 240 mL (100 mL contains 1.75 g magnesium citrate). **Pediatric:** 1/2 the adult dose.	Observe for magnesium intoxication. Do not give in case of poor renal function. *Administration:* Preferably, store in refrigerator to improve taste. *Nursing Considerations:* 1. Remain with patient and encourage drinking the entire solution at once. 2. Provide a cold solution of medication for this makes it taste best. 3. Assess for signs of magnesium toxicity. (For characteristics see Table 30, p. 1285.)
Magnesium hydroxide (M.O.M., Phillips' Milk of Magnesia, Phillips' Magnesia Tablets✱) (OTC)	**Suspension. Adults and children over 12 years:** 15–40 mL (10–20 mL of concentrate); **pediatric, 6–12 years:** 7.5–20 mL; **2–6 years:** 5–10 mL.	Suspension should be mixed with liquid (e.g., water, juice) to increase palatability.
Magnesium sulfate (Epsom Salt) (OTC)	**Granules. Adults:** 10–15 g; **pediatric:** 5–10 g.	Effective in 1–2 hr. *Administration:* Dissolve in glassful of ice water or other fluid to lessen the disagreeable taste.
Sodium phosphate and sodium biphosphate (Fleet Phosopho-Soda, Sodium Phosphates) (OTC)	**Solution. Adults:** 20–30 mL; **pediatric:** 5–15 mL.	These products contain 18 g of sodium phosphate and 48 g sodium biphosphate/ 100 mL. Doses should be mixed with 1/2 glass of cold water.

Dosage: Capsules, Tablets. Adults: 2–3 capsules or tablets t.i.d.; **pediatric, over 6 years:** 1–2 capsules or tablets b.i.d. **Powder. Adults:** 1–1.5 g t.i.d. **pediatric:** 1–1.5 g daily.

Citrucel Granules: Adults and children over 12 years of age, 1 19 g packet in 8 oz water 1–3 times daily; **children, 6–12 years:** 1 level teaspoon in 4 oz water t.i.d.–q.i.d. **Cologel Oral Solution: Adults,** 5–20 mL t.i.d. with a glass of water; **pediatric, over 6 years of age:** 5 mL b.i.d.

NURSING CONSIDERATIONS

See also *Nursing Considerations* for *Laxatives,* p. 1049, and *Bulk-Forming Laxatives,* p. 1055

Administration/Storage

Follow each dose of medication with a full glass of water or milk to prevent impaction.

PSYLLIUM HYDROPHILIC MUCILOID   (SILL-ee-um hi-droh-FILL-ik)

Effer-syllium, Fiberall, Hydrocil Instant, Karacil✾, Konsyl-D, Metamucil, Metamucil Instant Mix, Metamucil Instant Mix Orange Flavor, Metamucil Orange Flavor, Metamucil Strawberry Flavor, Metamucil Sugar Free, Modane Bulk, Prodiem Plain✾, Pro-Lax, Reguloid Natural, Reguloid Orange, Serutan, Versabran, V-Lax (OTC)

See also *Laxatives,* p. 1048.

Classification: Laxative, bulk-forming.

Action/Kinetics: This drug is obtained from the fruit of various species of plantago. The powder forms a gelatinous mass with water, which adds bulk to the stools and stimulates peristalsis. It also has a demulcent effect on an inflamed intestinal mucosa. These preparations may also contain dextrose, sodium bicarbonate, monobasic potassium phosphate, citric acid, and benzyl benzoate. Dependence may occur.

Uses: Prophylaxis of constipation in patients who should not strain during defecation. Short-term treatment of constipation; useful in geriatric patients with diminished colonic motor response and during pregnancy and postpartum to reestablish normal bowel function. To soften feces during fecal impaction.

Contraindications: Severe abdominal pain or intestinal obstruction.

Side Effects: Obstruction of the esophagus, stomach, small intestine, and rectum.

Drug Interactions: Psyllium should not be used concomitantly with salicylates, nitrofurantoin, or cardiac glycosides (e.g., digitalis).

Dosage: Dose depends on the product. General information on adult dosage follows. **Granules/Flakes:** 1–2 teaspoons 1–3 times/day spread on food or with a glass of water. **Powder:** 1 rounded teaspoon in 8 oz of liquid 1–3 times/day. **Effervescent powder:** 1 packet in water 1–3 times/day. **Chewable pieces:** 2 pieces followed by a glass of water 1–3 times/day.

NURSING CONSIDERATIONS

See *Nursing Considerations* for *Laxatives,* p. 1049, and *Bulk-Forming Laxatives,* p. 1055.

Administration/Storage

1. Laxative effects usually occur in 12–24 hr. The full effect may take 2–3 days.
2. The powder may be noxious and irritating to some personnel when removing from the packets or canister. Perform in a well-ventilated area and avoid inhaling particulate matter.

EMOLLIENT AND LUBRICANT LAXATIVES

Action/Kinetics: As their name implies, these laxatives promote defecation by softening the feces. These agents are useful when it is desirable to keep the feces soft or when straining at stool is undesirable. In addition to mineral oil (liquid petrolatum), this group of laxatives includes several surface-active agents that lower the surface tension of the feces and promote their penetration by water and fat. This increases the softness of the fecal mass.

Except for mineral oil, the compounds are not absorbed systemically and do not seem to interfere with the absorption of nutrients.

Uses: Prophylaxis of constipation in patients who should not strain during defecation (e.g., after rectal surgery, cardiovascular disease). Assist with defecation in geriatric patients with diminished colonic motor response. Treat constipation during pregnancy and postpartum. During fecal impaction to soften stools.

NURSING CONSIDERATIONS

Interventions

1. Observe elderly clients for signs of dehydration from diarrhea. Encourage increased fluid intake and report to the physician.
2. Observe for lipid pneumonias and lung abscesses that can occur when debilitated, immobile clients aspirate the oil. Report such signs to the physician immediately.
3. Observe the client for evidence of deficiency in vitamins A, D, K, and E. These are dissolved in and excreted in oil. Therefore, emollient laxatives should not be taken at meal time or in conjunction with foods high in these vitamins.

Client/Family Teaching

1. The unpleasant taste can be minimized by holding ice chips on the tongue prior to administration or by mixing with soda or juice.
2. Explain that the effects of the medication generally occurs in 6–8 hours.

DOCUSATE CALCIUM (DIOCTYL CALCIUM SULFOSUCCINATE)   (DOK-you-sayt)
Pro-Cal-Sof, Surfak (OTC)

DOCUSATE POTASSIUM (DIOCTYL POTASSIUM SULFOSUCCINATE)   (DOK-you-sayt)
Dialose, Diocto-K, Kasof (OTC)

DOCUSATE SODIUM (DIOCTYL SODIUM SULFOSUCCINATE)   (DOK-you-sayt)
Afko-Lube, Colace, Diocto, Dioeze, Diosuccin, Dio-Sul, Disonate, Di-Sosul, Doss, Doxinate, D-S-S, Duosol, Laxinate 100, Modane Soft, Molatoc, Pro-Sof, Pro-Sof Liquid Concentrate Regulex✦, Regulax SS, Regutol, Stulex, Therevac Plus, Therevac-SB (OTC)

See also *Laxatives,* p. 1048.

Classification: Laxative, emollient.

Action/Kinetics: These laxatives promote defecation by softening the feces. Useful when it is desirable to keep the feces soft or when straining at stool is undesirable. They act by lowering the surface tension of the feces and promoting their penetration by water and fat, thus increasing the softness of the fecal mass. Docusate is not absorbed systemically and does not seem to interfere with the absorption of nutrients.

Uses: To lessen strain of defecation in persons with hernia or cardiovascular diseases or other diseases in which straining at stool should be avoided. Megacolon or bedridden patients. Constipation associated with dry, hard stools.

Contraindications: Nausea, vomiting, abdominal pain, and intestinal obstruction.

Special Concerns: Pregnancy category: C.

Drug Interactions: Docusate may ↑ absorption of mineral oil from the GI tract.

Dosage: *Docusate calcium.* **Capsules. Adults:** 240 mg daily; **pediatric, over 6 years:** 50–150 mg daily. *Docusate potassium.* **Capsules. Adults,** 100–300 mg daily; **pediatric, over 6 years:** 100 mg at bedtime. *Docusate sodium.* **Capsules, Oral Solution, Syrup, Tablets. Adults and children over 12 years:** 50–500 mg; **pediatric, under 3 years:** 10–40 mg; **3–6 years:** 20–60 mg; **6–12 years:** 40–120 mg. **Rectal Solution.** *Flushing or retention enema:* 50–100 mg.

NURSING CONSIDERATIONS

See also *Nursing Considerations* for *Laxatives,* p. 1049, and *Emollient and Lubricant Laxatives,* p. 1058.

Administration/Storage

1. Administer oral solutions of docusate sodium with milk or fruit juices to help mask the bitter taste.

2. Because docusate salts are minimally absorbed, it may require 1–3 days to soften fecal matter.

MINERAL OIL

Agoral Plain, Fleet Mineral Oil, Fleet Enema Mineral Oil ✿, Kondremul✿, Kondremul Plain, Lansoyl✿, Milkinol, Neo-Cultrol, Nujol, Petrogalar Plain, Zymenol (OTC)

Classification: Emollient laxative.

Action/Kinetics: This mixture of liquid hydrocarbons obtained from petroleum lubricates the intestine; it also decreases absorption of fecal water from the colon. **Onset: PO,** 6–8 hr; **Enema,** 2–15 min.

Uses: Constipation, to avoid straining under certain conditions, such as rectal surgery, hemorrhoidectomy, and certain cardiovascular conditions. Short-term treatment of constipation; useful in geriatric patients with diminished colonic motor response and during pregnancy and postpartum to reestablish normal bowel function. To soften feces during fecal impaction.

Contraindications: Nausea, vomiting, abdominal pain, or intestinal obstruction.

Side Effects: Acute or chronic lipid pneumonia due to aspiration of mineral oil; young, elderly, and dysphagic patients are at greatest risk. Pruritus ani, which may interfere with healing following anorectal surgery. Use during pregnancy may decrease vitamin K absorption sufficiently to cause hypoprothrombinemia in the newborn.

Drug Interactions	
Anticoagulants, oral	↑ Hypoprothrombinemia by ↓ absorption of vitamin K from GI tract; also, mineral oil could ↓ absorption of anticoagulant from GI tract
Sulfonamides	↓ Effect of nonabsorbable sulfonamide in GI tract
Surface-active laxatives	↑ Absorption of mineral oil
Vitamins A, D, E, K	↓ Absorption following prolonged use of mineral oil

Dosage: Emulsion, Gel, Oral Suspension. Adults: 15–45 mL at bedtime; **children:** 5–20 mL at bedtime.

NURSING CONSIDERATIONS

See also *Nursing Considerations* for *Laxatives,* p. 1049, and *Emmolient and Lubricant Laxatives,* p. 1057.

Administration/Storage

1. Administer mineral oil at bedtime. Unless contraindicated, give the client orange juice or a piece of orange to suck on after taking the mineral oil.
2. The emulsion form is pleasant tasting and does not require anything to make it more palatable. However, when taken at bedtime, there is an increased risk of developing lipid pneumonia.
3. Store in the refrigerator to make the medication more palatable.
4. Administer mineral oil slowly to elderly, debilitated clients to prevent aspiration. Aspiration could result in lipid pneumonia.
5. Administer mineral oil carefully and slowly to children to prevent aspiration.
6. Do not administer mineral oil with food or vitamin preparations. The medication may delay digestion and prevent absorption of fat soluble vitamins, A, D, E, and K.

Assessment

Note if the client is of childbearing age and likely to be pregnant. Mineral oil may cause hypoprothrombinemia in the newborn and therefore should be avoided.

Interventions

If the client is taking more than 30 mL of mineral oil, check the perianal area for leakage of feces. These clients require more frequent cleansing and a perianal pad to prevent soiling of clothes and bedding.

Client/Family Teaching

1. Advise clients to sit upright when taking mineral oil to avoid the possibility of aspiration.
2. Caution the client of the potential problem of leakage of fecal matter if the client is taking mineral oil in large amounts and over extended periods of time.
3. Warn pregnant women not to take the medication to relieve constipation, but rather, to check with their physician for suitable alternatives.

MISCELLANEOUS LAXATIVES

GLYCERIN SUPPOSITORIES   (GLISS-er-in)

Fleet Babylax, Sani-Supp (OTC)

Classification: Miscellaneous laxative.

Action/Kinetics: Glycerin suppositories promote defecation by irritating the rectal mucosa as well as by a hyperosmotic action. Glycerin may also soften and lubricate fecal material. The suppository does not have to melt to be effective. **Onset:** 15–60 min.

Use: To establish normal bowel function in patients dependent on laxatives. To evacuate the colon prior to rectal and bowel examinations as well as colon surgery.

Contraindications: Should not be used in the presence of anal fissures, fistulas, ulcerative hemorrhoids, or proctitis.

Side Effects: Mucous membrane irritation.

Dosage: Suppository: Insert one adult or pediatric suppository high in the rectum and hold for 15 min. **Liquid:** 4 mL inserted gently with the tip of the applicator pointed toward the navel.

NURSING CONSIDERATIONS

See also *Nursing Considerations* for *Laxatives,* p. 1049.

Administration/Storage

1. Store in a tight container in the refrigerator below 25°C (77°F).
2. A small amount of liquid glycerin will remain in the applicator unit.
3. Anticipate onset of action within 1 hour.

LACTULOSE (LAK-tyou-lohs)

Chronulac (Rx)

See *Miscellaneous Drugs,* Chapter 72, p. 1377.

CHAPTER FIFTY-FIVE
Antidiarrheal Agents

Systemic Agents

Difenoxin Hydrochloride with Atropine
Sulfate *1062*
Diphenoxylate Hydrochloride with
Atropine *1064*

Loperamide Hydrochloride *1066*
Paregoric (Camphorated Opium
Tincture) *1067*

Local Agents—See Table 23.

General Statement: Diarrhea accompanies many different disorders and the physician should attempt to elucidate the underlying cause of its manifestations. When diarrhea is caused by an infectious organism, the physician may prescribe a specific antibiotic or chemotherapeutic agent to eradicate the causative agent.

Often diarrhea is a self-limiting natural defense reaction by means of which the body rids itself of a toxic or irritating substance. Dehydration and disturbance of the electrolyte balance can be a major complication of diarrhea. Symptomatic antidiarrheal therapy can prevent extreme dehydration.

Most antidiarrheal agents are used for symptomatic relief. Anticholinergic drugs (Chapter 47), p. 942, which reduce the excessive motility of the intestine, are also effective constipating agents.

Antidiarrheal agents fall into two categories: those that act locally on the intestine and its contents and those that act systemically.

SYSTEMIC AGENTS

DIFENOXIN HYDROCHLORIDE WITH ATROPINE SULFATE
Motofen (Rx)

Classification: Antidiarrheal.

Action/Kinetics: Difenoxin is related chemically to meperidine; thus, atropine sulfate is incorporated to prevent deliberate overdosage. Difenoxin is the active metabolite of diphenoxylate and is effective at one-fifth the dosage of diphenoxylate. Difenoxin slows intestinal motility by a local effect on the GI wall. **Peak plasma levels:** 40–60 min. The drug and its inactive metabolites are excreted through both the urine and feces.

Uses: Management of acute nonspecific diarrhea and acute episodes of chronic functional diarrhea.

Contraindications: Diarrhea caused by *Escherichia coli*, *Salmonella*, or *Shigella*; pseudomembranous colitis caused by broad-spectrum antibiotics; jaundice; children less than 2 years of age.

Special Concerns: Pregnancy category: C. Use with caution in ulcerative colitis, liver and kidney disease, lactation, and in patients receiving dependence-producing drugs or in those who are addiction-prone. Safety and effectiveness in children less than 12 years of age have not been determined.

Side Effects: *GI:* Nausea, vomiting, dry mouth, epigastric distress, constipation. *CNS:* Lightheadedness, dizziness, drowsiness, headache, tiredness, nervousness, confusion, insomnia. *Ophthalmic:* Blurred vision, burning eyes.

Symptoms of overdosage initially include dry skin and mucous membranes, hyperthermia, flushing, and tachycardia. These are followed by hypotonic reflexes, nystagmus, miosis, lethargy, coma, and respiratory depression (may occur up to 30 hr after overdose taken).

Drug Interactions	
Antianxiety agents	Potentiation or addition of CNS depressant effects
Barbiturates	Potentiation or addition of CNS depressant effects
Ethanol	Potentiation or addition of CNS depressant effects
Monoamine oxidase inhibitors	Precipitation of hypertensive crisis
Narcotics	Potentiation or addition of CNS depressant effects

Dosage: Tablets. Adults, initial: 2 tablets (2 mg difenoxin); **then,** 1 tablet (1 mg) after each loose stool or 1 tablet q 3–4 hr as needed. Total dose during a 24-hr period should not exceed 8 mg.

NURSING CONSIDERATIONS

Administration/Storage

1. Continued administration beyond 48 hr is not recommended, if clinical improvement is not noted.
2. Treatment beyond 48 hr is usually not necessary for acute diarrhea or acute exacerbation of functional diarrhea.
3. In cases of overdose, naloxone may be used to treat respiratory depression.

Assessment

1. Note the onset of the diarrhea and the frequency.
2. Discuss the possible precipitating factors with the client, e.g., travel, food, medication regimens.
3. Note evidence of dehydration such as weakness, weight loss, sunken eyes, poor skin turgor, elevated temperature, rapid weak pulse, or decreased urinary output.
4. Assess for evidence of electrolyte imbalance such as weakness, irritability, anorexia, nausea and dysrhythmias.
5. Note the client's skin and sclera color for evidence of hepatic disease.

Interventions

1. If the client has a history of heart disease, monitor closely and report any adverse effects to the physician immediately.
2. Monitor intake and output. Keep a record of the number and consistency of the stools. If the diarrhea persists, consult with the physician.

55

3. Monitor the client for changes in electrolyte balance. Document and report to the physician.

4. Check the client's gums for swelling and the extremities for numbness. If these occur, report to the physician.

5. If the client is also receiving Lomotil and other narcotics or barbiturates, observe closely for the potentiation of CNS depression.

6. If the client has a history of liver disease, observe for signs of impending coma, such as increased drowsiness, mental aberrations, motor disturbances, or a flapping tremor of the hands. Monitor liver function studies as drug may precipitate hepatic coma in clients with abnormal liver function.

7. Difenoxin contains atropine sulfate as an active ingredient; closely observe Down syndrome children receiving this drug for symptoms of atropinism.

8. Do not administer to clients receiving MAO inhibitors as concomitant use may precipitate hypertensive crisis.

9. Difenoxin has the potential to become addictive; monitor accordingly.

10. Overdosed clients should be hospitalized for observation since latent (12–30 hr later) respiratory depression may occur.

Client/Family Teaching

1. Provide the client and family with printed instructions concerning the recommended dosage schedule and side effects to be reported to the physician.

2. Caution clients not to perform tasks that require mental alertness until drug effects are realized.

3. Remind client to take only as directed and not to share medications with anyone, no matter what the symptoms.

4. Advise the client to suck on ice chips, chew sugarless gum, or suck on hard, sugarless candy if dry mouth is a problem.

5. Keep out of reach of children as drug may be fatal if ingested by children.

6. Drug should *not* be taken by mothers who are breast feeding.

DIPHENOXYLATE HYDROCHLORIDE WITH ATROPINE (dye-fen-OX-ih-layt, AH-troh-peen)

Diphenatol, Lofene, Logen, Lomanate, Lomotil, Lonox, Lo-Trol, Low-Quel, Nor-Mil (C-V) (Rx)

Classification: Antidiarrheal agent, systemic.

Action/Kinetics: Diphenoxylate is a systemic constipating agent chemically related to the narcotic analgesic drug meperidine, but without the analgesic properties. Diphenoxylate inhibits GI motility and has a constipating effect. High doses over prolonged periods can, however, cause euphoria and physical dependence. The preparation also contains small amounts of atropine sulfate, which is not present in sufficient quantities to decrease GI motility. However, the atropine will prevent abuse by deliberate overdosage. **Onset:** 45–60 min. **t½, diphenoxylate:** 2.5 hr; **diphenoxylic acid:** 12–24 hr. **Duration:** 2–4 hr. Diphenoxylate is metabolized in the liver to the active diphenoxylic acid and excreted through the urine.

Uses: Symptomatic treatment of chronic and functional diarrhea. Also, diarrhea associated with gastroenteritis, irritable bowel, regional enteritis, malabsorption syndrome, ulcerative colitis, acute infections, food poisoning, postgastrectomy, and drug-induced diarrhea. Therapeutic results for control of acute diarrhea are inconsistent. Also used in the control of intestinal passage time in patients with ileostomies and colostomies.

Contraindications: Obstructive jaundice, liver disease, diarrhea associated with pseudomembranous enterocolitis after antibiotic therapy, children under the age of 2.

Special Concerns: Use with caution during pregnancy (category: C) and lactation and in patients in whom anticholinergics may be contraindicated. Children (especially those with Down syndrome) are susceptible to atropine toxicity. Children and geriatric patients may be more sensitive to the respiratory depressant effects of diphenoxylate.

Side Effects: *GI:* Nausea, vomiting, anorexia, abdominal discomfort, paralytic ileus, megacolon. *Allergic:* Pruritus, angioneurotic edema, swelling of gums. *CNS:* Dizziness, drowsiness, malaise, restlessness, headache, depression, numbness of extremities, respiratory depression, coma. *Topical:* Dry skin and mucous membranes, flushing. *Other:* Tachycardia, urinary retention, hyperthermia.

Overdosage: Overdosage is characterized by flushing, lethargy, coma, hypotonic reflexes, nystagmus, pinpoint pupils, tachycardia, and respiratory depression.

Drug Interactions

Alcohol	Additive CNS depression
Barbiturates	Additive CNS depression
MAO inhibitors	↑ Chance of hypertensive crisis
Narcotics	↑ Effect of narcotics

Treatment: Gastric lavage and assisted respiration. IV administration of a narcotic antagonist. Administration may be repeated after 10–15 min. Observe patient and readminister antagonist if respiratory depression returns.

Dosage: Oral Solution, Tablets. Adults, initial: 2.5–5 mg (of diphenoxylate) t.i.d.–q.i.d.; **maintenance:** 2.5 mg b.i.d.–t.i.d. **Pediatric, 2–12 years:** 0.3–0.4 mg/kg/day (of diphenoxylate) in divided doses. Contraindicated in children under 2 years of age. See also below.

Pediatric/Dose

2–3 years	0.75–1.5 mg q.i.d.
3–4 years	1–1.5 mg q.i.d.
4–5 years	1–2 mg q.i.d.
5–6 years	1.25–2.25 mg q.i.d.
6–9 years	1.25–2.5 mg q.i.d.
9–12 years	1.75–2.5 mg q.i.d.

Based on 4 mL/tsp or 2 mg of diphenoxylate.

Each tablet or 5 mL of liquid preparation contains 2.5 mg diphenoxylate hydrochloride and 25 mcg of atropine sulfate. Dosage should be maintained at initial levels until symptoms are under control; then reduce to maintenance levels.

NURSING CONSIDERATIONS

See *Nursing Considerations* for *Difenoxin HCl with Atropine sulfate* p. 1063.

Administration/Storage

For liquid preparations, use only the plastic dropper supplied by the manufacturer to measure the dosage of drug.

LOPERAMIDE HYDROCHLORIDE   (loh-PER-ah-myd)

Imodium, Imodium A-D (Rx and OTC)

Classification: Antidiarrheal agent, systemic.

Action/Kinetics: Loperamide is a piperidine derivative that slows intestinal motility by acting on the nerve endings and/or intramural ganglia embedded in the intestinal wall. The prolonged retention of the feces in the intestine results in reducing the volume of the stools, increasing viscosity, and decreasing fluid and electrolyte loss. The drug is reported to be more effective than diphenoxylate. **Time to peak effect, capsules:** 5 hr; **oral solution:** 2.5 hr. **t½:** 9.1–14.4 hr.

Uses: Symptomatic relief of acute, nonspecific diarrhea, chronic diarrhea associated with inflammatory bowel disease, reduction of volume discharged from ileostomies.

Contraindications: Discontinue drug promptly if abdominal distention develops in patients with acute ulcerative colitis. In patients in whom constipation should be avoided.

Special Concerns: Safe use during pregnancy (pregnancy category: B) and in children under 2 years of age not established. Children less than 3 years of age are more sensitive to the narcotic effects of loperamide.

Side Effects: *GI:* Abdominal pain, distention, or discomfort. Constipation, dry mouth, nausea, vomiting, epigastric distress. Toxic megacolon in patients with acute colitis. *CNS:* Drowsiness, dizziness, fatigue. *Other:* Allergic skin rashes.

Dosage: Capsules, Oral Solution. *Acute diarrhea:* **Adults, initial:** 4 mg, followed by 2 mg after each unformed stool, up to maximum of 16 mg daily. *Day 1 doses, pediatric:* **8–12 years:** 2 mg t.i.d.; **5–8 years:** 2 mg b.i.d.; **2–5 years:** 1 mg t.i.d. After day 1, 1 mg/10 kg after a loose stool (total daily dosage should not exceed day 1 recommended doses).

Chronic diarrhea: **Adults,** 4–8 mg/day as a single or divided dose. Dosage not established for chronic diarrhea in children.

In acute diarrhea, discontinue drug after 48 hr if ineffective. In chronic diarrhea, discontinue if 16 mg daily for 10 days is ineffective.

Oral Solution, Tablets (OTC). *Acute diarrhea:* **Adults,** 2 mg after the first loose bowel movement followed by 2 mg after each subsequent bowel movement to a maximum of 8 mg daily. **Pediatric, 6–8 years:** 2 mg after the first bowel movement followed by 1 mg after each subsequent loose bowel movement, not to exceed 4 mg daily. **Pediatric, 9–11 years:** 2 mg after the first bowel movement followed by 1 mg after each subsequent loose bowel movement, not to exceed 6 mg daily.

NURSING CONSIDERATIONS

Assessment

Note any history of allergy to piperidine derivatives prior to administering drug.

Interventions

1. If the client has acute diarrhea, if the drug is not effective within the first 48 hours, and if 16 mg of the drug has been administered daily for 10 days, discontinue using it and report the problem to the physician.

2. If the client complains of nausea, vomiting, or abdominal pain, consult with the physician. Adjusting the dosage of medication may be indicated. If the symptoms persist a change in the medication may be in order.

Client/Family Teaching

1. Advise the client that loperamide may cause a dry mouth and provide instructions concerning relief.
2. Use caution while driving or in undertaking other tasks requiring alertness, because the drug may cause dizziness and drowsiness.
3. Instruct the client in recording the number and consistency of stools per day.
4. Contact physician if diarrhea lasts up to ten days without relief.
5. Advise the client to report to the physician if fever, abdominal pain, or abdominal distention occurs.
6. Remind parents that dietary treatment of diarrhea is preferred, if possible, in children.

PAREGORIC (CAMPHORATED OPIUM TINCTURE) (par-eh-GOR-ik)
(C-III, Rx)

See also *Narcotics,* p. 750.

Classification: Antidiarrheal agent, systemic.

Action/Kinetics: The active principle of the mixture is opium (0.04% morphine). The preparation also contains benzoic acid, camphor, and anise oil. Morphine increases the muscular tone of the intestinal tract, decreases digestive secretions, and inhibits normal peristalsis. The slowed passage of the feces through the intestines promotes desiccation, which is a function of the time the feces spend in the intestine. **t½:** 2–3 hr. **Duration:** 4–5 hr.

Uses: Acute diarrhea.

Contraindications: See *Morphine Sulfate,* p. 767. Do not use in patients with diarrhea caused by poisoning until toxic substance has been eliminated. Treatment of pseudomembranous colitis due to lincomycin, penicillins, and cephalosporins. Rubbing paregoric on the gums of a teething child is no longer recommended.

Special Concerns: Pregnancy category: C. Many physicians do not recommend use of paregoric in treating neonatal opioid dependence.

Side Effects: See *Morphine Sulfate,* p. 767.

Drug Interactions: See *Narcotic Analgesics,* p. 750.

Dosage: Liquid. Adult: 5–10 mL 1–4 times daily (5 mL contains 2 mg of morphine). **Pediatric:** 0.25–0.5 mL/kg 1–4 times daily.

NURSING CONSIDERATIONS

Administration/Storage

1. Administer paregoric with water to ensure that it will reach the stomach. The mixture will have a milky appearance.
2. Store the medication in a light-resistant container.
3. Carefully distinguish between paregoric and tincture of opium. Tincture of opium contains 25 times more morphine than paregoric.
4. Paregoric preparations are subject to the Controlled Substances Act and must be charted accordingly.
5. Have naloxone available to treat any overdosage.

Assessment

Note the length of time the client has been taking paregoric, the reasons for taking, and its level of effectiveness. Assess for evidence of drug dependence.

Client/Family Teaching

1. Advise the client to adhere to the prescribed regimen.
2. If the diarrhea persists, consult with the physician.
3. Stop medication once diarrhea has abated. Continued use of paregoric may result in constipation.

LOCAL AGENTS

General Statement: These are only moderately successful in the treatment of diarrhea, and their mode of action is not completely understood. A number of agents are found in such products. These include (a) aluminum hydroxide and bismuth salts for use as adsorbents and antacids; (b) attapulgite, kaolin and pectin for use as adsorbents (i.e., their large surface area adsorbs fluid and toxins) and to treat intestinal inflammation; (c) opium and codeine to decrease motility of the intestine; (d) belladonna alkaloids as atropine, hyoscyamine, and scopolamine to control excess acid secretion and intestinal motility; (e) zinc phenolsulfonate and zinc sulfocarbolate as intestinal astringents and antiseptics; and, (f) cultures of bacteria to change the intestinal flora. Most products contain one or more these ingredients. See Table 23.

Table 23   Locally Acting Antidiarrheal Agents

Drug	Dosage	Remarks
Atropine sulfate, hyoscyamine sulfate, kaolin, pectin, opium, scopolamine HBr (Amogel PG, Donnagel-PG, Donnapectolin-PG, Kapectolin PG, Quiagel PG) (C-V)	**Oral Suspension. Adults:** 30 mL initially; **then,** 15 mL q 3 hr as needed, up to a maximum of 4 doses in 24 hr. **Pediatric, over 6 years:** 10 mL initially; **then,** 5–10 mL q 3 hr as needed, up to 4 doses in 24 hr.	Each 30 mL contains atropine 0.0194 mg; hyoscyamine, 0.1037; kaolin, 6 g; pectin, 142.8 mg; opium, 24 mg; and, scopolamine, 0.0065 mg. **Duration:** 3–4 hr.
Atropine sulfate, hyoscyamine sulfate, kaolin, pectin, scopolamine HBr (Donnagel, Kapectolin Gel with Belladonna, Quiagel) (OTC)	**Suspension. Adults:** 30 mL; **then,** 15 mL q 3 hr.	These products contain the same amounts of drugs as above but without the opium.
Attapulgite, colloidal activated (Rheaban) (OTC)	**Rheaban Tablets:** 2 tablets after each bowel movement. **Diasorb Liquid: initial,** 20 mL; **then,** 20 mL after each bowel movement or q 2 hr.	Each tablet or 5 mL contains 750 mg attapulgite.
Attapulgite, activated (Diasorb) (OTC)		

Table 23 *(continued)*

Drug	Dosage	Remarks
	Diasorb Tablets: initial, 2 tablets; **then,** 4 tablets after each bowel movement or q 2 hr.	
Attapulgite, activated and pectin (Diar-Aid) (OTC)	**Tablets. Initial:** 2–4 tablets; **then,** 2 tablets after each bowel movement.	Each tablet contains 750 mg attapulgite and 150 mg pectin.
Bismuth subcarbonate, kaolin, pectin (K-C) (OTC)	**Suspension. Adults:** 10–20 mL q 6 hr.	Each 30 mL contains bismuth subcarbonate, 260 mg; kaolin, 3.9 g; and pectin, 260 mg.
Bismuth subcarbonate, calcium carbonate, opium (Diabismul) (C-III)	**Tablets. Adults:** 1–2 tablets q.i.d.	Each tablet contains bismuth subcarbonate 125 mg; calcium carbonate, 125 mg; and powderd opium, 1.23 mg.
Bismuth subcarbonate, kaolin, opium, pectin (KBP/O) (C-III)	**Capsules. Adults:** 2–4 capsules q 3–4 hr.	Each capsule contains bismuth subcarbonate, 60 mg in a pectin base; kaolin, 350 mg; and opium, 3 mg.
Bismuth subgallate and kaolin (Dia-Eze) (OTC)	**Suspension. Adults:** 30–60 mL q 2 hr.	Each 30 mL contains bismuth subgallate, 300 mg and kaolin, 11 g.
Bismuth subgallate, kaolin, opium, pectin, zinc phenolsulfonate (B.P.P.-Lemmon) (C-III)	**Tablets. Adults:** 4–6 tablets q 30 min for 3–4 doses; **then,** 2–4 tablets q 3 hr until symptom-free.	Each tablet contains bismuth subgallate, 120 mg; kaolin, 120 mg; opium, 1.2 mg; pectin, 1.2 mg; and zinc phenolsulfonate, 15 mg. The tablets may be chewed or swallowed whole.
Bismuth subsalicylate (Pepto-Bismol) (OTC)	**Suspension, Tablets. Adults:** 2 tablets or 30 mL. **Pediatric, 3–6 years:** 1/3 tablet or 5 mL; **6–9 years:** 2/3 tablet or 10 mL; **9–12 years:** 1 tablet or 15 mL. Dose may be repeated q 30–60 min as required up to 8 doses per day. Consult physician for use in children less than 3 years of age.	Each tablet or 15 mL contains bismuth subsalicylate, 262 mg. **Uses:** Indigestion, abdominal cramps, gas pains, prophylaxis and treatment of traveller's diarrhea. **Drug Interaction:** 1. The salicylate may increase the effect of anticoagulants and sulfonylureas. 2. Bismuth may decrease GI absorbtion of tetracyclines.

Table 23   (*continued*)

Drug	Dosage	Remarks
		Administration:
		1. Bismuth is radiopaque and may thus interfere with radiologic examinations.
		2. May cause short-term darkening of the stools.
		3. May cause impaction in debilitated patients and infants.
Bismuth subsalicylate, codeine phosphate, kaolin, pectin, sodium carboxymethylcellulose (Kaodene with Codeine) (C-V)	**Suspension. Adults:** 15 mL; **then,** 10 mL q 30 min as required.	Each 30 mL contains bismuth subsalicylate, 194.4 mg; codeine phosphate, 32.4 mg; kaolin, 3.9 g; pectin, 194.4 mg; and sodium carboxymethylcellulose, 194.4 mg.
Bismuth subsalicylate, kaolin, morphine (anhydrous), pectin, sodium carboxymethylcellulose (Kaodene with Paregoric) (C-V)	**Suspension. Adults:** 30 mL 1–4 times daily.	Each 30 mL contains anhydrous morphine, 1.5 mg and the same drug levels as Kaodene with Codeine (see above).
Bismuth subsalicylate, kaolin, pectin, sodium carboxymethylcellulose (Kaodene Non-Narcotic) (OTC)	**Suspension. Adults:** 45 mL 1–3 times day day; or, take after each loose stool.	Contains the same drug levels as Kaodene with Codeine but without the narcotic.
Bismuth subsalicylate, paregoric, pepsin, phenyl salicylate, zinc sulfocarbolate (Corrective Mixture with Paregoric) (C-V)	**Suspension. Adults:** 15 mL; **then,** 7.5 mL q 30 min as required.	Each 30 mL contains bismuth subsalicylate, 510 mg; pregoric, 3.6 mL; pepsin, 270 mg; phenylsalicylate, 132 mg; and zinc sulfo-carbolate, 60 mg.
Bismuth subsalicylate, opium, pectin, zinc phenolsulfonate (Banatol, Infantol Pink) (C-V)	**Liquid. Adults:** 30 mL q 15 min for 4 doses; **then,** 30 mL q 2 hr.	Each 30 mL contains opium, 15 mg.
Charcoal (Charcocaps) (OTC)	**Capsules, Tablets. Adults:** 520–975 mg after meals (or at the first signs of discomfort), up to 4.16 g daily.	**Uses:** Diarrhea, indigestion, gas, kidney dialysis to prevent pruritus. **Contraindications:** Children less than 3 years. **Note:** Activated charcoal is used for emergency

Table 23 *(continued)*

Drug	Dosage	Remarks
		treatment of a number of drug overdoses. It is part of the universal antidote.
Homatropine, opium, pectin (Dia-Quel) (C-V)	**Liquid. Adults:** 15–30 mL t.i.d.–q.i.d.	Each 30 mL contains homatropine, 0.9 mg; opium, 18 mg; and pectin, 144 mg.
Kaolin and pectin (Donnagel MB♣, Kao-Con♣, Kaopectate♣, Kao-tin, Kapectolin, K-C, K-P, K-Pek) (OTC)	**Oral Suspension.** Dose varies depending on the product. *K-P:* 60–120 mL after each bowel movement. *Kaopectate Concentrate:* 45–90 mL after each bowel movement. *All other products:* **Adults:** 60–120 mL after each loose bowel movement. **Pediatric, 3–6** years: 15–30 mL; **6–12** years: 30–60 mL.	Each 30 mL of *K-P* contains kaolin, 5.2 g and pectin, 260 mg. Each 30 mL of *Kaopectate Concentrate* contains: kaolin, 8.7 g and pectin, 195 mg. *All other products* contain (in each 30 mL): kaolin, 5.85 g and pectin, 130 mg
Kaolin, opium, pectin (Diabismul, Kapectolin with Paregoric, Parepectolin) (C-V)	**Suspension. Adults:** 15–30 mL after each loose bowel movement.	Each 30 mL of *Diabismul* contains: kaolin, 5 g in a pectin base and opium, 14 mg. Each 30 mL of either *Kapectolin with Paregoric* or *Parepectolin* contains: kaolin, 5.5 g, opium, 15 mg: and pectin, 162 mg.
Lactobacillus (Bacid, Lactinex, More-Dophilus) (OTC)	Dose varies depending on the product. *Bacid:* 2 capsules b.i.d.–q.i.d. (should take with milk). *Lactinex:* 1 packet of granules added to food (e.g., cereal, milk, juice, water) t.i.d.–q.i.d. *or* 4 chewable tablets t.i.d.–q.i.d. *More-Dophilus:* 5 mL daily with liquid.	**Uses:** Diarrhea due to antibiotic therapy. Fever blisters. **Content:** These products contain metabolic products produced by *Lactobacillus acidophilus* and *L. bulgaris*. **Contraindications:** Lactose intolerance. In presence of high fever or in children less than 3 years of age. **Administration:** No longer than 2 days.

Uses: Symptomatic treatment of diarrhea.

Contraindications: Pseudomembranous enterocolitis, toxigenic bacteria-induced diarrhea, in the presence of high fever, in children less than 3 years of age unless approved by physician.

Side Effects: Prolonged use may result in constipation or interfere with the proper absorption of nutrients.

NURSING CONSIDERATIONS

Administration/Storage

1. Local agents should not be given for more than 2 days. If there is no relief, the physician should be consulted.
2. These drugs should not be used for children under 3 years of age unless specifically approved by the physician.

Assessment

1. Note the number of times the client has had diarrhea in the past year. This could indicate an underlying problem not yet identified.
2. Record the frequency and character of the client's stools.
3. Note if the client has a fever, or if there have been tests made to determine the cause of the diarrhea.

Interventions

1. Record the client's intake and output and the frequency, character, and number of stools, once therapy has been initiated. For the elderly, dehydration can particularly pose a problem.
2. Analyze the stool record to evaluate the client's response to therapy.
3. Observe the client for any increase in diarrhea or development of constipation. Either symptom may require an adjustment in the dosage of medication.

Client/Family Teaching

1. Highly spiced foods and foods high in fat content should be eliminated from the diet.
2. Follow the directions provided by the physician. Following the prescribed regimen is important in the control of diarrhea.
3. Advise parents of infants and children under 5 years of age to consult with the physician before administering any antidiarrheal medications. Children are more susceptible to the consequences of severe fluid depletion or loss of electrolytes.
4. Advise elderly clients to report to the physician all incidences of diarrhea, the number of stools, the consistency and any foods that may have been ingested that could cause diarrhea. The cause may be minor, or it may be the result of a serious change in the client's physical condition.
5. Explain the constipation may occur. Therefore, it is important to stop taking the medication once the diarrhea is controlled.

CHAPTER FIFTY-SIX
Emetics /Antiemetics

EMETICS

General Statement: Emetics are used in cases of acute poisoning to induce vomiting when it is desirable to empty the stomach promptly and completely after ingestion of toxic materials.

Vomiting can be elicited either by direct action on the chemoreceptor trigger zone (CTZ) in the medulla or by indirect stimulation of the GI tract. Some agents act in both ways.

NURSING CONSIDERATIONS

56

Administration

1. Do not administer an emetic if the following conditions exist:
   - The client is semiconscious, unconscious or comatose.
   - The client has ingested a corrosive substance such as caustic soda, a strong acid or petroleum products such as kerosene.
   - The client has taken a convulsant poison such as strychnine.
2. Emetics are usually administered with water. Therefore, have available 200–300 mL of water at the time of administration.
3. For treating the ingestion of poison, have the following on hand:
   - gastric lavage equipment,
   - oxygen and positive pressure apparatus,
   - emergency drugs,
   - intravenous equipment and fluids.

Assessment

When possible, determine what the client has ingested, how much and under what conditions, and record on the client's chart.

Interventions

1. Position clients on their side after administering an emetic to prevent aspiration when the client vomits.
2. The telephone number of the poison control center serving your area should be prominently displayed at each nursing station (See Appendix 5, p. 1420.). The center should be consulted routinely for up-to-date information regarding the overall management of drug overdoses.

APOMORPHINE HYDROCHLORIDE (ah-poh-**MOR**-feen)

(Rx)

Classification: Emetic.

Action/Kinetics: Apomorphine is a synthetic derivative of morphine which produces emesis by stimulating the CTZ. The drug may also stimulate vestibular centers. **Onset after SC administration, Adults:** 5–10 min; **children:** 1–2 min. Not effective if given orally.

Use: Emergency use in drug overdose and in accidental poisonings.

Contraindications: Shock, drug-induced CNS depression, ingestion of corrosive substances, petroleum distillates, and lye, and for patients sensitive to morphine.

Special Concerns: Pregnancy category: C. Use with caution in patients with cardiac decompensation and debilitated persons. Use with caution during lactation. Children and geriatric patients may be more susceptible to apomorphine-induced respiratory depression.

Side Effects: *CNS:* Depression, euphoria, restlessness, tremors. *Other:* Tachypnea, cardiovascular collapse. Overdosage may result in excessive emesis, cardiac depression, and death.

Dosage: SC. Adults, 5–6 mg as a single dose; **pediatric:** 0.07–0.1 mg/kg as a single dose. **Do not repeat.**

NURSING CONSIDERATIONS

See also *Nursing Considerations* for *Emetics,* p. 1073.

Administration/Storage

1. Before administration, give the client 300 mL of water.
2. Do not use solutions with emerald-green hue, as this indicates that the drug has disintegrated.
3. Store solution in the dark in a closed container.
4. Have naloxone available.

Assessment

1. Note if the client has a sensitivity to morphine.
2. If possible, obtain information concerning what the client has taken, if it was accidental or intentional.
3. Determine if the client has a history of cardiovascular problems or if they are debilitated and document.

Interventions

1. Have the client drink 200–300 mL of water or evaporated milk immediately before or immediately after injection of drug.
2. Observe the client for evidence of respiratory distress for at least 1 hour following administration of apomorphine. Drug may depress the respiratory center.
3. Depending upon what the client has taken and why, direct the client to appropriate counselling.

IPECAC SYRUP (IP-eh-kak)

(OTC)

Classification: Emetic.

Action/Kinetics: The active principle of ipecac, an alkaloid extracted from Brazil root, acts both locally on the gastric mucosa and centrally on the chemoreceptor trigger zone. **Onset:** 20 min. **Duration:** 20–25 min. In contrast to apomorphine, a second dose may be given if necessary. **Ipecac syrup must not be confused with ipecac fluid extract, which is 14 times as potent.** Syrup of ipecac can be purchased without a prescription. It has been abused by patients suffering from bulimia.

Uses: To empty the stomach promptly and completely after oral poisoning or drug overdose.

Contraindications: With corrosives or petroleum distillates, in individuals who are unconscious or semicomatose, severely inebriated, or in shock. Infants under 6 months of age.

Special Concerns: Pregnancy category: C. If used in children less than 12 months of age, there is an increased risk of aspiration of vomitus.

Drug Interactions: Activated charcoal adsorbs ipecac syrup, thus decreasing its effect.

Dosage: Syrup. Adults and children over 12 years: 15–30 mL followed by 240 mL of water; **pediatric up to 1 year:** 5–10 mL preceded or followed by 120–240 mL of water; **pediatric, 1–12 years:** 15 mL preceded or followed by 120–240 mL water.

NURSING CONSIDERATIONS

Administration/Storage

1. Check label of medication closely so that the syrup and the fluid extract are not confused.
2. Dosage may be repeated once if vomiting does not occur within 30 min. Gastric lavage should be considered if vomiting does not occur within 15 minutes after the second dose.
3. Administer ipecac syrup with 200–300 mL of water.

Client/Family Teaching

1. Provide with the name and telephone number of the local poison control center or hospital (See Appendix 5, p. 1420.) and advise the client/parent to contact these before administering ipecac syrup.
2. Advise clients to have ipecac syrup available in the event of accidental poisoning.
3. Remind parents to be sure that ipecac syrup is kept in a locked closet, out of the reach of children.
4. If the drug is to be used as an expectorant, instruct the client as to the correct dosage and the

appropriate method of administration. Explain the difference between the dosage and methods used for expectorant purposes and emetic purposes.

5. Explain the potential for abuse, such as to induce vomiting after meals for weight reduction. (Some states have banned over-the-counter sales for this reason.)

ANTIEMETICS

General Statement: Nausea and vomiting can be caused by a variety of conditions, such as infections, drugs, radiation, motion, organic disease, or psychological factors. The underlying cause of the symptoms must be elicited before emesis is corrected.

The act of vomiting is complex. The vomiting center in the medulla responds to stimulation from many peripheral areas, as well as to stimuli from the CNS itself, the chemoreceptor trigger zone in the medulla, the vestibular apparatus of the ear, and the cerebral cortex.

The selection of an antiemetic depends on the cause of the symptoms, as well as on the manner in which the vomiting is triggered.

Many drugs used for other conditions, such as the antihistamines, phenothiazines, barbiturates and scopolamine, have antiemetic properties and can be so used. (For details see appropriate sections.) These agents often have serious side effects (mostly CNS depression) that make their routine use undesirable.

Drug Interaction: Because of their antiemetic and antinauseant activity, the antiemetics may mask overdosage caused by other drugs.

NURSING CONSIDERATIONS

Assessment

1. Take a complete client history, determining if this is an unusual occurrence or if it is a recurring phenomenon.
2. Determine the extent of the nausea and what event seems to have triggered it.
3. Note the number of times the client has had to take an antiemetic in the past and under what conditions.

Interventions

Assess for other untoward symptoms, such as increased intracranial pressure or intestinal obstruction. Antiemetic drugs may mask signs of underlying pathology or overdosage of other drugs. Report the symptoms to the physician.

Client/Family Teaching

Caution the client that the drug tends to cause drowsiness and dizziness. Advise the client to avoid driving or performing other hazardous tasks until individual response to the drug has been evaluated.

BENZQUINAMIDE HYDROCHLORIDE   (benz-KWIN-ah-myd)

Emete-Con (Rx)

Classification: Antiemetic.

Action/Kinetics: This drug has antiemetic, antihistaminic, anticholinergic, and sedative properties. It is a benzoquinoline derivative. **Onset:** rapid (15 min after parenteral administration). **t½:** 40 min. **Duration of effect:** 3–4 hr. Metabolized in liver, excreted in urine.

Uses: Prevention and treatment of nausea during anesthesia and surgery.

Contraindications: Hypersensitivity to drug. Pregnancy. IV for cardiac patients.

Special Concerns: Safety and efficacy have not been established for children.

Side Effects: *CNS:* Drowsiness, insomnia, restlessness, headache, excitement, dizziness, fatigue, nervousness. *GI:* Dry mouth, hiccoughs, salivation, anorexia, nausea. *CV:* Hypertension, hypotension, atrial fibrillation, premature atrial and ventricular contractions. *Other:* Shivering, sweating, flushing, blurred vision, hyperthermia, chills, muscle twitching/tremors, urticaria, skin rashes, weakness.

Drug Interaction: Use lower dose of benzquinamide in patients receiving epinephrine-like drugs or pressor agents.

Dosage: IM: 50 mg or 0.5–1 mg/kg. May be repeated after 1 hr, **then** q 3–4 hr. **IV:** 25 mg or 0.2–0.4 mg/kg. Inject slowly (30–60 sec); switch to **IM** after one **IV** dose.

NURSING CONSIDERATIONS

See also *Nursing Considerations* for *Antiemetics,* p. 1076.

Administration/Storage

1. Reconstituted solution is stable for 14 days at room temperature.
2. Store solution and unreconstituted powder in light-resistant containers.
3. For prophylaxis give 15 min prior to when client is expected to regain consciousness from anesthesia.
4. Use should be restricted to clients without cardiovascular disease.
5. Onset of action occurs in 15 minutes and lasts 3–4 hours.

Interventions

Monitor vital signs during administration. If the client complains of shivering, sweating, flushing, increased salivation, twitching or tremors and weakness, monitor for their severity. If they are severe or persist, withhold the next dose of medication, document and report these findings to the physician.

BUCLIZINE HYDROCHLORIDE (BYOU-klih-zeen)

Bucladin-S Softabs (Rx)

See also *Antiemetics,* p. 1076, and *Antihistamines,* p. 1003.

Classification: Antiemetic, antihistamine, piperazine type.

Action/Kinetics: Buclizine suppresses nausea and vomiting through an action on the CNS to decrease vestibular stimulation and depress labyrinthine function. The drug may also act on the chemoreceptor trigger zone to decrease vomiting. **Duration:** 4–6 hr.

Uses: Nausea, vomiting, dizziness of motion sickness.

Additional Contraindications: Hypersensitivity to drug, pregnancy, lactation.

Special Concerns: Pregnancy category: B. Safe use in children not established. Geriatric patients may be more susceptible to the usual adult dose.

Side Effects: Drowsiness, dry mouth, headache, nervousness.

Dosage: Chewable Tablets. Adults: 50 mg 30 min before travel; dosage may be repeated after 4–6 hr. *Severe nausea:* up to 150 mg daily.

NURSING CONSIDERATIONS

See *Nursing Considerations* for *Antiemetics,* p. 1076, and *Antihistamines,* p. 1007.

Administration/Storage

1. To prevent motion sickness, take medication 30 min before departure.
2. Tablets can be chewed, swallowed whole, or dissolved in the mouth.

CYCLIZINE HYDROCHLORIDE   (SYE-klih-zeen)
Marezine (OTC)

See *Antihistamines,* Chapter 51, p. 1011.

DIMENHYDRINATE   (dye-men-HY-drih-nayt)
Elixir, Syrup, Tablets, Chewable Tablets: Apo-Dimenhydrinate✻, Calm-X, Dimentabs, Dramamine, Gravol✻, Marmine, Motion-Aid, Nauseatol✻, Novodimenate✻, PMS-Dimenhydrinate✻, Travamine, Triptone (OTC). Injection: Dinate, Dommanate, Dramamine, Dramanate, Dramilin, Dramocen, Dramoject, Dymenate, Gravol✻, Hydrate, Marmine, Reidamine, Wehamine (Rx)

See *Antihistamines,* Chapter 51, p. 1003, and *Antiemetics,* p. 1076.

DIPHENHYDRAMINE HYDROCHLORIDE   (dye-fen-HY-drah-meen)
Allerdryl✻, AllerMax, Beldin Cough, Belix, Bena-D, Bena-D 50, Benadryl, Benadryl Complete Allergy, Benahist 10 and 50, Ben-Allergin-50, Benoject-10 and -50, Benylin Cough, Benaphen, Bydramine Cough, Diahist, Dihydrex, Diphenacen-10 and -50, Diphenadryl, Diphen Cough, Fenylhist, Fynex, Hydramine, Hydramine Cough, Hydril, Hyrexin-50, Noradryl, Nordryl, Nordryl Cough, Tusstat, Valdrene, Wehdryl (OTC and Rx).
    Sleep-Aids: Compoz, Dormarex 2, Insomnal✻, Nervine Nighttime Sleep-Aid, Nytol with DPH, Sleep-Eze 3, Sominex 2, Twilite (OTC)

See *Antihistamines,* Chapter 51, p. 1014.

DIPHENIDOL HYDROCHLORIDE   (dye-FEN-ih-dohl)
Vontrol (Rx)

Classification: Antiemetic.

Action/Kinetics: Diphenidol appears to depress labyrinth excitability and may also depress the chemoreceptor trigger zone. The drug is well absorbed from GI tract. **Peak plasma concentrations:** 1.5–3 hr. **Onset:** 30–45 min. **Duration:** 4 hr; **t½:** 4 hr. Metabolized, slowly excreted in urine.

Uses: Nausea, vomiting, and vertigo associated with infectious diseases, malignancies, radiation sickness, general anesthesia, motion sickness, labyrinthitis, and Meniere's disease.

Contraindications: Hypersensitivity to drug, anuria, pregnancy, children weighing less than 22.7 Kg.

Special Concerns: Administer with caution to patients with glaucoma, pyloric stenosis, pylorospasm, obstructive lesions of GI and urinary tract, and sinus tachycardia.

Side Effects: *CNS:* Confusion, disorientation, auditory and visual hallucinations; discontinue drug immediately if any of these symptoms occur. Also, drowsiness, malaise, headache, nervousness, excitation, depression, dizziness, sleep disturbances, weakness. *GI:* Dry mouth, GI irritation, nausea, indigestion, heartburn. *Other:* Skin rash, urticaria, mild jaundice, slight hypotension, blurred vision.

Symptoms of overdosage should be treated symptomatically with assurance that blood pressure and respiration are maintained. Gastric lavage may be indicated in oral overdosage.

Dosage: Tablets. Adults: 25–50 mg q 4 hr. **Pediatric.** *Nausea and vomiting only:* 0.88 mg/kg no more often than q 4 hr not to exceed 2.5 mg/lb/day. If symptoms persist after the first dose, a second dose can be given after 1 hr. The total daily dose should not exceed 5.5 mg/kg.

NURSING CONSIDERATIONS

See also *Nursing Considerations* for *Antiemetics,* p. 1076.

Assessment

1. Note any history of hypersensitivity to the drug.
2. Assess the client's general state of health. Determine the client's usual intake of fluid and output. Clients with anuria should not receive this drug.

Interventions

1. During the first three days of medication therapy, observe the client for disorientation, confusion or hallucinations. Apply side rails and put the bed in a low position. Withhold drug, document and report these symptoms to the physician.
2. If these side effects recur, apply side rails, keep night lights on and notify the physician.
3. Observe client closely for masking of symptoms related to undiagnosed pathology or toxicity.
4. Monitor BP and respirations, be prepared to assist with gastric lavage, and to provide supportive measures such as oxygen or mechanical ventilation in the event of drug overdose.

Client/Family

Discuss with the family the necessity for hospitalization and close medical supervision of the client while receiving the medication.

DRONABINOL (DELTA-9-TETRAHYDROCANNABINOL)   (droh-**NAB**-ih-nol)

Marinol (C-II, Rx)

Classification: Antinauseant.

Action/Kinetics: Dronabinol is the active component in marijuana and, as such, will manifest significant psychoactive effects. These include euphoria, anxiety, panic, depression, paranoia, decrement in memory and cognitive performance, decreased ability to control drives and impulses, and distortion in perception including time. In therapeutic doses, the drug also causes conjunctival injection and an increased heart rate. The antiemetic effect is thought to be due to inhibition of the vomiting center in the medulla. **Peak plasma levels:** 2–3 hr. Significant first-pass effect. The 11-hydroxytetrahydrocannabinol metabolite is active. **t½, biphasic:** 4 hr and 25–36 hr. **t½, 11-hydroxy-THC:** 15–18 hr. Metabolized in the liver and mainly excreted in the feces. Cumulative toxicity using clinical doses may occur.

Use: Nausea and vomiting associated with cancer chemotherapy, especially in patients who have not responded to other antiemetic treatment.

Contraindications: Nausea and vomiting from any cause other than cancer chemotherapy. Lactation. Hypersensitivity to sesame oil.

Special Concerns: Pregnancy category: B. Pediatric and geriatric patients should be monitored carefully due to an increased risk of psychoactive effects. Use with caution in patients with hypertension, heart disease, mania, depression, schizophrenia, and concomitantly with other psychoactive drugs.

Side Effects: *CNS:* Side effects are due mainly to the psychoactive effects of the drug and, in addition to those listed above, include dizziness, muddled thinking, coordination difficulties, irritability, weakness, headache, ataxia, paresthesia, hallucinations, visual distortions, depersonalization, confusion, nightmares, disorientation, and confusion. *CV:* Syncope, postural hypotension, tachycardia. *GI:* Diarrhea, dry mouth, fecal incontinence. *Other:* Facial flushing, tinnitus, speech difficulty, muscle pains.

Drug Interactions	
CNS depressants	Additive CNS depressant effects
Ethanol	During subchronic dronabinol use, lower and delayed peak alcohol blood levels

Dosage: Capsules. Adults and children, initial: 5 mg/m² 1–3 hr before chemotherapy; **then,** 5 mg/m² q 2–4 hr for a total of 4–6 doses per day. If ineffective, this dose may be increased by 2.5 mg/m² to a maximum of 15 mg/m² per dose. However, the incidence of serious psychoactive side effects increases dramatically at the higher dose levels.

NURSING CONSIDERATIONS

Administration/Storage

1. Due to its CNS effects, dronabinol should be used only when the client can be under close supervision.
2. Dronabinol can be abused. Therefore, prescriptions should be limited to one course of chemotherapy (i.e., several days).

Assessment

1. Note if the client has any history of allergic responses to sesame oil or seeds.
2. Determine if the client's nausea and vomiting are caused by anything other than cancer chemotherapy.

Interventions

If the client develops serious psychoactive side effects, the client should be placed in a quiet environment and provided with supportive care. Monitor vital signs and reassure client.

Client/Family Teaching

1. Discuss with the client and family the anticipated benefits to be derived from the therapy.
2. Advise the client to take the medication 1–3 hours before the scheduled cancer chemotherapy.
3. Instruct the client to use caution when sitting or standing suddenly because dizziness may occur.
4. Advise client not to drive or perform hazardous tasks that require mental acuity.
5. Discuss with the client the potential for psychoactive symptoms, visual distortions and mental confusion. Advise the family that these symptoms may be minimized by providing a quiet, supportive environment.

HYDROXYZINE   (hi-**DROX**-ih-zeen)

Atarax, Vistaril (Rx)

See *Antianxiety Agents,* Chapter 31, p. 624.

MECLIZINE HYDROCHLORIDE   (**MEK**-lih-zeen)

Antivert, Antivert/25 and /50, Antivert/25 Chewable, Antrizine, Bonamine✱, Bonine, Dizmiss, Meni-D, Ru-Vert-M (OTC and Rx)

See also *Antihistamines,* p. 1003, and *Antiemetics,* p. 1076.

Classification: Antihistamine (piperidine-type), antiemetic, antimotion sickness.

Action/Kinetics: The mechanism for the antiemetic effect is not known but may be due to a central anticholinergic effect to decrease vestibular stimulation and depress labyrinthine activity. The drug may also act on the chemoreceptor trigger zone to decrease vomiting.
   Onset: 30–60 min; **Duration:** 8–24 hr. **t¹/₂:** 6 hr.

Uses: Nausea, vomiting, dizziness of motion sickness, vertigo associated with diseases of the vestibular system.

Special Concerns: Pregnancy category: B. Safety for use during lactation and in children less than 12 years of age has not been determined. Pediatric and geriatric patients may be more sensitive to the anticholinergic effects of meclizine.

Side Effects: *CNS:* Drowsiness, excitation, nervousness, restlessness, insomnia, euphoria, vertigo, hallucinations (auditory or visual). *GI:* Nausea, vomiting, diarrhea, constipation, anorexia. *GU:* Urinary frequency or retention; difficulty in urination. *CV:* Hypotension, tachycardia, palpitations. *Miscellaneous:* Dry nose and throat, blurred or double vision, tinnitus, rash, urticaria.

Dosage: Capsules, Tablets, Chewable Tablets. *Motion sickness:* **Adults,** 25–50 mg 1 hr before travel; may be repeated q 24 hr during travel. *Vertigo:* **Adults:** 25–100 mg daily in divided doses.

NURSING CONSIDERATIONS

See also *Nursing Considerations* for *Antihistamines,* p. 1007, and *Antiemetics,* p. 1076.

Interventions

1. Assess the client for other adverse symptoms in addition to nausea. An antiemetic drug may

mask signs of drug overdose as well as signs of pathology such as increased intracranial pressure or intestinal obstruction.

2. Antiemetics tend to cause drowsiness and dizziness. Therefore, caution clients against driving or performing other hazardous tasks until individual response to the drug has been evaluated.

NABILONE (NAB-ih-lohn)

Cesamet (C-II, Rx)

Classification: Antinauseant.

Action/Kinetics: Nabilone is a synthetic cannabinoid producing effects similar to those of marijuana. These include euphoria, anxiety, panic, depression, paranoia, decrement in memory and cognitive performance, decreased ability to control drives and impulses, and distortions in perception of time. In addition, therapeutic doses cause dry mouth and hypotension. The antiemetic action may be due to inhibition of the vomiting center in the medulla. **Time to peak levels:** 2 hr. **Peak serum levels:** Approximately 10 ng/mL after oral administration. $t^{1/2}$, **nabilone:** 2 hr; $t^{1/2}$, **metabolites:** 35 hr. Nabilone and its metabolites are excreted mainly in the feces (via the bile), and to a lesser extent in the urine.

Uses: Nausea and vomiting associated with cancer chemotherapy, especially in patients who have not responded to other antiemetic treatment.

Contraindications: Nausea and vomiting from any cause other than cancer chemotherapy. During lactation.

Special Concerns: Use during pregnancy only if clearly needed. Safety and efficacy have not been determined in children less than 18 years of age. Geriatric patients may be more prone to the cardiac effects and orthostatic hypotension caused by nabilone. Use with caution in patients with hypertension, heart disease, mania, depression, schizophrenia, and concomitantly with other psychoactive drugs.

Side Effects: *CNS:* Untoward reactions are due mainly to the psychoactive effects of the drug and, in addition to those listed above, include: *CNS:* Drowsiness (most common), headache, increased awareness, impaired coordination, dizziness, tremors, seizures, irritability, ataxia, lapse in memory, hallucinations, depersonalization, confusion, sleep disturbances including nightmares, vertigo. *GI:* Nausea, anorexia, vomiting, constipation, increased appetite, gastritis, dyspepsia, mouth irritation, diarrhea. *CV:* Hypotension, fainting, tachycardia, postural hypotension, anemia, leukopenia, palpitations, arrhythmias, cerebral vascular accident, hypertension. *GU:* Urinary retention, increased or decreased urination. *Respiratory:* Cough, dyspnea, pharyngitis, nasal congestion, dry throat and nose, wheezing, nosebleeds. *Ear/Eye:* Ear "tightness," dry eyes, amblyopia, eye swelling, mydriasis, photophobia, effect on visual field. *Miscellaneous:* Tinnitus, paresthesia, muscular pain (back, neck, joint), perspiration, flushing of face, distortions of vision, speech difficulty, hot flashes, chills, malaise, fever, chest pain, facial edema, thirst.

Drug Interactions: Additive CNS depressant effects when used with other CNS depressants.

Dosage: Capsules. Adults: 1–2 mg b.i.d., up to a maximum of 6 mg daily in divided doses t.i.d.

NURSING CONSIDERATIONS

Administration/Storage

1. On the day of chemotherapy, the first dose of nabilone should be given 1–3 hr before the

antineoplastic agent. Also, administering 1–2 mg the night before chemotherapy may be helpful.

2. Can be given 2–3 times daily during the entire course of the chemotherapy cycle and, if necessary, for 2 days after the last dose of each chemotherapy cycle.

3. Start with the lower dose of drug to minimize side effects.

4. Due to its CNS effects, nabilone should be used only when the client can be under close supervision.

5. Nabilone can be abused. Therefore, prescriptions should be limited to one course of therapy (i.e., several days).

Assessment

1. Assess the client's mental attitude and whether or not he is taking any other CNS depressant drugs.

2. Check the client's blood pressure and pulse prior to initiating drug therapy.

Interventions

1. Monitor the blood pressure and pulse and compare with that taken prior to initiating drug therapy.

2. Observe the client closely for evidence of cardiovascular problems, such as hypotension, tachycardia, client complaints of palpitations, or urinary retention. Document and report to the physician.

3. If the client shows evidence of serious psychoactive side effects, place the client in a quiet environment and provide supportive treatment. Monitor closely and reassure client that symptoms will disappear once the drug is discontinued.

4. Note any evidence of the client developing psychological and/or physical dependence on the drug.

Client/Family Teaching

1. Advise the client to avoid ingestion of alcohol and any other unprescribed drugs.

2. Clients should be advised not to drive or perform hazardous tasks that require mental acuity due to the psychoactive effects of nabilone .

3. Discuss with the family the need for a family member to remain with the client while he is taking the drug so that any evidence of psychotic problems will be detected and reported to the physician immediately.

4. Explain that the psychotic episodes, if they occur, are the results of the drug. Client should not become unduly alarmed. Place the client in a quiet protected environment and be supportive. This is only a temporary effect and will disappear once drug therapy has been discontinued.

PHOSPHORATED CARBOHYDRATE SOLUTION

Calm-X, Emetrol, Naus-A-Way, Nausetrol (OTC)

Classification: Antiemetic.

Action/Kinetics: This product contains fructose, dextrose, and phosphoric acid with controlled hydrogen ion concentration. Claimed to relieve nausea and vomiting by direct action on the GI wall leading to a delay in gastric emptying time and a decrease in contraction of smooth muscles.

Uses: Symptomatic relief of nausea and vomiting due to a variety of causes, including vomiting due to psychogenic factors, morning sickness, nausea or vomiting due to drug therapy, and regurgitation in infants.

Contraindications: Diabetes, fructose intolerance.

Side Effects: *GI:* Diarrhea and abdominal pain, both due to fructose.

Dosage: Solution. *Morning sickness:* 15–30 mL on arising and q 3 hr thereafter if necessary. *Vomiting due to psychogenic factors:* **Adults,** 15–30 mL at 15 min intervals until vomiting subsides or until 5 doses have been taken; **pediatric,** 5–10 mL at 15 min intervals in same manner as adults. *Motion sickness, vomiting due to drug therapy, inhalation anesthesia:* **Adults and older children:** 15 mL; **young children:** 5 mL. *Regurgitation in infants:* 5–10 mL, 10–15 min before feeding (for refractory cases: 10–15 mL 30 min before feeding).

NURSING CONSIDERATIONS

Administration/Storage

1. *Do not* dilute.
2. Do not allow liquids PO for 15 min after administration.
3. In case of nausea, repeat at 15 min intervals until the condition is under control.
4. Regurgitating infants: 10–15 minutes before each feeding; refractory cases: 10–15 mL 30 min before feeding.
5. Morning sickness: On arising and q 3 hr thereafter or when nausea threatens.
6. There should be no toxicity or side effects associated with this medication, nor should it mask the symptoms of organic disease.

Assessment

Note if the client has a history of diabetes mellitus or fructose intolerance.

Interventions

1. If the client has diabetes, do not administer this concentrated carbohydrate solution.
2. Note if the client develops diarrhea or abdominal pain and report to the physician.

PROCHLORPERAZINE   (proh-klor-**PER**-ah-zeen)
Compazine (Rx)

PROCHLORPERAZINE EDISYLATE   (proh-klor-**PER**-ah-zeen)
Compazine (Rx)

PROCHLORPERAZINE MALEATE   (proh-klor-**PER**-ah-zeen)
Compazine, Compazine Spansules (Rx)

See *Phenothiazines,* Chapter 32, p. 639.

SCOPOLAMINE HYDROBROMIDE   (scoh-**POL**-ah-meen)
(Rx and OTC)

See *Anticholinergics,* Chapter 47, p. 947.

THIETHYLPERAZINE MALEATE   (thigh-eth-ill-**PER**-ah-zeen)

Torecan (Rx)

Classification: Antiemetic.

Action/Kinetics: Phenothiazine derivative that acts on both the chemoreceptor trigger zone and the vomiting center. **Onset, PO:** 30 min. **Duration:** 4 hr. For details, see *Phenothiazines,* Chapter 32, p. 627.

Uses: Control of nausea and vomiting of various origins. Possibly effective to treat vertigo.

Contraindications: Severe CNS depression, comatose states, pregnancy, children under 12 years of age. IV use (causes hypotension).

Special Concerns: Dosage has not been established for children less than 12 years of age. Administer with caution to patients with liver or kidney disease.

Side Effects: Drowsiness, dryness of mouth and nose, restlessness, hypotension, extrapyramidal complications.

Dosage: Tablets, Suppositories: 10–30 mg daily in divided doses. **IM:** 10 mg 1–3 times daily. **Do not use IV.**

NURSING CONSIDERATIONS

See also *Nursing Considerations* for *Antiemetics,* p. 1076, and for *Phenothiazines* p. 630.

Administration/Storage

1. Administer deep IM.
2. The onset of action occurs in 30 minutes and lasts for 4 hours.
3. Do not administer the medication if the respiratory rate is depressed, or if the client is comatose.
4. Have levarterenol and phenylephrine available to administer in the event of hypotension. Epinephrine is contraindicated.
5. Have caffeine sodium benzoate and IV diphenhydramine hydrochloride available to relieve extrapyramidal symptoms should they develop.

Interventions

1. Observe for postural hypotension manifested by weakness, dizziness, and faintness. Monitor the client's BP and advise the client to rise slowly from a prone to a sitting position before standing.
2. Assess for extrapyramidal symptoms, such as torticollis, dysphagia, random movements of the eyes, or convulsions. These adverse effects should be documented and reported to the physician so that medication can be administered for symptom relief.

TRIMETHOBENZAMIDE HYDROCHLORIDE   (try-meth-oh-**BENZ**-ah-myd)

Arrestin, Hymetic, Tebamide, T-Gen, Ticon, Tigan, Tiject-20 (Rx)

Classification: Antiemetic.

Action/Kinetics: Trimethobenzamide is an antiemetic related to the antihistamines but with weak antihistaminic properties. The drug is less effective than the phenothiazines but has fewer side effects. Not suitable as sole agent for severe emesis. Can be used rectally. Trimethobenzamide appears to control vomiting by depressing the chemoreceptor trigger zone of the medulla. **Onset: PO and IM,** 10–40 min. **Duration:** 3–4 hr. 30%–50% of drug excreted unchanged in urine in 48–72 hr.

Uses: Nausea and vomiting.

Contraindications: Hypersensitivity to drug, to benzocaine, or similar local anesthetics. Do not use suppositories for neonates; do not use IM in children.

Special Concerns: Use during pregnancy only if benefits outweigh risks. Use with caution during lactation.

Side Effects: *CNS:* Depression of mood, disorientation, headache, drowsiness, dizziness, seizures, coma, Parkinson-like symptoms, seizures. *Other:* Hypersensitivity reactions, hypotension, blood dyscrasias, jaundice, muscle cramps, opisthotonos, blurred vision, diarrhea, allergic skin reactions. *After IM injection:* Pain, burning, stinging, redness at injection site.

Drug Interactions: Concomitant use with atropine-like drugs and CNS depressants including alcohol should be avoided.

Dosage: Capsules. Adults: 250 mg t.i.d.–q.i.d.; **pediatric, 13.6–40.9 kg:** 100–200 mg t.i.d.–q.i.d. **Suppositories. Adults:** 200 mg t.i.d.–q.i.d.; **pediatric, under 13.6 kg:** 100 mg t.i.d.–q.i.d.; **13.6–40.9 kg:** 100–200 mg t.i.d.–q.i.d. **IM only. Adults:** 200 mg t.i.d.–q.i.d. (IM route not to be used in children.)

NURSING CONSIDERATIONS

See also *Nursing Considerations* for *Antiemetics,* p. 1076.

Administration/Storage

1. Inject drug IM deeply into the upper, outer quadrant of the gluteus muscle. Be careful to avoid escape of fluid from the needle so as to minimize local reaction.
2. Expect the onset of action to occur in 10–40 minutes after oral administration and to last 3–4 hours.
3. After IM injection, the action of the drug lasts 2–3 hours.
4. Do not administer suppositories to clients allergic to benzocaine or similar anesthetics.

Assessment

1. Note any history of sensitivity to benzocaine and document on the client's record.
2. Ask clients if they have experienced any local reaction to the suppositories and document.

Interventions

Observe the client for any evidence of skin reaction. Document, as this is the first sign of hypersensitivity to the drug.

CHAPTER FIFTY-SEVEN
Digestants

General Statement: Digestants are agents that replace or supplement one of the many enzymes or other chemical substances that participate in the digestion of food. They are rarely indicated for therapeutic reasons but may be required for elderly patients or those suffering from certain deficiency diseases of the GI tract. They may also be required after GI surgery.

Commonly used digestants include hydrochloric acid, bile salts, and the enzymes produced by the stomach and glands associated with digestion.

Nonprescription preparations also contain many of the same ingredients as prescription drugs; however, these are usually present at levels too low to be effective.

DEHYDROCHOLIC ACID   (dee-hy-droh-**KOH**-lik **AH**-sid)

Cholan-HMB, Decholin, Hepahydrin (Rx and OTC)

Classification: Digestant, laxative.

Action/Kinetics: Dehydrocholic acid is a derivative of bile acids. The drug has some laxative effect and appears to increase the flow of bile and facilitate evacuation of the gall bladder. Also, there is increased emulsification and absorption of fats.

Uses: Various conditions involving the biliary tract including recent or repeated surgery for biliary calculi or strictures, cholecystitis, cholangitis, biliary dyskinesia, to promote drainage of an infected bile duct, bile duct obstruction. Laxative.

Contraindications: Complete obstruction of the biliary, GI, or GU tracts. Also, hepatic insufficiency, jaundice, cholelithiasis. In presence of abdominal pain, nausea, or vomiting (i.e., symptoms of appendicitis).

Special Concerns: Use with caution in patients with a history of asthma and allergies as well as in children under 6 years, the elderly, and in prostatic hypertrophy.

Dosage: Tablets. Adults: 244–500 mg t.i.d. after meals for 4 to 6 weeks.

NURSING CONSIDERATIONS

Administration/Storage

1. Bile salts may be given concomitantly to ensure adequate digestion and absorption of nutrients.
2. If there is no improvement after 4 to 6 weeks, discontinue the drug.

57

Assessment

1. Obtain baseline liver function studies.
2. Note if the client has any evidence of biliary obstruction such as yellowing of the sclera, or if the client has abdominal pain.

Client/Family Teaching

Instruct client to consult the physician if pain persists or if severe nausea and pain develop.

GLUTAMIC ACID HYDROCHLORIDE (gloo-TAM-ik AH-sid)

Acidulin (OTC)

Classification: Digestant, gastric acidifier.

Action/Kinetics: On contact with water this compound releases hydrochloric acid, which acidifies the stomach. Thus, the drug has the same effect as hydrochloric acid but is easier to administer because it comes in capsule form. Also available combined with pepsin.

Uses: Hypochlorhydria, achlorhydria, as an adjunct in pernicious anemia or gastric cancer, certain allergies, chronic gastritis.

Contraindications: Hyperacidity and peptic ulcer.

Side Effects: An overdose may result in systemic acidosis.

Dosage: Capsules. Adults: 1–3 capsules (340 mg) t.i.d. before meals. *Note:* 340 mg contains about 1.8 mEq hydrochloric acid.

NURSING CONSIDERATIONS

Client/Family Teaching

1. Instruct the client to keep capsules dry.
2. Provide the client with a printed sheet describing the symptoms of systemic acidosis, such as weakness and deep, rapid breathing that may occur in the event of overdosage.
3. Advise the client to have sodium bicarbonate or sodium lactate solution available to treat overdosage and to notify the physician immediately if symptoms of overdosage are evident.

HYDROCHLORIC ACID, DILUTED

Classification: Digestant, gastric acidifier.

Action/Kinetics: Replacement of naturally occurring substance by diluted hydrochloric acid (10% w/v).

Uses: Hypochlorhydria, hydrochloric acid deficiency often occurring in the elderly (is frequently associated with pernicious anemia or gastric cancer).

Contraindications: Hyperacidity and peptic ulcer.

Side Effects: Prolonged administration may disturb electrolyte balance (depletion of sodium bicarbonate) and increase the levels of sodium chloride.

Dosage: Solution. Administer 2–8 mL of a 10% solution copiously diluted. Dilute each milliliter with at least 25 mL of water.

NURSING CONSIDERATIONS

Client/Family Teaching

1. Instruct the client to sip the medication through a plastic or paper straw to protect the tooth enamel. The client should take the medication with meals.
2. Rinse the mouth with an alkaline mouth wash if ingestion of hydrochloric acid solution will not be completed until after the meal has been completed.

OX BILE EXTRACT (BILE SALTS)   (OX BYEL)
Bilron (OTC)

Classification: Digestant (choleretic).

Action/Kinetics: Natural dried extract of ox bile, which allegedly increases the flow of bile as well as exerting a laxative effect. Effectiveness has not been shown, however.

Uses: Bile deficiency states. Laxative.

Contraindications: Severe jaundice, complete mechanical biliary obstruction. If symptoms of appendicitis are present (e.g., nausea, vomiting, abdominal pain).

Special Concerns: Use with caution in patients with obstructive jaundice.

Side Effects: Nausea, vomiting, diarrhea, and cramping.

Dosage: Bilron Capsules: 150–600 mg 1–3 times daily with or after meals. **Ox Bile Extract Enseal Tablets:** 324–648 mg (2 tablets) daily with meals, up to a total of 6 tablets daily.

NURSING CONSIDERATIONS

Interventions

Monitor liver function studies throughout therapy.

Client/Family Teaching

1. Instruct client not to chew tablets because they taste bitter.
2. Take the medication with water either with or after meals.

PANCREATIN   (PAN-kree-ah-tin)
Dizymes, Hi-Vegi-Lip (OTC)

Classification: Digestant.

Action/Kinetics: This mixture of enzymes (pancreatin, lipase, amylase, and protease) is obtained from hog pancreas. The preparation increases digestion, or predigestion of food.

Uses: Pancreatic deficiency diseases such as pancreatitis, cystic fibrosis of the pancreas, pancreatectomy.

Special Concerns: Give with caution to patients sensitive to hog protein. Use with caution in pregnancy and lactation.

Side Effects: *Allergic:* Rash, sneezing, lacrimation. Holding the tablets in the mouth may cause ulceration and stomatitis. High doses may cause hyperuricemia and hyperuricosuria.

Dosage: Tablets. 1–3 after meals.

NURSING CONSIDERATIONS

Assessment

Determine if the client is sensitive to hog enzymes.

Interventions

1. Assess the client for anorexia, and for bowel movements. Anorexia and constipation are indications of overdosage and the drug dosage should be reduced.
2. Follow-up to assure that the client understands and maintains the diet prescribed by the physician.

Client/Family Teaching

1. Advise client to swallow and not to chew the tablets.
2. Instruct the client to avoid using antacids while taking pancreatin.

PANCRELIPASE (pan-kree-**LIP**-ayz)

Cotazym, Cotazym-S, Creon, Entolase, Entolase-HP, Festal II, Ilozyme, Ku-Zyme HP, Pancoate, Pancrease, Pancrease MT 4, Pancrease MT 10, Pancrease MT 16, Protilase, Viokase, Zymase (OTC and Rx)

Classification: Digestant.

Action/Kinetics: Enzyme concentrate from hog pancreas, which contains lipase, amylase, and protease, enzymes that replace or supplement naturally occurring enzymes. The product is more active at neutral or slightly alkaline pH. Pancrelipase has 12 times the lipolytic activity and 4 times both the proteolytic and amylolytic activity of pancreatin.

Uses: Replacement therapy for patients with pancreatic insufficiency, chronic pancreatitis, cystic fibrosis, ductal obstructions due to pancreatic cancer, postpancreatectomy, steatorrhea or malabsorption syndrome, postgastrectomy. Also, for presumptive test for pancreatic function.

Contraindications: Hog protein sensitivity.

Special Concerns: Use with caution during pregnancy (pregnancy category: C). Safety for use during lactation and in children less than 6 months of age not established.

Side Effects: *GI:* Nausea, diarrhea, abdominal cramps. Inhalation of the powder is irritating to the skin and mucous membranes and may result in an asthma attack. High doses cause hyperuricemia and hyperuricosuria.

Drug Interactions: Antacids containing calcium carbonate or magnesium hydroxide may reverse the beneficial effect of pancrelipase.

Dosage: Capsules, Delayed-release Capsules, Powder, Tablets. Adults and children: Dosage should be calculated according to fat content of the diet. Products contain varying amounts of the enzymes. **Usual dose:** 1–3 capsules or tablets before or with meals and snacks (severe deficiencies may require up to 8 capsules or tablets if no GI side effects occur). The dose of the powder is 1 packet (containing 0.7 g) before or with meals and snacks. For treatment of steatorrhea, the dose may be increased up to 3 capsules with meals.

NURSING CONSIDERATIONS

Administration/Storage

1. When administering to young children, the contents of the capsule can be sprinkled on food.
2. After several weeks of use, the dosage should be adjusted according to the therapeutic response.
3. Unopened preparations should be stored in tight containers at a temperature not to exceed 25°C.
4. Enteric-coated products should not be crushed or chewed. Also, enteric-coated products that come in contact with foods with a pH greater than 5.5 will dissolve.

Assessment

1. Obtain a thorough nursing history.
2. Determine if the client has any sensitivity or allergy to hog protein. Hog protein is the main constituent of pancrelipase.

Interventions

Refer the client to a dietitian for appropriate dietary counseling and assistance in meal planning.

Client/Family Teaching

1. Instruct the client that the medication should be taken just before or with the meals.
2. Advise the client to report any nausea, cramping, or diarrhea. The dosage of medication may need to be adjusted.
3. Instruct the client to closely follow the prescribed diet.
4. Discuss the importance of reporting for follow-up laboratory studies as scheduled.

CHAPTER FIFTY-EIGHT

Insulin, Oral Antidiabetics, and Insulin Antagonists

58

INSULINS

10

General Statement: Diabetes mellitus is a disease in which the islets of Langerhans in the pancreas produce either no insulin or insufficient quantities of insulin. Diabetes mellitus is classified as insulin-dependent (Type I; formerly referred to as *juvenile-onset*) and noninsulin-dependent (Type II; formerly referred to as *maturity-onset*). Diabetes mellitus can be treated successfully by the administration of insulin isolated from the pancreas of cattle or hogs or of human insulin made either semisynthetically or derived from recombinant DNA technology.

The structure of insulin from pork sources more closely resembles human insulin than that from beef sources.

Proinsulin still remains the major impurity in insulin products. Such impurities may lead to local or systemic allergic reactions as well as antibody-mediated insulin resistance. In recent years, however, technology has improved so that insulin preparations currently marketed in the United States do not contain more than 25 parts per million (ppm) of proinsulin. Insulin products that contain less than 20 ppm of proinsulin are referred to as *improved single peak* insulins while those products that contain 10 ppm or less of proinsulin are referred to as *purified insulins*. In reality, purified pork insulins have approximate 1 ppm of proinsulin and human insulins made semisynthetically or from recombinant DNA have 1 and 0 ppm, respectively.

Insulin preparations with different times of onset, peak activity, and duration of action have been developed. Such products are prepared by precipitating insulin in the presence of zinc chloride to form zinc insulin crystals and/or by combining insulin with a protein such as protamine. Based on these modifications, insulin products are classified as fast-acting, intermediate-acting, and long-acting. These preparations permit the physician to select the preparation best suited to the lifestyle of the patient.

Rapid-Acting Insulin

1. Insulin injection (Regular Insulin, Crystalline Zinc Insulin, Unmodified Insulin)
2. Prompt insulin zinc suspension (Semilente)

Intermediate-Acting Insulin

1. Isophane insulin suspension (NPH)
2. Insulin zinc suspension (Lente)

Long-Acting Insulin

1. Protamine zinc insulin suspension (PZI)
2. Extended insulin zinc suspension (Ultralente)

Note: Insulin preparations with various times of onset and duration of action are often mixed to obtain optimum control in diabetic patients.

Action/Kinetics: Insulin, following combination with insulin receptors on cell plasma membranes, facilitates the transport of glucose into cardiac and skeletal muscle and adipose tissue. It also increases synthesis of glycogen in the liver. Insulin stimulates protein synthesis and lipogenesis and inhibits lipolysis and release of free fatty acids from fat cells.

This latter effect prevents or reverses the ketoacidosis sometimes observed in the diabetic. Insulin also causes intracellular shifts in magnesium and potassium.

Since insulin is a protein, it is destroyed in the GI tract. Thus, it must be administered subcutaneously so that it is readily absorbed into the bloodstream and distributed throughout the extracellular fluid. Insulin is metabolized mainly by the liver.

Uses: Replacement therapy in Type I diabetes; diabetic ketoacidosis. Insulin is also indicated in Type II diabetes when other measures have failed or with surgery, trauma, infection, fever, endocrine dysfunction, pregnancy, gangrene, Raynaud's disease, or kidney or liver dysfunction.

Regular insulin is used in IV hyperalimentation solutions, in IV dextrose to treat severe hyperkalemia, and IV as a provocative test for growth hormone secretion.

Diet: The dietary control of diabetes is as important as medication with appropriate drugs. The role of the nurse in teaching the patient how to eat properly cannot be underestimated.

As a first step, the physician must determine the individual patient's dietary requirements. Since there is a close relationship between carbohydrate (CHO), fat (F), and protein (P), intake of each of these nutrients must be regulated. The prescribed amount of CHO, P, and F eaten at each meal must remain constant.

The nurse and/or dietitian must teach the patient how to calculate exchange values of various foods. Food lists and food-exchange values published by the American Diabetes Association and the American Dietetic Association are valuable teaching aids.

Diabetic patients should adhere to a regular meal schedule. Patients taking large amounts of insulin will frequently be better controlled when they have four to six small meals daily rather than three large ones. The frequency of meals and the overall caloric intake vary with the type of drug taken. Diabetic children may be on a less restricted diet, adjusting the insulin dosage according to blood and urine glucose readings. Children with negative urine glucose tend to become hypoglycemic rapidly with exercise or decrease in appetite, and many physicians allow for glucose spilling.

Contraindication: Hypersensitivity to insulin.

Special Concerns: Pregnant diabetic patients often manifest decreased insulin requirements during the first half of pregnancy and increased requirements during the latter half.

Side Effects: *Hypoglycemia:* Due to insulin overdose, delayed or decreased food intake, too much exercise in relationship to insulin dose, or when transferring from one preparation to another. Even carefully controlled patients occasionally develop signs of insulin overdosage characterized by hunger, weakness, fatigue, nervousness, pallor or flushing, profuse sweating, headache, palpitations, numbness of mouth, tingling in the fingers, tremors, blurred and double vision, hypothermia, excess yawning, mental confusion, incoordination, tachycardia, and loss of consciousness.

Symptoms of hypoglycemia may mimic those of psychic disturbances. Severe prolonged hypoglycemia may cause brain damage, and in the elderly, may mimic stroke.

Allergic: Urticaria, angioedema, lymphadenopathy, bullae, anaphylaxis. Occurs mostly following intermittent insulin therapy or IV administration of large doses to insulin-resistant patients. Antihistamines or corticosteroids may be used to treat these symptoms. Patients who are highly allergic to insulin and cannot be treated with oral hypoglycemics may respond to human insulin products.

At site of injection: Swelling, stinging, redness, itching, warmth. These symptoms often disappear with continued use. Atrophy or hypertrophy of subcutaneous fat tissue (minimize by rotating site of injection).

Insulin resistance: Usual cause is obesity. Acute resistance may occur following infections, trauma, surgery, emotional disturbances, or other endocrine disorders.

Ophthalmologic: Blurred vision, transient presbyopia. Occurs mainly during initiation of therapy or in patients who have been uncontrolled for a long period of time.

Hyperglycemic rebound (Somogyi effect): Usually in patients who receive chronic overdosage.

Differentiation Between Diabetic Coma and Hypoglycemic Reaction (Insulin Shock)

Coma in diabetes may be caused by uncontrolled diabetes (high sugar content in blood or urine, ketoacidosis) or by too much insulin (insulin shock, hypoglycemia).

Diabetic coma and insulin shock can be differentiated in the following manner:

Diagnostic Feature	Hyperglycemia (Diabetic Coma)	Hypoglycemia (Insulin Shock)
Onset	Gradual (days)	Sudden (24–48 hr)
Medication	Insufficient insulin	Excess insulin
Food intake	Normal or excess	Probably too little
Overall appearance	Extremely ill	Very weak
Skin	Dry and flushed	Moist and pale
Infection	Frequent	Absent
Fever	Frequent	Absent
Mouth	Dry	Drooling
Thirst	Intense	Absent
Hunger	Absent	Occasional
Vomiting	Common	Absent
Abdominal pain	Frequent	Rare
Respiration	Increased, air hunger	Normal
Breath	Acetone odor	Normal
Blood pressure	Low	Normal
Pulse	Weak and rapid	Full and bounding
Vision	Dim	Diplopia
Tremor	Absent	Frequent
Convulsions	None	In late stages
Urine sugar	High	Absent in second specimen
Ketone bodies	High	Absent in second specimen
Blood sugar	High	Less than 60 mg/100 mL

Source: Adapted with permission from *The Merck Manual,* 11th ed.

Diabetic coma is usually precipitated by the patient's failure to take insulin. Hypoglycemia is often precipitated by the patient's unpredictable response, excess exertion, stress due to illness or surgery, errors in calculating dosage, or failure to eat.

Treatment of Diabetic Coma or Severe Acidosis

Administer 30–60 units of insulin. This is followed by doses of 20 units or more every 30 min. To avoid a hypoglycemic state, 1 g of dextrose is administered for each unit of insulin given. Treatment is often supplemented by electrolytes and fluids. Urine samples are collected for analysis, and vital signs are monitored as ordered.

Treatment of Hypoglycemia (Insulin Shock)

Mild hypoglycemia can be relieved by oral administration of carbohydrates such as orange juice, candy, or a lump of sugar. If the patient is comatose, adults may be given 10–30 mL of 50% dextrose solution IV; children should receive 0.5–1 mL/kg of 50% dextrose solution. Epinephrine, hydrocortisone, or glucagon may be used in severe cases to cause an increase in blood glucose.

Drug Interactions

Alcohol, ethyl	↑ Hypoglycemia → low blood sugar and shock
Anabolic steroids	↑ Hypoglycemic effect of insulin
Beta-adrenergic blocking agents	↑ Hypoglycemia due to insulin
Chlorthalidone	↓ Hypoglycemic effect of antidiabetics
Contraceptives, oral	↑ Dosage of antidiabetic due to impairment of glucose tolerance
Corticosteroids	↓ Effect of insulin due to corticosteroid-induced hyperglycemia
Dextrothyroxine	↓ Effect of insulin due to dextrothyroxine-induced hyperglycemia
Diazoxide	Diazoxide-induced hyperglycemia ↓ diabetic control
Digitalis glycosides	Use with caution, as insulin affects serum potassium levels
Epinephrine	↓ Effect of insulin due to epinephrine-induced hyperglycemia
Estrogens	↓ Effect of insulin due to impairment of glucose tolerance
Ethacrynic acid	↓ Hypoglycemic effect of antidiabetics
Fenfluramine	Additive hypoglycemic effects
Furosemide	↓ Hypoglycemic effect of antidiabetics
Glucagon	Glucagon-induced hyperglycemia ↓ effect of antidiabetics
Guanethidine	↑ Hypoglycemic effect of insulin
MAO inhibitors	MAO inhibitors ↑ and prolong hypoglycemic effect of antidiabetics
Oxytetracycline	↑ Effect of insulin
Phenothiazines	↑ Dosage of antidiabetic due to phenothiazine-induced hyperglycemia
Phenytoin	Phenytoin-induced hyperglycemia ↓ diabetic control
Propranolol	Propranolol inhibits rebound of blood glucose after insulin-induced hypoglycemia
Salicylates	↑ Effect of hypoglycemic effect of insulin
Tetracyclines	May ↑ hypoglycemic effect of insulin
Thiazide diuretics	↓ Hypoglycemic effect of antidiabetics
Thyroid preparations	↑ Dosage of antidiabetic due to thyroid-induced hyperglycemia
Triamterene	↓ Hypoglycemic effect of antidiabetic

Laboratory Test Interferences: Alters liver function tests and thyroid function tests. False + Coombs' test, ↑ serum protein, ↓ serum amino acids, calcium, cholesterol, potassium, and urine amino acids.

Dosage: Insulin is usually administered SC. Insulin injection (regular insulin) is the **only** preparation that may be administered IV. This route should be used only for patients with severe ketoacidosis or diabetic coma.

Dosage for insulin is always expressed in USP units.

Dosage is established and monitored by blood glucose (often using glucose monitoring machines in the home), urine glucose, and acetone tests. Dosage is highly individualized. Furthermore, since the requirements of patients may change with time, dosage must be checked at regular intervals. It is usually advisable to hospitalize patients while their daily insulin and caloric requirements are being established.

In pregnancy, insulin requirements may increase suddenly during the last trimester. After delivery, there may be a sudden drop in requirements to prepregnancy levels. To prevent the development of hypoglycemia, insulin is often discontinued on the day of delivery and glucose is administered IV.

The various insulin preparations can be mixed to obtain the combination best suited for the individual patient. However, mixing must be done according to the directions received from the physician and/or pharmacist.

NURSING CONSIDERATIONS

Applicable to all diabetic clients controlled by medication whether it is insulin or an oral hypoglycemic agent.

Administration/Storage

1. Read the product information brochure and any important notes inserted into the package of prescribed insulin.

2. Discard open vials that have not been used for several weeks or any whose expiration date has passed.

3. Refrigerate stock supply of insulin but avoid freezing. Freezing destroys the manner in which insulin is suspended in the formulation.

4. Store insulin vial in a cool place, avoiding extremes of temperature or exposure to sunlight.

5. The following guidelines should be followed with respect to mixing the various insulins:
   - Regular insulin may be mixed with NPH, PZI, or lente insulins. However to avoid transfer of the longer-acting insulin into the regular insulin vial, regular insulin should be drawn into the syringe first.
   - A mixture of regular insulin with NPH, lente, or PZI insulin should be administered within 15 min of mixing due to binding of regular insulin by excess protamine and/or zinc in the longer-acting preparations.
   - Lente, semilente, or ultralente insulins may be mixed with each other in any proportion; however, these insulins should not be mixed with NPH or PZI insulins.
   - When used in an insulin infusion, insulin may be mixed in any proportion with either 0.9% sodium chloride injection or water for injection. Due to stability changes, such mixtures should be used within 24 hr of their preparation.

6. Store compatible mixtures of insulin for no longer than 1 month at room temperature or 3 months at 2°C–8°C (36°F–46°F). However, bacterial contamination may occur.

7. To ensure a constant amount of precipitate in each dose, invert the vial several times to mix before the material is withdrawn. Avoid vigorous shaking and frothing of the material. (Regular and globin insulin are the only two insulins that do not have a precipitate.)

8. Discard any vial in which the precipitate is clumped or granular in appearance or which has formed a solid deposit of particles on the side of the vial.

9. In order to prevent dosage error, do not alter the order of mixing insulins or change the model or brand of syringe or needle.

10. Administer at a 90-degree angle when using a ½-inch needle and at a 45-degree angle when using a ⅝-inch needle for injection.

11. Provide an automatic injector for clients who are fearful of injecting themselves.

12. Assist the visually impaired diabetic to obtain information and devices for self-administration of insulin by consulting their local diabetes association or by writing to the New York Diabetes Association, 104 East 40th Street, New York, NY 10016, for *Devices for Visually Impaired Diabetics,* and to The Lighthouse, The New York Association for the Blind, 111 East 59th Street, New York, NY 10022, for *An Evaluation of Devices for Insulin Dependent Visually Handicapped Diabetics.*

13. Local atrophy may occur. This may appear as mild dimpling of the skin or as deep pits in young girls and women, and hypertrophy, appearing as well-developed muscle on the anterior and lateral thighs of young boys and men. To prevent this problem, rotate the sites of SC injections of insulin.
    * Make a chart indicating the injection sites (see Figure 6).
    * Allow 3–4 cm between injection sites.
    * Do not inject in the same site for at least 1 month.
    * Avoid injecting within 1 cm around the umbilicus because of the high vascularity in this area.
    * Avoid injections around the waist line because of the sensitive nerve supply to this area.
    * Use insulin at room temperature to prevent lipodystrophy.

14. If the insulin has been refrigerated, allow it to remain at room temperature for at least 1 hour before using.

15. Apply pressure for a minute after injection, but do not massage since this may interfere with the rate of absorption.

16. If breakfast must be delayed because of laboratory tests, delay administering the morning dose of insulin.

17. Care of reusable syringes and needles.
    * Do not use heavily chlorinated water or water with a high chemical content for sterilizing syringes. To sterilize, boil the syringe and needle for 5 min.
    * Needle and syringe can be sterilized by soaking in isopropyl alcohol for at least 5 min. The alcohol must evaporate from the equipment before use to prevent reduction in the strength (dilution) of the insulin.
    * Clean syringes covered by a precipitate with a cotton-tipped swab soaked in vinegar; then thoroughly rinse syringe in water and sterilize it. (Clean needles with a wire and sharpen with a pumice stone, if reusable.)

Assessment

1. Obtain a thorough nursing history from the client and/or family.

2. Assess the client for symptoms of hyperglycemia: thirst, polydypsia, polyuria, drowsiness, fruity odor to the breath, and flushed skin. Note state of consciousness.

3. Determine when the client first noticed changes in their physical condition and what these changes were.

4. Note if the client and/or family has noticed any psychological changes in the client and what they consisted of.

5. Identify and list other medications the client may be taking.

6. Weigh the client. This is especially important when working with elderly clients since the amount of hypoglycemic agent prescribed is determined by their weight.

Setting Up An Easy Rotation Cycle

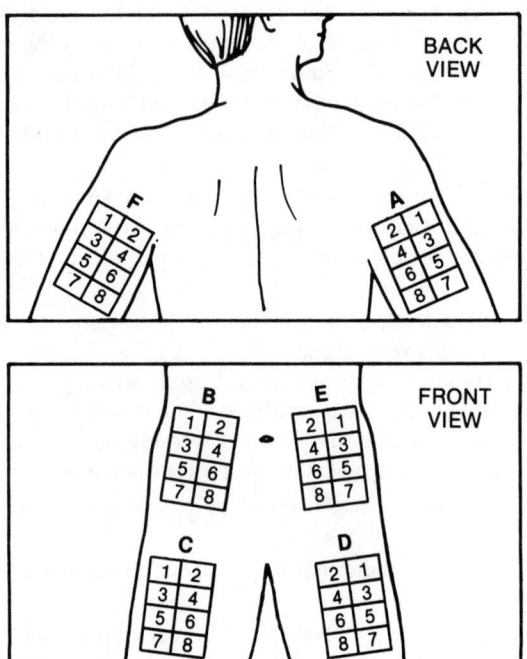

Injection Log

SITE		1	2	3	4	5	6	7	8
right arm	A								
right abdomen	B								
right thigh	C								
left thigh	D								
left abdomen	E								
left arm	F								

FIGURE 6   Pattern for varying insulin injection sites. If you follow the sketch, you will see that the right arm is marked A, the right side of the abdomen is B, and the right thigh is C. Crossing to the left side of the body, the left thigh is marked D, the abdomen E, and the left arm F. Each of these areas can be thought of as a rectangle that may be divided, as shown, into eight different squares more than one inch on each side. These squares are numbered, starting from the upper and outside corner, which is number one, to the lowest corner, which is number eight, with all even numbers toward the middle of the body. If you select square number one and inject into it at each of the six areas A through F, it will take you six days to return again to A. Then selecting square number two and injecting into it at each of the six areas again rotates you around your body, returning in six days to area A. Follow with square number three, and so forth. It is easy to see that this procedure provides 48 different places in which to make your injections. If you make one injection daily, it will be that many days before you return to the A-1 square ... almost seven weeks. (Figure and legend courtesy of Becton Dickinson and Company.)

Interventions

1. If the client has symptoms of a hyperglycemic reaction, obtain medical supervision as rapidly as possible.
   - Have regular insulin available for administration.
   - After administering the insulin, monitor the client closely.
   - Observe the client for further signs of hyperglycemia such as shortness of breath, facial flushing, air hunger, soft eyeballs, and acetone on the breath.
   - Check urine glucose, urine acetone, blood glucose and other related laboratory data.
2. Check the client for early symptoms of hypoglycemia, such as easy fatigue, hunger, headache, drowsiness, nausea, lassitude, and tremulousness.
   - More marked symptoms such as weakness, sweating, tremors, and/or nervousness may occur later.
   - Observe the client at night for excessive restlessness and profuse sweating.
   - Obtain a blood sugar level and promptly administer a carbohydrate (orange juice, candy, or a lump of sugar, if the client is conscious) and notify the physician.
   - If the client is conscious and has been taking long-acting insulin, also administer a slowly digestible carbohydrate, such as bread with corn syrup or honey. Provide additional carbohydrates such as crackers and milk for the next two hours.
   - If the client is in the hospital, have available 10%–20% dextrose solution for IV therapy or $D_{50\%}$ bristojets.
   - If the client is unconscious, apply honey or Karo syrup to the buccal membrane, or administer glucagon if available.
3. Some clients have a Somogyi effect and are often mistaken for clients who do not follow the prescribed methods of therapy. The Somogyi effect occurs when hypoglycemia triggers the release of epinephrine, glucocorticoids, and growth hormone, which stimulates glycogenesis and a resultant higher blood glucose level. Reduction in the dosage of insulin is necessary to stabilize the client. This should be anticipated in the client who has originally been treated for hypoglycemia.
4. Juveniles who have diabetes demand closer attention and observation for hypoglycemia. They are more susceptible to insulin shock than clients with diabetes in other age groups and have a more limited response to glucagon.
5. Assess juvenile diabetics more closely for infection or emotional disturbances that may increase their insulin requirements.
6. For the elderly client who has been newly diagnosed as having diabetes, the initial doses of insulin should be low, gradually increasing the dose until the desired effects have been achieved.
   - Be alert for signs of hypoglycemia such as slurred speech and mental confusion.
   - If the client is to be on NPO status for whatever reason, consult the physician about the dosage adjustment that will be required.
7. Review the client's entire medication regimen for drugs that may enhance or antagonize antidiabetic agents being used, and the dosage adjustment of antidiabetic agents that may be necessary.

Client/Family Teaching

1. Review with the client and family the nature of diabetes mellitus and its signs and symptoms.
2. Explain the necessity for close, regular medical supervision.

3. If the client is testing urine, explain how to test the urine for sugar and acetone and demonstrate how this test should be conducted. When testing the urine for glycosuria with Clinitest Tablets, Tes-Tape, Diastix, or Clinistix, as recommended by the physician, provide the client with printed instructions.

   - Test a fresh second-voided specimen.
   - Instruct the client to empty the bladder by voiding about 1 hr before mealtime.
   - As soon as the client can void again, obtain the specimen and test.
   - If the client is taking other medications, note what they are and determine if they may interfere with the test. Notify the lab and use appropriate tests if interference may be a problem.

4. If the client is performing finger sticks to monitor glucose levels demonstrate how this test should be conducted. If using a glucose monitoring machine have client perform a return demonstration to assure he/she knows the proper technique and proper calibration, operation and maintenance for the device. Some general principles may be followed.

   - Rotate sites.
   - Cleanse area with soap and water or alcohol prior to stabbing.
   - Stab finger and let a bead of blood form.
   - Wipe off with a cotton ball.
   - Then, let the bead of blood reform and apply to the test strip.
   - Follow specific guidelines for the individual equipment.

5. Discuss with the client the fact that regimes are specific to the individual client, based on age, the severity of the diabetes, weight, any other medical problems the client may have, as well as the philosophy of the health care team.

6. Instruct the client in administering insulin and have them perform a return demonstration.

7. Provide the client with a chart and instruct them in how to chart the injection sites and how to avoid either atrophy or hypertrophy of injection sites.

   - For self injection, instruct the client to brace the arm against a hard surface such as the wall or a chair.
   - Instruct the client to cleanse the area thoroughly, allow the area to dry, then, depending on the condition of the skin, either to pinch the skin between the thumb and forefingers of one hand, or to spread the skin using the thumb and fingers of one hand.
   - Insert the needle at a 45 degree angle into the subcutaneous tissue, and aspirate to be assured that the needle is not in a blood vessel.
   - Inject the insulin and withdraw the needle.

8. Explain the use and care of equipment, as well as the provision and storage of medication.

9. Advise the client always to have an extra vial of insulin and extra equipment on hand for administration when traveling, at home, or when hospitalized.

10. Instruct the client to always have regular insulin available for emergency use.

11. Explain the importance of exercise and the effect of exercise on the utilization of carbohydrates and increasing carbohydrate needs.

12. Stress the importance of adhering to the prescribed diet. Emphasize weight control and ingestion of food relative to the peak action of the insulin being used.

13. Provide the client with a food exchange list, explain it, and refer the client to a dietitian for assistance in meal planning.

14. Explain the importance of carrying candy or sugar at all times to counteract hypoglycemia should it occur.

15. Discuss with the client the possibility of allergic responses. Itching, redness, swelling, stinging

or warmth may occur at the site of injection. These will usually disappear after a few weeks of therapy. However, they should be reported to the physician because the type of insulin used may need to be changed.

16. Provide the client and family with a printed chart explaining symptoms of hypoglycemia and hyperglycemia and instructions concerning what to do for each. Also, instruct the client to notify the physician when either event occurs, explaining as specifically as possible what happened and what activity the client was engaged in. The dosage of insulin may need to be adjusted.

17. The client may have blurred vision at the beginning of insulin therapy. Advise the client that the condition should subside in 6–8 weeks. The effect is caused by the fluctuation of blood glucose levels which produce osmotic changes in the lens of the eye and within the ocular fluids. If the condition does not clear up in 8 weeks, the client should be advised to have an eye examination.

18. If the client feels ill and omits a meal because of fever, nausea, or vomiting, the next dose of insulin should be omitted unless the urine or finger stick test indicates that there is an increase in sugar levels. Report this problem to the physician immediately for guidance in regulating insulin and test glucose levels every 4 hours or as directed.

19. Advise the client that if they become ill the physician should be notified immediately. Explain that to prevent coma, the client should maintain adequate hydration by drinking 1 cup or more of noncaloric fluids such as coffee, tea, water, or broth every hour. The client or family member should conduct urine testing or finger sticks more frequently under these circumstances.

20. If foods have been omitted, replace them by a similar amount of carbohydrate such as orange juice or some other easily absorbed form of carbohydrate.

21. Instruct the client that if the supply of insulin is exhausted or the equipment is not available, to decrease the food intake by one-third and drink plenty of fluids. Omit the insulin and obtain the necessary supplies as soon as possible so as to be able to return to the prescribed diet and insulin dosage.

22. Explain the importance of good hygienic practices to prevent infection.

23. Advise the client to wear a Medic Alert bracelet or carry a card identifying the client as having diabetes, who to notify and what to do in the event the client is unable to respond for him/herself.

24. Advise the client to avoid alcoholic beverages. Alcohol can cause hypoglycemia. Excessive intake of alcohol may require a reduction in the dosage of insulin because alcohol potentiates the hypoglycemic effect of insulin.

25. Caution clients to use only the insulin prescribed and to check carefully each time they purchase insulin to be certain it is the correct form, brand and strength they have been taking. If there is any change in insulin purity, strength, type, source of the insulin or manufacturer, there may be a need to adjust the dosage of insulin.

26. Advise the client to check vials of insulin carefully before each dose is taken. Regular insulin should be clear, whereas other forms may be cloudy.

27. Two kinds of insulin can be mixed in the same syringe if the following guidelines are followed:
    - Regular insulin can be mixed with any other insulin.
    - Lente forms can be mixed with other lente insulins but cannot be mixed with other insulins with the exception of regular insulin.
    - A single form of insulin in a syringe can be stable for weeks or a month.
    - Except for commercially prepared mixtures, mixtures of insulin are not stable and should be administered within 5 minutes of preparation.
    - When insulins are mixed, regular (unmodified) insulin should always be drawn up in the

syringe first. Instruct the client to use the same procedure at all times when drawing up two insulins to avoid contamination of the two vials of insulin.

28. Refer the client and family to the American Diabetes Association and local support groups for additional information and support. This may also assist clients and families to understand and learn to cope with this disease.

Evaluation

1. Review with the client at each visit the goals of the therapy and determine the client's understanding of diabetes and coping strategies.
2. Monitor serum glucose and acetone levels to determine effectiveness of drug therapy.
3. Assess injection sites and skin to ensure that it remains healthy and intact.
4. Obtain weight to determine if any wide variations have occurred.

EXTENDED INSULIN ZINC SUSPENSION

Single Peak: Ultralente Iletin I (beef and pork), Ultralente Insulin (beef). Purified: Ultralente Purified Beef (OTC)

See also *Insulins,* p. 1094.

Classification: Long-acting insulin.

Action/Kinetics: Large crystals of insulin and a high content of zinc are responsible for the slow-acting properties of this preparation. Products containing both 40 units/mL and 100 units/mL are available. **Onset:** 4–8 hr. **Peak:** 18–24 hr. **Duration:** 36 hr or longer.

Uses: Mild to moderate hyperglycemia in stabilized diabetics. Not suitable for the treatment of diabetic coma or emergency situations.

Dosage: SC. *Individualized.* **Usual, initial:** 7–26 units as a single dose 30–60 min before breakfast. **Do not administer IV.**

> **NURSING CONSIDERATIONS**
> See *Nursing Considerations* for *Insulins,* p. 1098.

HUMAN INSULIN

Buffered Human Insulin: Humulin BR. Extended Insulin Zinc Suspension: Humulin U Ultralente. Human Insulin Zinc Suspension: Humulin L, Novolin L. Isophane Human Insulin Suspension: Humulin N, Insulatard NPH Human, Novolin N. Isophane Human Insulin Suspension and Insulin Human Injection: Humulin 70/30, Mixtard Human 70/30, Novolin 70/30. Regular Insulin Human: Humulin R, Novolin R, Velosulin Human.

See also *Insulins,* p. 1094.

Classification: Human insulin from semisynthetic or recombinant DNA sources.

Action/Kinetics: Human insulin derived from recombinant DNA technology utilizes genetically modified *Escherichia coli.* These organisms synthesize each chain of insulin into the same amino acid sequence as human insulin. The chains are then combined and purified to produce human insulin. Human insulin prepared semisynthetically undergoes a process whereby the terminal amino acid of porcine insulin is enzymatically substituted for an amino acid, making the product identical to human insulin. This product is then purified. *Note:* Human insulins are available as regular, insulin zinc, extended, and isophane; for the kinetics of these products, please refer to the appropriate products described elsewhere. Human insulins cause fewer allergic reactions and less insulin-induced antibody formation than insulins from animal sources.

Uses: Management of Type I diabetes mellitus. At this time, as long as the patient is well controlled on insulin from porcine or beef sources, transfer to human insulin may not be recommended. Human insulin may be preferred in the following situations: local or systemic allergic reactions to products from animal sources, lipoatrophy at injection site, Type II diabetes that requires short-term insulin treatment, in patients resistant to insulin from animal sources, in pregnancy, and in newly diagnosed diabetics.

Dosage: Dosage and routes of administration are similar to products from animal sources.

NURSING CONSIDERATIONS

See also *Nursing Considerations* for *Insulins,* p. 1098.

Client/Family Teaching

Remind clients that dose may have to be reduced, so it is particularly important to watch for signs and symptoms of hypoglycemia.

INSULIN INJECTION (CRYSTALLINE ZINC INSULIN, UNMODIFIED INSULIN, REGULAR INSULIN)

Single peak: Regular Iletin I (beef and pork), Regular Insulin (pork). Purified: Regular Iletin II (beef), Regular Iletin II (pork), Regular Insulin (pork), Velosulin (pork) (OTC)

See also *Insulins,* p. 1094.

Classification: Rapid-acting insulin.

Action/Kinetics: This product is rarely administered as the sole agent due to its short duration of action. Injections of 100 units/mL or less are clear; cloudy, colored solutions should not be used. Regular insulin is the only preparation suitable for IV administration. Is available in both 40 units/mL and 100 units/mL. **Onset, SC:** 30 min–1 hr; **IV:** 10–30 min. **Peak, SC:** 2–4 hr; **IV:** 15–30 min. **Duration, SC:** 5–7 hr; **IV:** 30–60 min.

Uses: Suitable for treatment of diabetic coma, diabetic acidosis, or other emergency situations. Especially suitable for the patient suffering from labile diabetes.

During acute phase of diabetic acidosis or for the patient in diabetic crisis, patient is monitored by serum glucose and serum ketone levels.

Dosage: SC, Individualized. Adults: usual, initial: 5–10 units; **pediatric:** 2–4 units. Injection is given 15–30 min before meals and at bedtime. *Diabetic ketoacidosis:* **Adults:** 0.1 unit/kg/hr given by continuous IV infusion.

NURSING CONSIDERATIONS

See *Nursing Considerations* for *Insulins,* p. 1098.

Administration/Storage

1. When used IV, the rate of insulin infusion should be decreased when plasma glucose levels reach 250 mg/dL.
2. Due to the short half-life of regular insulin, large single IV doses should not be administered.

INSULIN INJECTION, CONCENTRATED

Regular (Concentrated) Iletin II U-500 (Rx)

See also *Insulins,* p. 1094.

Classification: Insulin, concentrated.

Action/Kinetics: This concentrated preparation (500 units/mL) of insulin injection (see above) is indicated for patients with a marked resistance to insulin who require more than 200 units/day. Patients must be kept under close observation until dosage is established. Depending on response, dosage may be given SC or IM as a single or as 2 or 3 divided doses.

Not suitable for IV administration because of possible allergic or anaphylactoid reactions.

Uses: Diabetic patients requiring more than 200 units insulin per day.

Additional Side Effects: Deep secondary hypoglycemia 18 to 24 hr after administration.

NURSING CONSIDERATIONS

See *Nursing Considerations* for *Insulins,* p. 1098.

Administration/Storage

1. Administer only water clear solutions (concentrated insulin may appear straw-colored).
2. Use a tuberculin type syringe for accuracy of measurement.
3. Deep secondary hypoglycemia may occur 18–24 hr after administration. Therefore, have 10%–20% dextrose solution or D_{50}% bristojets available.
4. Keep insulin cool or refrigerated.

Interventions

1. Observe the client closely for signs and symptoms of hyper- or hypoglycemia during the period when the dosage is being established.
2. Monitor blood glucose levels frequently.

Client/Family Teaching

Teach the client to be alert for signs of hypoglycemia, which may indicate that responsiveness to insulin has been regained, and that a reduction in dosage is warranted.

INSULIN ZINC SUSPENSION

Single Peak: Lente Iletin I (beef and pork), Lente Insulin (beef). Purified: Lente Iletin II (beef), Lente Iletin II (pork), Lente Insulin (pork) (OTC)

See also *Insulins,* p. 1094.

Classification: Intermediate-acting insulin.

Action/Kinetics: Principal advantage is the absence of a sensitizing agent such as protamine. **Onset:** 1–3 hr. **Peak:** 8–12 hr. **Duration:** 18–28 hr.

Uses: Useful in patients allergic to other types of insulin and in patients disposed to thrombotic phenomena in which protamine may be a factor. Zinc insulin is not a replacement for regular insulin and is not suitable for emergency use.

Dosage: SC. Adults, initial: 7–26 units 30–60 min before breakfast. Dosage is then increased by daily or weekly increments of 2–10 units until satisfactory readjustment is established. A second smaller dose may be given prior to the evening meal or at bedtime.

Patients on NPH can be transferred to insulin zinc suspension on a unit-for-unit basis. Patients being transferred from regular insulin should begin zinc insulin at two-thirds to three-fourths the regular insulin dosage. If the patient is being transferred from protamine zinc insulin, the dose of zinc insulin should be about 50% of that required for protamine zinc insulin.

NURSING CONSIDERATIONS

See *Nursing Considerations* for *Insulins*, p. 1098.

ISOPHANE INSULIN SUSPENSION (NPH)   (EYE-so-fayn)

Single peak: NPH Iletin I (beef and pork), NPH Insulin (beef). Purified: NPH Iletin II (beef), NPH Iletin II (pork), Insulatard NPH, NPH Insulin (pork) (OTC)

See also *Insulins*, p. 1094.

Classification: Intermediate-acting insulin.

Action/Kinetic: Contains zinc insulin crystals modified by protamine, appearing as a cloudy or milky suspension. Not recommended for emergency use. Not suitable for IV administration. Not useful in the presence of ketosis. **Onset:** 3–4 hr. **Peak:** 6–12 hr. **Duration:** 18–28 hr.

Dosage: SC, individualized. Adult, usual, initial: 7–26 units as a single dose 30–60 min before breakfast. A second smaller dose may be given, if needed, prior to the evening meal or at bedtime. If necessary, the daily dose may be increased in increments of 2–10 units at daily or weekly intervals until desired control is achieved.

Patients on insulin zinc may be transferred directly to isophane insulin on a unit-for-unit basis. If patient is being transferred from regular insulin, the initial dose of isophane should be from two-thirds to three-fourths the dose of regular insulin.

NURSING CONSIDERATIONS

See *Nursing Considerations* for *Insulins*, p. 1098.

ISOPHANE INSULIN SUSPENSION AND INSULIN INJECTION   (EYE-so-fayn)

Mixtard (pork) (OTC)

See also *Insulins*, p. 1094.

Classification: Mixture of insulins to achieve variable duration of action.

Action/Kinetics: Contains 30% insulin injection and 70% isophane insulin. This combination allows for a rapid onset (30–60 min) due to insulin injection and a long duration (24 hr) due to isophane insulin. **Peak effect:** 4–8 hr.

NURSING CONSIDERATIONS

See *Nursing Considerations* for *Insulins*, p. 1098.

PROMPT INSULIN ZINC SUSPENSION (ZINK)

Single Peak: Semilente Iletin I (beef and pork), Semilente Insulin (beef). Purified: Semilente Insulin (pork) (OTC)

See also *Insulins,* p. 1094.

Classification: Fast-acting insulin.

Action/Kinetics: Contains small particles of zinc insulin in a nearly colorless suspension. Not suitable for emergency use. Cannot be injected IV. **Onset:** 1–3 hr. **Peak:** 2–8 hr. **Duration:** 12–16 hr.

Uses: In combination with insulin zinc or extended insulin zinc suspensions to control diabetes. May also be used alone for rapid control when initiating therapy.

Dosage: SC. Individualized. Adults, initial: 10–20 units 30 min before breakfast. A second daily dose is usually required.

NURSING CONSIDERATIONS

See *Nursing Considerations* for *Insulins,* p. 1098.

PROTAMINE ZINC INSULIN SUSPENSION (PZI INSULIN) (PROH-tah-meen)

Single Peak: Protamine, Zinc, & Iletin I (beef and pork). Purified: Protamine, Zinc & Iletin II (beef or pork) (OTC)

See also *Insulins,* p. 1094.

Classification: Long-acting insulin.

Action/Kinetics: Contains protamine, zinc, and insulin in a cloudy or milky suspension. Not suitable for use in emergency situations and not to be given IV. Due to its long onset and duration, this product is not as adaptable to dosage alterations as are other preparations. **Onset:** 4–6 hr. **Peak:** 14–24 hr. **Duration:** 36 hr.

Uses: Mild to moderate diabetes.

Dosage: SC. Individualized. Adults, initial: 7–26 units as a single dose 30–60 min before breakfast. If transferring from regular insulin, the initial dose should be approximately two-thirds that of regular insulin.

NURSING CONSIDERATIONS

See *Nursing Considerations* for *Insulins,* p. 1098.

ORAL ANTIDIABETIC AGENTS

General Statement: Several oral antidiabetic agents are available for patients with noninsulin-dependent diabetes. These agents are sulfonylureas, which are related chemically to sulfonamides; however, they are devoid of antibacterial activity. Oral hypoglycemic drugs are classified as either first- or second-generation. *Generation* refers to structural changes in the basic molecule. Second-generation oral hypoglycemic drugs are more lipophilic and, as such, have greater hypoglycemic potency. Also, second-generation drugs are bound to plasma protein by covalent bonds, whereas first-generation drugs are bound to plasma protein by ionic bonds. The implication is that the second-generation drugs are potentially less susceptible to displacement from plasma protein by drugs such as salicylates, oral anticoagulants, and others drugs

These agents are used chiefly for patients with maturity-onset, mild, nonketotic diabetes, usually associated with obesity, when the condition cannot be controlled by diet alone but the patient does not require insulin. The oral antidiabetics should not be used in unstable or brittle diabetes, whatever the patient's age.

Action/Kinetics: These drugs are believed to act by one or more of the following mechanisms: (1) the sensitivity of pancreatic islet cells is increased; (2) the pancreatic beta cell membrane is directly depolarized, leading to insulin secretion; or (3) the peripheral tissues become more sensitive to insulin due to an increase in the number of insulin receptors or an increased ability of circulating insulin to combine with receptors. The drugs are ineffective in the complete absence of functioning beta islet cells. All of the oral hypoglycemic drugs are significantly bound (90%) to plasma protein.

Patients whose condition is to be controlled by oral antidiabetics should be subjected to a 7-day therapeutic trial. A drop in blood sugar level, a decrease in glucosuria, and disappearance of pruritus, polyuria, polydipsia, and polyphagia indicate that the patient can probably be managed on oral antidiabetic agents. These drugs should not be used in patients with ketosis. If the patient is transferred from insulin to an oral antidiabetic drug, the hormone should be discontinued gradually over a period of several days. The sulfonylureas have similar pharmacologic actions but differ in their pharmacokinetic properties (see individual agents).

Uses: Non-insulin dependent diabetes mellitus (Type II) that does not respond to diet management alone. As an adjunct to stabilize insulin-dependent maturity-onset diabetes.

Contraindications: Stress before and during surgery, severe trauma, fever, infections, pregnancy, diabetes complicated by recurrent episodes of ketoacidosis or coma; juvenile, growth-onset, insulin-dependent, or brittle diabetes; impaired endocrine, renal, or liver function. Not indicated for patients whose diabetes can be controlled by diet alone. Relapse may occur with the sulfonylureas in undernourished patients. Long-acting products in geriatric patients.

Special Concerns: Use with caution during lactation since hypoglycemia may occur in the infant. Safety and effectiveness in children have not been established. Geriatric patients may be more sensitive to oral hypoglycemics and hypoglycemia may be more difficult to recognize in these patients. Use with caution in debilitated and malnourished patients.

Side Effects: Hypoglycemia is the most common side effect. *CV:* Chronic use of oral hypoglycemic drugs has been associated with an increased risk of cardiovascular mortality. *GI:* Nausea, heartburn, diarrhea, full feeling. *CNS:* Fatigue, dizziness, fever, headache, weakness, malaise. *Hepatic:* Cholestatic jaundice, aggravation of hepatic porphyria. *Dermatologic:* Skin rashes, urticaria, erythema, pruritus, eczema, photophobia. *Hematologic:* Thrombocytopenia, leukopenia, anemia, and eosinophilia are the most common. Also, agranulocytosis, hemolytic anemia, pancytopenia, aplastic anemia.

Resistance to drug action develops in a small percentage of patients.

Drug Interactions	
Acetazolamide	↑ Blood sugar in prediabetics and diabetics on oral hypoglycemics
Alcohol	Possible Antabuse-like syndrome, especially flushing of face and shortness of breath. Also, ↓ effect of oral hypoglycemic due to ↑ breakdown by liver
Anabolic steroids	↑ Hypoglycemic effect of oral antidiabetics

Drug Interactions

Anticoagulants, oral	↑ Effect of oral hypoglycemics by ↓ breakdown by liver and ↓ plasma protein binding
Beta-adrenergic blocking agents	↓ Hypoglycemic effect of oral hypoglycemics; also, symptoms of hypoglycemia may be masked
Calcium channel blockers	↑ Requirements for sulfonylureas
Chloramphenicol	↑ Effect of oral hypoglycemics by ↓ breakdown by liver and ↓ renal excretion
Cimetidine	↑ Effect of oral hypoglycemics due to ↓ breakdown by liver
Clofibrate	↑ Hypoglycemic effect of oral antidiabetics due to ↓ plasma protein binding
Corticosteroids	↑ Requirements for sulfonylureas
Diazoxide	Effects of both drugs decreased
Digitoxin	↓ Effect of digitoxin by ↑ breakdown by liver
Fenfluramine	Additive hypoglycemia
Guanethidine	↑ Effect of oral hypoglycemics
Isoniazid	↑ Requirements for sulfonylureas
Methyldopa	↑ Effect of sulfonylureas due to ↓ breakdown by liver
Miconazole	↑ Effect of oral hypoglycemics
Monoamine oxidase inhibitors	↑ Hypoglycemic effect of oral antidiabetics due to ↓ breakdown by liver
Nicotinic acid	↓ Effect of oral hypoglycemics
Nonsteroidal anti-inflammatory agents	↑ Hypoglycemic effect of oral antidiabetics
Oral contraceptives	↓ Hypoglycemic effect of oral antidiabetics
Phenobarbital	↓ Effect of oral hypoglycemics due to ↑ breakdown by liver
Phenothiazines	↑ Requirements for sulfonylureas due to ↓ release of insulin
Phenylbutazone	↑ Effect of oral hypoglycemics due to ↓ breakdown by liver, ↓ plasma protein binding, and ↓ renal excretion
Phenytoin	↓ Effect of sulfonylureas due to ↓ insulin release
Probenecid	↑ Effect of oral hypoglycemics
Ranitidine	↑ Effect of oral hypoglycemics
Rifampin	↓ Effect of sulfonylureas due to ↑ breakdown by liver
Salicylates	↑ Effect of oral hypoglycemics by ↓ plasma protein binding
Sulfonamides	↑ Effect of oral hypoglycemics by ↓ plasma protein binding and ↓ breakdown by liver
Sympathomimetics	↑ Requirements for sulfonylureas
Thiazides	↑ Requirements for sulfonylureas
Thyroid hormone	↑ Requirements for sulfonylureas

Laboratory Test Interference: ↑ BUN and serum creatinine.

Dosage: PO. See individual preparations. Adjust dosage according to needs of patient. Exercise and diet are of primary importance in the control of diabetes.

NURSING CONSIDERATIONS

See also *Nursing Considerations* for *Insulins (applicable to all diabetic clients controlled by medication whether insulin or an oral hypoglycemic)*, p. 1098.

Administration/Storage

1. These drugs may be taken with food to decrease the incidence of gastric upset.
2. If ketonuria, acidosis, increased glycosuria, or serious side effects occur, withdraw the medication.

Transfer from Insulin

1. If the client has been receiving 20 units or less of insulin daily, maintenance dosage of oral hypoglycemic agents may be instituted, and the insulin discontinued abruptly.
2. For clients receiving 20–40 units of insulin daily, institute a maintenance dosage of oral hypoglycemic agent and reduce insulin dose by 25–30%. Insulin should be discontinued gradually, using the absence of glucose in the urine as a guide.
3. For clients receiving more than 40 units of insulin daily, institute a maintenance dosage and reduce insulin by 20%. Discontinue insulin gradually, using glucose in the urine as a guide. It may be advisable to hospitalize clients on such high doses of insulin while they are being transferred to oral hypoglycemic agents.
4. Be prepared to begin treatment with IV dextrose solution if the client develops severe hypoglycemia.
5. Review the drugs with which oral hypoglycemic agents interact and determine if the client is taking any of them.

Transfer from One Oral Antidiabetic Agent to Another

1. Except for chlorpropamide, no conversion period is necessary. When transferring clients from chlorpropamide, caution should be exercised for 1–2 weeks due to the long half-life of chlorpropamide.
2. Mild symptoms of hyperglycemia may appear during the transfer period. Clients should perform finger sticks or test their urine for glucose and ketone bodies regularly (1 to 3 times daily) during the transfer period. Positive results must be reported to the physician.

Therapeutic Failure of Hypoglycemic Agents

Diabetic clients who do not respond to the sulfonylureas are said to be *primary failures*. Clients may respond to the sulfonylureas during the initial months of therapy, yet fail to respond thereafter. These clients are referred to as *secondary failures*.

Assessment

1. Note the amount of stress the client may be experiencing. Clients about to undergo surgical procedures, who have suffered severe trauma, who have a fever and infection or who are pregnant should not be placed on oral hypoglycemic agents.

2. Note the potential of the client to understand the complexities of the transfer process.

3. Assess the client as to their ability to adhere to the established protocol.

4. If the client is female, sexually active and of childbearing age, note if she is taking oral contraceptives. The effectiveness of oral contraceptive agents is lessened by oral hypoglycemic agents.

Interventions

1. Assess clients taking a sulfonylurea closely during the first 7 days of treatment to determine their therapeutic response.

2. Closely supervise and observe the client during the 3 to 5 days after the transfer.

Client/Family Teaching

1. Instruct the client in testing blood or urine at home for glucose and maintaining a written record of levels for review by the nurse and physician.

2. Explain the need to adhere to the prescribed diet if sulfonylurea is to be effective. Remind clients that most secondary failures are due to poor dietary compliance.

3. Explain that self-administering insulin may be necessary if complications occur. Instruct the client in self administration of insulin.

4. Advise the client to report to the physician when not feeling as well as usual, or if they develop pruritus, skin rash, jaundice, dark urine, fever, sore throat, or diarrhea.

5. If the client is scheduled for a thyroid test, report to the laboratory the fact that the client is taking a sulfonylurea. The drug interferes with the uptake of radioactive iodine.

6. Stress the need for close medical supervision for the first 6 weeks of therapy.

7. Stress the need for periodic laboratory tests as ordered by the physician. Oral hypoglycemic agents can cause blood dyscrasias.

Evaluation

1. Client displays an understanding of illness and cooperates in following prescribed regime.

2. Laboratory test results are within desired limits.

3. Freedom from complications with prescribed drug therapy.

ACETOHEXAMIDE   (ah-set-oh-**HEX**-ah-myd)

Dimelor✽, Dymelor (Rx)

See also *Oral Antidiabetic Agents,* p. 1108.

Classification: First-generation sulfonylurea.

Action/Kinetics: Onset: 1 hr. **t½:** 1.3 hr for acetohexamide and 6–8 hr for active metabolite. **Duration:** 12–24 hr. Metabolized in the liver to a potent active metabolite. Excreted through the kidney (80%) and feces (10%).

Special Concerns: Pregnancy category: C.

Additional Side Effects: Hair loss.

Dosage: PO. Adults, initial: 250 mg daily; **maintenance:** 500 mg daily, adjusting dosage thereafter until optimum control is achieved. Doses in excess of 1.5 g daily are not recommended. **Geriatric patients, initial:** 125–250 mg daily; **then,** adjust dosage gradually until desired effect is achieved.

NURSING CONSIDERATIONS

See *Nursing Considerations* for *Antidiabetic Agents, Oral,* p. 1111.

Administration/Storage

Doses of 1 g or over should be divided, usually before the morning and evening meals.

CHLORPROPAMIDE   (klor-**PROH**-pah-myd)

Apo-Chlorpropamide ✹, Diabinese, Glucamide, Novopropamide ✹ (Rx)

See also *Oral Antidiabetic Agents,* p. 1108.

Classification: First-generation sulfonylurea.

Action/Kinetics: Chlorpropamide may be effective in patients who do not respond well to other antidiabetic agents. **Onset:** 1 hr. **t½:** 35 hr. **Time to peak levels:** 2–4 hr. **Duration:** 24–48 hr (due to slow excretion). Eighty percent metabolized in liver; 80–90% excreted in the urine.

Additional Use: *Investigational:* Neurogenic diabetes insipidus.

Special Concerns: Pregnancy category: C. If the patient is susceptible to fluid retention or has impaired cardiac function, frequent monitoring is necessary.

Additional Side Effects: Untoward reactions occur frequently with chlorpropamide. Severe diarrhea is occasionally accompanied by bleeding in the lower bowel.

Severe GI distress may be relieved by dividing total daily dose in half. In older patients, hypoglycemia may be severe. May cause inappropriate antidiuretic hormone secretion, leading to hyponatremia, water retention, low-serum osmolality, and high-urine osmolality.

Additional Drug Interactions

Ammonium chloride	↑ Effect of chlorpropamide due to ↓ excretion by kidney
Disulfiram	More likely to interact with chlorpropamide than other oral antidiabetics
Probenecid	↑ Effect of chlorpropamide
Sodium bicarbonate	↓ Effect of chlorpropamide due to ↑ excretion by kidney

Dosage: PO. Adults, middle-aged patients: initial 250 mg daily as a single or divided dose; **geriatric: initial,** 100–125 mg daily. **All patients, maintenance:** 100–250 mg daily as single or divided doses. Severe diabetics may require 500 mg daily; doses greater than 750 mg daily are not recommended. *Neurogenic diabetes insipidus:* 125–250 mg daily, up to a maximum of 500 mg daily.

NURSING CONSIDERATIONS

See *Nursing Considerations* for *Antidiabetic Agents, Oral,* p. 1111.

Assessment

1. Note the age of the client. Elderly clients tend to be more sensitive to hypoglycemic agents and exhibit more side effects.
2. Determine if the client is pregnant. The drug is contraindicated in pregnancy.

Interventions

1. Monitor weight and blood pressure and assess for evidence of the inappropriate secretion of antidiuretic hormone. Clients may appear confused, complain of feeling dizzy, depressed, and complain of nausea.
2. Monitor the client's serum electrolytes and urine osmolality. Record intake and output.

GLIPIZIDE (GLIP-ih-zyd)

Glucotrol (Rx)

See also *Oral Antidiabetic Agents,:* p. 1108.

Classification: Second-generation sulfonylurea.

Action/Kinetics: Glipizide also has mild diuretic effects. **Onset:** 1–1.5 hr. **t½:** 2–4 hr. **Time to peak levels:** 1–3 hr. **Duration:** 12–24 hr. Metabolized in liver to inactive metabolites which are excreted through the kidneys.

Special Concerns: Pregnancy category: C.

Additional Drug Interaction: Cimetidine may ↑ effect of glipizide due to ↓ breakdown by liver.

Dosage: PO. Adults initial: 5 mg before breakfast; **then,** adjust dosage by 2.5–5 mg q few days until adequate control is achieved. **Maintenance:** 15–40 mg daily. Older patients should begin with 2.5 mg.

NURSING CONSIDERATIONS

See *Nursing Considerations* for *Antidiabetic Agents, Oral,* p. 1111.

Administration/Storage

1. Maintenance doses greater than 15 mg daily should be divided and given before the morning and evening meals.
2. For greatest effect, give 30 min before meals.

Interventions

1. Note client complaints of CNS side effects such as drowsiness or headache. Report these to the physician if they are persistent.
2. Some clients may suffer from anorexia, constipation or diarrhea, vomiting and gastralgia. Monitor the client's weight, and if the symptoms are severe, the intake and output. Document and report findings.
3. Note if the client reports skin reactions. Advise clients to avoid exposure to the sun, to use a sunscreen when in the sun, and to keep their arms and extremities covered.

Client/Family Teaching

Advise clients how to protect their skin when in the sun and to report any skin changes to the physician.

GLYBURIDE   (GLIB-your-yd)

Diabeta, Euglucon✳, Micronase (Rx)

See also *Oral Antidiabetic Agents,* p. 1108.

Classification: Second-generation sulfonylurea.

Action/Kinetics: Glyburide has a mild diuretic effect. **Onset:** 2–4 hr. **t½:** 10 hr. **Time to peak levels:** 4 hr. **Duration:** 24 hr. Metabolized in liver to weakly active metabolites. Excreted in bile (50%) and through the kidneys (50%).

Special Concerns: Pregnancy category: B.

Dosage: PO. Adults, initial: 2.5–5 mg daily given with breakfast (or the first main meal); **then,** increase by 2.5 mg at weekly intervals to achieve the desired response. **Maintenance:** 1.25–20 mg daily. Patients sensitive to sulfonylureas should start with 1.25 mg/day.

NURSING CONSIDERATIONS

See *Nursing Considerations* for *Antidiabetic Agents, Oral,* p. 1111.

Administration/Storage

1. For best results, administer prior to meals.
2. If daily dosage exceeds 15 mg, the dose should be divided and given before the morning and evening meals.

TOLAZAMIDE   (toe-LAZ-ah-myd)

Tolamide, Tolinase (Rx)

See also *Oral Antidiabetic Agents,* p. 1108.

Classification: First-generation sulfonylurea.

Action/Kinetics: Drug is effective in some patients who have a history of coma or ketoacidosis. Also, it may be effective in patients who do not respond well to other oral antidiabetic agents. Use with insulin is not recommended for maintenance. **Onset:** 4–6 hr. **t½:** 7 hr. **Time to peak levels:** 3–4 hr. **Duration:** 10 hr. Metabolized in liver to metabolites with minor hypoglycemic activity. Excreted through the kidneys (85%) and feces (7%).

Additional Contraindication: Renal glycosuria.

Special Concerns: Pregnancy category: C.

Additional Drug Interaction: Concomitant use of alcohol and tolazamide may → photosensitivity.

Dosage: PO. Adults, initial: 100 mg daily if fasting blood sugar is less than 200 mg/100 mL, or 250 mg daily if fasting blood sugar is greater than 200 mg/100 mL. Adjust dose to response not to exceed 1 g daily. If more than 500 mg daily is required, the dose should be given in 2 divided doses, usually before the morning and evening meals. **Elderly or debilitated patients:** 100 mg daily with breakfast, adjusting dose by increments of 50 mg daily each week. Doses greater than 1 g daily will probably not improve control.

NURSING CONSIDERATIONS

See *Nursing Considerations* for *Antidiabetic Agents, Oral,* p. 1111.

TOLBUTAMIDE (tohl-**BYOU**-ta-myd)

APO-Tolbutamide✱, Mobenol✱, Novobutamide✱, Oramide, Orinase (Rx)

TOLBUTAMIDE SODIUM (tohl-**BYOU**-ta-myd)

Orinase Diagnostic (Rx)

See also *Oral Antidiabetic Agents,* p. 1108.

Classification: First-generation sulfonylurea.

Action/Kinetics: Onset: 1 hr. **t½:** 4.5–6.5 hr. **Time to peak levels:** 3–4 hr. **Duration:** 6–12 hr. Changed in liver to inactive metabolites. Excreted through the kidney (75%) and feces (9%).

Additional Uses: Most useful for patients with poor general physical status who should receive a short-acting compound.

Tolbutamide sodium is used to diagnose pancreatic islet cell tumors. It causes blood glucose, in the presence of a tumor, to drop quickly after IV administration and remain low for 3 hr.

Special Concerns: Pregnancy category: C.

Additional Side Effects: Melena (dark, bloody stools) in some patients with a history of peptic ulcer. Relapse or secondary failure may occur a few months after therapy has been started. May cause hyponatremia and a mild goiter.

Additional Drug Interactions

Alcohol	Photosensitivity reactions
Sulfinpyrazone	↑ Effect of tolbutamide due to ↓ breakdown by liver

Dosage: PO. Adults, initial: 0.5–2 g/day; adjust dosage depending on response (usual maintenance: 0.25–3 g/day). Maximum daily dose should not exceed 3 g.

NURSING CONSIDERATIONS

See *Nursing Considerations* for *Antidiabetic Agents, Oral,* p. 1111.

Administration/Storage

Administer drug as a single dose before breakfast or as divided doses before the morning and evening meals.

INSULIN ANTAGONISTS

DIAZOXIDE ORAL   (dye-az-OX-yd)
Proglycem (Rx)

Classification: Insulin antagonist, hypotensive agent.

Action/Kinetics: Diazoxide inhibits the release of insulin from beta islet cells of the pancreas, leading to an increase in blood glucose levels. Effect is dose related. Diazoxide causes sodium, potassium, uric acid, and water retention. **Onset:** 1 hr. **t½:** 28 hr (up to 53 hr in patients with anuria). **Duration:** 8 hr. Metabolized in the liver although 50% is excreted through the kidneys unchanged.

Uses: Hypoglycemia caused by insulin overdosage or overproduction of insulin by malignant beta cells. The drug is used parenterally as an antihypertensive agent (see *Diazoxide,* p. 514).

Contraindications: Functional hypoglycemia, hypersensitivity to diazoxide or thiazides.

Special Concerns: Safe use during pregnancy not established (pregnancy category: C). Infants are particularly prone to development of edema. Use with extreme caution in patients with history of gout and in those in whom edema presents a risk (cardiac disease).

Side Effects: *CV:* Sodium and fluid retention (common), palpitations, increased heart rate, hypotension, transient hypertension. *Metabolic:* Hyperglycemia, glycosuria, diabetic ketoacidosis, hyperosmolar nonketotic coma. *GI:* Nausea, vomiting, diarrhea, transient taste loss, anorexia, ileus, abdominal pain. *CNS:* Weakness, headache, insomnia, extrapyramidal symptoms, dizziness, paresthesia, fever. *Hematologic:* Thrombocytopenia, purpura, eosinophilia, neutropenia, decreased hemoglobin. *Dermatologic:* Skin rashes, hirsutism, herpes, loss of hair from scalp, monilial dermatitis. *GU:* Hematuria, proteinuria, decrease in urine production, nephrotic syndrome (reversible). *Ophthalmologic:* Blurred or double vision, lacrimation, transient cataracts, ring scotoma, subconjunctival hemorrhage. *Other:* Pancreatitis, pancreatic necrosis, galactorrhea, gout, premature aging of bone, polyneuritis, enlargement of lump in breast.

Drug Interactions	
Alpha-adrenergic blocking agents	↓ Effect of diazoxide
Anticoagulants, oral	↑ Effect of anticoagulant due to ↓ plasma protein binding
Antihypertensives	Excessive ↓ blood pressure due to additive effects
Phenytoin	↓ Effect of phenytoin due to ↑ breakdown by liver
Sulfonylureas	↓ Effect of both drugs
Thiazide diuretics	↑ Hypoglycemic and hyperuricemic effects

Laboratory Test Interferences: ↑ Serum uric acid, SGOT, alkaline phosphatase; ↓ creatinine clearance.

Dosage: Capsules, Oral Suspension. Dosage is individualized on the basis of blood glucose level and response of patient. **Adults and children, usual, initial:** 1 mg/kg q 8 hr (adjust according to response); **maintenance:** 3–8 mg/kg/day divided into 2 or 3 equal doses q 8–12 hr. **Infants and**

newborns, initial: 3.3 mg/kg q 8 hr (adjust according to response); **maintenance:** 8–15 mg/kg/day divided into 2 or 3 equal doses q 8–12 hr.

NURSING CONSIDERATIONS

Administration/Storage

1. Blood glucose levels and urinary glucose and ketones must be monitored carefully until the client has stabilized, which usually takes 1 week. The drug is discontinued if a satisfactory effect has not been established within 2–3 weeks.
2. Have available insulin and IV fluids to counteract possible ketoacidosis.

Interventions

1. Determine the client's clinical response and assess laboratory test results. These are the basis for determining drug dosage.
2. If the client has a history of congestive heart failure, observe carefully for fluid retention which could precipitate heart failure.
3. If the client is already taking an antihypertensive agent, monitor blood pressure for potentiation of antihypertensive effect.
4. Monitor the client for ecchymosis, the development of petechiae, or frank bleeding. These symptoms should be reported to the physician and may require discontinuation of the drug.
5. If the client has had an overdosage of drug, observe closely for the first 7 days until blood sugar level is again within normal limits (80–120 mg/100 mL).
6. If the client develops hirsutism, reassure them that the condition should subside once the drug is discontinued.

GLUCAGON   (GLOO-kah-gon)
(Rx)

Classification: Insulin antagonist.

Action/Kinetics: Glucagon is a hormone produced by the alpha islet cells of the pancreas. The hormone increases blood glucose by increasing breakdown of glycogen to glucose, stimulating gluconeogenesis from amino acids and fatty acids, and inhibiting conversion of glucose to glycogen. Also, lipolysis is increased resulting in free fatty acids and glycerol for gluconeogenesis. The drug is effective in overcoming hypoglycemia only if the liver has a glycogen reserve. **Onset, hypoglycemia:** 5–20 min, **Maximum effect:** 30 min, **Duration:** 1–2 hr. $t^{1/2}$: 3–6 min. Metabolized in the liver, kidney, plasma membrane receptor sites, and in the plasma.

Uses: Used to terminate insulin-induced shock in diabetic or psychiatric patients. Patient usually regains consciousness 5–20 min after the parenteral administration of glucagon. The drug should only be used under medical supervision or in accordance with strict instructions received from the physician. Failure to respond may be an indication for IV administration of glucose—especially true in the juvenile diabetics. As a diagnostic aid in radiologic examination of the GI tract when a hypotonic state is desirable. *Investigational:* Inhibit bowel peristalsis in abdominal digital vascular imaging and in abdominal CT scanning to prevent misregistration artifact. Adjunct in diagnosis of GI bleeding. Treatment of toxicity due to beta-adrenergic blocking agents, quinidine, or tricyclic antidepressants.

Special Concerns: Pregnancy category: B. Use with caution in patients with renal or hepatic disease, in those who are undernourished and emaciated, and in patients with a history of pheochromocytoma or insulinoma.

Side Effects: *GI:* Nausea, vomiting. *Allergy:* Respiratory distress, urticaria, hypotension. Stevens-Johnson syndrome when used as diagnostic aid.

Drug Interactions	
Anticoagulants, oral	↑ Effect of anticoagulants by ↑ hypoprothrombinemia
Antidiabetic agents	Hyperglycemic effect of glucagon antagonizes hypoglycemic effect of antidiabetics
Corticosteroids, Epinephrine, Estrogens, Phenytoin	Additive hyperglycemic effect of drugs listed

Dosage: IM, IV, SC. *Hypoglycemia:* **Adults:** 0.5–1 mg; 1–2 additional doses may be given at 20 min intervals, if necessary. **Pediatric:** 0.025 mg/kg, up to a maximum of 1 mg; may be repeated in 20 min if needed. *Insulin shock therapy:* **IM, IV, SC,** 0.5–1 mg after 1 hr of coma; if no response, dose may be repeated. *Diagnostic aid for GI tract:* dose dependent on desired onset of action and duration of effect necessary for the examination: **IV,** 0.25–0.5 mg (onset: 1 min; duration: 9–17 min); 2 mg (onset: 1 min; duration 22–25 min). **IM,** 1 mg (onset: 8–10 min; duration: 12–27 min); 2 mg (onset: 4–7 min; duration: 21–32 min). *For colon examination:* **IM,** 2 mg 10 min prior to procedure. *Treatment of toxicity of beta-adrenergic blocking agents:* **Adults, IV, initial:** 2–3 mg given over 30 sec; may be repeated at the rate of 5 mg/hr until patient is stabilized.

NURSING CONSIDERATIONS

Administration/Storage

1. Once the hypoglycemic client responds, supplemental carbohydrates should be given to prevent secondary hypoglycemia.
2. Before reconstituting, the powder should be stored at room temperature.
3. Following reconstitution, the solution should be used immediately. However, if necessary, the solution may be stored at 5°C (41°F) for up to 2 days.
4. Doses higher than 2 mg should be reconstituted with sterile water for injection and used immediately.
5. Administer with dextrose solutions. A precipitate may form if saline solutions are used.

Interventions

1. Administer a carbohydrate after the client awakens following the administration of glucagon.
2. Have rapidly available sugar such as orange juice and Karo syrup in water to administer. If the shock was caused by a long-acting medication, administer slowly digestible carbohydrates such as bread with honey.

Client/Family Teaching

1. Instruct the family in the administration of glucagon SC or IM in the event the client has a hypoglycemic reaction and loses consciousness.
2. Discuss with the client and family the need to keep the physician informed of hypoglycemic reactions so that the dosage of insulin can be properly adjusted.
3. Advise the family not to try to administer fluids by mouth if the client has a reaction and is not fully conscious. The client could easily aspirate these fluids into the lungs.

CHAPTER FIFTY-NINE

Thyroid and Antithyroid Drugs

Thyroid Preparations

General Statement: The thyroid manufactures two active hormones: thyroxine and triiodothyronine, both of which contain iodine. These thyroid hormones are released into the bloodstream, where they are bound to protein.

Diseases involving the thyroid fall into two groups:

1. Hypothyroidism or diseases in which little or no hormone is produced. These can be subdivided into cretinism, resulting from a deficiency of thyroid hormone during fetal and early life, and myxedema, a deficiency of thyroid hormone in the adult. Cretinism is characterized by arrested physical and mental development, with dystrophy of the bones and soft parts and lowered basal metabolism. Myxedema is characterized by a dry, waxy swelling, with abnormal deposits of mucin in the skin. The edema is nonpitting and the facial changes are distinctive, with swollen lips and a thickened nose. Primary myxedema results from atrophy of the thyroid gland. Secondary myxedema may result from hypofunction of the pituitary gland or prolonged administration of antithyroid drugs.

2. Hyperthyroidism or conditions associated with an overproduction of hormones, as in Graves' or Basedow's disease (diffuse enlargement of the thyroid gland; often characterized by protruding eyes), and Plummer's disease, in which extra thyroid hormone is produced by a single "hot" thyroid nodule. These conditions are usually characterized by hypertrophy and hyperplasia of the thyroid and a state of extreme nervousness.

Euthyroid or Simple, Nontoxic Goiter (Endemic Goiter)

In these states, a normal or near-normal amount of hormone is produced by an enlarged thyroid gland. This condition can occur when the dietary intake of iodine is below normal. Today the disease is much rarer because iodine is added as a matter of routine to cooking salt.

The thyroid, in such patients, tends to become enlarged, especially during adolescent growth and pregnancy. Surgery may be necessary to alleviate the pressure on the trachea caused by the enlarged thyroid and to prevent the oxygen supply from being diminished.

Drugs used in the treatment of thyroid disease fall into two groups: (1) thyroid preparations used to correct thyroid deficiency diseases and (2) antithyroid drugs that reduce production of hormones by an overactive gland.

The external supply of thyroid hormones usually results in a reduction in the amount of natural hormone produced by the thyroid gland.

The accurate determination of thyroid function is crucial for the treatment of thyroid disease. Thyroid function can be evaluated by (1) total levothyroxine (T_4), (2) free levothyroxine, (3) serum liothyronine (T_3), (4) liothyronine resin uptake (RT_3U), (5) free thyroxine index, and (6) thyroid-stimulating hormone. The results of some of the tests are at times skewed by medications the patient is taking, so that the effect of these drugs must be considered when evaluating the test.

Thyroid conditions are often treated by fixed combinations of levothyroxine sodium and liothyronine sodium in a ratio of 4:1. Such a preparation is liotrix (Euthroid, Thyrolar). For all information regarding these drugs, see drug entries for levothyroxine sodium and liothyronine sodium.

Action/Kinetics: The thyroid hormones regulate growth by controlling protein synthesis and regulating energy metabolism by increasing the resting or basal metabolic rate (BMR). Other metabolic effects include increased conversion of cholesterol to bile acids, increase in protein bound iodine (PBI), increased carbohydrate utilization, and participation in the calcification of long bones.

The hormones also have a cardiostimulatory effect and can increase renal blood flow as well as the glomerular filtration rate (GFR) (diuresis). The thyroid gland is under the control of the hypothalamus and the pituitary gland, which produce thyroid-stimulating hormone releasing factor and thyrotropin (thyroid-stimulating hormone, TSH), respectively. Like other hormone systems, the thyroid, pituitary, and hypothalamus work together in a feedback mechanism. Excess thyroid hormone causes a decrease in TSH, and a lack of thyroid hormone causes an increase in the production and secretion of TSH.

59

Uses: Replacement therapy in primary and secondary myxedema, myxedemic coma, nontoxic goiter, hypothyroidism, some thyroid tumors, chronic thyroiditis, sporadic cretinism, and thyrotropin-dependent tumors. With antithyroid drugs for thyrotoxicosis (to prevent goiter or hypothyroidism).

Contraindications: Uncorrected adrenal insufficiency, myocardial infarction, hyperthyroidism, and thyrotoxicosis. Adrenal insufficiency unless treatment with adrenocortical steroids is initiated first. Not to be used to treat obesity or infertility in either males or females.

Special Concerns: Pregnancy category: A. Geriatric patients may be more sensitive to the usual adult dosage of these hormones. Use with extreme caution in the presence of angina pectoris, hypertension, and other cardiovascular diseases, renal insufficiency, and ischemic states.

Side Effects: Thyroid preparations have cumulative effects, and overdosage (i.e., symptoms of hyperthyroidism) may occur. *CV:* Arrhythmias, palpitations, angina, increased heart rate and pulse pressure, cardiac arrest, aggravation of congestive heart failure. *GI:* Cramps, diarrhea, nausea, appetite changes. *CNS:* Headache, nervousness, mental agitation, irritability, insomnia, tremors. *Miscellaneous:* Weight loss, hyperhidrosis, excessive warmth, irregular menses, heat intolerance, fever, dyspnea.

Drug Interactions

Anticoagulants	↑ Effect of anticoagulants by ↑ hypoprothrombinemia
Antidepressants, tricyclic	↑ Effect of antidepressants and ↑ effect of thyroid
Antidiabetic agents	Hyperglycemic effect of thyroid preparations may necessitate ↑ in dose of antidiabetic agent
Cholestyramine	↓ Effect of thyroid hormone due to ↓ absorption from GI tract
Corticosteroids	Thyroid preparations increase tissue demands for corticosteroids. Adrenal insufficiency must be corrected with corticosteroids before administering thyroid hormones. In patients already treated for adrenal insufficiency, dosage of corticosteroids must be increased when initiating therapy with thyroid drug
Digitalis compounds	↓ Effect of digitalis, with worsening of arrhythmias or congestive heart failure
Epinephrine	Cardiovascular effects ↑ by thyroid preparations
Estrogens	Estrogens may ↑ requirements for thyroid hormone
Ketamine	Concomitant use may result in severe hypertension and tachycardia
Levarterenol	Cardiovascular effects ↑ by thyroid preparations
Phenytoin	↑ Effect of thyroid hormone by ↓ plasma protein binding
Salicylates	Salicylates compete for thyroid-binding sites on protein

Laboratory Test Interferences: Alter thyroid function tests. ↑ Prothrombin time. ↓ Serum cholesterol.

Dosage: Thyroid drugs are started with a low dose that is gradually increased until a satisfactory response is achieved within safe dose limits. When necessary, a decrease in dosage and a more gradual upward adjustment relieve severe side effects.

NURSING CONSIDERATIONS

Administration

1. The treatment is initiated with small doses which are gradually increased.
2. The dose of medication for a child may be the same as the dosage for an adult.
3. When changing from one thyroid drug to another, follow the specific instructions to prevent overdosage or relapse.
4. Store thyroid preparations in a cool, dark place away from moisture and light.

Assessment

1. Take a complete nursing history.
2. Review all medications the client is currently receiving to be sure none interacts unfavorably with the thyroid medication.
3. Note if the client is taking antidiabetic agents or is on anticoagulant therapy and document.
4. Note the client's general physical condition and whether the client has a history of angina, cardiac problems or any other health problems.
5. Take a baseline ECG against which to compare subsequent ECG tracings once therapy has been instituted.

Interventions

1. Monitor the client's thyroid function studies closely.
2. Observe the client for side effects of the drug. Complaints of headache, insomnia and tremors should be documented and reported to the physician.
3. Observe the client on anticoagulant therapy for bleeding from any orifice or for purpura. Monitor PT/PTT closely as the action of anticoagulants is potentiated by thyroid preparations.
4. Clients with a history of angina or other cardiovascular disorders need to have their blood pressure and pulse monitored closely. If the pulse increases to more than 100 beats/min, withhold the drug and notify the physician, unless otherwise directed.
5. Take an ECG at regular intervals during the drug therapy and compare with the baseline tracing.
6. Note the client's general response to the therapy. Complaints of abdominal cramps, weight gain, dyspnea, palpitations, angina, fatigue, or observing increased pallor or edema may indicate that the client is experiencing cardiac problems and further assessment is indicated by the physician.
7. Observe for evidence of heat intolerance and if the client is losing weight. Document and report to the physician.

Client/Family Teaching

1. Stress that the drug must be taken only while the client is under medical supervision and that it must be taken for life.
2. Side effects of the medication may not appear for 4–6 weeks after the start of therapy. Therefore, explain to clients that they should notify the physician of any new signs or symptoms that may occur. The same is true if the dosage of drug is increased.
3. Instruct the client to report to the physician immediately any excessive weight loss, palpitations, leg cramps, nervousness, or insomnia. Provide the client with a printed list of the events that require immediate medical attention and a number to call to report these events.
4. If the client has diabetes, explain that thyroid preparations may require adjustment of the dosage of insulin. Therefore, it is important to monitor the urine and/or blood sugar levels closely and to report any changes to the physician.
5. Note that certain foods, such as cabbage, turnips, pears and peaches, are goitrogenic and may alter the requirements for thyroid hormone. Provide the client with a list of such foods and have the dietitian discuss diet and meal planning with the client.
6. Thyroid hormones increase the client's toxicity to iodine. Therefore explain the need to avoid using iodized salt preparations, multivitamins, dentifrices and other nonprescription medications that contain iodine.
7. Have the dietitian counsel clients regarding diet so that they will select foods according to the increased energy demands that should result from the medication therapy.
8. Thyroid preparations potentiate the action of anticoagulants; therefore, if the client is also

receiving anticoagulant therapy, explain the importance of reporting any excessive bruising or bleeding.

9. If the client is female, instruct her to keep a record of her menstrual periods and to report any changes.

10. Instruct the client to take the thyroid medication in a single morning dose to reduce the likelihood of nighttime insomnia.

11. Advise the client not to change brands of medication unless they have first consulted with the physician.

12. Encourage the client to keep all scheduled follow-up visits and scheduled laboratory tests.

Evaluation

1. Appropriate weight and normal sleep pattern are maintained.

2. Thyroid function studies are within normal range.

3. There is improvement in the client's hair and skin condition and they demonstrate increased mental alertness.

LEVOTHYROXINE SODIUM (T₄) (lee-voh-thigh-ROX-een)

Eltroxin✲, Levothroid, Levoxine, Synthroid, L-Thyroxine Sodium (Rx)

See also *Thyroid Drugs,* p. 1120.

Classification: Thyroid preparation.

Action/Kinetics: Levothyroxine is the synthetic sodium salt of the levoisomer of thyroxine (tetraiodothyronine). Levothyroxine from the GI tract is incomplete and variable, especially when taken with food. This hormone has a slower onset but a longer duration than sodium liothyronine. It is more active on a weight basis than thyroid. Is usually the drug of choice. Effect is predictable as thyroid content is standard. **Time to peak therapeutic effect:** 3–4 weeks. **t½:** 6–7 days in a euthyroid person, 9–10 days in a hypothyroid patient, and 3–4 days in a hyperthyroid patient. Is 99% protein bound. **Duration:** 1–3 weeks after withdrawal of chronic therapy.

Note: All levothyroxine products are not bioequivalent; thus, changing brands is not recommended.

Dosage: Tablets. *Mild hypothyroidism:* **Adults, initial,** 50 mcg as a single daily dose; **then,** increase by 25–50 mcg q 2–3 weeks until desired clinical response is attained; **maintenance, usual:** 75–125 mcg daily (although doses up to 200 mcg daily may be required in some patients). *Severe hypothyroidism:* **Adults, initial,** 12.5–25 mcg as a single daily dose; **then,** increase dose, as necessary, in increments of 25 mcg at 2–3 week intervals. *Hypothyroidism:* **Pediatric, 10 years and older:** 2–3 mg/kg daily as a single dose until the adult daily dose (usually 150 mcg) is reached. **6–10 years of age:** 4–5 mcg/kg daily or 100–150 mcg daily as a single dose. **1–5 years of age:** 3–5 mcg/kg daily or 75–100 mcg daily as a single dose. **6–23 months of age:** 5–6 mcg/kg daily or 50–75 mcg daily as a single dose. **Less than 6 months of age:** 5–6 mcg/kg daily or 25–50 mcg daily as a single dose.

IV. *Myxedematous coma without heart disease.* **Adults, initial,** 200–500 mcg even in geriatric patients. If there is no response in 24 hr, 100–300 mcg may be given on the second day. Smaller daily doses should be given until patient can tolerate oral medication. *Hypothyroidism:* **Adults,** 50–100 mcg as a single daily dose; **pediatric, IV, IM:** A dose of 75% of the usual oral pediatric dose should be given.

Transfer from liothyronine to levothyroxine: administer replacement drug for several days before discontinuing liothyronine. Transfer from levothyroxine to liothyronine: discontinue levothyroxine before starting patient on low daily dose of liothyronine.

NURSING CONSIDERATIONS

See also *Nursing Considerations* for *Thyroid Drugs,* p. 1122.

Administration/Storage

1. Prepare the solution for injection immediately before administration.
2. Add the prescribed amount of normal saline to the powder and shake the solution until it is clear.
3. Discard any unused portion of the IV medication.
4. Do not mix with other IV infusion solutions.

Assessment

1. Note the age of the client. Elderly clients are likely to have undetected cardiac problems. Therefore, a baseline ECG should be taken prior to initiating drug therapy.
2. Note if the client is pregnant. The woman must continue taking thyroid preparations throughout the pregnancy.

LIOTHYRONINE SODIUM (T₃)   (lye-oh-**THIGH**-roh-neen)

Cytomel, Sodium-L-Triiodothyronine (Rx)

See also *Thyroid Drugs,* p. 1120.

Classification: Thyroid preparation.

Action/Kinetics: Synthetic sodium salt of levoisomer of triiodothyronine. Liothyronine has more predictable effects due to standard hormone content. It may be preferred when a rapid effect or rapidly reversible effect is required. Drug has a rapid onset which may result in difficulty in controlling the dosage as well as the possibility of cardiac side effects and changes in metabolic demands. **t½:** 24 hr for euthyroid patients, approximately 34 hr in hypothyroid patients, and approximately 14 hr in hyperthyroid patients. **Duration:** Up to 72 hr. Is 99% protein bound.

Additional Contraindications: Use of liothyronine is not recommended in children with cretinism as there is some question about whether the hormone crosses the blood-brain barrier.

Dosage: Tablets. *Mild hypothyroidism: individualized:* **Adults,** 25 mcg daily. Increase by 12.5–25 mcg q 1–2 weeks until satisfactory response has been obtained. **Usual maintenance:** 25–75 mcg daily. Use lower initial dosage (5 mcg/day) for the elderly, children, and patients with cardiovascular disease. Increase gradually as adult dosage.
   Myxedema: **Adults, initial,** 2.5–5 mcg/day increased by 5–10 mcg daily q 1–2 weeks until 25 mcg/day is reached; **then,** increase q 1–2 weeks by 12.5–50 mcg. **Usual maintenance:** 50–100 mcg/day.
   Nontoxic goiter: **Initial,** 5 mcg/day; **then,** increase q 1–2 weeks by 5–10 mcg until 25 mcg daily is reached; **then,** dose can be increased by 12.5–25 mcg weekly until the maintenance dose of 50–100 mcg daily is reached.
   Transfer from other thyroid preparations to liothyronine: discontinue old preparation before starting on low daily dose of liothyronine. Transfer from liothyronine to another thyroid preparation: start therapy with replacement drug several days prior to complete withdrawal of sodium liothyronine.

NURSING CONSIDERATIONS
See also *Nursing Considerations* for *Thyroid Drugs,* p. 1122.

Administration
If symptoms of hyperthyroidism are noted, the drug can be withdrawn for 2–3 days after which therapy can be reinstituted, but at a lower dose.

LIOTRIX   (LYE-oh-trix)
Euthroid, Thyrolar (Rx)

See also *Thyroid Drugs,* p. 1120.

Classification: Thyroid preparation.

General Statement: Mixture of synthetic levothyroxine sodium (T_4) and liothyronine (T_3). The mixture contains the products in a 4:1 ratio by weight and in a 1:1 ratio by biologic activity. The two commercial preparations contain slightly different amounts of each component. Because of this discrepancy, a switch from one preparation to the other must be made cautiously. Liotrix has standard hormone content; thus, the effect is predictable.

Dosage: Tablets. Adults and children: initial, 50 mcg levothyroxine and 12.5 mcg liothyronine (Thyrolar) or 60 mcg levothyroxine and 15 mcg liothyronine (Euthroid) daily; **then,** at monthly intervals, increments of like amounts can be made until the desired effect is achieved. **Usual maintenance:** 50–100 mcg of levothyroxine and 12.5–25 mcg liothyronine daily.

NURSING CONSIDERATIONS
See also *Nursing Considerations* for *Thyroid Drugs,* p. 1122.

Administration/Storage
1. The initial dose for geriatric clients should be ¼–½ the usual adult dose; this dose can be doubled q 6–8 weeks until the desired effect is reached.
2. In children, dosing increments should be made q 2 weeks until the desired response has been attained.
3. Thyroid function tests should always be done before initiating dosage changes.
4. Administer as a single dose before breakfast.
5. Protect tablets from light, heat, and moisture.
6. Due to differences in the amounts of hormones between Euthroid and Thyrolar, once started on a particular brand, the client should not be switched.

THYROGLOBULIN   (thigh-roh-GLOB-you-lin)
Proloid (Rx)

See also *Thyroid Drugs,* p. 1120.

Classification: Thyroid preparation.

General Statement: Thyroid preparation containing levothyroxine (T_4) and liothyronine (T_3) in a ratio of 2.5 to 1. Drug is a natural product purified from hog thyroid glands. It has no clinical advantage over thyroid especially since the product contains varying amounts of the hormones. It has a slow onset of action that makes it unsuitable for the treatment of myxedematous coma.

Dosage: Tablets. *Hypothyroidism without myxedema, pediatric hypothyroidism:* **Adults, children, initial,** 32 mg, increased gradually at 1- to 2-week intervals until control is established. **Usual maintenance:** 65–160 mg daily. Therapy is aimed at maintaining a level of 5–9 mcg/100 mL protein-bound iodine. *Myxedema or hypothyroidism with cardiovascular disease, cretinism or severe hypothyroidism:* **Adults, initial,** 16–32 mg daily; **then,** the dose can be doubled q 2 weeks until the desired effect is obtained. **Usual maintenance:** 65–160 mg daily. Transfer from and to sodium liothyronine should be made gradually.

NURSING CONSIDERATIONS

See also *Nursing Considerations* for *Thyroid Drugs,* p. 1122.

THYROID DESICCATED   (THIGH-royd)
(Rx)

See also *Thyroid Drugs,* p. 1120.

Classification: Thyroid preparation.

Action/Kinetics: Due to variable content of both levothyroxine and liothyronine in the product, fluctuations in plasma levels of these hormones will be observed. The drug has a slow onset of action that makes it unsuitable for the treatment of myxedematous coma.

Dosage: Tablets. *Hypothyroidism without myxedema, pediatric hypothyroidism:* **Adults, children, initial,** 60 mg daily; **then,** increase by 30 mg q 30 days until the desired effect is reached. **Usual maintenance:** 60–120 mg daily. *Myxedema, hypothyroidism with cardiovascular disease, cretinism or severe hypothyroidism:* **Adults, children, initial,** 15 mg daily; **then** increase to 30 mg after 2 weeks and to 60 mg daily after an additional 2 weeks. The patient should be evaluated carefully after 30 and 60 days of treatment. If required, the dose can be further increased to 120 mg daily. **Usual maintenance:** 50–120 mg daily.

Transfer from liothyronine: Start thyroid several days before withdrawal. When transferring from thyroid, discontinue thyroid before starting with low daily dose of replacement drug.

NURSING CONSIDERATIONS

See also *Nursing Considerations* for *Thyroid Drugs,* p. 1122.

Administration/Storage

1. Store protected from moisture and light.
2. In geriatric clients, the initial dose should be 7.5–15 mg daily which can then be doubled q 6–8 weeks until desired effect has been attained.

THYROTROPIN   (thigh-roh-TROH-pin)
Thytropar, Thyroid Stimulating Hormone, TSH (Rx)

Classification: Thyroid preparation.

Action/Kinetics: Highly purified thyroid-stimulating hormone from bovine pituitary glands. Thyrotropin administration results in increased iodine uptake by the thyroid gland and increased formation and release of thyroid hormone. **Onset:** Within a few minutes. **Peak effect:** 1–2 days. **Duration:** Drug effects are terminated after the drug is withdrawn.

Uses: Diagnostic agent to evaluate thyroid function.

Contraindications: Untreated Addison's disease, coronary thrombosis.

Special Concerns: Safe use in pregnancy (pregnancy category: C), lactation, or children has not been established. Use with caution in patients with cardiac disease who cannot withstand stress.

Side Effects: *CV:* Tachycardia, hypotension. *GI:* Nausea, vomiting. *Miscellaneous:* Swelling of thyroid gland, urticaria, headache, anaphylaxis.

Dosage: IM, SC: Administer 10 IU daily for 1–3 days followed by radioiodine uptake study within 24 hours. **Note:** No response will occur if there is thyroid failure; however, a significant response will result in pituitary failure.

NURSING CONSIDERATIONS

See also *Nursing Considerations* for *Thyroid Drugs,* p. 1122.

Administration/Storage

The reconstituted solution may be stored in the refrigerator but for no longer than 2 weeks.

Assessment

Note any client history of coronary heart disease and document.

Interventions

1. Monitor the vital signs and observe closely for allergic reactions.
3. Note any evidence of urticaria, swelling of the thyroid gland, client complaint of headaches and symptoms of anaphylaxis. Document and report to the physician immediately.

IODINE SOURCES

POTASSIUM IODIDE
Pima, Thyro-Block ✦ (Rx)

SODIUM IODIDE
(Rx)

STRONG IODINE SOLUTION
Lugol's Solution (Rx)

Classification: Source of iodine.

Action/Kinetics: Small doses of iodine are concentrated by the thyroid gland resulting in an increased synthesis of thyroid hormones. However, large doses are capable of inhibiting thyroid hormone synthesis and release. This is the basis for the use of these drugs in treating hyperthyroidism. Iodine specifically produces involution of a hyperplastic thyroid gland, making it less friable and less vascular prior to surgery. Iodine also shortens the time required by other antithyroid drugs to reduce the output of natural hormone. **Onset:** 1–2 days. **Peak effects:** 10–15 days. **Duration:** Up to 6 weeks. Strong Iodine Solution contains 5% iodine and 10% sodium iodide.

Uses: Prophylaxis of simple and colloid goiters, exophthalmic goiter. As adjunct with antithyroid drugs to prepare thyrotoxic patients for thyroidectomy, to treat thyrotoxic crisis, or neonatal thyrotoxicosis. Also, for thyroid blocking in radiation emergency. *Investigational, Potassium Iodide:* Erythema nodosum, iodine deficiency.

Contraindications: Iodine is contraindicated in tuberculosis because it may cause breakdown of healing of lesions. Pulmonary edema. In patients hypersensitive to iodine.

Special Concerns: Pregnancy category: C.

Side Effects: *Acute poisoning:* Vomiting, abdominal pain, diarrhea, gastritis, swelling of glottis or larynx, shock syndrome. May be treated by soluble starch gastric lavage followed by milk to relieve irritation. *Chronic toxicity (iodism): Dermatologic:* Skin reactions including acneiform, vesicular, bullous, or maculopapular eruptions. *Mucous membranes:* Swelling and inflammation, conjunctivitis, bronchial irritation, coryza. *CV:* Edema, erythema, purpura. *Miscellaneous:* Fever, irritability.

Dosage: Sodium Iodide. IV. Thyroid crisis: 1–3 g/day.
   Potassium Iodide. Oral Solution, Syrup, Tablets. *Thyroid blocking in radiation emergency:* **Adults,** 100–150 mg daily 24 before and for 3–10 days after administration of or exposure to radiation. **Pediatric, 1 year and older:** 130 mg once daily for 10 days following administration of or exposure to radiation; **less than 1 year of age:** 65 mg once daily for 10 days following administration of or exposure to radiation. *To prepare patients for thyroidectomy:* **Adults,** 5 drops of the 1 g/mL oral solution (about 250 mg), 4 mL of the syrup (about 260 mg), or 2 tablets dissolved in a glass of water (about 260 mg) daily for 10 days before surgery usually with an antithyroid drug.
   Strong Iodine Solution. *Prior to thyroidectomy:* 2–6 drops t.i.d. for 10 days prior to surgery.

NURSING CONSIDERATIONS

See also *Nursing Considerations* for *Antithyroid Drugs,* p. 1122.

Administration/Storage

1. Measure iodine solutions carefully, using a calibrated dropper. This medication is potent and the dosing volume tends to be small.
2. Dilute iodine in 60 mL of chocolate milk, plain milk, or orange juice. The medication has a bitter taste.
3. To decrease the burning sensation in the mouth and to prevent discoloration of the teeth, use drinking straws when administering iodine solutions.
4. Do not store other than in the original brown, light-resistant container.

Assessment

1. Note if the client has any allergy to iodine preparations.
2. Ask the client if there have been any adverse reactions to medications or diagnostic tests where iodine has been used.
3. Obtain baseline data concerning the extent of the client's anxiety, nervousness, agitation, mood swings and irritability.
4. Note if the client has exophthalmos, tremors or increased tendon reflexes.

5. Obtain a baseline ECG, and measurement of blood pressure, pulse and respirations.
6. Check the client's medication history for the use of oral anticoagulants, insulin or anion exchange resins and document if in use.

Interventions

1. Monitor the client's blood pressure, temperature, respirations, weight. Determine glucose levels in the blood and urine as ordered.
2. Note if the client has a reduction in stress and changes in mood swings. Compare the client's responses with the baseline data obtained prior to initiating therapy.
3. If the client is receiving anticoagulants, monitor for increased bleeding tendencies.
4. Monitor the client's diet for excessive ingestion of goitrogenic foods that could cause symptoms of hypothyroidism.

Client/Family Teaching

1. Review with the client and family the purposes of the therapy.
2. Describe the symptoms of acute iodine poisoning. Provide printed information listing these symptoms.
3. Instruct the client to withhold the drug and report any evidence of toxicity to the physician immediately.
4. Advise the client to check with the physician before using iodized salt.
5. Instruct clients to sip the medication through a straw to avoid staining tooth enamel.
6. Dilute medication with water, juice, or milk to decrease gastric irritation.
7. Stress the importance of reporting for medical visits and follow-up laboratory tests.

Evaluation

1. There is an improvement in the client's psychological symptoms and sociability.
2. A reduction in the pulse rate, and a reduction in appetite and weight gain should be evident.
3. Within 3–8 weeks there is a decrease in tremors and a lessening of exophthalmos and a reduced diaphoresis.
4. Sensitivity to cold is eliminated.

ANTITHYROID DRUGS

Action/Kinetics: Antithyroid drugs include thiouracil derivatives and large doses of iodide. These drugs inhibit (partially or completely) the production of thyroid hormones by the thyroid gland. The drugs act by preventing the incorporation of iodide into tyrosine and coupling of iodotyrosines. Since these agents do not affect release or activity of preformed hormone, it may take several weeks for the therapeutic effect to become established.

Uses: Hyperthyroidism; prior to surgery or radiotherapy. Adjunct in treatment of thyrotoxicosis or thyroid storm.

Contraindications: Lactation (may cause hypothyroidism in the infant).

Special Concerns: Pregnancy category: D. Use with caution in the presence of cardiovascular disease.

Side Effects: *Hematologic:* Agranulocytosis, thrombocytopenia, granulocytopenia, hypoprothrombinemia. *GI:* Nausea, vomiting, taste loss, epigastric pain. *CNS:* Headache, paresthesia, drowsiness, vertigo. *Dermatologic:* Skin rash, urticaria, alopecia, skin pigmentation, pruritus, exfoliative dermatitis. *Miscellaneous:* Jaundice, arthralgia, myalgia, neuritis, edema, sialadenopathy, lymphadenopathy, vasculitis, lupus-like syndrome, drug fever, periarteritis, hepatitis, nephrotic syndrome.

NURSING CONSIDERATIONS

Assessment

1. Note if the client is taking any medications that may interact unfavorably with the antithyroid drug and document.
2. If the client is female and of childbearing age, determine if she is pregnant.

Interventions

1. Note any client complaint of unusual bleeding, nausea, loss of taste or epigastric pain. These symptoms should be reported to the physician.
2. Observe for the presence of skin rashes, urticaria, alopecia, changes in skin pigmentation or pruritus. Document and report to the physician.

Client/Family Teaching

1. Advise the client that it takes up to 12 weeks for the drug to produce the full effect. Stress that the drug must be taken regularly and exactly as directed. Hyperthyroidism may recur if the drug is not taken properly.
2. Explain that if the drug is taken as ordered for 1 or more years, more than half of the clients achieve a permanent remission.
3. Provide the client with a printed list of side effects and associated symptoms that require reporting immediately to the physician.
4. Advise the client to report any sore throat, enlargement of the cervical lymph nodes, GI disturbances, fever, rash, or jaundice. These symptoms may necessitate either a reduction of the dosage of drug or withdrawal of the drug by the physician.
5. Discuss with the client the potential loss of taste perception. If this occurs, advise them to increase the use of herbs and nonsodium seasonings.

METHIMAZOLE (meth-**IM**-ah-zohl)

Tapazole (Rx)

See also *Antithyroid Drugs,* p. 1130.

Classification: Antithyroid preparation.

Action/Kinetics: Onset is more rapid but effect is less consistent than that of propylthiouracil. Bioavailability may be affected by food. **t½:** 4–14 hr. **Onset:** 10–20 days. **Time to peak effect:** 2–10 weeks. Metabolized in the liver and excreted through the kidneys (7% unchanged).

Special Concerns: Incidence of hepatic toxicity may be greater than for propylthiouracil.

Dosage: Tablets. Adults, initial: *Mild hyperthyroidism:* 15 mg/day; *moderately severe hyperthyroidism:* 30–40 mg/day; *severe hyperthyroidism:* 60 mg/day. For hyperthyroidism, the dose may be given once daily or divided into 2 doses for 6–8 weeks (until patient becomes euthyroid). **Maintenance:** 5–30 mg daily as a single dose or divided into 2 doses. **Pediatric:** 0.4 mg/kg given once daily or divided into 2 doses; **maintenance:** 0.2 mg/kg. *Thyrotoxic crisis:* **Adults,** 15–20 mg q 4 hr during the first day as an adjunct to other treatments.

NURSING CONSIDERATIONS

See also *Nursing Considerations* for *Antithyroid Drugs,* p. 1131.

Interventions

1. Assess the client for changes in sensation of the extremities. For example, check if the client has any strange, tingling sensations of the fingers and toes. Some clients develop paresthesias. Document and report to the physician.
2. If the client is over 40 years of age, monitor for agranulocytosis. Question the client about sore throats, fever, chills and unexplained bleeding. Document and report any such incidence to the physician.
3. Note if the client complains of GI symptoms. Advise the client to take the medication with a snack to reduce gastric irritation. If it persists, notify the physician.
4. Observe for any evidence of hair loss and if evident, report to the physician.

Client/Family Teaching

1. Advise the client to take the medication at evenly spaced times and with evenly spaced doses during the day.
2. Instruct the client to report any unexpected symptoms to the physician immediately. The effects of the medication may not be evident for weeks after the therapy begins, and the physician may need to adjust the dosage of drug.

PROPYLTHIOURACIL   (proh-pill-thigh-oh-**YOUR**-ah-sill)

Propyl-Thyracil ✳ (Rx)

See also *Antithyroid Drugs,* p. 1130.

Classification: Antithyroid preparation.

Action/Kinetics: May be preferred for treatment of thyroid storm as the drug inhibits peripheral conversion of thyroxine to triiodothyronine. Rapidly absorbed from the GI tract. **Duration:** 2–3 hr. **t½:** 1–2 hr. **Onset:** 10–20 days. **Time to peak effect:** 2–10 weeks. Eighty percent is protein bound. Metabolized by the liver and excreted through the kidneys.

Special Concerns: Incidence of vasculitis is increased.

Drug Interactions: Propylthiouracil may produce hypoprothrombinemia, adding to the effect of anticoagulants.

Dosage: Tablets. *Hyperthyroidism:* **Adults, initial:** 300 mg/day (up to 900 mg/day may be required in some patients with severe hyperthyroidism) given as 1–4 divided doses; **maintenance:**

50–600 mg/day. **Pediatric, 6–10 years, initial:** 50–150 mg/day in 1–4 divided doses; **over 10 years, initial:** 50–300 mg/day in 1–4 divided doses. Maintenance for all pediatric use is based on response. *Thyrotoxic crisis:* **Adults,** 200–400 mg q 4 hr during the first day as an adjunct to other treatments. *Neonatal thyrotoxicosis:* 10 mg/kg daily in divided doses.

NURSING CONSIDERATIONS

See also *Nursing Considerations* for *Antithyroid Drugs,* p. 1131.

RADIOACTIVE AGENT

SODIUM IODIDE I 131

Iodotope Therapeutic, Sodium Iodide I 131 Therapeutic (Rx)

Classification: Radioactive agent.

Action/Kinetics: This compound is a radioactive iodide salt that is distributed throughout the extracellular fluid following oral ingestion. It concentrates in the thyroid gland, where it is incorporated into thyroid hormones which can then be visualized. Larger doses damage or destroy thyroid tissue. The drug emits both beta (90%) and gamma (10%) radiation. When given orally, the drug is rapidly absorbed. **Onset of effect:** 2–4 weeks. **Time to peak effect:** 2–4 months. **Time to radioactive visualization:** 4–24 hr. **t$\frac{1}{2}$:** 138 days. **Duration:** 8–10 weeks for thyroid function to return to normal. From 65%–90% excreted in the urine within 24 hr; 20% may appear in the breast milk within 24 hr.

Uses: *Therapeutic:* Hyperthyroidism, selected cases of thyroid cancer. *Diagnosis:* Thyroid function tests, uptake of thyroid tests, thyroid imaging.

Contraindications: Preexisting vomiting and diarrhea. Usually, patients under 30 years of age. Pregnancy, lactation.

Special Concerns: Pediatric patients may be at an increased risk of radiation exposure. The dose should be individualized if used in children.

Side Effects: The most severe effects are seen following use for thyroid carcinoma. *Hematologic:* Anemia, leukemia, bone marrow depression, leukopenia, thrombocytopenia. *Radiation sickness:* Nausea, vomiting. *Miscellaneous:* Acute thyroid crisis, chromosome abnormalities, cough, swelling or tenderness in neck, pain on swallowing, sore throat, alopecia (temporary).

Dosage: Capsules, Oral Solution. *Hyperthyroidism:* **Adults, usual,** 4–10 millicuries. *Thyroid cancer or metastases:* **Adults, usual,** 100–150 millicuries to destroy normal thyroid tissue followed by subsequent therapy of 100–200 millicuries. *Thyroid imaging:* **Adults,** 5–100 microcuries. *Localization of thyroid metastases:* **Adults,** 1–10 microcuries.

NURSING CONSIDERATIONS

Administration/Storage

1. Therapeutic dose is only given to hospitalized clients.

2. Upon standing, solution and glass storage containers may darken as a result of radiation. This does not affect efficacy of the product.
3. A stock solution may be prepared by diluting the oral solution with purified water containing 0.2% sodium thiosulfate.

Assessment

1. Prior to initiating therapy, determine if the client has a history of sensitivity to iodine preparations or iodine rich foods such as shell fish.
2. Ask the client about any adverse reactions to previous medications or diagnostic tests where iodine was used.
3. Determine if the client has had antithyroid medication within 2–3 days prior to the scheduled treatment.

Interventions

1. If the client has received antithyroid medication within the past 2–3 days, discuss with the physician and other health care team members.
2. If the treatment must be delayed, discuss the reasons with the client in order to allay any fears concerning the progression of the disease.
3. Institute appropriate measures for the protection of visitors and staff. Observe the institutional policy concerning proper care and disposal of the client's body fluids.
4. Instruct the client and visitors in the appropriate hospital procedure for protection from radiation.
5. Food may delay absorption. Encourage the client to increase fluid intake to promote excretion.
6. Provide printed guidelines for clients and family following dosage for treatment of cancer. Advise the client to avoid prolonged contact with small children for at least seven days following the treatment.

CHAPTER SIXTY
Calcitonin, Calcium Salts, and Calcium Regulators

General Statement: Appropriate calcium levels in the body are required to maintain homeostasis for many processes including blood coagulation, regulation of heart rhythm, and skeletal muscle contraction. Maintenance of extracellular calcium levels is controlled by parathyroid hormone utilizing a feedback mechanism similar to that for other hormones.

Dysfunction of the parathyroid may result in hypocalcemic tetany, seizures, and death. Administration of either parathyroid hormone obtained from animal sources or a synthetic compound restores calcium levels toward normal values. Because the response is slow, calcium salts are usually administered concomitantly.

60

CALCITONIN-HUMAN (kal-sih-**TOH**-nin)

Cibacalcin (Rx)

CALCITONIN-SALMON (kal-sih-**TOH**-nin)

Calcimar, Miacalcin (Rx)

Classification: Calcium regulator.

Action/Kinetics: Calcitonins are polypeptide hormones produced in mammals by the parafollicular cells of the thyroid gland. Calcitonin isolated from salmon has the same therapeutic effect as the human hormone, except for a greater potency per milligram and a somewhat longer duration of action. Calcitonin-human is a synthetic product that has the same sequence of amino acids as the naturally occurring calcitonin found in humans. Calcitonin is ineffective when administered orally. Calcitonin is beneficial in Paget's disease of bone by reducing the rate of turnover of bone; the drug acts to block initial bone resorption which decreases alkaline phosphatase levels in the serum and decreases urinary hydroxyproline excretion. Its effectiveness in treating osteoporosis or hypercalcemia is due to decreased serum calcium levels due to direct inhibition of bone resorption. **Time to peak effect, calcitonin-salmon:** 2 hr for hypercalcemia. **Duration, calcitonin-salmon:** 6–8 hr for hypercalcemia. **t½:** 60 min for calcitonin-human and 70–90 min for calcitonin-salmon. The onset of calcitonin-human in reducing serum alkaline phosphatase and urinary hydroxyproline excretion in Paget's disease may take 6–24 months. Calcitonin is metabolized to inactive compounds in the kidneys, blood, and peripheral tissues.

Uses: Moderate to severe Paget's disease characterized by polyostotic involvement with elevation of serum alkaline phosphatase and urinary excretion of hydroxyproline. For the early treatment of hypercalcemia. Calcitonin-salmon is used concomitantly with calcium and vitamin D to treat postmenopausal osteoporosis.

Contraindications: Allergy to calcitonin-salmon or its gelatin diluent.

Special Concerns: Use with caution during lactation and in pregnancy only if benefits outweigh risks (pregnancy category: C). Safe use in children not established.

Side Effects: *Allergic:* Due to foreign protein reaction to calcitonin or gelatin diluent. Skin rashes, systemic allergic reactions. *GI:* Nausea, vomiting, abdominal pain, diarrhea, anorexia, abdominal pain, salty taste. *Dermatologic:* Flushing of hands or face, inflammation at site of injection (salmon), foot edema. *CNS:* Headache, dizziness. *Other:* Antibody formation rendering the drug ineffective, increased urinary frequency, nocturia, eye pain, sensation of fever, chills, weakness, nasal congestion, shortness of breath, paresthesia.

Laboratory Test Alteration: Reduction of alkaline phosphatase and 24-hr urinary excretion of hydroxyproline are indicative of successful therapy. Monitor urine for casts (indicative of kidney damage).

Dosage: SC. *Calcitonin-Human. Paget's disease,* **Adults, initial,** 0.5 mg daily; **then,** depending on severity of disease, dosage may range from 0.5 mg 2–3 times weekly to 0.25 mg daily.
   IM, SC. *Calcitonin-Salmon. Paget's disease:* **Adults, initial,** 100 IU/day; **maintenance, usual:** 50 IU daily, every other day, or 3 times weekly. *Hypercalcemia;* **Adults, initial,** 4 IU/kg q 12 hr; **then,** increase the dose, if necessary, to 8 IU/kg q 12 hr up to a maximum of 8 IU/kg q 6 hr. *Postmenopausal osteoporosis:* **Adults,** 100 IU daily, once every other day, or 3 times a week given with calcium and vitamin D.

NURSING CONSIDERATIONS

Administration/Storage

1. Before initiating therapy, determine serum alkaline phosphatase and urinary hydroxyproline excretion.
2. Repeat the above studies at the end of 3 months, and every 3–6 months thereafter.
3. Store calcitonin-salmon at a temperature between 2°C–6°C (36°F–43°F).
4. Store calcitonin-human below 25°C (77°F).
5. When being used to treat Paget's disease, therapy for more than 1 year may be required to treat neurologic lesions.
6. Check for hypersensitivity reactions before administering either medication. Administer 1 IU in the forearm and observe for 15 min to ensure test is negative.
7. Have emergency drugs on hand for immediate use in the event of a hypersensitivity reaction.

Assessment

Note any history of client hypersensitivity to calcitonin-salmon or its gelatin diluent.

Interventions

1. Assess for systemic allergic reactions and be prepared to provide oxygen, epinephrine, and corticosteroids.
2. Report local inflammatory reactions at the site of injection.
3. Observe for facial flushing, which may occur with drug treatment. Document and report to the physician.
4. Observe client for hypocalcemic tetany. Clients will exhibit muscular fibrillation, twitching, tetanic spasms, and may go into convulsions. Have calcium available for emergency use should any of these symptoms occur. Remain with clients following the injection and check them at least every 10 min for the next 30 min.
5. Check the client for evidence of hypercalcemia. Complaints of increased thirst, anorexia, polyuria, nausea and vomiting should be reported to the physician.
6. Monitor the client for abdominal distress, anorexia, diarrhea, epigastric distress or changes in taste perception. Monitor and record the weight, intake and output, and notify the physician if these symptoms persist.
7. If the client has a good initial clinical response and then relapses, evaluate for antibody formation in response to serum calcitonin.

Client/Family Teaching

1. Teach how to make appropriate assessments of the client's condition and response to the therapy.
2. Instruct the client in aseptic methods of reconstituting the solution, proper injection technique, and the importance of alternating injection sites.
3. Explain that nausea and vomiting may occur at the onset of therapy. However, the problem should subside as the treatment continues. If it persists, notify the physician.
4. Stress the importance of returning for periodic urine sedimentation tests to assure that there is no kidney damage.
5. Suggest that the client take the doses of medication in the evening to minimize the problem of flushing.
6. Refer to a dietitian for counselling concerning adjustments in the diet that may be required.

Evaluation

1. Assess response to therapy by determining if a reduction in serum calcium, alkaline phosphatase and 24-hr urinary excretion of hydroxyproline are evident.
2. Freedom from complications of drug therapy.

CALCIUM SALTS

Classification: Electrolyte, mineral.

Action/Kinetics: Calcium is essential for maintenance of normal function of nerves, muscles, the skeletal system, and permeability of cell membranes and capillaries. For example, calcium is necessary for activation of many enzyme reactions and is required for nerve impulses; contraction of cardiac, smooth, and skeletal muscle, renal function, respiration, and blood coagulation. It has a role in the release of neurotransmitters and hormones; in the uptake and binding of amino acids, in vitamin B_{12} absorption, and in gastrin secretion.

The normal calcium serum concentration is 9–10.4 mg/dl (4.5–5.2 mEq/L). When the calcium level of the extracellular fluid falls below this level, calcium is first mobilized from bone. However, eventually blood calcium depletion may be significant. Hypocalcemia is characterized by muscular fibrillation, twitching, skeletal muscle spasms, leg cramps, tetanic spasms, cardiac arrhythmias, smooth muscle hyperexcitability, mental depression, and anxiety states. Excessive, chronic hypocalcemia is characterized by brittle, defective nails, poor dentition, and brittle hair.

The daily RDA for elemental calcium is 0.8 g/day for adults over 25 years of age and children 1–10 years of age, 1.2 g for pregnant or lactating women and both males and females 11–24 years of age, 0.6 g for children 6–12 months of age, and 0.4 g for infants less than 6 months of age. Calcium deficiency can be corrected by the administration of various calcium salts.

Calcium is well absorbed from the upper GI tract. However, severe low-calcium tetany is best treated by IV administration of calcium gluconate.

The presence of vitamin D is necessary for maximum calcium utilization. The hormone of the parathyroid gland is necessary for the regulation of the calcium level.

Uses: IV: Acute hypocalcemic tetany secondary to renal failure, hypoparathyroidism, premature delivery, maternal diabetes mellitus in infants, and poisoning due to magnesium, oxalic acid, radiophosphorus, carbon tetrachloride, fluoride, phosphate, strontium, and radium. To treat depletion of electrolytes. Also during cardiac resuscitation when epinephrine or isoproterenol has not improved myocardial contraction (may also be given into the ventricular cavity for this purpose). To reverse cardiotoxicity or hyperkalemia.

IM or IV: Reduce spasms in renal, biliary, intestinal, or lead colic. To relieve muscle cramps due to insect bites and to decrease capillary permeability in various sensitivity reactions.

PO: Osteoporosis, osteomalacia, chronic hypoparathyroidism, rickets, latent tetany, hypocalcemia secondary to use of anticonvulsant drugs. Myasthenia gravis, Eaton-Lambert syndrome, supplement for pregnant, postmenopausal, or nursing women. Also, prophylactically for primary osteoporosis.

Investigational: As an infusion to diagnose Zollinger-Ellison syndrome and medullary thyroid carcinoma. To antagonize neuromuscular blockade due to aminoglycosides.

Contraindications: Digitalized patients, sarcoidosis, renal or cardiac disease. Cancer patients with bone metastases.

Special Concerns: Calcium requirements decrease in geriatric patients; thus, dose may have to be adjusted. Also, low levels of active vitamin D metabolites may impair calcium absorption in older patients. Use with caution in cor pulmonale, respiratory acidosis, renal disease or failure, ventricular fibrillation, hypercalcemia.

Side Effects: Excess calcium may cause hypercalcemia characterized by lassitude, fatigue, depression of nervous and neuromuscular function (emotional disturbances, confusion, skeletal muscle weakness, and constipation), impairment of renal function (polyuria, polydipsia, and azotemia), renal calculi, arrhythmias, and bradycardia.

Following PO use: GI irritation, constipation.

Following IV use: Venous irritation, tingling sensation, feeling of oppression or heat, chalky taste. Rapid IV administration may result in vasodilation, decreased blood pressure and heart rate, cardiac arrhythmias, syncope, or cardiac arrest.

Following IM use: Burning feeling, necrosis, tissue sloughing, cellulitis, soft tissue calcification.

Note: If calcium is injected into the myocardium rather than into the ventricle, laceration of coronary arteries, cardiac tamponade, pneumothorax, and ventricular fibrillation may occur.

Drug Interactions	
Cephalocin	Incompatible with calcium salts
Corticosteroids	Interfere with absorption of calcium from GI tract
Digitalis	Increased digitalis arrhythmias and toxicity. Death has resulted from combination of digitalis and IV calcium salts
Milk	Excess of either may cause hypercalcemia, renal insufficiency with azotemia, alkalosis, and ocular lesions
Tetracyclines	↓ Effect of tetracyclines due to ↓ absorption from GI tract
Verapamil	Calcium antagonizes the effect of verapamil
Vitamin D	Enhances intestinal absorption of dietary calcium

Dosage: See individual agents: calcium carbonate, calcium glubionate, calcium gluceptate, calcium gluconate, calcium lactate, dibasic calcium phosphate dihydrate.

NURSING CONSIDERATIONS

Administration/Storage

Oral

1. Administer 1–1.5 hr after meals. Alkalis and large amounts of fat decrease the absorption of calcium.
2. If the client has difficulty swallowing large tablets, obtain a calcium in water suspension. Because calcium goes into suspension six times more readily in hot water than in cold water, the solution can be prepared by diluting the medication with *hot* water. Solution may then be cooled before administering to the client.

IV

1. Administer slowly, observing vital signs closely for evidence of bradycardia and hypotension.
2. Prevent leakage of medication into the tissues. These salts are extremely irritating.

IM

1. Rotate the injection sites because this medication may cause sloughing of tissue.
2. Do not administer IM calcium gluconate to children.

Assessment

1. Note if the client is receiving digitalis products. Document and report to the physician as the drug is contraindicated.
2. Obtain baseline renal function studies to determine if renal disease if present.

Interventions

If the client goes into hypocalcemic tetany, provide appropriate safety precautions to protect the client from injury.

Client/Family Teaching

1. Explain to the client and family that calcium requirements are best met by including milk in the diet.

2. Stress that multivitamin and mineral preparations are expensive and do not contain sufficient calcium to meet the daily calcium requirements.

3. Provide the client with printed instructions concerning prescribed diet. Have a dietitian work with them to assist with proper selection of foods and meal planning.

CALCIUM CARBONATE   (KAL-see-um)

Apocal✿, BioCal, Calcarb 600, Calci-Chew, Calciday 667, Calcite 500, Calsan✿, Caltrate 300✿, Caltrate 600, Caltrate Chewable✿, Gencalc, Mega-Cal✿, Nephro-Calci, Nu-Cal, Os-Cal 250 and 500, Os-Cal 500 Chewable, Oysco 500 Chewable, Oysco, Oyst-Cal 500, Oystercall 500, Super Calcium 1200 (OTC)

See also *Calcium Salts,* p. 1137, and *Antacids,* p. 1019.

Classification: Calcium salt.

Uses: Mild hypocalcemia, antacid, antihyperphosphatemic.

Special Concerns: Dosage has not been established in children.

Dosage: Capsules, Suspension, Tablets, Chewable Tablets. *Treat hypoglycemia, nutritional supplement:* **Adults,** 1.25–1.5 g 1–3 times daily with or after meals. *Antihyperphosphatemic:* **Adults,** 5–13 g daily in divided doses with meals. *Note:* The preparation contains 40% elemental calcium and 400 mg elemental calcium/g (20 mEq/g).

> **NURSING CONSIDERATIONS**
> See Antacids, p. 1019, and Calcium Salts, p. 1137.

CALCIUM CHLORIDE

(Rx)

See also *Calcium Salts,* p. 1137.

Classification: Calcium salt.

Uses: Mild hypocalcemia, latent tetany, severe hypocalcemic tetany, magnesium intoxication, cardiac resuscitation to reverse the harmful effects of hyperkalemia.

Special Concerns: Pregnancy category: C. Use usually restricted in children due to significant irritation and possible tissue necrosis and sloughing caused by IV calcium chloride.

Additional Side Effects: Peripheral vasodilation with moderate decreases in blood pressure.

Dosage: IV only. *Hypocalcemia, replenish electrolytes:* **Adults,** 0.5–1 g q 1–3 days (given at a rate not to exceed 13.6–27.3 mg/min). **Pediatric:** 25 mg/kg given slowly. *Magnesium intoxication:* 0.5 g; observe for recovery before other doses given. *Cardiac resuscitation:* 0.5–1 g IV or 0.2–0.4 g injected into the ventricular cavity as a single dose. *Hyperkalemia:* Sufficient amount to return ECG to normal. **Never administer IM.** *Note:* The preparation contains 27.2% calcium and contains 272 mg calcium/g (13.6 mEq/g).

CALCIUM CITRATE   (KAL-see-um)

Citracal (OTC)

See also *Calcium Salts,* p. 1137.

Additional Use: Renal osteodystrophy.

Special Concerns: Dosage has not been established in children.

Dosage: Tablets. *Treat hypocalcemia:* **Adults,** 0.9–1.9 g t.i.d.–q.i.d. after meals. *Nutritional supplement:* 3.8–7.1 g daily in 3–4 divided doses. Contains 21.1% elemental calcium and 211 mg calcium/g (10.5 mEq/g).

NURSING CONSIDERATIONS
See *Nursing Considerations* for *Calcium Salts,* p. 1139.

CALCIUM GLUBIONATE   (KAL-see-um)

Neo-Calglucon (OTC)

See also *Calcium Salts,* p. 1137.

Classification: Calcium salt.

Uses: Hypocalcemia, calcium deficiency, tetany of newborn, hypoparathyroidism, pseudohypoparathyroidism, osteoporosis, rickets, osteomalacia.

Special Concerns: Pregnancy category: C.

Dosage: Syrup. *Dietary supplement:* **Adults and children over 4 years,** 15 mL t.i.d.–q.i.d. **Pediatric (under 4 years):** 10 mL t.i.d. **Infants:** 5 mL 5 times/day. *Tetany of newborn:* On the basis of laboratory tests, usually 50–150 mg/kg/day in 3 or more divided doses. *Other calcium deficiencies:* **Adult:** 15–45 mL 1–3 times daily. *Note:* The preparation contains 6.5% elemental calcium and contains 65 mg/g calcium (3.2 mEq/g).

NURSING CONSIDERATIONS
See *Nursing Considerations* for *Calcium Salts,* p. 1139.

CALCIUM GLUCEPTATE   (KAL-see-um)

(Rx)

See also *Calcium Salts,* p. 1137.

Classification: Calcium salt.

Uses: Hypocalcemia, tetany, exchange transfusion in newborns. To replenish electrolytes. Antihypermagnesemic.

Special Concerns: Pregnancy category: C. Should only be given IM to infants and children in emergency situations when the IV route is not possible.

Dosage: IM. *Treat hypocalcemia:* **Adults, IM,** 0.44–1.1 g; **IV,** 1.1–4.4 g given slowly at a rate not exceeding 36 mg calcium ion/min. **Pediatric, IM, IV:** 0.44–1.1 g; if used IV, give as a single dose at a rate not to exceed 36 mg of calcium ion/min. *Antihypermagnesemic:* **Adults,** 1.2–2.4 given slowly at a rate not to exceed 36 mg calcium ion/min. *Exchange transfusions in newborns:* **IV,** 0.11 g after every 100 mL blood exchanged. The elemental calcium content is 8.2% and there is 82 mg calcium/g (4.1 mEq/g).

NURSING CONSIDERATIONS

See *Nursing Considerations* for *Calcium Salts,* p. 1139.

Administration/Storage

In adults if more than 5 mL must be used IM, the dose should be given in the gluteal area.

CALCIUM GLUCONATE   (KAL-see-um)

Kalcinate (Rx, injection; OTC, tablets)

See also *Calcium Salts,* p. 1137.

Classification: Calcium salt.

Uses: Latent hypocalcemic tetany, severe hypocalcemic tetany. Replenish electrolytes, antihyperkalemic, antihypermagnesemic, cardiotonic.

Contraindications: Intramuscular, intramyocardial, or subcutaneous use due to severe tissue necrosis, sloughing, and abscess formation.

Dosage: Tablets. *Treatment of hypocalcemia:* **Adults,** 8.8–16.5 g daily in divided doses; **pediatric,** 0.5–0.72 g/kg daily in divided doses. *Nutritional supplement:* **Adults,** 8.8–16.5 g daily in divided doses.

    IV only. *Treatment of hypocalcemia:* **Adults,** 0.97 g given slowly at a rate not to exceed 47.5 mg calcium ion/min; dose may be repeated if necessary. **Pediatric:** 0.2–0.5 g given at the same rate as adults. *Replenish electrolyte:* **Adults,** 0.97 g given slowly at a rate not to exceed 47.5 mg calcium ion/min. *Antihyperkalemic, antihypermagnesemic:* **Adults,** 1–2 g administered slowly at a rate not to exceed 47.5 mg calcium ion/min. *Exchange transfusions in newborns:* 97 mg as a single dose administered slowly. *Note:* The preparation contains 9% calcium; also, there are 90 mg calcium/g (4.5 Eq/g).

NURSING CONSIDERATIONS

See *Nursing Considerations* for *Calcium Salts,* p. 1139.

CALCIUM LACTATE

(OTC)

See also *Calcium Salts,* p. 1137.

Classification: Calcium salt.

Uses: Latent hypocalcemic tetany, hyperphosphatemia.

Dosage: Tablets. *Treatment of hypocalcemia:* **Adults:** 7.7 g daily in divided doses with meals. **Pediatric:** 0.34–0.5 g/kg daily in divided doses. *Note:* The preparation contains 13% calcium and contains 130 mg calcium/g (6.5 mEq/g).

> **NURSING CONSIDERATIONS**
>
> See *Nursing Considerations* for *Calcium Salts,* p. 1139.

DIBASIC CALCIUM PHOSPHATE DIHYDRATE
(OTC)

See also *Calcium Salts,* p. 1137.

Classification: Calcium salt.

Uses: Calcium deficiency states, dietary supplement.

Special Concerns: Increased risk of hypoparathyroidism or hyperphosphatemia in patients with renal insufficiency.

Dosage: Tablets. *Treatment of hypocalcemia:* **Adults:** 4.4 g daily in divided doses with or after meals; **pediatric:** 0.2–0.28 g/kg daily in divided doses with or after meals. *Note:* This preparation contains 23% calcium and contains 230 mg calcium/g (11.5 mEq/g).

> **NURSING CONSIDERATIONS**
>
> See *Nursing Considerations* for *Calcium Salts,* p. 1139.
>
> **Administration/Storage**
>
> Should be taken with meals in clients with achlorhydria or hypochlorhydria.

MISCELLANEOUS AGENTS

CELLULOSE SODIUM PHOSPHATE   (SELL-you-lohs)
Calcibind (Rx)

Classification: Calcium-binding agent.

Action/Kinetics: Sodium cellulose phosphate is a synthetic ion exchange substance that exchanges sodium for calcium and magnesium ions in the GI tract thus preventing absorption. The bound calcium, from both dietary and endogenous sources, is excreted in the feces. Thus, urinary calcium is decreased. There are small increases in urinary phosphorous and oxalate. Excreted through the feces as a calcium-cellulose phosphate complex.

Uses: Decrease incidence of new renal stone formation in absorptive hypercalciuria Type I. Diagnostic test for causes of hypercalciuria other than hyperabsorption.

Contraindications: Primary or secondary hyperparathyroidism, hypocalcemia, hypomagnesemia, enteric hyperoxaluria, osteoporosis, osteomalacia, osteitis, low intestinal absorption or renal excretion of calcium, when hypercalciuria is due to mobilization from bones. Children under age 16.

Special Concerns: Pregnancy category: C. Use with caution in congestive heart failure, or ascites.

Side Effects: *GI:* Diarrhea, dyspepsia, loose bowel movements. *Other:* Hyperparathyroid bone disease, hyperoxaluria, hypomagnesiuria, loss of copper, zinc, iron.

Dosage: Oral Suspension. *Urinary calcium greater than 300 mg/day:* 5 g with each meal; *urinary calcium less than 150 mg/day:* 2.5 g with breakfast and lunch and 5 g with dinner.

NURSING CONSIDERATIONS

Administration/Storage

1. Parathyroid hormone levels should be monitored at least once between 2 weeks and 3 months after therapy has been initiated.
2. A moderate calcium intake is recommended.
3. Mix each dose of sodium cellulose phosphate with water, juice, or soft drink, and take within 30 min of the meal.
4. Foods such as dark greens (e.g., spinach), rhubarb, chocolate, and brewed tea should be avoided as they contain oxalate. Vitamin C should also be avoided as it is metabolized to oxalate.
5. Sufficient fluid should be taken daily to ensure a minimum urine output of 2 L.
6. Magnesium gluconate supplements may be given as follows:
   - 1.5 g magnesium gluconate before breakfast and at bedtime for clients receiving 15 g of sodium cellulose phosphate daily,
   - 1 g magnesium gluconate, as above, in clients taking 10 g sodium cellulose phosphate daily.
   - To avoid binding, magnesium should be given either 1 hr before or 1 hr after sodium cellulose phosphate.
7. Treatment should be stopped if urinary oxalate is greater than 55 mg/day with moderate dietary oxalate restriction.
8. Magnesium, iron, and other trace-metal supplements may be ordered.

Client/Family Teaching

1. Advise the client to take the medication with meals to maximize the uptake of dietary calcium.
2. Advise the client to avoid ingesting calcium-containing foods such as milk, cheese, or ice cream.
3. Explain the need to avoid eating spinach and dark green vegetables, rhubarb, chocolate, and brewed tea. All of these contain oxalates, which may lead to calcium stone formation.
4. Advise the client to avoid taking vitamin C supplements, salt, and lightly salted foods.
5. Discuss the need to drink plenty of fluids. The urinary output should be 2 L/day.

ETIDRONATE DISODIUM (ORAL)   (eh-tih-**DROH**-nayt)

Didronel (Rx)

ETIDRONATE DISODIUM (PARENTERAL)   (eh-tih-**DROH**-nayt)

Didronel IV (Rx)

Classification: Bone growth regulator, antihypercalcemic.

Action/Kinetics: Paget's disease is characterized by bone resorption, compensatory new bone formation, and increased vascularization of the bone. Etidronate disodium slows bone metabolism, thereby decreasing bone resorption, bone turnover, and new bone formation; it also reduces bone vascularization. Renal tubular reabsorption of calcium is not affected. **Absorption:** Dose-dependent; after 24 hr, one-half of absorbed drug is excreted unchanged. **Onset:** 1 month for Paget's disease and within 24 hr for hypercalcemia. The drug remaining in the body is absorbed to bone, where therapeutic effects for Paget's disease persist 3–12 months after discontinuation of the drug. **Plasma t$^{1}/_{2}$:** 6 hr. Approximately 50% excreted unchanged in the urine; unabsorbed drug is excreted through the feces.

Uses: *Oral:* Paget's disease (osteitis deformans), especially of the polyostotic type accompanied by pain and increased urine levels of hydroxyproline and serum alkaline phosphatase. Heterotopic ossification due to spinal cord injury or total hip replacement.

Parenteral: Hypercalcemia due to malignancy, which is not responsive to hydration or dietary control.

Contraindications: Enterocolitis, fracture of long bones, hypercalcemia of hyperparathyroidism.

Special Concerns: Pregnancy category: B for tablets and C for parenteral form. Use with caution in the presence of renal dysfunction and during lactation. Dosage has not been established in children.

Side Effects: *GI:* Nausea, diarrhea, loose bowel movements. *Bones:* Increased incidence of bone fractures and increased or recurrent bone pain. Drug should be discontinued if fracture occurs and not restarted until healing takes place. *Allergy:* Angioedema, rash, pruritus, urticaria. Symptoms of rachitic syndrome have been reported in children receiving 10 mg or more/kg daily for long periods (up to 1 year) to treat heterotopic ossification or soft tissue calcification.

Dosage: Tablets. *Paget's disease:* **Adults, initial:** 5–10 mg/kg/day for 6 months or less; 11 mg/kg up to a maximum of 20 mg/kg/day for patients when bone metabolism suppression is highly advisable; treatment at this dose level should not exceed 3 months. Another course of therapy may be instituted after rest period of 3 months.

Heterotopic ossification due to spinal cord injury: **Adults:** 20 mg/kg/day for 2 weeks; **then** 10 mg/kg/day for 10 weeks. *Heterotopic ossification complicating total hip replacement:* 20 mg/kg/day for 30 days preoperatively; **then,** 20 mg/kg/day for 90 days postoperatively.

Hypercalcemia: **Adults:** 20 mg/kg daily for 30 days (up to a maximum of 90 days).

IV infusion. *Hypercalcemia due to malignancy:* 7.5 mg/kg daily for 3 successive days. If necessary, a second course of treatment may be instituted after a 3-day rest period. The safety and effectiveness of more than 2 courses of therapy has not been determined. Etidronate tablets may be started the day after the last infusion at a dose of 20 mg/kg daily for 30 days (treatment may be extended to 90 days if serum calcium levels are normal). Use for more than 90 days is not recommended.

NURSING CONSIDERATIONS

Administration/Storage

1. Administer as a single dose of medication with juice or water 2 hr before meals.
2. Urinary hydroxyproline excretion and/or serum alkaline phosphatase levels should be determined periodically when the drug is given for Paget's disease.
3. There are no indications to date that etidronate will affect mature heterotopic bone.
4. The IV dose must be diluted in at least 250 mL of sterile normal saline.
5. The IV dose, diluted, should be administered over a period of 2 hr.

Assessment

1. Note if the client has any evidence of renal dysfunction. Obtain baseline renal function studies and monitor during drug therapy.
2. If the client is of childbearing age and is sexually active, determine the possibility of pregnancy.

Client/Family Teaching

1. Assist the client and family in understanding the importance of maintaining a well-balanced diet with adequate intake of calcium and vitamin D.
2. Advise clients not to eat for 2 hr after taking medication because foods particularly high in calcium may reduce the absorption of the drug.

Evaluation

Determine levels of urinary hydroxyproline excretion and serum alkaline phosphatase because reduction in these levels is the first indication of a beneficial therapeutic response. Levels usually decrease 1–3 months after initiation of therapy.

TERIPARATIDE ACETATE   (ter-ih-**par**-ah-tyd)

Parathar (Rx)

Classification: Diagnostic agent, hypoparathyroidism.

Action/Kinetics: Teriparatide is a synthetic hormone consisting of the 1–34 fragment of human parathyroid hormone. The drug will initially cause an increased rate of calcium release from bone into blood. The most sensitive indicator for determining the type of hypoparathyroidism is the change in urinary cyclic AMP during the 0–30 minute postinfusion period. Patients with hypoparathyroidism will show up to a tenfold or greater increase over baseline of urinary cyclic AMP in the 0–30 minute postinfusion period. Over 90% of these patients will also show a threefold or greater increase in urinary phosphate excretion in the 0–60 minute postinfusion period. On the other hand, patients with pseudohypoparathyroidism will show less than a sixfold increase in urinary cyclic AMP excretion in the 0–30 minute postinfusion period and less than a threefold increase in urinary phosphate excretion in the 0–60 minute postinfusion period. **Time to peak excretion of AMP:** During the first 30 min after infusion; **time to peak excretion of phosphate:** during the second 30 min after infusion.

Uses: To determine the presence of either hypoparathyroidism or pseudohypoparathryoidism in patients manifesting hypocalcemia.

Special Concerns: Pregnancy category: C. Use with caution during lactation.

Side Effects: *Metabolic:* Hypercalcemia. *GI:* Nausea, diarrhea, abdominal cramps, urge to defecate. *Miscellaneous:* Metallic taste, tingling of extremities, pain at injection site (during or following infusion), allergic reactions.

Dosage: IV. Adults: 5 units/kg infused in 10 mL over 10 min up to a maximum of 200 units. **Pediatric, over than 3 years of age:** 3 units/kg, not to exceed 200 units, infused over 10 min.

NURSING CONSIDERATIONS

Administration/Storage

1. The test will distinguish between hypoparathyroidism and pseudohypoparathyroidism but not between these conditions and normal parathyroid function.

2. Clients should be fasting when the drug is administered. To maintain an active urine output during the test, 200 mL water should be ingested per hr for 2 hr before the study as well as during the study.

3. A baseline urine collection should be made during the 60-min period preceding infusion of the drug. Following infusion of the drug, urine should be collected during the 0–30, 30–60, and 60–120 min postinfusion periods.

4. Accuracy of the test will be affected by adequate hydration and urine flow, as well as complete collection of urine samples.

5. The reconstituted solution should be used within 4 hr.

6. Have epinephrine 1:1,000 available in the event of an allergic reaction.

Assessment

Assess baseline urinary output.

Interventions

Monitor the client's vital signs, especially the BP, during the test.

Client/Family Teaching

1. Instruct the client to fast for the test.

2. Provide printed guidelines for hydration and preparation for the test.

3. Explain that the client may experience a metallic taste in the mouth and pain at the site of the injection during administration of the drug.

CHAPTER SIXTY-ONE

Adrenocorticosteroids and Analogs

ADRENOCORTICOSTEROIDS AND ANALOGS

Action/Kinetics: The adrenocorticosteroids are a group of natural hormones produced by the adrenal cortex (outer shell of the adrenal gland). They are used for a variety of therapeutic purposes. Many slightly modified synthetic variants are available today, and some patients respond better to one substance than to another.

The hormones of the adrenal gland influence many metabolic pathways and all organ systems and are essential for survival.

The release of adrenocorticosteroids is controlled by hormones such as corticotropin-releasing factor, produced by the hypothalamus, and ACTH (corticotropin), produced by the anterior pituitary.

The adrenocorticosteroids play an important role in most major metabolic processes. They have the following effects:

1. **Carbohydrate metabolism.** Deposition of glucose as glycogen in the liver and the conversion of glycogen to glucose when needed. Gluconeogenesis (i.e., the transformation of protein into glucose).
2. **Protein metabolism.** The stimulation of protein loss from many organs (catabolism). This is characterized by a negative nitrogen balance.
3. **Fat metabolism.** The deposition of fatty tissue in facial, abdominal, and shoulder regions.
4. **Water and electrolyte balance.** Alteration of glomerular filtration rate; increased sodium and consequently fluid retention. Also affects the excretion rate of potassium, calcium, and phosphorus. Urinary excretion rate of creatine and uric acid increases.

The hormones have a marked anti-inflammatory effect by virtue of their ability to inhibit prostaglandin synthesis. These agents also inhibit accumulation of macrophages and leukocytes at sites of inflammation as well as inhibit phagocytosis and lysosomal enzyme release. They aid the organism to cope with various stressful situations (trauma, severe illness). The immunosuppressant effect is thought to be due to a reduction of the number of T-lymphocytes, monocytes, and eosinophils. Adrenocorticosteroids also decrease binding of immunoglobulin to receptors on the cell surface and inhibit the synthesis and/or release of interleukins which, in turn, decrease T-lymphocyte blastogenesis and reduce the primary immune response.

According to their chemical structure and chief physiologic effect, the adrenocorticosteroids fall into two subgroups, which have considerable functional overlap.

1. Those, like cortisone and hydrocortisone, that mainly regulate the metabolic pathways involving protein, carbohydrate, and fat. This group is often referred to as *glucocorticoids*. Glucocorticoids are qualitatively similar. Differences between these agents are due to duration of action and half-life (see individual agents).
2. Those, like aldosterone and desoxycorticosterone, that are more specifically involved in electrolyte and water balance. These are often referred to as *mineralocorticoids*. Hormones with mineralocorticoid activity result in reabsorption of sodium (and therefore water retention) and enhanced potassium and hydrogen excretion. Substances such as cortisone and hydrocortisone, although classified as glucocorticoids, possess significant mineralocorticoid activity.

Uses: When used for anti-inflammatory or immunosuppressant therapy, the corticosteroid should possess minimal mineralocorticoid activity. Therapy with glucocorticoids is not curative and in many situations should be considered as adjunctive rather than primary therapy.

1. **Replacement therapy.** Acute and chronic adrenal insufficiency, including Addison's disease,

61

congenital adrenal hyperplasia, adrenal insufficiency secondary to anterior pituitary insufficiency. However, not all drugs can be used for replacement therapy; some lack glucocorticoid effects while others lack mineralocorticoid effects. For replacement therapy, drugs must possess both effects.

2. **Rheumatic disorders.** Rheumatoid arthritis (including juveniles), ankylosing spondylitis, acute and subacute bursitis, acute nonspecific tenosynovitis, acute gouty arthritis, psoriatic arthritis, posttraumatic osteoarthritis, synovitis of osteoarthritis, epicondylitis.

3. **Collagen diseases.** Including systemic lupus erythematosus, acute rheumatic carditis, polymyositis, polyarteritis nodosa.

4. **Allergic diseases.** Control of severe allergic conditions refractory to conventional treatment as serum sickness, drug hypersensitivity reactions, anaphylaxis, urticarial transfusion reactions.

5. **Respiratory diseases.** Including bronchial asthma (and status asthmaticus), symptomatic sarcoidosis, seasonal or perennial rhinitis, berylliosis, aspiration pneumonitis.

6. **Ocular diseases.** Including allergic and inflammatory conjunctivitis, keratitis, herpes zoster ophthalmicus, iritis, iridocyclitis, chorioretinitis, diffuse posterior uveitis and choroiditis, optic neuritis, iritis, allergic corneal marginal ulcers.

7. **Dermatologic diseases.** Including severe erythema multiforme (Stevens-Johnson syndrome), exfoliative dermatitis, mycosis fungoides, severe seborrheic dermatitis, bullous dermatitis herpetiformis, severe psoriasis, angioedema or urticaria, contact dermatitis, atopic dermatitis, pemphigus. *Note:* See Table 24, p. 1154.

8. **Diseases of the intestinal tract.** Including chronic ulcerative colitis, regional enteritis, intractable sprue.

9. **Nervous system.** Myasthenia gravis.

10. **Malignancies.** Including leukemias and lymphomas in adults and acute leukemia in children.

11. **Nephrotic syndrome.**

12. **Hematologic diseases.** Including acquired hemolytic anemia, red blood cell anemia, idiopathic and secondary thrombocytopenic purpura, congenital hypoplastic anemia.

13. **Intra-articular or soft tissue administration.** To treat acute episodes of synovitis of osteoarthritis, rheumatoid arthritis, acute gouty arthritis, epicondylitis, acute nonspecific tenosynovitis, posttraumatic osteoarthritis.

14. **Intralesional administration.** To treat keloids, psoriatic plaques, granuloma annulare, lichen simplex chronicus, discoid lupus erythematosus, cystic tumors of an aponeurosis or ganglia, lesions of lichen planus.

15. **Miscellaneous.** Septic shock (use controversial), adult respiratory distress syndrome (use controversial), hirsutism, active and alcoholic hepatitis, certain types of cirrhosis. The effectiveness of corticosteroids in these situations remains unclear.

Contraindications: Corticosteroids are contraindicated in any situation where infection may be suspected, as these drugs may mask infections. Also peptic ulcer, psychoses, acute glomerulonephritis, herpes simplex infections of the eye, vaccinia or varicella, the exanthematous diseases, Cushing's syndrome, active tuberculosis, myasthenia gravis. Recent intestinal anastomoses, congestive heart failure or other cardiac disease, hypertension, systemic fungal infections, open-angle glaucoma. Also, hyperlipidemia, hyperthyroidism or hypothyroidism, osteoporosis, myasthenia gravis, tuberculosis. Lactation (if high doses are used).

Topical application in the treatment of eye disorders is contraindicated in dendritic keratitis, vaccinia, chickenpox, or other viral disease that may involve the conjunctiva or cornea. Also tuberculosis and fungal or acute purulent infections of the eye. Topical treatment of the ear is contraindicated in aural fungal infections and perforated eardrum. Topical use in dermatology contraindicated in tuberculosis of the skin, herpes simplex, vaccinia, varicella, and infectious conditions in the absence of anti-infective agents.

Special Concerns: Adrenoglucocorticoids should be used with caution in the presence of diabetes mellitus, hypertension, chronic nephritis, thrombophlebitis, convulsive disorders, infectious diseases, renal or hepatic insufficiency, pregnancy. Chronic use of corticosteroids may inhibit the growth and development of children or adolescents. Pediatric patients are also at greater risk for developing cataracts, osteoporosis, avascular necrosis of the femoral heads, and glaucoma. Geriatric patients are more likely to develop hypertension and osteoporosis (especially post-menopausal women).

Side Effects: Small physiologic doses given as replacement therapy or short-term high-dosage therapy during emergencies rarely cause side effects. Prolonged therapy may cause a Cushing-like syndrome with atrophy of the adrenal cortex and subsequent adrenocortical insufficiency. A steroid withdrawal syndrome may occur following prolonged use; symptoms include anorexia, nausea, vomiting, lethargy, headache, fever, joint pain, desquamation, myalgia, weight loss, hypotension.

Fluid and electrolyte: Edema, hypokalemic alkalosis, hypokalemia, hypertension, congestive heart failure. *Musculoskeletal:* Muscle wasting, muscle pain or weakness, osteoporosis, vertebral compression fractures, delayed wound healing. *GI:* Nausea, vomiting, anorexia or increased appetite, diarrhea or constipation, abdominal distention, pancreatitis, gastric irritation, ulcerative esophagitis. Development or exacerbation of peptic ulcers. *Endocrine:* Cushing's syndrome, amenorrhea, decreased glucose tolerance, hyperglycemia, diabetes mellitus. *CNS:* Headache, vertigo, insomnia, restlessness, increased motor activity, ischemic neuropathy, EEG abnormalities, seizures. Also, euphoria, mood swings, depression, anxiety, personality changes, psychoses. *Dermatologic:* Skin atrophy and thinning, acne, increased sweating, hirsutism, facial erythema, striae, petechiae, ecchymoses, easy bruising. *Allergic:* Allergic dermatitis, urticaria, angioedema, burning or tingling of perineal area following IV use. *Miscellaneous:* Hypercholesterolemia, atherosclerosis, thrombosis, thromboembolism, fat embolism, thrombophlebitis. **In children:** Suppression of linear growth; reversible pseudobrain tumor syndrome characterized by papilledema, oculomotor or abducens nerve paralysis, visual loss, or headache.

Intra-Articular

Postinjection flare, Charcot-like arthropathy. Due to reduction in inflammation and pain, patients may overuse the joint.

Eye Therapy

Application of corticosteroid preparations to the eye may reduce aqueous outflow and increase ocular pressure, thereby inducing or aggravating simple glaucoma. Ocular pressure therefore should be checked frequently in the elderly or in patients with glaucoma. Stinging, burning, dendritic keratitis (herpes simplex), corneal perforation (especially when the drugs are used for diseases that cause corneal thinning). Posterior subcapsular cataracts, especially in children. Exophthalmos, secondary fungal or viral eye infections.

Topical Use

Except when used over large areas, when the skin is broken, or with occlusive dressings, topically applied corticosteroids are not absorbed systemically in sufficiently large quantities to cause the untoward reactions noted in the previous paragraphs. Topically applied corticosteroids, however, may cause atrophy of the epidermis, drying of the skin, or atrophy of the dermal collagen. When used on the face, the agents may cause diffuse thinning and homogenization of the collagen, epidermal thinning, and striae formation. Topical corticosteroids should be used cautiously, or not at all, for infected lesions, and in that case, the use of occlusive dressings is contraindicated. Occasionally, topical corticosteroids may cause a sensitization reaction, which necessitates discontinuation of the drug.

Drug Interactions

Acetaminophen	↑ Risk of hepatotoxicity due to ↑ rate of formation of hepatotoxic acetaminophen metabolite
Alcohol	↑ Risk of GI ulceration or hemorrhage
Amphotericin B	Corticosteroids ↑ K depletion caused by amphotericin B
Aminoglutethimide	Aminoglutethimide ↓ adrenal response to corticotropin
Anabolic steroids	↑ Risk of edema
Antacids	↓ Effect of corticosteroids due to ↓ absorption from GI tract
Antibiotics, broad-spectrum	Concomitant use may result in emergence of resistant strains, leading to severe infection
Anticholinergics	Combination ↑ intraocular pressure; will aggravate glaucoma
Anticoagulants, oral	↓ Effect of anticoagulants by ↓ hypoprothrombinemia; also ↑ risk of hemorrhage due to vascular effects of corticosteroids
Antidiabetic agents	Hyperglycemic effect of corticosteroids may necessitate an ↑ dose of antidiabetic agent
Asparaginase	↑ Hyperglycemic effect of asparaginase and the risk of neuropathy and disturbances in erythropoiesis
Barbiturates	↓ Effect of corticosteroids due to ↑ breakdown by liver
Bumetanide	Enhanced K loss due to K-losing properties of both drugs
Carbonic anhydrase inhibitors	Corticosteroids ↑ K depletion caused by carbonic anhydrase inhibitors
Cholestyramine	↓ Effect of corticosteroids due to ↓ absorption from GI tract
Colestipol	↓ Effect of corticosteroids due to ↓ absorption from GI tract
Contraceptives, oral	Estrogen ↑ anti-inflammatory effect of hydrocortisone by ↓ breakdown by liver
Cyclophosphoramide	↑ Effect of cyclophosphoramide due to ↓ breakdown by liver
Cyclosporine	↑ Effect of both drugs due to ↓ breakdown by liver
Digitalis glycosides	↑ Chance of digitalis toxicity (arrhythmias) due to hypokalemia
Ephedrine	↓ Effect of corticosteroids due to ↑ breakdown by liver

Drug Interactions

Estrogens	Estrogens ↑ anti-inflammatory effect of hydrocortisone by ↓ breakdown by liver
Ethacrynic acid	Enhanced K loss due to K-losing properties of both drugs
Folic acid	Folic acid requirements may be increased
Furosemide	Enhanced K loss due to K-losing properties of both drugs
Heparin	Ulcerogenic effects of corticosteroids may → ↑ risk of hemorrhage
Immunosuppressant drugs	↑ Risk of infection
Indomethacin	↑ Chance of GI ulceration
Insulin	Hyperglycemic effect of corticosteroids may necessitate an ↑ dose of antidiabetic agent
Isoniazid	↓ Effect of isoniazid due to ↑ breakdown by liver and ↑ excretion
Mexiletine	↓ Effect of mexiletine due to ↑ breakdown by liver
Mitotane	Mitotane ↓ response of adrenal gland to corticotropin
Muscle relaxants, nondepolarizing	↓ Effect of muscle relaxants
Neuromuscular blocking agents	↑ Risk of prolonged respiratory depression or paralysis
Nonsteroidal anti-inflammatory agents	↑ Risk of GI hemorrhage or ulceration
Phenobarbital	↓ Effect of corticosteroids due to ↑ breakdown by liver
Phenytoin	↓ Effect of corticosteroids due to ↑ breakdown by liver
Potassium supplements	↓ Plasma levels of potassium
Rifampin	↓ Effect of corticosteroids due to ↑ breakdown by liver
Ritodrine	↑ Risk of maternal edema
Salicylates	Both are ulcerogenic; also, corticosteroids may ↓ blood salicylate levels
Somatrem, Somatropin	Glucocorticoids may inhibit effect of somatrem
Streptozocin	↑ Risk of hyperglycemia
Theophyllines	Corticosteroids ↑ effect of theophyllines
Thiazide diuretics	Enhanced K loss due to K-losing properties of both drugs
Tricyclic antidepressants	↑ Risk of mental disturbances
Vitamin A	Topical vitamin A can reverse impaired wound healing in patients receiving corticosteroids

Laboratory Test Interferences: ↑ Urine glucose, serum cholesterol, serum amylase. ↓ Serum potassium, triiodothyronine, serum uric acid. Alteration of electrolyte balance.

Dosage: Dosage is highly individualized, according to both the condition being treated and the response of the patient. Although the various adrenocorticosteroids are similar in their actions, patients may respond better to one type of drug than to another. It is most important that therapy not be discontinued abruptly. Except for replacement therapy, treatment should always involve the minimum effective dose and the shortest period of time. Long-term use often causes severe side effects. If corticosteroids are used for replacement therapy or high doses are used for prolonged periods of time, the dose must be *increased* if surgery is required.

For topical use, ointment, cream, lotion, solution, plastic tape, aerosol suspension, and aerosol cream are selected, depending on dermatologic condition to be treated. See Table 24.

Table 24   Corticosteroids Used Topically

Drug	Dosage/Administration
Alclometasone Dipropionate (Aclovate) (Rx)	Apply cream (0.05%) or ointment (0.05%) b.i.d.–t.i.d. on affected area. Massage gently until medication is gone. Occlusive dressings may be used for refractory psoriasis or deep-seated dermatoses.
Amcinonide (Cyclocort) (Rx)	Apply cream (0.1%), lotion (0.1%), or ointment (0.1%) b.i.d.–t.i.d. sparingly and rub in.
Betamethasone benzoate (Beben✿, Uticort) (Rx)	Apply cream, gel, or lotion (each 0.025%) sparingly b.i.d.–q.i.d. and rub in.
Betamethasone dipropionate (Alphalex, Diprolene✿, Diprosone, Maxivate) (Rx)	Apply aerosol (0.1%), cream (0.05%), lotion (0.5%), or ointment (0.05%) sparingly and rub in 1–2 times daily (t.i.d. for the aerosol).
Betamethasone dipropionate, augmented (Diprolene, Diprolene AF) (Rx)	Apply cream, lotion, or ointment (each 0.05%) sparingly b.i.d.–q.i.d. and rub in.
Betamethasone valerate (Betaderm✿, Betatrex, Beta-Val, Betnoate-1/2✿, Betnovate✿, Celestoderm-V✿, Celestoderm-V/2✿, Ectosone Mild✿, Ectosone Regular✿, Ectosone Scalp Lotion, Metaderm Mild✿, Metaderm Regular, Valisone, Valisone Valisone Reduced Strength, Valisone Scalp Lotion) (Rx)	Apply cream (0.01%, 0.1%), lotion (0.1%), or ointment (0.1%) sparingly and rub in.
Clobetasol propionate (Dermovate, Temovate) (Rx)	Apply cream or ointment (each 0.05%) to affected area b.i.d.–t.i.d. Treatment should be limited to 14 days. Not to be used with occlusive dressings.
Clocortolone pivalate (Cloderm) (Rx)	Apply cream (0.1%) sparingly t.i.d. and rub in.
Desonide (DesOwen, Tridesilon) (Rx)	**Adults:** Apply a thin film of cream or ointment (each 0.05%) b.i.d.–q.i.d. **Pediatric:** Apply to skin once daily.
Desoximetasone (Topicort, Topicort LP, Topicort Mild✿) (Rx)	Apply a thin film of cream (0.05% or 0.25%), gel (0.05%), or ointment (0.25%) b.i.d (for pediatrics, use once daily).

Table 24 *(continued)*

Drug	**Dosage/Administration**
Dexamethasone (Aeroseb-Dex, Decaderm, Decaspray) (Rx)	Apply aerosol (0.01%, 0.04%) or gel (0.1%) b.i.d.–q.i.d.
Dexamethasone ophthalmic (Maxidex) (Rx)	**Suspension** (0.1%): Apply 1–2 gtt to conjunctiva 4–6 times daily
Dexamethasone sodium phosphate (Decadron) (Rx)	Apply cream (0.1%) t.i.d.–q.i.d. (once daily. for children) and rub in lightly.
Dexamthasone sodium phosphate ophthalmic (AK-Dex Ophthalmic, Baldex, Decadron, Dexair, Dexotic, I-Methasone, Ocu-Dex) (Rx) (Rx)	**Solution** (0.1%): **initial,** 1–2 drops in conjunctival sac q hr during day and q 2 hr during night until a favorable response is obtained; **then,** decrease to 1 drop q 4 hr to 1 drop t.i.d.–q.i.d. **Ointment** (0.05%): **initial,** instill a small amount in conjunctival sac t.i.d.–q.i.d.; **then,** decrease to b.i.d. and then once daily.
Diflorasone diacetate (Florone, Florone E, Maxiflor, Psorcon) (Rx)	Apply cream (0.05%) or ointment (0.05%) sparingly 1–4 times daily and rub in.
Fluocinolone acetonide (Bio-Syn, Fluocet, Fluoderm✤, Fluolar✤, Fluonid, Fluonide✤, Fluosyn, Synalar, Synalar-HP, Synamol✤, Synemol) (Rx)	**Adults:** Apply cream (0.01%, 0.025%, 0.2%), ointment (0.025%) or solution (0.01%) b.i.d.–q.i.d. **Pediatric:** Apply 0.01% cream 1–2 times daily, 0.025 or 0.2% cream once daily, 0.025% ointment once daily, or 0.01% solution 1–2 times daily.
Fluocinonide (Fluocin, Licon, Lidemol✤, Lidex, Lidex-E, Lyderm✤, Metosyn Scalp Solution, Topsyn) (Rx)	Apply a thin film of cream, gel, ointment, or solution (each 0.05%) b.i.d.–q.i.d. (once daily for children).
Fluorometholone (Fluor-Op, FML Forte, FML Liquifilm, FML S.O.P.) (Rx)	**Suspension** (ophthalmic, 0.1%, 0.25%): **initially,** 1–2 drops into conjunctival sac q hr during day and q 2 hr at night until improvement is noted; **then,** reduce dose to 1 gtt q 4 hr and later to 1 gtt t.i.d.–q.i.d. **Ointment** (ophthalmic, 0.1%): **initial,** instill a small amount in conjunctival sac t.i.d.–q.i.d. until improvement noted; **then,** reduce to b.i.d. and then once daily.
Flurandrenolide (Cordran, Cordran SP, Drenison✤, Dremison-1/4) (Rx)	**Adults:** Apply cream (0.025%, 0.05%), lotion (0.05%), or ointment (0.025%, 0.05%) b.i.d.–t.i.d. (1–2 times daily for children). Tape (4 mcg/sq cm) is applied as occlusive dressing; change q 12 hr. Protect from light, heat, and freezing.

Table 24 *(continued)*

Drug	**Dosage/Administration**
Halcinoide (Halog, Halog-E) (Rx)	Apply cream (0.025%, 0.1%), ointment (0.1%), or solution (0.1%) b.i.d.–t.i.d. (once a day for children). Can be used with an occlusive dressing during night (12 hr); use without occlusion during day.

Hydrocortisone
    Cream, Rectal: Proctocort (Rx).
    Cream, Topical: Ala-Cort, Allercort, Bactine, Barriere-HC♣, Cort-Dome, Cortate♣, Cortifair, Dermacort, DermiCort, Dermolate Anti-Itch, Dermtex HC, Emocort♣, H₂Cort, Hi-Cor 1.0 and 2.5, Hydro-Tex, Hytone, Lemoderm, Nutricort, Penecort, Synacort, Unicort♣ (Rx and OTC).
    Lotion: Acticort 100, Ala-Cort, Ala-Scalp HP, Allercort, Cetacort, Cort-Dome, Cortate, Delacort, Dermacort, Dermolate Scalp-Itch, Emo-Cort, Gly-Cort, Hytone, LactiCare-HC, Lemoderm, Lexocort Forte, My Cort, Nutracort, Pentacort, Rederm, Sarna HC 1.0%, S-T Cort (Rx).
    Ointment: Allercort, Cortate, Cortef, Cortril, Dermolate Anal Itch, Hytone, Lemoderm, Penecort (Rx).
    Topical Solution: Emo-Cort Scalp Solution, Penecort, Texacort Scalp Solution (Rx).
    Topical Aerosol Solution: Aeroseb-HC, CaldeCORT Anti-Itch (Rx).
    Topical Spray Solution: Cortaid, Dermolate Anti-Itch (Rx).
	Apply cream (0.25%, 0.5%, 1%, 2.5%), lotion (0.25%, 0.5%, 1%, 2%, 2.5%), ointment (0.5%, 1%, 2.5%), topical solution (1%, 2.5%), topical aerosol (0.5%), topical spray (0.5%) 1–4 times daily depending on the dosage form. Medication should be rubbed in.

Hydrocortisone Acetate
    Cream, Rectal: Anusol HC, Corticaine (Rx).
    Cream, Topical: CaldeCORT Anti-Itch, CaldeCORT Light, Carmol-HC, Cortacet♣, Cortaid, Cortef Feminine Itch, Corticreme♣, FoilleCort, Gynecort, Hyderm♣, Lanacort, Novohydrocort♣, Pharma-Cort, Rhulicort (OTC and Rx).
    Lotion: Cortaid, Rhulicort (OTC).
    Ointment: Cortaid, Cortef Acetate, Cortoderm♣, Lanacort, Novohydrocort♣ (OTC and Rx).
    Rectal Suppositories: Anusol HC, Cort-Dome High Potency, Cortiment-10 and -40 (Rx).
    Topical Aerosol Foam: Epifoam (Rx).
	Apply cream (0.5%, 1%), lotion (0.5%), ointment (0.5%, 1%), or topical aerosol foam (1%) 1–4 times daily, depending on the dosage form.

Table 24 (*continued*)

Drug	Dosage/Administration
Hydrocortisone butyrate (Locoid) (Rx)	Apply cream (0.1% or ointment (0.1%) sparingly b.i.d.–t.i.d. (1–2 times daily for children) and rub in.
Hydrocortisone valerate (Westcort) (Rx)	Apply cream (0.2%) or ointment (0.2%) sparingly b.i.d.–t.i.d. (once daily for children) and rub in.
Medrysone (HMS Liquifilm) (Rx)	**Adults and children:** Apply suspension (1%) sparingly and rub in.
Methylprednisolone acetate (Medrol) (Rx)	Apply ointment (0.25%, 1%) sparingly 1–4 times daily and rub in.
Mometasone furoate (Elocon) (Rx)	Apply a thin film of the cream (0.1%) or ointment (0.1%) once daily to affected areas. Occlusive dressings should not be used.
Prednisolone acetate ophthalmic (AK-Tate Enconopred, Econopred Plus, Ocu-Pred-A, Predair A, Pred Forte, Pred Mild, Ultra Pred) (Rx)	Instill 1–2 gtt of the suspension (0.12%, 0.125%, 1%) into the conjunctival sac q hr during the day and q 2 hr during the night initially until a response is obtained; then, decrease dose to 1 gtt q 4 hr and then 1 gtt t.i.d.–q.i.d.
Prednisolone sodium phosphate ophthalmic (AK-Pred, Inflamase Forte, Inflamase Mild, I-Pred, Lite-Pred, Ocu-Pred, Ocu-Pred Forte, Predair, Predair Forte (Rx)	See *Prednisolone acetate ophthalmic.*
Triamcinolone acetonide **Cream:** Aristocort, Aristocort A, Aristocort C✿, Aristocort D✿, Aristocort R✿, Delat-Tritex, Flutex, Kenac, Kenalog, Kenalog-H, Kenonel, Triacet, Triaderm✿, Trianide Mild✿, Trianide Regular✿, Triderm, Trymex (Rx). **Dental Paste:** Kenalog in Orabase, Oracort, Oralone (Rx). **Lotion:** Kenalog, Kenonel (Rx). **Ointment:** Aristocort, Aristocort A, Aristocort D✿, Aristocort R✿, Kenac, Kenalog, Kenonel, Triaderm✿, Trymex (Rx). **Topical Aerosol:** Kenalog (Rx).	Apply cream (0.025%, 0.1%, 0.5%), lotion (0.025%, 0.1%), ointment (0.025%, 0.1%, 0.5%), or topical aerosol (0.015%) b.i.d.–q.i.d., depending on the dosage form. Apply dental paste (0.1%) b.i.d.–t.i.d. after meals and at bedtime.

*All products are Pregnancy Category: C.

Lotions are considered best for weeping eruptions, especially in areas subject to chafing (axilla, feet, and groin). Creams are suitable for most inflammations; ointments are preferred for dry, scaly lesions.

NURSING CONSIDERATIONS

Administration/Storage

1. Administer oral forms of drug with food to minimize ulcerogenic effect.
2. When corticosteroids are given chronically, use the smallest dose possible that will achieve the desired effect.
3. At frequent intervals, the dose of medication should be gradually decreased to determine if symptoms of the disease can be effectively controlled by the smaller amount of drug.
4. When treating clients with conditions such as asthma, ulcerative colitis, and rheumatoid arthritis, corticosteroids, given every other day, may maintain therapeutic effects while reducing or eliminating undesirable side effects.
5. Local administration of corticosteroids is preferred over systemic therapy in order to minimize systemic side effects.
6. Corticosteroids should be discontinued gradually if used chronically.

Administration of Topical Corticosteroids

1. Cleanse the area before applying the medication.
2. Apply the agent sparingly and rub gently into the area.
3. Apply an occlusive dressing to promote hydration of the stratum corneum and increase the absorption of the medication.
4. There are two methods of applying an occlusive type dressing:
   - Apply a large amount of medication to the cleansed area. Cover with a thin, pliable, nonflammable plastic film, which is then sealed to the surrounding tissue with skin tape or held in place with gauze. Change the dressing every 3–4 days.
   - Apply a small amount of medication to the area and cover with a damp cloth. Then cover with a thin, pliable, nonflammable plastic film and seal to the surrounding tissue with tape, or hold in place with gauze. Change dressing b.i.d.

Assessment

1. Obtain baseline data concerning the client's mental status and neurological function and record on the client's record.
2. Check the client's medication history for evidence of allergic reactions to corticosteroids or tartrazine, a coloring agent used in certain preparations.
3. Obtain baseline ECG, electrolytes, liver and renal function studies.
4. Document baseline blood pressure, pulse, temperature and weight.
5. List any medication the client is taking and identify those that may interact with corticosteroids. These include antidiabetic agents, cardiac glycosides, oral contraceptives, anticoagulants and drugs that are influenced by liver enzymes.
6. If the client is female, of childbearing age, and sexually active, discuss the possibility of pregnancy and notify the physician if pregnancy is determined.

Interventions

1. When the client is first placed on corticosteroids, take the blood pressure at least twice a day

until a maintenance dose has been established. Document and report any increases in blood pressure to the physician.

2. Repeatedly evaluate the client for increased sodium and fluid retention. Monitor the client's weight and observe for other evidences of edema. If fluid and salt retention are noted, adjust the client's diet to one that is low in sodium and high in potassium.

3. Assess the client for shortness of breath, distended neck veins, edema and easy fatigue. The client may be in congestive heart failure. Obtain a chest x-ray and ECG and compare with the baseline studies.

4. Conduct periodic blood glucose determinations and monitor serum electrolytes and platelet counts for clients on long-term therapy. Note any complaint of unusual bleeding, bruising, the presence of petechiae and any other skin changes.

5. Assess the client's muscles for weakness and wasting as these are signs of a negative nitrogen balance.

6. Report changes in the client's appearance especially those resembling Cushing's syndrome, such as rounding of the face, hirsutism, presence of acne, and thinning of the hair and nails.

7. If the client has diabetes, monitor the blood glucose levels frequently while on corticosteroid therapy. The client may develop hyperglycemia and a change in diet and insulin dosage may be necessary.

8. Assess the client for signs of depression, lack of interest in personal appearance, complaints of insomnia and anorexia. Document on the client's record, compare with prior data, and notify the physician.

9. Discuss with female clients the potential for menstrual difficulties and amenorrhea that may be caused by long-term therapy with corticosteroids.

10. Observe the client for signs and symptoms of other illnesses during therapy with adrenocortico-steroids as these drugs tend to mask the severity of most illnesses.

11. Weigh daily under standard conditions. Anticipate a small weight gain due to increased appetite, but sudden increases are probably due to edema and must be reported. Edema occurs most frequently with cortisone or desoxycorticosterone acetate and occurs less frequently with the new synthetic agents.

12. Check the height and weight of children regularly because growth suppression is a hazard of adrenocorticosteroid therapy.

13. GI bleeding may occur. Therefore, when the client is on long-term therapy periodically test the stools for the presence of occult blood.

Client/Family Teaching

1. Instruct clients to take the medication with food and to report to the physician any symptoms of gastric distress. To prevent the problem of gastric irritation, discuss the use of antacids and special diets. Suggest eating frequent small meals. If the symptoms persist, diagnostic x-rays may be ordered.

2. Caution clients and family members to report any changes in mood or affect to the physician.

3. Advise clients to weigh themselves daily at the same time, wearing clothing of approximately the same weight and using the same scales. Consistent weight gain may be evidence of fluid retention and should be reported to the physician immediately.

4. Assist the client and family in identifying foods high in potassium and low in sodium content. Explain how to supplement their diet with potassium-rich foods such as citrus juices, and bananas. Instruct the client in what to look for on labels of canned or processed foods.

5. Encourage clients to eat a diet high in protein to prevent the development of Cushing's syndrome.

6. Remind clients to be especially careful to avoid falls and other accidents. Steroids may cause osteoporosis, which makes the bones more susceptible to fractures. To reduce the possibility of falling and subsequent injury, advise clients to use a night light and to have a hand rail or other device for support when it is necessary to get up at night.

7. To decrease the possibility of osteoporosis, explain the need to exercise daily.

8. Instruct the client in how to monitor and record their weight, blood pressure, temperature and pulse for evidence of physiological changes that should be reported to the physician.

9. Provide a printed list of adverse drug reactions that should be reported to the physician should they occur.

10. Women who are using oral contraceptives need to be warned that corticosteroids can cause a loss of contraceptive action. Teach the client how to keep an accurate record of her menstrual periods. If pregnancy is suspected the physician should be notified immediately.

11. Males should be warned that corticosteroids may have an adverse effect on the sperm.

12. Explain that if there is a need to withdraw the medication, the process should proceed slowly so that the client's own adrenal cortex will gradually be reactivated and take over the production of hormones.

13. If there is a need to reduce the dosage of drug provide supportive measures and reassurance to clients who are having flare-ups. Explain that these symptoms are caused by the reduction of drug dosage.

14. Explain to clients with arthritis that they should not overuse the joint once it has become painless. Permanent joint damage may result from overuse, because underlying pathology is still present.

15. If the client has diabetes, discuss the need to monitor glucose levels frequently while taking steroids. If any change is noted, report to the physician and discuss the alterations in insulin and diet that may be necessary.

16. Explain that wounds may heal slowly because steroid therapy causes a delay in development of granulation tissue. There is also an increased potential for infection. Therefore, clients should observe any healing process carefully for signs of infection and report any injury to the physician so that appropriate medical supervision can be implemented.

17. Because antibody production is decreased by adrenocorticosteroids, clients are at risk for infection. Explain the need to maintain general hygiene and scrupulous cleanliness to avoid infection. Advise the client to notify the physician if he/she has a sore throat, cough, fever, malaise or an injury that does not heal.

18. Clients on long-term ophthalmic therapy are prone to developing cataracts, exophthalmus, and increased intraocular pressure. Advise these clients to have routine visits to the ophthalmologist for eye examinations.

19. Advise the client to delay any vaccination while receiving adrenocorticosteroid therapy because there is limited immune response during therapy with steroids.

20. If adverse side effects occur, remind the client not to discontinue therapy with the idea that the changes will be reversed. Any sudden change will provoke symptoms of adrenal insufficiency. List these symptoms and instruct the client to immediately report these findings to the physician.

21. Assist the client in establishing a means of maintaining a supply of medication on hand to avoid running out of the drug.

22. Stress the need for regular medical supervision to have the dosage of medication checked and adjusted as needed.

23. Remind the client to carry a card identifying the drug being used, the dosage, and who to contact in the event of an emergency.

24. Discuss with parents the fact that children may develop pseudotumor cerebri. Symptoms of this disorder include vertigo, headache, and convulsions. The physician should be notified immediately. These symptoms will disappear once the therapy is discontinued.

Topical Corticosteroids

1. Assess for local sensitivity reaction at the site of application. Withhold the medication and report any sensitivity response to the physician.

2. Observe the client closely for signs of infections since corticosteroids tend to mask the problem. Do not apply an occlusive dressing when an infection is present. Document the site of the infection, the nature of the infection and if there is any redness, swelling or drainage present and report to the physician.

3. If the client has a large occlusive dressing, take their temperature every 4 hours. If the temperature is elevated, remove the dressing and notify the physician.

4. Routinely assess the client for evidence of systemic absorption of the medication. Symptoms of systemic absorption may include, edema and transient inhibition of pituitary-adrenal cortical function as manifested by muscular pain, lassitude, depression, hypotension, and weight loss.

5. If a family member is to apply the topical ointment, advise them to wash their hands and to wear gloves or to apply the medication with a sterile applicator. Instruct them concerning what to expect in response to the prescribed therapy.

Evaluation

Review with the client and family the client's progress to date and note any need for modifications in diet, drug dosage or length of therapy.

BECLOMETHASONE DIPROPIONATE   (beh-kloh-**METH**-ah-zohn dye-**PROH**-pee-oh-nayt)

Aerosol: Beclovent, Vanceril (Rx). Intranasal: Beconase AQ, Beconase Nasal Inhaler, Vancenase AQ, Vancenase Nasal Inhaler (Rx). Topical: Propaderm✸

See also *Adrenocorticosteroids and Analogs,* p. 1149.

Classification: Adrenocorticosteroid, synthetic, glucocorticoid-type.

Action/Kinetics: Rapidly inactivated, thereby resulting in few systemic effects.
   Note: If a patient is on systemic steroids, transfer to beclomethasone may be difficult, since recovery from impaired renal function may be slow.

Uses: Inhalation therapy for chronic use in bronchial asthma. In glucocorticoid-dependent patients, beclomethasone often permits a decrease in the dosage of the systemic agent. Withdrawal of systemic corticosteroids must be carried out gradually.

Contraindications: Status asthmaticus, acute episodes of asthma, hypersensitivity to drug or aerosol ingredients.

Special Concerns: Safe use during pregnancy (category: C) and lactation, and in children under 6 years of age not established.

Dosage: Inhalation Aerosol. *Asthma*: **Adults,** 2 inhalations (total of 84 mcg beclomethasone) t.i.d.–q.i.d. *Severe asthma:* **initial,** 12–16 inhalations (504–672 mcg beclomethasone) daily; **then,** decrease dose according to response. **Maximum daily dose:** 20 inhalations (840 mcg beclomethasone). **Pediatric, 6–12 years:** 1–2 inhalations (42–84 mcg) t.i.d.–q.i.d., not to exceed 10 inhalations (420 mcg) daily.

Nasal Aerosol or Spray. *Rhinitis:* **Adults and children over 12 years,** 1 inhalation (42 mcg) in each nostril b.i.d.–q.i.d. (i.e., total daily dose: 168–336 mcg daily). If no response after 3 weeks, discontinue therapy.

In patients also receiving systemic glucocorticosteroids, beclomethasone should be started when condition of patient is relatively stable.

NURSING CONSIDERATIONS

See also *Nursing Considerations* for *Adrenocorticosteroids and Analogs,* p. 1158.

Administration/Storage

1. To administer beclomethasone use the following procedure:
   - Shake metal canister thoroughly immediately prior to use.
   - Instruct clients to exhale as completely as possible.
   - Have them place the mouthpiece of the inhaler into their mouth and instruct clients to tighten their lips around it.
   - Instruct clients to inhale deeply through their mouth while pressing the metal canister down with their forefinger.
   - Instruct clients to hold their breath for as long as possible.
   - Remove mouthpiece.
   - Instruct clients to exhale slowly.
2. A minimum of 60 sec must elapse between inhalations.
3. To prevent explosion of contents under pressure, do not store or use near heat or open flame, or throw in fire in incinerator. Keep secure from children.

Assessment

Note any history of sensitivity to the drug.

Interventions

1. For clients who are receiving systemic steroid therapy, initiate beclomethasone therapy *very* slowly, withdrawing the systemic steroids as ordered by the physician.
2. Observe the client for subjective signs of adrenal insufficiency, such as muscular pain, lassitude, and depression. Document and report to the physician even if the client's respiratory function has improved.
3. Note objective signs of adrenal insufficiency, such as hypotension and weight loss. This is an indication that the dosage of systemic steroid should be boosted temporarily, and then withdrawn more gradually.
4. Once the client has had a systemic steroid withdrawn, the client should be provided with a supply of oral glucocorticoids. These are to be taken immediately if the client is subjected to unusual stress or is having an asthmatic attack. Notify the physician immediately after the steroids have been taken.

Client/Family Teaching

1. Instruct the client in the use and care of the inhaler. Caution the client to wash the mouth piece and sprayer and to dry it after each use.

2. Explain that the inhaler is not to be used for asthmatic attacks.

3. Explain the importance of complying with the prescribed drug therapy even though it may take 1–4 weeks for any improvement in respiratory function to be realized.

4. More than 1 mg in adults or more than 500 mcg in children may precipitate hypothalamic-pituitary axis depression, resulting in adrenal insufficiency. Therefore, advise clients not to overuse the inhaler.

5. Instruct the client to observe for symptoms of localized fungal infections of the mouth. These must be reported immediately and will require antifungal medication and possibly discontinuation of the drug.

6. Advise clients also receiving bronchodilators by inhalation that they should use the bronchodilator for at least several minutes before using beclomethasone. This increases the penetration of steroid and reduces the potential toxicity from inhaled fluorocarbon propellants of both inhalers.

7. Instruct the client in relaxation techniques to use during stressful situations.

8. Advise the client to carry a card indicating the diagnosis, treatment, and the possible need for systemic glucocorticoids, in the event of exposure to unusual stress.

BETAMETHASONE   (bay-tah-**METH**-ah-sohn)

Betnesol✱, Celestone (Rx)

BETAMETHASONE ACETATE AND BETAMETHASONE SODIUM PHOSPHATE   (bay-tah-**METH**-ah-sohn)

Celestone Soluspan (Rx)

BETAMETHASONE BENZOATE   (bay-tah-**METH**-ah-sohn)

Topical: Beben✱, Uticort (Rx)

BETAMETHASONE DIPROPIONATE   (bay-tah-**METH**-ah-sohn)

Topical: Alphatrex, Diprolene, Diprosone, Maxivate (Rx)

BETAMETHASONE SODIUM PHOSPHATE   (bay-tah-**METH**-ah-sohn)

Betameth, Betnesol✱, Celestone Phosphate, Selestoject (Rx)

BETAMETHASONE VALERATE   (bay-tah-**METH**-ah-sohn **VAH**-ler-ayt)

Topical: Betacort✱, Betaderm✱, Betatrex, Beta-Val, Betnovate✱, Betnovate-1/2✱, Celestoderm-V✱, Celestoderm-V/2✱, Dermabet, Ectosone Mild✱, Ectosone Regular, Metaderm Regular✱, Novobetamet✱, Valisone, Valisone Reduced Strength, Valnac (Rx)

See also *Adrenocorticosteroids and Analogs,* p. 1149.

Classification: Adrenocorticosteroid, synthetic, glucocorticoid-type.

Action/Kinetics: Causes low degree of sodium and water retention, as well as potassium depletion. The injectable form contains both rapid-acting and repository forms of betamethasone (mixture of betamethasone sodium phosphate and betamethasone acetate). Not recommended for replacement therapy in any acute or chronic adrenal cortical insufficiency, because it does not have strong sodium-retaining effects. Long-acting. **t½:** over 300 min.

Additional Use: Prevention of respiratory distress syndrome in premature infants.

Special Concerns: Safe use during pregnancy and lactation have not been established.

Dosage: *Betamethasone.* **Syrup, Tablets.** 0.6–7.2 mg/day. *Betamethasone sodium phosphate:* **Parenteral (IV, local): initial,** up to 9 mg/day; then, adjust dosage at minimal level to reduce symptoms. *Betamethasone sodium phosphate and betamethasone acetate:* (contains 3 mg each of the acetate and sodium phosphate per mL). **IM:** initial, 0.5–9 mg/day. *Bursitis, peritendinitis, tenosynovitis:* 1 mL. *Rheumatoid arthritis and osteoarthritis:* 0.5–2 mL, depending on size of the joint. *Dermatologic:* **intradermally,** 0.2 mL/cm², not to exceed 1 mL/week. *Acute gouty arthritis:* 0.5–1 mL.

   Betamethasone benzoate, betamethasone dipropionate, betamethasone valerate: **Topical Aerosol, Cream, Gel, Lotion, Ointment:** Apply sparingly to affected areas and rub in lightly.

   Betamethasone sodium phosphate: **Ophthalmic or Otic Solution:** 2–3 drops in the ear or 1–2 drops in the eye q 2–3 hr; dosage should be decreased as inflammation improves.

NURSING CONSIDERATIONS

See *Nursing Considerations* for *Adrenocorticosteroids and Analogs,* p. 1158.

Administration/Storage

Avoid injection into deltoid muscle because SC atrophy of tissue may occur.

CORTICOTROPIN (ACTH, ADRENOCORTICOTROPIC HORMONE) (kor-tih-koh-**TROH**-pin)

Acthar (Rx)

CORTICOTROPIN REPOSITORY (ACTH GEL, CORTICOTROPIN GEL) (kor-tih-koh-**TROH**-pin)

Acthar Gel (H.P.)✳, H.P. Acthar Gel (Rx)

CORTICOTROPIN ZINC HYDROXIDE (kor-tih-koh-**TROH**-pin)

Cortrophin-Zinc (Rx)

See also *Adrenocorticosteroids and Analogs,* p. 1149.

Classification: Anterior pituitary hormone.

Action/Kinetics: Corticotropin is extracted from the anterior pituitary gland. The hormone stimulates the functional adrenal cortex to secrete its entire spectrum of hormones, including the corticosteroids.

   Thus, the overall physiologic effects of corticotropin are similar to those of cortisone. Since the latter is more easily obtainable, is more predictable, and has more prolonged activity, it is usually used for therapeutic purposes. Corticotropin is, however, useful for the diagnosis of Addison's disease and other conditions in which the functionality of the adrenal cortex is to be determined. *Corticotropin cannot elicit a hormonal response from a nonfunctioning adrenal gland.*

Uses: Diagnosis of adrenal insufficiency syndromes, severe myasthenia gravis, multiple sclerosis. For same diseases as glucocorticosteroids.

Additional Contraindications: Cushing's syndrome, psychotic or psychopathic patients, active TB, active peptic ulcers.

Special Concerns: Pregnancy category: C. Use with caution in patients who have diabetes and hypotension.

Additional Side Effects: In the treatment of myasthenia gravis, corticotropin may cause severe muscle weakness 2–3 days after initiation of therapy. Equipment for respiratory assistance must be on hand for such emergencies. Muscle strength returns and increases 2–7 days after cessation of treatment, and improvement lasts for about 3 months.

Dosage: SC, IM, or slow IV drip. *Highly individualized.* **Usual** (*aqueous solution*), **IM or SC:** 20 units q.i.d. **IV:** 10–25 units of aqueous solution in 500 mL 5% dextrose injection over period of 8 hr. Infants and young children require larger dose per body weight than do older children or adults.

  Repository gel (IM, SC) or aqueous suspension with zinc hydroxide (IM only): 40–80 units q 24–72 hr. A dose of 12.5 units q.i.d. causes little metabolic disturbance; 25 units q.i.d. causes definite metabolic alterations.

  As a general rule, patients are started on 10–12.5 units q.i.d. If no clinical effect is noted in 72–96 hr, dosage is increased by 5 units q few days to a final maximum of 25 units q.i.d.

  Multiple sclerosis, acute exacerbation: **IM,** 80–120 units daily for 2–3 weeks.

NURSING CONSIDERATIONS

See also *Nursing Considerations* for *Adrenocorticosteroids and Analogs,* p. 1158.

Administration/Storage

Check label carefully for IV administration. **The label must say that the product is for IV use.** IV administration should be slow, taking 8 hr.

Assessment

Before administering IV corticotropin, make sure that the client has been tested for any sensitivity to animal extracts and for sensitivity to the brand of corticotropin to be used.

Interventions

  1. Anticipate that the potassium requirements will be increased during IV administration of ACTH. Therefore, monitor serum potassium and sodium levels.
  2. Observe the client for exaggerated euphoria and nervousness or client complaints of insomnia and depression. These are indications that the dosage should be reduced or discontinued and the symptoms should be reported to the physician.
  3. Sedatives may be ordered p.r.n.
  4. Monitor BP, intake and output, and weight for any marked changes. Document and report these to the physician.

CORTISONE ACETATE (COMPOUND E)   (KOR-tih-sohn)

Cortone ✿, Cortone Acetate (Rx)

See also *Adrenocorticosteroids and Analogs,* p. 1149.

Classification: Adrenocorticosteroid, naturally occurring; glucocorticoid-type.

Action/Kinetics: Absorption: Slowly absorbed from IM injection site (24–48 hr). Short-acting. **Onset:** More rapid after PO administration. **Duration:** PO shorter than IM (effective, 24–48 hr). **t½:** 90 min.

Uses: Primarily used for replacement therapy in chronic cortical insufficiency. Also inflammatory or allergic disorders, but only for short-term use because the drug has a strong mineralocorticoid effect.

Special Concerns: Use during pregnancy only if benefits outweigh risks.

Dosage: Tablets or IM, initial *or during crisis:* 20–300 mg daily. Decrease gradually to lowest effective dose. *Anti-inflammatory:* 25–150 mg daily, depending on severity of the disease. *Acute rheumatic fever:* 200 mg b.i.d. day 1, thereafter, 200 mg daily. *Addison's disease:* **Maintenance, IM:** 0.25–0.35 mg/kg daily; **maintenance, PO:** 0.5–0.75 mg/kg daily.

NURSING CONSIDERATIONS

See *Nursing Considerations* for *Adrenocorticosteroids and Analogs,* p. 1158.

Administration/Storage

Single course of therapy should not exceed 6 weeks. Rest periods of 2–3 weeks are indicated between treatments.

COSYNTROPIN   (koh-sin-**TROH**-pin)
Cortrosyn (Rx)

Classification: Synthetic ACTH derivative.

Action/Kinetics: Cosyntropin is a synthetic ACTH derivative that causes effects similar to those of ACTH although fewer hypersensitivity reactions have been noted. The activity of 0.25 mg cosyntropin is equal to 25 units of ACTH.

Uses: Diagnosis of adrenocortical insufficiency.

Special Concerns: Pregnancy category: C.

Dosage: IM, rapid IV, IV infusion. Adults, Usual, IM: 0.25 mg dissolved in sterile saline. Range: 0.25–0.75 mg. **Pediatric, under 2 years:** 0.125 mg.

NURSING CONSIDERATIONS

See also *Nursing Considerations* for *Adrenocorticosteroids and Analogs,* p. 1158.

Administration/Storage

1. When given by IV infusion, 0.25 mg cosyntropin is added to dextrose or saline solution, and 40 mcg/hr is administered over 6 hr.
2. For IM use, the drug (usually 0.25 mg) should be dissolved in sterile saline.

DESOXYCORTICOSTERONE ACETATE   (des-ox-ee-kor-tih-koh-**STEER**-ohn)
DOCA Acetate (Rx)

DESOXYCORTICOSTERONE PIVALATE   (des-ox-ee-kor-tih-koh-**STEER**-ohn)
Percorten Pivalate (Rx)

See also *Adrenocorticosteroids and Analogs,* p. 1149.

Classification: Adrenocorticosteroid, naturally occurring; mineralocorticoid-type.

Action/Kinetics: Desoxycorticosterone, a mineralocorticoid, increases sodium and water retention and promotes potassium excretion by altering reabsorption by the renal tubules. It also decreases the sodium content of saliva, sweat, and gastric juices. By normalizing electrolyte balance and plasma volume, the hormone increases cardiac output, increases BP, increases fat and glucose absorption from the GI tract, and decreases nitrogen retention. Desoxycorticosterone does not affect protein or carbohydrate metabolism or skin pigmentation. **Duration:** 1–2 days for the acetate and 4 weeks for the pivalate product.

Uses: Primary and secondary adrenocortical insufficiency in Addison's disease and salt-losing adrenogenital syndrome.

Contraindication: Use with caution in patients with hypertension.

Special Concerns: Pregnancy category: C.

Side Effects: Serious adverse effects may result from excessive dosage or prolonged treatment. These include increased blood volume, edema, increased blood pressure, enlargement of heart, headaches, arthralgia, ascending paralysis, and low potassium syndrome (sudden attacks of weakness, changes in ECG).

Dosage: IM, maintenance: 2–5 mg daily with either hydrocortisone (10–30 mg daily) or cortisone (10–37.5 mg daily). Also available as a long-acting suspension (25–100 mg IM, q 4 weeks) or as implantable pellets lasting 8–12 months. The latter are implanted surgically under aseptic conditions.

Acute crisis: 10–15 mg b.i.d. for 1 or 2 days; supportive measures (whole adrenal cortical extract, cortisone or hydrocortisone, infusions of dextrose in isotonic sodium chloride solution, whole blood or plasma) may also be indicated.

Drug requirements and salt intake are inversely related. The higher the sodium intake, the lower are the requirements for the drug. Most patients need 3 mg of the drug when ingesting 3–6 g of sodium chloride in addition to a normal diet. Potassium intake has no effect.

NURSING CONSIDERATIONS

See also *Nursing Considerations* for *Adrenocorticosteroids and Analogs,* p. 1158.

Administration/Storage

IM: Use a 20-gauge needle and inject into upper, outer quadrant of buttock.

DEXAMETHASONE   (dex-ah-**METH**-ah-sohn)

Oral: Decadron, Deronil ✹, Dexameth, Dexamethasone Intensol, Dexasone ✹, Dexone, Hexadrol, Mymethasone, Oradexon ✹ (Rx). Topical: Aeroseb-Dex, Decaderm, Decaspray (Rx). Ophthalmic: Maxidex Ophthalmic (Rx)

See also *Adrenocorticosteroids and Analogs,* p. 1149.

Classification: Adrenocorticosteroid, synthetic; glucocorticoid-type.

Action/Kinetics: Long-acting. Low degree of sodium and water retention. Diuresis may ensue when patients are transferred from other corticosteroids to dexamethasone. Not recommended for replacement therapy in adrenal cortical insufficiency. **t½:** over 300 min.

Additional Use: In acute allergic disorders, oral dexamethasone may be combined with dexamethasone sodium phosphate injection. This combination is used for 6 days. Used to test for adrenal cortical hyperfunction. Cerebral edema due to brain tumor, craniotomy, or head injury. Diagnosis of depression. Antiemetic in cisplatin-induced vomiting. Prophylaxis or treatment of acute mountain sickness.

Special Concerns: Use during pregnancy only if benefits outweigh risks.

Additional Drug Interaction: Ephedrine ↓ the effect of dexamethasone due to ↑ breakdown by the liver.

Dosage: Oral Solution, Tablets. Initial, 0.75–9 mg/day; **maintenance:** gradually reduce to minimum effective dose (0.5–3 mg/day). *Suppression test for Cushing's syndrome:* 0.5 mg q 6 hr for 2 days for 24-hr urine collection (or 1 mg at 11 P.M. with blood withdrawn at 8 A.M. for blood cortisol determination). *Suppression test to determine cause of pituitary ACTH excess:* 2 mg q 6 hr for 2 days (for 24-hr urine collection).

   Topical Aerosol, Cream, Gel: Apply sparingly as a light film to affected area b.i.d.–t.i.d.
   Ophthalmic Ointment, Solution: 1–2 gtt in the conjunctival sac q hr during day and q 2 hr during night until a satisfactory response obtained; **then,** 1 gtt q 4 hr and finally 1 gtt q 6–8 hr.
   For allergic disorders, either self-limited or acute worsening of chronic conditions: Combination of oral and parenteral therapy. **Day 1:** 4–8 mg of dexamethasone sodium phosphate, **IM. Days 2 and 3:** Two 0.75 mg dexamethasone tablets b.i.d. **Day 4:** One 0.75-mg dexamethasone tablet b.i.d. **Days 5 and 6:** One 0.75-mg dexamethasone tablet. **Day 8:** Follow-up visit to physician.

NURSING CONSIDERATIONS
See *Nursing Considerations* for *Adrenocorticosteroids and Analogs,* p. 1158.

DEXAMETHASONE ACETATE   (dex-ah-**METH**-ah-sohn)

Dalalone D.P., Dalalone L.A., Decadron-LA, Decaject-L.A., Dexacen LA-8, Dexasone-LA, Dexone LA, Solurex-LA (Rx)

See also *Adrenocorticosteroids and Analogs,* p. 1149.

Classification: Adrenocorticosteroid, synthetic; glucocorticoid-type.

Action/Kinetics: This ester of dexamethasone is practically insoluble and provides the prolonged activity suitable for repository injections. Not for IV use.

Special Concerns: Use during pregnancy only if benefits outweigh risks.

Dosage: Repository injection. IM: 8–16 mg q 1–3 weeks, if necessary. **Intralesional:** 0.8–1.6 mg. **Soft tissue and intra-articular:** 4–16 mg repeated at 1- to 3-week intervals.

NURSING CONSIDERATIONS
See *Nursing Considerations* for *Adrenocorticosteroids and Analogs,* p. 1158.

DEXAMETHASONE SODIUM PHOSPHATE   (dex-ah-**METH**-ah-sohn)

Systemic: AK-Dex, Dalalone, Decadrol, Decadron Phosphate, Decaject, Dexacen-4, Dexone, Hexadrol Phosphate, Solurex (Rx). Inhaler: Decadron Phosphate Respihaler (Rx). Nasal: Decadron Turbinaire (Rx).

Ophthalmic: AK-Dex, Baldex, Decadron Phosphate, Dexair, Dexotic, I-Methasone, Maxidex, Ocu-Dex (Rx). Otic: AK-Dex, Decadron, I-Methasone (Rx). Topical: Decadron Phosphate (Rx)

See also *Adrenocorticosteroids and Analogs,* p. 1149.

Classification: Adrenocorticosteroid, synthetic; glucocorticoid-type.

Additional Uses: For IV or IM use in emergency situations when dexamethasone cannot be given PO. Routes of administration include inhalation (especially for bronchial asthma), ophthalmic, topical, intrasynovial, and intra-articular.

Contraindications: Acute infections, persistent positive sputum cultures of *Candida albicans.*

Special Concerns: Use during pregnancy only if benefits outweigh risks.

Dosage: Elixir, Oral Solution, Tablets. Initial, 0.5–9 mg daily (usually one-third to one-half the oral dose); **then,** adjust dose if required (some may require high doses in life-threatening situations). *Cerebral edema:* **initial, IV:** 10 mg; **then, IM,** 4 mg q 6 hr until maximum effect obtained. Switch to oral therapy (1–3 mg t.i.d.) as soon as feasible and then slowly withdraw over 5–7 days. **Pediatric: PO** 0.2 mg/kg daily in divided doses. *Shock, unresponsive:* **IV, initial,** either 1–6 mg/kg or 40 mg; **then,** repeat IV dose q 2–6 hr as long as necessary. *Intralesional, intra-articular, soft tissue injections:* 0.4–6 mg, depending on the site.

    Inhalation: *Bronchial asthma:* **Adults, initial,** 3 inhalations (84 mcg dexamethasone/inhalation) t.i.d.–q.i.d.; **maximum:** 3 inhalations/dose; 12 inhalations/day. **Pediatric: initial,** 2 inhalations t.i.d.–q.i.d.; **maximum:** 2 inhalations/dose; 8 inhalations/day.

    Intranasal: *Allergies, nasal polyps:* **Adults,** 2 sprays (total of 168 mcg dexamethasone) in each nostril b.i.d.–t.i.d. (maximum: 12 sprays/day); **pediatric, 6–12 years:** 1–2 sprays (total of 84–168 mcg dexamethasone) in each nostril b.i.d. (maximum: 8 sprays/day).

    Ophthalmic Ointment, Solution: Instill a small amount into the conjunctival sac t.i.d.–q.i.d. As response is obtained, reduce the number of applications. **Ophthalmic solution:** Instill 1–2 drops into the conjunctival sac q hr during the day and q 2 hr at night until response obtained; **then,** reduce to 1 gtt q 6–8 hr.

    Otic Solution: 3–4 drops into the ear canal b.i.d.–t.i.d.

    Topical cream: Apply sparingly to affected areas and rub in.

NURSING CONSIDERATIONS

See also *Nursing Considerations* for *Adrenocorticosteroids and Analogs,* p. 1158.

Administration/Storage

Do not use preparation containing lidocaine IV.

FLUDROCORTISONE ACETATE   (flew-droh-**KOR**-tih-sohn)

Florinef (Rx)

See also *Adrenocorticosteroids and Analogs,* p. 1149.

Classification: Adrenocorticosteroid, synthetic; mineralocorticoid type.

Action/Kinetics: Produces marked sodium retention and inhibits excess adrenocortical secretion. Should not be used systemically for its anti-inflammatory effects. Supplementary potassium may be indicated.

Uses: Addison's disease and adrenal hyperplasia.

Special Concerns: Pregnancy category: C.

Dosage: Tablets. *Addison's disease:* 0.1–0.2 mg daily to 0.1 mg 3 times/week, usually in conjunction with hydrocortisone or cortisone. *Salt-losing adrenogenital syndrome:* 0.1–0.2 mg/day.

NURSING CONSIDERATIONS

See *Nursing Considerations* for *Adrenocorticosteroids and Analogs,* p. 1158.

FLUNISOLIDE   (flew-**NISS**-oh-lyd)

Inhalation: AeroBid, Bronalide✻ (Rx). Intranasal: Nasalide, Rhinalar✻ (Rx)

See also *Adrenocorticosteroid and Analogs,* p. 1149.

Classification: Intranasal and inhalation corticosteroid.

Action/Kinetics: Produces anti-inflammatory effects intranasally with minimal systemic effects. Several days may be required for full beneficial effects. After inhalation, there is a significant first-pass effect through the liver and the drug is rapidly metabolized. **t½:** 1.8 hr.

Uses: Inhalation: Bronchial asthma in combination with other therapy. Not used when asthma can be relieved by other drugs, in patients where systemic corticosteroid treatment is infrequent, and in nonasthmatic bronchitis. **Intranasal:** Seasonal or perennial rhinitis, especially if other treatment has proven unsatisfactory.

Contraindications: Active or quiescent tuberculosis, especially of the respiratory tract. Untreated fungal, bacterial, systemic viral infections. Ocular herpes simplex. Do not use until healing occurs following recent ulceration of nasal septum, nasal surgery, or trauma. Lactation.

Special Concerns: Pregnancy category: C. Safety and effectiveness in children less than 6 years of age have not been determined.

Additional Side Effects: *Respiratory:* Hoarseness, coughing, throat irritation; *Candida* infections of nose, larynx, and pharynx. *GI:* Dry mouth. Systemic corticosteroid effects, especially if recommended dose is exceeded.

Dosage: Inhalation. Adults: 2 inhalations (total of 500 mcg flunisolide) in A.M. and P.M., not to exceed 4 inhalations b.i.d. (i.e., total daily dose of 2 mg). **Pediatric, 6–15 years:** 2 inhalations b.i.d.
   Intranasal. Adults: initial, 50 mcg (2 sprays) in each nostril b.i.d.; may be increased to 2 sprays t.i.d. up to maximum daily dose of 400 mcg (i.e., 8 sprays in each nostril). **Children, 6–14 years: initial,** 25 mcg (1 spray) in each nostril t.i.d. or 50 mcg (2 sprays) in each nostril b.i.d. Up to maximum daily dose of 200 mcg (i.e., 4 sprays in each nostril). **Maintenance, adults, children:** smallest dose necessary to control symptoms. Some patients are controlled on 1 spray in each nostril daily.

NURSING CONSIDERATIONS

See also *Nursing Considerations* for *Adrenocorticosteroids and Analogs,* p. 1158.

Administration/Storage

1. When initiating the inhalant in clients receiving corticosteroids systemically, the aerosol should be used concomitantly with the systemic steroid for one week. Then, slowly withdraw the systemic corticosteroid over several weeks.

2. If nasal congestion is present, use a decongestant before administration to ensure the drug reaches the site of action.

3. If beneficial effects do not occur within 3 weeks, discontinue therapy.

Interventions

Assess the oral mucosa closely for any evidence of fungal infections.

Client/Family Teaching

1. Instruct client and family how to administer nasal spray.

2. Remind clients to rinse their mouth with water after inhalation to prevent alterations in taste and to maintain adequate oral hygiene.

HYDROCORTISONE (CORTISOL) (hy-droh-**KOR**-tih-sohn)

Rectal: Dermolate Anal-Itch, Proctocort, Rectocort✷. Tablets: Cortef, Hydrocortone. Parenteral: Sterile Hydrocortisone Suspension. Topical Aerosol Solution: Aeroseb-HC, CaldeCORT Anti-Itch. Topical Cream: Ala-Cort, Allercort, Alphaderm, Bactine, Barriere-HC✷, Cortate✷, Cort-Dome, Cortifair, Dermacort, DermiCort, Dermolate Anti-Itch, Dermtex HC, Emo-Cort✷, H₂Cort, Hi-Cor 1.0 and 2.5, Hydro-Tex, Hytone Lemoderm, Nutracort, Penecort, Synacort, Unicort✷. Topical Lotion: Acticort 100, Ala-Cort, Ala-Scalp HP, Allercort, Cetacort, Cortate✷, Cort-Dome, Delacort, Dermacort, Dermolate Scalp-Itch, Emo-Cort✷, Gly-Cort, Hytone, LactiCare-HC, Lemoderm, Lexocort Forte, My Cort, Nutracort, Pentacort, Rederm, Sarna HC 1.0%✷, S-T Cort. Topical Ointment: Allercort, Cortril, Dermolate Anal-Itch, Hytone, Lemoderm, Penecort. Topical Solution: Penecort, Emo-Cort Scalp Solution, Texacort Scalp Solution. Topical Spray: Cortaid, Dermolate Anti-Itch. (OTC, Rx)

HYDROCORTISONE ACETATE (hy-droh-**KOR**-tih-sohn)

Dental Paste: Orabase-HCA. Ophthalmic/Otic: Cortamed✷. Parenteral: Hydrocortone Acetate. Rectal: Anusol HC, Cort-Dome High Potency, Cortenema, Corticaine, Cortifoam, Cortiment-10 and -40✷. Topical Aerosol Foam: Epifoam. Topical Cream: Anusol-HC, CaldeCORT Anti-Itch, CaldeCORT Light, Carmol-HC, Cortacet✷, Cortaid, Cortef Feminine Itch, Corticaine, Corticreme✷, FoilleCort, Gynecort, Hyderm✷, Lanacort, Novohydrocort✷, Pharma-Cort, Rhulicort. Topical Lotion: Cortaid, Rhulicort. Topical Ointment: Cortaid, Cortef Acetate, Cortoderm✷, Lanacort, Novohydrocort. (OTC, Rx)

HYDROCORTISONE BUTYRATE (hy-droh-**KOR**-tih-sohn)

Topical Cream: Locoid (Rx)

HYDROCORTISONE CYPIONATE (hy-droh-**KOR**-tih-sohn)

Oral Suspension: Cortef (Rx)

HYDROCORTISONE SODIUM PHOSPHATE (hy-droh-**KOR**-tih-sohn)

Parenteral: Hydrocortone Phosphate (Rx)

HYDROCORTISONE SODIUM SUCCINATE (hy-droh-**KOR**-tih-sohn)

Parenteral: A-hydroCort, Solu-Cortef (Rx)

HYDROCORTISONE VALERATE (hy-droh-**KOR**-tih-sohn)

Topical Cream/Ointment: Westcort (Rx)

See also *Adrenocorticosteroids and Analogs,* p. 1149.

Classification: Adrenocorticosteroid, naturally occurring; glucocorticoid-type.

Action/Kinetics: Short-acting. **t½:** 90 min.

Dosage: *Hydrocortisone.* **PO:** 20–240 mg/day, depending on disease. **IM only:** one-third to one-half the oral dose q 12 hr. **Rectal:** 100 mg in retention enema nightly for 21 days (up to 2 months of therapy may be needed; discontinue gradually if therapy exceeds 3 weeks). **Topical (ointment, cream, gel, lotion, solution, spray):** Apply sparingly to affected area and rub in lightly t.i.d.–q.i.d.

Hydrocortisone acetate. **Intralesional, intra-articular, soft tissue:** 5–50 mg, depending on condition. **Topical:** See *Hydrocortisone.*

Hydrocortisone butyrate. **Topical:** See *Hydrocortisone.*

Hydrocortisone cypionate (as suspension). 20–240 mg/day, depending on the severity of the disease.

Hydrocortisone sodium phosphate. **IV, IM, SC: initial,** 15–240 mg/day depending on use and on severity of the disease. Usually, one-half to one-third of the oral dose is given q 12 hr. *Adrenal insufficiency, acute.* **IV, adults: initial,** 100 mg; **then,** 100 mg q 8 hr in an IV fluid; **older children: initial, IV bolus,** 1–2 mg/kg; **then,** 150–250 mg/kg daily **IV** in divided doses; **infants: initial, IV bolus,** 1–2 mg/kg; **then,** 25–150 mg/kg daily in divided doses.

Hydrocortisone sodium succinate. **IM, IV, initial:** 100–500 mg; **then,** adjust dosage depending on response and severity of condition.

Hydrocortisone valerate. **Topical (cream):** See *Hydrocortisone.*

NURSING CONSIDERATIONS

See also *Nursing Considerations* for *Adrenocorticosteroids and Analogs,* p. 1158.

Administration/Storage

1. Check label of parenteral hydrocortisone to verify route that can be used for a particular preparation, because IM and IV routes are not necessarily interchangeable.
2. When using topical products, washing the area prior to application may increase the penetration of the drug.
3. Topical products should not come in contact with the eyes.
4. Prolonged use of topical products should be avoided near the genital/rectal areas, eyes, on the face, and in creases of the skin.

METHYLPREDNISOLONE   (meth-ill-pred-**NISS**-oh-lohn)

Tablets: Medrol, Meprolone (Rx)

METHYLPREDNISOLONE ACETATE   (meth-ill-pred-**NISS**-oh-lohn)

Enema: Medrol Enpak (Rx). Parenteral: depMedalone-40 and -80, Depoject-40 and -80, Depopred-40 and -80, Depo-Medrol, Depo-Predate 40 and 80, Duralone-40 and -80, Medralone-40 and -80, Rep-Pred 40 and 80 (Rx). Topical Ointment: Medrol (Rx)

METHYLPREDNISOLONE SODIUM SUCCINATE   (meth-ill-pred-**NISS**-oh-lohn)

Parenteral: A-methaPred, Solu-Medrol (Rx)

See also *Adrenocorticosteroids and Analogs,* p. 1149.

Classification: Adrenocorticosteroid, synthetic, glucocorticoid-type.

Action/Kinetics: Low incidence of increased appetite, peptic ulcer, and psychic stimulation. Also, low degree of sodium and water retention. May mask negative nitrogen balance. **Onset:** Slow, 12–24 hr. **Duration:** Long, up to 1 week.

Special Concerns: Use during pregnancy only if benefits outweigh risks.

Additional Drug Interactions

| Erythromycin | ↑ Effect of methylprednisolone due to ↓ breakdown by liver |
| Troleandomycin | ↑ Effect of methylprednisolone due to ↓ breakdown by liver |

Laboratory Test Interference: ↓ Immunoglobulins A, G, M.

Dosage: *Highly individualized. Methylprednisolone,* **Tablets:** *Rheumatoid arthritis,* 6–16 mg daily. Decrease gradually when condition is under control. **Pediatric:** 6–10 mg daily. *Systemic lupus erythematosus:* **acute:** 20–96 mg daily; **maintenance:** 8–20 mg daily. *Acute rheumatic fever:* 1 mg/kg body weight daily. Drug is always given in 4 equally divided doses after meals and at bedtime.

Methylprednisolone acetate, **not for IV use. IM:** *Adrenogenital syndrome:* 40 mg q 2 weeks. *Rheumatoid arthritis:* 40–120 mg/week. *Dermatologic lesions, dermatitis:* 40–120 mg/week for 1–4 weeks; for severe cases, a single dose of 80–120 mg should provide relief. *Seborrheic dermatitis:* 80 mg/week. *Asthma, rhinitis:* 80–120 mg. **Intra-articular, soft tissue and intralesional injection:** 4–80 mg, depending on site. **Retention enema:** 40 mg 3 to 7 times/week for 2 or more weeks. **Topical, ointment:** 0.25%–1% applied sparingly b.i.d.–q.i.d.

Methylprednisolone sodium succinate. **IV: initial,** 10–40 mg, depending on the disease; **then,** adjust dose depending on response, with subsequent doses given either **IM, IV.** *Severe conditions:* 30 mg/kg infused IV over 10–20 min; may be repeated q 4–6 hr for 2–3 days only. **Pediatric:** not less than 0.5 mg/kg/day.

NURSING CONSIDERATIONS

See also *Nursing Considerations* for *Adrenocorticosteroids,* p. 1158.

Administration/Storage

Solutions of methylprednisolone sodium succinate should be used within 48 hr after preparation.

PARAMETHASONE ACETATE (par-ah-**METH**-ah-sohn)

Haldrone (Rx)

Classification: Adrenocorticosteroid, synthetic.

Action/Kinetics: Approximately two and one-half times as potent as prednisone. **Onset:** (rapid), 30 min. **Duration:** 8–10 hr. **Plasma t½:** Approximately 5 hr.

Dosage: Tablets. Initial: 2–24 mg daily; **maintenance:** 1–8 mg daily.

NURSING CONSIDERATIONS

See also *Nursing Considerations* for *Adrenocorticosteroids,* p. 1158.

PREDNISOLONE   (pred-**NISS**-ah-lohn)

Syrup: Prelone. Tablets: Delta-Cortef (Rx)

PREDNISOLONE ACETATE   (pred-**NISS**-ah-lohn)

Parenteral: Articulose 50, Key-Pred 25 and 50, Predaject-50, Predalone 50, Predcor-25 and -50, Predicort-50 (Rx). Ophthalmic Suspension: AK-Tate, Econopred, Econopred Plus, Ocu-Pred-A, Predair A, Pred Forte, Pred Mild, Ultra Pred (Rx)

PREDNISOLONE ACETATE AND PREDNISOLONE SODIUM PHOSPHATE   (pred-**NISS**-ah-lohn)

(Rx)

PREDNISOLONE SODIUM PHOSPHATE   (pred-**NISS**-ah-lohn)

Oral Solution: Pediapred (Rx). Ophthalmic Solution: AK-Pred, Inflamase✹, Inflamase Forte, Inflamase Mild, I-Pred, Lite Pred, Ocu-Pred, Ocu-Pred Forte, Predair, Predair Forte (Rx). Parenteral: Hydeltrasol, Key-Pred-SP, Predate S, Predicort-RP (Rx)

PREDNISOLONE TEBUTATE   (pred-**NISS**-ah-lohn **TEB**-you-tayt)

Hydeltra-T.B.A., Nor-Pred T.B.A., Predalone T.B.A., Predate TBA, Predcor-TBA (Rx)

See also *Adrenocorticosteroids and Analogs,* p. 1149.

Classification: Adrenocorticosteroid, synthetic.

Action/Kinetics: Intermediate-acting. Prednisolone is five times more potent than hydrocortisone and cortisone. Side effects are minimal except for GI distress. **t½:** over 200 min.

Contraindications: Lactation.

Special Concerns: Use during pregnancy only if benefits outweigh risks. Use with particular caution in diabetes.

Dosage: *Prednisolone.* **PO:** 5–60 mg/day, depending on disease being treated. *Multiple sclerosis (exacerbation):* 200 mg/day for 1 week; **then,** 80 mg on alternate days for 1 month.
  Prednisolone acetate. **IM:** 4–60 mg daily. **Not for IV use. Intralesional, intra-articular, soft tissue injection:** 5–100 mg (larger doses for large joints). *Multiple sclerosis (exacerbation):* See *Prednisolone.* **Ophthalmic** (0.12%–1% suspension): 1–2 drops in the conjunctival sac q hr during the day and q 2 hr during the night; **then,** after response obtained, decrease dose to 1 drop q 6–8 hr.
  Prednisolone acetate and prednisolone sodium phosphate. Systemic. **IM only:** 20–80 mg acetate and 5–20 mg sodium phosphate q several days for 3–4 weeks. **Intra-articular, intrasynovial:** 20–40 mg prednisolone acetate and 5–10 mg prednisolone sodium phosphate.
  Prednisolone sodium phosphate. **Oral Solution:** 5–60 mg daily in single or divided doses. *Adrenocortical insufficiency:* **Pediatric,** 0.14 mg/kg (4 mg/m²) daily in 3–4 divided doses. *Other uses:* **Pediatric:** 0.5–2 mg/kg (15–60 mg/m²) daily in 3–4 divided doses.
  IM, IV: 4–60 mg/day. *Multiple sclerosis (exacerbation):* See *Prednisolone.* **Intralesional, intra-articular, soft tissue injection:** 2–30 mg, depending on site and severity of disease. **Ophthalmic** (0.125%–1% solution): See *Prednisolone Acetate.*
  Prednisolone tebutate. **Intra-articular, intralesional, soft tissue injection:** 4–30 mg, depending on site and severity of disease.

NURSING CONSIDERATIONS

See also *Nursing Considerations* for *Adrenocorticosteroids and Analogs,* p. 1158.

Administration/Storage

1. Before administering prednisolone, check spelling and dose carefully; this drug is frequently confused with prednisone.
2. Check to see if physician wants oral form of drug administered with an antacid.

PREDNISONE   (PRED-nih-sohn)

Oral Solution: Prednisone Intensol (Rx). Syrup: Liquid Pred (Rx). Tablets: Apo-Prednisone✶, Deltasone, Meticorten, Orasone 1, 5, 10, and 50, Prednicen-M, Sterapred, Sterapred DS, Winpred✶ (Rx)

See also *Adrenocorticosteroids and Analogs,* p. 1149.

Classification: Adrenocorticosteroid, synthetic.

Action/Kinetics: Drug is three to five times as potent as cortisone or hydrocortisone. May cause moderate fluid retention. Prednisone is metabolized in the liver to prednisolone, the active form.

Special Concerns: Use during pregnancy only if benefits outweigh risks.

Dosage: *Highly individualized.* **Oral Solution, Syrup, Tablets: (acute, severe conditions): initial,** 5–60 mg daily, in 4 equally divided doses after meals and at bedtime. Decrease gradually by 5–10 mg q 4–5 days to establish minimum maintenance dosage (5–10 mg) or discontinue altogether until symptoms recur. **Pediatric:** *Replacement,* 0.1–0.15 mg/kg daily.

NURSING CONSIDERATIONS

See *Nursing Considerations* for *Adrenocorticosteroids and Analogs,* p. 1158.

TRIAMCINOLONE   (try-am-SIN-oh-lohn)

Dental Paste: Kenalog in Orabase, Oracort, Oralone (Rx). Tablets: Aristocrat, Kenacort (Rx)

TRIAMCINOLONE ACETONIDE   (try-am-SIN-oh-lohn)

Inhalation Aerosol: Azmacort (Rx). Parenteral: Cenocort A-40, Cinonide 40, Kenaject-40, Kenalog-10 and -40, Tac-3, Triam-A, Triamonide 40, Tri-Kort, Trilog (Rx). Topical Aerosol: Kenalog (Rx). Topical Cream: Aristocort, Aristocort A, Aristocort C✶, Aristocort D✶, Aristocort R✶, Delta-Tritex, Flutex, Kenac, Kenalog, Kenalog-H, Kenonel, Triacet, Triaderm✶, Trianide Mild, Trianide Regular, Triderm, Trymex (Rx). Topical Lotion: Kenalog, Kenonel (Rx). Topical Ointment: Aristocort, Aristocort A, Aristocort D✶, Aristocort R✶, Kenac, Kenalog, Kenonel, Triaderm✶, Trymex (Rx)

TRIAMCINOLONE DIACETATE   (try-am-SIN-oh-lohn)

Parenteral: Amcort, Aristocort Forte, Aristocort Intralesional, Articulose-LA, Cenocort Forte, Cenalone 40, Triam-Forte, Triamolone 40, Trilone, Tristoject (Rx). Syrup: Aristocort, Kenacort Diacetate (Rx)

TRIAMCINOLONE HEXACETONIDE   (try-am-SIN-oh-lohn)

Aristospan Intra-Articular, Aristospan Intralesional (Rx)

See also *Adrenocorticosteroids and Analogs,* p. 1149.

Classification: Adrenocorticosteroid, synthetic.

Action/Kinetics: More potent than prednisone. Intermediate-acting. **Onset:** several hours. **Duration:** 1 or more weeks. **t½:** Over 200 min.

Additional Uses: Pulmonary emphysema accompanied by bronchospasm or bronchial edema. Diffuse interstitial pulmonary fibrosis. With diuretics to treat refractory CHF or cirrhosis of the liver with ascites. Multiple sclerosis. Inflammation following dental procedures. Triamcinolone hexacetonide is restricted to intra-articular or intralesional treatment of rheumatoid arthritis and osteoarthritis.

Special Concerns: Use during pregnancy only if benefits clearly outweigh risks. Use with special caution in patients who have decreased renal function or renal disease.

Additional Side Effects: Intra-articular, intrasynovial, or intrabursal administration may cause transient flushing, dizziness, local depigmentation, and, rarely, local irritation. Exacerbation of symptoms has also been reported. A marked increase in swelling and pain and further restricted joint movement may indicate septic arthritis. Intradermal injection may cause local vesicular ulceration and persistent scarring.

Syncope and anaphylactoid reactions have been reported with triamcinolone regardless of route of administration.

Dosage: *Highly individualized. Triamcinolone.* **Tablets.** *Adrenocortical insufficiency (with mineralocorticoid therapy):* 4–12 mg/day. *For treating other disease states:* 8–60 mg/day. *Acute leukemias (children):* 1–2 mg/kg. *Acute leukemia or lymphoma (adults):* 16–40 mg daily (up to 100 mg daily may be necessary). *Edema:* 16–20 mg (up to 48 mg may be required). *Tuberculosis meningitis:* 32–48 mg.

Triamcinolone acetonide. **IM only (not for IV use):** *Systemic,* 2.5–60 mg daily, depending on the disease and its severity. **Intra-articular, intrabursal, tendon sheaths:** 2.5–5 mg for smaller joints and 5–15 mg for larger joints, although up to 40 mg has been employed. **Intradermal:** 1 mg per injection site (use 10 mg/mL suspension only). **Topical** (0.025%, 0.1%, 0.5% ointment or cream; 0.025%, 0.1% lotion; aerosol—to deliver 0.2 mg): Apply sparingly to affected area b.i.d.–q.i.d. and rub in lightly. **Respiratory inhalant. Adults, usual:** 2 inhalations (about 200 mcg) t.i.d.–q.i.d, not to exceed 1,600 mcg daily. **Pediatric, 6–12 years:** 1–2 inhalations (100–200 mcg) t.i.d.–q.i.d., not to exceed 1,200 mcg daily.

Triamcinolone diacetate. **IM,** 40 mg weekly. **Intra-articular/intrasynovial:** 5–40 mg. **Intralesional/sublesional:** 5–48 mg (no more than 12.5 mg per injection site and 25 mg per lesion). **Syrup.** *Adrenocortical insufficiency:* **Adults,** 4–12 mg daily as a single or as divided doses; **pediatric,** 0.117 mg/kg (3.3 mg/m²) daily as a single or as divided doses. *Other uses:* **Adults,** 4–48 mg daily as a single or as divided doses; **pediatric,** 0.416–1.7 mg/kg (12.5–50 mg/m²) daily as a single or as divided doses (for leukemia, the initial dose may be as high as 2 mg/kg daily).

Triamcinolone hexacetonide. **Intra-articular:** 2–6 mg for small joints and 10–20 mg for large joints. **Intralesional/sublesional:** up to 0.5 mg per square inch of affected area. **Not for IV use.**

NURSING CONSIDERATIONS

See also *Nursing Considerations* for *Adrenocorticosteroids and Analogs,* p. 1158.

Client/Family Teaching

1. Instruct client to ingest a liberal amount of protein, because with this drug clients experience gradual weight loss, associated with anorexia, muscle wasting, and weakness.
2. Remind client to lie down if feeling faint. If syncopal episodes persist and interfere with daily activities, then report to physician.
3. Report immediately any new onset of symptoms of depression as well as aggravation of existing symptoms.

MISCELLANEOUS AGENTS

AMINOGLUTETHIMIDE   (ah-meen-oh-glue-**TETH**-ih-myd)

Cytadren (Rx)

Action/Kinetics: This drug decreases the synthesis of glucocorticoids and mineralocorticoids in the adrenal cortex by inhibiting the enzymatic conversion of cholesterol to delta-5-pregnenolone (a precursor to the steroids). **t½:** 5–9 hr (after 1–2 wk use). **Time to peak levels:** 1.5 hr. **Onset to suppress adrenal function:** 3–5 days. **Duration:** 36–72 hr after withdrawing aminoglutethimide and hydrocortisone. Approximately 50% excreted unchanged and 20%–50% is excreted as the acetylated metabolite (approximately one-fifth the activity of aminoglutethimide).

Uses: Cushing's syndrome. *Investigational:* Advanced breast carcinoma in postmenopausal patients; metastatic prostate carcinoma.

Contraindications: Hypersensitivity to aminoglutethimide or glutethimide (Doriden). Can cause harm to the fetus if administered to pregnant women (pregnancy category: D).

Special Concerns: Safety and effectiveness in children not known although the drug in rare cases may induce precocious sexual development in males and masculinization and hirsutism in females. Assess benefits versus risks for use during lactation. Geriatric patients may manifest a higher incidence of CNS effects (including lethargy).

Side Effects: *Most common:* Drowsiness, morbilliform skin rash, nausea, anorexia. *GI:* Vomiting. *CNS:* Headache, dizziness. *Hematologic:* Anemia, pancytopenia, thrombocytopenia, agranulocytosis. *Endocrine:* Adrenal insufficiency, hypothyroidism, masculinization and hirsutism in females, precocious sex development in males. *CV:* Hypotension including orthostatic, tachycardia. *Dermatologic:* Rash, pruritus, urticaria. *Miscellaneous:* Fever, myalgia, cholestatic jaundice (due to hypersensitivity), hepatotoxicity.

Drug Interaction	
Alcohol	↑ Effects of aminoglutethimide
Coumarin	↓ Effect of coumarin due to ↑ rate of breakdown by liver
Dexamethsone	↑ Biotransformation of dexamethasone
Digitoxin	↓ Effect of digitoxin due to ↑ rate of breakdown by liver
Medroxyprogesterone	↓ Effect of medroxyprogesterone due to ↑ rate of breakdown by liver
Theophylline	↓ Effect of theophylline due to ↑ rate of breakdown by liver
Warfarin	↓ Effect of warfarin due to ↑ rate of breakdown by liver

Laboratory Test Interferences: Abnormal liver function tests. ↑ SGOT, alkaline phosphatase.

Dosage: Tablets. Adults: initial, 250 mg b.i.d.–t.i.d. for 2 weeks; **maintenance:** 250 mg q.i.d. *Breast cancer, prostatic cancer:* **Adults,** 250 mg b.i.d.–t.i.d. for 2 weeks in combination with hydrocortisone, 40 mg daily; **maintenance:** 250 mg q 6 hr in combination with hydrocortisone, 40 mg daily.

NURSING CONSIDERATIONS

Administration/Storage

1. Dosage should be initiated in a hospital setting until a stable regimen is reached.
2. Therapy may have to be discontinued or modified in the event of adverse reactions. For example, terminate therapy if skin rash persists for more than 5 to 8 days.
3. When used in combination with hydrocortisone for breast or prostatic carcinoma, 10 mg hydrocortisone should be given in the morning, 10 mg at 5:00 p.m., and 20 mg at bedtime.
4. It may be necessary to initiate mineralocorticoid or glucocorticoid (e.g., hydrocortisone, 20–30 mg PO in the morning) replacement therapy.

Interventions

1. Observe for evidence of suppression of the adrenal cortical function, especially if the client is having surgery, is faced with trauma, or an acute illness.
2. Monitor blood pressure and observe for evidence of hypotension. This results from the suppression of the production of aldosterone.
3. Check the client for hypothyroidism. This is manifested by an enlargement of the thyroid gland and reduced plasma levels of thyroid hormone.
4. Conduct complete blood counts throughout the therapy.

Client/Family Teaching

1. Instruct the client to be alert for symptoms of hypotension, such as weakness, dizziness, and headaches. Sit down or lie down if symptoms occur.
2. Remind client to report any persistent drowsiness, nausea, anorexia, headache, dizziness, weakness, or skin rash.
3. Use caution when driving a car or operating machinery that require mental alertness, because drowsiness or dizziness may occur.

METYRAPONE   (meh-**TEER**-ah-pohn)

Metopirone (Rx)

Classification: Adrenocorticosteroid inhibitor, synthetic.

Action: Metyrapone inhibits cortisol synthesis by the adrenal cortex at the 11-β-hydroxylation step. This results a compensatory increase in ACTH release in persons who have normal hypothalamic-pituitary function followed by a two- to fourfold increase in 17-hydroxycorticoids and a twofold increase in 17-ketosteroid excretion. In hypopituitarism, a subnormal response to metyrapone is seen. **t½:** 1–2.5 hr.

Use: To test for hypothalamicopituitary function. *Investigational:* Control cortisol secretion in Cushing's syndrome.

Contraindications: Adrenocortical insufficiency; hypersensitivity to drug.

Special Concerns: Safe use in pregnancy not established (pregnancy category: C). Assess benefit versus risk for use during lactation.

Side Effects: *GI:* Nausea, abdominal discomfort. *CNS:* Sedation, headache, dizziness. *Dermatologic:* Rashes.

Drug Interactions	
Cyproheptadine	Erroneous results for pituitary function up to 2 weeks following cessation of cyproheptadine therapy
Estrogens	↓ Response to metyrapone
Phenytoin	Erroneous results for pituitary function up to 2 weeks following cessation of phenytoin therapy

Dosage: Tablets. Adults: 750 mg q 4 hr for 6 doses. **Pediatric:** 15 mg/kg q 4 hr for 6 doses (minimal single dose: 250 mg). After a 24-hr control measurement of 17-hydroxycorticoids and 17-ketosteroids (day 1) followed by administration of ACTH to assess cortical function (day 2), metyrapone is given on day 5. On day 6, another 24-hr steroid determination is made.

NURSING CONSIDERATIONS

Administration/Storage

1. Corticosteroid therapy must be discontinued before and during testing.
2. Administer with milk or food, to decrease gastric irritation.

Client/Family Teaching

1. Instruct client to report any drowsiness, nausea, dizziness, or skin rash.
2. Caution client not to perform tasks that require mental alertness until drug effects become apparent.

TRILOSTANE   (TRYE-loh-stayn)

Modrastane (Rx)

Classification: Adrenal corticosteroid inhibitor.

Action/Kinetics: Trilostane inhibits the synthesis of steroids by the adrenal cortex resulting in a decrease in circulating levels of corticosteroids. The drug is effective following the first few days of therapy. Response to the drug is not uniform among patients and is not curative. Results in increased urinary 17-ketosteroids.

Uses: Cushing's syndrome, especially for initial therapy until other approaches can be undertaken (use no longer than 3 months).

Contraindications: Adrenal insufficiency. Kidney or liver disease, pregnancy (pregnancy category: X).

Special Concerns: Use with caution during lactation and in patients receiving other drugs that suppress adrenocortical activity. Safety and efficacy in children have not been established.

Side Effects: *GI:* Diarrhea (common), nausea, GI upset, abdominal pain or discomfort, cramps, bloated feeling, flatulence, belching. *CNS:* Headache, fever, fatigue, fainting. *Dermatologic:* Skin rash, erythema, numbness, tingling. *Other:* Flushing, burning sensation of nasal or oral membranes, pain in muscles and joints, lacrimation, rhinorrhea, nasal stuffiness.

Drug Interactions	
Aminoglutethimide	Severe hypofunction of the adrenal cortex
Loop diuretics (bumetanide, ethacrynic acid, furosemide)	Use with trilostane ↓ potassium loss due to the diuretic
Mitotane	Severe hypofunction of the adrenal cortex
Thiazide diuretics	Use with trilostane ↓ potassium loss due to the diuretic

Dosage: Capsules. Adults: initial, 30 mg q.i.d.; **then,** slowly increase the dose q 3–4 days up to usual of 360 mg/day. Doses above 480 mg/day are not recommended. If no response within 2 weeks, therapy should be discontinued.

NURSING CONSIDERATIONS

Administration/Storage

1. To establish a dosage regimen, therapy should be started in the hospital.
2. In times of severe stress (i.e., illness, surgery), administration of corticosteroids may be necessary.
3. The client must be carefully monitored for corticosteroid levels and plasma electrolytes.

Client/Family Teaching

1. Advise client that barrier-type or other nonhormonal contraception should be practiced during treatment.
2. If pregnancy is suspected, advise the client to report to the physician immediately.

CHAPTER SIXTY-TWO

Estrogens, Progestins, and Oral Contraceptives

ESTROGENS

62

General Statement: Estrogens are first produced in large quantities during puberty and are responsible for the development of primary and secondary female sex characteristics. From puberty on, estrogens are secreted primarily by the ovarian follicles during the early phase of the menstrual cycle. Their production decreases sharply at menopause, but small quantities continue to be produced. Men also produce some estrogens. During each menstrual cycle, estrogens trigger the proliferative phase of the endometrium, affect the vaginal tract mucosa and breast tissue, and increase uterine tone. During adolescence, estrogens cause closure of the epiphyseal junction. Large doses inhibit the development of the long bones by causing premature closure and inhibiting endochondral bone formation. In adult women, estrogens participate in bone maintenance by aiding the deposition of calcium in the protein matrix of bones. They increase elastic elements in the skin, tend to cause sodium and fluid retention, and produce an anabolic effect by enhancing the turnover of dietary nitrogen and other elements into protein. Furthermore, they tend to keep plasma cholesterol at relatively low levels.

All natural estrogens, including estradiol, estrone, and estriol, are steroids. These compounds are either obtained from the urine of pregnant mares or prepared synthetically. Nonsteroidal estrogens, including diethylstilbestrol and chlorotrianisene, are prepared synthetically.

Action/Kinetics: Estrogens combine with receptors in the cytoplasm of the cell, resulting in an increase in protein synthesis. For example, estrogens are required for development of secondary sex characteristics, development and maintenance of the female genital system and breasts. They also produce effects in the pituitary and hypothalamus. Natural estrogens are generally administered parenterally because they are either destroyed in the GI tract or have a significant first-pass effect; hence, adequate plasma levels are never reached. Synthetic derivatives can be given PO and are rapidly absorbed, distributed, and excreted. Estrogens are metabolized in the liver and excreted in urine (major portion) and feces.

Uses: Systemic: Primary ovarian failure, female hypogonadism or castration, menopausal symptoms (especially flushing, sweating, chills), atrophic vaginitis, kraurosis vulvae, abnormal uterine bleeding (progestins are preferred), postpartum breast engorgement. Adjunct to diet and calcium for prophylaxis of osteoporosis. Palliative treatment in advanced, inoperable, metastatic breast carcinoma in postmenopausal women and in men. Advanced inoperable carcinoma of the prostate. Certain estrogens are used as postcoital contraceptives. Mestranol or ethinyl estradiol in combination with a progestin are components of oral contraceptives.

Vaginal: Atrophic vaginitis, atrophic dystrophy of the vulva due to menopause or ovariectomy.

Contraindications: Cancerous or precancerous lesions of the breast (until 5 years after menopause) and of the genital tract. Administer with caution, if at all, to patients with a history of thrombophlebitis, thromboembolism, asthma, epilepsy, migraine, cardiac failure, renal insufficiency, diseases involving calcium or phosphorus metabolism, or a family history of mammary or genital tract cancer. Estrogen therapy may be contraindicated in patients with blood dyscrasias, hepatic disease, or thyroid dysfunction. Prolonged therapy is inadvisable in women who plan to become pregnant. Undiagnosed abnormal genital bleeding.

Estrogens are also contraindicated in patients who have not yet completed bone growth. Estrogens should not be used during pregnancy because they may damage the fetus (pregnancy category: X). Use during lactation.

Special Concerns: Safety and effectiveness have not been determined in children, and estrogens should be used with caution in adolescents in whom bone growth is incomplete.

Side Effects: Systemic use. Untoward reactions to estrogens are dose-dependent. *CV:* Potentially, the most serious side effects involve the cardiovascular system. Thromboembolism, thrombophlebitis, myocardial infarction, pulmonary embolism, retinal thrombosis, mesenteric thrombosis, subarachnoid hemorrhage, postsurgical thromboembolism. Hypertension, edema, stroke. *GI:* Nausea, vomiting, abdominal cramps, bloating, diarrhea, changes in appetite. *Dermatologic:* Most common are chloasma or melasma. Also, erythema multiforme, erythema nodosom, hirsutism, alopecia, hemorrhagic eruptions. *Hepatic:* Cholestatic jaundice, aggravation of porphyria, benign (most common) or malignant liver tumors. *Genitourinary:* Breakthrough bleeding, spotting, changes in amount and/or duration of menstrual flow, amenorrhea (following use), dysmenorrhea, premenstrual-like syndrome. Increased incidence of *Candida* vaginitis. *CNS:* Mental depression, dizziness, changes in libido, chorea, headache, aggravation of migraine headaches, fatigue, nervousness. *Ocular:* Steepening of corneal curvature resulting in intolerance of contact lenses. Optic neuritis or retinal thrombosis, resulting in sudden or gradual, partial or complete loss of vision, double vision, papilledema. *Hematologic:* Increase in prothrombin and blood coagulation factors VII, VIII, IX, and X. Decrease in antithrombin III. *Miscellaneous:* Breast tenderness, enlargement, or secretions. Increased risk of gallbladder disease. Premature closure of epiphyses in children. Increased frequency of benign or malignant tumors of the cervix, uterus, vagina, and other organs. Weight gain. Increased risk of congenital abnormalities. Hypercalcemia in patients with metastatic breast carcinoma.

In males, estrogens may cause gynecomastia, loss of libido, decreased spermatogenesis, testicular atrophy, and feminization. Prolonged use of high doses may inhibit the function of the anterior pituitary. Estrogen therapy affects many laboratory tests.

Vaginal use. *GU:* Vaginal bleeding, vaginal discharge, endometrial withdrawal bleeding, serious bleeding in ovariectomized women with endometriosis. *Miscellaneous:* Breast tenderness.

Drug Interactions	
Anticoagulants, oral	↓ Anticoagulant response by ↑ activity of certain clotting factors
Anticonvulsants	Estrogen-induced fluid retention may precipitate seizures. Also, contraceptive steroids ↑ effect of anticonvulsants by ↓ breakdown in liver and ↓ plasma protein binding
Antidiabetic agents	Estrogens may impair glucose tolerance and thus change requirements for antidiabetic agent
Barbiturates	↓ Effect of estrogen by ↑ breakdown by liver
Phenytoin	See *Anticonvulsants*
Rifampin	↓ Effect of estrogen due to ↑ breakdown by liver
Succinylcholine	Estrogens may ↑ effects of succinylcholine
Tricyclic antidepressants	Possible increased effects of tricyclic antidepressants

Laboratory Test Interferences: Alter liver function tests and thyroid function tests. False + urine glucose test. ↓ Serum cholesterol, total serum lipids, pregnanediol excretion, serum folate. ↑ Serum triglyceride levels, thyroxine-binding globulin, sulfobromophthalein retention, prothrombin; factors VII, VIII, IX, X. Impaired glucose tolerance, reduced response to metyrapone.

Dosage: PO, IM, SC, vaginal, topical, or by implantation.
The dosage of estrogens is highly individualized and is aimed at the minimal effective amount.

NURSING CONSIDERATIONS

Administration/Storage

1. Estrogens may be administered orally, parenterally, intravaginally, or by implanting pellets.
2. The dose is highly individualized and is aimed at the minimal amount that will be effective.
3. Most orally administered estrogens are metabolized rapidly and, with the exception of chlorotrianisene, must be administered daily.
4. Parenterally administered estrogens are released more slowly from their aqueous suspensions or oily solutions. When administered by injection, the drug should be administered slowly and deeply.
5. To avoid continuous stimulation of reproductive tissue, cyclic therapy consisting of 3 weeks on and 1 week off is usually recommended.
6. To reduce postpartum breast engorgement, doses are administered during the first few days after delivery.

Assessment

1. Obtain a health history of the client, noting any history of thromboembolic problems before administering the drug.

2. Note if the client has diabetes.

3. Obtain baseline serum glucose level if client is diabetic and liver function studies if long term therapy is anticipated.

4. List any history of depression, migraine headaches or attempted suicide, document and report to the physician.

Interventions

1. Observe the client for alterations in mental attitude. Signs of depression, withdrawal, complaints of insomnia or anorexia, or a lack of attention to personal appearance should be documented and called to the attention of the physician.

2. Monitor liver function studies.

3. If the client has diabetes, monitor serum glucose and triglyceride levels and report any elevations to the physician.

4. If the client has a history of problems with blood coagulation factors, monitor these and the prothrombin time routinely and report any increase to the physician.

Client/Family Teaching

1. Medical supervision is essential during prolonged estrogen therapy. Advise the client to notify the physician if any new changes occur in her condition.

2. Advise the client who is receiving cyclical therapy to take the medication for 3 weeks and then to omit it for 1 week. Menstruation may then occur, but pregnancy will not occur because ovulation is suppressed. Instruct the client to keep a record of menstruation and any problem encountered such as missed menses, spotting, or irregularity, and report these to the physician.

3. Notify the physician immediately if pregnancy is suspected.

4. Explain to the client that breast tenderness may occur. Also, there may be enlargement or breast secretion. Instruct the client in self breast examination and encourage her to perform this exam monthly. Any continued problems or changes in the breasts should be reported to the physician.

5. If the client has a history of thromboembolic problems, instruct her in how to take her blood pressure and pulse, and how to keep an accurate written record to share with the physician at her next visit.

6. Instruct the client to report to the physician if there are leg pains, sudden onset of chest pain, dizziness, shortness of breath, weakness of the arms or legs or any evidence of numbness.

7. Advise the client to report any unusual vaginal bleeding. This may be caused by excessive amounts of estrogen and the dosage may need to be reduced.

8. Warn the client that nausea, bloating, abdominal cramping, changes in appetite and vomiting may occur. These usually disappear with the continuation of therapy. Taking medication with meals or a light snack will prevent gastric irritation and usually eliminate the nausea. If the medication is to be taken once a day, taking it at bedtime may eliminate the problem.

9. Some clients may develop changes in the curvature of the cornea, making it difficult to wear contact lenses. The client who wears contact lenses needs to be made aware of this potential problem and advised to consult the ophthalmologist if a problem develops.

10. Advise the client to report any skin changes such as alopecia or melasma. The dose of drug may need to be changed or the physician may elect to use a different drug.

11. If the client has diabetes, estrogen can alter glucose tolerance. Advise particularly close monitoring of blood and urine to detect hyperglycemia and glycosuria, and to report any

increase immediately to the physician. The dose of antidiabetic medication may need to be changed.

12. Discuss with male clients who are receiving estrogen therapy the fact that they may develop feminine characteristics or suffer from impotence. These symptoms usually disappear once the course of therapy has been completed.

13. If the treatment demands the use of vaginal suppositories, teach the client how to correctly insert the suppository. Advise the client to wear a perineal pad if there is an increase in vaginal discharge during the treatment. Remind the client to store the suppositories in the refrigerator.

14. Sometimes estrogen ointments may cause systemic reactions to occur. Explain this to the client using the ointment and direct her to notify the physician of these findings.

15. If the client is to apply a vaginal preparation it is best done at bedtime. Advise the client to wear a sanitary napkin when vaginal preparations are being used. Remind her to avoid the use of tampons.

16. If the client is pregnant and is planning to breast-feed her baby, she should notify her physician. A woman who is planning to breast feed should not take estrogens and should consult with her physician for alternative forms of contraception.

17. If the client smokes, explain the added dangers in combination with this drug therapy and assist her in her efforts to stop smoking.

18. Explain that some potential risks have been associated with estrogen therapy, such as endometrial cancer. Check with the physician to ensure that the client is aware of these.

CHLOROTRIANISENE   (klor-oh-try-**AN**-ih-seen)

Tace (Rx)

Classification: Estrogen, synthetic, nonsteroidal.

Action/Kinetics: The long-lasting effect of this synthetic estrogen is attributed to its storage in adipose tissue, which then acts as a reservoir.

Dosage: Capsules. *Prostatic cancer:* 12–25 mg daily (given chronically). *Breast engorgement:* The following regimens are used: (a) 12 mg q.i.d. for 7 days or (b) 50 mg q 6 hr for 6 doses. For each regimen, the first dose should be given within 8 hr after delivery. *Atrophic vaginitis, kraurosis vulvae:* 12–25 mg daily given cyclically for 30 to 60 days. *Female hypogonadism:* 12–25 mg/day cyclically for 21 days; give PO progestin for last 5 days of therapy or IM progesterone (100 mg). Begin next course on day 5 of menstrual flow. *Vasomotor symptoms associated with menopause:* 12–25 mg daily given cyclically for 30 days; additional courses of treatment may be necessary.

NURSING CONSIDERATIONS
See *Nursing Considerations* for *Estrogens,* p. 1183.

DIENESTROL   (dye-en-**ESS**-trohl)

DV, Ortho Dienestrol (Rx)

Classification: Estrogen, synthetic.

Use: Dienestrol is available only as a cream and is used for atrophic vaginitis and kraurosis vulvae.

Side Effect: Vaginal bleeding and/or discharge; breast tenderness, estrogen withdrawal bleeding.

Dosage: Vaginal cream: initial, 1–2 applicatorfuls daily for 1–2 weeks; **then,** 1 applicatorful (or one-half the initial dose) every other day for an additional 1–2 weeks. Once vaginal mucosa is restored, a maintenance dose of 1 applicatorful 1–3 times a week may be used.

NURSING CONSIDERATIONS
See *Nursing Considerations* for *Estrogens,* p. 1183.

DIETHYLSTILBESTROL DIPHOSPHATE (DES)   (dye-eth-ill-still-**BESS**-trohl)

Honvol ✿, Stilphostrol (Rx)

See also *Estrogens,* p. 1181, and *Antineoplastic Agents,* p. 287.

Classification: Estrogen, synthetic, nonsteroidal.

Action/Kinetics: As an antineoplastic agent for prostatic carcinoma, estrogens inhibit the release of LH which, in turn, decreases testosterone levels. Thus further growth of the neoplasm is inhibited. Metabolized in the liver.

Uses: Palliative treatment of prostatic cancer and inoperable breast cancer in men and postmenopausal women.

Contraindications: Active thrombophlebitis, thromboembolic disease, markedly impaired liver function. **Not to be used during pregnancy because of the possibility of vaginal cancer in female offspring.**

Special Concerns: Use with caution in presence of hypercalcemia, epilepsy, migraine, asthma, cardiac and renal disease.

Side Effects: Thrombophlebitis, pulmonary embolism, cerebral thrombosis, neuro-ocular lesions. *GI:* Nausea, vomiting, anorexia. *CNS:* Headaches, malaise, irritability. *Skin:* Allergic rash, itching. *GU:* Gynecomastia, changes in libido. *Other:* Porphyria, backache, pain and sterile abscess at injection site, postinjection flare.

Dosage: Tablets. *Prostatic carcinoma, inoperable and progressive:* 50 mg t.i.d. up to 200 mg t.i.d., not to exceed 1 g daily. **IV.** *Prostatic carcinoma, inoperable and progressive:* 500 mg (in 250 mL 5% dextrose or saline) on day 1 followed by 1 g (in 250–500 mL 5% dextrose or saline) daily for 5 days. **Maintenance, IV:** 250–500 mg 1 to 2 times weekly. Maintenance dose may also be given orally.

NURSING CONSIDERATIONS
See also *Nursing Considerations* for *Estrogens,* p. 1183, and *Antineoplastic Agents,* p. 303.

Administration/Storage
1. Administer the diphosphate slowly by drip, 20–30 drops per minute for first 10–15 minutes. Then adjust the flow for a total administration period of 1 hour.
2. If stored away from direct light, the disphosphate solutions are stable at room temperature for five days.
3. Do not use the solution if it appears cloudy or if a precipitate has formed.
4. Have IV fluids, diuretics, adrenocorticosteroids and phosphate supplements available in the event of severe hypercalcemia.

Assessment

1. Take a complete client history, noting any past occurrences of thrombophlebitis, thromboembolic conditions or impaired liver function.
2. If the client is of childbearing age, identify the possibility of pregnancy. The drug is contraindicated in pregnancy.
3. Note any history of poor cardiac function. Obtain a baseline ECG against which to measure subsequent tests.

Interventions

1. If the client has a history of poor cardiac function, check routinely for the presence of edema.
2. The combined effect of the drug and osteolytic metastases may result in hypercalcemia. Assess client for symptoms of hypercalcemia some of which may include insomnia, lethargy, anorexia, nausea, vomiting, coma, and vascular collapse. Withhold the drug, obtain serum calcium levels and report to the physician if high.
3. Encourage a high fluid intake to minimize hypercalcemia.
4. If the client is resuming therapy after a drug-induced hypercalcemia has been corrected, monitor her closely.
5. Gynecomastia may be prevented in men by administering low doses of radiation prior to initiating diethylstilbestrol therapy. If this is a concern, it should be discussed with the physician.

Client/Family Teaching

1. Encourage the client to report any lumps or sores that do not heal. These may be sterile abscesses and require the attention of the physician.
2. Advise the client to report any nausea, vomiting, abdominal pain, or painful swelling of the breasts to the physician.
3. Advise clients that eating solid food often relieves nausea.
4. Discuss with clients who have a history of poor cardiac function the need to be weighed daily, noting any gradual increase in weight. This could be an indication of edema. Instruct the client in how to check the extremities for edema and some of the less obvious signs of its presence. If they occur, they should be reported to the physician immediately.

ESTERIFIED ESTROGENS (es-TER-ih-fyd ES-troh-jens)

Estratab, Menest, Neo-Estrone ❋ (Rx)

See also *Estrogens,* p. 1181.

Classification: Estrogen, natural.

Action/Kinetics: This product is a mixture of sodium salts of sulfate esters of natural estrogenic substances: 75%–85% estrone sodium sulfate and 6%–15% equilin sodium sulfate. Less potent than estrone.

Uses: Replacement therapy in primary ovarian failure, following castration, or hypogonadism. Prostatic or breast carcinoma. Vasomotor symptoms, atrophic vaginitis, and kraurosis vulvae due to menopause. Prophylaxis of osteoporosis.

Dosage: Tablets. *Menopausal symptoms:* 0.3–1.25 mg daily, up to 3.75 mg daily if necessary, given cyclically. *Atrophic vaginitis, kraurosis vulvae:* 0.3–1.25 mg/day; use cyclically for short-term.

Hypogonadism: 2.5–7.5 mg/day in divided doses for 20–21 days, followed by a 7- to 10-day rest period. *Primary ovarian failure, castration:* 1.25 mg/day in divided doses for 20 days with the addition of a progestin the last 5 days. *Prostatic carcinoma:* 1.25–2.5 mg t.i.d. for several weeks. *Breast carcinoma in men and postmenopausal women:* 10 mg t.i.d. for 3 months. *Prophylaxis of osteoporosis:* 0.3–1.25 mg daily for 20 or 21 days (a progestin should be given concurrently for 10–14 days of each cycle).

NURSING CONSIDERATIONS

See *Nursing Considerations* for *Estrogens,* p. 1183.

ESTRADIOL ORAL   (ess-trah-**DYE**-ohl)

Estrace (Rx)

Classification: Estrogen, naturally derived, steroidal.

Dosage: Tablets. *Vasomotor symptoms, kraurosis vulvae, atrophic vaginitis, hypogonadism, primary ovarian failure:* **initial,** 1–2 mg daily; **then,** adjust dosage to control symptoms. Give cyclically (3 weeks on, 1 week off). *Prostatic carcinoma:* 1–2 mg t.i.d. chronically. *Breast carcinoma in males and females:* 10 mg t.i.d. for a minimum of 3 months.
   Vaginal Cream. *Atrophic vaginitis, kraurosis vulvae:* 2–4 g/day for 2 weeks; **then,** slowly reduce to one-half initial dose for 2 weeks. **Maintenance:** 1 g 1–3 times a week.

NURSING CONSIDERATIONS

See also *Nursing Considerations* for *Estrogens,* p. 1183.

Administration/Storage

When used vaginally, the medication should be inserted high into the vagina (2/3 the length of the applicator).

Evaluation

Determine effectiveness in clients with prostatic carcinoma by determining phosphatase levels along with symptomatic improvements.

ESTRADIOL CYPIONATE IN OIL   (ess-trah-**DYE**-ohl)

depGynogen, Depo-Estradiol Cypionate, Depogen, Dura-Estrin, Estra-D, Estro-Cyp, Estroject-LA, Estronol-LA (Rx)

Uses: Female hypogonadism, vasomotor symptoms associated with menopause.

Dosage: IM only. *Menopausal symptoms:* 1–5 mg q 3–4 weeks. *Hypogonadism:* 1.5–2.0 mg at monthly intervals. Supplied in cottonseed oil.

NURSING CONSIDERATIONS

See also *Nursing Considerations* for *Estrogens,* p. 1183.

Administration/Storage

1. Injectable solutions of the esters should be protected from light and stored at room temperature to prevent separation of crystals from oil solutions.

2. For IM administration of estradiol in oil, heat the unopened vial in warm water for a few minutes to decrease the viscosity of the oil.

3. Agitate the vial to resuspend the medication. When no more particles are visible on the sides or bottom of the vial, the drug has been adequately suspended in solution.

4. Draw up the correct dosage in a syringe that has been fitted with a 19–21 gauge needle, and administer immediately before the oil cools.

5. Inject the drug into the buttocks, thigh or ventrogluteal region, using slow, even pressure. Injecting the medication too rapidly may cause the needle and syringe to separate and spilling of the drug, resulting in an inaccurate dosage.

6. Establish a record for documentation of sites and rotate injection sites.

7. Never administer oil preparations IV.

Assessment

1. Determine if the client has an allergy to tartrazine, a yellow dye used in some brands of preparation.

2. Determine if the client has a sensitivity to cottonseed oil before initiating therapy.

ESTRADIOL TRANSDERMAL SYSTEM   (ess-trah-**DYE**-ohl)

Estraderm (Rx)

See also *Estrogens,* p. 1181.

Classification: Estrogen.

Action/Kinetics: This transdermal system allows a constant low dose of estradiol to reach the systemic circulation directly. It is believed that this system overcomes certain of the problems associated with oral use, including first-pass hepatic metabolism, GI upset, and induction of liver enzymes. The system is available in surface areas of 10 cm² (4 mg estradiol with a release rate of 0.05 mg/24 hr) and 20 cm² (8 mg estradiol with a release rate of 0.1 mg/24 hr).

Uses: Menopausal symptoms, female hypogonadism or castration, atrophic vaginitis, kraurosis vulvae, primary ovarian failure.

Dosage: Dermal System. Initial: One 0.05 mg system applied to the skin two times each week; **then,** dose is adjusted to control symptoms. Attempts should be made to decrease the dose or withdraw the medication every 3–6 months.

NURSING CONSIDERATIONS

See also *Nursing Considerations* for *Estrogens,* p. 1183.

Administration/Storage

1. If the client has been taking oral estrogens, withdraw the oral therapy and wait 1 week before applying the system.

2. For clients who have not undergone a hysterectomy, the system is usually used for 3 weeks, followed by 1 week of rest.

3. Place the system on a clean, dry area of the skin on the trunk of the body (preferably the abdomen).

4. The system should not be applied to the breasts or the waistline.

5. The application site should be rotated. Allow at least a 1-week interval between reapplication to a particular site.

6. Addition of a progestin for 7 or more days may reduce the incidence of endometrial hyperplasia.

Client/Family Teaching

1. If the client is to use a transdermal patch, instruct her to cleanse the area, usually on the abdomen, and apply the patch.

2. Instruct the client to avoid using areas of the body with excessive amounts of hair.

3. Advise the client to apply the system immediately after opening the pouch and removing the protective liner. Instruct her to press the system firmly in place by holding for 10 sec.

4. Instruct the client that if the patch falls off it should be replaced by a new one and the days of dosage administration should be readjusted. If the client has difficulty following the instructions, stress the importance of contacting the nurse or physician to review the instructions.

5. The drug is usually prescribed to be used twice a week. Discuss with the client the importance of administering the drug only as prescribed.

6. Explain the importance of rotating the patch sites and teach the client how to record them so that one area is not overused.

ESTRADIOL VALERATE IN OIL   (ess-trah-**DYE**-ohl)

Deladiol-40, Delestrogen, Dioval, Dioval XX, Dioval 40, Duragen-10, -20, and -40, Estradiol L.A. 10, 20 and 40, Estra-L-20 and -40, Femogex✿, Gynogen L.A. 10, 20, and 40, L.A.E. 20, Valergen-10, 20-, and -40 (Rx)

Uses: Severe vasomotor symptoms, atrophic vaginitis, or kraurosis vulvae associated with menopause. Female hypogonadism, primary ovarian failure, female castration. Prophylaxis of postpartum breast engorgement. Prostatic carcinoma.

Dosage: IM Only. *Menopause, atrophic vaginitis, kraurosis vulvae, hypogonadism, primary ovarian failure:* 10–20 mg q 4 weeks. *Postpartum breast engorgement:* 10–25 mg as a single injection at end of first stage of labor. *Prostatic carcinoma:* 30 mg (or more) q 1–2 weeks. Supplied in sesame oil.

NURSING CONSIDERATIONS

See also *Nursing Considerations* for *Estrogens,* p. 1183.

Assessment

Determine if the client has a sensitivity to sesame oil prior to initiating therapy.

ESTROGENIC SUBSTANCES, AQUEOUS

Estroject-2, Gynogen, Kestrin Aqueous, Wehgen (Rx)

See also *Estrogens,* p. 1181.

Classification: Estrogen, steroidal.

Action/Kinetics: These preparations contain a mixture of steroidal estrogens, mostly estrone, in an aqueous suspension.

Dosage: IM only. *Menopause, kraurosis vulvae, atrophic vaginitis:* 0.1–0.5 mg 2–3 times/week. *Hypogonadism, primary ovarian failure, castration:* **Initial:** 0.1–1 mg/week in single or divided doses. Up to 2 mg/week may be necessary. *Prostatic carcinoma (inoperable):* 2–4 mg 2–3 times/week. Response to therapy should become apparent within 3 months after initiation of therapy.

NURSING CONSIDERATIONS

See *Nursing Considerations* for *Estrogens,* p. 1183.

ESTROGENS CONJUGATED, ORAL (CONJUGATED ESTROGENIC SUBSTANCES) (ES-troh-jens)

C.E.S.✿, Conjugated Estrogens C.S.D.✿, Premarin, Progens (Rx)

ESTROGENS CONJUGATED, PARENTERAL (ES-troh-jens)

Premarin IV (Rx)

ESTROGENS CONJUGATED, VAGINAL (ES-troh-jens)

Premarin (Rx)

See also *Estrogens,* p. 1181, and *Esterified Estrogens,* p. 1187.

Classification: Estrogen, natural.

Action/Kinetics: This preparation contains 50–65% sodium estrone sulfate and 20–35% sodium equilin sulfate.

Uses: Oral: Menopausal symptoms, atrophic vaginitis, kraurosis vulvae, hypogonadism in females, primary ovarian failure, female castration, palliation in mammary or prostatic carcinoma, osteoporosis, prophylaxis of postpartum breast engorgement. **Parenteral:** Abnormal bleeding due to imbalance of hormones and in the absence of disease. **Vaginal:** Atrophic vaginitis and kraurosis vulvae associated with menopause.

Dosage: Tablets. *Menopausal symptoms, primary ovarian failure, female castration:* 1.25 mg daily. *Atrophic vaginitis, kraurosis vulvae:* 0.3–1.25 mg daily (higher doses may be necessary, depending on the response). *Hypogonadism in females:* 2.5–7.5 mg daily in divided doses followed by a 10-day rest period. *Palliation of mammary carcinoma:* 10 mg t.i.d. for at least 90 days. *Palliation of prostatic carcinoma:* 1.25–2.5 mg t.i.d. *Prophylaxis of postpartum breast engorgement:* 3.75 mg q 4 hr for a total of 5 doses (alternate regimen: 1.25 mg q 4 hr for 5 days). *Prophylaxis of osteoporosis:* 0.625 mg daily (given cyclically).
   IM, IV: 25 mg, which may be repeated after 6–12 hr if necessary.
   Vaginal cream: 2–4 g daily given for 3 weeks on and 1 week off.

NURSING CONSIDERATIONS

See also *Nursing Considerations* for *Estrogens,* p. 1183.

Administration/Storage

1. For all uses, except postpartum breast engorgement and palliation of mammary and prostatic

carcinoma, oral conjugated estrogens are administered cyclically—3 weeks of hormone therapy and 1 week off.

2. Parenteral solutions of conjugated estrogens are compatible with normal saline, invert sugar solutions, and dextrose solutions.

3. Parenteral solutions are incompatible with acid solutions, ascorbic acid solutions, and protein hydrolysates.

4. Reconstituted parenteral solutions should be used within a few hours after mixing if kept at room temperatures. Put the date and time of reconstitution on the solution label.

5. If the solution is refrigerated it will remain stable for 60 days.

6. When used vaginally, the cream should be inserted high into the vagina (2/3 the length of the applicator).

Evaluation
When the client has been treated with conjugated estrogens the effectiveness in palliation of prostatic carcinoma can be assessed by determining the serum phosphatase levels.

ESTRONE AQUEOUS SUSPENSION   (ESS-trohn)
Estrone 5, Estronol, Kestrone-5, Theelin Aqueous (Rx)

See also *Estrogens,* p. 1181.

Classification: Estrogen, natural.

Uses: Hypogonadism, primary ovarian failure, female castration, atrophic vaginitis, kraurosis vulvae, abnormal uterine bleeding due to hormone imbalance. Inoperable and progressive prostatic cancer and breast cancer (in men and postmenopausal women).

Dosage: IM only. *Menopausal symptoms, atrophic vaginitis, kraurosis vulvae:* 0.1–0.5 mg 1–3 times weekly. *Hypogonadism, primary ovarian failure, castration:* 0.1–1 mg/week in single or divided doses (up to 2 mg/week may be necessary). *Abnormal uterine bleeding due to hormone imbalance:* 2–5 mg for several days. *Prostatic carcinoma (inoperable):* 2–4 mg 2–3 times/week; response should be apparent within 3 months of initiating therapy. *Breast cancer (inoperable):* 5 mg 3 or more times weekly (dose determined on severity of pain).

NURSING CONSIDERATIONS
See *Nursing Considerations* for *Estrogens,* p. 1183.

ESTROPIPATE (PIPERAZINE ESTRONE SULFATE)   (ESS-troh-pip-ayt)
Ogen (Rx)

See also *Estrogens,* p. 1181.

Classification: Estrogen, steroidal, natural or synthetic.

Action/Kinetics: This product contains solubilized crystalline estrone stabilized with piperazine.

Uses: Oral: Vasomotor symptoms, atrophic vaginitis, kraurosis associated with menopause. Primary ovarian failure, female castration, female hypogonadism.

Vaginal: Atrophic vaginitis and kraurosis vulvae associated with menopause.

Dosage: Tablets. *Vasomotor symptoms, atrophic vaginitis, kraurosis vulvae:* 0.625–5 mg/day for short-term therapy (give cyclically). *Hypogonadism, primary ovarian failure, castration:* 1.25–7.5 mg/day for first 3 weeks; **then,** rest period of 8–10 days. A progestin can be given during the third week if withdrawal bleeding does not occur. **Vaginal cream:** 1–2 applicatorsful/day; then, reduce dose gradually. **Vaginal Cream:** 2–4 g daily (depending on severity of condition) for 3 weeks followed by a 1 week rest period.

NURSING CONSIDERATIONS
See *Nursing Considerations* for *Estrogens,* p. 1183.

ETHINYL ESTRADIOL   (ETH-in-ill)
Estinyl, Feminone (Rx)

See also *Estrogens,* p. 1181.

Classification: Estrogen, steroidal, synthetic.

Action/Kinetics: This synthetic steroid is a derivative of estradiol. It is effective orally and is a component of many oral contraceptives.

Uses: Vasomotor symptoms associated with menopause, female hypogonadism. Inoperable, progressive carcinoma of the breast and prostate.

Dosage: Tablets. *Menopausal symptoms:* 0.02 or 0.05 mg daily (up to 1.5 mg daily may be necessary). Give cyclically (3 weeks on followed by a 7 day rest period); a progestin may be added during last 5 days of cycle. *Female hypogonadism:* 0.05 mg 1–3 times/day for first 2 weeks of theoretical menstrual cycle; then, administer progesterone for the second half of the cycle. Continue for 3–6 months after which patient is not treated for 2 months. Additional cycles may be necessary. *Carcinoma of the female breast (inoperable):* 1 mg t.i.d. chronically. *Carcinoma of prostate:* 0.15–2 mg daily, given chronically.

NURSING CONSIDERATIONS
See *Nursing Considerations* for *Estrogens,* p. 1183.

POLYESTRADIOL PHOSPHATE   (poll-ee-es-trah-DYE-ol)
Estradurin (Rx)

See *Antineoplastic Agents,* Chapter 18, p. 373.

QUINESTROL   (kwin-ESS-trohl)
Estrovis (Rx)

Classification: Estrogen, steroidal.

Action/Kinetics: Orally active estrogen is stored in body fat, is slowly released, and is subsequently metabolized in the blood to the active ethinyl estradiol. Ethinyl estradiol is excreted unchanged in the feces and by the kidneys.

Uses: Vasomotor symptoms associated with menopause, female hypogonadism, atrophic vaginitis, kraurosis vulvae, primary ovarian failure, female castration.

Dosage: Tablets. *Menopausal symptoms, atrophic vaginitis, replacement therapy, kraurosis vulvae:* **Initial,** 100 mcg daily for 7 days; **then,** 100 mcg weekly beginning 2 weeks after starting therapy. Some patients may require 200 mcg/week. At 3–6 month intervals, attempts should be made to discontinue or reduce the dosage of the drug.

NURSING CONSIDERATIONS
See *Nursing Considerations* for *Estrogens,* p. 1183.

PROGESTERONE AND PROGESTINS

General Statement: Progesterone is a natural female ovarian steroid hormone produced in large amounts during pregnancy. It is chiefly secreted by the corpus luteum during the second half of the menstrual cycle and is produced by the placenta during pregnancy.

The hormone acts on the thick muscles of the uterus (myometrium) and on its lining (endometrium). It prepares the latter for the implantation of the fertilized ovum. Under the influence of progesterone, the estrogen-primed endometrium enters its "secretory phase" during which it thickens and secretes large quantities of mucus and glycogen. The myometrium relaxes under the effect of progesterone. During puberty, progesterone participates in the maturation of the female body, acting on the breasts and the vaginal mucosa.

Progesterone interacts, by a feedback mechanism, with the hormones FSH and LH produced by the anterior pituitary. When progesterone and estrogen are high, there is a decrease in the production of FSH and LH. This inhibits ovulation and accounts for the fact that progesterone is an effective contraceptive. Natural progesterone has to be injected, but a whole series of compounds with progesterone-type activity (collectively called *progestins*) can be taken orally. These substances are now routinely substituted for natural progesterone. Progesterone is essential for the maintenance of pregnancy.

Although progesterone stimulates the development of alveolar mammary tissue during pregnancy, it does not initiate lactation. On the contrary, it suppresses the lactogenic hormone; lactation starts postpartum only when progesterone and estrogen levels have decreased.

Action/Kinetics: Physiologic doses are used for replacement therapy and to suppress gonadotropin production, which inhibits ovulation. Pharmacologic doses have several uses (see below). Progesterone must be administered parenterally because of major inactivation in the liver (first-pass effect). The hormones are metabolized in the liver and a major portion is excreted in the urine (urinalysis is used to monitor progesterone levels).

Uses: Abnormal uterine bleeding, primary or secondary amenorrhea (used with an estrogen), endometriosis, premenstrual tension. Alone or with an estrogen for contraception. May also be used in combination with an estrogen for endometriosis and hypermenorrhea. Certain types of cancer. *Note:* Not to be used to prevent habitual abortion or to treat threatened abortion.

Contraindications: Genital malignancies, thromboembolic disease, vaginal bleeding of unknown origin, impaired liver function. Pregnancy, especially during the first four months. Cancer of the breast, missed abortion, as a diagnostic test for pregnancy. Lactation.

Special Concerns: Use with caution in case of asthma, epilepsy, depression, and migraine.

Side Effects: Occasionally noted with short-term dosage, frequently observed with prolonged high dosage. *Genitourinary:* Spotting, irregular periods, amenorrhea, changes in amount and/or duration of menstrual flow, changes in cervical secretions and cervical erosion, breast tenderness or secretions. *Dermatologic:* Allergic rashes, pruritus, acne, melasma, chloasma, alopecia, hirsutism. *CNS:* Depression, pyrexia, insomnia. *Miscellaneous:* Weight gain or loss, cholestatic jaundice, masculinization of the female fetus, nausea, edema, precipitation of acute intermittent porphyria, photosensitivity.

Drug Interactions: Rifampin and possibly phenobarbital ↓ the effect of progesterone by ↑ breakdown by the liver.

Dosage: Progesterone must be administered parenterally. Other progestins can be administered PO and parenterally. The usual schedule of administration for *functional uterine bleeding, amenorrhea, infertility, dysmenorrhea, premenstrual tension and contraception* is days 5 through 25 of the menstrual cycle, with day 1 being the first day of menstrual flow.

NURSING CONSIDERATIONS

Assessment

1. Assess the client's history for evidence of thrombophlebitis, pulmonary embolism, or cerebrovascular accidents.
2. Obtain a baseline blood pressure, pulse, and weight and document.
3. Determine if the client has a history of psychic depression and record on the client's record.
4. Note if the client has diabetes mellitus.

Interventions

1. Monitor the blood pressure and pulse and report any changes from the baseline findings.
2. Observe the client's extremities for evidence of edema, document and report to the physician.
3. Check the client for changes such as yellowing of the sclera and report if evident.

Client/Family Teaching

1. Teach the client the symptoms of thrombic disorders such as pains in the legs, sudden onset of chest pain, shortness of breath, and coughing for no apparent reason. Instruct the client to report these symptoms to the physician immediately.
2. Advise the client to weigh him/herself at least twice a week and to report any unusual weight gain. Rapid weight gain may indicate the presence of edema.
3. Discuss with the client the need to report any yellowing of the skin or sclera. This indicates jaundice and may necessitate the discontinuation of the medication or a change in the dosage.
4. To avoid gastric irritation and nausea, advise the client to take the medication with a light snack, in the evening.
5. Explain to the client that gastric distress usually subsides after the first few cycles of the drug. However, if these symptoms persist, they should be reported to the physician.
6. If any episodes of bleeding occur, they should be reported to the physician.
7. Discuss with the client and family the fact that progestins may reactivate or worsen a psychic depression. Advise them to take particular note of any psychic changes the client may undergo, the circumstance of the depression, and to report this to the physician.
8. Advise clients with diabetes that progesterone may alter glucose tolerance. Instruct them to

report positive urine tests for glucose and abnormal finger stick results promptly because the dosage of antidiabetic medication may need to be adjusted.

9. Instruct the client to report early symptoms of ophthalmic pathology, such as headaches, dizziness, blurred vision, or partial loss of vision.

10. If the client smokes, advise her to stop smoking. Offer assistance and suggest an antismoking program that has proven successful.

11. Emphasize the need to report to the physician regularly for medical follow-up.

HYDROXYPROGESTERONE CAPROATE IN OIL (hi-drok-see-proh-JESS-ter-ohn)
Duralutin, Gesterol L.A.250, Hydrogest 250, Hylutin, Pro-Depo (Rx)

Classification: Progestational hormone, synthetic.

Action/Kinetics: Hydroxyprogesterone is a synthetic progestin devoid of androgenic effects. It is suitable for prolonged therapy; priming with estrogens may be necessary to obtain desired response. **Duration:** 9–17 days.

Additional Side Effects: Rarely, dyspnea, chest constriction, coughing, allergic reactions.

Dosage: IM. *Amenorrhea and other menstrual disorders:* 375 mg, started anytime during cycle. If no menses after 21 days, cyclic therapy should be initiated repeating every 4 weeks and stopping after 4 cycles. Wait for 2–3 cycles after cessation of therapy to determine whether normal cyclic function has occurred. *Adenocarcinoma of uterine corpus (advanced):* **Initially,** 1 g; **then,** 1–7 g/week. If no response after 12 weeks, therapy should be terminated. *Test for endogenous estrogen production:* 250 mg, anytime during the cycle; repeat after 4 weeks for confirmation.

NURSING CONSIDERATIONS
See also *Nursing Considerations* for *Progesterone and Progestins,* p. 1195.

Administration/Storage

1. A wet syringe and needle may cause the solution to become cloudy. This does not affect the potency of the drug.
2. Store at room temperature.

INTRAUTERINE PROGESTERONE CONTRACEPTIVE SYSTEM
Progestasert (Rx)

Classification: Contraceptive system (intrauterine device).

Action/Kinetics: Progestasert is an intrauterine contraceptive device (IUD) impregnated with a reservoir of 38 mg progesterone. Its contraceptive effectiveness is 12 months and it is considered superior to conventional IUDs, because of its smaller size. It can, however, be expelled from the uterine cavity inadvertently.

The mechanism of action is uncertain. It is believed to change the uterine milieu to prevent nidation and/or alter capacitation (ability of sperm to fertilize egg). Releases 65 mcg progesterone/day into the uterine cavity.

Uses: Contraception in parous and nulliparous women. *Investigational:* Menorrhagia.

Contraindications: Pregnancy or suspicion thereof, previous ectopic pregnancy, presence or history of pelvic inflammatory disease (PID), venereal disease, postpartum endometriosis, previous pelvic surgery, suspicion of malignant uterine disease, genital bleeding of unknown origin, acute cervicitis.

Special Concerns: Use with caution in presence of coagulopathy. Use with caution in patients with a history of metrorrhagia or menorrhagia following IUD use, valvular or congenital heart disease.

Side Effects: Increased incidence of septic abortion; increased likelihood of ectopic pregnancy occurs with device in place. Transitory bleeding and cramps during initial weeks after insertion. Also, endometriosis, spontaneous abortion, septicemia, perforation of uterus and cervix, pelvic infection, cervical erosion, vaginitis, leukorrhea, uterine embedment, difficult removal, intermenstrual spotting, increased duration of menstruation, anemia, amenorrhea, delayed menses, dysmenorrhea, backaches, dyspareunia (painful coitus), neurovascular episodes including bradycardia and syncope following insertion, perforation of abdomen resulting in abdominal adhesions, intestinal penetration, intestinal obstruction, cystic masses in the pelvis.

Drug Interaction: Use with caution in patients receiving anticoagulants.

Dosage: One Progestasert system inserted into the uterine cavity; must be replaced once a year after insertion.

NURSING CONSIDERATIONS

Administration/Storage
The drug should be inserted during or shortly after menses, since the system may cause the fetus to abort if the woman is pregnant.

Assessment
1. Note if the client has a history of syncope, bradycardia, or other neurovascular episodes. These problems may occur during the insertion or removal of an IUD.
2. Obtain a Papanicolaou (Pap) smear, a culture for gonococcus infection and tests for other venereal diseases before insertion of an IUD.
3. Determine if the client suspects pregnancy, is postpartum or has had previous pelvic surgery.

Interventions
1. Note any client complaint of transitory bleeding and cramps during the first weeks after insertion. Document and report these to the physician.
2. Observe for any evidence of pelvic infection, such as elevation of temperature, cramping, vaginitis or leukorrhea. Report these to the physician immediately.

Client/Family Teaching
1. Instruct the client to read the instructions and package insert carefully and to ask the nurse or physician if she does not understand the directions.
2. Plan for insertion during menstruation to reduce the possibility of insertion during pregnancy.
3. Advise the client that bleeding and cramping may occur for a few weeks after insertion. However, these should subside and if not, the problem should be reported to the physician.
4. Explain to the client the schedule for reexamination and replacement:
   - Preferably after the first menses following the insertion, and definitely by the third month after insertion.
   - An annual examination is necessary.

- An annual replacement, if this form of contraception is to be continued, since the progesterone supply of the device will then have been depleted.

5. Explain how to recognize the symptoms of an ectopic pregnancy. These may include a delayed menses, excessive bleeding, pelvic pain, weakness and fatigue.

6. Review with the client the symptoms of septicemia. Septicemia is usually characterized by "flu-like" symptoms, such as fever, abdominal cramping, pain, bleeding, or abnormal vaginal discharge. Symptoms of ectopic pregnancy and septicemia should be reported to the physician immediately.

7. Explain to the client how to check for proper placement of the IUD.

8. If the client notices that the threads of the IUD do not protrude from the cervix after menstruation, she should suspect that there has been partial expulsion. The client should then return for removal or replacement of the IUD.

MEDROXYPROGESTERONE ACETATE   (meh-drok-see-proh-JESS-ter-ohn)

Amen, Curretab, Cycrin, Depo-Provera, Provera (Rx)

See also *Progesterone/Progestins,* p. 1194, and *Antineoplastic Agents,* p. 287.

Classification: Progestational hormone, synthetic.

Action/Kinetics: Medroxyprogesterone acetate, a synthetic progestin, is devoid of estrogenic and androgenic activity. The drug prevents stimulation of endometrium by pituitary gonadotropins. Also available in depot form. Priming with estrogen is necessary before response is noted.

Additional Uses: Secondary amenorrhea, abnormal uterine bleeding due to hormonal imbalance (no organic pathology). Adjunct in palliative treatment of inoperable, recurrent, or metastatic endometrial or renal carcinoma. *Investigational:* Premenopausal and menopausal symptoms (injection). To stimulate respiration in obesity—hypoventilation syndrome (oral). The depot form has been used as a long-acting contraceptive and to treat advanced breast cancer.

Contraindications: Patients with or a history of thrombophlebitis, thromboembolic disease, cerebral apoplexy. Liver dysfunction. Known or suspected malignancy of the breasts or genital organs. Missed abortion; as a diagnostic for pregnancy. Undiagnosed vaginal bleeding.

Dosage: Tablets. *Secondary amenorrhea:* 5–10 mg/day for 5–10 days, with therapy beginning at any time. If endometrium has been estrogen primed: 10 mg medroxyprogesterone per day for 10–13 days (beginning on day 16–13, respectively). *Abnormal uterine bleeding with no pathology:* 5–10 mg/day for 5–10 days, with therapy beginning on day 16 or 21 of the menstrual cycle. If endometrium has been estrogen primed: 10 mg/day for 10 days, beginning on day 16 of the menstrual cycle. Bleeding usually begins within 3–7 days. **IM.** *Endometrial or renal carcinoma:* **initial,** 400–1,000 mg weekly; **then, if improvement noted,** 400 mg monthly. Medroxyprogesterone is not intended to be the primary therapy. *Long-acting contraceptive:* 150 mg of depot form q 3 months or 450 mg of depot form q 6 months.

NURSING CONSIDERATIONS

See *Nursing Considerations* for *Antineoplastic Agents,* p. 303, and *Progesterone and Progestins,* p. 1195.

Administration

Have IV fluids, diuretics, corticosteroids and phosphate supplements available in the event the client develops severe hypercalcemia.

Interventions

1. The combined effect of the drug and osteolytic metastases may result in hypercalcemia. Therefore, note especially client complaints of insomnia, lethargy, anorexia, nausea, and vomiting. Withhold the drug, obtain serum calcium levels and report if high to the physician.
2. Encourage a high fluid intake to minimize hypercalcemia.
3. Closely monitor the client who has resumed therapy after drug-induced hypercalcemia has been corrected.

MEGESTROL ACETATE   (meh-JESS-trohl)
Megace (Rx)

See also *Progesterone/Progestins,* p. 1194, and *Antineoplastic Agents,* p. 287.

Classification: Synthetic progestin.

Action/Kinetics: The antineoplastic activity is due to suppression of gonadotropins (antiluteinizing effect). Drug contains tartrazine, which can cause allergic-type reactions, including asthma, often occurring in patients sensitive to aspirin.

Uses: Palliative treatment of endometrial or breast cancer. Should not be used as sole treatment.

Additional Contraindications: Not to be used for diagnosis of pregnancy. Pregnancy.

Side Effects: *Few:* Abdominal pain, headache, nausea, vomiting, breast tenderness, carpal tunnel syndrome (soreness, weakness, and tenderness of muscles of thumbs), deep vein thrombosis, alopecia.

Dosage: Tablets. *Breast cancer:* 40 mg q.i.d. *Endometrial cancer:* 40–320 mg/day in divided doses. To determine efficacy, treatment should be continued for at least 2 months.

NURSING CONSIDERATIONS
See *Nursing Considerations* for *Antineoplastic Agents,* p. 303, *Progesterone and Progestins,* p. 1195, and *Medroxyprogesterone Acetate,* p. 1198.

NORETHINDRONE   (nor-ETH-in-drohn)
Norlutin (Rx)

NORETHINDRONE ACETATE   (nor-ETH-in-droh)
Aygestin, Norlutate (Rx)

Classification: Progestational hormone, synthetic.

Action/Kinetics: Norethindrone is twice as potent and norethindrone acetate is four times as potent as parenteral progesterone. Both synthetic progestins have estrogenic and androgenic properties and should not be used during pregnancy (masculinization of female fetus).

Uses: Amenorrhea, abnormal uterine bleeding due to hormone imbalance, endometriosis. Norethindrone or norethindrone acetate, in combination with mestranol or ethinyl estradiol, are widely used for oral contraception.

Dosage: Tablets. *Norethindrone: Amenorrhea, abnormal uterine bleeding,* 5–20 mg daily beginning on day 5 and ending on day 25 of menstrual cycle. *Endometriosis:* 10 mg/day for 2 weeks; **then,** increase in 5-mg increments every 2 weeks until a dose of 30 mg/day is reached (therapy maintained for 6–9 months).

Tablets. *Norethindrone acetate: Amenorrhea, abnormal uterine bleeding,* 2.5–10 mg daily beginning on day 5 and ending on day 25 of menstrual cycle. *Endometriosis:* 5 mg/day for 2 weeks; **then,** increase in 2.5-mg increments q 2 weeks until a dose of 15 mg/day is reached (therapy maintained for 6–9 months).

NURSING CONSIDERATIONS

See *Nursing Considerations* for *Progesterone and Progestins,* p. 1195.

PROGESTERONE IN OIL

Femotrone in Oil, Gesterol 50, Progestaject (Rx)

PROGESTERONE POWDER

(Rx)

Classification: Progestational hormone, natural.

Action/Kinetics: This natural progestational hormone has minimal androgenic effects. IM injection of an oil solution acts more rapidly than SC injection of aqueous suspension. Pain and swelling at injection site are common. Progesterone powder is available for prescription compounding.

Dosage: IM. Oil. *Amenorrhea,* 5–10 mg for 6–8 consecutive days. If effective, withdrawal bleeding will occur within 2–3 days after the last injection. *Functional uterine bleeding:* 5–10 mg daily for 6 days (or a single dose of 50–100 mg). After 6 days, bleeding should stop.

NURSING CONSIDERATIONS

See *Nursing Considerations* for *Progesterone and Progestins,* p. 1195.

Administration/Storage

1. If progesterone is used with estrogen, begin progesterone after 2 weeks.
2. When menses begins, therapy should be terminated.

ORAL CONTRACEPTIVES: ESTROGEN-PROGESTERONE COMBINATIONS

General Statement: The majority of oral contraceptives contain both an estrogen and a progestin in each tablet; such products are referred to as *combination oral contraceptives*. There are three types of combination products: (1) Monophasic—contain the same amount of estrogen and progestin in each tablet; (2) biphasic—contain the same amount of estrogen in each tablet but the progestin content is lower for the first 10 days of the cycle and higher for the last 11 days; (3) triphasic—the estrogen content may be the same or may vary throughout the medication cycle; the progestin content varies. The purpose of the biphasic and triphasic products is to provide hormones in a manner similar to that occurring physiologically. This is said to decrease breakthrough bleeding during the medication cycle. Combination oral contraceptive products are listed in Tables 25 and 26.

Table 25   Combination Oral Contraceptive Preparations Available In The United States

Trade Name	Estrogen	Progestin
	MONOPHASIC	
Brevicon 21-day	Ethinyl estradiol (35 mcg)	Norethindrone (0.5 mg)
Brevicon 28-day	Ethinyl estradiol (35 mcg)	Norethindrone (0.5 mg)
Demulen 1/35–21	Ethinyl estradiol (35 mcg)	Ethynodiol diacetate (1 mg)
Demulen 1/35–28	Ethinyl estradiol (35 mcg)	Ethynodiol diacetate (1 mg)
Demulen 1/50–21	Ethinyl estradiol (50 mcg)	Ethynodiol diacetate (1 mg)
Demulen 1/50–28	Ethinyl estradiol (50 mcg)	Ethynodiol diacetate (1 mg)
Genora 0.5/35 21 Day	Ethinyl estradiol (35 mcg)	Norethindrone (0.5 mg)
Genora 0.5/35 28 Day	Ethinyl estradiol (35 mcg)	Norethindrone (0.5 mg)
Genora 1/35 21 Day	Ethinyl estradiol (35 mcg)	Norethindrone (1 mg)
Genora 1/35 28 Day	Ethinyl estradiol (35 mcg)	Norethindrone (1 mg)
Genora 1/50 21 Day	Mestranol (50 mcg)	Norethindrone (1 mg)
Genora 1/50 28 Day	Mestranol (50 mcg)	Norethindrone (1 mg)
Levlen 21	Ethinyl estradiol (30 mcg)	Levonorgestrel (0.15 mg)
Levlen 28	Ethinyl estradiol (30 mcg)	Levonorgestrel (0.15 mg)
Loestrin 21 1/20	Ethinyl estradiol (20 mcg)	Norethindrone acetate (1 mg)
Loestrin 21 1.5/30	Ethinyl estradiol (30 mcg)	Norethindrone acetate (1.5 mg)
Loestrin Fe 1/20 (28 day)	Ethinyl estradiol (20 mcg)	Norethindrone acetate (1 mg)
Loestrin Fe 1.5/30 (28 day)	Ethinyl estradiol (30 mcg)	Norethindrone acetate (1.5 mg)
Lo/Ovral-21	Ethinyl estradiol (30 mcg)	Norgestrel (0.3 mg)
Lo/Ovral-28	Ethinyl estradiol (30 mcg)	Norgestrel (0.3 mg)
Modicon 21	Ethinyl estradiol (35 mcg)	Norethindrone (0.5 mg)
Modicon 28	Ethinyl estradiol (35 mcg)	Norethindrone (0.5 mg)
N.E.E. 1/35 21 Day	Ethinyl estradiol (35 mcg)	Norethindrone (1 mg)
N.E.E. 1/35 28 Day	Ethinyl estradiol (35 mcg)	Norethindrone (1 mg)
Nelova 0.5/35E 21 Day	Ethinyl estradiol (35 mcg)	Norethindrone (0.5 mg)
Nelova 0.5/35E 28 Day	Ethinyl estradiol (35 mcg)	Norethindrone (0.5 mg)
Nelova 1/35E 21 Day	Ethinyl estradiol (35 mcg)	Norethindrone 1 mg)
Nelova 1/35E 28 Day	Ethinyl estradiol (35 mcg)	Norethindrone 1 mg)
Nelova 1/50M 21 Day	Mestranol (50 mcg)	Norethindrone (1 mg)
Nelova 1/50M 28 Day	Mestranol (50 mcg)	Norethindrone (1 mg)
Norcept-E 1/35 21 Day	Ethinyl estradiol (35 mcg)	Norethindrone (1 mg)
Norcept-E 1/35 28 day	Ethinyl estradiol (35 mcg)	Norethindrone (1 mg)
Nordette-21	Ethinyl estradiol (35 mcg)	Levonorgestrel (0.15 mg)
Nordette-28	Ethinyl estradiol (35 mcg)	Levonorgestrel (0.15 mg)
Norethin 1/35E	Ethinyl estradiol (35 mcg)	Norethindrone (1 mg)
Norethin 1/50M 21 Day	Mestranol (50 mcg)	Norethindrone (1 mg)
Norethin 1/50M 28 Day	Mestranol (50 mcg)	Norethindrone (1 mg)
Norinyl 1 + 35 21-day	Ethinyl estradiol (35 mcg)	Norethindrone (1 mg)
Norinyl 1 + 35 28-day	Ethinyl estradiol (35 mcg)	Norethindrone (1 mg)
Norinyl 1 + 50 21-day	Mestranol (50 mcg)	Norethindrone (1 mg)
Norinyl 1 + 50 28-day	Mestranol (50 mcg)	Norethindrone (1 mg)
Norlestrin 21 1/50	Ethinyl estradiol (50 mcg)	Norethindrone acetate (1 mg)
Norlestrin 28 1/50	Ethinyl estradiol (50 mcg)	Norethindrone acetate (1 mg)
Norlestrin Fe 1/50	Ethinyl estradiol (50 mcg)	Norethindrone acetate (1 mg)
Norlestrin 21 2.5/50	Ethinyl estradiol (50 mcg)	Norethindrone acetate (2.5 mg)

Table 25   (*continued*)

Trade Name	Estrogen	Progestin
Norlestrin Fe 2.5/50	Ethinyl estradiol (50 mcg)	Norethindrone acetate (2.5 mg)
Ortho Novum 1/35–21	Ethinyl estradiol (35 mcg)	Norethindrone (1 mg)
Ortho Novum 1/35–28	Ethinyl estradiol (35 mcg)	Norethindrone (1 mg)
Ortho Novum 1/50–21	Mestranol (50 mcg)	Norethindrone (1 mg)
Ortho Novum 1/50–28	Mestranol (50 mcg)	Norethindrone (1 mg)
Ovcon-35 21 Day	Ethinyl estradiol (35 mcg)	Norethindrone (0.4 mg)
Ovcon-35 28 Day	Ethinyl estradiol (35 mcg)	Norethindrone (0.4 mg)
Ovcon-50 21 Day	Ethinyl estradiol (50 mcg)	Norethindrone (1 mg)
Ovcon-50 28 Day	Ethinyl estradiol (50 mcg)	Norethindrone (1 mg)
Ovral 21 day	Ethinyl estradiol (50 mcg)	Norgestrel (0.5 mg)
Ovral 28 day	Ethinyl estradiol (50 mcg)	Norgestrel (0.5 mg)

BIPHASIC

Trade Name	Estrogen	Progestin
Nelova 10/11–21	Ethinyl estradiol (35 mcg in each tablet)	Norethindrone (10 tablets of 0.5 mg followed by 11 tablets of 1 mg)
Nelova 10/11–28	See Nelova 10/11–21	
Ortho-Novum 10/11–21	Ethinyl estradiol (35 mg in each tablet)	Norethindrone (10 tablets of 0.5 mg followed by 11 tablets of 1 mg)
Ortho-Novum 10/11–28	See Ortho-Novum 10/11–21	

TRIPHASIC

Trade Name	Estrogen	Progestin
Ortho-Novum 7/7/7 (21 or 28 days)	Ethinyl estradiol (35 mg in each tablet)	Norethindrone (0.5 mg the first 7 days, 0.75 the next 7 days, and 1 mg the last 7 days)
Tri-Levlen-21 and Tri-Levlen-28	1st 6 days: Ethinyl estradiol (30 mg)	Levonogestrel (0.05 mg)
	Next 5 days: Ethinyl estradiol (40 mg)	Levonorgestrel (0.075 mg)
	Last 10 days: Ethinyl estradiol (30 mg)	Levonorgestrel (0.125 mg)
Tri-Norinyl (21 or 28 day)	Ethinyl estradiol (35 mg in each tablet)	Norethindrone (0.5 mg the first 7 days, 1 mg the next 9 days, and 0.5 mg the last 5 days)
Triphasil-21 (21 or 28 day)	1st 6 days: Ethinyl estradiol (30 mg)	Levonorgestrel (0.05 mg)
	Next 5 days: Ethinyl estradiol (40 mg)	Levonorgestrel (0.075 mg)
	Last 10 days: Ethinyl estradiol (30 mg)	Levonorgestrel (0.125 mg)

All combination oral contraceptives are Rx and Pregnancy Category: X.

Table 26   Oral Contraceptives Used for Hypermenorrhea or Endometriosis

Trade Name	Content	Dosage
Enovid 5 mg	Mestranol: 75 mcg Norethynodrel: 5 mg	*Endometriosis:* **initial,** 5–10 mg norethynodrel daily for 2 weeks (begin
Enovid 10 mg	Mestranol: 150 mcg Norethynodrel: 9.86 mg	on day 5 of menstrual cycle); **then,** increase 5–10 mg at 2 week intervals until the dose is 20 mg daily. Continue without interruption for 6–9 months. In severe cases, norethynodrel, 40 mg/day, can be used. *Hypermenorrhea:* **initial,** beginning on day 5 of cycle, 20–30 mg norethynodrel/day until bleeding is controlled; **then,** decrease to 10 mg/day until day 24 of cycle and withdraw medication. Cycles may then be regulated by giving 5–10 mg norethynodrel daily from day 5–day 24 of the next 2–3 cycles.

Both products are Rx and Pregnancy Category: X.

The other type of oral contraceptive is the progestin-only ("mini-pill") product, which contains small amounts of a progestin in each tablet (see Table 27).

Action/Kinetics: The combination oral contraceptives are thought to act by inhibiting ovulation due to an inhibition (through negative feedback mechanism) of LH and FSH, which are required for development of ova. These products also act to alter the cervical mucus so that it is not conducive to sperm penetration, as well as to render the endometrium less suitable for implantation of the blastocyst should fertilization occur.

Although oral contraceptives may be associated with serious side effects, a number of noncontraceptive health benefits have been confirmed. These include increased regularity of the menstrual cycle, decreased incidence of dysmenorrhea, decreased blood loss, decreased incidence of functional ovarian cysts and ectopic pregnancies, and decreased incidence of diseases such as fibroadenomas, fibrocystic disease, acute pelvic inflammatory disease, endometrial cancer, and ovarian cancer.

The progestin-only products do not consistently inhibit ovulation. However, these products also alter the cervical mucus, render the endometrium unsuitable for implantation, and may alter tubal transport of the ovum. This method of contraception is less reliable than combination therapy.

Table 27   Progestin-Only Contraceptive Preparations Available in the United States

Trade Name	Manufactuer	Progestin
Micronor	Ortho	Norethindrone (0.35)
Nor QD	Syntex	Norethindrone (0.35 mg)
Ovrette	Wyeth	Norgestrel (0.075 mg)

Dosage: 1 tablet daily every day of the year. These products are each Rx and Pregnancy Category: X.

Uses: Contraception, menstrual irregularities, menopausal symptoms. High doses are used for endometriosis and hypermenorrhea.

Contraindications: History of cerebrovascular disease (e.g., coronary artery disease, myocardial infarction, angina pectoris, cerebral vascular disease), thrombophlebitis, and/or pulmonary embolism, hypertension, ocular proptosis, partial or complete loss of vision, defects in the visual field, diplopia, carcinoma of the breast or genital tract, adolescents with incomplete epiphyseal closure, impaired hepatic function, undiagnosed genital bleeding. Smoking.

Special Concerns: Pregnancy category: X. Use with caution in patients with asthma, epilepsy, migraine, diabetes, metabolic bone disease, renal or cardiac disease, and a history of mental depression. Use with caution in patients taking ampicillin, antiepileptic drugs, phenylbutazone, and rifampin, since intermittent bleeding (spotting) and unwanted pregnancy may result.

Side Effects: The oral contraceptives have wide-ranging effects. These are particularly important, since the drugs are given for long periods of time to healthy women. Many authorities have voiced concern about the long-term safety of these agents. Some advise discontinuing therapy after 18–24 months of continuous use. The majority of untoward reactions of oral contraceptives are due to the estrogen component. These are listed under *Estrogens*.

Other untoward reactions include: Auditory disturbances, Raynaud's syndrome, pancreatitis, rhinitis, hemolytic uremic syndrome, and a possible association with systemic lupus erythematosus. Also, there is an increased risk of congenital abnormalities if oral contraceptives are given to pregnant women. Oral contraceptives decrease the quantity and quality of breast milk. Selected studies have concluded that the risk of breast cancer may be increased in patients who started long-term use of oral contraceptives before age 25 and in long-term users of oral contraceptives before their first pregnancy.

Drug Interactions	
Acetaminophen	↓ Hepatotoxicity of acetaminophen due to ↑ breakdown by liver; this effect ↓ therapeutic effect
Anticoagulants, oral	↓ Effect of anticoagulants by increasing levels of certain clotting factors
Ascorbic acid	↑ Effect of oral contraceptives due to ↓ breakdown by liver
Barbiturates	↓ Effect of oral contraceptives due to ↑ breakdown by liver
Benzodiazepines	↑ or ↓ Effect of benzodiazepines due to changes in breakdown by liver
Caffeine	↑ Effect of caffeine due to ↓ breakdown by liver
Carbamazepine	↓ Effect of oral contraceptives due to ↑ breakdown by liver
Clofibrate	↑ Excretion of the active form of clofibrate (clofibric acid)
Corticosteroids	↑ Effect of corticosteroids due to ↓ breakdown by liver
Griseofulvin	Griseofulvin may ↓ effect of oral contraceptives
Guanethidine	↓ Effect of guanethidine
Hypoglycemics	Oral contraceptives ↓ effect of hypoglycemics

Drug Interactions (continued)

Insulin	Oral contraceptives may ↑ insulin requirements
Isoniazid	↓ Effect of oral contraceptives due to ↑ breakdown by liver
Lorazepam	↑ Clearance of lorazepam due to ↑ breakdown by liver
Metoprolol	↑ Effect of metoprolol due to ↓ breakdown by liver
Neomycin	↓ Effect of oral contraceptive due to ↑ breakdown by liver
Oxazepam	↑ Clearance of oxazepam due to ↑ breakdown by liver
Penicillins	Penicillins may ↓ effect of oral contraceptives
Phenylbutazone	↓ Effect of contraceptives due to ↑ breakdown by liver
Phenytoin	↓ Effect of oral contraceptives due to ↑ breakdown by liver
Rifampin	↓ Effect of contraceptives due to ↑ breakdown by liver
Temazepam	↑ Clearance of temazepam due to ↑ breakdown by liver
Tetracyclines	↓ Effect of contraceptives due to tetracycline-induced inhibition of gut bacteria that hydrolyze steroid conjugates
Theophyllines	Oral contraceptives ↑ effect of theophyllines due to ↓ breakdown by liver
Tricyclic antidepressants	Oral contraceptives ↑ effect of antidepressants due to ↓ breakdown by liver
Troleandomycin	↑ Chance of jaundice

Laboratory Test Interferences: Altered liver and thyroid function tests. ↓ Prothrombin time, 17-hydroxycorticosteroids, 17-ketosteroids, and 17-ketogenic steroids. (Therapy with ovarian hormones should be discontinued 60 days before performance of laboratory tests.) ↑ Gamma globulins.

Dosage: See *Administration/Storage*.

NURSING CONSIDERATIONS

See also *Nursing Considerations* for *Estrogens,* p. 1183, and *Progesterone and Progestins.* p. 1195.

Administration/Storage

1. Tablets should be taken at approximately the same time each day (e.g., with a meal or at bedtime).
2. Spotting or breakthrough bleeding may occur for the first 1–2 cycles; if it continues past this time, consult the physician.
3. For the initial cycle, an **additional** form of contraception should be used for the first week.
4. The type of oral contraceptive preparation will determine the precise manner in which the drug is taken:

- For the 21-day regimen, one tablet is taken daily beginning on day 5 of menses (day 1 is the first day of menstrual flow). No tablets are taken for 7 days.
- For a 28-day regimen, hormone-containing tablets are taken for the first 21 days, followed by 7 days of inert or iron-containing tablets.
- Certain products, including the biphasic and selected triphasic oral contraceptives, are termed *Sunday start*. The first tablet should be taken the Sunday following the beginning of menses (if menses begins on Sunday, the first tablet should be taken that day). *Note:* The biphasic and triphasic products have varying amounts of estrogen and/or progestin, depending on the stage of the cycle; the client should understand fully how these preparations are to be taken and which tablets are to be taken at various times during the medication cycle.
- For progestin-only products, the first tablet is taken on the first day of menses; thereafter, one tablet is taken every day of the year.

5. It is recommended that for a women beginning combination oral contraceptive therapy, a product be chosen that contains the least amount of estrogen for that particular client.
6. If a woman fails to take one or more tablets, the following recommendations should be followed:
   - If one tablet is missed, it should be taken as soon as it is remembered. Alternatively, two tablets can be taken the following day.
   - If two tablets are missed, two tablets can be taken each day for two days; alternatively, two tablets can be taken on the day the missed tablets are remembered, with the second missed tablet being discarded.
   - If three tablets are missed, a new medication cycle should be initiated 7 days after the last tablet was taken, and an additional form of contraception should be used until the start of the next menstrual period.

Note: With each succeeding tablet missed, the possibility increases that ovulation will occur.

Assessment

Determine the client's beliefs and needs concerning contraception and instruct them accordingly.

Client/Family Teaching

1. Advise the client to take the tablets exactly as prescribed to prevent pregnancy.
2. Remind the client if she misses taking 1 tablet she should take the tablet as soon as the oversight has been detected.
3. If 2 consecutive tablets have been missed, the dosage must be doubled for the next 2 consecutive days. The regular schedule may then be resumed. However, the client or her partner should use additional contraceptive measures for the remainder of the cycle.
4. If 3 tablets are missed, discontinue the therapy and start a new course as indicated by the type of medication. Alternative contraceptive measures should be used when the tablets are not taken, and should be continued for 7 days after a new course has been started.
5. Advise the client that if she develops pain in the legs or chest, respiratory distress, an unexplained cough, severe headaches, dizziness, or blurred vision to discontinue the therapy and notify the physician.
6. Oral contraceptives decrease the viscosity of cervical mucus, increasing the susceptibility to vaginal infections. These are difficult to treat successfully; therefore, advise that good hygienic practice is essential.
7. If the client has persistent nausea, edema, and skin eruptions beyond the four cycles, advise the client to consult with the physician for a possible adjustment of drug dosage or for a different combination.

8. Instruct the client to report symptoms of eye pathology, such as headaches, dizziness, blurred vision, or partial loss of sight.

9. Alterations in thought processes, depression or fatigue should be reported to the physician since a medication preparation with less progesterone activity may be indicated.

10. If the client is disturbed by androgenic effects such as weight gain, increased oiliness of the skin, acne, or hirsutism, notify the physician as a change in medication or dosage may be in order.

11. Advise the client to report any missed menstrual periods. If two consecutive periods are missed, discontinue the therapy until pregnancy has been ruled out.

12. Advise the client not to take the tablets longer than 18 months without consulting her physician.

13. Explain the need to practice another form of contraception if she is receiving ampicillin, anticonvulsants, phenylbutazone, rifampin, or tetracycline. These drugs may cause intermittent bleeding and the drug interactions could result in an unwanted pregnancy.

14. Contraceptives interfere with the elimination of caffeine. Therefore, advise clients to limit their caffeine consumption to prevent insomnia, irritability, tremors, and cardiac irregularities that may result.

15. If the woman is breast feeding her infant, another form of contraception should be used until lactation is well established.

16. All clients using oral contraceptives should be advised to avoid smoking. Offer encouragement and assist the client to quit. Suggest participation in smoking cessation programs that have proven effective.

17. Advise the client that a potential risk of endometrial cancer has been identified with this drug therapy and there is controversy as to the possibility of an increased risk of breast cancer. Ensure that the client is made aware of these potential inherent risks prior to initiating drug therapy.

18. Stress the importance for the client to report for a yearly Pap smear and physical examination.

CHAPTER SIXTY-THREE

Ovarian Stimulants and Inhibitor

Ovarian Stimulants

Chorionic Gonadotropin (HCG)   *1208*
Clomiphene Citrate   *1210*
Gonadorelin Acetate   *1211*

Menotropins   *1213*
Nafarelin Acetate   *1215*
Urofollitropin for Injection   *1216*

Ovarian Inhibitor

Danazol   *1218*

OVARIAN STIMULANTS

General Statement: Ovarian stimulants are potent drugs to be used only in carefully selected patients. The fertility of the husband must be established prior to the treatment of the wife. A thorough clinical evaluation must also precede each new course of treatment.

CHORIONIC GONADOTROPIN (HCG)   (kor-ee-**ON**-ik go-nad-oh-**TROH**-pin)

A.P.L., Chorex-5 and -10, Chorigon, Choron 10, Corgonject-5, Follutein, Glukor, Gonic, Pregnyl, Profasi HP (Rx)

Classification: Gonadotropic hormone.

Action/Kinetics: The actions of human chorionic gonadotropin (HCG), produced by the trophoblasts of the fertilized ovum and then by the placenta, resemble those of luteinizing hormone (LH).

In males, HCG stimulates androgen production by the testes, the development of secondary sex characteristics, and testicular descent when no anatomic impediment is present. In women, HCG stimulates progesterone production by the corpus luteum and completes expulsion of the ovum from a mature follicle.

Uses: *Males:* Prepubertal cryptorchidism, hypogonadism due to pituitary insufficiency. *Females:* Infertility (together with menotropins).

Contraindications: Precocious puberty, prostatic cancer or other androgen-dependent neoplasm, hypersensitivity to drug. Development of precocious puberty is cause for discontinuance of therapy.

Special Concerns: Pregnancy category: C. Since HCG increases androgen production, drug should be used with caution in patients in whom androgen-induced edema may be harmful (epilepsy, migraines, asthma, cardiac or renal diseases).

Side Effects: *CNS:* Headache, irritability, restlessness, depression, fatigue. *Miscellaneous:* Edema, precocious puberty, gynecomastia, pain at injection site.

Dosage: IM only. *Prepubertal cryptorchidism, not due to anatomical obstruction:* various regimens including (1) 4,000 USP units 3 times/week for 3 weeks; (2) 5,000 USP units q other day for 4 injections; (3) 15 injections over a period of 6 weeks of 500–1,000 units/injection; (4) 500 USP units 3 times/week for 4–6 weeks; may be repeated after 1 month using 1,000 USP units. *Hypogonadism in males:* The following regimens may be used: (1) 500–1,000 USP units 3 times/week for 3 weeks; **then,** same dose twice weekly for 3 weeks; (2) 4,000 USP units 3 times/week for 6–9 months; then, 2,000 USP units 3 times/week for 3 more months; (3) 1,000–2,000 USP 3 times weekly. *Induction of ovulation (used with menotropins):* 5,000–10,000 USP units one day after the last dose of menotropins. *Stimulation of spermatogenesis (used with menotropins):* 5,000 units 3 times a week for 4–6 weeks; reduce dose of 2,000 units twice weekly when menotropin therapy is begun.

NURSING CONSIDERATIONS

Administration/Storage

1. Reconstituted solutions are stable for 1–3 months, depending on manufacturer, when stored at 2° C–8° C (35.6° F–46.4° F).
2. Have emergency drugs and equipment available in the event of an acute allergic response.

Assessment

1. Note any client history of hypersensitivity to the drug.
2. Assess the prepubescent male client for the appearance of secondary sex characteristics. The drug is contraindicated in this instance.

Interventions

1. Once started on the therapy, periodically examine the client for the beginning of secondary sex characteristics. This is an indication of sexual precocity and the drug should be withdrawn.
2. Note client complaints of headache, easy fatigue and restlessness, or if the family complains that the client has become increasingly irritable and depressed. Note if there is any change in the client's attention to physical appearance. Document and report these to the physician as the drug may have to be withdrawn.
3. When treating clients for cryptorchidism, examine them once a week for testicular descent to evaluate the response to therapy.
4. Because edema is common, monitor the client's weight and extent of edema at regular intervals and report to the physician.
5. Observe the client for gynecomastia and offer emotional support. This is especially important for young male clients.
6. In female clients being treated for corpus luteum deficiency, question about the occurrence of bleeding after the 15th day of therapy. If bleeding occurs, withhold the drug and notify the physician.

Client/Family Teaching

1. Instruct clients in how to assess for edema and advise them to report any occurrence to the physician.
2. Explain that delayed menses, excessive menstrual bleeding, pain in the pelvic region, weakness,

63

and fatigue are signs and symptoms of ectopic pregnancy and should be reported to the physician immediately.

3. Discuss with the client the possibility of multiple births when the drug is used with menotropins.

4. Encourage the client to return for scheduled follow-up visits to monitor the effectiveness of the drug therapy.

CLOMIPHENE CITRATE   (KLOH-mih-feen)

Clomid, Milophene, Serophene (Rx)

Classification: Ovarian stimulant.

Action/Kinetics: The drug acts by combining with estrogen receptors, thus decreasing the number of available receptor sites. Through negative feedback, the hypothalamus and pituitary are thus stimulated to increase secretion of LH and FSH. Under the influence of increased levels of these hormones, an ovarian follicle develops, followed by ovulation and corpus luteum development. Most patients ovulate after the first course of therapy. Further treatment may be inadvisable if pregnancy fails to occur after ovulatory responses. It is readily absorbed from the GI tract and is excreted in the feces. **t½:** 5–7 days. **Time to peak effect:** 4–10 days after the last day of treatment for ovulation.

Uses: Selected cases of female infertility in which normal endogenous estrogen levels have been observed. *Investigational:* Male infertility, insufficiency of the corpus luteum, diagnosis of hypothalamic-pituitary-gonadal axis function in males and in ovarian function studies.

Contraindications: Pregnancy, liver disease or history thereof, abnormal bleeding of undetermined origin. Ovarian cysts. The absence of neoplastic disease should be established before treatment is initiated. Therapy is ineffective in patients with ovarian or pituitary failure.

Side Effects: *Ovarian:* Ovarian overstimulation and/or enlargement and subsequent symptoms resembling those of premenstrual syndrome. *Ophthalmologic:* Blurred vision, spots, or flashes, probably due to intensification of after images. *GI:* Abdominal distention, pain, or soreness; nausea, vomiting. *GU:* Abnormal uterine bleeding, breast tenderness. *CNS:* Insomnia, nervousness, headache, depression, fatigue, lightheadedness, dizziness. *Other:* Hot flashes, increased urination, allergic symptoms, weight gain, alopecia (reversible).

Laboratory Test Interferences: ↑ Serum thyroxine and thyroxine-binding globulin.

Dosage: Tablets. *First course:* 25–50 mg daily for 5 days. *Second course:* same dosage if ovulation has occurred. In absence of ovulation, dose may be increased to 100 mg/day for 5 days (some patients may require up to 250 mg daily to induce ovulation).

NURSING CONSIDERATIONS

Administration

1. Therapy may be started any time in clients who have had no recent incidence of uterine bleeding.

2. If the client has had recent uterine bleeding, start the therapy on the fifth day of the cycle.

3. If the client has had a previous course of therapy to which she did not respond, start the new therapy after 30 days have elapsed.

Note: Most clients will respond following the first course of therapy. Further therapy is not recommended if pregnancy does not result following 3 or 4 ovulatory responses.

Assessment

1. Note if the client has a history of hepatic dysfunction.
2. Determine if the client has had a history of abnormal bleeding of undetermined origin.
3. If the client is sexually active, determine the possibility of pregnancy.

Client/Family Teaching

1. Instruct the client in taking basal body temperature and show client how to chart her temperature on the graph to determine if ovulation has occurred.
2. Explain that if the client develops pain in the pelvic area or abdominal distention she should discontinue the drug and report the symptoms to the physician. These symptoms indicate ovarian enlargement and the possible presence of an ovarian cyst.
3. Explain to the client that if she develops blurred vision, has spots or flashes in the eyes, the retina of the eye may be affected. Advise the client to discontinue taking the medication and to have an ophthalmologic examination.
4. Instruct the client to avoid performing hazardous tasks involving body coordination or mental alertness because the drug may cause lightheadedness, dizziness, or visual disturbances.
5. Advise the client to discontinue taking the medication and check with the physician if pregnancy is suspected, because the drug may have teratogenic effect.

GONADORELIN ACETATE   (go-nad-oh-**RELL**-in)

Lutrepulse (Rx)

Classification: Gonadotropin-releasing hormone.

Action/Kinetics: Gonadorelin is a synthetic hormone which is identical in amino acid sequence to the naturally occurring gonadotropin-releasing hormone. Thus, gonadorelin stimulates the synthesis and release of FSH and LH from the adenohypophysis. FSH and LH then stimulate the ovaries to synthesize estrogen and progesterone which are necessary for development and release of an ovum. $t^{1/2}$, **initial:** 2–10 min; **final:** 10–40 min. Gonadorelin is metabolized to inactive peptide fragments which are excreted in the urine.

Uses: Primary hypothalamic amenorrhea.

Contraindications: Sensitivity to gonadorelin acetate or gonadorelin HCl (used for determining gonadotropic function of the pituitary). Pituitary prolactinoma, causes of anovulation other than those of hypothalamic origin (e.g., ovarian cysts), hormone-dependent tumors.

Special Concerns: Pregnancy category: B. There is no indication for use of gonadorelin acetate during lactation. Safety and efficacy have not been determined in children less than 18 years of age.

Side Effects: *Ovarian hyperstimulation:* Ovarian enlargement, ascites with or without pain, pleural effusion. *Local, due to use of infusion pump:* Inflammation, infection, mild phlebitis, hematoma at site of catheter. *Anaphylaxis:* Bronchospasm, flushing, tachycardia, urticaria, induration at injection site. *Miscellaneous:* Multiple pregnancy.

Drug Interactions: Gonadorelin should not be used with ovarian stimulators.

Dosage: IV: 5 mcg q 90 min (range: 1–20 mcg) delivered by Lutrepulse pump using the 0.8 mg solution at 50 mcL per pulse. The recommended treatment interval is 21 days. If there is no response after three treatment intervals, the dose should be increased cautiously and in stepwise fashion.

NURSING CONSIDERATIONS

Administration/Storage

1. The kit contains the lyophilized powder for injection, diluent, catheter and tubing, alcohol swabs, IV cannula units, syringe and needle, elastic belt, batteries, the Lutrepulse pump, physician pump manual, and package insert.
2. Gonadorelin is reconstituted with 8 mL of diluent immediately prior to use and then transferred to the plastic reservoir.
3. The presterilized bag with the infusion catheter set supplied is filled with the reconstituted solution for IV administration.
4. The drug is then administered IV using the "Lutrepulse" pump which can deliver 25 or 50 mcL of solution over a period of 1 min and at a pulse frequency of 90 min. Depending on the concentration of the solution and the volume/pulse, the pump can deliver 2.5, 5, 10, or 20 mcg of gonadorelin.
5. The 8 mL of solution will last for approximately 7 consecutive days.
6. The cannula and IV site should be changed every 48 hr.
7. Have emergency drugs and equipment available in the event of an anaphylactic reaction.

Assessment

1. Perform a thorough nursing history. Proper diagnosis is critical for treatment to be successful.
2. Determine that hypothalamic amenorrhea or hypogonadism is due to a deficiency in quantity or pulsing of endogenous gonadotropin-releasing hormone.
3. Note any history of ovarian cysts or pituitary tumors as drug is contraindicated under these circumstances.
4. Obtain baseline ovarian ultrasound, pelvic exam and mid-luteal phase serum progesterone level prior to initiating therapy.

Client/Family Teaching

1. Demonstrate the appropriate method for drug administration. Provide detailed instructions both orally and in writing regarding the proper use and care of the Lutrepulse infusion pump.
2. Stress the importance of using aseptic technique.
3. Have client return demonstrate so that any problems or questions may be identified prior to leaving the office. Provide client with a phone number where assistance may be found 24 hr a day.
4. Instruct the client in how to assess the infusion site for evidence of inflammation, phlebitis, erythema, infection or hematoma and to report these findings to the physician, as the site will need to be changed.
5. Provide the client with a list of symptoms of hyperstimulation of the ovaries and advise the client to avoid having intercourse if these symptoms occur. A rupture of an ovarian cyst could occur resulting in hemoperitoneum.
6. Explain the importance of careful record keeping in relation to menses, basal temperatures and graph recordings, medication administration and any side effects that may be noted, which should always be reported to the physician.
7. Explain to the client that if ovulation occurs with the pump in place, to notify the physician as the therapy should be continued for 2 more weeks in order to maintain the corpus luteum.
8. Explain that clinical response to gonadorelin acetate therapy is generally monitored by ovarian ultrasound, mid-luteal phase serum progesterone levels, and regularly scheduled physical

exams including a pelvic. Additionally, the infusion site will be examined and changed every 48 hr. Stress the importance of complying with these frequently scheduled tests. This therapy may require a relatively long-term commitment by the client.

Evaluation

1. Response to gonadorelin usually occurs within 2–3 weeks after initiation of therapy. Assess for evidence of ovum.
2. Observe for freedom from complications of drug therapy.

MENOTROPINS   (men-oh-**TROH**-pinz)

Pergonal (Rx)

Classification: Ovarian stimulant.

Action/Kinetics: Menotropins is a mixture of follicle-stimulating hormone (FSH) and luteinizing hormone (LH), which cause growth and maturation of ovarian follicles. For ovulation to occur, HCG is administered the day following menotropins. **Time to peak effect, females:** 18 hr. In men, menotropins with HCG given for a minimum of 3 months induce spermatogenesis. Eliminated through the kidneys.

Uses: *Females:* In combination with HCG to induce ovulation in patients with anovulatory cycles not due to primary ovarian failure. *Males:* In combination with HCG to induce spermatogenesis in males with primary or secondary hypogonadotropic hypogonadism.

Contraindications: *Women:* Pregnancy. Primary ovarian failure as indicated by high levels of urinary gonadotropins, ovarian cysts, intracranial lesions, including pituitary tumors. *Men:* Normal gonadotropin levels, primary testicular failure, disorders of fertility other than hypogonadotropic hypogonadism. Thyroid or adrenal dysfunction. Absence of neoplastic disease should be established before treatment is initiated.

Special Concerns: Pregnancy category: X.

Side Effects: *Women:* Ovarian overstimulation, hyperstimulation syndrome (maximal 7–10 days after discontinuation of drug), ovarian enlargement (20% of patients), ruptured ovarian cysts, hemoperitoneum, thromboembolism, multiple births (20%). Fever, hypersensitivity. *Men:* Gynecomastia.

Dosage: Women, IM. *individualized:* **initial,** 75 IU of FSH and 75 IU of LH for 9–12 days, followed by 5,000–10,000 USP units of HCG one day after last dose of menotropins. *Subsequent courses:* same dosage schedule for two more courses, if ovulation has occurred. **Then,** dose may be increased to 150 IU of FSH and 150 IU of LH for 9 to 12 days, followed by HCG as above for 2 or more courses.

Men, IM: To increase serum testosterone levels, it may be necessary to give HCG alone, 5,000 IU 3 times weekly, for 4–6 months prior to menotropins; **then,** 75 IU FSH and 75 IU LH **IM** 3 times weekly and HCG 2,000 IU 2 times weekly for at least 4 months. If no response after 4 months, double each dose of menotropins with the HCG dose unchanged.

NURSING CONSIDERATIONS

Administration/Storage

1. Menotropins are destroyed in the GI tract, therefore, they must be administered parenterally.
2. Reconstituted solutions must be used immediately.

3. Discard any unused portions of the reconstituted drug.

4. Have emergency drugs and equipment available to treat allergic reactions should they occur.

Assessment

1. Determine if the client has been tested for high levels of urinary gonadrotropins or evaluated for the presence of ovarian cysts. The drug is contraindicated in these instances.

2. Obtain baseline peripheral pulse assessments as data against which to compare future findings.

Interventions

1. Take the client's urinary estrogen excretion levels daily. If they are greater than 100 μg, or if the daily estriol excretion is greater than 50 μg, *withhold HCG* and notify the physician. These levels are signs of an impending hyperstimulation syndrome.

2. An occasional client will develop erythrocytosis. Therefore, monitor the complete blood count on a routine basis.

3. Observe the client for complaints of unexplained fever or abdominal pain. Withhold the medication and report these findings to the physician.

4. If the client requires hospitalization for hyperstimulation, the following interventions should be performed:
   - Place the client on bed rest.
   - Monitor intake and output and weigh client daily.
   - Monitor the specific gravity of the urine. Monitor hematocrit and serum and urinary electrolytes.
   - Assess for hemoconcentration. If the hematocrit rises to critical levels, have sodium heparin on hand for administration.
   - Increase the client's fluid intake and anticipate electrolyte replacement therapy.
   - Provide analgesics if the client needs them for comfort.

Client/Family Teaching

1. Instruct the client to report any pain in the extremities, if an extremity is cool to the touch or if an extremity becomes pale blue. This is a sign of arterial thromboembolism and must be reported to the physician immediately.

2. Explain that fever or the development of lower abdominal pain may be the result of overstimulation of the ovaries that has caused cysts to form, a loss of fluid into the peritoneum or bleeding and must be reported to the physician immediately. Discuss the need for examination for this phenomenon at least every other day during drug therapy and for 2 weeks thereafter. If overstimulation occurs, hospitalization is necessary for close monitoring.

3. Explain the need to collect a 24-hr urine daily, to be analyzed for estrogen and provide a suitable container for collection. Provide the client with printed instructions concerning the delivery of a 24-hr urine sample to the appropriate laboratory facility.

4. Instruct the client in taking her basal body temperature and charting it on a graph.

5. Describe the signs that indicate ovulation, such as an increase in the basal body temperature, and an increase in the appearance and volume of cervical mucus. Also, discuss the significance of the urinary excretion of estriol.

6. Advise the client to engage in daily intercourse from the day before chorionic gonadotropin is administered and until ovulation occurs.

7. If symptoms indicate overstimulation of the ovaries, a significant ovarian enlargement may have

occurred. Instruct client to abstain from intercourse because of the increased possibility of rupturing the ovarian cysts.

8. Discuss with the client and family that with this therapy there is an increased possibility of multiple births.

9. Explain that pregnancy usually occurs 4–6 weeks after the completion of therapy.

NAFARELIN ACETATE   (NAF-ah-reh-lin)

Synarel (Rx)

Classification: Gonadotropin-releasing hormone.

Action/Kinetics: Nafarelin is a hormone produced through biotechnology; it differs by only one amino acid from naturally occurring gonadotropin-releasing hormone. The drug stimulates the release of luteinizing hormone (LH) and follicle-stimulating hormone (FSH) from the adenohypophysis. These hormones cause estrogen and progesterone synthesis in the ovary which result in the maturation and subsequent release of an ovum. With repeated use of the drug, however, the pituitary becomes desensitized and no longer produces endogenous LH and FSH; thus endogenous estrogen is not produced leading to a regression of endometrial tissue, cessation of menstruation, and a menopausal-like state. The drug is broken down by the enzyme peptidase. **Peak serum levels:** 10–40 min. **t½:** 3 hr. 80% is bound to plasma proteins.

Uses: Endometriosis (including reduction of endometriotic lesions) in patients aged eighteen or older; use restricted to no more than six months.

Contraindications: Hypersensitivity to gonadotropin-releasing hormone or analogs. Abnormal vaginal bleeding of unknown origin. Pregnancy or possibility of becoming pregnant. Lactation.

Special Concerns: Pregnancy category: X. Use of nafarelin in pregnancy is not recommended; pregnancy should be ruled out before initiating therapy. Safety and effectiveness in children have not been established.

Side Effects: *Due to hypoestrogenic effects:* Hot flashes (common), decreased libido, vaginal dryness, headaches, emotional lability, insomnia. *Due to androgenic effects:* Acne, myalgia, reduced breast size, edema, seborrhea, weight gain, increased libido, hirsutism. *Musculoskeletal:* Decrease in vertebral trabecular bone density and total vertebral bone mass. *Miscellaneous:* Nasal irritation, depression, weight loss.

Laboratory Test Interference: ↑ Cholesterol and triglyceride levels, plasma phosphorus, eosinophils. ↓ Serum calcium, white blood cell counts.

Dosage: Nasal spray: 200 mcg into one nostril in the morning and 200 mcg into the other nostril at night (400 mcg b.i.d. may be required by some women).

NURSING CONSIDERATIONS

Administration/Storage

1. Treatment with nafarelin should be initiated between days 2 and 4 of the menstrual cycle.

2. Use for longer than 6 months is not recommended due to the lack of safety data.

3. The product should be stored at room temperature in an upright position protected from light.

Assessment

1. Perform a complete client history and note any evidence of chronic alcohol, tobacco or corticosteroid use. Query about any family history of osteoporosis. Conditions such as these are major risk factors for loss of bone mineral content and would deter repeated courses of treatment with this drug.

2. Note client description of menstrual cycles. Document any incidence of abnormal vaginal bleeding of unknown origin as drug is contraindicated in this event.

3. Determine if the client is pregnant prior to administering therapy as drug is teratogenic.

4. Review the method of contraception being practiced. A nonhormonal method should be advised and practiced during drug therapy.

Client/Family Teaching

1. Instruct client that the treatment should begin between the second and fourth day of the menstrual cycle. Stress the importance of accurate record keeping in relation to menstrual patterns and cycles.

2. Teach the client how to administer the nasal spray and remind her to use only as directed. The client should be encouraged to take the spray upon arising and just before bedtime. Stress the importance of alternating the nostrils to decrease mucosal irritation.

3. Explain to the client that menses should cease while on nafarelin therapy. If regular menses continues the physician should be notified.

4. Remind the client that breakthrough bleeding may occur if she misses successive doses.

5. Stress the importance of using a nonhormonal form of contraception. Explain the potential hazards to the fetus should one become pregnant during therapy with nafarelin acetate.

6. If a topical nasal decongestant is required during treatment with nafarelin, advise client that the decongestant should be used at least 30 minutes after nafarelin in order to decrease the chances of reducing the absorption of nafarelin.

7. Provide the client with a printed list of the hypoestrogenic and androgenic side effects that may occur with this drug therapy. Instruct the client to report these symptoms to the physician as a change in drug dosage or drug therapy may be indicated.

Evaluation

1. Determine if normal function of the pituitary-gonadal system is restored in 4–8 weeks.

2. Assess for a reduction in the number of endometriotic lesions.

UROFOLLITROPIN FOR INJECTION   (YOU-roh-foal-ih-troh-pin)

Metrodin (Rx)

Classification: Ovarian stimulant.

Action/Kinetics: Urofollitropin is prepared from the urine of postmenopausal women. The drug is a gonadotropin that stimulates follicular growth in the ovaries of women without primary ovarian failure. Since treatment with urofollitropin only causes growth and maturation of a follicle, human chorionic gonadotropin (HCG) must also be given to effect ovulation. **Time to peak effect:** 32–36 hr after HCG.

Uses: To cause ovulation in patients with polycystic ovarian disease; such patients should have an elevated LH/FSH ratio and should have failed to respond to therapy with clomiphene. In conjunction with HCG to stimulate development of several ova in patients undergoing in vitro fertilization.

Contraindications: Primary ovarian failure (as indicated by high levels of both LH and FSH), renal dysfunction, thyroid dysfunction, pituitary tumor, abnormal uterine bleeding of unknown cause, ovarian cysts, enlarged ovaries (not as a result of polycystic disease), infertility due to causes other than failure to ovulate. Pregnancy.

Special Concerns: Pregnancy category: X. Use with caution in lactation.

Side Effects: *Ovarian:* Hyperstimulation resulting in ovarian enlargement, abdominal distention or pain, ascites, pleural effusion. *GI:* Nausea, vomiting, diarrhea, bloating, abdominal cramps. *Pyrogenic or allergic reaction:* Chills, fever, muscle aches or pains, fatigue, malaise. *Dermatologic:* Hives, dry skin, loss of hair, rash. *Other:* Headache, ectopic pregnancy, breast tenderness.

Dosage: IM. *Polycystic ovary syndrome:* **Adults, initial,** 75 IU urofollitropin daily for 7–12 days followed by 5,000–10,000 IU HCG 24 hr after the last dose of urofollitropin. If ovulation has occurred but pregnancy has not resulted, this dosage regimen may be repeated for 2 more courses of therapy. If pregnancy still has not resulted, the dose of urofollitropin may be increased to 150 IU daily for 7–12 days followed by 5,000–10,000 IU HCG 24 hr after the last dose of urofollitropin. This regimen may be repeated for 2 additional courses if pregnancy has not occurred. *In vitro fertilization:* **Adults,** 150 IU once daily beginning on day 2 or 3 of the cycle followed by 5,000–10,000 IU of HCG 1 day after the last dose of urofollitropin. Treatment is usually limited to 10 days.

NURSING CONSIDERATIONS

Administration/Storage

1. The powder for injection should be reconstituted by dissolving in 1–2 mL of sterile saline immediately before use.
2. Any unused drug should be discarded.
3. Urofollitropin should be protected from light and stored at 37°–77°F (3°–25°C).

Assessment

1. A thorough gynecologic and endocrinologic evaluation and examination should be completed before initiating urofollitropin therapy.
2. Note any history of renal dysfunction, thyroid dysfunction, or abnormal uterine bleeding from an unknown cause.

Client/Family Teaching

1. Instruct client to report any sudden abdominal pain or tenderness to the physician.
2. Explain that the treatment usually consists of daily injections for 7–12 days.
3. Advise the couple to engage in daily intercourse, beginning one day prior to the administration of HCG until ovulation occurs.
4. During the treatment and for 2 weeks thereafter, the client should be examined at least every other day for hyperstimulation of the ovaries. Explain that if evidence of hyperstimulation occurs, the drug will be stopped immediately by the physician.
5. Provide the client with a list of symptoms of hyperstimulation of the ovaries and advise the

client to avoid having intercourse if these symptoms occur. A rupture of an ovarian cyst could occur resulting in hemoperitoneum.

6. Explain that the use of this drug enhances the risk of multiple births.

7. Stress the importance of reporting all side effects to the physician and reporting for all examinations as scheduled.

OVARIAN INHIBITOR

DANAZOL   (DAN-ah-zohl)

Cyclomen ✣, Danocrine (Rx)

Classification: Gonadotropin inhibitor.

Action/Kinetics: This synthetic androgen inhibits the release of gonadotropins (FSH and LH) by the anterior pituitary. In women this action arrests ovarian function, induces amenorrhea, and causes atrophy of normal and ectopic endometrial tissue. Has weak androgenic effects. **Onset, fibrocystic disease:** 4 weeks. **Time to peak effect, amenorrhea and anovulation:** 6–8 weeks; **fibrocystic disease:** 2–3 months to eliminate breast pain and tenderness and 4–6 months for elimination of nodules. **t½:** 4.5 hr. **Duration:** Ovulation and menstruation usually resume 60–90 days after cessation of therapy.

Uses: Endometriosis amenable to hormonal management in patients who cannot tolerate or who have not responded to other drug therapy. Fibrocystic breast disease. Hereditary angioedema in males and females. *Investigational:* Gynecomastia, menorrhagia, precocious puberty.

Contraindications: Undiagnosed genital bleeding, markedly impaired hepatic, renal, and cardiac function, pregnancy and lactation.

Special Concerns: Use with caution in children treated for hereditary angioedema due to the possibility of virilization in females and precocious sexual development in males. Geriatric patients may have an increased risk of prostatic hypertrophy or prostatic carcinoma.

Side Effects: *Androgenic:* Acne, decrease in breast size, oily hair and skin, weight gain, deepening of voice and hair growth, clitoral hypertrophy, testicular atrophy. *Estrogen deficiency:* Flushing, sweating, vaginitis, nervousness, changes in emotions. *GI:* Nausea, vomiting, constipation, gastroenteritis. *Hepatic:* Jaundice, dysfunction. *CNS:* Fatigue, tremor, headache, dizziness, sleep problems, paresthesia, anxiety, depression, appetite changes. *Miscellaneous:* Allergic reactions, muscle cramps or spasms, joint swelling or lock-up, hematuria, increased blood pressure, chills, pelvic pain, carpal tunnel syndrome, hair loss, change in libido.

Drug Interactions	
Insulin	Danazol ↑ insulin requirements
Warfarin	Danazol ↑ prothrombin time in warfarin-stabilized patients

Dosage: Capsules. *Endometriosis:* 400 mg b.i.d. (moderate to severe) or 100–200 mg b.i.d. (mild) for 3–6 months (up to 9 months may be required in some patients). Begin therapy during menses, if possible, to be sure that patient is not pregnant. *Fibrocystic breast disease:* 50–200 mg b.i.d. beginning on day 2 of menses. *Hereditary angioedema:* **Initial,** 200 mg b.i.d.–t.i.d.; after desired response, decrease dosage by 50% (or less) at 1- to 3-month intervals. Subsequent attacks can be treated by giving up to 200 mg/day. No more than 800 mg daily should be given to adults.

NURSING CONSIDERATIONS

Assessment

1. Discuss with the client the presence of undiagnosed genital bleeding and determine onset, frequency, extent and any precipitating factors.
2. Obtain renal and hepatic function studies to serve as baseline data.
3. If the client is female, sexually active and of child-bearing age, determine if she is pregnant.

Interventions

1. Observe the client closely for signs of virilization such as hirsutism, reduced breast size, deepening of the voice, acne, increased oiliness of the skin, and clitoral enlargement. Some androgenic side effects may not be reversible and may require a change in drug dosage or discontinuation of the drug.
2. Observe clients with a history of epilepsy, migraines, cardiac or renal dysfunction for fluid retention. Danazol may cause fluid retention with resultant edema and if this occurs it may be necessary to have the drug discontinued.

Client/Family Teaching

1. Describe the signs of virilization that may occur with drug therapy. Advise the client to report these symptoms to the physician so that the dosage of drug can be adjusted.
2. Explain that the hypoestrogenic side effects usually disappear after the therapy is discontinued.
3. Ovulation will resume 60–90 days after the drug has been discontinued.
4. Advise client that wearing cotton underwear and paying careful attention to hygiene may diminish the incidence of vaginitis associated with danazol therapy.

CHAPTER SIXTY-FOUR

Abortifacients

General Statement: Several agents are used to terminate pregnancy during the second trimester of pregnancy. These include the prostaglandins F_2 alpha and E_2 or highly concentrated solutions of sodium chloride (20%).

After administration, most of these agents induce evacuation of the uterus within a predictable number of hours. If uterine contractions fail to start or are not strong enough to expel the fetus, the same abortifacient is readministered. If this measure is again unsuccessful, the pregnancy must be terminated by another means, such as the administration of a different abortifacient, oxytocin, or surgery.

Second-trimester abortions are usually carried out by a physician trained in amniocentesis and in a hospital in which intensive care and surgical facilities are available.

Sodium chloride is administered intra-amniotically while carboprost is given by IM injection and dinoprostone by vaginal suppository. Oxytocin is sometimes administered concurrently, with both prostaglandins and sodium chloride.

NURSING CONSIDERATIONS

Administration (Intra-amniotic)

1. To prevent the injection of abortifacient into the bladder, have the client void before the procedure begins.
2. Prepare the abdomen with an antiseptic solution.
3. Be prepared to assist while the physician administers local anesthetic and inserts a needle through the abdominal wall. A 14-gauge spinal needle with stylet is suitable for amniocentesis. One milliliter of amniotic fluid is withdrawn to check the position of the needle.
4. If the fluid withdrawn contains blood, the needle must be repositioned.
5. If no blood is noted in the fluid, a Teflon catheter is threaded through the needle. The needle is withdrawn and administration of the abortifacient is started once designated amount of amniotic fluid has been removed.
6. An amount of amniotic fluid approximately equivalent to the volume of the abortifacient to be injected is withdrawn through the catheter.
7. The abortifacient is slowly injected, in order to determine the sensitivity of the client.
8. To facilitate repeat administration of the drug, the catheter may be left in place for 24–48 hours.
9. Have antibiotics available for prophylactic administration through the catheter.
10. When the catheter is withdrawn, apply a small surgical dressing to the abdomen.
11. Have RhoGam available for administration after delivery to unsensitized Rh-negative women.

Assessment

1. Obtain a thorough nursing history. Identify the reasons for performing this abortion.
2. Determine if the client has a support system and what psychological preparation will be required.

Interventions

1. Explain the abortion procedure, the administration of drug, labor and delivery. Provide an opportunity for the client to ask questions and answer them as factually as possible.
2. Offer emotional support to the client receiving an abortifacient because she is in great need of reassurance and acceptance and often lacks a good support system.
3. Have the client empty the bladder.
4. To minimize vomiting, have antiemetics available and administer before the procedure.
5. Provide support to the client during the administration of the abortifacient.
6. Assess client for the onset of labor.
7. Monitor the progress of labor, noting the frequency, length, and strength of contractions.
8. Monitor BP, temperature, pulse rate, and respirations to determine the presence of hypertension, hemorrhage, dyspnea, bradycardia, and changes in CNS function.
9. Observe the client for nausea, vomiting, and diarrhea. Try to minimize the discomfort, medicate as needed, and note any evidence of electrolyte imbalance.
10. If oxytocin is also to be administered, determine that contractions have ceased before initiating therapy. If contractions exceed 50 mm Hg as measured on an electronic monitor, or if contractions last longer than 70 seconds without a period of complete relaxation of the uterus between contractions, discontinue oxytocin and notify the physician. Otherwise, there is a danger of rupturing the uterus and causing cervical lacerations. Remain with the client receiving oxytocin for induction of labor.
11. Closely monitor the client during the fourth stage of labor.
12. Monitor vital signs and assess the client for hemorrhage, fever, and signs of infection. These may indicate that placenta was retained after the delivery of the fetus.
13. Observe the perineal area for trickles of blood from the vagina. This may indicate the presence of an undetected cervical laceration.

Client/Family Teaching

1. Instruct the client concerning signs and symptoms of infection and/or hemorrhage. Advise the client to report any of these findings immediately to the physician.
2. Advise the client to report any change or increase in vaginal discharge.
3. Explain the need to avoid having vaginal intercourse, using tampons, or taking douches for at least 2 weeks after delivery.
4. Stress the importance of the client returning for an examination in 2 to 4 weeks.
5. Discuss with the client and family the symptoms of depression, which are common after delivery. Provide a telephone number of someone to call for assistance if the need arises.
6. Advise the client to wear a supporting bra if lactation occurs after the abortion.
7. After the postpartum examination, provide information concerning methods of contraception if the client desires family planning and/or if family planning is medically indicated.

64

PROSTAGLANDINS

Action/Kinetics: These hormone-like substances induce uterine contractions similar to normal labor, usually resulting in expulsion of the fetus in 12–48 hr. The drugs also facilitate dilation and softening of the cervix. Due to their effect on smooth muscle, prostaglandins may also increase GI tract motility, cause bronchospasms, vasoconstriction, and changes in blood pressure. The drugs differ with respect to route of administration, number of weeks after gestation when they can be used, and the intensity of side effects.

Uses: See individual drugs.

Contraindications: Hypersensitivity to drug. Acute pelvic inflammatory disease. Acute cardiovascular, pulmonary, renal, or hepatic disease.

Special Concerns: Use with caution for patients with history of asthma, epilepsy, hypo-or hypertension, anemia, jaundice, diabetes, cervicitis, infected endocervical lesions, acute vaginitis, history of uterine surgery (e.g., cesarean section).

Side Effects: *GI:* Nausea, vomiting, diarrhea, hiccoughs. *CNS:* Headache, weakness, anxiety, drowsiness, dizziness, paresthesia, lethargy. *GU:* Laceration or perforation of uterus or cervix, rupture of uterus, endometritis, urinary tract infections, profuse bleeding, pain. *CV:* Chest tightness or pain, hypo- or hypertension, cardiac arrhythmias. *Respiratory:* Wheezing, dyspnea, coughing, hyperventilation, epistaxis. *Other:* Sweating, backache, skin rash, breast tenderness, eye pain, fever, chills.

Note: Since prostaglandins do not directly affect the fetal placental unit, it is possible that a live fetus may be born.

Dosage: See individual drugs.

NURSING CONSIDERATIONS

See also *Nursing Considerations* for *Abortifacients,* p. 1220.

Interventions

1. Monitor the client for pyrexia for at least 3 days after the abortion.
2. Determine if the postabortion pyrexia is caused by endometritis or is prostaglandin-induced.
   - Drug-induced pyrexia is usually manifested 1–16 hours after the first injection. The temperature returns to pretreatment levels once the therapy has been discontinued.
   - With endometritis, the pyrexia usually occurs the third day after the abortion and an infection occurs, unless the client is treated.
3. If the pyrexia is drug-induced, sponge the client with cool water or alcohol and maintain adequate hydration.
4. Do not administer aspirin to the client.
5. Be prepared for a live birth.

CARBOPROST TROMETHAMINE   (KAR-boh-prost troh-METH-ah-meen)

Hemabate, Prostin/15 M (Rx)

See also *Prostaglandins,* p. 1222.

Action/Kinetics: Synthetic analog of prostaglandin F_2 alpha which may act directly on the myometrium. The drug also enhances cervical dilation and softening. Carboprost may be preferred over other prostaglandin abortifacients since IM injection is less difficult to administer, and it may be used without fear of expulsion of vaginal suppositories in presence of excess vaginal bleeding. **Time to peak levels:** 30 min. **Mean time to abortion:** 16 hr.

Uses: To induce abortion from weeks 13–20 of pregnancy. Postpartum hemorrhage due to atonic uterus. *Investigational:* Induction of labor, treatment of hydatidiform mole, ripen cervix prior to vacuum currettage.

Additional Side Effects: *CNS:* Sleep disorders, nervousness, vertigo. *GI:* Dry mouth and throat, hematemesis, alterations in taste, epigastric pain, excessive thirst, gagging or fullness of throat, sensation of choking. *Opthalmologic:* Blurred vision, twitching eyelids. *Respiratory:* Asthma, respiratory distress, upper respiratory tract infections. *CV:* Flushing, vasovagal syndrome, palpitations. *Miscellaneous:* Muscle pain, leg cramps, dystonia, tinnitus, septic shock, torticollis, thyroid storm, retained placenta fragment, uterine sacculation, pain at injection site.

Drug Interaction: Carboprost may ↑ activity of other oxytocic agents.

Dosage: IM only. *Abortion:* **initial,** 0.25 mg deep in the muscle; **then,** repeat at intervals of 1.5 and 3.5 hr depending on response. Dose may be increased to 0.5 mg if response inadequate after several 0.25 mg doses. Total dose should not exceed 12 mg or be administered for more than 2 days. *Refractory postpartum bleeding:* **initial,** 0.25 mg deep in the muscle; **then,** if necessary, additional doses may be given at 15–90 min intervals but total dose should not exceed 2 mg.

NURSING CONSIDERATIONS

See *Nursing Considerations* for *Abortifacients,* p. 1220, and *Prostaglandins,* p. 1222.

Interventions

Pretreatment or concurrent use of an antiemetic and/or antidiarrheal agent will decrease the GI side effects.

DINOPROSTONE (PROSTAGLANDIN E₂)   (DYE-noh-prost-ohn)
Prostin E2 (Rx)

See also *Prostaglandins,* p. 1222.

Action/Kinetics: Dinoprostone is a naturally occurring prostaglandin derivative. It is thought to act directly on the myometrium to stimulate myometrial contractions which are usually of sufficient magnitude to cause abortion. The drug also has a softening effect on the cervix thus enhancing cervical dilation. The response of the uterus increases slowly during pregnancy. **Onset:** Contractions begin within 10 min following insertion of the vaginal suppository. **Mean time to abortion:** 17 hr.

Uses: To induce abortion in weeks 12–20. To evacuate the uterus in intrauterine fetal death, hydatidiform mole, anencephalic fetus, missed abortion, elective abortion (from weeks 12–20), and in uterine perforation before completion of suction curettage. *Investigational:* Low doses to initiate labor and to induce cervical ripening before induction of labor.

Additional Side Effects: *CV:* Flushing, hot flashes. *Musculoskeletal:* Joint inflammation, arthralgia, muscle cramps or pain, nocturnal leg cramps, myalgia, stiff neck. *GU:* Vulvitis, vaginitis, urine retention, vaginismus. *Miscellaneous:* Blurred vision, dehydration, hearing impairment, tremor, pharyngitis, laryngitis, skin discoloration.

Dosage: Vaginal suppository: *Abortifacient:* One 20 mg suppository inserted high in the vagina. Repeat, if necessary, q 3–5 hr until abortion occurs. Should not be given for more than 2 days. *Induction of labor, cervical ripening:* Specially prepared vaginal suppository containing 0.2–5 mg dinoprostone.

NURSING CONSIDERATIONS

See *Nursing Considerations* for *Abortifacients,* p. 1220, and *Prostaglandins,* p. 1222.

Administration/Storage

1. Client should remain supine for 10 min after insertion.
2. The number of suppositories used should be determined by client tolerance and uterine contractility.
3. Suppositories should be stored at 20° C or below.
4. Allow suppositories to warm to room temperature before unwrapping and inserting.

OTHER AGENT

SODIUM CHLORIDE 20% SOLUTION
(Rx)

Classification: Abortifacient.

Action/Kinetics: Hypertonic sodium chloride may release prostaglandins that cause uterine contractions. Abortion may be incomplete in 25–40% of all cases and must be completed by other means. **Onset:** 12–24 hr for labor to begin. Usually induces termination of pregnancy within 36 hr (97% abort within 72 hr). IV oxytocin may be used concomitantly to decrease time to abortion.

Uses: Termination of pregnancy during second trimester (weeks 16 to 24).

Contraindications: Increased intra-amniotic pressure, as in actively contracting or hypertonic uterus. Suspected pelvic adhesions. Patients sensitive to sodium chloride overload (cardiovascular and renal disorders, hypertension and epilepsy), or suffering from blood disorders. Previous uterine surgery. Pregnancies less than 15 or more than 24 weeks gestation.

Side Effects: *CV:* Cardiovascular shock, hemolysis, and cortical necrosis of the kidney if inadvertent intravascular injection occurs. Flushing, severe hemorrhage. *GU:* Necrosis of uterine musculature, retention of placental tissue. *Miscellaneous:* Water intoxication, fever, pneumonia, pulmonary embolism, infection at site of injection.

If hypertonic sodium chloride is inadvertently injected intravascularly, severe, life-threatening hypernatremia may occur.

Drug Interactions: Terbutaline may prolong the time to abortion when used with hypertonic sodium chloride.

Dosage: Transabdominal intra-amniotic: Following transabdominal tap of amniotic sac, introduce 20% sodium chloride solution in a volume equal to that removed of amniotic fluid. If labor has not begun within 48 hr after instillation, the patient should be reassessed by the physician.

NURSING CONSIDERATIONS

See also *Nursing Considerations* for *Abortifacients,* p. 1220.

Administration

1. The 20% sodium chloride solution should be slowly administered over 20–30 min.
2. Oxytocin (in 5% dextrose in water) may be used as an adjunct to hasten onset of abortion.

Interventions

1. Encourage client to drink at least 2 L of water on the day of the procedure, to facilitate the excretion of salt.
2. During the instillation of saline pay close attention to client complaints such as sensation of heat, thirst, severe headache, mental confusion, vague distress, lower back, pelvic or abdominal pain, tingling sensations, numbness of fingertips, a feeling of warmth about the lips and tongue, extreme nervousness, or tinnitus. These symptoms may indicate that the drug is not being instilled into the amniotic sac. Be prepared to assist with 5% dextrose infusion and other supportive therapy to prevent hypernatremic shock.
3. Observe the client for 1–2 hr after instillation of hypertonic saline for adverse reactions and the onset of labor.
4. Continue to assess for symptoms of hypernatremia following the injection. Symptoms of hypernatremia may include thirst, rough dry tongue, flushed skin, elevated temperature, excitement, hypo- or hypertension, tachycardia, and numbness of fingertips. Obtain appropriate lab data, document and report these findings to the physician.

Evaluation

Determine if intended response was obtained following drug administration.

CHAPTER SIXTY-FIVE

Androgens and Anabolic Steroids

Anabolic Steroids

Androgens

ANABOLIC STEROIDS

Information on specific anabolic steroids is listed in Table 28.

Action/Kinetics: Anabolic steroids are synthetic derivatives of testosterone and thus have minimal androgenic effects but retain anabolic (tissue-building) effects. Thus, these drugs cause a reverse of catabolism and cause a positive nitrogen balance. They stimulate appetite if there is proper intake of proteins and calories. The drugs also are effective in various types of anemias by increasing production of erythropoietin. All of the anabolic steroids are about equal in efficacy; differences in drugs are due to incidence of side effects, route of administration, and duration of action.

Uses: Reverse catabolism in chronic infections, extensive surgery, burns, or severe trauma. Treatment of anemias due to bone marrow failure, deficient red cell production, or associated with renal disease. Prophylaxis of hereditary angioedema. Treatment of breast cancer in postmenopausal women.

Contraindications: Use for osteoporosis. Use of anabolic steroids by athletes is not recommended.

Special Concerns: Pregnancy category: X. Use with caution in children and adolescents due to the possibility of premature epiphyseal closure, virilization in females, and precocious sexual development in males.

Side Effects: When used by athletes, there is a risk of serious side effects including suppression of spermatogenesis, testicular atrophy, hepatotoxicity, and hepatic cancer. Use in women may cause virilization (e.g., deepening of the voice, acne, unnatural growth of hair) and menstrual difficulties. Other side effects in males include frequent urination (due to bladder irritation), gynecomastia, breast soreness, and priapism. See also *Side Effects* for *Testosterone,* p. 1231.

Dosage: See individual drugs, Table 28.

Table 28 Androgens and Anabolic Steroids

Drug	Uses	Dosage	Remarks
Ethylestrenol (Maxibolin) (Rx) Pregnancy category: X.	Treat catabolism due to chronic infections, surgery, severe trauma, use of corticosteroids.	**Elixir, Tablets. Adults: Usual,** 4 mg daily up to 8 mg daily for severe catabolic stress. Dosage not established in children.	Synthetic anabolic steroid. *Administration:* Therapy should not exceed 6 weeks. *Nursing Considerations:* 1. Therapy may be reinstituted after a 4-week rest period. 2. Androgenic effects are less marked than other drugs in adults; however, androgenic effects may be marked in children. 3. Periodic liver function tests are indicated since the drug may affect liver function. 4. Growth may occur for up to 6 months after drug has been terminated.
Fluoxymesterone (Android-F, Halotestin, Ora-Testryl) (Rx) Pregnancy category: X.	Hypogonadism or delayed puberty in males; inoperable breast carcinoma in women. *Investigational:* Anemias due to deficient red cell production.	**Tablets.** *Males: Hypogonadism,* 5–20 mg daily. *Delayed puberty,* **usual,** 2.5–10 mg daily for 4–6 months (up to 20 mg may be used). *Females: Inoperable breast carcinoma,* 20–50 mg daily for 1 month (up to 2–3 months for objective response). *Anemias:* 20–50 mg daily or a minimum of 2–6 months.	Synthetic androgen. *Notes:* 1. Does not cause full sexual maturation in patients with prepubertal testicular failure. 2. GI disturbances more common than with other androgens. 3. Greater potency than testosterone when used for hypogonadism or delayed puberty.
Methyltestosterone (Android-5, -10, and -25; Metandren, Oreton, Testred, Virilon) (Rx) Pregnancy category: X.	**Capsules, Buccal Tablets, Tablets.** impotence, androgen deficiency, postpubertal cryptorchidism. *Females:* Breast carcinoma.	**PO.** *Males: Hypogonadism, Replacement therapy: climacteric, impotence, hypogonadism:* 10–50 mg daily (buccal: 5–25 mg). *Postpubertal cryptorchidism:* 10 mg t.i.d. (buccal: 5 mg t.i.d.). *Delayed puberty in males:* 5–25 mg daily for 4–6 months (buccal: 2.5–12.5 mg daily). *Breast cancer in females:* 50 mg 1–4 times daily (buccal: 25 mg 1–4 times daily).	Semisynthetic androgen. *Administration:* Buccal use provides twice the androgenic effect as oral tablets. *Note:* Ineffective in producing full sexual maturation in patients with prepubertal testicular failure.

65

1227

Table 28 (continued)

Drug	Uses	Dosage	Remarks
Nandrolone Decanoate (Anabolin LA-100, Androlone 50, Androlone D, Deca-Durabolin, Hybolin Decanoate, Nandrobolic L.A., Neo-Durabolic) (Rx) Pregnancy category: X.	Anemia due to renal disease *Investigational:* Catabolism due to inoperable conditions, inoperable metastatic breast cancer in postmeno-pausal women.	**IM.** *Males:* 50–200 mg at 1–4 week intervals. *Females:* 50–100 mg at 1–4 week intervals. **Pediatric, 2–13 years:** 25–50 mg q 3–4 weeks.	Synthetic anabolic steroid. *Administration:* 1. Give deep IM, preferably into the gluteal muscle. 2. Treatment should be intermittent with duration of therapy dependent on extent of untoward reactions. 3. Adequate iron intake is necessary for maximum response.
Nandrolone Phenpropionate (Anabolin, Androlone, Durabolin, Hybolin-Improved, Nandrobolic) (Rx) Pregnancy category: X.	Metastatic breast carcinoma in postmenopausal women.	**IM. Adults:** 25–100 mg weekly up to 12 weeks. Cycle may be repeated after a 4 week rest period. Dosage has not been established in children.	Synthetic anabolic steroid. *Administration:* 1. Give deep IM, preferably into the gluteal muscle. 2. Treatment should be intermittent with duration of therapy dependent on extent of untoward reactions.
Oxandrolone (Anavar) (Rx) Pregnancy category: X.	Enhance weight gain in patients with chronic infections, after severe trauma, or after extensive surgery. *Investigational:* Turner's syndrome in women.	**Tablets. Adults, usual:** 2.5 mg b.i.d.–q.i.d. (up to 20 mg may be used). **Pediatric:** 0.25 mg/kg/day. *Turner's syndrome:* 0.05–0.125 mg/kg daily.	Synthetic anabolic steroid. *Administration:* 1. Therapy is continued for 2–4 weeks, not to exceed 3 months. 2. A course of therapy may be repeated, as necessary. 3. Children may be particularly sensitive to the androgenic effects of oxandrolone. 4. When used for Turner's syndrome, the lowest possible dose should be used, to prevent side effects.

Oxymetholone (Anadrol, Anapolon 50◆) (Rx) Pregnancy category: X.

Anemias including deficient red blood cell production, acquired or congenital aplastic anemia, hypoplastic anemias and myelofibrosis due to use of myelotoxic drugs. Prophylaxis of hereditary angioedema.

Tablets. Usual: 1–2 mg/kg/day (up to 5 mg/kg/day may be given) for a period of 3–6 months. **Premature infants and neonates:** 0.175 mg/kg (5 mg/m$_2$) daily as a single dose.

Synthetic anabolic steroid. *Administration:*
1. Dosage should be individualized and effect is not often immediate.
2. When in remission, some patients may require lower maintenance doses of the drug.
3. Continuous therapy is usually indicated for congenital aplastic anemia.

Stanozolol (Winstrol) (Rx) Pregnancy category: X.

To decrease frequency and severity of attacks of hereditary angioedema (used prophylactically). *Investigational:* Treatment of antithrombin III deficiency and excess fibrinogen. Treatment of hereditary angioedema.

Tablets. Adults: 2 mg t.i.d. to 4 mg q.i.d. for 5 days; **then,** individualize according to response. After a favorable response, dose should be decreased at intervals of 1–3 months to a maintenance of 2 mg daily or 2 mg every other day. **Pediatric, up to 6 years:** 1 mg daily given only during an attack of angioedema. **Pediatric, 6–12 years:** 2 mg daily given only during an attack of angioedema.

Synthetic anabolic steroid. *Administration:*
1. The dose used prior to stressful situations may be higher than listed.
2. May cause premature epiphyseal closure in children; thus, long-term use is not recommended, especially since frequency of attacks in children is not high.

NURSING CONSIDERATIONS

See *Nursing Considerations* for *Testosterone,* p. 1232.

Client/Family Teaching

Teach the client that anabolic steroid therapy should be accompanied by a well-balanced diet which provides adequate proteins and calories.

ANDROGENS

Since the principal male hormone manufactured by the interstitial cells of the testes is testosterone, this hormone will be discussed in detail. All other androgens are listed in Table 28, p. 1227.

TESTOSTERONE AQUEOUS SUSPENSION   (tess-**TOSS**-teh-rohn)

Andro 100, Andronaq-50, Histerone 50 and 100, Malogen ✹, Testamone 100, Testaqua, Testoject-50 (Rx)

TESTOSTERONE CYPIONATE IN OIL   (tess-**TOSS**-teh-rohn)

Andro-Cyp 100 and 200, Andronaq-LA, Andronate 100 and 200, dep-Andro 100 and 200, Depotest, Depo-Testosterone, Depo-Testosterone Cypionate ✹, Duratest-100 and -200, T-Cypionate, Testa-C, Testoject LA, Testred Cypionate 200, Virilon IM (Rx)

TESTOSTERONE ENANTHATE   (tess-**TOSS**-teh-rohn)

Andro LA 200, Andropository 100, Andryl 200, Delatest, Delatestryl, Durathate-200, Everone, Malogex ✹, Testone LA 100 and 200, Testrin PA (Rx)

TESTOSTERONE PROPIONATE IN OIL   (tess-**TOSS**-teh-rohn)

Malogen ✹, Testex (Rx)

Classification: Androgen, natural hormone and salts of natural hormone.

Action/Kinetics: Testosterone, its degradation products, and synthetic substitutes are collectively referred to as the *androgens* (from the Greek *andros,* man). Like the primary female hormones, estrogen and progesterone, the production of testosterone is controlled by the gonadotropins: follicle-stimulating hormone (FSH), and the interstitial cell-stimulating hormone (ICSH), both of which are produced by the anterior pituitary.

At puberty, these gonadotropins initiate the production of testosterone, which in turn stimulates the development of primary sex organs and secondary sexual characteristics. Testosterone also stimulates bone and skeletal muscle growth, increases the retention of dietary protein nitrogen (anabolism), and slows down the breakdown of body tissues (catabolism). The anabolic effect is due to stimulation of RNA polymerase activity and specific RNA synthesis which results in increased protein production. Androgens promote retention of sodium, potassium, nitrogen, and phosphorus and the excretion of calcium. Toward the end of puberty, testosterone hastens the conversion of cartilage into bone, thereby terminating linear growth.

Treatment with testosterone and its congeners is complicated by the fact that the exogenous supply of the hormone may depress secretion of the natural hormone through inhibitory effects on the pituitary. Too large a dose may cause permanent damage. Treatment is usually associated with a feeling of well-being. In addition to testosterone and its various esters, several synthetic variants are available commercially.

Uses: Replacement therapy in males for congenital or acquired primary hypogonadism, congenital or acquired hypogonadotropic hypogonadism, delayed puberty. In postmenopausal females to treat inoperable metastatic breast carcinoma or in premenopausal females following oophorectomy. Postpartum breast engorgement. *Investigational:* Treat various anemias.

Contraindications: Prostatic or breast (males) carcinoma. Pregnancy (masculinization of female fetus) and lactation. Discontinue if hypercalcemia occurs.

Special Concerns: Pregnancy category: X. Use with caution in young males and females who have not completed their growth (because of premature epiphyseal closure). Androgens may also cause virilization in females or precocious sexual development in males. Geriatric patients may manifest an increased risk of prostatic hypertrophy or prostatic carcinoma. Also use with caution in patients with cardiac, renal, or hepatic disorders (because of edema caused by androgen administration).

Side Effects: *Hepatic:* Liver toxicity is the most serious side effect. Jaundice, cholestasis, alterations in BSP retention, SGOT, and SPGT. Rarely, hepatic necrosis, hepatocellular neoplasms, peliosis hepatis. *GI:* Nausea, vomiting, diarrhea, anorexia, symptoms of peptic ulcer. *CNS:* Headache, anxiety, increased or decreased libido, insomnia, excitation, paresthesias, sleep apnea syndrome, CNS hemorrhage, chills, choreiform movements, habituation, confusion (toxic doses). *GU:* Testicular atrophy with inhibition of testicular function, impotence, chronic priapism, epididymitis, irritable bladder, oligospermia, prepubertal phallic enlargement, decreased volume of ejaculate. *Electrolyte:* Retention of sodium, chloride, calcium, potassium, phosphates. Edema. *Miscellaneous:* Acne, flushing, suppression of clotting factors (II, V, VII, X), polycythemia, leukopenia, rashes, dermatitis, anaphylaxis (rare), muscle cramps. Hypercalcemia, especially in immobilized patients or those with metastatic breast carcinoma.

In females, menstrual irregularities, virilization, clitoral enlargement, hirsutism, increased libido, baldness (male pattern), virilization of external genitalia of female fetus.

In children, disturbances of growth, premature closure of epiphyses, precocious sexual development.

Buccal preparations may cause stomatitis. Inflammation and pain at site of IM or SC injection.

Note: Side effects of the cypionate and enanthate products are not readily reversible due to the long duration of action of these dosage forms.

Drug Interactions	
Anticoagulants, oral	Anabolic steroids ↑ effect of anticoagulants
Antidiabetic agents	Additive hypoglycemia
Barbiturates	↓ Effect of androgens due to ↑ breakdown by liver
Corticosteroids	↑ Chance of edema
Phenylbutazone	Certain androgens ↑ effect of phenylbutazone

Laboratory Test Interferences: Alter thyroid function tests. False + or ↑ BSP, alkaline phosphatase, bilirubin, cholesterol, and acid phosphatase (in women). Alteration of glucose tolerance tests.

Dosage: *Testosterone and testosterone propionate,* **IM only.** *Replacement therapy:* 25–50 mg 2–3 times/week. *Postpartum breast engorgement:* 25–50 mg daily for 3–4 days beginning at the time of delivery. *Breast cancer:* 50–100 mg 3 times/week. *Delayed puberty in males:* 12.5–25 mg 2–3 times a week for no more than 4–6 months.

Testosterone enanthate and cypionate, **IM only.** *Hypogonadism, replacement therapy, impotence:* 50–400 mg q 2–4 weeks. *Delayed puberty:* 25–200 mg q 2–4 weeks for no more than 4–6 months. *Breast cancer in women:* 200–400 mg q 2–4 weeks.

NURSING CONSIDERATIONS

Administration/Storage

1. Crystals of testosterone enanthate or cypionate may be redissolved by warming and shaking the vial.
2. Pellets for subcutaneous injection can be inserted surgically or with a specially designed injector. The procedure may be done in the doctor's office. Two or more pellets may be injected at one time. The drug will be slowly absorbed over 4–6 months.
3. Proper dosage of pellets for the client is determined first by administering oral medication before administration of the pellets SC.
4. For IM oil-based suspensions, warm the unopened vial in warm water to decrease the viscosity of the oil. Vigorously rotate the vial to resuspend the medication in the oil. A film may appear on the sides of the vial. When no more suspended particles are observed on the bottom or sides of the vial, the drug has been suspended appropriately. Administer the needle deep into the muscle, and administer the medication slowly.
5. When parenteral injection is to be used, testosterone propionate is more effective than testosterone because it is released more slowly.
6. Continue the therapy for at least 2 months for a satisfactory response, and for 5 months for an objective response.

Assessment

1. Review the client's general health history for evidence of existing cardiac, renal or hepatic dysfunction.
2. Obtain baseline data concerning the client's neurological status, blood pressure, respirations, heart sounds, and GU function.
3. Note the client's hair distribution and skin texture.
4. Check the client's medication history for interacting drugs such as anticoagulants, hypoglycemic agents and mineralocorticoids.
5. If the client is female, of childbearing age and sexually active, note the potential for pregnancy.
6. Obtain a baseline complete blood count, serum glucose level, electrolyte levels and liver and renal function studies.

Interventions

1. Monitor the client for signs of mental depression such as insomnia, lack of interest in personal appearance and a general withdrawal from social contacts.
2. Note any client complaints of tingling of the fingers and toes, or complaint of loss of appetite. Document and report to the physician.
3. Monitor the client's weight, blood pressure, pulse and serum electrolytes. Note any evidence of edema, such as distension of the jugular veins. Auscultate the lung sounds and report any signs of edema to the physician, since diuretics may be ordered to control the edema.
   - Monitor and record the client's weight at least twice a week.
   - Monitor the client's intake and output.
4. Assess for relaxation of the skeletal muscles and note if client complains of pain deep in the

bones. The discomfort in the bones is caused by a honeycombing of the bones. These complaints are often a first indication of an increase in the client's calcium levels and must be further investigated.

5. If client complains of flank pain this may be caused by kidney stones, which may result from excessively high serum calcium levels.

6. Normal serum calcium levels are 4.5–5.5 mEq/L. If the client has a high serum calcium level, withdraw the drug, notify the physician and administer large amounts of fluids to prevent renal calculi. If the hypercalcemia is the result of metastases, other appropriate therapy should be instituted.

7. Observe the client for jaundice, malaise, complaints of right upper quadrant pain, pruritus or a change in the color or consistency of the stools. Obtain liver function studies, document and report to the physician.

8. Observe the client for easy bruising, reports of bleeding, or client complaints of sore throat or the development of fever. Obtain a CBC, white cell count and differential to rule out polycythemia and leukopenia.

9. If the client is a child, monitor closely for growth retardation and development of precocious puberty.
   - Review the program of therapy with the parents. Often therapy will be intermittent to allow for periods of normal bone growth.
   - Discuss with the physician the advisability of regular x-rays of the wrists and hands to monitor the maturation of bone.
   - Monitor and record the child's height and weight.

10. If the client is female, report the onset of signs of virilization, such as deepening of the voice and clitoral enlargement.

11. Discuss with female clients any changes in libido. Provide emotional support and report this problem to the physician. Increased libido may be an early sign of serious drug toxicity.

12. Note the presence of acne and other skin changes. If the acne is severe, consult the physician. It may be necessary to change the dose of medication.

Client/Family Teaching

1. Instruct the client to report any unusual incidents of bleeding or bruising. Androgens suppress clotting factors and polycythemia and leukopenia may also occur.

2. If the client has received the drug via pellets, sloughing can occur. Instruct the client to notify the physician immediately if this occurs.

3. Discuss with the client the potential for bladder irritation to occur. Review the symptoms that may occur as a result of this irritation and advise the client to report these findings to the physician.

4. Instruct parents of children receiving testosterone to weigh the child at least twice a week and to measure the child's length at least every 2–3 months. These measurements should be reported to the physician.

5. Discuss with the client the importance of reporting to the laboratory for tests of serum calcium levels and serum cholesterol. If the serum cholesterol level is high, the physician may wish to change the dosage of drug. Also, discuss with the client the need to follow a low-cholesterol diet and refer to a dietician for further assistance in meal planning.

6. Reassure female clients that any growth in facial hair and the development of acne are reversible once the drug is withdrawn.

7. Explain to premenopausal female clients that the medication may cause irregularities in the menstrual cycle. In postmenopausal women the medication may cause withdrawal bleeding.

- Advise women to keep a written record of their menstrual periods.
- For sexually active women, discuss with them the advisability of consulting the physician regarding birth control measures during the first few weeks of androgen therapy and for several weeks after the androgen therapy has been withdrawn.
- Advise women to notify the physician immediately if pregnancy is suspected. There is an increased risk of fetal abnormalities with this drug.

8. Instruct male clients to report priapism. The physician may withdraw the drug at least temporarily.

9. Unless contraindicated, recommend that the client follow a diet high in calories, proteins, vitamins, minerals, and other nutrients.

10. Discuss with young clients and their parents if possible, the potential for drug abuse. Explain the long-term effects and the permanent physical damage that is caused by indiscriminate use of these agents.

CHAPTER SIXTY-SIX

Posterior Pituitary Hormone and Related Drugs/Growth Hormone

The two important hormones secreted by the posterior pituitary are oxytocin and vasopressin (ADH, antidiuretic hormone) each of which contains eight amino acids. Oxytocin is formed in the paraventricular nuclei of the hypothalamus while vasopressin is formed in the supraoptic nuclei. Once synthesized the hormones are carried by a protein, named neurophysin, down nerve endings to the posterior pituitary where they are stored. Oxytocin acts on the smooth muscle of the uterus and alveoli of the breast. Vasopressin controls reabsorption of water from the glomerular filtrate and increases blood pressure by causing contraction of the vascular bed and increased peripheral resistance (pressor effect). Except for posterior pituitary injection, which has oxytocic, vasopressor, and ADH activity, the drugs belonging to this group are used either for obstetric or antidiuretic purposes.

POSTERIOR PITUITARY HORMONE

POSTERIOR PITUITARY INJECTION
Pituitrin (Rx)

Classification: Posterior pituitary hormone.

Action/Kinetics: The natural extract of the posterior pituitary has oxytocic, vasopressor, and antidiuretic hormone properties. The rapid pressor effect of this drug may make its use hazardous. Most physicians now use more refined agents with specific oxytocic or antidiuretic properties.

Uses: In the past posterior pituitary injection has been used for postoperative ileus, to stimulate expulsion of gas prior to pyelography, to achieve hemostasis in presence of esophageal varices, and in the treatment of postpartum hemorrhage.

Contraindications: Toxemia of pregnancy, cardiac disease, hypertension, epilepsy, advanced arteriosclerosis, first stage of labor.

Special Concerns: Pregnancy category: C. Use with great caution at any stage of delivery. Use with caution in patients under barbiturate sedation.

Side Effects: *Common:* Facial pallor, increased GI motility, uterine cramps. *Miscellaneous:* Tinnitus, anxiety, proteinuria, unconsciousness, eclamptic attacks, mydriasis, anaphylaxis, angioneurotic edema, urticaria, blindness, diarrhea.

Drug Interactions	
Barbiturates	↑ Risk of coronary insufficiency and cardiac arrhythmias
Carbamazepine	↑ Antidiuretic effect of posterior pituitary hormones
Chlorpropamide	↑ Antidiuretic effect of posterior pituitary hormones
Clofibrate	↑ Antidiuretic effect of posterior pituitary hormones

Dosage: IM (preferred) and SC. *Postoperative ileus:* 5–20 units (usual: 10 units). *Hemostasis:* 10–20 USP units. *Postpartum hemorrhage:* 10 USP units.

NURSING CONSIDERATIONS

Assessment

1. Note any client past history of cardiac disease, hypertension or arteriosclerosis.
2. List medications currently being used to determine if any interact with posterior pituitary injection.

Interactions

1. Observe the client closely for allergic responses following administration of the drug. Have emergency supportive medications and equipment readily available.
2. Monitor BP closely for ½ hour following administration of the medication. The drug reduces cardiac output and may diminish coronary blood flow.
3. Posterior pituitary injection is short-acting. Consult with the physician about supplementing with another drug after the primary use of posterior pituitary injection to control postpartum hemorrhage.

OXYTOCICS

General Statement: The uterus consists mainly of two types of tissues: (1) the *endometrium,* or mucous membrane lining the inner surface, whose function is governed chiefly by the ovarian hormones, and (2) the *myometrium,* a thick wall of smooth muscle heavily interlaced with blood vessels. The latter are necessary to supply the placenta and fetus with oxygen and nutrients.

An understanding of the different stages of labor is essential for the judicious use of drugs in obstetrics. Premature use of any agent might be harmful to mother and child.

Labor is divided into 3 stages. Stage I is characterized by the onset of strong regular contractions of the myometrium and complete dilatation of the cervix. Stage II begins with the complete dilatation of the cervix and ends with the delivery of the baby. Stage III begins after delivery, involves placental separation, and terminates with birth of the placenta.

Immediately after delivery, the smooth muscles of the uterus are completely relaxed (uterine atony), and during this time the patient may bleed heavily. This period of smooth muscle relaxation is followed by renewed contractions, which produce placental separation and also clamp shut the countless blood vessels exposed when the placenta separates from the uterus. The average amount of blood lost during this stage is 200–300 mL.

The drugs discussed in this section assist the uterus during the various stages of labor. The oxytocic drugs, like oxytocin and ergotamine, promote contraction. These agents are used occasionally to induce labor and to promote incomplete abortions.

As a rule, oxytocic agents are not used during the first or second stage of labor. The premature use of oxytocic agents may cause severe laceration and trauma to the mother (rupture of the uterus), and trauma—even death—to the infant.

Action/Kinetics: Oxytocics cause contraction of uterine musculature by combining with specific receptors in the myometrium. Although the exact mechanism is not known, it may involve calcium, prostaglandins, and cyclic AMP. Uterine sensitivity to oxytocics increases gradually during gestation with a sharp increase in sensitivity just before parturition. Oxytocics also cause contraction of the myoepithelium of the lacteal glands resulting in lactation.

Drug Interactions

Anesthetics, local	See *Vasoconstrictors*
Cyclophosphamide	↑ Effect of oxytocics
Vasoconstrictors (e.g., in anesthetics)	May have synergistic and additive effects with oxytocics. Concomitant use may result in severe, persistent hypertension and rupture of cerebral blood vessels

---

ERGONOVINE MALEATE   (er-go-**NO**-veen)

Ergotrate Maleate (Rx)

METHYLERGONOVINE MALEATE   (meth-ill-er-go-**NO**-veen)

Methergine (Rx)

Classification: Oxytocic agents.

Action/Kinetics: Ergonovine is a natural alkaloid obtained from ergot (a fungus that grows on rye), while methylergonovine is a closely related synthetic drug. These drugs stimulate the rate, tone, and amplitude of uterine contractions. The uterus becomes more sensitive to the drug toward the end of pregnancy. Ergonovine maleate also stimulates smooth muscle surrounding certain blood vessels by interacting with adrenergic, dopaminergic, and tryptaminergic receptors. *Ergonovine.* **Onset** (uterine contractions): **PO,** 5–15 min; **IM,** 2–3 min; **IV,** 60 sec. **Duration: PO, IM,** 3 or more hr; **IV,** 45 min. *Methylergonovine.* **Onset** (uterine contractions): **PO,** 5–10 min; **IM,** 2–5 min; **IV,** immediate. **t½, IV:** 2–3 min (initial) and 20–30 min (final). **Duration, PO, IM:** 3 hr; **IV:** 45 min.

Uses: Management and prevention of postpartum and postabortal hemorrhage by producing firm uterine contractions and decreasing uterine bleeding. Migraine headaches (ergonovine). Incomplete abortion (methylergonovine). *Investigational:* Ergonovine has been used to diagnose Prinzmetal's angina (variant angina).

Contraindications: Pregnancy, toxemia, hypertension. Ergot hypersensitivity. Should be given with caution in sepsis, obliterative vascular disease, impaired renal or hepatic function. To induce labor or threatened spontaneous abortions. Administration prior to delivery of the placenta.

Side Effects: *Ergonovine. GI:* Nausea, vomiting, diarrhea. *Miscellaneous:* Allergic reactions, headache, increased blood pressure. *Ergotism:* In overdosage. Nausea, vomiting, diarrhea, changes in blood pressure, chest pain, hypercoagulability, numb and cold extremities, gangrene of fingers and toes, dyspnea, weak pulse, excitability to convulsions, delirium, hallucinations, death. Treatment is symptomatic as well as to decrease drug absorption.

Methylergonovine. GI: Nausea, vomiting. *CNS:* Dizziness, headache, tinnitus. *Miscellaneous:* Sweating, chest pain, dyspnea, palpitations, transient hypertension.

Note: Use of these agents during labor may result in uterine tetany with rupture, cervical and perineal lacerations, embolism of amniotic fluid as well as hypoxia and intracranial hemorrhage in the infant.

Dosage: *Ergonovine. Uterine stimulant:* **IM, IV (emergencies only),** 0.2 mg no more often than q 2–4 hr, up to 5 doses. *Diagnosis of angina pectoris:* **IV,** 0.05 mg q 5 min until chest pain occurs or a total dose of 0.4 mg has been given.

Tablets, oral or sublingual: 0.2–0.4 mg q 6–12 hr for 48 hr or until danger of uterine atony has passed. *Note:* Severe cramping is indicator of effectiveness. IV calcium salts may be required to enhance effectiveness in calcium-deficient patients.

Methylergonovine. **IM, IV (emergencies only):** 0.2 mg q 2–4 hr following delivery of placenta, of the anterior shoulder, or during the puerperium. **Tablets.** 0.2–0.4 mg b.i.d.–q.i.d. until danger of hemorrhage and uterine atony is over (usually within 2 days, although treatment for up to 7 days may be necessary).

NURSING CONSIDERATIONS

Administration/Storage

1. IV methylergonovine should be administered slowly over 1 minute.
2. Ergonovine ampules must be stored in a cold place away from light.
3. Since ergonovine loses its potency, if kept in the delivery room, it must be discarded after 60 days.
4. Ampules of discolored methylergonovine should be discarded.

Assessment

1. Determine the location of the fundus, its height, and consistency.
2. Observe and record the amount of lochia.

Interventions

1. Note the character and amount of lochia, document and report to the physician if the amount is abnormal.
2. Monitor the uterus and palpate the fundus and note findings.
3. Monitor the blood pressure, pulse and respirations. If there is any abnormal elevation or decrease in blood pressure, or if the pulse and respirations assume a pattern unusual for the client, document and report to the physician.
4. If the client complains of severe cramping, report to the physician. This adverse effect suggests the need for a reduction in dosage of the drug.
5. Question the client about the presence of dizziness, headache, or ringing in the ears. Note if the client has nausea, complains of drowsiness, or has diarrhea, and if they appear to be confused. These are early signs of accidental ergotism as the drug is a derivative of lysergic acid. GI and CNS effects may occur before disturbances to the circulation of the hands and feet. Document and report to the physician immediately.
6. After administration, check the client's vital signs for evidence of shock or hypertension. Have emergency drugs available.

OXYTOCIN, PARENTERAL   (ox-eh-**TOE**-sin)

Pitocin (Rx)

OXYTOCIN, SYNTHETIC, NASAL   (ox-eh-**TOE**-sin)

Syntocinon (Rx)

Classification: Oxytocic agent.

Action/Kinetics: These products are synthetic compounds identical to the natural hormone isolated from the posterior pituitary. Oxytocin has uterine stimulant, vasopressive, and antidiuretic properties. It acts by an indirect effect to mimic contractions of normal labor. Uterine sensitivity to oxytocin, as well as amplitude and duration of uterine contractions, increases gradually during gestation and just before parturition increases rapidly. The hormone facilitates ejection of milk from the breasts by stimulating smooth muscle. **Onset, IV:** immediate; **IM,** 3–5 min; **Nasal,** several minutes. **Peak effects:** 40 min. **t½:** 1–6 min (decreased in late pregnancy and lactation). **Duration, IV:** 20 min after infusion is stopped; **IM:** 30–60 min; **nasal:** 20 min. Eliminated through the urine, liver, and functional mammary gland.

Uses: *Antepartum:* Induction or stimulation of labor at term. Used to overcome true primary or secondary uterine inertia. Induction of labor with oxytocin is indicated only under certain *specific* conditions and is not usual because serious toxic effects can occur.
 Oxytocin is indicated

1. for uterine inertia.
2. for induction of labor in cases of erythroblastosis fetalis, maternal diabetes mellitus, preeclampsia, and eclampsia.
3. for induction of labor after premature rupture of membranes in last month of pregnancy when labor fails to develop spontaneously within 12 hr.
4. for routine control of postpartum hemorrhage and uterine atony.
5. to hasten uterine involution.
6. to complete inevitable abortions after the 20th week of pregnancy.
7. intranasally for initial letdown of milk.

Investigational: Breast engorgement, oxytocin challenge test for determining antepartum fetal heart rate.

Contraindications: Hypersensitivity to drug, cephalopelvic disproportion, malpresentation of the fetus, undilated cervix, overdistention of the uterus, hypotonic uterine contractions, and history of cesarean section or other uterine surgery. Also, predisposition to thromboplastin and amniotic fluid embolism (dead fetus, abruptio placentae), history of previous traumatic deliveries, or patients with four or more deliveries. Oxytocin should never be given IV undiluted or in high concentrations. Oxytocin citrate is contraindicated in severe toxemia, cardiovascular or renal disease. Intranasal oxytocin is contraindicated during pregnancy (pregnancy category: X).

Side Effects: *Mother:* Tetanic uterine contractions, rupture of the uterus, hypertension, tachycardia, and electrocardiographic changes after IV administration of concentrated solutions. Also, rarely, anxiety, dyspnea, precordial pain, edema, cyanosis or reddening of the skin, and cardiovascular spasm. Water intoxication from prolonged IV infusion, maternal deaths due to hypertensive episodes, subarachnoid hemorrhage, or uterine rupture.
 Fetus: Death, premature ventricular contractions, bradycardia, tachycardia, hypoxia, intracranial hemorrhage due to overstimulation of the uterus during labor leads to uterine tetany with marked impairment of uteroplacental blood flow.
 Note: Hypersensitivity reactions occur rarely. When they do, they occur most often with natural oxytocin administered IM or in concentrated IV doses and least frequently after IV infusion or diluted doses. Accidental swallowing of buccal tablets is not harmful.

Drug Interactions: Severe hypertension and possible stroke when used with sympathomimetic pressor amines.

Dosage: IV infusion, IM. *Induction or stimulation of labor:* **IV infusion,** dilute 10 units (1 mL) to 1,000 mL isotonic saline or 5% dextrose. **Initial:** 0.001–0.002 unit/min (0.1–0.2 mL/min); dose can be gradually increased at 15–30 min intervals by 0.001 unit/min (0.1 mL/min) to maximum of 0.02 unit/min (2 mL/min). *Reduction of postpartum bleeding:* **IV infusion,** dilute 10–40 units (1–4 mL) to 1,000 mL with isotonic saline or 5% dextrose. Administer at a rate to control uterine atony, usually at a rate of 0.02–0.1 unit/min. *Incomplete or therapeutic abortion:* **IV infusion,** 10 units at a rate of 0.02–0.04 unit/min. **IM:** 10 units after placental delivery.

Synthetic, nasal (*for milk letdown*): one spray into one or both nostrils 2–3 min before nursing or pumping breasts.

NURSING CONSIDERATIONS

Administration/Storage

1. For *IV* use: Use Y-tubing system, with one bottle containing IV solution and oxytocin, and the other containing only the IV solution. This allows for the discontinuation of the drug while maintaining the patency of the vein when it is decided to change to the drug-free infusion bottle. Parenteral oxytocin infusions should be administered only with an electric infusion device.
2. As a *nasal spray:* Have the client sit upright and hold the bottle upright. Apply gentle pressure while spraying medication into the nostril. The nasal spray may be administered in drop form by applying gentle pressure to the bottle.
3. Oxytocin is rapidly broken down by sodium bisulfite. Have magnesium sulfate immediately available.
4. The physician should be immediately available during the administration of the drug.

Assessment

1. Note if the client has any history of hypersensitivity to the drug.
2. Check for dilation of the uterus and time the length and frequency of the uterine contractions.
3. Carefully review the client's history for any contraindications prior to administering oxytocin.

(For induction and stimulation of labor and/or oxytocin challenge test):

Interventions

1. Before initiating therapy, inform the client of the rationale for using oxytocic agents and reassure the client that the procedure is not unusual.
2. Remain with the client during the induction period and throughout the stimulation of labor. The client must be attended by a qualified registered nurse.
3. Take the vital signs and check the intake and output every 15 minutes.
4. Check the resting uterine tone and assess the uterine contractions for frequency, length of time of the contraction, and the strength.
5. Monitor the fetal heart rate and rhythm at least every 10 minutes, document and report immediately any alterations from the normal pattern.
6. Prevent uterine rupture and fetal damage by clamping off IV oxytocin, starting medication-free IV fluids, providing oxygen, and notifying the physician when the following events occur:
   - If the contractions occur more frequently than every 2 minutes and last longer than 60 sec with no period of uterine relaxation between contractions.
   - If the contractions are excessively strong and/or exceed 50 mm Hg, as measured either on an external monitor or by an internal uterine catheter with an electronic monitor.

- If the fetal heart rate indicates bradycardia, tachycardia, or irregularities of rhythm, as measured by the fetoscope, Dopptone, or other type of electronic monitor.
7. Assess for water intoxication following prolonged administration of oxytocin. Monitor the client's intake and output closely.
8. Observe the client for lethargy, confusion, and stupor. Note if the client has developed neuromuscular hyperexcitability with increased reflexes and muscular twitching. These symptoms should be reported immediately since convulsions and coma may occur if left untreated. Magnesium sulfate should be readily available.

(During the fourth stage of labor when oxytocin is administered for prevention or control of hemorrhage):

Interventions

1. Describe the location, size, and firmness of the uterus. Report to the physician if the uterus is displaced or boggy and follow designated hospital protocol.
2. Note the amount and color of the lochia. Report any bright red lochia, excessive bleeding, or the passage of clots.
3. Monitor the client's vital signs until they remain stable.
4. Closely monitor intake and output.
5. Observe the client for signs of water intoxication, document and report to the physician immediately.

Evaluation

1. Assess for a positive clinical response.
2. Evaluate for freedom from complications of drug therapy.

ANTIDIURETIC HORMONE AND ANALOGS

Vasopressin (or antidiuretic hormone) controls the reabsorption of water from the glomerular filtrate. Diabetes insipidus results from deficiency of this hormone. Patients suffering from a mild form of the disease can be treated by intranasal application of suitable substances (desmopressin, lypressin), whereas patients with severe disease may require systemic treatment with vasopressin or vasopressin tannate.

Treatment requires individual dosage adjustment. Overdosage may cause fluid retention and hypernatremia. Another common adverse reaction is contraction of the smooth muscles of the intestine, uterus, and blood vessels. Animal proteins that may be present in the extracts of the pituitary glands may result in allergic reactions. Thus, synthetic preparations are preferred.

DESMOPRESSIN ACETATE   (des-moh-**PRESS**-in)
DDAVP, Stimate (Rx)

Classification: Antidiuretic hormone, synthetic.

Action/Kinetics: Desmopressin is a synthetic antidiuretic devoid of vasopressor and oxytocic effects. The drug acts to increase absorption of water in the kidney by increasing permeability of cells in the collecting ducts. **Onset:** 1 hr. **Peak:** 1–5 hr. **Duration:** 8–20 hr. **t½:** initial, 8 min; final: 75 min. Effect ceases abruptly. It also increases factor VIII levels (**onset:** 30 min; **peak:** 1.5–2 hr) and von Willebrand's factor activity.

Uses: *Parenteral:* Neurogenic diabetes insipidus, hemophilia A with factor VIII levels more than 5%, Type I von Willebrand's disease with factor VIII levels greater than 5%. *Intranasal:* Central diabetes insipidus (drug of choice due to low incidence of side effects, ease of administration, effectiveness, and long duration of action). To manage temporary polydipsia and polyuria due to trauma or surgery in the pituitary area. Primary nocturnal enuresis.

Contraindications: Hypersensitivity to drug. Children under 3 months for hemophilia A or severe classic von Willebrand's disease (type III). Parenteral administration for diabetes insipidus in children under 12 years and intranasal administration in children less than 3 months. Nephrogenic diabetes insipidus, polyuria due to psychogenic diabetes insipidus, renal disease, hypercalcemia, hyperkalemia, or administration of demeclocycline or lithium.

Special Concerns: Safety during pregnancy (pregnancy category: B) and lactation not established. Use with caution and with restricted fluid intake in infants due to an increased risk of hyponatremia and water intoxication. Geriatric patients may have a greater risk of developing hyponatremia and water intoxication.

Side Effects: Rare. High doses may cause dose-dependent transient headaches, nausea, nasal congestion, rhinitis, flushing, mild abdominal cramps and vulval pain. Side effects can be reduced by a reduction in dosage.

Drug Interaction: Chlorpropamide, clofibrate, and carbamazepine may potentiate the effects of desmopressin.

Dosage: SC, direct IV. *Antidiuretic:* **Adults, SC, IV, usual,** 0.002–0.004 mg/day in 2 doses given in the morning and evening. Then, adjust dosage depending on response. *Antihemorrhagic:* **Adults, IV,** 0.0003 mg/kg diluted in 50 mL 0.9% sodium chloride injection infused over 15–30 min; dose may be repeated, if necessary. **Pediatric, 3 months or older, weighing 10 kg or less, IV:** 0.0003 mg/kg diluted in 10 mL of 0.9% sodium chloride injection and given over 15–30 min; repeat if necessary. **Pediatric, 3 months or older, weighing 10 kg or more, IV:** 0.0003 mg/kg diluted in 50 mL of 0.9% sodium chloride injection and given over 15–30 min; repeat if necessary.

Intranasal. *Antidiuretic:* **Adults, initial,** 0.01 mg at bedtime; dose may be increased nightly in increments of 0.0025 mg until a satisfactory response is obtained. If urine volume is still large, 0.01 mg can be given in the morning. **Maintenance:** 0.01–0.04 mg daily in 1–3 doses. **Pediatric, 3 months–12 years:** 0.005 mg at bedtime; dose may be increased by 0.0025 mg nightly until a satisfactory response is obtained. A 0.005 mg morning dose may be added if the urine volume remains large. **Maintenance:** 0.002–0.004 mg/kg daily to 0.005–0.03 mg daily in 1–3 divided doses. *Nocturnal enuresis:* **Age 5 years and older, initial,** 0.02 mg (0.2 mL) at bedtime with one-half the dose in each nostril; if no response, the dose may be increased to 0.04 mg.

NURSING CONSIDERATIONS

Administration/ Storage

1. Measure the dosage exactly because the drug is potent.
2. Cleanse and dry the tube appropriately.
3. Note the three graduation marks on the soft flexible plastic nasal tube: 0.2, 0.1, and 0.05 mL. The 0.05 level is not designated by number.

4. Refrigerate the solution and injection at 4°C (39.2°F).

5. If the drug is used for hemophilia A or von Willebrand's disease, do not use it more often than every 2 days. Tachyphylaxis may occur if used more often.

Assessment

1. Note any client history of hypersensitivity to the drug.

2. Determine if the client is taking any medications that could be potentiated by the use of desmopressin acetate.

Interventions

1. Monitor the client's intake and output and record.

2. Observe for early signs of water intoxication, such as drowsiness, headache, and vomiting.

3. Adjust the client's fluid intake to avoid water intoxication and hyponatremia.

4. If there is excessive fluid retention, this may be treated with a diuretic such as furosemide.

5. Monitor the duration of sleep. The amount of sleep, together with the client's daily intake and output provide parameters to estimate the clinical response to drug therapy.

Client/Family Teaching

1. If a spray is used, instruct the client in the appropriate administration technique.

2. Provide recommendations concerning fluid intake.

3. Explain how to measure intake and output and stress the importance of keeping an accurate record of fluid status.

4. Provide the client with printed instructions indicating the symptoms of water intoxication and hyponatremia.

5. Impress upon the client the importance of notifying the physician at the earliest signs of trouble, such as a decrease in urinary output, the development of headaches, or severe nasal congestion. The latter two can be mistaken for an upper respiratory infection.

LYPRESSIN   (lye-PRESS-in)

Diapid (Rx)

Classification: Antidiuretic hormone, synthetic.

Action/Kinetics: Lypressin is a synthetic antidiuretic, similar to vasopressin, for intranasal use only. This drug increases reabsorption of water from kidney by increasing the permeability of the collecting ducts. It has minimal vasopressor and oxytocic effects. **Onset:** Within 1 hr. **Time to peak effect:** 30–120 min. **Duration:** 3–4 hr. t^{1}/$_2$: 15 min. The drug is metabolized in the kidney and liver and excreted in urine.

Uses: Diabetes insipidus of neurohypophyseal origin. Particularly suitable for patients allergic or refractory to vasopressin of animal origin.

Special Concerns: Use during pregnancy (pregnancy category: C) only if benefits clearly outweigh risks.

Side Effects: *Nasal:* Congestion, pruritus, irritation, or ulceration of nasal passages. Rhinorrhea. *GI:* Increased bowel movements, abdominal cramps. *Miscellaneous:* Periorbital edema with itching.

Fluid retention (overdose). Heartburn (due to dripping into pharynx). Headache, conjunctivitis, hypersensitivity. Inhalation has resulted in coughing, transient dyspnea, substernal tightness.

Drug Interactions: Chlorpropamide, clofibrate, or carbamazepine may potentiate the effects of lypressin.

Dosage: Topical (intranasal), adults and children: 1 (2 USP units) or more sprays 3–4 times daily. Two or three sprays in each nostril is maximum that can be absorbed at any one time. (Each spray contains approximately 7 μg lypressin.)

NURSING CONSIDERATIONS

Administration/Storage

1. Encourage the client to clear nasal passages before use.
2. Hold the bottle upright and insert the nozzle into the client's nostril with the head in a vertical position.
3. Apply gentle pressure to the bottle while spraying medication into the nostril.

Interventions

1. Check the client's skin turgor and the condition of the mucous membranes for evidence of dehydration.
2. Observe the client for early signs of water intoxication, such as drowsiness, headaches, and vomiting and document.

Client/Family Teaching

1. Explain and demonstrate the appropriate technique for drug administration.
2. Discuss with the client the need to take the medication only as directed and not to increase the number of sprays. If a change is indicated, the frequency of administration is usually increased, rather than increasing the number of sprays administered at one time.
3. Report feelings of drowsiness, listlessness, headaches, shortness of breath, heartburn, nausea, abdominal cramps, or severe nasal congestion to the physician. These are symptoms of water intoxication and demand immediate attention.
4. Provide the client with printed instructions including recommended fluid intake levels. Explain how to measure intake and output, and instruct client to keep a written record for review at each follow-up visit.
5. Instruct client that if increased thirst occurs or frequency of urination increases, 1 or 2 sprays may be administered to control the symptoms. This occurrence should be noted and reported to the physician.

VASOPRESSIN   (vay-so-PRESS-in)

Pitressin Synthetic (Rx)

VASOPRESSIN TANNATE INJECTION   (vay-so-PRESS-in TAN-nayt)

Pitressin Tannate in Oil (Rx)

Classification: Pituitary (antidiuretic) hormone.

Action/Kinetics: The antidiuretic hormone ADH, more often referred to as vasopressin, is released from the anterior pituitary gland. The hormone regulates water conservation by promoting reabsorption of water by increasing the permeability of the collecting ducts in the kidney.

Insufficient output of ADH results in neurogenic or central diabetes insipidus, characterized by the excretion of large quantities of normal but dilute urine and excessive thirst. These symptoms result from primary (no organic lesion) or secondary (injury) malfunction of posterior pituitary. Vasopressin is effective in the treatment of the condition. It is ineffective when the diabetes insipidus is of renal origin (nephrogenic diabetes insipidus).

In addition to its diuretic properties, vasopressin also causes vasoconstriction (pressor effect) of the splanchnic and portal vessels (and to a lesser extent of peripheral, cerebral, pulmonary, and coronary vessels). Vasopressin also increases the smooth muscular activity of the bladder, GI tract, and uterus. *Vasopressin*. **IM, SC: Onset,** variable; **duration,** 2–8 hr. **t½:** 10–20 min. **Effective plasma levels:** 4.5–6 microunits. *Vasopressin tannate*. **Duration:** 24–96 hr. Hormone metabolized by the liver and kidney.

Use: Vasopressin: Neurogenic diabetes insipidus, relief of postoperative intestinal gaseous distention, to dispel gas shadows in abdominal roentgenography. *Investigational:* Bleeding esophageal varices. **Vasopressin tannate:** Neurogenic diabetes insipidus. *Investigational:* Diagnosis of diabetes insipidus, diagnosis of renal function.

Contraindications: Vascular disease, especially when involving coronary arteries; angina pectoris. Chronic nephritis until reasonable blood nitrogen levels are attained. Never give the tannate IV.

Special Concerns: Pregnancy category: C. Pediatric and geriatric patients have an increased risk of hyponatremia and water intoxication. Use caution in the presence of asthma, epilepsy, migraine, and congestive heart failure.

Side Effects: *GI:* Nausea, vomiting, increased intestinal activity (e.g., belching, cramps, urge to defecate), flatus. *Miscellaneous:* Facial pallor, tremor, sweating, allergic reactions, vertigo, bronchoconstriction, anaphylaxis, "pounding" in head, water intoxication (drowsiness, headache, coma, convulsions).

IV use of vasopressin may result in severe vasoconstriction; local tissue necrosis if extravasation occurs. IM use of tannate may cause pain and sterile abscesses at site of injection.

Drug Interactions: Carbamazepine, chlorpropamide, or clofibrate may ↑ antidiuretic effects of vasopressin.

Dosage: Vasopressin, IM, SC. *Diabetes insipidus.* **Adults,** 5–10 units b.i.d.–t.i.d.; **pediatric:** 2.5–10 units t.i.d.–q.i.d. *Abdominal distention.* **Adults, initial, IM,** 5 units; **then,** 10 units q 3–4 hr; **pediatric:** dose should be individualized (usual: 2.5–5 units). *Abdominal roentgenography.* **IM, SC:** 2 injections of 10 units each 2 hr and ½ hr before films exposed.

Vasopressin tannate, IM only. *Diabetes insipidus.* **Adults,** 1.5–5 units q 1–3 days; **pediatric:** 1.25–2.5 units q 1–3 days. *Diagnosis of diabetes insipidus.* **Adults,** 5 units during the evening followed by collection of urine samples for comparison of osmolality. *Diagnosis of renal function.* **Adults,** 5–10 units 2 hr before collecting urine samples for determination of specific gravity.

NURSING CONSIDERATIONS

Administration/Storage

1. Administration of 1–2 glasses of water prior to use for diabetes insipidus will reduce side effects such as nausea, cramps, and blanching of the skin.
2. Warm the vial of vasopressin tannate in oil in the hands and mix until the hormone is distributed throughout the solution before withdrawing the dose.

Assessment

1. Note any client history of vascular disease, especially any involving the coronary arteries.
2. Determine if the client has any history of asthma or migraine headaches and document.

Interventions

1. Monitor intake and output to evaluate the client's response to therapy.
2. Check skin turgor, the condition of mucous membranes, and assess for the presence of thirst to determine if dehydration is present.
3. When the drug is used to improve bladder activity, check for increased continence and decreased urinary frequency.
4. If the drug is used to improve peristalsis in the GI tract, check the client for bowel sounds, the passage of flatus, and the resumption of bowel movements.
5. Take the BP at least 2 times/day while the client is on a regimen of vasopressin, and report to the physician any adverse reactions, such as an excessive elevation of BP or lack of response to the drug as characterized by a lowering of BP.
6. Weigh the client daily and record.

GROWTH HORMONE

SOMATREM   (SO-mah-trem)
Protropin (Rx)

SOMATROPIN   (SO-mah-TROH-pin)
Humatrope (Rx)

Classification: Growth hormone.

Action/Kinetics: Both somatrem and somatropin are derived from recombinant DNA technology. Somatrem contains the same sequence of amino acids (191) as human growth hormone derived from the pituitary gland plus one additional amino acid (methionine). Somatropin, on the other hand, has the identical sequence of amino acids as does human growth hormone of pituitary origin. These agents stimulate linear growth by increasing somatomedin-C serum levels, which, in turn, increases the incorporation of sulfate into proteoglycans thereby stimulating skeletal growth. These hormones also increase the number and size of muscle cells, increase synthesis of collagen, increase protein synthesis, and increase internal organ size. Serum insulin levels increase (indicative of insulin resistance), and there is acute mobilization of lipid.

Uses: Stimulate linear growth of children who suffer from lack of adequate levels of endogenous growth hormone.

Contraindications: In patients in whom epiphyses have closed. Active intracranial lesions, sensitivity to benzyl alcohol (somatrem); sensitivity to m-cresol or glycerin (somatropin). **Note:** Hypothyroidism (which may be induced by the drug) decreases the response to somatrem.

Special Concerns: Concomitant use of glucocorticoids may decrease the response to growth hormone.

Side Effects: Development of persistent antibodies to growth hormone (30%–40% of patients taking somatrem and 2% of patients taking somatropin). Development of insulin resistance. Adults have experienced headache, weakness, glucosuria, muscle pain, edema. Leukemia has developed in a small number of children.

Drug Interactions: Glucocorticoids inhibit the effect of somatrem on growth.

Dosage: Somatrem. IM. Individualized. Usual: Up to 0.1 mg/kg (0.2 IU/kg) 3 times weekly. The incidence of side effects increases if the dose is greater than 0.1 mg/kg.

    Somatropin. IM, SC. Individualized. Usual: Up to 0.06 mg/kg (0.16 IU/kg) 3 times weekly. Side effects increase if the dose exceeds 0.06 mg/kg.

NURSING CONSIDERATIONS

Administration/Storage

1. Somatrem should be administered only by a physician experienced in the diagnosis and treatment of pituitary disorders.
2. Due to the development of insulin resistance, clients should be evaluated for possible glucose intolerance.
3. The powder for injection for somatrem should be reconstituted *only* with bacteriostatic water for injection (benzyl alcohol preserved).
4. If somatrem is to be used in newborns, it should be reconstituted with water for injection since benzyl alcohol can be toxic to newborns.
5. Somatropin should be reconstituted only with the diluent provided; if sensitivity occurs, sterile water for injection can be used.
6. If somatropin is reconstituted with sterile water for injection, the following guidelines must be followed.
   - Use only one dose per reconstituted vial.
   - The solutions should be refrigerated if not used immediately after reconstitution.
   - The reconstituted dose should be used within 24 hr.
   - After the dose is administered, any unused portion should be discarded.
7. When reconstituting somatrem or somatropin, the vial should not be shaken. Rather, it should be swirled with a gentle rotary motion.
8. Only reconstituted somatrem solution that is clear and without particulate matter should be injected.
9. The needle used for injection should be at least 1 inch or greater in length to ensure that the injection reaches the muscle layer.
10. Reconstituted somatrem should be used within 7 days and should not be frozen.

Assessment

Note if the client is receiving glucocorticoids. These inhibit the effect of somatrem on growth.

Interventions

1. Measure the client's height monthly and record.
2. Monitor thyroid function studies routinely for evidence of hypothyroidism.
3. Routinely assess clients with diabetes for evidence of hyperglycemia and acidosis.

PART ELEVEN

Agents Affecting Water and Electrolytes

11

CHAPTER SIXTY-SEVEN

Diuretics

67

Carbonic Anhydrase Inhibitor Diuretics

Loop Diuretics

Osmotic Diuretics

Potassium-Sparing Diuretics

Thiazides and Related Diuretics

DIURETICS

General Statement: The kidney is a complex organ with three main functions:

1. Elimination of waste materials and return of useful metabolites to the blood.
2. Maintenance of the acid-base balance.
3. Maintenance of an adequate electrolyte balance, which in turn governs the amount of fluid retained in the body.

Malfunction of one or more of these regulatory processes may result in the retention of excessive fluid by various tissues (edema). The latter can be an important manifestation of many conditions, for example, congestive heart failure, pregnancy, and premenstrual tension.

Action: Diuretic drugs increase the urinary output of water and sodium (prevention or correction of edema), mostly through one of the following mechanisms:

1. Increasing the glomerular filtration rate.
2. Decreasing the rate at which sodium is reabsorbed from the glomerular filtrate by the renal tubules; therefore water is excreted along with sodium.
3. Promoting the excretion of sodium, and therefore water, by the kidney.

Some of the commonly used diuretics, especially the thiazides, also have an antihypertensive effect. Diuretic drugs can enhance the normal function of the kidney but cannot stimulate a failing kidney into functioning. According to their mode of action and chemical structure, the diuretics fall into the following classes: thiazides (benzothiadiazides), carbonic anhydrase inhibitors (used mainly for glaucoma), osmotic diuretics, loop diuretics, and potassium-sparing drugs.

Uses: Edema, congestive heart failure, hypertension, pregnancy, and premenstrual tension. See also individual agents.

NURSING CONSIDERATIONS

Administration

1. If a diuretic is to be taken daily, administer it in the morning so that the major diuretic effect will occur before bedtime.
2. Liquid potassium preparations are bitter. Therefore, when they are to be used, administer with fruit juice or milk to make them more palatable.

Assessment

1. Obtain baseline serum electrolyte levels as well as client weight, intake and output and record.
2. Determine the extent of the client's edema.
3. Review drugs the client has been taking to identify those with which diuretics interact.
4. Conduct baseline studies of renal and hepatic function.

Interventions

1. Weigh the client each morning after the client has voided and before the client has eaten or taken fluids. Record the weight and report any sudden increase in weight to the physician.
2. Monitor the client's intake and output. Report any absence of or decrease in diuresis.

3. Check ambulatory clients for edema in the extremities. Check clients on bed rest for edema in the sacral area. Measure daily, document the extent of edema or ascites and report to the physician.

4. Monitor for serum electrolyte levels and the following *signs of electrolyte imbalance:*
   - *Hyponatremia* (low-salt syndrome)—characterized by muscle weakness, leg cramps, dryness of mouth, dizziness, and GI disturbances.
   - *Hypernatremia* (excessive sodium retention in relation to body water)—characterized by CNS disturbances such as confusion, loss of sensorium, stupor, and coma. Poor skin turgor or postural hypotension are not as prominent as when there are combined deficits of sodium and water.
   - *Water intoxication* (caused by defective water diuresis)—characterized by lethargy, confusion, stupor, and coma. Neuromuscular hyperexcitability with increased reflexes, muscular twitching, and convulsions if water intoxication is acute.
   - *Metabolic acidosis*—characterized by weakness, headache, malaise, abdominal pain, nausea, and vomiting. Hyperpnea occurs in severe metabolic acidosis. Signs of volume depletion, such as poor skin turgor, soft eyeballs, and a dry tongue may also be observed.
   - *Metabolic alkalosis*—characterized by irritability, neuromuscular hyperexcitability, and, in severe cases, tetany.
   - *Hypokalemia* (deficiency of potassium in the blood)—characterized by muscular weakness, failure of peristalsis, postural hypotension, respiratory embarrassment, and cardiac arrhythmias.
   - *Hyperkalemia* (excess of potassium in the blood)—characterized by early signs of irritability, nausea, intestinal colic and diarrhea; and by later signs of weakness, flaccid paralysis, dyspnea, difficulty in speaking, and arrhythmias.

5. All signs of electrolyte imbalance should be reported to the physician, and documented in the chart. Electrolyte levels should be monitored and the physical safety of the client should be safeguarded.

6. If the client is receiving enteric-coated potassium tablets, monitor for the presence of abdominal pain, distention, or GI bleeding. These tablets can cause small bowel ulceration. If these symptoms occur, discontinue the tablets. Also, monitor the client's stool to ensure that the tablets have not passed through intact.

7. If the client is also receiving antihypertensive drugs, monitor for excessively low blood pressure. Diuretics potentiate the effects of antihypertensive agents.

8. Diuretics may precipitate symptoms of diabetes mellitus in clients with latent or mild diabetes. Therefore, test the urine or perform finger sticks routinely in diabetic clients and observe for signs of hyperglycemia.

9. If the client is taking digitalis, check the apical pulse. Hyper-or hypokalemia associated with diuretic therapy may potentiate the toxic effects of digitalis and precipitate cardiac arrhythmias.

10. Assess the client for complaints of sore throat, the presence of a skin rash and yellowing of the skin or sclera. These may be signs of blood dyscrasias due to drug hypersensitivity.

11. If the client has a history of liver disease, be alert for electrolyte imbalances that could cause stupor, coma, and death.

12. If the client has a history of gout, note any increase in the frequency of acute attacks that may be precipitated by diuretics. Document and report to the physician.

Client/Family Teaching

1. Advise the client that the drug may cause frequent, copious voiding. Assist the client in planning activities to accommodate this occurrence. Assure the client that there is no need to be alarmed by the diuresis.

2. Advise clients who need additional potassium intake to include foods in the diet that are high in potassium. Eating such foods is preferable to taking potassium chloride supplements. Provide the client with a list of foods high in potassium such as citrus, grape, cranberry, apple, pear, and apricot juices; bananas; meat, fish, or fowl; cereals; and tea and cola beverages. Refer the client to a dietician for assistance in shopping and planning appropriate menus.

3. Unless the client has a preexisting condition such as gastric ulcer or diabetes, clients who are taking diuretics and who require potassium supplements should be encouraged to drink a large glass of orange juice daily.

4. Advise the client to use caution in driving a car or operating other hazardous machinery until drug effects become apparent. Weakness and/or dizziness may occur with diuresis.

5. Caution the client to rise slowly from bed and to sit down or lie down if feeling faint or dizzy.

6. Instruct the client in taking blood pressure and pulse, recording the measurements and how to determine if adverse effects have occurred that need to be reported to the physician. These measurements may assist the physician to determine if symptoms are drug related and if the dosage of drug is appropriate.

7. Advise the client to maintain a written record of weight. Explain that there may be some weight loss from the diuresis related to the drug therapy.

CARBONIC ANHYDRASE INHIBITOR DIURETICS

General Statement: The carbonic anhydrase inhibitor diuretics are related chemically to sulfonamides, but they are devoid of anti-infective activity. They may, however, cause the same hypersensitivity reactions as other sulfonamides. Although widely used as diuretics in the past, today they are particularly useful in the treatment of glaucoma, certain types of seizures, and altitude sickness.

Patients may respond to one carbonic anhydrase inhibitor and not to another. Failures in therapy may result from overdosage or from too frequent use.

Action/Kinetics: The mechanism for the antiglaucoma effect is due to a decrease in aqueous humor production as a result of a decrease in bicarbonate ion levels in ocular fluid. They do not affect outflow of aqueous humor. As an anticonvulsant, these drugs are thought to act by inhibition of carbonic anhydrase in the CNS which increases carbon dioxide tension and a decrease in neuronal conduction. Manifestation of systemic metabolic acidosis (as a result of decreased plasma bicarbonate levels and increased plasma chloride levels) may also play a role in the anticonvulsant action. The effectiveness of carbonic anhydrase inhibitors in altitude sickness is thought to be due to metabolic acidosis resulting in an increase in respiratory drive and arterial oxygen tension as well as diuresis. The diuretic effect results from decreased formation of hydrogen and bicarbonate ions from carbon dioxide and water; this reduces the availability of these ions for active transport. The decrease in hydrogen ion concentration produces an alkaline diuresis which increases the solubility of weakly acidic drugs in the urine, thus promoting their excretion. An alkaline urine also increases the solubility of uric acid and cystine which decreases the formation of either uric acid- or cystine-containing renal stones.

Uses: Glaucoma (open-angle, angle-closure, secondary, malignant). Epilepsy (tonic-clonic seizure patterns, absence seizures, mixed seizures, simple partial seizures, myoclonic seizures). Prophylaxis and treatment of altitude sickness. *Investigational:* Treat toxicity of weakly acidic drugs, prophylaxis and treatment of uric acid or cystine renal calculi, treatment of familial periodic paralysis.

Contraindications: Idiopathic renal hyperchloremic acidosis, renal failure, hepatic insufficiency, and conditions associated with depressed sodium and potassium levels, such as Addison's disease and all other types of adrenal failure. In the presence of mild acidosis, hepatic cirrhosis, advanced pulmonary disease. Severe or absolute glaucoma; chronic, noncongestive angle-closure glaucoma.

Special Concerns: Use during pregnancy only if benefits clearly outweigh risks. Use with caution during severe respiratory acidosis, pulmonary obstruction, emphysema.

Side Effects: *Electrolyte imbalance:* Metabolic acidosis characterized by nausea; dizziness; numbness of fingers, toes, and lips; fatigue; drowsiness; headache; dry mouth; irritability; diarrhea; tinnitus; disorientation; dysuria; ataxia; and weight loss. Hypokalemia. *GI:* Nausea, vomiting, constipation, anorexia, melena. *CNS:* Drowsiness, depression, dizziness, tremor, confusion, ataxia, malaise, fatigue, nervousness, globus hystericus, seizures, weakness, headache, vertigo, disorientation. *Musculoskeletal:* Flaccid paralysis, paresthesias of the extremities, tongue, and mucocutaneous junction of the anus, lips, and mouth. *Dermatologic:* Pruritus, urticaria, erythema multiforme, Stevens-Johnson syndrome, photosensitivity. *Renal:* Crystalluria, polyuria, hematuria, glycosuria, urinary frequency, renal colic, renal calculi. *Hematologic:* Thrombocytopenia, hemolytic anemia, bone marrow depression, leukopenia, pancytopenia, agranulocytosis. *Miscellaneous:* Tinnitus, hepatic insufficiency, transient myopia, weight loss, fever.

Untoward reactions may be dose related and are often relieved by decrease in dosage. Alternate day therapy or rest periods allow kidney to recover.

Drug Interactions	
Amphetamine	↑ Effect of amphetamine by ↑ renal tubular reabsorption
Digitalis	↑ Risk of hypokalemia which sensitizes the heart to digitalis
Ephedrine	↑ Effect of ephedrine by ↑ renal tubular reabsorption
Flecainide	↑ Effect of flecainide by ↑ renal tubular reabsorption
Lithium carbonate	↓ Effect of lithium by ↑ renal excretion
Methotrexate	↓ Effect of methotrexate due to ↑ renal excretion
Primidone	↓ Effect of primidone due to ↓ GI absorption
Pseudoephedrine	↑ Effect of pseudoephedrine by ↑ renal tubular reabsorption
Quinidine	↑ Effect of quinidine by ↑ renal tubular reabsorption
Salicylates	Severe metabolic acidosis; also, salicylates may ↑ effect of carbonic anhydrase inhibitors by ↓ plasma protein binding and ↓ renal excretion

Dosage: See individual agents below.

NURSING CONSIDERATIONS

See also *Nursing Considerations* for *Diuretics,* p. 1250.

Administration/Storage

1. Because of the self-inhibitory metabolic acidosis produced by the carbonic anhydrase drugs,

they are usually administered for 3 consecutive days each week or every other day. Since kidney recovery does not play a role, intermittent administration is not necessary when drugs are used for glaucoma or epilepsy.

2. Due to possible differences in bioavailability, brands should not be interchanged.

3. Five with food if GI upset occurs.

Assessment

1. Determine if the client has a history of allergic responses to sulfonamide antibacterial drugs, thiazide diuretics or other sulfonamide-derivative diuretics. Cross-sensitivity to carbonic anhydrase inhibitors can occur.

2. Obtain renal and hepatic function studies to serve as baseline data against which to compare client response while undergoing therapy.

3. Obtain serum electrolytes, vital signs, an ECG and blood urea nitrogen prior to initiating therapy.

4. Note any drugs the client has been taking for evidence of possible drug interactions.

Interventions

1. Monitor the client's blood pressure regularly, noting any changes from the baseline data obtained prior to initiating therapy.

2. Observe for signs of depression, sedation or complaints of fatigue and weakness. Clients may attribute these symptoms to aging or physical condition as opposed to the side effects of the drug. Document and report to the physician.

3. Report the development of any client fever to the physician.

4. Monitor the client's platelet and complete blood cell count on a regular basis.

5. Encourage the client to drink from 2500–3000 mL of fluid daily unless contraindicated, to avoid constipation.

6. Weigh the client daily and observe for signs of dehydration. Client complaints of constant thirst, nausea, lightheadedness and weakness should be followed up. Check for a decrease in blood pressure, an increase in pulse and a decrease in skin turgor and report these findings to the physician.

7. Monitor the client for an alteration in electrolytes. Muscle weakness, apathy, abdominal distension and paralytic ileus, or ECG changes such as flattened or inverted T waves, prolonged QT intervals and a prominent U wave should be noted and reported to the physician immediately.

8. If the client is being treated for glaucoma, note and report any complaints of eye pain. The drug may not be effective and the intraocular pressure may be unrelieved or increasing.

9. Anticipate that carbonic anhydrase inhibitors should be administered at least once daily in the treatment of glaucoma or epilepsy; whereas, the drug is administered intermittently for the treatment of edema.

Client/Family Teaching

1. In order to maintain effectiveness of the drug and to prevent the development of metabolic acidosis, caution the client to specifically follow the dosage schedule prescribed by the physician.

2. Advise the client to report any unexpected bleeding or bruising. This could be the result of thrombosis.

3. Explain the importance of reporting rashes, fever or sore throat which could be signs of agranulocytosis.

4. If potassium supplements are ordered, advise the client to take them as ordered. Provide the client with printed material listing the foods that are high in potassium and those that are borderline potassium rich that can provide important increases in potassium intake.

5. If the client is taking carbonic anhydrase inhibitors for glaucoma, stress the importance of reporting for follow-up eye examinations to evaluate the effectiveness of the drug therapy.

ACETAZOLAMIDE   (ah-see-tah-ZOHL-ah-myd)

Acetazolam ✿, AK-Zol, Apo-Acetazolamide ✿, Daranide, Dazamide, Diamox, Diamox Sequels, Neptazane (Rx)

ACETAZOLAMIDE SODIUM   (ah-see-tah-ZOHL-ah-myd)

Diamox (Rx)

See also *Anticonvulsants,* p. 714, and *Carbonic Anhydrous Inhibitors,* p. 1252.

Classification: Anticonvulsant (miscellaneous), diuretic (carbonic anhydrase inhibitor).

Action/Kinetics: Acetazolamide is a sulfonamide derivative possessing carbonic anhydrase inhibitor activity. As an anticonvulsant, beneficial effects may be due to inhibition of carbonic anhydrase in the CNS which increases carbon dioxide tension resulting in a decrease in neuronal conduction. Systemic acidosis may also be involved. As a diuretic, the drug inhibits carbonic anhydrase in the kidney which decreases formation of bicarbonate and hydrogen ions from carbon dioxide thus reducing the availability of these ions for active transport. Use as a diuretic is limited because the drug promotes metabolic acidosis, which inhibits diuretic activity. This may be partially circumvented by giving acetazolamide on alternate days. Acetazolamide also reduces intraocular pressure.

Absorbed from the GI tract and widely distributed throughout the body, including the CNS. Excreted unchanged in the urine. **Tablets: Onset,** 60–90 min; **peak:** 2–4 hr; **duration:** 8–12 hr. **Sustained-release capsules: Onset,** 2 hr; **peak:** 8–12 hr; **duration:** 18–24 hr. **Injection (IV): Onset,** 2 min; **peak:** 15 min; **duration:** 4–5 hr. The drug is eliminated mainly unchanged through the kidneys.

Uses: Adjunct in clonic-tonic, myoclonic seizures, absence seizures (petit mal), mixed seizures, simple partial seizure patterns. Open-angle, secondary, angle-closure, or malignant glaucoma. Prophylaxis or treatment of acute mountain sickness. *Investigational:* Hypokalemic and hyperkalemic forms of familial periodic paralysis; to induce forced alkaline diuresis to increase excretion of certain weakly acidic drugs; prophylaxis of uric acid or cystine renal calculi.

Contraindications: Low serum levels of sodium and potassium. Renal and hepatic dysfunction. Hyperchloremic acidosis, adrenal insufficiency, hypersensitivity to thiazide diuretics. Not to be used chronically in presence of noncongestive angle-closure glaucoma.

Special Concerns: Use with caution in the presence of mild acidosis, advanced pulmonary disease, and pregnancy.

Side Effects: *Short-term therapy* (minimal adverse reactions): Anorexia, polyuria, drowsiness, confusion, paresthesia. *Long-term therapy:* Acidosis, transient myopia. *Rarely:* Urticaria, glycosuria, hepatic insufficiency, melena, flaccid paralysis, convulsions. Also, side effects similar to those produced by sulfonamides.

Drug Interactions: Also see *Diuretics,* p. 1249.

Drug Interactions	
Amphetamine	↑ Effect of amphetamine by ↑ renal tubular reabsorption
Ephedrine	↑ Effect of ephedrine by ↑ renal tubular reabsorption
Lithium carbonate	↓ Effect of lithium by ↑ renal excretion
Methotrexate	↓ Effect of methotrexate due to ↑ renal excretion
Primidone	↓ Effect of primidone due to ↓ GI absorption
Pseudoephedrine	↑ Effect of pseudoephedrine by ↑ renal tubular reabsorption
Quinidine	↑ Effect of quinidine by ↑ renal tubular reabsorption
Salicylates	↓ Effect of salicylates by ↑ renal excretion

Dosage: Extended-release capsules, Tablets. *Seizures.* **Adults/children:** 4–30 mg/kg/day in divided doses. Optimum daily dosage: 375–1,000 mg (doses higher than 1,000 mg do not increase therapeutic effect). *If used as adjunct to other anticonvulsants:* **initial,** 250 mg once daily; dose can be increased up to 1,000 mg/day if necessary.

Glaucoma, simple open angle: 0.25–1 g daily in divided doses. *Glaucoma, closed angle prior to surgery or secondary:* 0.25 g q 4 hr, 0.25 g b.i.d., or 0.5 g followed by 0.125–0.25 g q 4 hr. **Extended-release capsules:** 500 mg b.i.d. in the morning and evening. **Pediatric:** 8–30 mg/kg (usual: 10–15 mg/kg or 300–900 mg/m^2) daily in divided doses.

Acute mountain sickness. 250 mg b.i.d.–q.i.d. (500 mg 1–2 times daily of extended-release capsules). During rapid ascent, 1 g daily is recommended.

NURSING CONSIDERATIONS

See also *Nursing Considerations* for *Diuretics,* p. 1250, and *Sulfonamides,* p. 205, and *Carbonic Anhydrous Inhibitors,* p. 1253.

Administration/Storage

1. Change from other anticonvulsant therapy to acetazolamide should be gradual.
2. Use parenteral solutions within 24 hr after reconstitution.
3. IV administration is preferred; IM administration is painful due to alkalinity.
4. Reconstitute with at least 5 mL of sterile water for injection.
5. Tolerance after prolonged use may necessitate dosage increase.
6. Do not administer the sustained-release dosage form as an anticonvulsant.
7. When used for prophylaxis of mountain sickness, dosage should be initiated 1–2 days before ascent and should be continued for at least 2 days while at high altitudes.
8. Due to possible differences in bioavailability, brands should not be interchanged.

Assessment

1. Obtain a complete nursing history.
2. Evaluate laboratory findings for levels of electrolytes, uric acid and glucose. Obtain labs for and document any evidence of liver and renal dysfunction prior to administering the medication.
3. Obtain a complete client drug history to assure that the client is not receiving any drug therapy that interacts with the medication.

Client/Family Teaching

1. Taking the drug with food may decrease gastric irritation and GI upset.
2. The drug increases the frequency of voiding. Therefore, take the medication early in the day to avoid interrupting sleep.
3. Clients with diabetes should be warned that the drug may increase blood glucose levels. Therefore, they should monitor serum glucose levels carefully and report increases as the dose of hypoglycemic agent may require adjustment.
4. If nausea, dizziness, muscle weakness, or cramps occur, report these to the physician.
5. Note any changes in the color of stools and report.
6. Stress the importance of reporting for scheduled laboratory studies.

DICHLORPHENAMIDE   (dye-klor-**FEN**-ah-myd)

Daranide (Rx)

See also *Carbonic Anhydrase Inhibitors,* p. 1252.

Classification: Carbonic anhydrase inhibitor.

Action/Kinetics: Onset: Within 60 min. **Peak effect:** 2–4 hr. **Duration:** 6–12 hr.

Uses: Glaucoma, especially open-angle glaucoma, secondary glaucoma, and preoperatively in acute angle-closure glaucoma.

Special Concerns: Dosage has not been established in children.

Dosage: Tablets. Adults, initial: 100–200 mg; **then,** 100 mg q 12 hr until desired response occurs. **Maintenance:** 25–50 mg 1–3 times daily.

NURSING CONSIDERATIONS

See also *Nursing Considerations* for *Carbonic Anhydrase Inhibitor Diuretics,* p. 1253.

Administration/Storage

For acute angle-closure glaucoma, dichlorphenamide is used with miotics and osmotic agents to reduce intraocular pressure quickly.

METHAZOLAMIDE   (meth-ah-**ZOH**-lah-myd)

Neptazane (Rx)

See also *Carbonic Anhydrase Inhibitors,* p. 1252.

Classification: Carbonic anhydrase inhibitor.

Action/Kinetics: Onset: 2–4 hr. **Peak effect:** 6–8 hr. **Duration:** 10–18 hr.

Uses: Glaucoma, especially open-angle glaucoma, secondary glaucoma, and preoperatively in acute angle-closure glaucoma.

Dosage: Tablets. Adults, 25–100 mg b.i.d.–t.i.d.

NURSING CONSIDERATIONS
See *Nursing Considerations* for under *Carbonic Anhydrase Inhibitor Diuretics,* p. 1253.

Administration/Storage
Methazolamide may be used with a miotic and osmotic agent.

LOOP DIURETICS

BUMETANIDE   (byou-MET-ah-nyd)
Bumex (Rx)

See also *Diuretics,* p. 1249.

Classification: Loop diuretic.

Action/Kinetics: Bumetanide inhibits reabsorption of both sodium and chloride in the ascending loop of Henle. It may also have some activity in the proximal tubule especially to promote phosphate excretion. **Onset, PO:** 30–60 min. **Peak effect, PO:** 1–2 hr. **Duration, PO:** 4–6 hr (dose-dependent). **Onset, IV:** Several minutes. **Peak effect, IV:** 15–30 min. **Duration, IV:** 3.5–4 hr. **t½:** 1–1.5 hr. Metabolized in the liver although 45% excreted unchanged in the urine.

Uses: Edema associated with congestive heart failure, nephrotic syndrome, hepatic disease. Adjunct to treat acute pulmonary edema. Especially useful in patients refractory to other diuretics. *Investigational:* In combination with other drugs to treat mild to moderate hypertension. Hypercalcemia.

Contraindications: Anuria, hepatic coma, severe electrolyte depletion, hypersensitivity to the drug.

Special Concerns: Safety during pregnancy (category: C) and lactation and children under 18 has not been established. Geriatric patients may be more sensitive to the hypotensive and electrolyte effects and are at greater risk in developing thromboembolic problems and circulatory collapse.

Side Effects: *Electrolyte and fluid changes:* Excess water loss, dehydration, electrolyte depletion including hypokalemia, hypochloremia, hyponatremia; hypovolemia, thromboembolism, circulatory collapse. *Otic:* Hearing loss, ear discomfort, tinnitus, ototoxicity. *GI:* Nausea, abdominal pain, vomiting, dry mouth, diarrhea, gastric upset, anorexia, jaundice, acute pancreatitis. *CNS:* Dizziness, headache, vertigo, blurred vision, asterixis, encephalopathy (with preexisting liver disease). *Allergic:* Pruritus, urticaria, rashes. *GU:* Premature ejaculation, difficulty in maintaining an erection, renal failure. *Hematologic:* Agranulocytosis, thrombocytopenia. *Miscellaneous:* Rash, pain following parenteral use, hypotension, hyperglycemia, ECG changes, joint and muscle pain, chest pain, sweating, hyperventilation, pruritus, hives, nipple tenderness. Cross-sensitivity may be seen in patients allergic to sulfonamides.

Drug Interactions	
Aminoglycosides	Additive ototoxicity
Antihypertensive drugs	Potentiation of antihypertensive effect

Drug Interactions (continued)

Cisplatin	↑ Chance of ototoxicity
Digitalis glycosides	Bumetanide produces excess K loss with ↑ chance of cardiac arrhythmias
Indomethacin	↓ Effect of bumetanide
Lithium	↑ Risk of lithium toxicity due to ↓ renal excretion
Probenecid	↓ Effect of bumetanide

Laboratory Test Interferences: Alterations in LDH, SGOT, SGPT, alkaline phosphatase, creatinine clearance, total serum bilirubin, serum proteins.

Dosage: Tablets. Adults, 0.5–2 mg once daily; if response is inadequate, a second or third dose may be given at 4- to 5-hr intervals up to a maximum of 10 mg daily. **IV, IM:** 0.5–1 mg; if response is inadequate, a second or third dose may be given at 2- to 3-hr intervals up to a maximum of 10 mg daily. Oral dosing should be started as soon as possible.

NURSING CONSIDERATIONS

See also *Nursing Considerations* for *Diuretics,* p. 1250.

Administration/Storage

1. Solutions for IM or IV use should be freshly prepared and used within 24 hr.
2. Ampules may be reconstituted with 5% dextrose in water, 0.9% sodium chloride, or lactated Ringer's solution.
3. IV solutions should be administered slowly over 1–2 min.
4. IV or IM administration should be reserved for clients in whom oral use is not practical or in whom absorption from the GI tract is impaired.
5. The recommended oral medication schedule is on alternate days or for 3–4 days with a 1- to 2-day rest period in between.
6. Bumetanide, at a 1:40 ratio of bumetanide to furosemide, may be ordered for clients allergic to furosemide.

Interventions

1. Monitor BP and pulse regularly. Rapid diuresis may cause dehydration and circulatory collapse. Hypotension may also occur when drug is administered with antihypertensive drugs.
2. Observe for ototoxicity, especially if the client is receiving other ototoxic drugs.
3. Monitor hepatic and renal function studies as well as serum electrolyte levels.

ETHACRYNATE SODIUM   (eth-ah-**KRIH**-nayt)

Sodium Edecrin (Rx)

ETHACRYNIC ACID   (eth-ah-**KRIH**-nik **AH**-sid)

Edecrin (Rx)

See also *Diuretics,* p. 1249.

Classification: Loop diuretic.

Action/Kinetics: Ethacrynic acid inhibits the reabsorption of sodium and chloride in the loop of Henle; the drug also decreases reabsorption of sodium and chloride and increases potassium excretion in the distal tubule. It also acts directly on the proximal tubule to enhance excretion of electrolytes. Large quantities of sodium and chloride and smaller amounts of potassium and bicarbonate ion are excreted during diuresis. **Onset: PO,** 30 min; **IV,** 5–15 min. **Peak: PO,** 2 hr; **IV,** 15–30 min. **Duration: PO,** 6–8 hr. **IV,** 2 hr. Metabolites are excreted through the urine. Diuresis and electrolyte loss are more pronounced with ethacrynic acid than with thiazide diuretics. Ethacrynic acid is often effective in patients refractory to other diuretics. Careful monitoring of the diuretic effects is necessary.

Uses: Of value in patients resistant to less potent diuretics. Congestive heart failure, pulmonary edema, edema associated with nephrotic syndrome, ascites due to idiopathic edema, lymphedema, malignancy. Short-term use for ascites as a result of malignancy, lymphedema, or idiopathic edema; also, for short-term use in pediatric patients (except infants) with congenital heart disease. *Investigational.* **Ethacrynic acid:** Nephrogenic diabetes insipidus unresponsive to vasopressin. In combination with other drugs to treat mild to moderate hypertension. **Ethacrynate sodium:** Hypercalcemia, bromide intoxication, and with mannitol in ethylene glycol poisoning.

Contraindications: Pregnancy. Not recommended for use in neonates. Anuria and severe renal damage. Patients with history of gout should be watched closely.

Special Concerns: Geriatric patients may be more sensitive to the usual adult dose. To be used with caution in diabetic patients and those with hepatic cirrhosis (who are particularly susceptible to electrolyte imbalance).

Side Effects: Electrolyte imbalance (hypokalemia). The drug may also cause dehydration, reduction in blood volume, vascular complications, tetany, and metabolic alkalosis. *GI* (frequent): Anorexia, nausea, diarrhea, vomiting, acute pancreatitis, jaundice, dysphagia. Severe, watery diarrhea is an indication for permanent discontinuance of drug. GI bleeding, especially in patients on IV therapy or receiving heparin concomitantly. *CNS:* Tinnitus, hearing loss (permanent), vertigo, headache, blurred vision, apprehension, confusion, fatigue, malaise, dizziness. *Hematologic:* Agranulocytosis, thrombocytopenia, neutropenia. *Miscellaneous:* Skin rashes, abnormal liver function tests in seriously ill patients, fever, chills, hematuria. Ethacrynic acid increases uric acid levels and may precipitate attacks of gout. The drug may also produce changes in glucose metabolism (hyperglycemia and glycosuria).

Drug Interactions

Alcohol	↑ Orthostatic hypotension
Aminoglycoside antibiotics	Additive ototoxicity and nephrotoxicity
Anticoagulants, oral	↑ Effect of anticoagulants by ↓ plasma protein binding
Antidiabetic agents	Ethacrynic acid antagonizes hypoglycemic effect of antidiabetics
Antihypertensive agents	↑ Antihypertensive effect
Barbiturates	↑ Orthostatic hypotension
Cephaloridine	↑ Risk of ototoxicity and nephrotoxicity
Cisplatin	↑ Risk of ototoxicity
Corticosteroids	Enhanced K loss due to K-losing properties of both drugs
Digitalis glycosides	Ethacrynic acid produces excess K and Mg loss with ↑ chance of cardiac arrhythmias

Drug Interactions

Furosemide	Combination may result in hypokalemia, tachycardia, deafness, hypotension—**do not use together**
Indomethacin	↓ Effect of ethacrynic acid
Lithium	↑ Risk of lithium toxicity due to ↓ renal clearance
Narcotics	↑ Orthostatic hypotension
Skeletal muscle relaxants, nondepolarizing	↑ Muscle relaxation
Warfarin	↑ Effect of warfarin due to ↓ plasma protein binding

Dosage: Ethacrynic acid: Oral Solution, Tablets. Adults, initial: 50–100 mg daily in single or divided doses; can increase by 25–50 mg daily if needed. **Maintenance:** Usually 50–200 mg (up to a maximum of 400 mg) daily once dry weight is reached. **Pediatric, initial:** 25 mg daily; can increase by 25 mg daily if needed. **Maintenance:** Adjust dose to needs of patient.

Ethacrynate sodium: IV. Adults: 50 mg (base) (or 0.5–1 mg/kg); may be repeated in 2–4 hr if needed; **then,** administer q 4–6 hr if patient is responding, to a maximum of 100 mg daily. **Pediatric:** 1 mg/kg.

NURSING CONSIDERATIONS

See also *Nursing Considerations* for *Diuretics,* p. 1250.

Administration/Storage

1. Due to local pain and irritation, the drug should not be given SC or IM.
2. IV administration should be at a slow rate over a 30-min period given either directly or through IV tubing.
3. If a second IV injection is necessary, a different site should be used to prevent thrombophlebitis.
4. When used orally, administer after meals.
5. Reconstitute the powder for injection by adding 50 mL of 5% dextrose injection or sodium chloride injection.
6. When reconstituted with 5% dextrose injection, the resulting solution may be hazy or opalescent. Such solutions should not be used. Also, this solution should not be mixed with whole blood or its derivatives.
7. Use reconstituted solutions within 24 hr.
8. Ammonium chloride or arginine chloride may be prescribed for clients who are at a higher risk of developing metabolic acidosis.

Assessment

1. Note if the client has diabetes mellitus or hepatic cirrhosis.
2. Check the client's urinary output to determine that anuria has not occurred.
3. List the drugs the client is taking to identify any with which the drug interacts unfavorably.

Interventions

1. Observe the client for excessive diuresis or a weight loss of up to 2 lb daily, because electrolyte imbalance may develop quickly.
2. Assess clients with rapid excessive diuresis for pain in their calves, in the pelvic area, or in the chest. Rapid hemoconcentration may cause thromboembolic effects.

3. Observe clients for GI effects that may necessitate discontinuing the drug. The drug should be withdrawn if the client manifests severe, watery diarrhea.
4. Monitor for occult blood in the urine and the stools.
5. Observe the client for vestibular disturbances. Do not administer the drug IV concomitantly with any other ototoxic agent.
6. Monitor the serum potassium levels and consult with the physician regarding the need for supplementary potassium.
7. Since ethacrynic acid has such a profound effect on sodium excretion, dietary salt restriction is not necessary; if sodium is restricted, hyponatremia may result.

FUROSEMIDE (fur-**OH**-seh-myd)

Apo-Furosemide ✴, Furoside ✴, Lasix, Lasix Special ✴, Myrosemide, Novosemide ✴, Uritol ✴ (Rx)

See also *Diuretics,* p. 1249.

Classification: Loop diuretic.

Action/Kinetics: Furosemide inhibits the reabsorption of sodium and chloride in the ascending loop of Henle, resulting in the excretion of sodium, chloride, and, to a lesser degree, potassium and bicarbonate ions. The drug also decreases reabsorption of sodium and chloride and increases the excretion of potassium in the distal tubule. The resulting urine is more acid. Diuretic action is independent of changes in patients' acid-base balance. Furosemide has a slight antihypertensive effect. **Onset: PO, IM:** 30–60 min; **IV:** 5 min. **Peak: PO, IM:** 1–2 hr; **IV:** 20–60 min. **Duration: PO, IM:** 6–8 hr; **IV:** 2 hr. Metabolized in the liver and excreted through the urine.

The drug may be effective for patients resistant to thiazides and for those with reduced glomerular filtration rates.

Uses: Edema associated with congestive heart failure, nephrotic syndrome, hepatic cirrhosis, and ascites. Hypertension alone or as an adjunct. IV for acute pulmonary edema. Furosemide can be used in conjunction with spironolactone, triamterene, and other diuretics *except* ethacrynic acid. *Investigational:* Hypercalcemia.

Contraindications: Never use with ethacrynic acid. Anuria, hypersensitivity to drug, severe renal disease associated with azotemia and oliguria, hepatic coma associated with electrolyte depletion. Lactation.

Special Concerns: Use during pregnancy (category: C) only when benefits clearly outweigh risks. Use with caution in premature infants and neonates due to prolonged half-life in these patients (dosing interval must be extended). Geriatric patients may be more sensitive to the usual adult dose.

Side Effects: *Electrolyte and fluid effects:* Fluid and electrolyte depletion leading to dehydration, hypovolemia, thromboembolism. Hypokalemia and hypochloremia may cause metabolic alkalosis. Hyperuricemia, azotemia, hyponatremia. *GI:* Nausea, GI irritation, vomiting, anorexia, diarrhea (especially in children) or constipation, cramps. *Otic:* Tinnitus, hearing impairment (may be reversible or permanent), reversible deafness. Usually following rapid IV or IM administration of high doses. *CNS:* Vertigo, headache, dizziness, lightheadedness, blurred vision, weakness, restlessness, paresthesias, xanthopsia. *CV:* Orthostatic hypotension, thrombophlebitis, chronic aortitis. *Hematologic:* Anemia, thrombocytopenia, neutropenia, leukopenia, agranulocytosis, purpura. Rarely, aplastic anemia. *Allergic:* Rashes, pruritus, urticaria, photosensitivity, exfoliative dermatitis, vasculitis, erythema multiforme. *Miscellaneous:* Hyperglycemia, glycosuria, exacerbation of, aggravation of, or worsening of systemic lupus erythematosus, increased perspiration, muscle spasms, urinary bladder spasm, urinary frequency.

Following IV use: Thrombophlebitis, cardiac arrest. *Following IM use:* Pain at injection site, cardiac arrest.

Because this drug is resistant to the effects of pressor amines and potentiates the effects of muscle relaxants, it is recommended that the oral drug be discontinued 1 week before surgery and the IV drug 2 days before surgery.

Drug Interactions

Adrenergic blocking agents	Potentiation of effects
Alcohol	↑ Orthostatic hypotension
Aminoglycoside antibiotics	Additive ototoxicity and nephrotoxicity
Anticoagulants	↑ Effect of anticoagulant due to ↓ plasma protein binding
Antidiabetic agents	Furosemide antagonizes hypoglycemic effect of antidiabetics
Antihypertensive agents	Potentiation of antihypertensive effect
Barbiturates	↑ Orthostatic hypotension
Cephalosporins	↑ Renal toxicity of cephalosporins
Cisplatin	↑ Risk of ototoxicty
Corticosteroids	Enhanced K loss due to K-depleting properties of both drugs
Digitalis glycosides	Furosemide produces excess K and Mg loss with ↑ chance of cardiac arrhythmias
Ethacrynic acid	Combination may result in hypokalemia, tachycardia, deafness, hypotension—**do not use together**
Ganglionic blocking agents	Potentiation of effects
Indomethacin	↓ Diuretic and antihypertensive effects of furosemide
Lithium	↓ Renal clearance of lithium leading to ↑ risk of toxicity
Metolazone	↑ Diuresis and electrolyte loss
Narcotics	↑ Orthostatic hypotension
Phenytoin	↓ Diuretic effect of furosemide due to ↓ absorption
Salicylates	↑ Risk of salicylate toxicity due to ↓ renal excretion
Succinylcholine	Effect of succinylcholine is ↑ by low doses and ↓ by high doses of furosemide.
Theophylline	Furosemide may ↑ or ↓ the effect of theophyllines
d-Tubocurarine	Effect of tubocurarine is ↑ by low doses and ↓ by high doses of furosemide

Dosage: Oral Solution, Tablets. *Diuretic.* **Adults, initial:** 20–80 mg daily as a single dose. For resistant cases, dosage can be increased by 20–40 mg q 6–8 hr until desired diuretic response is attained. Maximum daily dose should not exceed 600 mg. **Pediatric, initial:** 2 mg/kg as a single dose; **then,** dose can be increased by 1–2 mg/kg q 6–8 hr until desired response is attained (up to 5 mg/kg may be required in children with nephrotic syndrome; maximum dose should not exceed 6 mg/kg). *Hypertension:* **Adults, initial:** 40 mg b.i.d. Adjust dosage depending on response. *Antihypercalcemic:* **Adults:** 120 mg daily in 1–3 doses.

IV, IM. *Diuretic:* **Adults, initial:** 20–40 mg; if response inadequate after 2 hr, increase dose in 20-mg increments. **Pediatric, initial:** 1 mg/kg given slowly; if response inadequate after 2 hr, increase dose by 1 mg/kg. Doses greater than 6 mg/kg should not be given. **IV.** *Acute pulmonary edema:* **Adults:** 40 mg slowly over 1–2 min; if response inadequate after 1 hr, give 80 mg slowly over 1–2 min. Concomitant oxygen and digitalis may be used. *Hypertensive crisis, normal renal function:* **Adults, IV:** 40–80 mg. *Hypertensive crisis with pulmonary edema or acute renal failure:* **Adults, IV:** 100–200 mg. *Antihypercalcemic:* **Adults, IM, IV:** 80–100 mg for severe cases; dose may be repeated q 1–2 hr if needed.

NURSING CONSIDERATIONS

See also *Nursing Considerations* for *Diuretics,* p. 1250.

Administration/Storage

1. The drug should be given 2–4 days/week.
2. If used IV, furosemide should not be mixed with solutions with a pH below 5.5.
3. When high doses of the medication are required parenterally, administer by infusion at a rate not to exceed 4 mg/min.
4. Food decreases the bioavailability of furosemide and ultimately the degree of diuresis.
5. Discoloration resulting from light does not affect potency.
6. Store in light-resistant containers.

Interventions

1. Monitor serum electrolytes and observe client for signs and symptoms of hypokalemia.
2. In clients with rapid diuresis, observe for dehydration and circulatory collapse. Monitor BP and pulse and document.
3. When the client has renal impairment or is receiving other ototoxic drugs, observe for ototoxicity.
4. Observe for signs of vascular thrombosis and embolism, particularly in the elderly.

Client/Family Teaching

1. Assure the client that any pain after IM injection will be transitory.
2. Advise the client to take medication in the morning to avoid interruption of sleep.
3. Assist clients to establish the timing of the diuretic so that they can participate in social activities.
4. Advise client to consult with the physician before taking aspirin for any reason. Salicylate intoxication occurs at lower levels than normal because of competition at the renal excretory sites.
5. Instruct clients to use sunscreens and protective clothing when exposed to the sun to minimize the effects of drug-induced photosensitivity.
6. Discuss the need for a diet high in potassium. Instruct clients to supplement their diet with vegetables and fruits high in potassium.

OSMOTIC DIURETICS

Action/Kinetics: Osmotic diuretics increase the osmotic pressure of the glomerular filtrate inside the renal tubules. This decreases the amount of fluid and electrolytes that are reabsorbed by the tubules, thereby increasing the loss of fluid, chloride, sodium, and, to a lesser extent, potassium. The osmotic diuretics maintain their effectiveness even when renal circulation is acutely compromised, such as in hypovolemic shock, trauma, and dehydration.

NURSING CONSIDERATIONS

See also *Nursing Considerations* for *Diuretics,* p. 1250.

Interventions

1. Maintain the client on strict intake and output.
2. If the client is comatose, incontinent, or unable to void, anticipate an order to insert a Foley catheter. Drug therapy is based on strict evaluation of intake and output.
3. Observe for signs and symptoms of water intoxication and for electrolyte imbalance.
4. Assess the IV site for edema due to extravasation into SC tissue and for thrombophlebitis due to local irritation from the drug. Sloughing may occur.
5. Monitor vital signs at least hourly while client is being treated for an acute episode.
6. Observe the client for dyspnea, distended neck veins, or labored respirations. Auscultate for rales, and note any increase in agitation. These are signs of pulmonary congestion and/or congestive heart failure. They should be documented and reported to the physician immediately.
7. Weigh the client daily and record. If the client's urinary output is less than 30–50 mL/hour or if the weight gain is more than 3 lb/day, notify the physician.

GLYCERIN   (GLISS-er-in)

Glyrol, Osmoglyn (Rx)

Classification: Osmotic diuretic.

Action/Kinetics: Glycerin increases the osmolarity of the blood plasma which causes a flow of water from extravascular spaces into the plasma. In glaucoma, removal of fluid from the eye by osmosis causes a reduction in intraocular pressure. Also, withdrawal of fluid from the brain and CSF results in reduced intracranial pressure and CSF volume and pressure. **Onset:** 10–30 min. **Peak effect:** 60–90 min. **Duration:** 4–5 hr. $t^{1/2}$: 30–45 min. Excreted through the kidney (7–14% unchanged).

Uses: Acute attack of glaucoma, prior to ocular surgery to decrease intraocular pressure. *Investigational:* To lower intracranial pressure due to various causes.

Contraindications: Hypersensitivity, severe dehydration, anuria, acute pulmonary edema, severe cardiac decompensation.

Special Concerns: Pregnancy category: C. Use with caution during lactation, in confused mental states, congestive heart failure, diabetes, senility, geriatric patients, and in hypervolemia.

Side Effects: *CNS:* Confusion, disorientation, headache. *GI:* Nausea, vomiting. *Electrolyte:* Hyperosmolar nonketotic coma, severe dehydration. *CV:* Arrhythmias.

Dosage: Oral Solution. Adults, 1–1.5 g/kg; additional doses of 0.5 g/kg may be given at 6 hr intervals. **Pediatric:** 1–1.5 g/kg (40 g/m²); the dose may be repeated in 4–8 hr if needed.

NURSING CONSIDERATIONS

See also *Nursing Considerations* for *Diuretics,* p. 1250.

Interventions

1. Have the client lie down during oral administration to prevent or to relieve headache associated with cerebral dehydration.
2. Observe closely for dehydration, especially in elderly, senile, or severely ill clients.

MANNITOL   [MAN-nih-tol]

Osmitrol (Rx)

Classification: Diuretic, osmotic.

Action/Kinetics: Mannitol increases the osmolarity of the glomerular filtrate which decreases the reabsorption of water while increasing excretion of sodium and chloride. It also increases the osmolarity of the plasma which causes enhanced flow of water from tissues into the interstitial fluid and plasma. Thus, cerebral edema, increased intracranial pressure, and CSF volume and pressure are decreased. **Onset, IV:** 1–3 hr for diuresis and within 15 min for reduction of cerebrospinal and intraocular pressure. **Peak:** 30–60 min for reduction of intraocular pressure. **Duration:** 4–8 hr for reduction of intraocular pressure. **t½:** 100 min. Over 90% excreted through the urine unchanged. A test dose is given in patients with impaired renal function or oliguria.

Uses: Acute renal failure, cerebral edema, reduction of intracranial pressure, glaucoma (when other measures have failed). To enhance urinary excretion of toxic substances. As a urinary irrigant to prevent hemolysis and hemoglobin buildup during transurethral prostatic resection. *Investigational:* Prevent hemolysis during cardiopulmonary bypass surgery.

Contraindications: Anuria, pulmonary edema, dehydration, intracranial bleeding, progressive heart failure or pulmonary congestion after mannitol therapy, progressive renal damage following mannitol therapy.

Special Concerns: Pregnancy category: B or C. Use with caution during lactation.

Side Effects: *Electrolyte:* Hypernatremia, acidosis, loss of electrolytes, dehydration. *GI:* Nausea, vomiting, dry mouth, thirst, diarrhea. *CV:* Edema, hypotension or hypertension, increase in heart rate, angina-like chest pain, thrombophlebitis. *CNS:* Dizziness, headaches, blurred vision, seizures. *Miscellaneous:* Urinary retention, pulmonary congestion, marked diuresis, rhinitis, chills, fever, urticaria, pain in arms, skin necrosis.

Drug Interaction: May cause deafness when used in combination with kanamycin.

Laboratory Test Interference: ↑ or ↓ Inorganic phosphorus. ↑ Ethylene glycol values because mannitol also is oxidized to an aldehyde during test.

Dosage: IV infusion only. *Test dose (oliguria or reduced renal function):* Either 50 mL of a 25% solution, 75 mL of a 20% solution, or 100 mL of a 15% solution infused over 3–5 min. If urine flow is 30–50 mL/hr, therapeutic dose can be given. If no response, give a second test dose; if still no response, patient must be reevaluated. *Diuretic:* **Adults,** 50–100 g, as a 5–25% solution, given at a rate to maintain urine flow of at least 30–50 mL/hr. **Pediatric:** 2 g/kg (60 g/m²) as a 15–20%

solution given over a period of 2–6 hr. *Glaucoma, elevated intracranial pressure, cerebral edema:* **Adults,** 1.5–2 g/kg as a 15–25% solution given over 30–60 min. In small or debilitated patients, 0.5 mg/kg may be sufficient. **Pediatric:** 1–2 g/kg (30–60 g/m²) as a 15–20% solution given over 30–60 min. *Antidote to remove toxic substances:* **Adults,** 50–200 g as a 5–25% solution given at a rate to maintain urine flow of 100–150 mL/hr. **Pediatric:** Up to 2 g/kg (60 g/m²) as a 5–10% solution. *Antihemolytic:* **Adults,** Use as a 2.5% irrigating solution for the bladder.

NURSING CONSIDERATIONS

See also *Nursing Considerations* for *Diuretics,* p. 1250.

Administration/Storage

1. If concentrated mannitol is used, a filter should be used on the administration set.
2. If the concentration of mannitol is greater than 15%, it may crystallize. To redissolve, warm the bottle in a hot water bath or autoclave. Then cool to body temperature before administering to the client.
3. IV administration can reduce cerebrospinal and intraocular pressure within 15 minutes. Onset of diuresis occurs in about 1–3 hours.
4. Mannitol should not be added to other IV solutions nor should it be mixed with other medications.
5. If blood is to be administered at the same time, add 20 mEq of sodium chloride to each liter of mannitol to prevent pseudoagglutination.

Assessment

Note other medications the client may be taking that can be affected by mannitol. Lithium, for example can be excreted more rapidly than normal, thereby impairing the therapeutic effects of the drug.

Interventions

1. Monitor and record vital signs, intake and output.
2. Observe the client for signs of electrolyte imbalances and dehydration.
3. Monitor serum electrolytes and renal function throughout the drug therapy.
4. Observe for signs and symptoms of pulmonary edema manifested by dyspnea, cyanosis, rales, and frothy sputum. Slow the rate of infusion, and notify the physician immediately.

UREA   (you-REE-ah)

Ureaphil (Rx)

Classification: Diuretic, osmotic.

Action/Kinetics: Due to an increase the plasma osmolarity, water flows from tissues into the interstitial fluid and plasma. Thus, elevated intracranial pressure, cerebral edema, and intraocular pressure are reduced. **Onset:** Within 10 min for reduction of intraocular and intracranial pressure. **Peak effect:** 1–2 hr. **Duration:** 3–10 hr after infusion stopped for diuresis and reduction in cerebrospinal pressure; 5–6 hr for reduction in intraocular pressure.

Uses: To decrease intraocular and intracranial pressure.

Contraindications: Impaired renal function, dehydration, liver failure, intracranial bleeding. Not for use in lower extremities of geriatric patients due to possible phlebitis and thrombosis.

Special Concerns: Pregnancy category: C. Use with caution during lactation and renal impairment. A rebound increase in intraocular and intracranial pressure may be observed within 12 hr after administration of urea.

Side Effects: *CNS:* Disorientation, headaches, syncope, confusion, nervousness. *GI:* Nausea, vomiting, dehydration. *Miscellaneous:* Hypotension, hyperthermia, pain, skin irritation.

Note: Phlebitis, thrombosis, infection, or extravasation at the injection site may be observed.

Drug Interactions	
Anticoagulants	↑ Effect of anticoagulants
Lithium carbonate	↓ Lithium effect by ↑ renal excretion

Dosage: Slow IV infusion. Adults and children over 2 years of age: 0.5–1.5 g/kg as a 30% solution in 5 or 10% dextrose injection or 10% invert sugar injection; give at a rate of about 4–6 mL/min over 30–120 min. Maximum daily dose: 2 g/kg. **Pediatric: up to 2 years of age,** 0.1–1.5 g/kg given the same as the adult dose.

NURSING CONSIDERATIONS

See also *Nursing Considerations* for *Diuretics,* p. 1250.

Administration/Storage

1. The rate of infusion should not exceed 4 mL/min of the 30% solution.
2. Dextrose or invert sugar (osmotic concentrations) are given with urea to prevent hemolysis caused by pure urea.
3. Only freshly prepared solutions should be used; any unused solution should be discarded after 24 hr.
4. Because of its fibrinolytic effect, do not administer urea into the lower extremities of elderly clients. It may cause thrombosis.
5. Do not mix urea with blood or other drugs in the same syringe.

Assessment

1. Review drugs the client is currently taking to identify those with which urea may interact unfavorably.
2. Obtain renal and liver function studies prior to initiating therapy.

Interventions

1. Observe for redness, swelling and pain at the site of infusion. If extravasation occurs there may be skin and tissue damage that may result in necrosis. Restart IV and notify physician.
2. Observe the client for nervousness or confusion. This can occur if the medication is administered too rapidly. Slow down the rate of infusion and notify the physician.
3. Monitor vital signs closely and check the client for any evidence of pulmonary edema. The increase in plasma volume resulting from the injection of urea may precipitate pulmonary edema.
4. Note if the client becomes mentally confused, exhibits personality changes or develops hypotension. Document and report these findings to the physician.
5. Provide close supervision and safety measures such as side rails during drug therapy.

POTASSIUM-SPARING DIURETICS

AMILORIDE HYDROCHLORIDE   (ah-MILL-oh-ryd)
Midamor (Rx)

Classification: Diuretic, potassium-sparing.

Action/Kinetics: Amiloride acts on the distal tubule to inhibit sodium exchange for potassium which results in increased secretion of sodium and water and conservation of potassium. The drug also has weak diuretic and antihypertensive activity. **Onset:** 2 hr. **Peak effect:** 6–10 hr. **Peak plasma levels:** 3–4 hr. **Duration:** 24 hr. **t½:** 6–9 hr. 23% is bound to plasma protein. Approximately 50% is excreted unchanged by kidney and 40% by the feces unchanged.

Uses: Adjunct with thiazides or other kaliuretic diuretics in the treatment of hypertension or edema due to congestive heart failure, hepatic cirrhosis, and nephrotic syndrome to help restore normal serum potassium or prevent hypokalemia. *Investigational:* Prophylaxis and treatment of hypokalemia in patients for whom other treatments are inappropriate.

Contraindications: Hyperkalemia (greater than 5.5 mEq potassium/L). In patients receiving other potassium-sparing diuretics or potassium supplements. Impaired renal function. Diabetes mellitus.

Special Concerns: Pregnancy category: B. Use with caution in metabolic or respiratory acidosis; during lactation. Geriatric patients may have a greater risk of developing hyperkalemia.

Side Effects: *Electrolyte:* Hyperkalemia, hyponatremia and hypochloremia if used with other diuretics. *CNS:* Headache, dizziness, encephalopathy, tremors, paresthesias, mental confusion, insomnia, decreased libido, depression, sleepiness, vertigo, nervousness. *GI:* Nausea, anorexia, vomiting, diarrhea, changes in appetite, gas and abdominal pain, dry mouth, flatulence, abdominal fullness, GI bleeding, thirst, dyspepsia, heartburn. *Respiratory:* Dyspnea, cough, shortness of breath. *Musculoskeletal:* Weakness, muscle cramps, fatigue; joint, neck and back pain; pain in extremities. *GU:* Impotence, polyuria, dysuria, bladder spasms, urinary frequency. *CV:* Angina, palpitations, arrhythmias, orthostatic hypotension. *Miscellaneous:* Aplastic anemia, neutropenia, visual disturbances, nasal congestion, tinnitus, increased intraocular pressure, skin rash, itching, pruritus, alopecia.

Drug Interactions	
Angiotensin-converting enzyme inhibitors	↑ Risk of significant hyperkalemia
Lithium	↓ Renal excretion of lithium → ↑ chance of toxicity
Potassium products	Hyperkalemia with possibility of cardiac arrhythmias or cardiac arrest
Spironolactone, Triamterene	Hyperkalemia, hyponatremia, hypochloremia

Dosage: Tablets. *As single agent or with other diuretics:* **Adults, initial,** 5 mg/day; 10 mg/day may be necessary in some patients. Doses as high as 20 mg/day may be used, if needed, with careful monitoring of electrolytes.

NURSING CONSIDERATIONS

See also *Nursing Considerations* for *Diuretics,* p. 1250.

Administration/Storage

Administer with food to reduce chance of GI upset.

Interventions

1. Monitor renal function studies, intake and output.
2. Monitor serum electrolytes. Assess for hyperkalemia and for indications to withdraw the drug. Cardiac irregularities may be precipitated.
3. Do not encourage potassium supplementation or foods rich in potassium because drug does not promote potassium excretion.
4. Do not administer with other potassium-sparing diuretics.

SPIRONOLACTONE   (speer-on-oh-**LAK**-tohn)

Aldactone, Novospiroton ✳, Sincomen ✳ (Rx)

See also *Diuretics,* p. 1249.

Classification: Diuretic, potassium-sparing.

Action/Kinetics: Spironolactone is a mild diuretic that acts on the distal tubule to inhibit sodium exchange for potassium which results in increased secretion of sodium and water and conservation of potassium. It is also an aldosterone antagonist. The drug manifests a slight antihypertensive effect. It also interferes with synthesis of testosterone and may increase formation of estradiol from testosterone thus leading to endocrine abnormalities. **Onset:** Urine output increases over 1–2 days. **Peak:** 2–3 days. **Duration:** 2–3 days, and declines thereafter. It is metabolized to an active metabolite (canrenone). **t½:** 13–24 hr for canrenone. The drug is almost completely bound to plasma protein. Spironolactone is also found in Aldactazide.

Uses: Edema due to congestive heart failure, cirrhosis of the liver, nephrotic syndrome. Primary hyperaldosteronism, essential hypertension, hypokalemia (especially in patients taking digitalis). Frequently used as adjunct with potassium-losing diuretics when it is important to avoid hypokalemia. *Investigational:* Polycystic ovary syndrome.

Contraindications: Acute renal insufficiency, progressive renal failure, hyperkalemia, and anuria. Patients receiving potassium supplements.

Special Concerns: Use during pregnancy only if benefits clearly outweigh risks. Use with caution in impaired renal function. Geriatric patients may be more sensitive to the usual adult dose.

Side Effects: *Electrolyte:* Hyperkalemia, hyponatremia (characterized by lethargy, dry mouth, thirst, tiredness). *GI:* Diarrhea, cramps, ulcers, gastritis, gastric bleeding, vomiting. *CNS:* Drowsiness, ataxia, lethargy, confusion, headache. *Endocrine:* Gynecomastia, menstrual irregularities, impotence, bleeding in postmenopausal women, deepening of voice, hirsutism. *Miscellaneous:* Skin rashes, drug fever, urticaria, breast carcinoma, hyperchloremic metabolic acidosis in hepatic cirrhosis (decompensated), agranulocytosis. **Note:** Spironolactone has been shown to be tumorigenic in chronic rodent studies.

Drug Interactions

Anesthetics, general	Additive hypotension
Angiotensin-converting enzyme inhibitors	Significant hyperkalemia
Anticoagulants, oral	Inhibited by spironolactone
Antihypertensives	Potentiation of hypotensive effect of both agents. Reduce dosage, especially of ganglionic blockers, by one-half

Drug Interactions (continued)

Captopril	↑ Risk of significant hyperkalemia
Digitalis	The potassium-conserving effect of spironolactone may decrease effectiveness of digitalis. Though severe consequences have occurred in patients with impaired kidney function, drugs are often given concomitantly. Monitor closely
Diuretics, others	Often administered concurrently because of potassium-sparing effect of spironolactone. Severe hyponatremia may occur. Monitor closely
Lithium	↑ Chance of lithium toxicity due to ↓ renal clearance
Norepinephrine	↓ Responsiveness to norepinephrine
Potassium salts	Since spironolactone conserves potassium excessively, hyperkalemia may result. Rarely used together
Salicylates	Large doses may ↓ effects of spironolactone
Triamterene	Hazardous hyperkalemia may result from combination

Laboratory Test Interference: Interference with radioimmunoassay for digoxin. False + plasma cortisol (as determined by fluorometric assay of Mattingly).

Dosage: Tablets. *Diuretic:* **Adults, initial,** 100 mg/day (range: 25–200 mg/day) in 2–4 divided doses for at least 5 days; **maintenance:** 75–400 mg daily in 2–4 divided doses. **Pediatric:** 1–3 mg/kg/day as a single dose or as 2–4 divided doses. *Antihypertensive:* **Adults, initial,** 50–100 mg/day as a single dose or as 2–4 divided doses—give for at least 2 weeks; **maintenance:** adjust to individual response. **Pediatric:** 1–3 mg/kg in a single dose or in 2–4 divided doses. *Treat hypokalemia:* **Adults,** 25–100 mg/day as a single dose or 2–4 divided doses. *Diagnosis of primary hyperaldosteronism:* **Adults,** 400 mg/day for either 4 days or 3–4 weeks (depending on test used). *Hyperaldosteronism, prior to surgery:* 100–400 mg/day in 2–4 doses prior to surgery.

NURSING CONSIDERATIONS

See also *Nursing Considerations* for *Diuretics,* p. 1250.

Administration/Storage

1. When used as the sole drug to treat edema, the initial dose should continue for at least 5 days. After that adjustments may be made. If the dosage is not effective, a second diuretic may be added, especially one that acts in the proximal tubules.
2. When administered to small children, the tablets may be crushed and given as a suspension in cherry syrup.
3. Food may increase the absorption of spironolactone.
4. Protect the drug from light.

Assessment

Obtain serum electrolyte levels prior to starting therapy. If the client's potassium level is greater than 5.5 mEq of potassium/L, withhold the medication and notify the physician.

Interventions

1. Monitor the client's serum electrolytes, liver and renal function studies and arterial blood gases. Compare with the baseline data and report any abnormalities.

2. Note if the client develops deep, rapid respirations, complains of headaches, or appears to be slower mentally. This may indicate the development of metabolic acidosis. Document and report these findings to the physician.

3. Record vital signs, intake, output and weight.

4. Note if the client develops dysuria, urinary frequency, or renal spasm. Take a urine culture, check for sensitivity, request a urinalysis and consult with the physician. It may be necessary to stop the medication.

5. Assess the client for tolerance to the drug, which may be characterized by edema and reduced urine output.

6. If the client has a history of cardiac disease, be alert to cardiac side effects.

7. If the client develops jaundice, tremors or appears mentally confused, report to the physician. If hepatic disease already exists, clients may develop hepatic encephalopathy.

8. Administer the drug with a snack or meals to relieve the symptoms of gastric distress. If nausea, bloating, anorexia, vomiting or diarrhea persist, notify the physician. The dosage of drug may need to be changed or the drug may need to be discontinued.

Client/Family Teaching

1. Instruct the client in how to take his BP and assist him to develop a method to maintain a written record for review by the physician.

2. Advise the client to avoid foods high in potassium, because spironolactone is potassium-sparing.

3. Caution clients taking large doses of medication not to drive a car and not to operate dangerous machinery until drug effects become apparent, because drowsiness or ataxia may occur.

TRIAMTERENE   (try-**AM**-ter-een)

Dyrenium (Rx)

See also *Diuretics,* p. 1249.

Classification: Diuretic, potassium-sparing.

Action/Kinetics: Triamterene is a mild diuretic that acts directly on the distal tubule. It promotes the excretion of sodium—which is exchanged for potassium or hydrogen ions—bicarbonate, chloride, and fluid. The drug increases urinary pH. It is also a weak folic acid antagonist. **Onset:** 2–4 hr. **Peak effect:** 1 to several days. **Duration:** 7–9 hr. $t^{1/2}$: 1.5–2 hr. From one-half to two-thirds of the drug is bound to plasma protein. About 20% is excreted unchanged through the urine. Triamterene is also found in Dyazide.

Uses: Edema due to congestive heart failure, hepatic cirrhosis, nephrotic syndrome, steroid therapy, secondary hyperaldosteronism. Also, idiopathic edema. May be used alone or with other diuretics. *Investigational:* Prophylaxis and treatment of hypokalemia, adjunct in the treatment of hypertension.

Contraindications: Hypersensitivity to drug, severe renal insufficiency, severe hepatic disease, anuria, hyperkalemia, hyperuricemia, gout, history of nephrolithiasis. Lactation.

Special Concerns: Pregnancy category: B. Safety and efficacy have not been determined in children.

Side Effects: *Electrolyte:* Hyperkalemia, electrolyte imbalance. *GI:* Nausea, vomiting (may also be indicative of electrolyte imbalance), diarrhea, dry mouth. *CNS:* Dizziness, drowsiness, fatigue, weakness, headache. *Hematologic:* Megaloblastic anemia, thrombocytopenia. *Miscellaneous:* Anaphylaxis, photosensitivity, hypokalemia, jaundice, muscle cramps, rash.

Drug Interactions	
Amantadine	↑ Toxic effects of amantadine due to ↓ renal excretion
Angiotensin-converting enzyme inhibitors	Significant hyperkalemia
Antihypertensives	Potentiated by triamterene
Captopril	↑ Risk of significant hyperkalemia
Digitalis	Inhibited by triamterene
Indomethacin	↑ Risk of nephrotoxicity
Lithium	↑ Chance of lithium toxicity due to ↓ renal clearance
Potassium salts	Additive hyperkalemia
Spironolactone	Additive hyperkalemia

Laboratory Test Interference: Triamterene may impart blue fluorescence to urine, interfering with fluorometric assays (e.g., lactic dehydrogenase, quinidine).

Dosage: Capsules, Tablets. *Diuretic:* **Adults, initial:** 25–100 mg daily after meals; **maximum daily dose:** 300 mg. **Maintenance:** 100 mg q other day. **Pediatric:** 2–4 mg/kg (120 mg/m^2) daily or on alternate days; **maintenance:** Up to 6 mg/kg daily to a maximum of 300 mg daily in divided doses.

NURSING CONSIDERATIONS

See also *Nursing Considerations* for *Diuretics,* p. 1250.

Administration/Storage

1. Minimize nausea by giving the drug after meals.
2. Triamterene dosage is usually reduced by one-half when another diuretic is added to the regimen.

Assessment

1. Take a complete drug history, noting drugs with which triamterene interacts.
2. Obtain baseline serum electrolytes, renal function studies and uric acid levels before administering the drug.
3. Determine that a CBC with differential and an ECG have been performed prior to initiating therapy.

Interventions

1. Monitor serum electrolytes, BUN, uric acid and CBC. Report any variations from the baseline studies to the physician.
2. If the client has a history of heart disease, obtain an ECG and be alert to the development of cardiac arrhythmias.
3. If the client has a history of alcoholism, megaloblastic anemia may occur, as triamterene is a weak antagonist of folic acid. Monitor the CBC and WBC differential periodically.

4. Observe for hyperkalemia, as this is an indication to withdraw the drug, because cardiac irregularities may result.

5. Note client complaints of sore throat, rash, or fever. These may be signs of blood dyscrasias and may require the withdrawal of the drug.

6. Observe the client for evidence of lethargy, complaints of headache, drowsiness, vomiting, restlessness, mental wandering, and foul breath. These are signs of uremia. Document and report immediately to the physician.

7. Avoid using potassium supplements, because the drug is potassium-sparing.

THIAZIDES AND RELATED DIURETICS

Action/Kinetics: The thiazide diuretics are related chemically to the sulfonamides. They are devoid of anti-infective activity but can cause the same hypersensitivity reactions as the sulfonamides.

The thiazides and related diuretics promote diuresis by decreasing the rate at which sodium and chloride are reabsorbed by the distal renal tubules of the kidney. By increasing the excretion of sodium and chloride, they force excretion of additional water. They also increase the excretion of potassium and, to a lesser extent, bicarbonate, as well as decrease the excretion of calcium and uric acid. Sodium and chloride are excreted in approximately equal amounts. The thiazides do not affect the glomerular filtration rate.

The antihypertensive mechanism of action of the thiazides is attributed to direct dilation of the arterioles, as well as to a reduction in the total fluid volume of the body and altered sodium balance. *Diuretic effect:* Usual, **Onset:** 1–2 hr. **Peak:** 4–6 hr. **Duration:** 6–24 hr. *Antihypertensive effect:* **Onset:** several days. *Optimal therapeutic effect:* 3–4 weeks.

Most thiazides are absorbed from the GI tract; a large fraction is excreted unchanged in urine.

Uses: Edema due to congestive heart failure, nephrosis, nephritis, renal failure, premenstrual syndrome, hepatic cirrhosis, corticosteroid or estrogen therapy. Hypertension. *Investigational:* Alone or in combination with allopurinol (or amiloride) for prophylaxis of calcium nephrolithiasis. Nephrogenic diabetes insipidus.

Contraindications: Hypersensitivity to drug, anuria, renal decompensation. Impaired renal function and advanced hepatic cirrhosis.

Drugs should not be used indiscriminately in patients with edema and toxemia of pregnancy, even though they may be therapeutically useful, because the thiazides may have adverse effects on the newborn (thrombocytopenia and jaundice).

Thiazides and related diuretics may precipitate myocardial infarctions in elderly patients with advanced arteriosclerosis, especially if the patient is also receiving therapy with other antihypertensive agents.

Patients with advanced heart failure, renal disease, or hepatic cirrhosis are most likely to develop hypokalemia.

Thiazides may activate or worsen systemic lupus erythematosus.

Special Concerns: Geriatric patients may manifest an increased risk of hypotension and changes in electrolyte levels. Administer with caution to debilitated patients or to those with a history of hepatic coma or precoma, gout, diabetes mellitus, or during pregnancy and lactation. Particular care must be exercised when thiazides are administered concomitantly with drugs that also cause potassium loss, such as digitalis, corticosteroids, and some estrogens.

Side Effects: *Electrolyte imbalance:* Hypokalemia (most frequent) characterized by cardiac arrhythmias. Hyponatremia characterized by weakness, lethargy, epigastric distress, nausea, vomiting. Hypokalemic alkalosis. *GI:* Dry mouth, thirst, stomach pain or upset, sore throat, diarrhea, bitter taste, anorexia. *CNS:* Mood changes, vertigo, paresthesias, weakness, restlessness, anxiety, depression, nervousness, neuropathy, tiredness, fever, syncope, dizziness. *CV:* Irregular heart rate, orthostatic hypotension, venous thrombosis, excessive volume depletion, palpitations, cold extremities, allergic myocarditis. *Allergic:* Skin rashes, urticaria, photosensitivity, purpura, vasculitis, necrotizing angiitis, anaphylaxis, pruritus, hives, dry skin, pneumonitis, pulmonary edema. *Hematologic:* Agranulocytosis, thrombocytopenia, aplastic anemia, leukopenia, neutropenia, hemolytic anemia. *Endocrine:* Hyperglycemia, aggravation of preexisting diabetes mellitus, hyperuricemia, electrolyte imbalance. *GU:* Frequent urination, polyuria, nocturia, impotence, reduced libido, crystalluria. *Respiratory:* Respiratory distress, dyspnea, pneumonitis, sinus congestion, epistaxis, cough, sore throat. *Miscellaneous:* Muscle cramps, joint pain and swelling, impaired liver function, pancreatitis, jaundice, hepatic coma, acute attacks of gout, blurred vision, rhinorrhea, flushing, chills, weight loss.

Drug Interactions

Anticholinergic agents	↑ Effect of thiazides due to ↑ amount absorbed from GI tract
Anticoagulants, oral	↑ Effect of anticoagulants by concentrating circulating clotting factors and ↑ clotting factor synthesis in liver
Antidiabetic agents	Thiazides antagonize hypoglycemic effect of antidiabetic agents
Antihypertensive agents	Thiazides potentiate the effect of antihypertensive agents
Cholestyramine	↓ Effect of thiazides due to ↓ absorption from GI tract
Colestipol	↓ Effect of thiazides due to ↓ absorption from GI tract
Corticosteroids	Enhanced potassium loss due to potassium-losing properties of both drugs
Diazoxide	Enhanced hypotensive effect. Also, ↑ hyperglycemic response
Digitalis glycosides	Thiazides produce ↑ potassium and magnesium loss with ↑ chance of digitalis toxicity
Ethanol	Additive orthostatic hypotension
Fenfluramine	↑ Antihypertensive effect of thiazides
Furosemide	Profound diuresis and electrolyte loss
Guanethidine	Additive hypotensive effect
Indomethacin	↓ Effect of thiazides, possibly by inhibition of prostaglandins
Lithium	Increased risk of lithium toxicity due to ↓ renal excretion
Muscle relaxants, nondepolarizing	↑ Effect of muscle relaxants due to hypokalemia
Norepinephrine	Thiazides ↓ arterial response to norepinephrine

Drug Interactions

Quinidine	↑ Effect of quinidine due to ↑ renal tubular reabsorption
Reserpine	Additive hypotensive effect
Sulfonamides	↑ Effect of thiazides due to ↓ plasma protein binding
Tetracyclines	↑ Risk of azotemia
Tubocurarine	↑ Muscle relaxation and ↑ hypokalemia
Vasopressors (sympathomimetics)	Thiazides ↓ responsiveness of arterioles to vasopressors

Laboratory Test Interferences: Hypokalemia, hypercalcemia, hyponatremia, hypomagnesemia, hypochloremia, hypophosphatemia, hyperuricemia. ↑ BUN, creatinine, glucose in blood and urine. ↓ Serum PBI levels (no signs of thyroid disturbance). Initial ↑ in total cholesterol, LDL cholesterol, and triglycerides.

Dosage: Drugs are preferentially given **PO,** but some preparations can be given parenterally. They are usually given in the morning, so the peak effect occurs during the day. See drugs listed below and those in Table 29.

NURSING CONSIDERATIONS

See also *Nursing Considerations* for *Diuretics,* p. 1250.

Administration/Storage

1. May be taken with food or milk if GI upset occurs.
2. Clients resistant to one type of thiazide may respond to another.
3. Thiazides should not be taken with any other medication (including OTC drugs for asthma, cough and colds, hay fever, weight control) unless approved by the physician.
4. To minimize electrolyte imbalance, thiazides may be taken every other day or on a 3–5 day basis for treatment of edema.
5. To prevent excess hypotension, the dose of other antihypertensive agents should be reduced when beginning thiazide therapy.

Assessment

1. Note if the client has any history of hypersensitivity to the drug.
2. Obtain renal and liver function tests prior to initiating therapy.
3. Note any history of heart disease. This is an indication that the client will require close monitoring once the drug has been administered.

Interventions

1. If the client is to undergo surgery, anticipate that the drug will be stopped at least 48 hr before the procedure. Thiazide inhibits the pressor effects of epinephrine.
2. Evaluate dietary potassium intake. Potassium chloride supplements should be given only when dietary measures are inadequate.
3. If potassium supplements are required, use liquid preparations to avoid ulcerations that may be produced by potassium.
4. If the client has diabetes, monitor blood glucose levels more frequently after beginning thiazide therapy. It may be necessary to change the dose of insulin or oral hypoglycemic agent.

Table 29 Thiazides and Related Diuretics

Drug	Dosage	Remarks			
		Onset	**Peak**	**Duration**	**t½**
Bendroflumethiazide (Naturetin) (Rx)	**Tablets.** *Edema,* **initial:** 2.5–10 mg 1–2 times daily, once every other day, or once daily for 3–5 days a week; **maintenance:** 2.5–5 mg daily, every other day, or once daily for 3–5 days a week. **Pediatric:** 0.4 mg/kg (12 mg/m^2) daily in 1–2 doses; **maintenance:** 0.05–0.1 mg/kg (1.5–3 mg/m^2) once daily. *Hypertension,* 2.5–20 mg daily in 1–2 doses. **Pediatric:** 0.05–0.4 mg/kg (1.5–12 mg/m^2) daily in 1–2 doses.	1–2 hr	6–12 hr	>18 hr	8.5 hr
Benzthiazide (Exna, Hydrex) (Rx) Pregnancy category: B.	**Tablets.** *Edema,* **initial:** 50–200 mg daily; **maintenance:** 50–150 mg daily. If daily dose exceeds 100 mg, divide dose and administer after breakfast and the evening meal. *Hypertension,* **initial:** 25–50 mg after breakfast and lunch; **maintenance:** according to patient response, up to a maximum daily dose of 200 mg. **Pediatric:** 0.9–3.9 mg/kg (30–120 mg/m^2) daily in single or divided doses.	2 hr	4–6 hr	12–18 hr	
Cyclothiazide (Anhydron, Fluidil) (Rx) Pregnancy category: C.	**Tablets.** *Edema,* **adults:** 1–2 mg once daily in the morning. Dose may be reduced depending on patient response (e.g., 1 or 2 mg every other day or 2–3 times weekly). *Hypertension,* 2 mg once daily, up to 4–6 mg. **Pediatric:** 0.02–0.04 mg/kg (0.6–1.2 mg/m^2) once daily.	2–4 hr	7–12 hr	18–24 hr	

Table 29 (continued)

Drug	Dosage	Remarks			
		Onset	Peak	Duration	t½
Hydroflumethiazide (Diucardin, Saluron) (Rx) Pregnancy category: D.	**Tablets.** *Edema*, **initial:** 50 mg 1–2 times daily; **maintenance:** 25–200 mg daily. Divide dose when it exceeds 100 mg daily. May also be given once every other day or once daily for 3–5 days a week. *Hypertension*, **initial:** 50 mg b.i.d.; **maintenance:** 50–100 mg daily, up to a maximum of 200 mg daily. **Pediatric:** 1 mg/kg (30 mg/m²) once daily.	1–2 hr	3–4 hr	18–24 hr	17 hr
Methylclothiazide (Aquatensen, Duretic❖, Enduron) (Rx) Pregnancy category: C.	**Tablets.** *Edema*, **adults:** 2.5–10 mg once daily, once every other day, or once daily for 3–5 days q week. Maximum effective dose is 10 mg. *Hypertension*, **adults:** 2.5–10 mg once daily. An additional antihypertensive agent should be added to the regimen if satisfactory control is not achieved within 8–12 weeks with 5 mg daily. **Pediatric:** 0.05–0.2 mg/kg (1.5–6 mg/m²) once daily.	2 hr	4–6 hr	24 hr	
Metolazone (Diulo, Zaroxolyn❭ (Rx) Pregnancy category: B.	**Prompt Tablets.** *Hypertension*, **adults, initial,** 0.5 mg once daily; **maintenance:** 0.5–1 mg daily. **Extended-release tablets.** *Edema*, **adults,** 5–20 mg once daily. *Hypertension*, **adults,** 2.5–5 mg once daily. Geriatric patients may be more sensitive to the usual adult dose.	1 hr	2 hr	12–24 hr	14 hr
	Additional contraindications: Prehepatic and hepatic coma. Use in children.				
	Additional untoward reactions: Chest pain, chills, bloating, palpitations.				
Polythiazide (Renese) (Rx)	**Tablets.** *Edema*, **adults,** 1–4 mg daily, once every other day, or once daily for 3–5 days a week. *Hypertension*: **adults,** 2–4 mg once daily. **Pediatric:** 0.02–0.08 mg/kg (0.5–2.5 mg/m²) once daily.	2 hr	6 hr	24–28 hr	Approximately 25 hr

Drug	Dosage	Onset	Peak	Duration	Half-life
Quinethazone (Hydromox) (Rx)	**Tablets.** *Edema or hypertension*: 50–200 mg daily in 1–2 doses. Geriatric patients may be more sensitive to the usual adult dose.	2 hr	6 hr	18–24 hr	
Trichlormethiazide (Metahydrin, Naqua) (Rx) Pregnancy category: B.	**Tablets.** *Edema,* **adults,** 1–4 mg a day, every other day or once daily for 3–5 days a week. *Hypertension,* **adults,** 2–4 mg once daily. **Pediatric:** 0.07 mg/kg (2 mg/m^2) daily in 1–2 doses. Geriatric patients may be more sensitive to the usual adult dose.	2 hr	6 hr	24 hr	Approximately 5.3 hr

Client/Family Teaching

1. Advise the client to avoid alcoholic beverages, because alcohol, in combination with thiazides, causes severe hypotension.
2. Advise the client to avoid eating licorice. Licorice may precipitate severe hypokalemia.
3. Encourage clients to eat a diet high in potassium. Encourage them to include orange juice and bananas.
4. Suggest the client take thiazide in the morning to avoid interrupting sleep with the frequent need to void.
5. If the client has a history of gout, advise them to reduce their intake of purines. Provide a list of foods to avoid.
6. If the client has diabetes, discuss the importance of more careful monitoring of urine and finger sticks for glucose determinations. Advise the client how to adjust the hypoglycemic agent in accordance with the physician's prescribed orders, and to keep the physician informed of any changes in blood glucose levels or the effectiveness of the hypoglycemic agent being used.
7. Explain the importance of taking thiazides as directed and stress the importance of reporting for scheduled follow up visits to evaluate the effectiveness of drug therapy. Provide the client with a list of side effects that should be reported to the physician should they occur.

ALDACTAZIDE   (al-**DAK**-tah-zyd)
(Rx)

Content/Classification: This drug is a combination of a thiazide and potassium-sparing diuretic.
Diuretic: Spironolactone, 25 or 50 mg.
Diuretic/antihypertenisve: Hydrochlorothiazide, 25 or 50 mg.
Also see information on individual components, p. 1270, and p. 1282.

Contraindications: Use in pregnancy only if benefits outweigh risks.

Uses: Congestive heart failure, essential hypertension, edema, or ascites in cirrhosis of the liver.

Dosage: Tablets. *Edema.* **Adults, usual:** 100 mg of each drug daily (range: 25–200 mg), given as single or divided doses. **Pediatric, usual:** equivalent to 1.65–3.3 mg/kg spironolactone. *Hypertension.* **Adults, usual:** 50–100 mg of each drug daily in single or divided doses.

NURSING CONSIDERATIONS

See *Nursing Considerations* for *Diuretics,* p. 1250, *Spironolactone,* p. 1271, and *Thiazide and Related Diuretics,* p. 1276.

CHLOROTHIAZIDE   (klor-oh-**THIGH**-ah-zyd)
Diuril (Rx)

CHLOROTHIAZIDE SODIUM   (klor-oh-**THIGH**-ah-zyd)
Sodium Diuril (Rx)

See also *Diuretics,* p. 1249, and *Thiazide and Related Diuretics,* p. 1274.

Classification: Diuretic, thiazide type.

Action/Kinetics: Onset: 1–2 hr; **Peak effect:** 4 hr; **Duration:** 6–12 hr. **t½:** 13 hr. Incompletely absorbed from the GI tract. Produces a greater diuretic effect if given in divided doses. Also found in Diupres.

Special Concerns: Pregnancy category: C. Geriatric patients may be more sensitive to the usual adult dose.

Dosage: Oral Suspension, Tablets, IV. *Antidiuretic, diabetes insipidus,* **Adults,** 250 mg q 6–12 hr. *Antihypertensive:* **Adults, PO,** 250 mg–1 g daily in one or more divided doses; **Adults, IV,** 0.5–1 g daily in one or more divided doses. **Pediatric, 6 months and older:** 10–20 mg/kg daily in a single dose or in 2 divided doses; **6 months and younger:** 10–30 mg/kg daily in a single dose or in 2 divided doses.

NURSING CONSIDERATIONS

See *Nursing Considerations* for *Diuretics,* p. 1250, and *Thiazides and Related Diuretics,* p. 1276.

Administration/Storage

1. To obtain an isotonic solution for injection, add 18 mL sterile water for injection to 500 mg powder.
2. IV use is not recommended for children and should be reserved for those adults unable to take oral medication or in emergency situations.
3. Unused reconstituted solutions should be discarded after 24 hr.
4. Simultaneous administration of whole blood or derivatives with chlorothiazide should be avoided.
5. The IV solution is compatible with sodium chloride or dextrose solutions.
6. Extravasation into SC tissues should be avoided.

CHLORTHALIDONE   (klor-**THAL**-ih-dohn)

Apo-Chlorthalidone ✿, Hygroton, Novo-Thalidone ✿, Thalitone, Uridon ✿ (Rx)

See also *Diuretics,* p. 1249, and *Thiazide and Related Diuretics,* p. 1274.

Classification: Diuretic, thiazide.

Action/Kinetics: Onset: 2 hr. **Peak effect:** Within 2–6 hr. **Duration:** 24–72 hr. **t½:** 35–50 hr.

Additional Uses: Particularly good for potentiation of and for reducing dosage of other antihypertensive agents.

Special Concerns: Pregnancy category: B. Geriatric patients may be more sensitive to the usual adult dose.

Dosage: Tablets. *Antidiuretic:* **Adults,** 25–100 mg daily or 100–200 mg 3 times/week. **Maximum daily dose:** 200 mg. **Pediatric:** all uses, 2 mg/kg (60 mg/m²) 3 times weekly. *Hypertension:* **initial,** 25–50 mg once daily up to 100 mg daily; **maintenance;** usually lower than initial dose but determined by patient response.

NURSING CONSIDERATIONS

See *Nursing Considerations* for *Diuretics,* p. 1250, and *Thiazides and Related Diuretics,* p. 1276.

Administration/Storage

Administer in the morning with food.

DYAZIDE   (DYE-ah-zyd)
(Rx)

Classification/Content: This drug is a combination of hydrochlorothiazide and a potassium-sparing diuretic (triamterene).

Antihypertensive/diuretic: Hydrochlorothiazide, 25 mg. *Diuretic:* Triamterene, 50 mg. See also individual components, p. 1282, and p. 1272.

Uses: Adjunct in treatment of edema due to congestive heart failure, hepatic cirrhosis, nephrotic syndrome, and estrogen or corticosteroid usage. Also used in idiopathic edema. May also be used in hypertension.

Special Concerns: Use during pregnancy only if benefits outweigh risks. Use in children not recommended. Geriatric patients may be more sensitive to the usual adult dose.

Dosage: Capsules. Individualized. Adults, usual: 1–2 capsules b.i.d. after meals, not to exceed 4 capsules daily.

NURSING CONSIDERATIONS

See also *Nursing Considerations* for *Diuretics,* p. 1250, and *Thiazides and Related Diuretics,* p. 1276.

Administration/Storage

1. If another antihypertensive drug is to be used concurrently, the dose of the other antihypertensive should be one-half the usual dose.
2. If potassium supplements are being used with other diuretics, they should be discontinued when using Dyazide due to the potassium-sparing effects of triamterene.
3. Some clients may be maintained on one capsule of Dyazide daily or every other day.

HYDROCHLOROTHIAZIDE   (hy-droh-klor-oh-THIGH-ah-zyd)
Apo-Hydro✳, Diuchlor H✳, Esidrex, Hydro-DIURIL, Neo-Codema✳, Novo-Hyrazide✳, Oretic, Urozide✳
(Rx)

See also *Diuretics,* p. 1249, and *Thiazide and Related Diuretics,* p. 1276.

Classification: Diuretic, thiazide type.

Action/Kinetics: Onset: 2 hr. **Peak effect:** 4–6 hr. **Duration:** 6–12 hr. **t½:** Approximately 15 hr. Hydrochlorothiazide is also found in Aldactazide, Aldoril, Apresazide, Dyazide, Hydropres, and Ser-Ap-Es.

Special Concerns: Pregnancy category: B. Geriatric patients may be more sensitive to the usual adult dose.

Dosage: Oral Solution, Tablets. *Antidiuretic, diabetes insipidus:* **Adults:** 25–100 mg once or twice daily, once every other day, or once a day for 3–5 days a week. *Antihypertensive:* **Adults:** 25–100 mg/day as a single dose or in two divided doses. **Pediatric, all uses:** 1–2 mg/kg (30–60 mg/m²) daily as a single dose or 2 divided doses. Infants up to 6 months of age may require up to 3 mg/kg daily.

NURSING CONSIDERATIONS

See also *Nursing Considerations* for *Diuretics,* p. 1250, and *Thiazides and Related Diuretics,* p. 1276.

Administration/Storage

1. Divide daily doses in excess of 100 mg.
2. Give b.i.d. at 6- to 12-hr intervals.

INDAPAMIDE   (in-**DAP**-ah-myd)

Lozide ✽, Lozol (Rx)

See also *Diuretics,* p. 1249, and *Thiazide and Related Diuretics,* p. 1274.

Classification: Diuretic, thiazide type.

Action/Kinetics: Onset: 1–2 weeks after multiple doses. **Peak levels:** 2 hr. **Duration:** Up to 8 weeks with multiple doses. **t½:** 14 hr. Nearly 100% is absorbed from the GI tract. Excreted through the kidneys (70% with 7% unchanged) and the GI tract (23%).

Uses: Alone or in combination with other drugs for treatment of hypertension. Edema in congestive heart failure.

Special Concerns: Pregnancy category: B. Dosage has not been established in children. Geriatric patients may be more sensitive to the hypotensive and electrolyte effects.

Dosage: Tablets. *Edema, hypertension,* **adults:** 2.5 mg in the morning. If necessary, may be increased to 5 mg daily after 1 week if treating edema and 4 weeks if treating hypertension.

NURSING CONSIDERATIONS

See *Nursing Considerations* for *Diuretics,* p. 1250, and *Thiazides and Related Diuretics,* p. 1276, .

Administration/Storage

1. May be combined with other antihypertensive agents if the response is inadequate. Initially, the dose of other agents should be reduced by 50%.
2. Doses greater than 5 mg daily do not increase effectiveness but may increase hypokalemia.

CHAPTER SIXTY-EIGHT

Electrolytes and Caloric Agents

General Statement: Water, electrolytes, and nutrients are used as adjuncts in the management of a great variety of disorders and conditions. Since there is a close link between fluid volume and electrolyte balance, these two subjects will be discussed together.

The electrolyte levels in the body vary within extremely narrow limits (see appendix 1). Any major deviation from normal quickly results in physiologic changes manifested by dehydration, fluid retention, and disturbance of the acid-base balance. Severe illness (chronic or acute), shock, trauma, poisoning, burns, and certain medications often affect the fluid and electrolyte balance of the body. The administration of suitable replacements to prevent or correct disequilibration of the fluid and electrolyte balance is an important aspect of patient care.

Fluid and electrolytes can be supplied orally, subcutaneously (rare), or IV. The oral route should be chosen whenever possible. Parenteral therapy should be discontinued at the earliest possible time.

Numerous single and multiple electrolyte replacement solutions with or without carbohydrates are commercially available. The electrolytes and nutrients in these products are indistinguishable by the body from the same materials supplied in the diet and are metabolized in the same manner. Drugs are often added to parenterally administered solutions, and the nurse must be aware of possible interactions and incompatibilities. Unless specifically instructed to do otherwise, it is advisable to add only one drug at a time to the IV assembly.

Fluid balance can also be manipulated with diuretics. These drugs are discussed in Chapter 67, p. 1249; Calcium, an electrolyte, is discussed in Chapter 60, p. 1135. Blood volume expanders are discussed in Chapter 21, p. 414. Characteristic clinical symptoms of electrolyte imbalance are summarized in Table 30, p. 1285.

Table 30   Clinical Symptoms of Electrolyte Imbalance

Calcium

Hypocalcemia
CNS: Mental depression, anxiety states
CV: Arrhythmias
GI: Abdominal cramps
Neuromuscular: Peripheral numbness, tingling of
  fingers, muscular fibrillation, facial muscle
  cramping, skeletal muscle cramps, leg cramps,
  tetany, smooth muscle irritablility
Other: Abnormal blood coagulation, fractures

Hypercalcemia (Acute Crisis)
CNS: Stupor, coma
CV: Cardiac arrest
GI: Nausea, vomiting, dehydration
Neuromuscular: Weakness (long-term)
GU: Flank pain (renal calculi)
Other: Deep pain over bony areas

Magnesium

Hypomagnesemia
CV: Arrhythmias, vasodilation, ↓ BP
Neuromuscular: Hyperirritability, leg and foot
  cramps, ↑ deep tendon reflexes, involuntary
  muscle twitching and movements, weakness,
  spasticity, tetany, tremors, convulsions

Hypermagnesemia
CNS: Depression, lethargy; slow, shallow
  breathing
CV: ↓ BP, slow weak pulse
Neuromuscular: ↓ Deep tendon reflexes
Other: Flushing of skin

Potassium

Hypokalemia
CNS: Dizziness, mental confusion
CV: Arrhythmias; weak, irregular pulse; hypotension,
  cardiac arrest
GI: Abdominal distention, anorexia
Neuromuscular: Weakness, paresthesia
Other: Malaise

Hyperkalemia
CV: Bradycardia, then tachycardia, cardiac arrest
GI, GU: Abdominal cramps, oliguria or anuria,
  nausea, diarrhea
Neuromuscular: Weakness, tingling, paralysis

Sodium

Hyponatremia
CNS: Anxiety, lassitude
GI, GU: Rough, dry tongue; abdominal cramps,
  ↓ specific gravity of urine
Neuromuscular: Tremors, progressing to
  convulsions

Hypernatremia
CNS: Headaches, convulsions, ↑ body
  temperature
GI, GU: Nausea, vomiting, ↓ specific gravity
  of urine
Neuromuscular: ↓ Reflexes, weakness
Other: Thirst, restlessness, dry mucous
  membranes

Chloride

Hypochloremia
CNS: ↓ Respiration
Neuromuscular: Hypertonicity, tetany

Hyperchloremia
CNS: Stupor; rapid, deep breathing; weakness
  leading to coma

68

Note: The dosage of IV solutions is highly individualized especially for infants, children, elderly, or debilitated patients and those suffering from cardiovascular diseases.

ELECTROLYTES

MAGNESIUM SULFATE   (mag-**NEE**-see-um)
Epsom Salts (OTC and Rx)

See also *Anticonvulsants,* p. 714, and *Laxatives,* p. 1048.

Classification: Anticonvulsant, electrolyte, saline laxative.

Action/Kinetics: Magnesium is an important cation present in the extracellular fluid at a concentration of 1.5–2.5 mEq/L. Magnesium is an essential element for muscle contraction, certain enzyme systems, and nerve transmission.

Magnesium depresses the CNS and controls convulsions by blocking release of acetylcholine at the myoneural junction. Also, the drug decreases the sensitivity of the motor end plate to acetylcholine and decreases the excitability of the motor membrane. **Therapeutic serum levels:** 4–6 mEq/L (normal Mg levels: 1.5–3.0 mEq/L). **Onset: IM,** 1 hr; **IV,** immediate. **Duration: IM,** 3–4 hr; **IV,** 30 min. Magnesium is excreted by the kidneys.

Uses: Seizures associated with toxemia of pregnancy, epilepsy, or when abnormally low levels of magnesium may be a contributing factor in convulsions, such as in hypothyroidism or glomerulonephritis. Acute nephritis in children. Uterine tetany. Replacement therapy in magnesium deficiency. Adjunct in total parenteral nutrition (TPN). Laxative.

Contraindications: In the presence of heart block or myocardial damage.

Special Concerns: Pregnancy category: A. Use with caution in patients with renal disease because magnesium is removed from the body solely by the kidneys.

Side Effects: Magnesium intoxication. *CNS:* Depression. *CV:* Flushing, hypotension, circulatory collapse, depression of the myocardium. *Other:* Sweating, hypothermia, muscle paralysis, respiratory paralysis. Suppression of knee jerk reflex can be used to determine toxicity. Respiratory failure may occur if given after knee jerk reflex disappears.

Treatment of Magnesium Intoxication:

1. Use artificial ventilation immediately.
2. Have 5–10 mEq of calcium (e.g., 10–20 mL of 10% calcium gluconate) readily available for IV injection.

Drug Interactions	
CNS depressants (general anesthetics, sedative-hypnotics, narcotics)	Additive CNS depression
Digitalis	Heart block when Mg intoxication is treated with calcium in digitalized patients
Neuromuscular blocking agents	Possible additive neuromuscular blockade

Dosage: IM. *Anticonvulsant:* 1–5 g of a 25–50% solution up to 6 times daily. **Pediatric:** 20–40 mg/kg using the 20% solution (may be repeated if necessary). **IV:** 1–4 g using 10–20% solution, not to exceed 1.5 mL/min of the 10% solution. **IV infusion:** 4 g in 250 mL 5% dextrose at a rate not to exceed 3 mL/min.

Hypomagnesemia, mild, **IM:** 1 g as a 50% solution q 6 hr for 4 times (or total of 32.5 mEq/24 hr). *Severe,* **IM:** up to 2 mEq/kg over 4 hr or **IV:** 5 g (40 mEq) in 1,000 mL dextrose 5% or sodium chloride solution by **slow** infusion over period of 3 hr. *Hyperalimentation,* **adults:** 8–24 mEq/day; **infants:** 2–10 mEq/day.

Laxative. **PO. Adults:** 10–15 g; **pediatric:** 5–10 g.

NURSING CONSIDERATIONS

See also *Nursing Considerations* for *Anticonvulsants,* p. 720, and *Laxatives,* p. 1049.

Administration/Storage

1. For IV injections, administer only 1.5 mL of 10% solution per minute. Discontinue administration when convulsions cease.
2. For IV infusion, administration should not exceed 3 mL/min. IV: dilute as specified by manufacturer.
3. Dilutions for IM: deep injection of 50% concentrate is appropriate for adults. A 20% solution should be used for children.
4. When used as a laxative, dissolve in a glassful of ice water or other fluid to lessen the disagreeable taste.
5. Have available emergency equipment and IV calcium gluconate or IV calcium gluceptate to use as an antidote for magnesium intoxication.

Assessment

1. Determine if the client has a history of kidney disease.
2. Obtain baseline serum magnesium levels.
3. Note the purpose for which magnesium sulfate is being administered.
4. Note the client's cardiac condition. Assess the ECG for evidence of any abnormality prior to administering drug IV. Magnesium sulfate is usually contraindicated in the presence of myocardial damage or heart block.

Interventions

1. Observe the client for depression of patellar reflexes, hypothermia, or the presence of flaccid paralysis. Monitor the levels of magnesium sulfate throughout the therapy and report any adverse reactions to the physician.
2. Observe the client for flushing, hypotension and depressed cardiac function, all signs of magnesium intoxication. If the respirations fall below 16/min, or if the urinary output is less than 100 mL during the past 4 hours, withhold the drug and report to the physician.
3. Monitor the blood pressure and pulse. If the client is pregnant, monitor the fetal heart rate and quality, and assess the status of the fetus.
4. Do not administer magnesium sulfate for 2 hours preceding the delivery of a baby.
5. If a mother has received continuous IV therapy of magnesium sulfate during 24 hr prior to delivery, assess the newborn for neurologic and respiratory depression.
6. Anticipate that the dose of CNS depressants administered to the client receiving magnesium sulfate will be adjusted.
7. If the client is receiving digitalis preparations and magnesium sulfate, monitor the client closely. Toxicity treated with calcium is extremely dangerous and may result in heart block.

POTASSIUM SALTS
POTASSIUM ACETATE, PARENTERAL

(Rx)

POTASSIUM ACETATE, POTASSIUM BICARBONATE, AND POTASSIUM CITRATE (TRIKATES)

Oral Solution: Tri-K (Rx)

POTASSIUM BICARBONATE AND CITRIC ACID

Effervescent Tablets: K+Care ET, Klor-Con/EF (Rx)

POTASSIUM BICARBONATE AND POTASSIUM CHLORIDE

Effervescent Granules: Klorvess Effervescent Granules, Neo-K✹ (Rx). Effervescent Tablets: Klorvess, K-Lyte/Cl, K-Lyte/Cl 50, Potassium-Sandoz✹ (Rx)

POTASSIUM BICARBONATE AND POTASSIUM CITRATE

Effervescent Tablets: K-Lyte, K-Lyte DS (Rx)

POTASSIUM CHLORIDE

Extended-release Capsules: K-Norm, Micro-K, Micro-K 10 (Rx).Oral Solution: Cena-K, K-10✹, Kaochlor-10 and -20✹, Kaochlor 10%, Kaochlor S-F 10%, Kaon-Cl 20% Liquid, Kay Ciel, KCl 5%✹, Klorvess 10% Liquid, Potachlor 10% and 20%, Potasalan, Roychlor-10% and -20%, Rum-K (Rx). Powder for Oral Solution: Kato, Kay Ciel, K+Care, K-Lor, Klor-Con Powder, Klor-Con/25 Powder, K-Lyte/Cl Powder, Potage (Rx). Extended-release Tablets: Apo-K✹, K+10, Kalium Durules✹, Kaon-Cl, Kaon-Cl-10, K-Dur, K-Long✹, Klor-Con 8 and 10, Klotrix, K-Tab, Novolente-K✹, Slow-K, Slo-Pot 600✹, Slow-K✹, Ten-K (Rx)

POTASSIUM CHLORIDE, POTASSIUM BICARBONATE, AND POTASSIUM CITRATE

Effervescent Tablets: Kaochlor-Eff (Rx)

POTASSIUM GLUCONATE

Elixir: Kaon, Kaylixir, K-G Elixir, Potassium-Rougier✹, Royonate✹ (Rx). Tablets: Kaon✹ (Rx)

POTASSIUM GLUCONATE AND POTASSIUM CHLORIDE

Oral Solution and Powder for Oral Solution: Kolyum (Rx)

POTASSIUM GLUCONATE AND POTASSIUM CITRATE

Oral Solution: Twin-K (Rx)

POTASSIUM GLUCONATE, POTASSIUM CITRATE, AND AMMONIUM CHLORIDE

Oral Solution: Twin-K-Cl (Rx)

Classification: Electrolyte.

General Statement: Potassium is the major cation of the body's intracellular fluid. It is essential for the maintenance of important physiologic processes, including cardiac, smooth, and skeletal muscle function, acid-base balance, gastric secretions, renal function, protein and carbohydrate metabolism. Symptoms of hypokalemia include weakness, cardiac arrhythmias, fatigue, ileus, hyporeflexia or areflexia, tetany, polydipsia, and, in severe cases, flaccid paralysis and inability to concentrate urine. Loss of potassium is usually accompanied by a loss of chloride resulting in hypochloremic metabolic alkalosis.

The usual adult daily requirement of potassium is 40–80 mg. In adults, the normal plasma concentration of potassium ranges from 3.5 to 5 mEq/L. Concentrations of up to 5.6 mEq/L are normal in children.

Both hypokalemia and hyperkalemia, if uncorrected, can be fatal; thus, potassium must always be administered cautiously.

Potassium is readily and rapidly absorbed from the GI tract. Though a number of salts can be used to supply the potassium cation, potassium chloride is the agent of choice since hypochloremia frequently accompanies potassium deficiency. Dietary measures (bananas, orange juice) can often prevent and even correct potassium deficiencies.

Potassium is excreted by the kidney and is partially reabsorbed from the glomerular filtrate.

Uses: Correction of potassium deficiency caused by vomiting, diarrhea, excess loss of GI fluids, hyperadrenalism, malnutrition, debilitation, prolonged negative nitrogen balance, dialysis, metabolic alkalosis, diabetic acidosis, certain renal conditions, cardiac arrhythmias, cardiotonic glycoside toxicity, and myasthenia gravis (experimentally).

Long-term electrolyte replacement regimen or total parenteral nutrition with potassium-free solutions. Correction of potassium deficiency possibly caused by certain drugs, including many diuretics, adrenal corticosteroids, testosterone, or corticotropin.

Prophylaxis after major surgery when urine flow has been reestablished.

Contraindications: Severe renal function impairment, postoperatively before urine flow has been reestablished. Crush syndrome, Addison's disease, hyperkalemia from any cause, oliguria or azotemia, anuria, heat cramps, acute dehydration, severe hemolytic reactions, adynamia episodica hereditaria.

Special Concerns: Safety during pregnancy (pregnancy category: C) and lactation and in children has not been established. Geriatric patients are at greater risk of developing hyperkalemia due to age-related changes in renal function. Administer with caution in the presence of cardiac and renal disease and in patients receiving potassium-sparing drugs.

Side Effects: Hypokalemia. *CNS:* Dizziness, mental confusion. *CV:* Arrhythmias; weak, irregular pulse; hypotension, heart block, ECG abnormalities, cardiac arrest. *GI:* Abdominal distention, anorexia, nausea, vomiting, diarrhea. *Neuromuscular:* Weakness, paresthesia of extremities, flaccid paralysis, areflexia, muscle or respiratory paralysis, weakness and heaviness of legs. *Other:* Malaise.

Hyperkalemia. *CV:* Bradycardia, then tachycardia, cardiac arrest. *GI:* Nausea, vomiting, diarrhea, abdominal cramps, GI bleeding or obstruction. Ulceration or perforation of the small bowel from enteric-coated potassium chloride tablets. *GU:* Oliguria, anuria. *Neuromuscular:* Weakness, tingling, paralysis. *Other:* Skin rashes, hyperkalemia.

Treatment of Overdosage: (Plasma potassium levels greater than 6.5 mEq/L.) All measures must be monitored by electrocardiogram. Measures consist of actions taken to shift potassium ions from plasma into cells by

1. **Sodium bicarbonate:** IV infusion of 50–100 mEq over period of 5 min. May be repeated after 10–15 minutes if ECG abnormalities persist.
2. **Glucose and Insulin:** IV infusion of 3 g glucose to 1 unit regular insulin in order to shift potassium into cells.
3. **Calcium gluconate—or other calcium salt** (only for patients not on digitalis or other cardiotonic glycosides): IV infusion of 0.5–1 g (5–10 mL of a 10% solution) over period of 2 min. Dosage may be repeated after 1–2 minutes if ECG remains abnormal. When ECG is approximately normal, the excess potassium should be removed from the body by administration of polystyrene sulfonate, hemodialysis or peritoneal dialysis (patients with renal insufficiency), or other means.

4. **Sodium polystyrene sulfonate, hemodialysis, peritoneal dialysis:** To remove potassium from the body.

Drug Interactions

Angiotensin-converting enzyme (ACE) inhibitors	May cause potassium retention → hyperkalemia
Digitalis glycosides	Cardiac arrhythmias
Potassium-sparing diuretics	Severe hyperkalemia with possibility of cardiac arrhythmias or arrest

---

Dosage: Highly individualized. Oral administration is preferred because the slow absorption from the GI tract prevents sudden, large increases in plasma potassium levels. Dosage is usually expressed as mEq/L of potassium. The bicarbonate, chloride, citrate, and gluconate salts are usually administered orally. The chloride, acetate, and phosphate may be administered by **slow IV** infusion.

IV infusion. *Serum K less than 2.0 mEq/L:* 400 mEq/day at a rate not to exceed 40 mEq/hr. *Serum K more than 2.5 mEq/L:* 200 mEq/day at a rate not to exceed 20 mEq/hr.

PO. Pediatric, IV infusion: Up to 3 mEq potassium/kg (or 40 mEq/m^2) daily.

Prophylaxis of hypokalemia: 16–24 mEq/day. *Potassium depletion:* 40–100 mEq/day. **Note:** Usual dietary intake of potassium is 40–250 mEq/day.

For patients with accompanying metabolic acidosis, an alkalizing potassium salt (potassium bicarbonate, potassium citrate, or potassium acetate) should be selected.

NURSING CONSIDERATIONS

Administration/Storage

PO

1. Dilute or dissolve liquid potassium in fruit or vegetable juice if not already in flavored base.
2. Chill to increase palatability.
3. Instruct the client to swallow enteric-coated tablets and not to dissolve them in the mouth.
4. Give oral doses 2–4 times daily. Hypokalemia should be corrected slowly over a period of 3–7 days to minimize the development of hyperkalemia.
5. Salt substitutes should not be used concomitantly with potassium preparations.
6. Administer dilute liquid solutions of potassium rather than tablets to clients with esophageal compression.

Parenteral

1. Administer slowly as ordered by the physician for each individual client.
2. Potassium should not be administered IV undiluted. Usual method is to administer by slow IV infusion in dextrose solution at a concentration of 40–80 mEq/L.
3. Ensure uniform distribution of potassium by inverting container during addition of potassium solution and then by agitating container. Squeezing the plastic container will not prevent potassium chloride from settling to the bottom.
4. Check site of administration frequently for pain and redness because drug is extremely irritating.
5. In critical clients, potassium chloride may be given slow IV in a solution of saline (unless

contraindicated) since dextrose may lower serum potassium levels by producing an intracellular shift.

6. Administer all concentrated potassium infusions and riders with an infusion control device.
7. Have available sodium bicarbonate, calcium gluconate, and regular insulin for parenteral use to treat clients who develop hyperkalemia.
8. Have sodium polystyrene sulfonate (Kayexalate) available for oral/rectal administration in the event of hyperkalemia.

Assessment

1. Obtain baseline serum electrolyte levels and ECG.
2. Note any prior history of impaired renal function.
3. Monitor the client's intake and output for adequate urinary flow before administering potassium. Impaired renal function can lead to hyperkalemia.

Interventions

1. Once parenteral potassium administration is initiated, discontinue administering potassium-rich foods and oral potassium medication to the client.
2. If the client develops abdominal pain, distention, or GI bleeding, withhold oral potassium medication and report to the physician.
3. Note client complaints of weakness, fatigue, or the presence of cardiac arrhythmias. These may be symptoms of hypokalemia indicating a low *intracellular* potassium level, although the serum potassium level may appear to be within normal limits.
4. Monitor intake and output. If the client develops oliguria, anuria, or azoturia, withhold the drug, document and report to the physician.
5. Observe the client for symptoms of adrenal insufficiency or extensive tissue breakdown. Withhold potassium, document findings and report to the physician.
6. Note client complaints of weakness or heaviness of the legs, the presence of a gray pallor, cold skin, listlessness, mental confusion, flaccid paralysis, hypotension, or cardiac arrhythmias. These are symptoms of hyperkalemia. The medication should be stopped and the physician notified immediately, as the client may go into cardiovascular collapse.
7. While the client is on parenteral potassium, monitor ECG for signs of hyperkalemia, as evidenced by peaked T waves and a widened QRS.
8. Monitor the serum potassium levels while the client is receiving parenteral potassium. The normal level is 3.5–5.0 mEq/L. Any variation should be reported to the physician.

Client/Family Teaching

1. Clients receiving potassium-sparing diuretics, such as spironolactone or triamterene should not take potassium supplements or eat foods high in potassium unless specifically designated by the physician.
2. Provide the client with printed information explaining the symptoms of hypo- and hyperkalemia and when to call the physician.
3. Review with the client the importance of potassium in the diet and its importance to other medications prescribed for the client.
4. Explain that once the parenteral potassium is discontinued it is important to ingest potassium-rich foods such as citrus juices, bananas, apricots, raisins, and nuts. The daily requirement is

usually 3–4 g or 40 to 60 mEq/L. Have a dietician work with the client to assure a proper dietary regimen and to assist with meal planning.

Evaluation

1. Review with the client the regimen prescribed and assess the client's ability to adhere to this regimen.
2. Determine clinical response to therapy by assessing serum potassium levels.

SODIUM CHLORIDE

Tablets: Slo-Salt. Topical: Ayr Saline, HuMIST Saline Nasal, NaSal Saline Nasal, Ocean Mist, Salinex Nasal Mist. Ophthalmic: Adsorbonac Ophthalmic, AK-NaCl, Hypersal 5%, Muro-128 Ophthalmic. Parenteral: Sodium Chloride IV Infusions (0.2%, 0.45%, 0.9%, 3%, 5%), Sodium Chloride Injection for Admixtures (50, 100, 625 mEq/vial), Sodium Chloride Diluent (0.9%), Concentrated Sodium Chloride Diluents (14.6%, 23.4%) (Parenteral is Rx; Topical and ophthalmic are OTC)

Classification: Electrolyte.

Action/Kinetics: Sodium is the major cation of the body's extracellular fluid. It plays a crucial role in maintaining the fluid and electrolyte balance. Excess retention of sodium results in overhydration (edema, hypervolemia), which is often treated with diuretics. Abnormally low levels of sodium result in dehydration. Normally, the plasma contains 136–145 mEq sodium/L and 98–106 mEq chloride/L. The average daily requirement of salt is approximately 5 g.

Uses: PO: Prophylaxis of heat prostration or muscle cramps, chloride deficiency due to diuresis or salt restriction. **Parenteral:** Fluid and electrolyte replacement. **Topical:** Relief of inflamed, dry, or crusted nasal membranes; irrigating solution. **Ophthalmic:** Use hypertonic solutions to decrease corneal edema due to bullous keratitis; as an aid to facilitate ophthalmoscopic examination in gonioscopy, biomicroscopy, and funduscopy.

Contraindications: Congestive heart failure, severely impaired renal function. Administer with caution to patients with cardiovascular, cirrhotic, or renal disease, in presence of hyperproteinemia, and in patients receiving corticosteroids or corticotropin.

Special Concerns: Pregnancy category: C.

Side Effects: Hypernatremia, postoperative intolerance of sodium chloride characterized by cellular dehydration, asthenia, disorientation, anorexia, nausea, oliguria, and increased BUN levels.

Dosage: Tablets (including extended release and enteric coated): *Heat cramps/dehydration:* 0.5–1 g with 8 oz water up to 10 times/day; total daily dose should not exceed 4.8 g.

IV: *Individualized* as required. *Hypotonic* (0.11%–0.45% NaCl) solutions are used when fluid losses exceed electrolyte depletion. *Isotonic* (0.9% NaCl) provides approximately physiologic concentrations of sodium and chloride ions. *Hypertonic* (3% or 5%) when sodium loss exceeds fluid loss.

Ophthalmic. *Solution:* 1–2 gtt in eye q 3–4 hr. *Ointment:* Instill once (or more often, if necessary) daily.

NURSING CONSIDERATIONS

Administration/Storage

Hypertonic injections of NaCl must be given slowly and cautiously in an amount not to exceed 100 mL/hr. Plasma electrolyte levels should be determined before additional sodium chloride is given.

Interventions

1. Observe the client for flushed skin, elevated temperature, rough dry tongue, and edema. These are symptoms of hypernatremia; document and report to the physician.
2. Monitor vital signs for evidence of hypertension, hypotension, or tachycardia. Document and report.
3. Monitor urine specific gravity and serum sodium levels. If the urine specific gravity is above 1.02, and if the serum sodium level is above 146 mEq/L, report to the physician and anticipate that the drug will be discontinued.
4. Record intake and output.
5. Monitor electrolyte levels and hepatic and renal function studies.
6. Note level of consciousness and periodically assess heart sounds.

CALORIC AGENTS

CARBOHYDRATES

Classification: Caloric agents.

Action/Kinetics: The simplest and most easily absorbed caloric agents are dextrose (D-glucose) and fructose, or an equimolar mixture of the two (invert sugar). Fructose and dextrose are monosaccharides that can replace and supplement orally absorbed food and water. They decrease excess ketone formation and spare body proteins and electrolytes.

Uses: One liter of a 10% solution of any of the above provides 340–380 calories. Five percent solutions are approximately isotonic. Both 5% and 10% solutions are used to correct dehydration and supply calories. More concentrated solutions also have a diuretic effect. *Note:* Solutions without NaCl should not be used as diluents for blood.

Contraindications: Do not use concentrated (hypertonic) solutions in the presence of intracranial or intraspinal hemorrhages or delirium tremens in dehydrated patients.

NURSING CONSIDERATIONS

Administration/Storage

1. The amount of fluid to be administered in a specific amount of time is to be ordered by the physician. The amount is highly individualized, especially in children.
2. Administer concentrated solutions into a large, central vein to prevent irritation.

Interventions

1. Assess and record the client's vital signs, weight, intake and output.
2. Monitor renal function, pH, phosphorus, magnesium and glucose levels and report any abnormal values to the physician.
3. If the client is receiving isotonic parenteral therapy, observe for signs of cerebral edema, as evidenced by a slow pulse rate, high blood pressure, and headaches. *Reduce* the rate of flow and report these findings to the physician.
4. If the client is receiving hyperosmolar (hypertonic) parenteral therapy, observe for signs of

dehydration, such as a rapid pulse rate, low blood pressure, and restlessness. In this event, *reduce* the rate of flow and report to the physician.

- To prevent further electrolyte imbalance, monitor the rate of flow of the hyperosmolar solutions so that they do not run faster that 3–4 mL/minute.
- Observe the infusion area for redness and pain. Hyperosmolar solutions can cause sclerosis and thrombophlebitis.

5. If there is an abrupt withdrawal of hypertonic dextrose solution, anticipate that a 5% or 10% dextrose solution will be administered to prevent rebound hypoglycemia.

ALCOHOL IN DEXTROSE INFUSIONS   (DEX-trohs)

5% Alcohol and 5% Dextrose in Water, 10% Alcohol and 5% Dextrose in Water (Rx)

See also information on *Dextrose,* p. 1295.

Classification: Caloric agent, carbohydrate.

Action/Kinetics: Alcohol provides 5.6 calories/mL whereas dextrose provides 3.4 calories/gm of d-glucose monohydrate.

Uses: To increase caloric intake and to replenish fluids. *Investigational:* Premature labor (10% solution of alcohol IV).

Contraindications: Diabetic coma, infections of the urinary tract, alcoholism, epilepsy.

Special Concerns: Pregnancy category: C. Use with caution (due to the alcohol) in shock, after cranial surgery, liver or kidney impairment, postpartum hemorrhage, acute intermittent porphyria. Use with caution (due to dextrose) in diabetes mellitus.

Side Effects: *CNS:* Alcohol intoxication if infusion is too rapid, vertigo, disorientation, fever, sedation. *CV:* Venous thrombosis or phlebitis, hypervolemia, extravasation. *Other:* Infection at injection site; alcohol may precipitate gout; reduction in milk-ejecting response (due to alcohol). *Note:* Administration of alcohol during labor may cause depression and intoxication of the infant.

Drug Interactions: Drug interactions due to alcohol in dextrose infusion are due to the alcohol component.

Drug Interactions	
Antidiabetic sulfonylureas	See *Disulfiram;* also, either hypo- or hyperglycemia
Antihypertensives	↑ Vasodilating effect of alcohol
Aspirin	↑ Risk of gastric bleeding
Cefamandole	See *Disulfiram*
Cefoperazone	See *Disulfiram*
CNS depressants	Additive CNS depression
Disulfiram	Acute alcohol intolerance (e.g., flushing, nausea, vomiting, tachycardia, sweating)
Furosemide	↑ Vasodilating effect of alcohol
Metoclopramide	Additive CNS depression
Metronidazole	See *Disulfiram*
Moxalactam	See *Disulfiram*
Phenytoin	Alcohol ↓ half-life of phenytoin by 50–75%
Tolazoline	See *Disulfiram*
Tolbutamide	Alcohol ↓ half-life of tolbutamide by 50–75%

Dosage: Slow IV infusion only. *Individualized depending on age, weight, and clinical state.* **Adults, usual:** 1–2 liters of the 5% solution daily. **Pediatric:** 40 mL/kg/day (from 350–1,000 mL).

NURSING CONSIDERATIONS

See also *Nursing Considerations* for *Carbohydrates,* p. 1293.

Administration/Storage

1. These solutions should be given at a rate that produces neither intoxication nor glycosuria (from 0.5–0.85 gm/kg/hr).
2. Use only clear solutions with the seal intact.
3. Solutions should be protected from extreme heat or freezing.

Assessment

1. Note medications the client is taking to determine if any of them have the potential to interact with the alcohol in the dextrose infusion.
2. Obtain hepatic and renal function studies prior to initiating therapy.

Interventions

1. Determine the client's level of consciousness during the therapy. If any changes occur, slow the rate of infusion and notify the physician.
2. If the client receives the drug during labor, monitor the newborn closely and observe for evidence of intoxication and CNS depression.

DEXTROSE   (DEX-trohs)

Dextrose in Water Injection (D-2½-W, D-5-W, D-10-W, D-20-W, D-25-W, D-30-W, D-38.5-W, D-40-W, D-50-W, D-60-W, D-70-W) (Rx)

Classification: Caloric agent, carbohydrate.

Action/Kinetics: Dextrose provides 3.4 calories/gm of d-glucose monohydrate. Dextrose may result in decreased nitrogen and protein loss, cause increased glycogen storage, and prevent or reduce ketosis. It may also cause diuresis. Dextrose, 5% solution, is isotonic.

Uses: *Up to 10%:* To supply calories and water when nonelectrolytic fluid and caloric replacement are necessary. Also, to spare proteins and minimize loss of electrolytes. *20%:* Provide calories in a minimum amount of water. *25%:* To treat hypoglycemia in neonates or infants. *50%:* To restore blood glucose levels in insulin shock or hyperinsulinemia. *10%–70%:* Used as a source of glucose for central IV infusions.

Additional Contraindications: Hyperglycemia. Concentrated solutions in presence of intraspinal or intracranial hemorrhage, in dehydrated patients with delirium tremens, and in glucose-galactose malabsorption syndrome.

Special Concerns: Pregnancy category: C. Use with caution in infants of diabetic mothers.

Side Effects: Hyperglycemia and glycosuria (especially with rapid injection of hypertonic solutions). *CNS:* Fever, mental confusion, unconsciousness. *CV:* Thrombosis or phlebitis from site of injection, extravasation, hypo- or hypervolemia, dehydration. *Hypertonic solutions:* Irritation to veins, significant hyperglycemia, glycosuria, hyperosmolar syndrome.

Drug Interactions

Corticosteroids/Corticotropin	↑ Retention of sodium ions, especially if parenteral solution contains sodium
Vitamin B complex	Deficiency of vitamin B complex

Dosage: IV. *Individualized,* depending on the age, weight, and condition of the patient. *Insulin-induced hypoglycemia:* **adults and children, IV, usual,** 10–25 g. **neonates/infants, IV, usual,** 250–500 mg/kg/dose (5–10 mL of 25% dextrose in a 5 kg infant). *Older infants or severe cases:* 10–12 mL of 25% dextrose; continuous IV infusion of 10% glucose may be required to stabilize blood glucose levels.

NURSING CONSIDERATIONS

See also *Nursing Considerations* for *Carbohydrates,* p. 1293.

Administration/Storage

1. Maximum rate of administration to avoid hyperglycemia: 0.5 g/kg/hr.
2. Concentrated solutions should not be given IM or SC.
3. Dextrose solutions are available in percentages ranging from 2.5–70%. These solutions should only be used if clear; they should not be frozen or exposed to extreme heat.
4. Concentrations of glucose over 12.5% should only be administered by a central vein after appropriate dilution.
5. Potassium-free solutions may cause significant hypokalemia.
6. Pseudoagglutination may occur if blood is given simultaneously with dextrose through the same infusion set.
7. Additives may be incompatible with dextrose solutions.

Interventions

1. Monitor the client's level of consciousness and serum glucose levels throughout therapy.
2. Assess clients receiving digitalis therapy for hypokalemia, hypophosphatemia and hypomagnesemia. Monitor serum levels periodically and report abnormal findings to the physician.

DEXTROSE AND ELECTROLYTES   (DEX-trohs)

Lytren, Pedialyte, Rehydralyte, Resol (Rx)

Classification: Electrolyte replenisher.

Action/Kinetics: These oral products containing varying amounts of sodium, potassium, chloride, citrate and dextrose (Lytren and Resol contain 20 g/L whereas Pedialyte and Rehydralyte contain 25 g/L). In addition, Resol contains magnesium, calcium, and phosphate. **Time to peak effect:** 8–12 hr.

Uses: Diarrhea. Prophylaxis and treatment of electrolyte depletion in diarrhea or in continuing fluid loss. Maintenance of hydration.

Contraindications: Anuria, oliguria. Severe dehydration including severe diarrhea (IV therapy is necessary for prompt replacement of fluids and electrolytes). Malabsorption of glucose. Severe and sustained vomiting when the patient is unable to drink. Intestinal obstruction, perforated bowel, paralytic ileus.

Special Concerns: Use with caution in premature infants.

Side Effects: Overhydration indicated by puffy eyelids. Hypernatremia, vomiting (usually shortly after treatment has started).

Dosage: Oral Solution. *Mild dehydration:* **Adults and children over 10 years, initial:** 50 mL/kg over 4–6 hr; **maintenance:** 100–200 mL/kg over 24 hr until diarrhea stops. *Moderate dehydration:* **Adults and children over 10 years, initial:** 100 mL/kg over 6 hr; **maintenance:** 15 mL/kg q hr until diarrhea stops. *Moderate to severe dehydration:* **Pediatric, 2–10 years, initial:** 50 mL/kg over the first 4–6 hr followed by 100 mL/kg over the next 18–24 hr; **less than 2 years of age, initial:** 75 mL/kg during the first 8 hr and 75 mL/kg during the next 16 hr.

NURSING CONSIDERATIONS

Administration/Storage

1. No more than 1,000 mL/hr should be given to adults and no more than 100 mL of fluid should be given to children over a 20-min period.
2. The amount and rate of solution should be adjusted depending on need, thirst, and response.
3. Infants and small children should be assisted in drinking the solution slowly and frequently in small quantities and, if necessary, being fed by a spoon.
4. Rehydration solutions should not be diluted with water.

Client/Family Teaching

1. Instruct parents and clients that soft foods such as bananas, cereal, cooked peas, beans and potatoes should be given to maintain nutrition.
2. Explain to parents and clients that if output of fluid exceeds intake, if there is no weight gain, or if clinical symptoms of dehydration persist, client should be seen by the physician immediately.
3. Instruct that if vomiting occurs after oral therapy is initiated, continue therapy but use small amounts of solution administered frequently and slowly.
4. If dehydration is severe, instruct parents and client to seek medical attention immediately. IV fluids and electrolytes should be started since the onset of action of oral solution is too slow. Explain that the oral solution should not be discarded as it can be used for maintenance.

FRUCTOSE (LEVULOSE) IN WATER   (FROOK-tose)

(Rx)

Classification: Caloric agent, carbohydrate.

Action/Kinetics: More rapidly metabolized and converted to glycogen than dextrose. When necessary can be administered more quickly than dextrose (100 g in 1 hr). Suitable for diabetic patients because it does not require insulin to be metabolized.

Uses: To supply calories and water if nonelectrolyte fluids are not required.

Contraindications: Acute hypoglycemia (use dextrose instead), hereditary fructose intolerance. Gout.

Special Concerns: Pregnancy category: C. Safety and effectiveness have not been determined in patients less than 12 years of age.

Side Effects: *CNS:* Fever. *CV:* Hypervolemia, venous thrombosis or phlebitis, extravasation. *Other:* Infection at injection site.

In infants, rapid administration has caused an increase in pulse and respiratory rate and liver size, accompanied by a decrease in blood pH value and CO_2.

Dosage: IV. *individualized depending on weight, age, and clinical condition,* **usual daily dose,** 1–3 liters of 10% solution. **Infants:** 100–1,000 mL of 10% solution; **children:** 200–2,000 mL of 10% solution. Each 10 mL of solution contains approximately 1 g of fructose.

NURSING CONSIDERATIONS

See also *Nursing Considerations* for *Carbohydrates,* p. 1293.

Administration/Storage

1. Use IV only. Unless otherwise instructed, administer slowly, especially in children. The rate should not exceed 1 g/kg/hr.
2. Use only clear solutions with the seal intact.
3. Solutions should be protected from extreme heat or freezing.

INVERT SUGAR

Travert (Rx)

See also information on *Dextrose,* p. 1295, and *Fructose,* p. 1297.

Classification: Caloric agent, carbohydrate.

Action/Kinetics: Equimolar mixture of dextrose and fructose; the combination is more rapidly utilized than dextrose alone. A 5% solution is sometimes administered together with amino acids.

Dosage: IV. *Individualized depending on age, weight, and clinical condition of the patient.* **IV: usual,** 1–3 liters of 10% solution daily.

NURSING CONSIDERATIONS

See also *Nursing Considerations* for *Carbohydrates,* p. 1293.

Administration/Storage

The rate is determined by the reaction of the client.

INTRAVENOUS NUTRITIONAL THERAPY

Action/Kinetics: Intravenous nutrition is an important treatment regimen for patients in whom oral feeding is not possible or is inadequate. There are a large number of products available that provide one or more of the following nutrients: dextrose, electrolytes, amino acids, fat emulsion, vitamins, minerals, and fluids. These preparations are administered IV either peripherally or via a central venous catheter. Such regimens are often referred to as total parenteral nutrition (TPN). The success of TPN is gauged by weight gain and positive nitrogen balance.

The proper administration of TPN products requires a thorough knowledge of the nutritional needs of the patients, as well as of their fluid and electrolyte balance. Central administration, via a central venous catheter, is used in patients requiring long-term parenteral nutrition or in those patients who are severely debilitated. Peripheral parenteral administration is used for short-term parenteral nutrition (up to 12 days), in situations where the caloric requirements are not excessive, or as a supplement to oral feeding. Patients receiving TPN must be frequently evaluated by means of complete laboratory tests.

Uses: In situations where GI absorption of nutrients is impaired due to disease, obstruction, or other drug therapy (e.g., cancer chemotherapy). Following GI surgery or in situations where nutrient requirements are increased as in trauma, burns, or severe infections.

Special preparations are available for use in renal failure, hepatic failure or encephalopathy, or in acute metabolic stress.

Contraindications: Hypersensitivity to specific proteins or inborn errors of amino acid metabolism. Products for general nutritional purposes (e.g., crystalline amino acid infusions) should not be used in severe kidney or liver disease, hyperammonemia, hepatic coma, or encephalopathy. Also, severe uncorrected acid-base imbalance.

Special Concerns: Use with caution in pregnancy. Sodium-containing products should be used with caution in patients with congestive heart failure, renal insufficiency, or edema. Potassium-containing products should be used cautiously in patients with severe renal failure or hyperkalemia. Products containing acetate should be used with care in alkalosis and hepatic insufficiency.

Side Effects: *Metabolic:* Metabolic acidosis or alkalosis, hyperammonemia, ketosis, dehydration, hypo- or hypervitaminosis, elevated hepatic enzymes, electrolyte imbalances, hypophosphatemia, hypocalcemia, osteoporosis, glycosuria, hypervolemia, osmotic diuresis. Rapid withdrawal of concentrated dextrose solutions may result in hypoglycemia. Essential fatty acid deficiency following long-term use of products that are fat free (symptoms include dry, scaly skin, rash resembling eczema, alopecia, slow wound healing, and fatty infiltration of the liver). *Dermatologic:* Skin rashes, flushing, sweating. *Other:* Nausea, vertigo, fever, headache, dizziness. *At site of catheter:* Venous thrombosis, phlebitis.

Drug Interactions	
Folic acid	Precipitation of calcium as calcium folate
Sodium bicarbonate	Precipitation of calcium and magnesium carbonate; ↓ effect of insulin and vitamin B complex with C
Tetracyclines	↓ Effect of amino acids to conserve protein

Dosage: The dose, route of administration, and content of the infusion are determined individually for each patient depending on the nutritional need, physical state, and length of therapy anticipated.

NURSING CONSIDERATIONS

See also *Nursing Considerations* for *Central Parenteral Administration* in Chapter 6, p. 44.

Administration/Storage

1. Appropriate laboratory monitoring with baseline values and evaluation is required before and during administration.
2. Dextrose, 12.5% or greater should not be utilized in peripheral venous infusions.
3. Blood should not be administered through the same infusion site. An exception would be a multi-lumen catheter in the subclavian (or large central) vein.
4. Solutions must be prepared aseptically under a laminar flow hood in the pharmacy.
5. Solutions should be used as soon as possible after preparation. No more than 24 hours should elapse for administration of a single bottle.
6. The IV administration set should be replaced daily.
7. Appropriate guidelines must be followed for clients in whom indwelling catheters will be in place for a long period of time.

8. Administer TPN (total parenteral nutrition) solutions utilizing an electronic infusion device.

9. If the infusion must be discontinued, do not stop the infusion abruptly. Infuse dextrose 10% at the TPN rate until the next bag/bottle is available.

Assessment

1. Obtain a thorough nursing history.

2. Determine that a nutritional assessment is performed by the dietician prior to initiating therapy.

3. Obtain baseline laboratory data including hepatic and renal function studies, blood glucose level, electrolyte levels, pH, protein level and albumin level prior to initiating therapy.

4. Consult the nutritional support team.

5. Determine if the client has a history of allergic responses to protein hydrolysate. This is characterized by pruritus, urticaria, and wheals. Report positive responses and observations to the physician.

Interventions

1. Monitor blood glucose levels at least every 6 hours initially; utilize urine, finger sticks or serum determinations. Generally blood glucose levels over 200 mg/100 mL or fractional urine determinations of 3^+-4^+ indicate the need for insulin to be added to the TPN.

2. Obtain written parameters and guidelines from the physician for controlling hyperglycemia.

3. If the blood glucose level exceeds 1,000 mg/100 mL discontinue TPN and substitute a hypo-osmolar solution to prevent neurologic dysfunction and coma.

4. Monitor and record vital signs, intake and output throughout the therapy.

AMINO ACID FORMULATION FOR HEPATIC FAILURE OR HEPATIC ENCEPHALOPATHY (ah-MEE-no AH-sid)

HepatAmine (Rx)

Classification: Nutritional agent.

Action/Kinetics: This product contains both essential and nonessential amino acids with high levels of branched chain amino acids as leucine, isoleucine, and valine. The branched chain amino acids improve mental status and EEG patterns. Fat emulsion, dextrose, electrolytes, and vitamins may be added if required.

Use: To normalize amino acid levels and improve nitrogen balance in patients with cirrhosis and hepatitis who manifest hepatic encephalopathy.

Additional Contraindication: Anuria.

Special Concerns: Pregnancy category: C.

Dosage: IV: 80–120 g amino acids (equivalent to 12–18 g nitrogen) daily.

NURSING CONSIDERATIONS

See also *Nursing Considerations* for *Intravenous Nutritional Therapy,* p. 1299.

Administration/Storage

1. The total daily fluid intake is usually 2–3 L given over a period of 8–12 hr.

2. Infusion rates should be slow to start and gradually increased from 60–125 mL/hr.

3. The product may be given either peripherally or by central venous indwelling catheter.

AMINO ACID FORMULATION FOR HIGH METABOLIC STRESS   (ah-MEE-no AH-sid)

Aminosyn-HBC 7%, 4% BranchAmin, FreAmine HBC 6.9% (Rx)

Classification: Nutritional agent.

Action/Kinetics: This preparation has similar content as that for hepatic failure.

Use: Acute metabolic stress characterized by increased urinary excretion of nitrogen, hyperglycemia, and decreased concentration or plasma branched chain amino acids.

Additional Contraindications: Anuria, electrolyte imbalance, acid-base imbalance, hepatic coma.

Special Concerns: Pregnancy category: C.

Dosage: IV. *Adults with adequate calories:* 1.5 g/kg (approximate).

NURSING CONSIDERATIONS

See also *Nursing Considerations* for *Intravenous Nutritional Therapy,* p. 1299.

Administration/Storage

This product may be administered either peripherally or by central venous indwelling catheter.

AMINO ACID FORMULATIONS FOR RENAL FAILURE   (ah-MEE-no AH-sid)

Aminess 5.2%, Aminosyn-RF 5.2%, 5.4% NephrAmine, RenAmin (Rx)

Classification: Nutritional agent.

Action/Kinetics: The nutritional requirements for patients with renal disease are different from those for patients with normal renal function. Administration of minimal amounts of essential amino acids enhances utilization of urea. Administration of nonessential amino acids should be restricted. These products promote protein synthesis and improve cellular metabolic balance.

Use: Uremia patients requiring parenteral nutrition.

Additional Contraindications: Acid-base imbalance, electrolyte imbalance, hyperammonemia.

Special Concerns: Pregnancy category: C. Use with caution in children with acute renal failure and in infants with low birth weight.

Dosage: IV. Adults: *Aminess 5.2%,* 400 mL mixed with 500 mL of 70% dextrose (solution contains 2.3% essential amino acids and 30% dextrose). *Aminosyn-RF 5.2%,* 300 mL (up to 600 mL may be used) mixed with 500 mL of 70% dextrose (solution contains 1.96% essential amino acids and 44% dextrose). *5.4% NephrAmine,* 250 mL (up to 500 mL may be used) mixed with 500 mL of 70% dextrose (solution contains 1.8% essential amino acids and 47% dextrose). *RenAmin,* 250–500 mL.
   Pediatric: *Individualized,* **usual,** 0.5–1 g/kg/day (initial doses should be lower and then slowly increased).

NURSING CONSIDERATIONS

See also *Nursing Considerations* for *Intravenous Nutritional Therapy,* p. 1299.

Administration/Storage

1. These products should be given through a central venous catheter at an initial rate not to exceed 20–30 mL/hr for the first 6–8 hr. Then the rate can be increased by 10 mL/hr each 24 hr to a maximum of 60–100 mL/hr.

2. Use of Aminess or NephrAmine in infants may increase the chance of hyperammonemia as these products do not contain arginine.

3. If the hypertonic dextrose solution is discontinued, rebound hypoglycemia may be prevented by giving 5% or 10% dextrose solutions.

CRYSTALLINE AMINO ACID INFUSION   (ah-**MEE**-no **AH**-sid)

Aminosyn 3.5%, 3.5%M, 5%, 8.5%, and 10%; Aminosyn (pH 6) 7% and 8.5%; Aminosyn 7% and 8.5% with Electrolytes; Aminosyn 3.5% with 5% Dextrose; Aminosyn 3.5% or 4.25% with 25% Dextrose; Aminosyn II 3.5%, 5%, 7%, 8.5%, 10%; Aminosyn II 7%, 8.5%, or 10% with Electrolytes; Aminosyn II 3.5% or 3.5%M with 5% Dextrose; Aminosyn II 3.5%, 4.25%, or 5% in 25% Dextrose; Aminosyn II 3.5% or 4.25% with Electrolytes in 25% Dextrose; Aminosyn II 4.25%M in 10% Dextrose; Aminosyn-PF 7% or 10%; Freamine III 8.5% and 10%; Freamine III 3% with Electrolytes; Novamine 11.4% or 15%; Novamine without Electrolytes; Procalamine; Travasol 10%; Travasol 5.5% or 8.5% with Electrolytes; Travasol 5.5% or 8.5% without Electrolytes; 3.5% Travasol with Electrolytes; TrophAmine 6% (Rx)

See information on *Intravenous Nutritional Therapy,* p. 1298.

Classification: Nutritional agent.

Action/Kinetics: These products contain both essential and nonessential amino acids as well as various electrolytes. Dextrose, IV fat emulsion, vitamins, and minerals may be added as required. Percentage refers to the amino acid concentration. The amino acids present in the products either conserve protein or induce protein synthesis by providing the necessary amino acids.

Special Concerns: Pregnancy category: C.

NURSING CONSIDERATIONS

See also *Nursing Considerations* for *Intravenous Nutritional Therapy,* p. 1299.

Administration/Storage

The initial rate of infusion should not exceed 2 mL/min. The rate may then be increased slowly depending on laboratory values of urinary and blood glucose.

INTRAVENOUS FAT EMULSION

Intralipid 10% and 20%, Liposyn 10% and 20%, Liposyn II 10% and 20%, Soyacal 10% and 20%, Travamulsion 10% and 20% (Rx)

Classification: Nutritional agent.

Action/Kinetics: These products contain either soybean oil or safflower oil in a concentration of 10% or 20%, egg yolk phospholipids (1.2%), glycerin (2.21%–2.5%), and water for injection. The fatty acids present in these preparations (linoleic, linolenic, oleic, palmitic, and stearic) provide essential fatty acids to maintain normal cellular membrane function. The products provide from 1.1 cal/mL (10% oil) to 2.0 cal/mL (20% oil). Since it is isotonic, it can be administered into a peripheral vein. The preparations increase heat production, oxygen consumption, and decrease the respiratory quotient (ratio of CO_2/O_2; normal: 0.77–0.90).

Uses: Source of calories and essential fatty acids for prolonged parenteral nutrition (longer than 5 days). Fatty acid deficiency.

Contraindications: Disturbances of fat metabolism (e.g., lipoid nephrosis, pathologic hyperlipidemia, acute pancreatitis with hyperlipemia). Sensitivity to egg yolk.

Special Concerns: Safe use in pregnancy not established (pregnancy category: B for Soyacal 10%; pregnancy category: C for all others). Caution should be exercised when used in premature or jaundiced premature infants. Use with caution in patients with hepatic damage, anemia, respiratory disease, coagulation problems, or possibility of fat embolism.

Side Effects: *Premature infants:* Deaths due to intravascular fat accumulation in the lungs. **Acute untoward reactions.** *GI:* Nausea, vomiting. *CNS:* Headache, fever, drowsiness, dizziness. *Other:* Hyperlipemia, dyspnea, increased coagulation, flushing, sweating, cyanosis, back and chest pain, pressure over eyes, hypersensitivity reactions with urticaria, increases in liver enzymes (transient). Neonates may manifest thrombocytopenia. **Long-term untoward reactions.** *Hepatic:* Jaundice, hepatomegaly, alterations in liver function tests. *Overloading syndrome:* Splenomegaly, focal seizures, fever, leukocytosis, shock. *Other:* Deposition of pigment (brown) in reticuloendothelial system.
   Sepsis and thrombophlebitis due to contamination or procedure.

Dosage: IV. *Total parenteral nutrition,* **Maximum:** 3 g/kg/day. **Pediatric maximum:** 4 g/kg/day. The product should not exceed 60% of daily caloric intake. *Fatty acid deficiency:* Approximately 8%–10% of caloric intake.

NURSING CONSIDERATIONS

See also *Nursing Considerations* for *Intravenous Nutritional Therapy,* p. 1299.

Administration/Storage

1. Discard if oiling out occurs before administration.
2. May be given parenterally or centrally using a separate line, though it can be administered into same peripheral vein as carbohydrate-amino acid solutions using a Y-connection located near the infusion site. Flow rate of each solution should be controlled separately by an infusion pump. Do not use filters.
3. May be mixed with certain nutrient solutions (check package insert).
4. The rate of infusion should be: **Adults: 10% products, initial,** 1 mL/min for first 15–30 min; **then,** if no untoward reactions, increase to 83–125 mL/hr up to 500 mL the first day. Amount may be increased the second day. **Adults: 20% products, initial,** 0.5 mL/min for first 15–30 min; **then,** if no untoward reactions, increase to 62.5 mL/hr up to 250–500 mL (depending on product) the first day. Amount may be increased the second day. Total daily dose should not exceed 3 g/kg. **Pediatric: 10% products, initial,** 0.1 mL/min for first 10–15 min; **then,** if no untoward reactions, increase to maximum of 1 g/kg/4 hr (100 mL/hr). **Pediatric: 20% products, initial,** 0.05 mL/min over the first 10–15 min; **then,** if no untoward reactions, increase to maximum of 1 g/4 hr (50 mL/hr). Total daily dose should not exceed 4 g/kg.
5. Carefully review and follow institutional guidelines for administration of fats.
6. Store in refrigerator at 4°C–8°C (39.2°F–46.4°F) if so designated on product literature.

Interventions

Observe the client closely for the first 10 to 15 minutes of the administration for signs of allergic reaction to the medication. Document and report to the physician immediately and stop the infusion.

CHAPTER SIXTY-NINE
Acidifying and Alkalinizing Agents

Acidifying Agent

Ammonium Chloride *1304*

Alkalinizing Agents

Sodium Bicarbonate *1306*   Tromethamine *1307*
Sodium Lactate *1306*

Potassium-Removing Resin

Sodium Polystyrene Sulfonate *1308*

General Statement: Acidifying and alkalinizing agents are used to alter the pH of the blood, stomach, or the urine for the purpose of correcting acid-base balance, increasing or decreasing the absorption or excretion of certain drugs, or as an adjunct in drug therapy. Caution must be exercised to prevent excesses in changes in pH.

ACIDIFYING AGENT

AMMONIUM CHLORIDE (ah-**MOH**-nee-um)

Ammonium Muriate ✽ (Rx)

Classification: Urinary acidifying agent, diuretic.

Action/Kinetics: The ammonium ion is metabolized to urea liberating hydrogen ions that acidify the urine and decrease the pH of the extracellular fluid and blood. Ammonium chloride also induces diuresis. Ammonium chloride is rapidly absorbed from the GI tract even though the full effect of the drug becomes apparent only after several days.

Uses: Systemic acidifier used for the prevention or correction of metabolic alkalosis due to chloride ion loss caused by vomiting (especially in infants with pyloric obstruction), gastric fistula drainage, gastric suction; to acidify the urine to decrease or promote the excretion of certain drugs. Urinary calculi to promote solubility of calcium and phosphate. Diuretic. Expectorant.

Contraindications: Marked renal and hepatic impairment. Respiratory acidosis. Administration by the SC, rectal, or IP route.

Side Effects: Symptoms are due to overdosage. Severe metabolic acidosis especially in patients with impaired renal function. *Electrolyte:* Hypokalemia, hyperchloremic acidosis. *CV:* Arrhythmias, bradycardia. *GI:* Nausea, vomiting, thirst. *CNS:* Headache, drowsiness, confusion, tonic seizures, twitching, coma. *Other:* Sweating, pallor. *Rapid IV:* Pain, irritation at site or along the vein.

Treatment of Overdosage: Sodium bicarbonate, sodium acetate, or sodium lactate, IV, is used to reverse acidosis or loss of electrolytes. Potassium supplements, PO, will reverse hypokalemia.

Drug Interactions	
Aminosalicylic acid	↑ Chance of aminosalicylic acid crystalluria
Amphetamine	↓ Effect of amphetamine by ↓ renal tubular reabsorption
Antidepressants, tricyclic	↓ Effect of tricyclics by ↓ renal tubular reabsorption
Salicylates	↑ Effect of salicylates by ↑ renal tubular reabsorption

Dosage: Tablets: 1 g daily t.i.d. for no more than 6 days. Drug is more effective as diuretic when rest periods of a few days are part of regimen (i.e., 3 days on, 2 days off).

   IV Infusion. *Metabolic alkalosis:* **Highly individualized,** and based on blood chemistry determinations (CO_2 combining power or chloride ion deficit). Always start with minimal dosage. **Usual, Adults and children:** 10 mL/kg of 2.14% solution at a rate of 0.9–1.3 mL/minute up to 2 mL/minute.

NURSING CONSIDERATIONS

Administration/Storage

1. To minimize GI effects, give the medication after meals or as enteric-coated tablets.
2. Administer the liquid form with acid juices, raspberry, or cherry syrup to mask the saline taste.
3. Do not administer with milk or any other alkaline solution. These are not compatible with ammonium chloride.
4. When administered parenterally for metabolic alkalosis the dose is highly individualized and based on the client's blood chemistry.
5. Have sodium bicarbonate or sodium lactate available for treatment of electrolyte loss and/or metabolic acidosis.

Assessment

1. Obtain baseline serum ammonium levels and serum electrolyte levels prior to beginning therapy.
2. Note if the client is taking any salicylates, antidepressants, quinidine or amphetamines.
3. Determine if the client has any history of impaired renal or hepatic function. The drug should not be administered to clients with a history of hepatic impairment.

Interventions

1. Monitor serum electrolyte levels, pH, and carbon dioxide combining power periodically during therapy to assure that serious acidosis does not occur.
2. Monitor the client's urinary pH, hepatic and renal function studies.
3. Observe the client for twitching, hand flapping tremors (asterixis) or development of tonic seizures. Monitor the level of consciousness and notify the physician immediately if there is any change. This is especially important when the client is receiving ammonium chloride IV.

69

4. Observe the client for an increase in pallor, sweating, irregular breathing, and cardiac arrhythmias. These are signs of possible ammonium toxicity and should be documented and reported to the physician.

5. If the client develops hypokalemia, anticipate that potassium supplements will be ordered.

6. Note if the client develops any alteration in voiding patterns and report if evident.

7. If the drug is being used as a diuretic, anticipate intermittent administration.

ALKALINIZING AGENTS

SODIUM BICARBONATE

Arm and Hammer Pure Baking Soda, Bell/ans, Citrocarbonate, Neut, Soda Mint (Rx and OTC)

See information on *Sodium Bicarbonate,* Chapter 52, p. 1029.

SODIUM LACTATE

(Rx)

Classification: Systemic alkalinizing agent.

Action/Kinetics: The alkalinizing effect occurs due to metabolism of sodium lactate to bicarbonate (usually takes 1–2 hr) in the liver with removal of both lactate and hydrogen. The lactate ion is eventually metabolized to carbon dioxide and water. However, sodium bicarbonate is usually preferred as an alkalinizing agent.

Uses: Metabolic acidosis.

Contraindications: Congestive heart failure, edema, oliguria, anuria, in patients receiving cortcosteroids, pulmonary edema, metabolic or respiratory alkalosis, severe hepatic insufficiency, shock, hypoxia, hypernatremia. Lactic acidosis.

Side Effects: Metabolic acidosis (from overtreatment). Reactions at the injection site including infection, thrombosis, phlebitis, extravasation.

Dosage: IV Infusion. *Highly individualized* and based on blood level of sodium ion. The following formula can be used to estimate correct dose:

$$\text{Dose in mL of } \tfrac{1}{6} \text{ M sodium lactate (167 mEq/liter each of sodium and lactate ions)} = \frac{(60 - \text{plasma } CO_2) \times}{(0.8 \text{ body weight in pounds})}$$

Alkalinization of urine: 30 mL/kg/day in divided doses.

NURSING CONSIDERATIONS

Administration/Storage

Administration rate should not exceed 300 mL/hour of 1/6 M solution.

Interventions

1. Monitor serum electrolytes, glucose and pH levels routinely.
2. Monitor and evaluate client's hepatic and renal function studies during prolonged therapy.
3. Record intake and output. Weigh the client and monitor vital signs. Note any abnormal readings or evidence of fluid retention and report to the physician.
4. This drug is *not* indicated for the treatment of lactic acidosis.

TROMETHAMINE (troh-**METH**-ah-meen)
Tham, Tham-E (Rx)

Classification: Systemic alkalinizing agent.

Action/Kinetics: Tromethamine, an organic amine, is a buffering and systemic alkalinizing agent. It actively binds hydrogen ions, thereby decreasing and correcting acidosis. It promotes the excretion of acids, carbon dioxide, and electrolytes and is thought to be able to neutralize some intracellular acid. It acts as an osmotic diuretic, increasing urine flow. Seventy-five percent of the drug is eliminated within 8 hr, the remainder within 3 days.

Uses: Prevention and correction of systemic acidosis, especially that accompanying cardiac bypass surgery and cardiac arrest.

Contraindications: Uremia and anuria, pregnancy.

Special Concerns: Pregnancy category: C. Use with caution in newborns and infants. Administer with caution to patients with renal disorders.

Side Effects: *Respiratory:* Respiratory depression. *Other:* Fever, hypervolemia, transient decrease of blood glucose. *At injection site:* Extravasation, phlebitis, venous thrombosis, infection. *In newborn:* Hemorrhagic liver necrosis when given by umbilical vein.

Dosage: Slow IV. Minimum amount to correct acid-base imbalance. The amount of tromethamine can be estimated using the buffer base deficit of the extracellular fluid:

$$\text{mL of 0.3 M tromethamine solution required} = \text{body weight (kg)} \times \text{base deficit (mEq/L)} \times 1.1$$

Dose of tromethamine without electrolyte. *Acidosis in cardiac bypass surgery:* **Adults,** 500 mL (150 mEq). Severe cases may require 1,000 mL. *Acidosis in cardiac arrest* (given at the same time other standard procedures are being applied): **if chest is open, Adults,** 65–185 mL (2–6 g) into the ventricular cavity (not into the cardiac muscle); **if chest closed,** 111–333 mL (3.6–10.8 g) into a large peripheral vein. *For acidity in acid citrate dextrose (ACD) blood:* 15–77 mL (0.5–2.5 g) added to each 500 mL of ACD blood.

Dose of tromethamine with electrolytes. *Acidosis in cardiac bypass surgery:* **Adults, usual,** 694 mL (25 g) given at a rate of 0.14 mL/kg/min. *Acidosis in cardiac arrest* (given at the same time as other standard procedures are being applied): **if chest is open, Adults,** 55–165 mL (2–6 g) into the ventricular cavity (not into the cardiac muscle); **if chest closed, Adults,** 100–300 mL (3.6–10.8 g) into a large peripheral vein. *For acidity in acid citrate dextrose (ACD) blood:* 14–70 mL (0.5–2.5 g) added to each 500 mL of ACD blood.

NURSING CONSIDERATIONS

Administration/Storage

1. Tests on blood pH, pCO_2, bicarbonate, glucose, and electrolytes should be determined before, during, and after administration of tromethamine.

2. Concentration of solution administered *must not* exceed 0.3 M.

3. Prepare a 0.3-M solution of tromethamine by adding 1,000 mL of sterile water for injection to 36 g of lyophilized tromethamine.

4. Infuse slowly.

5. Administer into the largest antecubital vein through a large needle or indwelling catheter and elevate limb.

6. For treatment of cardiac arrest, the drug may be injected into the ventricular cavity if the chest is open. If the chest is not open, the drug may be injected into a large peripheral vein.

7. Do not administer longer than 1 day unless acute life-threatening situation exists.

8. Discontinue administration *immediately,* if extravasation occurs.

   • Administer 1% procaine hydrochloride with hyaluronidase to reduce venospasm and to dilute the drug in the tissues.

   • Phentolamine mesylate (Regitine) has been used for local infiltration for its adrenergic blocking properties.

   • If necessary, a nerve block of the autonomic fibers may be done.

Assessment

1. Note if the client has any history of urinary or bladder problems.

2. Obtain renal and hepatic function studies prior to administration of the medication to serve as baseline data against which to compare once medication therapy has been initiated.

3. If the client is female and of childbearing age, check to determine if she is pregnant.

Interventions

1. Observe for respiratory depression and have mechanical ventilation equipment available.

2. Observe the client for complaints of weakness, the presence of moist pale skin, tremors, and a full bounding pulse. These are symptoms of hypoglycemia which can occur after a rapid or high dose of the drug has been administered. Document and report immediately to the physician.

3. Assess the client for nausea, diarrhea, tachycardia, oliguria, weakness, numbness or tingling sensations. These are symptoms of hyperkalemia and are more likely to occur in clients with impaired renal function.

4. Maintain an accurate record of intake and output.

5. Monitor serum electrolytes, blood glucose levels, pH, and hepatic and renal function studies periodically throughout drug therapy. Report any abnormal findings to the physician.

6. Observe the client closely for extravasation. The drug is extremely irritating to the vein.

POTASSIUM-REMOVING RESIN

SODIUM POLYSTYRENE SULFONATE   (pol-ee-STY-reen SUL-fon-ayt)

Kayexalate (Rx)

Classification: Potassium ion exchange resin.

Action/Kinetics: Sodium polystyrene sulfonate is a resin that exchanges sodium ions for potassium ions primarily in the large intestine. Thus, excess amounts of potassium (as well as calcium and magnesium) may be removed. Therapy is governed by daily monitoring of serum potassium levels. Discontinue therapy when serum potassium levels have reached 4–5 mEq/L. Patients should also be monitored for serum calcium and magnesium levels. **Onset, PO:** 2–12 hr.

Uses: Hyperkalemia.

Special Concerns: Use with caution in geriatric patients as they are more likely to develop fecal impaction. Use with caution in patients sensitive to sodium overload (e.g., in cardiovascular disease) or for those receiving digitalis preparations since the action of these agents is potentiated by hypokalemia.

Side Effects: *GI:* Nausea, vomiting, constipation, anorexia, gastric irritation, diarrhea (rarely). Fecal impaction in geriatric patients. *Electrolyte:* Sodium retention, hypokalemia, hypocalcemia, hypomagnesemia. *Other:* Overhydration, pulmonary edema.

Drug Interactions	
Aluminum hydroxide	↑ Risk of intestinal obstruction
Calcium- or magnesium-containing antacids or laxatives	↑ Risk of metabolic alkalosis

Dosage: Powder for Suspension, Suspension. Adults, PO: 15 g resin suspended in 20–100 mL water or syrup (to increase palatability) 1–4 times daily. Up to 40 g daily have been used. **Pediatric:** To calculate dose, use an exchange ratio of 1 mEq potassium/g resin (usually, 1 g/kg per dose). **Enema:** 25–100 g suspended in 100 mL sorbitol or 20% dextrose in water q 6 hr.

NURSING CONSIDERATIONS

Administration/Storage

1. To treat or to prevent constipation, 10–20 mL of 70% sorbitol may be given PO q 2 hr (or as necessary) to produce 1–2 watery stools each day.
2. For oral administration, give the resin suspended in water or syrup (3–4 mL/g resin). If necessary, the resin can be administered through a nasogastric tube, either as an aqueous suspension, mixed with dextrose, or as a peanut or olive oil emulsion.
3. Rectal administration:
   - First, administer a cleansing enema.
   - To administer medication, insert a large-size rubber tube (e.g., French 28) into the rectum for a distance of 20 cm until it is well into the sigmoid colon and tape in place.
   - Suspend resin in appropriate vehicle (see *Dosage*) at body temperature. Administer by gravity while stirring suspension.
   - Flush suspension that remains in the container with 50–100 mL fluid, clamp the tube, and leave in place.
   - Elevate client's hips, or ask the client to assume a knee-chest position, for a short time if there is back-leakage.
   - The enema should be kept in the colon as long as possible (3–4 hr).
   - Resin is removed by colonic irrigation with 2 quarts of a *nonsodium*-containing solution warmed to body temperature. Returns are drained constantly through a Y-tube.
4. Retention enemas of the resin are less effective than oral administration.
5. Use freshly prepared solutions within 24 hr. Do not heat resin.
6. Oral suspension products contain sorbitol and sodium.

7. Orders for the drug should designate the grams of powder and the percent sorbitol and volume to be used or the amount of premixed suspension. The frequency and route of administration should also be specified.

Assessment

Determine if the client has a history of cardiovascular disease and/or is taking digitalis preparations. These clients are at risk for having hypokalemia potentiated by this drug.

Interventions

1. Monitor renal function studies and the level of serum potassium, sodium, magnesium, and calcium. Observe the client for any signs of electrolyte imbalance.
2. The administration of calcium- or magnesium-containing antacids during oral administration of sodium polystyrene sulfonate may predispose the client to metabolic alkalosis. Therefore, administer antacids cautiously.
3. Monitor vital signs and intake and output. If the client has an increase in urinary output, report this finding to the physician.
4. Encourage clients receiving the medication rectally to retain the medication for several hours to ensure effectiveness of drug therapy.

Evaluation

Obtain serum potassium level to determine effectiveness of drug therapy.

PART TWELVE
Miscellaneous Agents

12

CHAPTER SEVENTY
Vitamins

70

Vitamin A   *1313*

General Statement: Vitamins are divided into fat-soluble (A, D, E, K) and water-soluble (B complex, C) vitamins. Vitamins are necessary for the normal metabolic functioning of the body. Although a normal diet usually provides sufficient vitamins, supplemental vitamins are of value in certain disease states (e.g., malabsorption syndrome, blood dyscrasias), during pregnancy, and for

1311

children during maximum periods of growth. However, there is no advantage of giving patients excessive amounts of vitamins and, in fact, this practice may be dangerous if fat soluble vitamins are given in excess.

The Recommended Daily Allowances (RDA) have been determined for vitamins (see Table 31, p. 1314.) and serve as a guide to ensure adequate nutrition for various age groups. The body also requires small amounts of certain minerals as iodine, magnesium, iron, calcium, phosphorus, copper, zinc, and manganese.

NURSING CONSIDERATIONS

Assessment

1. Obtain a complete dietary history of the client. Refer client to the dietician for a baseline nutritional assessment.
2. Observe clients for symptoms of vitamin deficiency, such as an inflamed tongue, cracks at the corners of the mouth and blunted, turned down fingernails.
3. Evaluate for a history of any infections or inflammatory conditions that would cause prolonged diarrhea, anorexia, or drug induced malabsorption that could lead to poor absorption of food.
4. Determine if the client has a history of renal disease, cirrhosis of the liver or a genetic defect that would lessen the ability of the body to utilize vitamins and minerals.
5. Note if the client is receiving hemodialysis or has some physical condition that tends to increase the loss of nutrients.
6. Assess the client's age, physical activity, and whether or not the client is pregnant. These states increase the individual's nutrition requirements.
7. Note the client's educational level, earning capacity, and general ability to provide nutrition for self and family.

Client/Family Teaching

1. Provide the client with printed materials explaining the recommended daily allowances for vitamins and minerals. Review with clients and discuss any problems they may have in meeting the nutritional needs of self and family. Where necessary, direct the client to a dietitian for help in understanding basic concepts in nutrition and meal planning. When economically necessary refer to a state or federal agency for assistance in obtaining adequate food supplies.
2. Advise clients in how to read labels to ensure they are purchasing nutritious foods for themselves and family.
3. Discuss with the clients low-cost foods that will meet their nutritional needs.
4. Discuss cultural foods, their nutritional value, and how they may be used to encourage eating where anorexia may be a problem.
5. Explain the uses of vitamin preparations, how to read the labels, and how to determine that vitamins purchased will meet the client's daily requirements. Assure clients that unless the physician has ordered larger doses of vitamin supplements, they likely do not need them.
6. Advise clients that overdosing of vitamins is dangerous and can cause severe health problems. Minerals should be taken only on the advice of the physician.
7. Vitamins should be stored in a cool, dry place and should be in light-resistant containers. These measures are to minimize the loss of vitamin potency.
8. Advise clients who take mineral oil that they should not take this at the same time as they take fat-soluble vitamins. Vitamins A, D, E, and K will be dissolved in the oil and will not be absorbed by the body.
9. Explain the need to keep all vitamins out of the reach of children. Overdosage of vitamins for a child can be lethal.

10. If the vitamins are to be used for a child, discuss the use of vitamins especially designed for them and explain why adult dosages are inappropriate. Encourage the parent to consult with the physician. If the situation is such that the client has no physician, advise the client to consult with the pharmacist.

VITAMIN A

Alphalin, Aquasol A (Rx and OTC)

Classification: Fat-soluble vitamin.

Action/Kinetics: The active principle of vitamin A is retinol. One international unit or USP unit of vitamin A is equivalent to 0.3 mcg of retinol, 0.6 mcg of beta-carotene, or 12 mcg of carotenoid provitamins. Beta-carotene, known as provitamin A, is converted to retinol after absorption from the GI tract. Vitamin A has an important role in night vision, the physiology of the epithelial tissue (prevention of follicular keratosis), and bone growth and regeneration. It may also function as a cofactor in various biochemical reactions. Vitamin A deficiency can result in night-blindness (xerophthalmia), blindness, growth retardation, thickening of bone, lowered resistance to infection, hyperkeratinization, and tooth malformation. Excess vitamin A can result in hypervitaminosis A, which can be reversed by withdrawal of the vitamin. Regular intake of normal doses of vitamin A or its precursors seems to increase protection from cancer.

Retinol combines with opsin (red protein moiety of visual pigment), forming rhodopsin, necessary for darkness adaptation. Absorption of vitamin A requires bile acids, dietary fat, and pancreatic lipase. It is mainly stored in the liver both in parenchymal cells and nonparenchymal fat-storing cells with small amounts stored in the lung and kidney. Serum levels of vitamin A range from 80–130 IU/mL.

Uses: Vitamin A deficiency and prophylaxis during periods of high requirement, such as infancy, pregnancy, and lactation. Supplements may also be required in patients with cirrhosis of the liver, partial gastrectomy, biliary tract disease, sprue, colitis, celiac disease, pancreatic disease, regional enteritis, cystic fibrosis, and steatorrhea.

Contraindications: Pregnancy (pregnancy category: X). Hypervitaminosis A, IV use, orally in malabsorption syndrome. Systemically for treatment of acne.

Special Concerns: Young children are more sensitive to high doses of vitamin A.

Side Effects: Hypervitaminosis A, characterized by the following symptoms: *CNS:* Increased intracranial pressure/pseudotumor cerebri manifested by bulging fontanels, exophthalmos, papilledema, headache, vertigo, irritability, fatigue, malaise, lethargy. *GI:* Anorexia, vomiting, abdominal discomfort. *Dermatologic:* Inflammation of the tongue, lips, and gums; pruritus, erythema, alopecia, drying and cracking of skin, lip fissures, desquamation, scaling, increased pigmentation. *Skeletal:* Slow growth, bone pain, premature epiphyseal closure, arthralgia, cortical thickening over radius and tibia. *Miscellaneous:* Night sweats, hypomenorrhea, jaundice, leukopenia, edema of legs, hepatosplenomegaly. High plasma levels also manifest hypercalcemia, polydipsia, and polyuria.

Drug Interactions	
Anticoagulants	Large doses of vitamin A → hypoprothrombinemia when taken with anticoagulants
Cholestyramine	↓ Absorption of vitamin A from the intestine
Colestipol	↓ Absorption of vitamin A from the intestine

Table 31   Vitamins and Related Substances

Substance*/RDA	Use	Good Food Source	Usual Therapeutic Dose
Vitamin A 4,000–5,000 IU; Retinol equivalents (RE): 800–1,000 mcg; Children, 1–10 years: 400–700 mcg RE: Infants up to 1 year: 375 mcg RE	Helps form and maintain healthy function of eyes, skin, hair, teeth, gums, various glands, and mucous membranes. It is also involved in fat metabolism. *Deficiency symptoms*: night blindness, hyperkeratosis of skin, xerophthalmia.	Whole milk, eggs, dark green or deep yellow vegetables (e.g., spinach, kale, broccoli, turnip greens, brussel sprouts, carrots, squash), melons, berries.	Up to 100,000 units/day
Vitamin B₁ (thiamine): 1.0–1.5 mg; Children, 1–10 years: 0.7–1 mg; Infants up to 1 year: 0.3–0.4 mg	Helps get energy from food by promoting proper metabolism of sugars. *Deficiency symptoms*: beriberi, peripheral neuritis, cardiac disease.	Milk; chicken; fish; red meat; liver; whole grain bread; green, leafy vegetables.	5–30 mg/day
Vitamin B₂ (riboflavin): 1.2–1.8 mg; Children, 1–10 years: 0.8–1.2 mg; Infants up to 1 year: 0.4–0.5 mg	Functions in the body's use of carbohydrates, proteins and fats, particularly to release energy to cells. *Deficiency symptoms*: cheilosis, angular stomatitis, dermatitis, photophobia, growth retardation in the young.	Milk; eggs; red meat; liver; whole grain enriched bread; green, leafy vegetables; nuts; seeds.	10–30 mg/day
Vitamin B₆ (pyridoxine): 1.4–2.0 mg; Children, 1–10 years: 1–1.4 mg; Infants up to 1 year: 0.3–0.6 mg	Has many important roles in protein metabolism. Also aids in the formation of red blood cells and in the proper function of the nervous system, including brain cells. *Deficiency symptoms*: seborrhea-like skin lesions; nerve inflammations, anemias, epileptiform convulsions in infants.	Green, leafy vegetables; red meat; whole grains; green beans.	25–100 mg/day
Vitamin B₁₂ (cyanocobalamin): 2.0 mcg; Children, 1–10 years: 0.7–1.4 mcg; Infants up to 1 year: 0.3–0.5 mcg	Helps to build vital genetic material (nucleic acids) for cell nuclei, and to form red blood cells. Essential for normal function of all body cells, including brain and other nerve cells as well as tissues that make red cells. *Deficiency symptoms*: megaloblastic anemia, pernicious anemia.	Milk, fish (saltwater), red meat, liver, oysters, kidneys.	1–2 mg/day

1314

Folate: 0.15–0.2 mg; Children, 1–10 years: 0.05–0.1 mg; Infants up to 1 year: 0.025–0.035 mg	Assists in the formation of certain body proteins and genetic materials for the cell nucleus, and in the formation of red blood cells with cyanocobalamin. *Deficiency symptoms*: macrocytic anemia (nutritional).	Green, leafy vegetables; liver.	1–15 mg/day
Pantothenic acid: 10 mg	Is a key substance in body metabolism involved in changing carbohydrates, fats, and proteins into molecular forms needed by the body. Is also required for formation of certain hormones and nerve-regulating substances. *Deficiency symptoms* (rare): fatigue, malaise, headache, sleep disturbance, cramps, tenderness in heels.	Eggs; green, leafy vegetables; nuts; liver; kidneys.	5–10 mg/day
Niacin (niacinamide B_3): 13–20 mg; Children, 1–10 years: 9–13 mg; Infants up to 1 year: 5–6 mg	Is present in all body tissues and is involved in energy-producing reactions in cells. Essential for synthesis of fatty acids and cholesterol. *Deficiency symptoms*: pellagra.	Eggs, red meat, liver, whole grain, whole grain enriched bread.	100–1,000 USP units/day
Biotin: 0.30 mg	Is involved in the formation of certain fatty acids and the production of energy from the metabolism of glucose. Is essential for the working of many chemical systems in the body. *Deficiency symptoms*: dermatitis, glossitis, depression, muscle pains.	Eggs; green, leafy vegetables; string beans; kidneys; liver.	

Table 31 (continued)

Substance*/RDA	Use	Good Food Source	Usual Therapeutic Dose
Vitamin C: 50–60 mg; Children, 1–10 years: 40–45 mg; Infants up to 1 year: 30–35 mg	Helps form and keep bones, teeth, and blood vessels healthy. Is also important in the formation of collagen, a protein that helps support body structures such as skin, bone, and tendon. Prevents excessive oxidation of vitamins A and E and polyunsaturated fats; converts folacin to folinic acid. May assist in resistance to infection, carcinogenesis, and tumor growth. *Deficiency symptoms*: scurvy (hemorrhage, loose teeth, gingivitis).	Potatoes; dark green, leafy vegetables; tomatoes; green peppers; broccoli; cabbage; citrus fruits and juices; melons; berries.	100–1,000 mg/day
Vitamin D (including D$_2$ and D$_3$): 200–400 IU; 10 mcg cholecalciferol = 400 IU vitamin D; Children, 1–10 years: 400 IU; Infants, up to 1 year: 300–400 IU	Is essential for strong teeth and bones and helps the body use calcium and phosphorus properly. *Deficiency symptoms*: infantile rickets, infantile tetany, osteomalacia.	Milk, egg yolks, tuna, salmon, cod liver oil.	400–1,600 USP units/day
Vitamin E (tocopherol): 12–15 IU; (1.49 IU = 1 mg d-alpha-tocopherol); Children, 1–10 years: 9–10 IU; Infants up to 1 year: 4–6 IU	Protects fat in the body's tissue from abnormal breakdown. *Deficiency symptoms*: abnormal fat deposits, creatinuria, macrocytic anemia (when associated with protein deficiency). Hemolytic anemia in low-birth-weight babies.	Vegetable oil, whole grains.	Not established
Vitamin K: 45–80 mcg; Children, 1–10 years: 15–30 mcg; Infants up to 1 year: 5–10 mcg	Is essential for normal blood clotting. *Deficiency symptoms*: hemorrhages, prolonged clotting time. Hemorrhagic disease in newborns.	Green, leafy vegetables.	See drug entry.
Calcium: 800–1,200 mg; Children, 1–10 years: 800 mg; Infants up to 1 year: 400–600 mg	Helps build strong bones and teeth. Is also required for activity of nerve and muscle cells, including the heart, and for normal blood clotting.	Milk, egg yolks, tuna, salmon, cheese.	

Copper 2.0 mg	Is present in many organs, including the brain, liver, heart, and kidneys. Occurs as part of important proteins, including certain enzymes involved in brain and red blood cell function. Also needed for making red blood cells.	Kidneys, nuts, raisins, chocolate, mushrooms.
Iodine: 150 mcg; Children, 1–10 years: 70–120 mcg Infants up to 1 year: 40–50 mcg	Forms an integral part of hormones produced by the thyroid gland, which is involved in the regulation of cell metabolism.	Seafood (shrimp, oysters, fish) and iodized salt.
Iron: 10–15 mg; Children, 1–10 years: 10 mg; Infants up to 1 year: 6–10 mg	An essential part of hemoglobin, it is the protein substance that enables red blood cells to carry oxygen throughout the body. Is also part of certain important enzymes.	Red meat, egg yolks, liver, green vegetables (e.g., spinach, kale, broccoli, chard, turnip greens, brussels sprouts), raw oysters, sardines, tuna fish, walnuts, beans.
Magnesium: 270–400 mg; Children, 1–10 years: 80–170 mg; Infants up to 1 year: 40–60 mg	Is an important constituent of all soft tissues and bones. Helps trigger many vital enzyme reactions in humans.	Broccoli, whole grain enriched bread, meat.
Phosphorus: 800–1,200 mg; Children, 1–10 years: 800 mg; Infants up to 1 year: 300–500 mg	Is essential in building and maintaining strong teeth and bones, in quick release of energy, in muscle contraction, and in nerve function.	Milk, fish, meat, whole grains, cottage cheese, swiss cheese, yogurt.
Chromium Cobalt Fluorine Manganese Molybdenum Selenium: 40–70 mcg; Children, 1–10 years: 20–30 mcg Infants up to 1 year: 10–15 mcg	Zinc is considered essential every day for normal skeletal growth and tissue repair. Fluorine makes the teeth harder. Cobalt is an integral part of the vitamin B_{12} molecule. The others are needed in a wide variety of body functions.	Whole grains, broccoli, liver, meat, strawberries, oranges.
Zinc: 12–15 mg; Children, 1–10 years: 10 mg; Infants up to 1 year: 5 mg		

*Unless indicated otherwise, values given are *Recommended Daily Allowances* for individuals 11 years of age and older. National Academy of Science, 1989.

Drug Interactions

Corticosteroids	Impairment of wound healing in patients receiving topical vitamin A—systemic vitamin A may inhibit anti-inflammatory effect of systemic corticosteroids
Isotretinoin	Additive toxic effects
Mineral oil	↓ Absorption of vitamin A from intestine
Neomycin (oral)	↓ Absorption of vitamin A from intestine
Oral contraceptives	Oral contraceptives ↑ plasma vitamin A levels
Sucralfate	↓ Absorption of vitamin A from intestine
Vitamin E	↑ Absorption, storage, and use of vitamin A → ↓ toxicity

Dosage: Capsules, Oral Solution, Tablets. *Deficiency:* **Adults,** 10,000–25,000 daily for 1–2 weeks or until improvement occurs. **Pediatric:** 5,000 Units/kg daily. *Deficiency with xerophthalmia:* **Adults,** 25,000–50,000 Units daily. **Pediatric:** 5,000 Units/kg daily for 5 days; **then,** combine with IM vitamin A (25,000 Units/day) until recovery.

IM. *Deficiency:* **Adults and children over 8 years of age,** 50,000–100,000 Units/day for 3 days; **then,** 50,000 Units/day for 2 weeks. **Pediatric, up to 1 year:** 5,000–10,000 Units/day for 10 days (if severe deficiency, 7,500–15,000 Units/day for 10 days). **Pediatric, 1–8 years:** 5,000–15,000 Units/day for 10 days (if severe deficiency, 17,500–35,000 Units/day for 10 days).

NURSING CONSIDERATIONS

See also *Nursing Considerations* for *Vitamins,* p. 1312.

Assessment

1. Note if the client has malabsorption syndrome.
2. Determine if the client has night blindness.
3. Observe the client for dryness of mucous secreting cells of the mouth, eye, and skin. Assess the client's tendency for increased infections and the development of skin lesions.
4. Determine if the client has cirrhosis. Impaired hepatic function decreases the ability to absorb vitamin A.

Client/Family Teaching

1. Advise clients to avoid excessive intake of vitamin A because of the danger of toxicity.
2. Instruct the client about foods that are high in vitamin A and suggest that they include these in larger amounts in their daily diet.
3. Women of childbearing age and pregnant clients should only take the prescribed dose. Drug safety at higher dosage levels has not been established.
4. Instruct clients taking retinoic acid to avoid excessive exposure to ultraviolet light and/or sunlight.

VITAMIN B COMPLEX

Action/Kinetics: The B vitamins are *coenzymes;* they have a crucial role in the tricarboxylic (TCA, Krebs or citric acid) cycle—the main metabolic pathways that convert carbohydrates (e.g., glucose) to energy (high-energy phosphate bonds).

Drug Interaction: Anticoagulants (oral) may interact with B complex vitamins and cause hemorrhage.

NURSING CONSIDERATIONS

See *Nursing Considerations* for *Vitamins,* p. 1312.

Assessment

Determine if the client is taking oral anticoagulants. These may interact with vitamin B complex and cause hemorrhage.

CYANOCOBALAMIN (VITAMIN B₁₂) (sye-**AN**-oh-koh-**BAL**-ah-min)

Oral: Kaybovite. Parenteral: Anacobin✤, Bedoz✤, Berubigen, Betalin 12, Cyanabin✤, Kaybovite-1000, Redisol, Rubion✤, Rubramin✤, Rubramin PC (OTC, Rx)

Classification: Vitamin B_{12}.

Action/Kinetics: Cyanocobalamin (vitamin B_{12}) is a cobalt-containing vitamin essential to growth. The vitamin can also be isolated from liver and is identical to that of the antianemic factor of liver. This vitamin is required for hematopoiesis, cell reproduction, nucleoprotein and myelin synthesis. Plasma vitamin B_{12} levels: 150–750 pg/mL.

Intrinsic factor is required for adequate absorption of oral vitamin B_{12} and in pernicious anemia and malabsorption diseases intrinsic factor is administered simultaneously. This vitamin is rapidly absorbed following IM or SC administration. Following absorption, vitamin B_{12} is carried by plasma proteins to the liver where it is stored until required for various metabolic functions.

Products containing less than 500 mcg vitamin B_{12} are nutritional supplements and are not to be used for the treatment of pernicious anemia. **$t^{1/2}$:** 6 days (400 days in the liver). **Time to peak levels, after PO:** 8–12 hr.

Uses: Vitamin B_{12} deficiency due to pernicious anemia, cancer of the bowel or pancreas, sprue, total or partial gastrectomy, accompanying folic acid deficiency, GI surgery or pathology, gluten enteropathy, fish tapeworm infestation, bacterial overgrowth of the small intestine.

Also, in conditions with an increased need for vitamin B_{12} such as thyrotoxicosis, hemorrhage, malignancy, pregnancy, and in liver and kidney disease. Vitamin B_{12} is particularly suitable for the treatment of patients allergic to liver extract.

Investigational: Diagnosis of vitamin B_{12} deficiency.

Note: Folic acid is not a substitute for vitamin B_{12} although concurrent folic acid therapy may be required.

Contraindications: Hypersensitivity to cobalt, Leber's disease.

Special Concerns: Pregnancy category: C. Use with caution in patients with gout.

Side Effects: Untoward reactions are manifested following parenteral use. *Allergic:* Urticaria, itching, exanthema, anaphylaxis, shock, death. *CV:* Peripheral vascular thrombosis, congestive heart failure, pulmonary edema. *Other:* Polycythemia vera, optic nerve atrophy in patients with hereditary optic nerve atrophy, diarrhea, hypokalemia, body feels swollen.

Note: Benzyl alcohol, which is present in certain products, may cause a fatal "gasping syndrome" in premature infants.

Drug Interactions	
Alcohol	↓ Vitamin B_{12} absorption
Aminosalicylic acid	↓ Vitamin B_{12} absorption

Drug Interactions (continued)	
Chloramphenicol	Chloramphenicol ↓ response to vitamin B_{12} therapy
Cholestyramine	↓ Vitamin B_{12} absorption
Cimetidine	↓ Digestion and release of Vitamin B_{12}
Colchicine	↓ Vitamin B_{12} absorption
Neomycin	↓ Vitamin B_{12} absorption
Potassium, timed-release	↓ Vitamin B_{12} absorption

Laboratory Test Interferences: Antibiotics may interfere with the microbiologic assay for serum and erythrocyte vitamin B_{12}.

Dosage: Tablets, Soluble Tablets. *Nutritional supplement:* **Adults,** 1 mcg daily (up to 25 mcg for increased requirements). **Pediatric, up to 1 year:** 0.3 mcg daily; **over 1 year:** 1 mcg daily.

   IM, Deep SC. *Treatment of deficiency:* **Adults,** 100 mcg daily for 6–7 days; **then,** 100 mcg every other day for 7 doses. If improvement is noted along with a reticulocyte response, 100 mcg q 3–4 days for 2–3 weeks; **maintenance, IM:** 100–200 mcg once a month. **Pediatric, initial:** 30–50 mcg daily for 2 or more weeks (total dose of 1–5 mg); **maintenance:** 100 mcg once a month. *Diagnosis of vitamin B_{12} deficiency:* **Adults, IM,** 1 mcg/day for 10 days plus low dietary folic acid and vitamin B_{12}. Loading dose for the Schilling test is 1,000 mcg given IM.

NURSING CONSIDERATIONS

See also *Nursing Considerations* for *Vitamins,* p. 1312.

Administration/Storage

1. Protect cyanocobalamin crystalline injection from light.
2. The medication should not be frozen.
3. Have epinephrine, antihistamines and steroids available in the event of an adverse drug reaction.
4. Note that if the client is being treated for pernicious anemia, the drug cannot be administered orally.

Assessment

1. Determine if the client is allergic to cobalt.
2. Note if the client has been taking chloramphenicol. This drug antagonizes the hematopoietic response to vitamin B_{12}.
3. Determine if the client is taking any other drugs that could cause an unfavorable response to vitamin B_{12}.
4. Perform a baseline assessment of the client's peripheral pulses.

Interventions

1. Observe the client for urticaria, complaints of itching, and evidence of anaphylaxis. Report these findings to the physician immediately.
2. If the client complains of diarrhea, monitor the frequency and consistency of stools. If the diarrhea is severe or persists, a change in drug may be required.
3. Monitor serum potassium levels if the client is being treated for megaloblastic anemia.

Client/Family Teaching

1. If the client is being treated for pernicious anemia, stress that vitamin B$_{12}$ *must* be taken for life.
2. Advise the client that when repository vitamin B$_{12}$ is used, it will provide medication for at least 4 weeks.
3. Explain that the stinging, burning sensation that may occur after injection is transitory. However, remind the client that if the burning sensation occurs anywhere except where the needle is, to call it to the nurse's attention immediately. The needle should be withdrawn and a different site selected for injection.
4. Where vitamin B$_{12}$ is the result of dietary deficiency, discuss diet with the client. Provide printed material concerning appropriate foods and review with the client methods of achieving a balanced diet. Refer to a dietician for additional assistance as needed.
5. Advise clients to avoid alcohol while they are taking vitamin B$_{12}$ as it will interfere with the absorption of the medication.

FOLIC ACID   (FOH-lik AH-sid)

Apo-Folic ✴, Folvite, Novofolacid ✴ (Rx and OTC)

Classification: Vitamin B complex.

Action/Kinetics: Folic acid (which is converted to tetrahydrofolic acid) is necessary for normal production of red blood cells and for synthesis of nucleoproteins. Synthetic folic acid is absorbed from the GI tract even if the patient suffers from malabsorption syndrome. Is stored in the liver.

Uses: Prophylaxis and treatment of folic acid deficiency (e.g., sprue, pregnancy, infancy or childhood, nutritional causes). Diagnosis of folate deficiency.

Contraindications: Use in aplastic, normocytic, or pernicious anemias (is ineffective). Folic acid injection that contains benzyl alcohol should not be used in neonates or immature infants.

Side Effects: Allergies.

Drug Interactions	
Corticosteroids (chronic use)	↑ Folic acid requirements
Methotrexate	Is a folic acid antagonist
Oral contraceptives	↑ Risk of folate deficiency
Phenytoin	Folic acid ↑ seizure frequency; also, phenytoin ↓ serum folic acid levels.
Pyrimethamine	Folic acid ↓ effect of pyrimethamine in toxoplasmosis; also, pyrimethamine is a folic acid antagonist
Sulfonamides	↓ Absorption of folic acid
Triamterene	↓ Utilization of folic acid as it is a folic acid antagonist
Trimethoprim	↓ Utilization of folic acid as it is a folic acid antagonist

Dosage: Tablets. *Dietary supplement:* **Adults and children:** 100 mcg daily (up to 1 mg in pregnancy); may be increased to 500–1,000 mcg if requirements increase. *Treatment of deficiency:* **Adults, initial:** 250–1,000 mcg daily until a hematologic response occurs; **maintenance:** 400 mcg daily (800 mcg during pregnancy and lactation). **Pediatric, initial:** 250–1,000 mcg daily until a hematologic response occurs. **Maintenance, infants:** 100 mcg daily; **children up to 4 years:** 300 mcg daily; **children 4 years and older:** 400 mcg daily.

IM, IV, Deep SC. *Treatment of deficiency:* **Adults and children:** 250–1,000 mcg daily until a hematologic response occurs. *Diagnosis of folate deficiency:* **Adults, IM:** 100–200 mcg daily for 10 days plus low dietary folic acid and vitamin B_{12}.

NURSING CONSIDERATIONS

See also *Nursing Considerations* for *Vitamins,* p. 1312.

Administration/Storage

1. Folic acid is given orally unless there is severe malabsorption in which case it can be given either IV or SC.
2. Regardless of age, the dosage should never be less than 0.1 mg daily.
3. Folic acid will remain stable in solution if the pH is kept above 5.
4. The drug may be administered IM or by direct IV push or added to infusions. However, if administered by IV, the rate should not exceed 5 mcg/min.
5. When parenteral forms are used, have drugs and equipment available to treat potential allergic drug reactions.

HYDROXOCOBALAMIN (VITAMIN B₁₂ₐ) (hi-drok-so-koh-**BAL**-ah-min)

Acti-B12✦, AlphaRedisol, Codroxomin, Droxomin (Rx)

Classification: Vitamin B complex.

For all information on Hydroxocobalamin, see *Cyanocobalamin,* p. 1319.

Uses: May be preferred to treat vitamin B_{12} deficiency.

Side Effects: Pain at injection site, transient diarrhea; rarely, allergic reaction.

Special Concerns: Pregnancy category: C.

Dosage: IM, Deep SC. *Treatment of deficiency:* **Adults and children,** 30–50 mcg daily (100 mcg if severe megaloblastic anemia) for 5–10 days (2 or more weeks for children for a total dose of 1–5 mg); **maintenance:** 100–200 mcg once a month. *Diagnosis of vitamin B_{12} deficiency:* **Adults, IM,** 1 mcg daily for 10 days plus low dietary folic acid and vitamin B_{12}. The loading dose for the Schilling test of 1,000 mcg.

NURSING CONSIDERATIONS

See *Nursing Considerations* for *Cynocobalamin,* p. 1320, and *Vitamins,* p. 1312.

LEUCOVORIN CALCIUM (CITROVORUM FACTOR, FOLINIC ACID) (loo-koh-**VOR**-in)

Wellcovorin (Rx)

Classification: Folic acid derivative.

Action/Kinetics: Leucovorin is a formyl derivative (reduced form) of folic acid. It does not require reduction by dihydrofolate reductase in order to be active in intracellular metabolism; thus, it is not affected by dihydrofolate inhibitors. Leucovorin is rapidly absorbed following oral administration.

Peak serum levels, PO: Approximately 1.7 hr; **after IM:** approximately 0.7 hr. **Onset, PO:** 20–30 min; **IM:** 10–20 min; **IV:** Less than 5 min. **t½:** 3.5 hr (PO) and 3.7 hr (IM). **Duration:** 3–6 hr. The drug is excreted by the kidney.

Uses: Megaloblastic anemias due to nutritional deficiency, sprue, pregnancy, and infancy. When oral folic acid is not appropriate. Prophylaxis and treatment of toxicity due to methotrexate, pyrimethamine, and trimethoprim. Leucovorin rescue following high doses of methotrexate. *Investigational:* Adjunct with 5-fluorouracil to treat metastatic colorectal carcinoma.

Contraindications: Pernicious anemia or megaloblastic anemia due to vitamin B_{12} deficiency.

Special Concerns: Pregnancy category: C, although it is recommended for megaloblastic anemia caused by pregnancy. Use with caution during lactation. May increase the frequency of seizures in susceptible children.

Side Effects: *Allergic:* Erythema, skin rash, itching, malaise, respiratory difficulties, bronchospasms. High doses may cause: *GI:* Anorexia, nausea, distention, flatulence, bad taste in mouth. *CNS:* Excitement, altered sleep patterns, difficulty in concentration, irritability, overactivity, mental depression, confusion, and impaired judgment.

Drug Interactions	
Aminosalicylic acid	↓ Serum folate levels → folic acid deficiency
Phenytoin	↓ Effect of phenytoin due to ↑ rate of breakdown by liver; also, phenytoin may ↓ plasma folate levels
Primidone	↓ Serum folate levels → folic acid deficiency
Sulfasalazine	↓ Serum folate levels → folic acid deficiency

Dosage: For Oral Solution, Tablets, IM, IV. *Overdose of folic acid antagonists—leucovorin rescue following methotrexate:* **Adults and children:** 10 mg/m² q 6 hr until methotrexate blood level falls to less than 5 x 10⁻⁸ M; if after 24 hr serum creatinine level is 50% greater than premethotrexate serum creatinine levels, increase the dose of leucovorin to 100 mg/m² q 3 hr IV until serum methotrexate is less than 5 x 10⁻⁸ M. *Leucovorin rescue following trimethoprim or pyrimethamine:* **Adults and children,** 5–15 mg daily. *Treatment following pyrimethamine or trimethoprim:* **Adults and children,** 400 mcg–5,000 mcg (5 mg) with each dose of the folic acid antagonist. *Megaloblastic anemia:* **Adults and children,** 1 mg daily.

NURSING CONSIDERATIONS

See also *Nursing Considerations* for *Vitamins,* p. 1312.

Administration/Storage

1. If leucovorin is used for methotrexate rescue purposes, the client should be well hydrated and the urine should be alkalinized in order to reduce nephrotoxicity.
2. Leucovorin calcium injection should be diluted with 5 mL bacteriostatic water for injection and used within one week. If water for injection is employed, the solution should be used immediately.
3. The oral solution is stable for 14 days if refrigerated or for 7 days if stored at room temperature.
4. Doses higher than 25 mg should be given parenterally as oral absorption is saturated.
5. Leucovorin calcium injection containing benzyl alcohol should not be used for doses greater than 10 mg/m².

Assessment

Note if the client has a history of vitamin B_{12} deficiency that has resulted in pernicious anemia or megaloblastic anemia and report.

Interventions

1. Anticipate that leucovorin rescue is used in conjunction with methotrexate therapy.
2. Note any client complaints of skin rash, itching, malaise, or difficulty breathing. Document and report to the physician immediately.
3. If the client is receiving the drug for rescue therapy, it should be administered promptly following a high dose of folic acid antagonists. The prescribed method must be followed exactly in order to be effective.
4. Parenteral therapy generally is utilized following chemotherapy because nausea and vomiting may prevent oral absorption.
5. Leucovorin may obscure the diagnosis of pernicious anemia if previously undiagnosed.
6. Monitor appropriate renal and hematologic values.
7. When high-dose therapy is used be alert for the client exhibiting mental confusion and impaired judgment.

NIACIN (NICOTINIC ACID)   (NYE-ah-sin, nih-koh-TINick AH-sid)

Nia-Bid, Niac, Niacels, Nico-400, Nicobid, Nicolar, Nicotinex, Slo-Niacin, Span-Niacin, Tega-Span, Tri-B3�֍ (Rx and OTC)

NIACINAMIDE   (NYE-ah-SIN-ah-myd)

(Rx: Injection; OTC: Tablets)

Classification: Vitamin B complex.

Action/Kinetics: Niacin (nicotinic acid) and niacinamide are water-soluble, heat-resistant vitamins prepared synthetically. Niacin (after conversion to the active niacinamide) is a component of the coenzymes NAD and NADP, which are essential for oxidation-reduction reactions involved in lipid metabolism, glycogenolysis, and tissue respiration. Deficiency of niacin results in pellagra, the most common symptoms of which are dermatitis, diarrhea, and dementia. In high doses niacin also produces vasodilation and a reduction in serum lipids. **Peak serum levels:** 45 min; **t½:** 45 min.

Uses: Prophylaxis and treatment of pellagra; niacin deficiency. Niacin is also used to treat hyperlipidemia in patients not responding to either diet or weight loss.

Contraindications: Hypotension, hemorrhage, liver dysfunction, peptic ulcer. Use with caution in diabetics, gallbladder disease, and patients with gout.

Special Concerns: Pregnancy category: C. The extended-release tablets and capsules are not recommended for use in children.

Side Effects: *GI:* Nausea, vomiting, diarrhea, peptic ulcer activation, abdominal pain. *Dermatologic:* Flushing, warm feeling, skin rash, pruritus, dry skin, itching and tingling feeling, keratosis nigricans. *Other:* Hypotension, headache, macular cystoid edema, amblyopia. **Note:** Megadoses are accompanied by serious toxicity including the symptoms listed above as well as liver damage, hyperglycemia, hyperuricemia, arrhythmias, tachycardia, and dermatoses.

Drug Interactions	
Chenodiol	↓ Effect of chenodiol
Probenecid	Niacin may ↓ uricosuric effect of probenecid

Drug Interactions (continued)	
Sulfinpyrazone	Niacin ↓ uricosuric effect of sulfinpyrazone
Sympathetic blocking agents	Additive vasodilating effects → postural hypotension

Dosage: *Niacin.* **Extended-release Capsules, Oral Solution, Tablets, Extended-release Tablets.** *Vitamin:* **Adults,** Up to 500 mg daily; **pediatric,** Up to 300 mg daily. *Antihyperlipidemic:* **Adults, initial,** 1 g t.i.d.; **then,** increase dose in increments of 500 mg daily q 2–4 weeks as needed. **Maintenance:** 1–2 g t.i.d. (up to a maximum of 6 g daily). **IM, IV.** *Pellagra:* **Adults, IM,** 50–100 mg 5 or more times daily; **IV, slow,** 25–100 mg 2 or more times daily. **Pediatric, IV slow,** Up to 300 mg daily.

Niacinamide. **Capsules, Tablets.** *Vitamin:* **Adults,** Up to 500 mg daily. **Pediatric:** Up to 300 mg daily. Capsules not recommended for use in children. **IM, IV.** *Pellagra:* **Adults, IM,** 50–100 mg 5 or more times daily; **IV, slow,** 25–100 mg 2 or more times daily. **Pediatric, IV, slow:** Up to 300 mg daily.

NURSING CONSIDERATIONS

See also *Nursing Considerations* for *Vitamins,* p. 1312.

Administration/Storage

1. Nicotinic acid should be taken orally only with cold water (no hot beverages).
2. Can be taken with meals if GI upset occurs.

Client/Family Teaching

1. Advise the client that he/she may feel a warm flushing in the face and ears within 2 hours after taking the medication.
2. Clients who feel weak and dizzy after taking niacin should be instructed to lie down until this feeling passes and to inform the physician of this occurrence.
3. Instruct clients to report for scheduled lab studies.
4. Clients who have diabetes mellitus should not take niacin unless specifically ordered. Then the blood glucose levels must be closely monitored for hyperglycemia. Clients must also be monitored for ketonuria and glucosuria. Advise clients taking antidiabetic agents that they may require an increase in dosage of these agents when taken in combination with niacin.
5. Instruct clients with hepatic dysfunction to report any skin color change or yellowing of the sclera.
6. Clients who are predisposed to gout may experience flank, joint or stomach pains. Instruct client to report this to the physician immediately.
7. Advise that some clients may develop blurred vision. If this occurs they should remain out of direct sunlight.

PANTOTHENIC ACID (VITAMIN B₅) (PAN-toe-THEHN-nic)
Calcium Pantothenate, Dexol T.D. (OTC)

Classification: Vitamin B complex.

Action/Kinetics: Pantothenic acid is a precursor of coenzyme A, which is a cofactor required for oxidative metabolism of carbohydrates, synthesis and breakdown of fatty acids, sterol synthesis, gluconeogenesis, and steroid synthesis. Pantothenic acid is found in many foods; thus, deficiency in humans has not been observed.

Uses: There is no therapeutic indication for pantothenic acid alone as deficiency has not been observed. However, it is included in vitamin preparations for the prophylaxis and treatment of vitamin deficiency.

Contraindications: Hemophilia. Should not be used to treat diabetic neuropathy, increasing GI peristalsis, Addison's disease, allergies, respiratory disorders, improvement of mental processes, prevention of birth defects, or treatment of toxicity due to salicylate or streptomycin.

Side Effects: Allergic symptoms have occurred occasionally.

Dosage: Tablets. Adults and children: Up to 100 mg daily have been used.

NURSING CONSIDERATIONS

See also *Nursing considerations* for *Vitamins,* p. 1312.

Client/Family Teaching

Instruct the client to report any adverse side effects to the physician.

PYRIDOXINE HYDROCHLORIDE (VITAMIN B₆) (peer-ih-**DOX**-een)

Beesix, Hexa-Betalin, Pyroxine, Rodex, TexSix T.R. (Rx: Injection; OTC: Tablets)

Classification: Vitamin B complex.

Action/Kinetics: Pyridoxine hydrochloride is a water-soluble, heat-resistant vitamin which is destroyed by light. It is prepared synthetically. It acts as a coenzyme in the metabolism of protein, carbohydrates, and fat. As the amount of protein increases in the diet, the pyridoxine requirement increases. $t^{1/2}$: 2–3 weeks. Metabolized in the liver and excreted through the urine.

Uses: Pyridoxine deficiency including poor diet, drug-induced (e.g., oral contraceptives, isoniazid), and inborn errors of metabolism. *Investigational:* Hydrazine poisoning, premenstrual tension, high urine oxalate levels.

Special Concerns: Pregnancy category: A. Dosage has not been established in children for the extended-release capsules.

Side Effects: *CNS:* Unstable gait; decreased sensation to touch, temperature, and vibration; paresthesia, sleepiness, numbness of feet, perioral numbness. **Note:** Abuse and dependence have been noted in adults administered 200 mg/day.

Drug Interactions	
Chloramphenicol	↑ Pyridoxine requirements
Contraceptives, oral	↑ Pyridoxine requirements
Cycloserine	↑ Pyridoxine requirements
Ethionamide	↑ Pyridoxine requirements
Hydralazine	↑ Pyridoxine requirements
Immunosuppressants	↑ Pyridoxine requirements
Isoniazid	↑ Pyridoxine requirements
Levodopa	Daily doses exceeding 5 mg pyridoxine antagonize the therapeutic effect of levodopa
Penicillamine	↑ Pyridoxine requirements

Dosage: Extended-release Capsules, Tablets. *Dietary supplement:* **Adults,** 10–20 mg daily for 2 weeks; **then,** 2–5 mg daily as part of a multivitamin preparation for several weeks. **Pediatric,** 2.5–10 mg daily for 3 weeks; **then,** 2–5 mg daily as part of a multivitamin preparation for several weeks. *Pyridoxine dependency syndrome:* **Adults and children, initial,** 30–600 mg daily; **maintenance,** 50 mg daily for life. **Infants, maintenance:** 2–10 mg daily for life. *Drug-induced deficiency:* **Adults, prophylaxis,** 10–50 mg daily for penicillamine or 100–300 mg daily for cycloserine, hydralazine, or isoniazid. **Adults, treatment,** 50–200 mg daily for 3 weeks followed by 25–100 mg daily to prevent relapse. **Adults, alcoholism,** 50 mg daily for 2–4 weeks; if anemia responds, continue pyridoxine indefinitely. *Hereditary sideroblastic anemia:* **Adults,** 200–600 mg daily for 1–2 months; **then,** 30–50 mg daily for life.

IM, IV. *Pyridoxine dependency syndrome:* **Adults,** 30–600 mg daily. **Pediatric:** 10–100 mg. *Drug-induced deficiency:* **Adults,** 50–200 mg daily for 3 weeks followed by 25–100 mg daily as needed. *Cycloserine poisoning:* **Adults,** 300 mg daily. *Isoniazid poisoning:* **Adults,** 1 g for each gram of isoniazid taken.

NURSING CONSIDERATIONS

See also *Nursing Considerations* for *Vitamins,* p. 1312.

Administration/Storage

If the client is also receiving levodopa, preparations of vitamins containing vitamin B$_6$ should be avoided since vitamin B$_6$ decreases the availability of levodopa to the brain.

Assessment

Take a complete drug history. If the client is taking cycloserine, isoniazid, or oral contraceptives, consult with the physician before administering vitamin B$_6$. These drugs increase pyridoxine requirements.

Interventions

Observe the client for changes in dermatitis around the eyes, nose and mouth and document. These could indicate an appropriate response to the drug therapy.

Client/Family Teaching

1. Provide the client with a printed list of foods high in vitamin B$_6$.
2. If the client is taking levodopa, advise him/her to avoid taking vitamin supplements containing vitamin B$_6$. More than 5 mg of the vitamin antagonizes the effect of levodopa. At the same time, concomitant administration of carbidopa will prevent the effect of vitamin B$_6$ on levodopa.
3. If the client is also taking phenobarbital and/or phenytoin, advise the client to report for serum levels on a routine basis since pyridoxine alters serum concentrations of these drugs.
4. If the client is a nursing mother, advise her that pyridoxine may inhibit lactation.

RIBOFLAVIN (VITAMIN B$_2$)   (RYE-boh-flay-vin)

(OTC)

Classification: Vitamin B complex.

Action/Kinetics: Riboflavin is a water-soluble, heat-resistant substance which is sensitive to light. Riboflavin acts as a coenzyme for various tissue respiration reactions. Riboflavin deficiency is characterized by characteristic lesions of the tongue, lips and face, photophobia, itching, burning and keratosis of the eyes. Riboflavin deficiency often accompanies pellagra.

Uses: Prophylaxis or treatment of riboflavin deficiency. Adjunct, with niacin, in the treatment of pellagra.

Side Effects: Large doses may cause urine to have a yellow discoloration.

Drug Interactions	
Alcohol	Impairs absorption of riboflavin
Antidepressants, tricyclic	↑ Requirements of riboflavin
Chloramphenicol	Riboflavin may counteract bone marrow depression and optic neuritis due to chloramphenicol
Phenothiazines	↑ Requirements for riboflavin
Probenecid	↑ Requirements for riboflavin
Tetracyclines	Antibiotic activity ↓ by riboflavin

Dosage: Tablets. *Deficiency states:* 5–30 mg daily for several days; **then,** 1–4 mg daily.

NURSING CONSIDERATIONS

See *Nursing Considerations* for *Vitamins,* p. 1312.

THIAMINE HYDROCHLORIDE (VITAMIN B₁)   (THIGH-ah-meen)

Betalin S, Bewon, Biamine (Rx: Injection; OTC: Tablets)

Action/Kinetics: Water-soluble vitamin, stable in acid solution. The vitamin is decomposed in neutral or acid solutions. Thiamine is required for the synthesis of thiamine pyrophosphate, a coenzyme required in carbohydrate metabolism.

Uses: Prophylaxis and treatment of thiamine deficiency states and associated neurologic and cardiovascular symptoms. Prophylaxis and treatment of beriberi. Alcoholic neuritis, neuritis of pellagra, and neuritis of pregnancy. To correct anorexia due to thiamine insufficiency. *Investigational:* Treatment of subacute necrotizing encephalomyelopathy, maple syrup urine disease, pyruvate carboxylase deficiency, hyperalaninemia.

Special Concerns: Use with caution during lactation.

Side Effects: Serious hypersensitivity reactions can occur; thus, intradermal testing is recommended if sensitivity is suspected. *Dermatologic:* Pruritus, urticaria, sweating, feeling of warmth. *CNS:* Weakness, restlessness. *Other:* Nausea, tightness in throat, angioneurotic edema, cyanosis, hemorrhage into the GI tract, pulmonary edema, cardiovascular collapse. Death has been reported. *Following IM use:* Induration, tenderness.

Drug Interaction: Since vitamin B₁ is unstable in neutral or alkaline solutions, the vitamin should not be used with substances such as citrates, barbiturates, or carbonates that yield alkaline solutions.

Dosage: Elixir, Tablets. *Mild beriberi or maintenance following severe beriberi:* **Adults,** 5–10 mg daily (as part of a multivitamin product); **infants:** 10 mg daily. *Treatment of deficiency:* **Adults,** 5–10 mg daily; **pediatric:** 10–50 mg daily. *Alcohol-induced deficiency:* **Adults,** 40 mg daily. *Dietary supplement:* **Adults,** 1–2 mg daily; **pediatric:** 0.3–0.5 mg daily for infants and 0.5 mg daily for children. *Genetic enzyme deficiency disease:* 10–20 mg daily (up to 4 g daily has been used in some patients).
   IM, Slow IV. *Severe beriberi:* **Adults,** 5–100 mg t.i.d.; **pediatric:** 10–25 mg.

NURSING CONSIDERATIONS

NURSING CONSIDERATIONS

See also *Nursing Considerations* for *Vitamins*, p. 1312.

Administration/Storage

The drug may enhance the effects of neuromuscular blocking agents. Have epinephrine available to treat clients for anaphylactic shock if a large parenteral dose of thiamine is ordered.

VITAMIN C

ASCORBATE SODIUM   (as-KOR-bayt)

Cenolate, Cetane, Cevita (Rx)

ASCORBIC ACID   (as-KOR-bic AH-sid)

Ascorbicap, Cebid, Cecon, Cemill, Cetane, Cevalin, Cevi-Bid, Ce-Vi-Sol, Cevita, C-Span, Flavorcee, Kamu Jay✹, Redoxon✹, Sunkist (OTC)

Action/Kinetics: Vitamin C (ascorbic acid) is a specific antiscorbutic substance. The vitamin is unstable and easily destroyed by air, light, and heat. Vitamin C is essential to the maintenance of the connective and supporting tissue of the body; for the synthesis of catecholamines, steroids, and carnitine; for tyrosine metabolism; and for conversion of folic acid to folinic acid. Vitamin C deficiency leads to scurvy, which is characterized by changes in the fibrous tissues, the matrix of dentine, bone, cartilage, and the vascular endothelium.

The stores of vitamin C in the body are depleted rapidly and patients on IV feeding may develop ascorbic acid deficiency. This may cause a delay in healing in patients who have undergone surgery. Due to an increased rate of oxidation during infectious diseases, the daily requirements of vitamin C rise.

Uses: Prophylaxis and treatment of scurvy. Vitamin C supplementation is indicated for burn victims, debilitated patients, and as an adjunct in iron therapy and in patients on prolonged IV feedings. *Investigational:* Large doses of vitamin C have been indicated for treating cancer, asthma, atherosclerosis, wounds, schizophrenia and to prevent the common cold. Also, as a urinary acidifier in methenamine therapy, adjunct to treat chronic iron toxicity, and adjunct to treat methemoglobinemia.

Contraindications: Excessive doses in diabetics, in patients with a history of renal calculi, those on anticoagulant therapy or sodium restricted diets.

Special Concerns: Pregnancy category: C. Use with caution during lactation.

Side Effects: *Large or megadoses:* Diarrhea, renal stones (oxalate, urate). *Rapid IV administration:* Transitory faintness and dizziness. *SC, IM use:* Mild, transient soreness.

Drug Interactions	
Acidic drugs	Large doses of ascorbic acid ↑ reabsorption of acid drugs in kidney → ↑ effect
Amphetamine	↓ Effect of amphetamine due to ↓ renal tubular reabsorption

Drug Interactions	
Antidepressants, tricyclic	↓ Effect of tricyclics due to ↓ renal tubular reabsorption
Basic drugs	↓ Effect of basic drugs due to ↓ renal tubular reabsorption
Dicumarol	Ascorbic acid may influence the intensity and duration of action
Digitalis	Calcium ascorbate may cause cardiac arrhythmias in patients receiving digitalis
Disulfiram	Ascorbic acid may interfere with the action of disulfiram
Erythromycin, parenteral	Decomposition of erythromycin due to ↓ pH
Ethinyl estradiol	↑ Effect of ethinyl estradiol due to ↑ plasma concentrations
Salicylates	↑ Effect of salicylates due to ↑ renal tubular reabsorption
Smoking	↑ Requirements for vitamin C
Sulfonamides	↑ Chance of crystallization of sulfonamides in urine
Warfarin	Ascorbic acid ↓ effect of warfarin

Laboratory Test Interference: Megadoses may cause false − urine glucose determinations (glucose oxidase method) or false + (copper reductase or Benedict's solution).

Dosage: Syrup, Tablets, Chewable Tablets, Effervescent Tablets, Extended-release Capsules or Tablets, Oral Solution. *Dietary supplement:* **Adults,** 50–100 mg daily (100–200 mg in chronic dialysis). **Pediatric, less than 4 years:** 20–50 mg daily. *Treatment of deficiency:* **Adults,** 100–250 mg 1–3 times daily (500 mg b.i.d. for extended-release capsules and oral solution). **Pediatric:** 100–300 mg daily in divided doses. *Urinary acidifier:* **Adults,** 4–12 g daily in divided doses q 4 hr. *Adjunct to treat idiopathic methemoglobinemia:* **Adults,** 300–600 mg daily in divided doses.

IM, IV: Ascorbic Acid or Sodium Ascorbate. *Treatment of deficiency:* **Adults,** 100–250 mg 1–3 times daily; **pediatric:** 100–300 mg daily in divided doses.

NURSING CONSIDERATIONS

See also *Nursing Considerations* for *Vitamins,* p. 1312.

Assessment

1. Take a drug history, noting the drugs the client may be taking that interact with ascorbic acid.
2. Note if the client has been on a fad diet or if the client has been on a therapeutic diet where vitamin C was deficient.
3. Note if clients on prolonged IV therapy, parenteral hyperalimentation or chronic hemodialysis exhibit symptoms of marginal vitamin C deficiency.

Interventions

1. Be alert to the many drug interactions that are possible when the client is taking vitamin C.
2. Note if the client receiving prolonged IV therapy is becoming increasingly debilitated.
3. Determine if clients bruise easily, have sensitive, swollen, bleeding gums, and nosebleeds.

Document and report to the physician. Investigate the possibility that the client may not be receiving adequate amounts of vitamin C.

Client/Family Teaching

1. If clients have been taking large doses of vitamin C, advise them to taper off vitamin C rather than stop taking the drug abruptly.
2. To ensure potency, instruct client to protect the drug from contact with copper, light, heat, and exposure to air.
3. If the client is of childbearing age or pregnant, advise her *not* to exceed the recommended dosage.
4. If the vitamin C is for infants advise parents not to heat the orange juice or formula since heat destroys vitamin C. Instruct them to serve these fluids at room temperature.

VITAMIN D

Classification: Fat-soluble vitamin.

General Statement: Vitamin D, the antirachitic factor, has a key role in controlling calcium and phosphorus metabolism. The regulating (homeostatic) effect on calcium serum levels is such that it is now considered to have hormonal activity.

In the presence of sunlight (UV irradiation) humans can synthesize vitamin D in the skin from a variety of plant and animal sterols. Under ideal circumstances intake of exogenous vitamin D may not be necessary. Irradiated milk and fish liver oils, however, are excellent sources of the vitamin.

Vitamin D deficiency is characterized by inadequate absorption of calcium and phosphate. During periods of active growth, vitamin D deficiency may lead to rickets. In adults, vitamin D deficiency may result in osteomalacia (adult rickets).

Several compounds have vitamin D activity. The most important of these are calcitriol, calcifediol, cholecalciferol (D_3), dihydrotachysterol, and ergocalciferol (D_2).

Action/Kinetics: Vitamin D analogs, along with parathyroid hormone and calcitonin, regulate serum calcium levels by increasing absorption of calcium (and phosphorus), increasing resorption of calcium by bone, and increasing reabsorption of calcium and phosphate by the kidney. In addition, dihydrotachysterol increases absorption of calcium from the intestine and mobilizes calcium in the absence of parathyroid hormone. Vitamin D is rapidly absorbed from the small intestine and is stored mainly in the liver. It is bound to plasma alpha globulins and albumin. Vitamin D is excreted mainly through the bile.

Uses: Treatment of chronic hypocalcemia, hypophosphatemia, osteodystrophy, rickets. Prophylaxis and treatment of tetany, vitamin D deficiency. See also individual agents.

Contraindications: Impaired renal or cardiac function, arteriosclerosis, concomitantly with digitalis glycosides, hypercalcemia, hyperphosphatemia. Vitamin D toxicity, hypercalcemia, malabsorption syndrome, sarcoidosis.

Special Concerns: Pregnancy category: C. Infants may be overly sensitive even to small doses. Use with caution in impaired renal function.

Side Effects: Physiologic doses are virtually without adverse effects. However, excessive doses produce both acute and chronic toxicity. **Acute toxicity.** *GI:* Nausea, vomiting, dry mouth, constipation, metallic taste. *CNS:* Sleepiness, headache. *Miscellaneous:* Muscle and bone pain, weakness. **Chronic.** *GI:* Anorexia, weight loss. *CV:* Hypertension, cardiac arrhythmias. *GU:* Polydipsia, polyuria, nocturia, albuminuria. *Metabolic:* Hypercholesteremia, hypercalcemia, elevated BUN, SGOT, and SGPT. *CNS:* Irritability, psychoses (rare). *Miscellaneous:* Conjunctivitis, pancreatitis, photophobia, hyperthermia, pruritus, decreased libido, ectopic calcification, rhinorrhea.

Treatment of Overdose: Immediate discontinuation of therapy, institution of a low calcium diet, and withdrawal of any calcium supplements. To increase excretion of calcium, give IV fluids, acidify urine, or administer a loop diuretic (e.g., ethacrynic acid, furosemide, others).

In acute accidental overdosage, induction of emesis or gastric lavage is beneficial if the overdose is discovered within a short time; also, administration of mineral oil may increase fecal excretion of the drug.

Drug Interactions	
Antacids (magnesium-containing)	↑ Risk hypermagnesemia
Barbiturates	↓ Effect of vitamin D by ↑ breakdown by liver
Calcitonin	↓ Effect of calcitonin in hypercalcemia
Cholestyramine	↓ Effect vitamin D due to ↓ absorption from GI tract
Colestipol	↓ Effect of vitamin D due to ↓ absorption from GI tract
Corticosteroids	↓ Effects of vitamin D
Digitalis	Hypercalcemia may ↑ risk of arrhythmias
Mineral oil	Chronic use of mineral oil ↓ absorption of fat-soluble vitamins from the GI tract
Phenobarbital	↓ Effect of vitamin D due to ↑ breakdown by liver
Phenytoin	↓ Effect of vitamin D due to ↑ breakdown by liver
Sucralfate	↓ Effect of vitamin D due to ↓ absorption from GI tract
Thiazides	↑ Risk of hypercalcemia
Verapamil	Hypercalcemia may ↑ risk of atrial fibrillation

Laboratory Test Interference: Toxic doses of vitamin D analogs may ↑ urinary calcium, phosphate, albumin: also, ↑ BUN, serum cholesterol, SGOT, SGPT. ↓ Serum alkaline phosphatase.

Dosage: See individual agents.

NURSING CONSIDERATIONS

See also *Nursing Considerations* for *Vitamins,* p. 1312.

Assessment

1. Note if the client has a history of renal disease.
2. Determine if the client has a history of vitamin D toxicity.
3. Document if the client has a history of cardiac dysfunction and also note if they are taking digitalis glycosides.
4. List the drugs the client is currently taking to determine if any of them interact unfavorably with vitamin D.

Interventions

1. Observe the client for complaints of nausea, vomiting, dry mouth, constipation or a metallic

taste in the mouth. Document and report to the physician. Check the amount of vitamin D the client is taking and inquire to determine if they are taking vitamins not prescribed by the physician.

2. If the client continues to have symptoms of overdose, discontinue the therapy, institute a diet low in calcium and withdraw any calcium supplements. Administer IV fluids and acidify the urine or administer a loop diuretic to increase the excretion of calcium.

3. If the client has an acute accidental overdosage that is discovered within a short time, induce emesis or conduct a gastric lavage. Administer mineral oil to increase the excretion of drug via the feces.

Client/Family Teaching

1. Encourage the client to have periodic laboratory studies done to evaluate calcium, magnesium, phosphorus, alkaline phosphatase levels, and hepatic and renal function.

2. Advise the client to avoid taking antacids that contain magnesium.

3. Explain the need to withhold the drug and to report to the physician if the client feels weak, has nausea and vomiting, a dry mouth, develops constipation, muscle pain, bone pain, or a metallic taste in the mouth. These are symptoms of vitamin D intoxication and demand immediate attention.

4. Instruct the client to take the medication only as prescribed by the physician since the dosage for each person is highly individualized.

5. Review the prescribed diet and need for calcium supplementation.

6. Advise the client to avoid nonprescription medications unless advised to take them by the physician.

7. Explain the necessity of eating a light diet, drinking plenty of fluids, and using laxatives in the event of constipation. These measures facilitate elimination of excessive calcium from the body.

8. Instruct women of childbearing age *not* to exceed the prescribed dose of medication.

CALCIFEDIOL   (kal-sih-feh-**DYE**-ol)

Calderol (Rx)

Action/Kinetics: Absorbed from the intestine. **t½:** 16 days. **Time to peak serum levels:** About 4 hr. **Duration:** 15–20 days. Excreted mainly by the bile.

Uses: Metabolic bone disease, hypocalcemia in patients on chronic renal dialysis.

Special Concerns: Pregnancy category: C.

Dosage: Capsules. Adults and children over 10 years: initial, 300–350 mcg/week in divided daily or alternate daily dosage; if no response, increase at 4-week intervals. Patients with normal serum calcium may respond to 20 mcg q other day. **Usual doses:** 50–100 mcg daily or 100–200 mcg every other day. **Pediatric, 2–10 years:** 50 mcg daily; **up to 2 years:** 20–50 mcg daily.

NURSING CONSIDERATIONS

See also *Nursing Considerations* for *Vitamins,* p. 1312, and *Vitamin D,* p. 1332.

Client/Family Teaching

To ensure potency, advise client to protect the drug from light, heat and moisture.

CALCITRIOL   (cal-sih-**TRY**-ol)

Calcijex, Rocaltrol (Rx)

Action/Kinetics: Onset: 2–6 hr. **Time to peak serum levels:** About 2 hr. **Duration:** 1–2 days. **t½:** 3–8 hr.

Uses: Hypocalcemia in patients on chronic renal dialysis. Hypoparathyroidism or pseudohypoparathyroidism. Renal osteodystrophy.

Special Concerns: Pregnancy category: C.

Dosage: Capsules. *Hypocalcemia in renal dialysis:* **Adults, initial,** 0.25 mcg/day; **then,** if necessary, increase by 0.25 mcg/day at 2–4 week intervals. Some may respond to 0.25 mcg on alternate days. (Range: 0.25–3 mcg daily). **Pediatric:** 0.25–2 mcg daily. *Hypoparathyroidism:* **Adults,** 0.25–2.7 mcg daily; **pediatric:** 0.04–0.08 mcg/kg daily. *Renal osteodystrophy:* **Adults,** 0.25 mcg q other day–3 mcg (or more) daily; **pediatric:** 0.014–0.041 mcg/kg daily.

    IV, rapid. *Antihypocalcemic:* **Adults,** 0.5 mcg/kg three times weekly; dose may be increased by increments of 0.25–0.5 mcg q 2–4 weeks. **Maintenance:** 0.5–3 mcg three times weekly.

NURSING CONSIDERATIONS

See also *Nursing Considerations* for *Vitamins,* p. 1312, and *Vitamin D,* p. 1332.

Administration/Storage

To be most effective, calcitriol may have to be given in divided doses 2–3 times daily.

Interventions

Monitor serum calcium levels monthly once the maintenance dose has been established.

CHOLECALCIFEROL (VITAMIN D₃)   (kohl-eh-kal-**SIF**-er-ohl)

Delta-D (OTC)

Action/Kinetics: Bile is necessary for maximum absorption. Excreted primarily by the bile. One mg provides 40,000 IU of vitamin D activity.

Uses: Prophylaxis or treatment of vitamin D deficiency (i.e., osteomalacia, rickets), dietary supplement.

Special Concerns: Pregnancy category: C.

Dosage: Tablets. 400–1,000 IU daily.

NURSING CONSIDERATIONS

See *Nursing Considerations* for *Vitamins,* p. 1312, and *Vitamin D,* p. 1332.

DIHYDROTACHYSTEROL   (dye-hi-droh-tak-**ISS**-ter-ohl)

DHT, DHT Intensol, Hytakerol (Rx)

Action/Kinetics: Onset: slow, 7–10 days. Maximum effect occurs up to 2 weeks after daily administration. **Duration:** Up to 9 weeks. One milligram dihydrotachysterol equals 3 mg ergocalciferol (vitamin D₂).

Uses: Hypocalcemic tetany, hypoparathyroidism. *Investigational:* Familial hypophosphatemia, renal osteodystrophy.

Special Concerns: Pregnancy category: C.

Dosage: Capsules, Oral Solution, Tablets. *Hypocalcemic tetany:* **Adults, initial,** 250 mcg–2.5 mg (depending on the severity) daily for 3 days; **maintenance:** 250 mcg/week–1 mg/day as required by the patient. *Hypoparathyroidism:* **Adults, initial,** 750 mcg–2.5 mg daily for several days; **maintenance,** 200 mcg–1 mg daily. **Pediatric, initial:** 1–5 mg/day for 4 days after which dose may be reduced to ¼; **maintenance:** 500 mcg–1.5 mg daily. *Familial hypophosphatemia:* **Adults and children, initial,** 500 mcg–2 mg daily; **maintenance:** 200 mcg–1.5 mg daily. *Renal osteodystrophy:* **Adults,** 100–250 mcg daily; **maintenance:** 200 mcg–1 mg daily.

Note: Oral calcium may be used to supplement dihydrotachysterol.

ERGOCALCIFEROL (VITAMIN D₂) (er-go-kal-**SIF**-er-ohl)

Calciferol, Deltalin, Drisdol, Ostoforte ✿, Radiostol ✿, Radiostol Forte ✿ (Rx and OTC)

Action/Kinetics: Serum calcium levels should be maintained between 9–10 mg/dl. **Onset (PO, IM):** 10–24 hr. **Peak effect:** 4 weeks after daily dosage. **Duration:** Up to 6 months (cumulative effects). **t½:** 24 hr. Bile is required for absorption. Excreted mainly by the bile. One milligram ergocalciferol is equivalent to 40,000 IU units of vitamin D activity.

Uses: Refractory rickets, familial hypophosphatemia, hypoparathyroidism, dietary supplement. *Investigational:* Renal osteodystrophy, impaired renal function.

Special Concerns: Pregnancy category: C. Prolonged use in children (more than 1,800 units daily) may arrest growth.

Dosage: Capsules, Oral Solution, Tablets. *Vitamin D deficiency:* **Adults,** 1,000–2,000 Units daily, reduced to 400 Units daily when appropriate; **pediatric:** 1,000–4,000 Units daily, reduced to 400 Units daily when appropriate. *Vitamin D-resistant rickets:* **Adults,** 12,000–500,000 Units daily. *Vitamin-D dependent rickets:* **Adults,** 10,000–60,000 Units daily (up to 500,000 may be required in some patients); **pediatric:** 3,000–10,000 Units daily (some may require 50,000 Units daily). *Familial hypophosphatemia:* **Adults,** 50,000–100,000 Units daily. *Hypoparathyroidism:* **Adults,** 50,000–150,000 Units daily; **pediatric:** 50,000–200,000 Units daily. *Osteomalacia due to prolonged anticonvulsant use:* **Adults,** 1,000–4,000 Units daily; **pediatric:** 1,000 Units daily. *Renal osteodystrophy:* **Adults, initial,** 20,000 Units daily; **maintenance:** 10,000–300,000 Units daily. **Pediatric:** 4,000–40,000 Units daily. *Impaired renal function:* **Adults,** 40,000–100,000 Units daily.

IM. Adults and children: *Malabsorption,* 10,000 Units daily.

NURSING CONSIDERATIONS

See also *Nursing Considerations* for *Vitamins,* p. 1312, and *Vitamin D,* p. 1332.

Interventions

Anticipate that clients with GI, hepatic or biliary disease associated with malabsorption of vitamin D will have the drug administered IM only.

VITAMIN E (TOCOPHEROL, TOCOPHEROL ACETATE)

PO: Aquasol E, Chew-E, E-Ferol, Eprolin, Epsilan-M, Pheryl-E, Viterra E. Topical: E-Ferol, Gordo-Vita E, Vitec (OTC)

Action/Kinetics: Vitamin E refers to a group of fat-soluble substances, including the powerful antioxidants alpha-, beta-, gamma-, and delta-tocopherol. The exact physiologic function of vitamin E is not known; however, its actions are probably related to its antioxidant effects. Vitamin E preserves the integrity of red blood cell walls, enhances vitamin A utilization, may act as a cofactor in various enzyme systems, stabilizes cell membranes thus protecting them against peroxidation, and may suppress platelet aggregation.

Uses: Prophylaxis and treatment of vitamin E deficiency. *Topical:* Dry, chapped skin. Also, minor skin disorders such as burns, diaper rash, sunburn, abrasions, itching; deodorant. *Investigational:* Premature infants to reduce toxicity of oxygen therapy on the lung parenchyma and retina. Decrease severity of hemolytic anemia in infants. The vitamin has also been used to treat cancer, sexual dysfunction, heart disease, nocturnal leg cramps, premenstrual syndrome, the aging process, and increase athletic performance.

Contraindications: IV use. Iron deficiency anemia (vitamin E may impair the hematologic response to iron products). Hypoprothrombinemia.

Side Effects: Large doses over prolonged periods may cause hypervitaminosis: *GI:* Nausea, diarrhea, flatulence. *CNS:* Fatigue, weakness, headache. *Miscellaneous:* Blurred vision, dermatitis.

Drug Interactions

Antacids	↓ Absorption of vitamin E from the GI tract
Anticoagulants, oral	Vitamin E ↑ effect of anticoagulants
Cholestyramine	↓ Absorption of vitamin E from the GI tract
Colestipol	↓ Absorption of vitamin E from the GI tract
Iron Therapy	Vitamin E ↓ response to iron therapy
Mineral oil	↓ Absorption of vitamin E from the GI tract
Sucralfate	↓ Absorption of vitamin E from the GI tract
Vitamin A	Vitamin E may ↑ absorption, storage, and utilization of vitamin A → ↓ vitamin A toxicity

Dosage: Capsules, Oral Solution, Tablets, Chewable Tablets. *Prophylaxis of deficiency:* **Adults,** 30 Units daily. *Treatment of deficiency:* **Adults,** 60–75 Units daily; **pediatric:** 1 Unit/kg daily. *Premature infants receiving formulas high in polyunsaturated fats:* 15–25 Units daily (7 Units/liter of formula).

Topical: Creams, Liquids, Oils, Ointments. Apply as needed and rub in lightly.

NURSING CONSIDERATIONS

See also *Nursing Considerations* for *Vitamins,* p. 1312.

Assessment

1. Note if the client is receiving anticoagulant therapy. Vitamin E increases the effects of anticoagulants.
2. Assess client's skin to determine if there is evidence of dry, chapped skin, abrasions and/or itching and document.

Client/Family Teaching

1. Advise the client not to exceed the recommended dose.
2. Instruct the client to report any side effects such as nausea, diarrhea, flatulence, fatigue, weakness and headaches to the physician.

VITAMIN K

Classification: Fat-soluble vitamin, blood clotting factor.

Action/Kinetics: Vitamin K is essential for the hepatic synthesis of factors II, VII, IX, and X, all of which are essential for blood clotting. The chief manifestation of vitamin K deficiency is an increase in bleeding tendency. This is demonstrated by ecchymoses, epistaxis, hematuria, GI bleeding, postoperative and intracranial hemorrhage.

Vitamin K is available as phytonadione (vitamin K_1), a synthetic lipid-soluble analog, and menadiol sodium diphosphate (vitamin K_4), a water-soluble synthetic analog.

Uses: Primary and drug-induced hypoprothrombinemia, especially that caused by anticoagulants of the coumarin and phenindione type. Vitamin K cannot reverse the anticoagulant activity of heparin.

Parenteral use for vitamin K malabsorption syndromes. Adjunct during whole blood transfusions. Preoperatively to prevent the danger of hemorrhages in surgical patients who may require anticoagulant therapy.

Certain forms of liver disease. Hemorrhagic states associated with obstructive jaundice, celiac disease, ulcerative colitis, sprue, biliary fistula, cystic fibrosis of the pancreas, regional enteritis, resection of intestine.

Contraindications: Severe liver disease.

Special Concerns: Use in infants. Use with caution during lactation. Use with caution in patients with sulfite sensitivity.

Side Effects: *Allergic:* Rash, urticaria, anaphylaxis. *After PO use:* Nausea, vomiting, stomach upset, headache. *After parenteral use:* Flushing, alteration of taste, sweating, hypotension, dizziness, rapid and weak pulse, dyspnea, cyanosis, delayed skin reactions. Pain, swelling, and tenderness at injection site. *Newborns:* Hyperbilirubinemia and fatal kernicterus.

Drug Interactions	
Antibiotics	Antibiotics may inhibit the body's production of vitamin K and may lead to bleeding. Vitamin K supplements should be given
Anticoagulants, oral	Vitamin K antagonizes anticoagulant effect
Cholestyramine	↓ Effect of phytonadione and menadione due to ↓ absorption from GI tract
Colestipol	↓ Effect of phytonadione and menadione due to ↓ absorption from GI tract
Hemolytics	↑ Potential for toxicity (especially with menadione)
Mineral oil	↓ Effect of phytonadione and menadione due to ↓ absorption from GI tract
Quinidine, Quinine	↑ Requirement for vitamin K
Salicylates	High doses of salicylates → ↑ requirements for vitamin K.
Sucralfate	↓ Effect of phytonadione and menadione due to ↓ absorption from GI tract
Sulfonamides	↑ Requirements for vitamin K.

Dosage: See individual drugs.

NURSING CONSIDERATIONS

See also *Nursing Considerations* for *Vitamins,* p. 1312.

Assessment

1. Determine if client has any sensitivity to sulfites and document.
2. Note drugs the client is taking to determine how they may interact with vitamin K.
3. Obtain baseline PT/PTT, liver and hematologic values prior to initiating therapy.
4. Determine if client has any history or laboratory evidence of advanced liver disease.

Interventions

Monitor liver function studies and hematologic values during drug therapy.

MENADIOL SODIUM DIPHOSPHATE (VITAMIN K₄) (men-ah-DYE-ohl)

Synkayvite (Rx)

Classification: Vitamin K.

Action/Kinetics: Precursors of blood-clotting factors. Menadiol sodium diphosphate is water soluble and is converted to menadione in the body. Both may be absorbed directly into the bloodstream even in the absence of bile. **Onset, IM, SC:** 8–24 hr. **Duration:** (normal prothrombin time), 8–24 hr. **IV,** onset faster than IM, SC; **duration:** shorter.

Uses: Not as safe as phytonadione in treating hemorrhagic disease of the newborn. Ineffective in treating oral anticoagulant-induced hypoprothrombinemia.

Contraindications: Last weeks of pregnancy or during labor as a prophylaxis against hypoprothrombinemia or hemorrhagic disease of the newborn. Use in infants.

Special Concerns: Pregnancy category: C. Use with caution in children due to an increased risk of hepatotoxicity and hemolytic anemia.

Additional Side Effects: Hemolysis of red blood cells in patients with glucose 6-phosphate dehydrogenase deficiency.

Laboratory Test Interference: Falsely elevated urinary 17-hydroxycorticosteroid levels (Reddy, Thorn, and Jenkins procedure).

Dosage: Tablets. *Hypoprothrombinemia due to obstructive jaundice and biliary fistulas:* **Adults,** 5 mg/day. *Hypoprothrombinemia due to antibacterial/salicylate use:* **Adults,** 5–10 mg/day. **Pediatric, all uses:** 5–10 mg daily.

   IM, SC. *Hypoprothrombinemia,* **Adults:** 5–15 mg, 1–2 times/day; **children:** 5–10 mg, 1–2 times/day.

NURSING CONSIDERATIONS

See also *Nursing Considerations* for *Vitamins,* p. 1312, and *Vitamin K,* p. 1338.

Administration/Storage

Although the response following IV use is faster, IM or SC use leads to a more sustained effect.

Interventions

1. Monitor liver function studies and hematologic values.

2. If the client is sensitive to sulfites, caution them to avoid taking menadiol sodium diphosphate and menadione.

3. Large doses of menadione may decrease client response to oral anticoagulants.

4. If the client has decreased bile secretion, administer bile salts to ensure the absorption of vitamin K_4 taken orally.

PHYTONADIONE (VITAMIN K_1) (fye-toe-nah-DYE-ohn)

Aqua-Mephyton, Konakion, Mephyton (Rx)

Classification: Fat soluble vitamin.

Action/Kinetics: Phytonadione is similar to natural vitamin K. Its has a more rapid and more prolonged effect than menadiol sodium diphosphate and is generally more effective. GI absorption requires the presence of bile salts. Heparin may be used to reverse overdosage of phytonadione. Frequent determinations of prothrombin time are indicated during therapy. **IM: Onset,** 1–2 hr. *Control of bleeding:* Parenteral, 3–6 hr. *Normal prothrombin time:* 12–14 hr. **PO, Onset,** 6–12 hr.

Additional Uses: Prophylaxis of hemorrhagic disease of the newborn.

Special Concerns: Pregnancy category: C.

Additional Side Effects: IV administration may cause severe reactions leading to death. May be transient flushing of the face, sweating, a sense of constriction of the chest, and weakness. Cramp-like pain, weak and rapid pulse, convulsive movements, chills and fever, hypotension, cyanosis, or hemoglobinuria have been reported occasionally. Shock, cardiac, and respiratory failure may be observed.

Dosage: Tablets. *Hypoprothrombinemia, drug-induced:* **Adults,** 2.5–10 mg (up to 25 mg); dose may be repeated after 12–48 hr if needed. *Vitamin supplement, prothrombogenic, drug-induced hypoprothrombinemia:* **Pediatric:** 5–10 mg.
  IM, SC. *Vitamin supplement, prothrombogenic, drug-induced hypoprothrombinemia:* **Adults,** 2.5–10 mg (up to 25 mg) which may be repeated after 6–8 hr if needed. **Infants:** 1–2 mg; **children:** 5–10 mg. *Prophylaxis of hypoprothrombinemia during prolonged TPN:* **Adults, IM,** 5–10 mg once weekly; **pediatric:** 2–5 mg once weekly. *Infants receiving milk substitutes or who are breast fed:* 1 mg monthly if vitamin K in diet is less than 0.1 mg/liter. *Prevention of hemorrhagic disease in the newborn:* 0.5–1 mg immediately after delivery; dose may be repeated in 6–8 hr if needed. Higher doses may be required for infants whose mothers took anticonvulsants or anticoagulants during pregnancy.

NURSING CONSIDERATIONS

See also *Nursing Considerations* for *Vitamins,* p. 1312, and *Vitamin K,* p. 1338.

Administration/Storage

1. Store injectable emulsion or colloidal solutions in cool, 5° C–15° C (41° F–59° F), dark place.
2. Do not freeze.
3. Protect vitamin K from light.
4. Mix emulsion only with water or D_5W.
5. Mix colloidal solution with D_5W, isotonic sodium chloride injection, or dextrose and sodium chloride injection.

Interventions

1. Monitor liver function studies and prothrombin time while the client is receiving drug therapy.

2. Observe the client during parenteral administration for evidence of sweating, transient facial flushing, client complaints of weakness and constriction of the chest. Notify the physician, especially if the client develops tachycardia and hypotension as this may progress to shock, cardiac arrest, and respiratory failure.

3. If the client has decreased bile secretion, administer bile salts to ensure the absorption of oral phytonadione.

CHAPTER SEVENTY-ONE
Heavy Metal Antagonists

General Statement: Heavy metals are toxic because they bind to reactive sites, thus inactivating important substances, such as enzymes. Heavy metal antagonists have the ability to bind (chelate) the metal ions to form a nontoxic complex that is eliminated by the kidneys.

Heavy metal poisoning occurs as a consequence of overdosage from drugs such as gold compounds (used to treat rheumatoid arthritis) and iron (used to treat anemias) as well as accidental ingestion of substances such as lead-containing paint, arsenic-containing weed-killers, and pesticides.

DEFEROXAMINE MESYLATE   (deh-fer-**OX**-ah-meen)

Desferal (Rx)

Classification: Heavy metal antagonist (iron chelator).

Action/Kinetics: Deferoxamine, a complex organic molecule, binds to trivalent iron forming ferrioxamine which is a water-soluble chelate excreted by the kidneys (urine is a reddish color) as well as in the feces via the bile. Iron is removed from ferritin, hemosiderin and to a lesser extent from transferrin, but iron is not removed from hemoglobin, myoglobin, or cytochromes. The drug must be given parenterally for systemic activity. Adequate renal function is necessary for effectiveness. $t^{1}/_{2}$, **IV:** 60 min. The drug may be quickly eliminated by the kidneys without binding to iron.

Uses: Adjunct in treatment of acute iron intoxication. Chronic iron overload including thalassemia. *Investigational:* Accumulation of aluminum in renal failure and in encephalopathy due to aluminum.

Contraindications: Severe renal disease, anuria. Should *not* be used to treat primary hemochromatosis.

Special Concerns: Use in pregnancy only if clearly necessary. Use with caution for patients with pyelonephritis. Should not be used in children under the age of 3 years unless mobilization of 1 mg iron/day or more can be shown. Deferoxamine and ascorbic acid should be used with caution in geriatric patients due to a greater risk of cardiac decompensation.

Side Effects: *Allergic:* Rash, itching, wheal formation, anaphylaxis. *GI:* Abdominal discomfort, diarrhea. *Other:* Dysuria, blurred vision, leg cramps, fever, tachycardia, high-frequency hearing loss. *Ophthalmologic:* Rarely, impaired peripheral, night, or color vision; cataracts, decreased visual acuity. *Following rapid IV use:* Hypotension, urticaria, erythema. *Following SC use:* Local pain, erythema, swelling, pruritus, skin irritation.

Dosage: IM, IV, SC. *Acute iron intoxication:* **Adults and children over three years of age, IM (preferred), initial,** 1 g; **then,** 0.5 g q 4 hr for 2 doses; if necessary, then give 0.5 g q 4–12 hr, not to exceed 6 g/day. **IV infusion** (*only in emergencies as cardiovascular collapse:*) Same as IM at a rate not to exceed 15 mg/kg/hr. Begin IM therapy as soon as possible. *Chronic iron overload:* **IM,** 0.5–1.0 g/day; **SC,** 1–2 g (20–40 mg/kg/day) given by mini-infusion pump over an 8–24-hr period; **IV,** 2 g (given separately but at same time as each unit of blood and in addition to IM administration); IV rate not to exceed 15 mg/kg/hr.

NURSING CONSIDERATIONS

Administration/Storage

1. Dissolve deferoxamine mesylate by adding 2 mL of sterile water to each ampule.
2. For IV administration use physiologic saline, glucose in water, or Ringer's lactated solution and administer *slowly* at a rate not exceeding 15 mg/kg/hour.
3. Discard dissolved drug if not used within 1 week.
4. Pain and induration may occur at IM injection site.
5. Have epinephrine available to treat allergic reactions.
6. In the event of iron intoxication and/or acidosis, have gastric lavage equipment, suction, IV fluids, blood and equipment to maintain a patent airway readily available.

Assessment

1. Conduct renal function studies and determine if the client has an adequate flow of urine before initiating therapy.
2. Take a client history, noting if the client has any history of pyelonephritis.
3. Obtain baseline ophthalmologic and audiometry examinations.
4. If the client is female and of childbearing age, determine if pregnant.

Interventions

1. In clients with a history of pyelonephritis, note the development of hematuria or pain. These may be caused by deferoxamine, which may induce an exacerbation of the disease.

2. Observe the client for evidence of shock and report to the physician. Anticipate that the client may be placed on IM administration or a slow IV infusion after recovery from shock.

3. Note any client complaints of visual disturbances such as changes in color vision or altered visual acuity. These may be caused by the drug and should be documented and reported to the physician.

4. Observe and report any evidence of adverse otic effects as these too may be drug related.

Client/Family Teaching

1. Explain to the client the likelihood of pain and induration occurring at the site of administration.

2. Advise the client that the drug may give the urine a reddish color.

3. Instruct the client to report for periodic ophthalmologic and audiometric examinations.

4. Advise women of childbearing age to practice birth control while on drug therapy.

DIMERCAPROL   (dye-mer-**KAP**-rohl)

BAL In Oil (Rx)

Classification: Chelating agent for heavy metals.

Action/Kinetics: Dimercaprol forms a chelate by binding sulfhydryl groups with arsenic, mercury, lead, and gold, thus increasing both urinary and fecal excretion of the metals. Thus, because the drug has a higher affinity for the metal than it does for sulfhydryl groups on protein in the body, BAL reverses enzyme inhibition by regenerating free sulfhydryl groups. To be fully effective, the drug should be administered 1–2 hr after exposure. **Peak plasma concentration: IM,** 30–60 min. Mostly distributed to extracellular fluid. **Time to peak levels:** 30–60 min.
Rapidly metabolized to inactive product and completely excreted in urine and feces in 4 hr.

Uses: Acute arsenic, mercury and gold poisoning. With EDTA in acute lead poisoning. Not effective for chronic mercury poisoning.

Contraindications: Iron, cadmium, silver, uranium, or selenium poisoning. Hepatic insufficiency. Poisoning from arsine gas.

Special Concerns: Use during pregnancy (pregnancy category: C) only if poisoning is life-threatening. Use with caution in the presence of renal insufficiency and in patients with glucose 6-phosphate dehydrogenase deficiency. The drug is of questionable value in poisoning by bismuth or antimony.

Side Effects: *CV:* Most common including hypertension and tachycardia. *GI:* Nausea, vomiting, salivation, abdominal pain, burning feeling of the lips, mouth and throat. *CNS:* Anxiety, weakness, restlessness, headache. *Other:* Constriction and pain in the throat, chest, or hands; sweating of the hands and forehead, conjunctivitis, blepharal spasm, lacrimation, rhinorrhea, tingling of hands, burning feeling in the penis, sterile abscesses.
Children may also develop fever. At high doses dimercaprol may cause coma or convulsions and metabolic acidosis.

Drug Interactions: Dimercaprol may increase the toxicity of cadmium, iron, selenium, or uranium salts.

Laboratory Test Interference: Iodine-131 thyroidal uptake ↓ during and immediately after dimercaprol therapy.

Dosage: Deep IM only. *Mild arsenic and gold poisoning:* **Adults,** 2.5 mg/kg q 4 hr for day 1; 2.5 mg/kg q 6 hr on day 2; b.i.d. on day 3; once daily for 10 days thereafter or until recovery is complete. *Severe arsenic or gold poisoning:* **Adults,** 3 mg/kg q 4 hr for days 1 and 2; q.i.d. on day 3; b.i.d. for 10 days. *Mercury poisoning, mild:* **Adults, initial,** 5 mg/kg; **then,** 2.5 mg/kg 1 or 2 times daily for 10 days. Alternate dosing regimen: 2.5 mg/kg q 4 hr on day 1, q 6 hr on day 2, q 12 hr on day 3, and thereafter, once daily for the next 10 days or until recovery occurs. *Mercury poisoning, severe:* **Adults,** 5 mg/kg for the first dose followed by 2.5 mg/kg q 3 hr for the first 24 hr; **then,** 2 mg/kg q 4 hr on day 2; 3 mg/kg q 6 hr on day 3; and, 3 mg/kg q 12 hr for the next 10 days or until recovery. *Mild lead encephalopathy:* **Adults,** 4 mg/kg alone initially; **then,** 3 mg/kg q 4 hr in combination with calcium EDTA administered in a separate site. Treatment should be continued for 2–7 days only if the blood level at the end of the first course of combined BAL-CaEDTA therapy exceeds 80–90 mcg/dl. *Severe lead encephalopathy:* **Adults,** 4 mg/kg alone initially; **then,** 4 mg/kg q 4 hr in combination with calcium EDTA administered in a separate site. Treatment should be continued for 2–7 days and repeated after an interval of 2 days for 5 additional days only if the blood lead level at the end of the first course of combined BAL-CaEDTA therapy exceeds 80–90 mcg/dl. *Lead toxicity in symptomatic children, acute encephalopathy:* 75 mg/m² q 4 hr (up to 450 mg/m² in 24 hr). After the first dose, give calcium EDTA, 1,500 mg/m² over a 24 hr period in divided doses q 4 hr at a separate IM site; maintain treatment for five days and after an interval of 2 days, the treatment may be repeated for 5 additional days. *Lead toxicity in children, other symptoms:* 50 mg/m² q 4 hr. After the first dose, give calcium EDTA, 1,000 mg/m² over a 24 hr period in divided doses q 4 hr at a separate IM site; maintain treatment for 5 days and after an interval of 2 days, the treatment may be repeated for 5 more days if the lead levels are still high.

NURSING CONSIDERATIONS

Administration/Storage

1. Check with the physician whether a local anesthetic may be given with IM injection to minimize pain at the injection site.
2. Inject IM deeply into muscle and massage after injection. Do not allow the fluid to come in contact with the skin as it may cause a skin reaction.
3. Have ephedrine and/or an antihistamine available for premedication or for later use if the client should experience any adverse effects from the drug.
4. Do not administer iron therapy until at least 24 hours after the last dose of dimercaprol.

Assessment

1. Obtain baseline liver and renal function studies against which to compare similar studies throughout drug therapy.
2. Assess the client for adequate flow of urine prior to initiating therapy.
3. Determine if women of childbearing age are pregnant.

Interventions

1. Monitor the urinary pH throughout drug therapy. Urine should be kept alkaline to protect the kidneys during drug therapy.
2. Record blood pressure, pulse, and temperature and monitor readings to assist in evaluating the client's response to the medication.

3. If the client develops adverse GI or CNS symptoms during drug therapy, reassure them that these symptoms will pass within 30–90 minutes. Provide emotional support to the client.

4. The drug imparts a strong, unpleasant garlic-like odor to the client's breath. Offer mouth rinses as needed.

EDETATE CALCIUM DISODIUM (CALCIUM EDTA) (ED-eh-tayt)

Calcium Disodium Versenate (Rx)

Classification: Heavy metal chelator.

Action/Kinetics: The calcium in calcium EDTA is replaced by lead and cadmium from the body tissues to form stable complexes which are excreted through the urine. It also combines with free heavy metal ions in the extracellular fluid. Lead excretion: **Onset:** 1 hr after IV therapy. **Peak lead excretion:** 24–48 hr. **t½, IV:** 20–60 min; **IM,** 1.5 hr. Calcium EDTA is mainly distributed in extracellular fluid and excreted unchanged or as metal chelate in urine.

Uses: Acute and chronic lead poisoning; lead encephalopathy. The preferred therapy for lead encephalopathy in children is combined therapy with dimercaprol. It is ineffective in mercury or arsenic poisoning. *Investigational:* Determination of lead mobilization.

Contraindications: Anuria, severe oliguria.

Special Concerns: Use during pregnancy only if benefits clearly outweigh risks. Use with caution in hypercalcemia and impaired renal function.

Side Effects: Few side effects are noted when drug is administered at prescribed dosage levels. The greatest danger is renal tubular necrosis that may occur when drug is given at too high dosage and increased intracranial pressure following rapid IV administration in patients with cerebral edema.

Other side effects include: malaise, fatigue, excessive thirst, numbness and tingling, followed by sudden fever and shaking chills, myalgia, arthralgia, headache, GI disturbances, and transitory allergic manifestations. Thrombophlebitis.

Prolonged administration may cause kidney damage, transient bone marrow depression, GI disturbances, and mucocutaneous lesions.

Dosage: IM (preferred), IV. *Lead toxicity:* **Adults,** 30–50 mg/kg (1–1.75 g/m²) daily in 2 divided doses q 12 hr for 3–5 days. If necessary a second course of treatment can be given for 5 additional days after a rest period of at least 2 days (but preferably 2 weeks). **Pediatric, IM:** 15–35 mg/kg (0.5–1 g/m²) daily in 2 divided doses 8–12 hr apart for 3–5 days (up to 75 mg/kg can be given in 24 hr). A second course of treatment can be given after a drug-free period of at least 4 days (but preferably 2 weeks). *Lead mobilization test:* **Adults, IM,** UP to 50 mg/kg in a single dose or 0.5 g q 12 hr for 2 doses. **Pediatric, IM:** 50 mg/kg in 2 doses 12 hr apart.

NURSING CONSIDERATIONS

Administration/Storage

1. **IV.** Administer to asymptomatic adults over a period of 1 hour b.i.d. and to symptomatic adults over a period of 2 hours b.i.d. For symptomatic adults, excess fluids should be avoided.

2. **IM.** Procaine (to achieve a concentration of 0.5%) can be added to IM injections to reduce pain at the injection site.

3. If the client is dehydrated from vomiting, urine flow should be established by IV infusion prior to the initiation of calcium EDTA therapy. Once the drug has been administered, fluids should be kept to basal levels.

4. If administered together for lead encephalopathy, calcium EDTA and dimercaprol should be given at separate deep IM sites.

5. IV infusions of drug should be well diluted to minimize irritation and the accompanying thrombophlebitis.

6. Avoid rapid IV administration during the management of lead encephalopathy.

7. Check that an x-ray film has been taken before initiating calcium EDTA therapy to determine if all lead has been removed from the gut.

8. **Never exceed the recommended daily dose of drug. Calcium EDTA may produce toxic and potentially fatal reactions.**

Interventions

1. Monitor complete blood count, liver and renal function studies throughout drug therapy.

2. Record intake and output. If anuria occurs, withhold the drug and report to the physician.

3. Analyze the lab results of daily urine specimens for proteinuria, hematuria, and renal casts. If any of these are detected, withhold the medication and report to the physician.

4. Monitor the pulse regularly for evidence of cardiac arrhythmias. These may be caused by the medication and should be documented and reported to the physician.

5. If lead has been ingested, give the client large amounts of milk to facilitate the removal of lead salts from the intestines.

6. Enemas are also indicated in lead ingestion to hasten the removal of lead.

7. Unless contraindicated (as in lead encephalopathy), encourage a high fluid intake to facilitate the excretion of lead.

8. Avoid contact of calcium EDTA with the contaminated skin of the client. Such contact increases systemic absorption.

9. Determine serum lead levels periodically to evaluate the client's response to the drug. Children with lead levels above 40 mcg/100 mL of blood require treatment.

Evaluation

Obtain serum lead level to evaluate clinical response to drug therapy.

EDETATE DISODIUM (EDTA)   (ED-eh-tayt)
Chealamide, Disotate, Endrate (Rx)

Classification: Heavy metal chelator.

Action/Kinetics: Edetate disodium has a great affinity for calcium, forming a soluble chelate in the blood. The chelate is then excreted through the urine. This leads to a lowering of serum calcium and a mobilization of calcium stores, especially from bone. When used to treat digitalis toxicity, edetate disodium exerts a negative inotropic effect on the heart and thus the chronotropic and inotropic effects of digitalis on the heart are antagonized. The drug also forms chelates with magnesium, zinc, and other trace elements. When used ophthalmically, calcified corneal deposits are dissolved from the conjunctiva, corneal epithelium, and anterior layers of the stroma.

Uses: *Systemic:* Treatment of hypercalcemia, digitalis glycoside toxicity. Anticoagulant for blood drawn for hematological studies. *Investigational:* Ophthalmically to treat corneal calcium deposits, eye burns from calcium hydroxide, and eye injury by zinc chloride.

Contraindications: Use with caution in patients with heart disease (e.g., congestive heart failure) or hypokalemia. Anuric patients; patients with ventricular arrhythmias. Not to be used to treat arteriosclerosis, atherosclerotic vascular disease, lead poisoning, or renal calculi by retrograde irrigation.

Special Concerns: Use during pregnancy only if the benefits clearly outweigh the risks.

Side Effects: *Metabolic:* Electrolyte imbalance including hypocalcemia, hypokalemia, hypomagnesemia, hyperuricemia may occur during treatment. *CV:* Decrease in both systolic and diastolic pressure, thrombophlebitis, anemia. *GI:* Nausea, vomiting, diarrhea. *CNS:* Headache, numbness, circumoral paresthesia, fever. *Other:* Exfoliative dermatitis, nephrotoxicity, reticuloendothelial system damage with hemorrhagic tendencies.

Rapid injection may produce hypocalcemic tetany and convulsions, respiratory arrest, and severe arrhythmias.

Laboratory Test Interference: ↓ Alkaline phosphatase levels.

Dosage: IV. *Hypercalcemia, digitalis toxicity:* **Adults,** Individualized and depending on degree of hypercalcemia. Usual: 50 mg/kg over 24 hr (up to 3 g/day may be prescribed); dose may be repeated for 4 consecutive days followed by a 2 day rest period with repeated courses, if needed, up to 15 doses. **Pediatric:** 40 mg/kg over 24 hr up to a maximum of 70 mg/kg/day. **Ophthalmic:** *Calcium deposits, calcium hydroxide burns,* **Adults and children:** 0.35–1.85% solution as an irrigation for 15–20 min. *Zinc chloride injury:* **Adults and children:** 1.7% solution as an irrigation for 15 min.

NURSING CONSIDERATIONS

Administration/Storage

1. Administer to client while in a Fowler's position.
2. Check label on vial carefully to determine that drug is disodium edetate and not calcium disodium edetate.
3. For use in adults, dilute medication in 500 mL of 5% dextrose solution or isotonic saline solution as ordered. For pediatric use, the final concentration should not exceed 3%.
4. Record which vein is used for site of administration because repeated use of the same vein is likely to result in thrombophlebitis. Greater dilution of the solution and slower administration reduces the incidence of thrombophlebitis if the same vein must be used.
5. Infuse slowly over 3 to 4 hours, being careful not to exceed the cardiac reserve of the client.
6. Do not exceed the recommended dose, concentration, or rate of administration.
7. There is no ophthalmic product available in the U.S.; however, the injection can be used to prepare the ophthalmic dosage form.

Interventions

1. Monitor Ca, Mg, electrolyte levels, and renal function studies. Assess urinalysis, before and during drug therapy.
2. Monitor BP during infusion because a transitory hypotension may occur. This would necessitate lowering the client from a Fowler's position until hypotension has passed and BP has stabilized.
3. Be alert to a generalized systemic reaction that may occur from 4–8 hours after infusion of the drug and that usually subsides within 12 hours. Report such a reaction and provide supportive care for fever, chills, back pain, vomiting, muscle cramps, or urinary urgency should these symptoms occur.
4. Use cautiously in clients who have heart disease, a history of seizures and/or tuberculosis.

Client/Family Teaching

1. Advise clients with diabetes mellitus that the drug may cause hypoglycemia. The client should consult with the physician concerning whether to reduce insulin dosage or increase food intake in the event of hypoglycemia.

2. Clients with diabetes should be instructed to test the urine or finger sticks regularly. If urine is negative for glucose or, if the finger sticks reveal low glucose levels, the clients should consult with the physician concerning management of their diabetes.

PENICILLAMINE (pen-ih-**SILL**-ah-meen)

Cuprimine, Depen (Rx)

Classification: Heavy metal antagonist, antiarthritic, to treat cystinuria.
See Chapter 39, p. 828.

CHAPTER SEVENTY-TWO
Miscellaneous Agents

72

ADENOSINE PHOSPHATE (ADENOSINE 5-MONOPHOSPHATE, AMP)   (ah-**DEN**-oh-seen)

Cobalasine, Kaysine (Rx)

Action/Kinetics: The adenosine phosphates are essential to the energy economy of muscle tissue. The therapeutic effects of adenosine phosphate in reducing tissue edema and inflammation are believed to result from increasing levels of adenosine triphosphate (ATP) or from its vasodilator effect and ability to decrease edema and inflammation. Adenosine phosphate may also act as a neurotransmitter.

Uses: Adjunct in treatment of varicose vein ulcers with stasis dermatitis. *Investigational:* Herpes infections, supraventricular tachycardia, increase flow of blood to brain tumors.

Contraindications: Myocardial infarction, cerebral hemorrhage.

Special Concerns: Use during pregnancy only if benefits clearly outweigh risks. Safe use in children has not been determined. Use with caution in patients with a history of asthma.

Side Effects: *CNS:* Dizziness, headaches. *GI:* Nausea, epigastric distress, diarrhea. *Other:* Flushing, diuresis, palpitations, rash, hypotension, dyspnea, increased symptoms of bursitis or tendinitis. Local reaction at injection site.

Dosage: IM only. Initial: 25–50 mg 1–2 times daily; **maintenance:** 25 mg 2–3 times/week.

NURSING CONSIDERATIONS

Assessment

1. Take a complete client history, noting if there is any history of asthma, cardiovascular disease or cerebral hemorrhage.
2. Document serum calcium, magnesium and electrolyte levels prior to initiating therapy.
3. Obtain renal function studies and urinalysis before starting therapy.

Interventions

1. Observe the client for generalized systemic reactions such as fever, chills, back pain, vomiting, muscle cramps or urinary urgency. Document and report to the physician.
2. Monitor the serum calcium, magnesium and electrolyte levels and conduct urinalysis periodically during the therapy.
3. Clients with diabetes should be observed closely for the development of hypoglycemia. Consult with the physician to determine whether to reduce the insulin dosage or to increase the client's food intake.

ALPHA₁-PROTEINASE INHIBITOR (HUMAN) (ALPHA₁-PI)   (AL-fa-1-PROH-tee-in-ayz)

Prolastin (Rx)

Classification: Alpha₁-proteinase inhibitor.

Action/Kinetics: Alpha₁-PI is the enzyme that is deficient in alpha₁-antitrypsin disease. This disease causes a progressive breakdown of elastin tissues in the alveoli, resulting in emphysema. Often fatal, alpha₁-antitrypsin disease is usually manifested in the third and fourth decades of life. Prolastin is a sterile, lyophilized product obtained from pooled human plasma that is nonreactive for the human immunodeficiency virus (HIV) antibody and the hepatitis B surface antigen. $t^{1/2}$: 4.5 days. **Therapeutic serum levels:** Approximately 80 mg/dl, although such levels may not reflect actual functional alpha₁-PI levels.

Use: Panacinar emphysema due to congenital alpha₁-proteinase deficiency.

Contraindications: Patients with PiMZ or PiMS phenotypes of alpha₁-antitrypsin deficiency.

Special Concerns: Use during pregnancy (category: C) only if benefits clearly outweigh risks. Safety and efficacy for use in children not determined. Use with caution in patients at risk for circulatory overload.

Side Effects: Although precautions are taken during the manufacture of this product, it is possible that hepatitis and other infectious viruses may be present. *Miscellaneous:* Delayed fever up to 12 hr following treatment, dizziness, lightheadedness, mild transient leukocytosis.

Dosage: IV only. Adults: 60 mg/kg each week at a rate of 0.08 mL/kg/min (or greater).

NURSING CONSIDERATIONS

Administration/Storage

1. Administer within 3 hr after reconstitution.
2. Administer only via IV. Follow recommended procedures for reconstitution.
3. Prolastin should be stored at 2° C–8° C and should not be frozen.
4. When reconstituted, Prolastin is equal to or greater than 20 mg/mL and has a pH of 6.6–7.4.
5. The reconstituted drug should not be mixed with other diluents except for normal saline.
6. Clients should be immunized against hepatitis B prior to using Prolastin. If time does not permit adequate immunization, a single dose of Hepatitis B Immune Globulin (Human), 0.06 mL/kg IM, should be given at the time of the initial dose of Prolastin.
7. Equipment used and any unused reconstituted Alpha 1-Proteinase Inhibitor (Human) should be appropriately discarded.

Assessment

1. Obtain a complete nursing history.
2. Obtain a hepatitis profile. If the client has not received hepatitis B immunization, document and provide predrug therapy.

Interventions

1. Observe the client for delayed fever which may occur within 12 hr. This is usually resolved in 24 hr.
2. Note any complaints of lightheadedness or dizziness and report to the physician.

Client/Family Teaching

1. Advise the client that cigarette smoking may accelerate and aggravate the client's condition by causing an increase of elastin secretion.
2. Discuss with the client and family the fact that there is a familial tendency to alpha$_1$-antitrypsin deficiency and explain the need for all relatives to be screened and provided appropriate counseling.
3. Stress the importance of reporting weekly for medication to maintain an adequate antielastase barrier.
4. Explain that the therapy must continue throughout the client's lifetime.
5. Discuss that the product is prepared from human plasma, and explain the associated risks.

Evaluation

1. Levels of Prolastin should be within therapeutic range (80 mg/dl).
2. ABGs within acceptable range and client experiences less difficulty and effort with breathing.
3. Freedom from complication of drug therapy.
4. Appropriate family members identified and screened.

ALPROSTADIL (PGE$_1$)   (al-PROSS-tah-dill)
Prostin VR Pediatric (Rx)

Classification: Prostaglandin.

Action/Kinetics: Alprostadil is one of the prostaglandins that is a naturally occurring acidic lipid. Alprostadil relaxes smooth muscle of the ductus arteriosus leading to increased pulmonary blood flow with increased blood oxygenation and lower body perfusion. Patients with low pO$_2$ values respond best. The drug may also cause vasodilation, inhibit platelet aggregation, and stimulate both intestinal and uterine smooth muscle. When injected intracavernosally, alprostadil relaxes the trabecular cavernous smooth muscles and causes dilation of penile arteries. This results in increased arterial blood flow to the corpus cavernosa and thus swelling and elongation of the penis. **Onset, systemic:** 1.5–3 hr for acyanotic congenital heart disease and 15–30 min for cyanotic congenital heart disease. **Time to peak effect:** 3 hr for coarctation of the aorta and 1.5 hr for interruption of aortic arch. **Duration:** Closure of the ductus arteriosus usually begins 1–2 hr after infusion discontinued. Alprostadil is rapidly metabolized (80% in one pass) by oxidation in the lung, and metabolites are excreted by the kidney.

Uses: For temporary maintenance of patency of the ductus arteriosus (until surgery can be performed) in neonates with congenital heart defects. *Investigational:* Diagnosis and treatment of impotence.

Contraindications: Respiratory distress syndrome (hyaline membrane disease). Use with caution in neonates with bleeding tendencies. History of priapism, sickle cell disease.

Side Effects: *Respiratory:* Apnea (in 10–12% of neonates), especially in neonates less than 2 kg at birth; bronchial wheezing, bradypnea, hypercapnia, respiratory depression. *CNS:* Fever, seizures, hypothermia, jitteriness, lethargy, cerebral bleeding, stiffness, hyperextension of the neck, irritability. *CV:* Flushing, especially after intra-arterial dosage, bradycardia, hypotension, tachycardia, cardiac arrest, edema, congestive heart failure, shock, arrhythmias. *GI:* Diarrhea, hyperbilirubinemia, gastric regurgitation. *Renal:* Hematuria, anuria. *Skeletal:* Cortical proliferation of long bones. *Hematologic:*

Disseminated intravascular coagulation, thrombocytopenia, anemia, bleeding. *Miscellaneous:* Sepsis, peritonitis, hypoglycemia, hypokalemia or hyperkalemia.

Laboratory Test Interferences: ↑ Bilirubin. ↓ Glucose, serum calcium. ↑ or ↓ Potassium.

Dosage: Continuous IV infusion or umbilical artery: Initial, 0.05–0.1 mcg/kg/min; **then,** after response achieved, decrease infusion rate to lowest dose that will maintain response (e.g., 0.1–0.05 to 0.025–0.01 mcg/kg/min). *Note:* If 0.1 mcg/kg/min is insufficient, dosage can be increased up to 0.4 mcg/kg/min. **Intracavernosal:** 2.5–20 mcg (up to 40 mcg) with dose adjusted according to response; should not be given more than 3 times a week or for 2 days in succession.

NURSING CONSIDERATIONS

Administration/Storage

1. Administer only in pediatric intensive care facilities.
2. Dilute 500 mcg with either sodium chloride injection or dextrose injection in volumes appropriate for the infant's fluid intake and suitable for the type of infusion pump available.
3. Use a Y setup.
4. Discard unused solutions and prepare a fresh infusion solution every 24 hr.
5. Sterile solutions should be infused for the shortest time and at the lowest dose that will produce the desired effect.
6. Have a respirator available at the cribside.
7. Store ampules at 2°C–8°C (36°F–46°F).

Assessment

1. Assess the client's cardiac function, blood pressure, and respiratory function and document prior to administering the medication.
2. Determine if the neonate has restricted pulmonary blood flow.

Interventions

1. Monitor arterial pressure intermittently by umbilical artery catheter, auscultation, Dinemapp or with a Doppler transducer. If the arterial pressure falls significantly, decrease the rate of flow immediately. Obtain written guidelines for arterial pressures from the physician.
2. Observe the infant for apnea, bradycardia, pyrexia, flushing and hypotension. These are symptoms of overdosage. The following guidelines are appropriate:
   - If the infant develops apnea or bradycardia, stop the administration of drug, change to the unmedicated solution, start resuscitation and report to the physician.
   - If the infant develops pyrexia or hypotension, reduce the rate of IV flow and report to the physician. The rate of IV flow will likely be reduced until the temperature and blood pressure return to baseline values.
   - If flushing occurs, report to the physician. This symptom indicates an incorrect intra-arterial placement of the catheter. The catheter requires repositioning.
3. If the infant has restricted pulmonary blood flow, monitor the blood gases. A positive response to alprostadil is indicated by at least a 10 mm Hg increase in blood pO_2.
4. If the infant has restricted systemic blood flow, monitor the systemic blood pressure and serum pH. If the infant has acidosis, a positive response to alprostadil would be indicated by an increased pH, an increase in blood pressure, and a decreased ratio of pulmonary artery pressure to aortic pressure.

AZATHIOPRINE   (ay-zah-**THIGH**-oh-preen)
Imuran (Rx)

Classification: Immunosuppressant.

Action/Kinetics: Antimetabolite that is quickly split to form mercaptopurine. To be effective, the drug must be given during the induction period of the antibody response. The precise mechanism in depressing the immune response is unknown, but it suppresses cell-mediated hypersensitivities, causing changes in antibody production. The drug inhibits synthesis of DNA, RNA, and proteins and may interfere with miosis and cellular metabolism. Is readily absorbed from the GI tract. The anuric patient manifests increased effectiveness and toxicity (up to twofold). **Onset:** 6–8 weeks for rheumatoid arthritis. **t½:** 3 hr.

Uses: Prophylaxis to prevent rejection of kidney transplants. Rheumatoid arthritis (adults only). *Investigational:* Chronic ulcerative colitis, chronic active hepatitis, systemic lupus erythematosus, nephrotic syndrome, glomerulonephritis, biliary cirrhosis, inflammatory myopathy, myasthenia gravis, pemphigoid, pemphigus, systemic dermatomyositis.

Contraindications: Treatment of rheumatoid arthritis in pregnancy or in patients previously treated with alkylating agents. Pregnancy and lactation.

Side Effects: *Hematologic:* Leukopenia, thrombocytopenia. *GI:* Nausea, vomiting, diarrhea, steatorrhea. *Other:* Increased risk of carcinoma, severe infections, and hepatotoxicity are major side effects. Less frequent: Skin rashes, fever, alopecia, arthralgias, negative nitrogen balance.

Drug Interactions	
Allopurinol	↑ Pharmacologic effect of azathioprine due to ↓ breakdown in liver
Corticosteroids	With azathioprine, it may cause muscle wasting after prolonged therapy
Tubocurarine	Azathioprine ↓ effect of tubocurarine

Dosage: Tablets, IV. *Immunosuppression:* **Adults and children, initial,** 3–5 mg/kg (120 mg/m²), 1–3 days before or on the day of transplantation; **maintenance:** 1–2 mg/kg (45 mg/m²) daily. *Rheumatoid arthritis, systemic lupus erythematosus:* **Adults and children, tablets: initial,** 1 mg/kg; **then,** increase dose by 0.5 mg/kg/day after 6–8 weeks and thereafter every 4 weeks up to maximum of 2.5 mg/kg/day; **maintenance:** lowest effective dose. Dosage should be reduced in patients with renal dysfunction. *Investigational Uses:* **Adults and children, tablets, initial:** 1 mg/kg; **then,** increase the dose by 0.5 mg/kg daily after 6–8 weeks and q 4 weeks thereafter up to a maximum of 2.5 mg/kg daily.

NURSING CONSIDERATIONS

Administration/Storage
Reconstitute the drug with sterile water for injection and use within 24 hr.

Assessment
Take a drug history to determine if the client is taking any drugs with which azathioprine interacts unfavorably.

Interventions
1. Observe the client for symptoms of hepatic dysfunction. If the client develops jaundice, discontinue the drug and report to the physician.

2. Monitor intake and output and weigh client daily.

3. Observe the client for any decreases in urine volume and creatinine clearance. These are symptoms of rejection of kidney transplant.

4. Report any oliguria to the physician.

5. Encourage the client to increase fluid intake.

Evaluation

1. Assess for positive clinical response to drug therapy in the prevention of kidney transplant rejections.

2. When used for rheumatoid arthritis, the client should be considered refractory if no beneficial effect is noted after 12 weeks.

BETA-CAROTENE   (BAY-tah-KAR-oh-teen)

Max-Caro, Provatene, Solatene (Rx)

Classification: Vitamin A precursor.

Action/Kinetics: Beta-carotene eliminates the photosensitivity reaction (burning sensation, edema, erythema, pruritus, and/or cutaneous lesions) in patients suffering from erythropoietic protoporphyria (edema produced by exposure to sunlight). Patients receiving beta-carotene develop yellowing of the skin, but not of the sclera. The protective effect of the drug becomes apparent 2–6 weeks after initial administration and persists 1–2 weeks after discontinuing therapy.

Uses: Erythropoietic protoporphyria (EPP).

Contraindications: Hypersensitivity to drug, pregnancy (pregnancy category: C).

Special Concerns: Use with caution in patients with impaired renal and hepatic function and during lactation.

Side Effects: Yellowing of skin starting with palms of hands, soles of feet and face. Loose stools, ecchymoses.

Dosage: Capsules. Adults, individualized: 30–300 mg daily as single or divided dose; **children under 14 years:** 30–150 mg daily.

NURSING CONSIDERATIONS

Administration/Storage

1. Administer the drug with meals.

2. For clients unable to swallow capsules, empty the contents of the capsule into orange juice or tomato juice and mix.

Assessment

1. Check for any prior known hypersensitivity to the drug.

2. Obtain baseline liver and renal function studies.

3. If the client is female and of childbearing age, determine if pregnant.

Client/Family Teaching

1. Instruct the client not to take additional vitamin preparations of vitamin A because beta-carotene fulfills the normal vitamin A requirements.

2. Advise the client to avoid exposure to the sun for 2–6 weeks after the start of drug therapy. The palms of the hands and soles of the feet and the face will turn yellow as the client becomes carotemic. Then the client may expose him/herself to the sun gradually. Advise that the protective effect is not complete, and each individual must establish their own limits of exposure.

3. Explain that pretreatment hypersensitivity to ultraviolet light or sunlight usually returns once the drug therapy ceases.

BROMOCRIPTINE MESYLATE   (broh-moh-**KRIP**-teen)

Parlodel (Rx)

Classification: Prolactin secretion inhibitor; dopamine receptor agonist.

Action/Kinetics: Bromocriptine is a nonhormonal agent that inhibits the release of the hormone prolactin by the pituitary. The drug should be used only when prolactin production by pituitary tumors has been ruled out. Its effect in parkinsonism is due to a direct stimulating effect on dopamine type 2 receptors in the corpus striatum. Less than 30% of the drug is absorbed from the GI tract. **Onset, lower prolactin:** 2 hr; **antiparkinson:** 30–90 min; **decrease growth hormone:** 1–2 hr. **Peak plasma concentration:** 1–3 hr. **t½, plasma:** 3 hr; **terminal:** 15 hr. **Duration, lower prolactin:** 24 hr (after a single dose); **decrease growth hormone:** 4–8 hr. Significant first-pass effect. Metabolized in liver, excreted mainly through bile and thus the feces.

Uses: Short-term treatment of amenorrhea/galactorrhea associated with hyperprolactinemia. Prevention of physiologic lactation. Acromegaly. Parkinsonism. Female infertility associated with hyperprolactinemia. *Investigational:* Hyperprolactinemia due to pituitary adenoma; male infertility.

Contraindications: Sensitivity to ergot alkaloids. Pregnancy, lactation, children under 15 years of age. Peripheral vascular disease, ischemic heart disease.

Special Concerns: Geriatric patients may manifest more CNS effects. Use with caution in liver or kidney disease.

Side Effects: The type and incidence of untoward reactions depend on the use of the drug. *When used for hyperprolactinemia. GI:* Nausea, vomiting, abdominal cramps, diarrhea, constipation. *CNS:* Headache, dizziness, fatigue, drowsiness, lightheadedness, psychoses. *Other:* Nasal congestion, mild hypotension.

When used to prevent physiological lactation. GI: Nausea, vomiting, cramps, diarrhea. *CNS:* Headaches, dizziness, fatigue, syncope. *CV:* Decreased blood pressure (transient).

When used for acromegaly. GI: Nausea, vomiting, anorexia, dry mouth, dyspepsia, indigestion, GI bleeding. *CNS:* Dizziness, syncope, drowsiness, tiredness, headache; rarely, lightheadedness, lassitude, vertigo, sluggishness, paranoia, insomnia, decreased sleep requirement, delusional psychosis, visual hallucinations. *CV:* Orthostatic hypotension, digital vasospasm, worsening of Raynaud's syndrome; rarely, arrhythmias, ventricular tachycardia, bradycardia, vasovagal attack; *Other:* Rarely, potentiation of effects of alcohol, hair loss, shortness of breath, paresthesia, tingling of ears, muscle cramps, facial pallor, reduced tolerance to cold.

When used for Parkinsonism. GI: Nausea, vomiting, abdominal discomfort, constipation, anorexia, dry mouth, dysphagia. *CNS:* Confusion, hallucinations, fainting, drowsiness, dizziness, insomnia, depression, vertigo, anxiety, fatigue, headache, lethargy, nightmares. *GU:* Urinary incontinence, urinary retention, urinary frequency. *Other:* Abnormal involuntary movements, asthenia, visual disturbances, ataxia, hypotension, shortness of breath, edema of feet and ankles, blepharospasm, erythromelalgia, skin mottling, nasal stuffiness, paresthesia, skin rash, signs and symptoms of ergotism.

Drug Interactions

Alcohol	↑ Chance of GI toxicity; alcohol intolerance
Antihypertensives	Additive ↓ in blood pressure
Butyrophenones	↓ Effect of bromocriptine because butyrophenones are dopamine antagonists
Diuretics	Should be avoided during bromocriptine therapy
Phenothiazines	↓ Effect of bromocriptine because phenothiazines are dopamine antagonists

Laboratory Test Interference: ↑ BUN, SGOT, SGPT, GGPT, CPT, alkaline phosphatase, uric acid.

Dosage: Capsules, Tablets. *Amenorrhea/galactorrhea/female or male infertility due to hyperprolactinemia:* **Adults, initial,** 1.25–2.5 mg daily with meals; **then,** increase dose by 2.5 mg q 3–7 days until optimum response observed (usual: 5–7.5 mg daily; range: 2.5–15 mg daily). For amenorrhea/galactorrhea, do not use for more than 6 months. *Prevention of physiological lactation:* (begin no sooner than 4 hr after delivery) usual, 2.5 mg b.i.d. with meals; therapy should be continued for 14–21 days. *Parkinsonism:* **Initial,** 1.25 mg (one-half tablet) b.i.d. with meals while maintaining dose of levodopa, if possible. Dosage may be increased q 14–28 days by 2.5 mg/day with meals. Dose should not exceed 100 mg/day. *Acromegaly:* **initial,** 1.25–2.5 mg for 3 days with food and on retiring; **then,** increased by 1.25–2.5 mg q 3–7 days until optimum response observed. Usual optimum therapeutic range: 20–30 mg daily, not to exceed 100 mg daily. Patients should be reevaluated monthly and dosage adjusted accordingly.

NURSING CONSIDERATIONS

Administration/Storage

1. Before administering the first dose of drug, have the client lie down. This is due to the possibility of fainting or dizziness.
2. For doses less than 5 mg, tablets should be used.

Assessment

1. In taking a drug history, inquire about any sensitivity to ergot alkaloids.
2. Note the age of the client, if she is female and sexually active and likely to become pregnant.
3. If the client has any history of liver or kidney dysfunction, obtain baseline liver and renal function studies.
4. List other drugs the client is taking to determine the potential for drug interactions.

Interventions

Observe the client for complaints of fatigue, headache, nausea, drowsiness, cramps or diarrhea. Document and report these findings to the physician.

Client/Family Teaching

1. Advise client to take the drug with food to minimize GI upset.
2. Caution that drug may cause dizziness, drowsiness or syncope. If clients experience syncope or dizziness, instruct them to lie down. Advise clients to avoid activities that require mental alertness.
3. If the client is using oral contraceptives, advise her to use other contraceptive measures while taking bromocriptine.

4. When a menstrual period is missed, schedule the sexually active client for pregnancy tests every 4 weeks during the period of amenorrhea and after resumption of menses.

5. Discuss with the client the signs and symptoms of pregnancy. If there is a likelihood of pregnancy, advise withholding the drug and reporting to the physician. Explain that pregnancy tests may fail to diagnose early pregnancy and the medication may harm the fetus.

CAPSAICIN (kap-**SAY**-ih-sin)

Axsain, Zostrix (Rx)

Classification: Topical drug used to relieve pain.

Action/Kinetics: Capsaicin is derived from natural sources from plants of the solanaceae family. It is believed the drug depletes and prevents the reaccumulation of substance P. Substance P is believed to be the main mediator of pain impulses from the periphery to the CNS. Two products are available: Axsain (0.075% cream) and Zostrix (0.025% cream).

Uses: *Axsain:* Relief of neuralgias due to painful diabetic neuropathy and postsurgical pain. *Zostrix:* Temporary relief of pain (neuralgia) after open skin lesions have healed following herpes zoster infections. *Investigational:* Capsaicin is being studied for possible use in psoriasis, intractable pruritus, reflex sympathetic dystrophy, postmastectomy and postamputation neuroma.

Side Effects: *Skin:* Transient burning following application.

Dosage: Cream. Apply to affected area no more than 3–4 times daily.

NURSING CONSIDERATIONS

Client/Family Teaching

1. Advise that the drug is for external use only.
2. Instruct client to avoid getting the medication in the eyes or on broken or irritated skin.
3. If the medication is applied with the fingers, advise clients to wash their hands immediately after application.
4. Remind the client not to bandage the affected area tightly.
5. Instruct the client to consult the physician if the condition worsens, if symptoms persist more than 14–28 days, or if the symptoms clear but then occur again within a few days.

CHENODIOL (CHENODEOXYCHOLIC ACID) (kee-noh-**DYE**-ohl)

Chenix (Rx)

Classification: Naturally occurring human bile acid.

Action/Kinetics: Chenodiol, by reducing hepatic synthesis of cholesterol and cholic acid, replaces both cholic and deoxycholic acids in the bile acid pool. This effect helps desaturation of biliary cholesterol and leads to dissolution of radiolucent cholesterol gallstones. The drug is ineffective on calcified gallstones or on radiolucent bile pigment stones. Fifty percent of patients have stone recurrence within 5 years. The drug also increases low-density lipoproteins and inhibits absorption of fluid from the colon. Chenodiol is well absorbed following oral administration. It is metabolized by bacteria in the colon to lithocholic acid, most of which is excreted in the feces.

Uses: Patients with radiolucent cholesterol gallstones in whom surgery is a risk due to age or systemic disease. The drug is ineffective in some patients and has potential liver toxicity. The best results have been seen in thin females with a serum cholesterol not higher than 227 mg/dl and who have a small number of radiolucent cholesterol gallstones.

Contraindications: Known hepatic dysfunction or bile ductal abnormalities. Colon cancer. Pregnancy or in those who may become pregnant (pregnancy category: X).

Special Concerns: Safety and efficacy in lactation and in children have not been established.

Side Effects: Hepatotoxicity including increased SGPT in one-third of patients, intrahepatic cholestasis. *GI:* Diarrhea (common), anorexia, constipation, dyspepsia, flatulence, heartburn, cramps, epigastric distress, nausea/vomiting, abdominal pain. *Hematologic:* Decreased white cell count. Chenodiol may contribute to colon cancer in susceptible patients.

Drug Interactions

Antacids, aluminum	↓ Effect of chenodiol due to ↓ absorption from GI tract
Cholestyramine	See *Antacids*
Clofibrate	↓ Effect of chenodiol due to ↑ biliary cholesterol secretion
Colestipol	See *Antacids*
Estrogens, oral contraceptives	↓ Effect of chenodiol due to ↑ biliary cholesterol secretion

Dosage: Tablets. Adults, initial: 250 mg b.i.d. for 2 weeks; **then,** increase by 250 mg weekly until maximum tolerated or recommended dose is reached (13–16 mg/kg/day in 2 divided doses morning and night with milk or food). *Note:* Doses less than 10 mg/kg are usually ineffective and may result in increased risk of cholecystectomy.

NURSING CONSIDERATIONS

Assessment

1. Obtain liver and renal function studies prior to initiating therapy.
2. Take a complete drug history, noting any potential drug interactions.
3. Determine if women in childbearing years are pregnant.

Interventions

1. Obtain periodic liver function tests such as serum aminotransferase levels, serum cholesterol, and monitor for stone dissolution.
2. Note any client complaint of severe, sudden upper quadrant pain that radiates to the shoulder, nonspecific abdominal pain, nausea or vomiting. Report these symptoms to the physician immediately. These may be symptoms that the client has developed gallstone complications.
3. If the client develops diarrhea, the dose of medication may be reduced temporarily and antidiarrheal agents may be administered.

Client/Family Teaching

1. Advise the client that the drug may need to be taken for 24 months before gallstones are dissolved.
2. Discuss with the client the likelihood that gallstones may recur even after successful treatment.

3. Pregnancy should be avoided during drug therapy. Oral contraceptives may decrease the effectiveness of chenodiol. Therefore, advise women of childbearing age to practice alternative methods of birth control.

4. Advise women to report to the physician if there is any possibility that conception has occurred.

5. Stress the importance of having periodic liver function tests performed and cholecystograms or gallbladder ultrasonography to evaluate the effectiveness of the drug therapy.

6. Advise the client to consult with the physician if there is a need to use antacids. Most antacids have an aluminum base which absorbs the drug.

7. Instruct the client to report any incidence of diarrhea. This may be related to the dose of drug and can be relieved by appropriate changes in the dosage.

CHYMOPAPAIN FOR INJECTION   (KYE-moh-pah-payn)
Chymodiactin, Discase ❀ (Rx)

Classification: Proteolytic enzyme.

Action/Kinetics: Chymopapain is a proteolytic enzyme derived from the crude latex of *Carica papaya*. The nanoKatal (nKat) is used as the unit of chymopapain activity (1 mg of chymopapain is equivalent to at least 0.52 nKat units). The preparation also contains sodium L-cysteinate hydrochloride as a reducing agent to keep the sulfur in the sulfhydryl form.

Chymopapain is injected into the herniated lumbar intervertebral disc (nucleus pulposus), where it hydrolyzes the noncollagenous proteins or polypeptides that maintain the structure of the chondromucoprotein of the nucleus pulposus. As a result of hydrolysis, the osmotic activity is decreased, leading to a decreased fluid absorption thus reducing intradiscal pressure.

Although chymopapain acts locally in the disc, it does appear in the plasma, where it is inactivated. Small amounts are excreted in the urine.

Uses: Chymopapain should be used only in a hospital setting by physicians and supportive personnel trained in the diagnosis and treatment of herniated lumbar intervertebral disc disease that has not responded to more conservative therapy.

Contraindications: Sensitivity to chymopapain, papaya, or its derivatives. Severe spondylolisthesis, significant spinal stenosis, spinal cord tumor or a cauda equina lesion, or in progressing paralysis manifested by rapidly progressing neurologic dysfunction. Patients previously treated with chymopapain. Injection into any location other than lumbar area.

Special Concerns: Use during pregnancy only when benefits outweigh risks (pregnancy category: C). Safety and efficacy have not been established for use in children.

Side Effects: *Neuromuscular:* Back pain, stiffness, soreness, back spasm, paraplegia, acute transverse myelitis or myelopathy characterized by onset of paraplegia or paraparesis (without prior symptoms) within 2–3 weeks. Also, sacral burning, leg pain, hyperalgesia, leg weakness, tingling/numbness in legs/toes, cramping in both calves, paresthesia, pain in opposite leg, postinjection pain, bacterial and aseptic discitis. *Allergic:* Anaphylaxis (more common in females). Complications secondary to anaphylaxis including staphylococcal meningitis with disc abscess. Rash, itching, urticaria, pilomotor erection, vasomotor rhinitis, conjunctivitis, angioedema, GI disturbances. *Other:* Cerebral hemorrhage, nausea, itching, paralytic ileus, urinary retention, headache, dizziness.

Drug Interactions: Possible arrhythmias if used with halothane or epinephrine.

Dosage: A single injection of 2–4 nKat units/disc (usual is 3 nKat units/disc in a volume of 1.5 mL). Maximum dose with multiple disc herniation is 10 nKat units.

NURSING CONSIDERATIONS

Administration/Storage

1. An open IV line must always be available in the event of anaphylaxis. Epinephrine is the drug of choice to treat anaphylaxis.
2. Sterile water for injection should be used for reconstitution, as bacteriostatic water for injection inactivates the enzyme. The reconstituted drug must be used within 2 hr. Any unused, reconstituted drug should be discarded promptly.
3. Automatic filling syringes should not be used since a residual vacuum is present in the vial.
4. Alcohol should be used to cleanse the vial stopper before inserting the needle; since alcohol inactivates the enzyme, it should be allowed to dry before continuing with reconstitution.
5. The package literature should be consulted for the specific procedures for administration.
6. Prior to use, the client should be treated with histamine receptor H_1 and H_2 antagonists to decrease the severity of an anaphylactic reaction (e.g., cimetidine, 300 mg PO, q 6 hr and diphenhydramine, 50 mg PO, q 6 hr, both for 24 hr prior to therapy).

Interventions

Monitor the client's blood pressure and respiratory status. The drug can cause hypotension and bronchospasms.

Client/Family Teaching

1. Advise clients that back pain and muscle spasms may occur within several days to several weeks following treatment.
2. Discuss with the client the possibility of paraplegia and paresis occurring suddenly, several weeks after treatment. This should be reported immediately to the physician.
3. Explain the need to report to the physician if there is leg weakness, tingling or numbness of the legs and/or toes, or cramping in the calves of the legs.

CYCLOSPORINE (SYE-kloh-spor-een)

Sandimmune (Rx)

Classification: Immunosuppressant.

Action/Kinetics: Cyclosporine is an immunosuppressant thought to act by inhibiting the immunocompetent lymphocytes in the G_o or G_1 phase of the cell cycle. T-lymphocytes are specifically inhibited. Cyclosporine also inhibits interleukin 2 or T-cell growth factor production and release. **Peak plasma levels:** 3.5 hr. **t½:** Approximately 19 hr for adults and 7 hr in children. Metabolized by the liver. Inactive metabolites are excreted mainly through the bile.

Uses: In combination with corticosteroids for prophylaxis of rejection in kidney, liver, and heart transplants. Treatment of chronic rejection in patients previously treated with other immunosuppressants.

A number of other diseases have been treated with cyclosporine including aplastic anemia, myasthenia gravis, atopic dermatitis, Crohn's disease, Graves ophthalmology, severe psoriasis, multiple sclerosis, polymyositis, dermatomyositis, uveitis, biliary cirrhosis, and others.

Contraindications: Hypersensitivity to cyclosporine or polyoxyethylated castor oil. Lactation.

Special Concerns: Use with caution during pregnancy (category: C), and in patients with impaired renal or hepatic function. Safety and efficacy have not been established in children.

Side Effects: *GI:* Nausea, vomiting, diarrhea, gum hyperplasia, anorexia, gastritis, hiccoughs, peptic ulcer, abdominal discomfort. *Hematologic:* Leukopenia, lymphoma, thrombocytopenia. *Allergic:* Anaphylaxis (rare). *CV:* Hypertension, edema, myocardial infarction. *CNS:* Headache, tremor, confusion, fever, seizures, anxiety, depression, weakness, lethargy. *Other:* Nephrotoxicity, hepatotoxicity, acne, hirsutism, flushing, paresthesia, sinusitis, gynecomastia, conjunctivitis, brittle fingernails, hearing loss, tinnitus, hyperglycemia, muscle pain, infections, hematuria.

Drug Interactions	
Aminoglycosides	↑ Risk of nephrotoxicity
Amphotericin B	↑ Risk of nephrotoxicity
Carbamazepine	↓ Plasma level of cyclosporine due to ↑ breakdown by liver
Cimetidine	↑ Plasma level of cyclosporine due to ↓ breakdown by liver
Danazol	↑ Plasma level of cyclosporine due to ↓ breakdown by liver
Diltiazem	↑ Plasma level of cyclosporine due to ↓ breakdown by liver
Erythromycin	↑ Plasma level of cyclosporine due to ↓ breakdown by liver and ↓ excretion
Imipenem-cilastatin	↑ Plasma level of cyclosporine due to ↓ breakdown by liver
Isoniazid	↓ Plasma level of cyclosporine due to ↑ breakdown by liver
Ketoconazole	↑ Plasma level of cyclosorine due to ↓ breakdown by liver
Melphalan	↑ Risk of nephrotoxicity
Methylprednisolone	↑ Risk of seizures
Methyltestosterone	↑ Plasma level of cyclosporine due to ↓ breakdown by liver
Metoclopramide	↑ Plasma level of cyclosporine due to ↑ absorption from GI tract
Nephrotoxic drugs	Additive nephrotoxicity
Oral contraceptives	↑ Plasma level of cyclosporine due to ↓ breakdown by liver
Phenobarbital	↓ Plasma level of cyclosporine due to ↑ breakdown by liver
Phenytoin	↓ Plasma level of cyclosporine due to ↑ breakdown by liver
Prednisolone	↑ Plasma level of cyclosporine due to ↓ breakdown by liver
Rifampin	↓ Plasma level of cyclosporine due to ↑ breakdown by liver
Sulfamethoxazole and/or trimethoprim	↑ Risk of nephrotoxicity
Sulfatrimethoprim	↓ Plasma level of cyclosporine due to ↑ breakdown by liver
Verapamil	↑ Degree of immunosuppression

Laboratory Test Interferences: ↑ Serum creatinine, BUN, total bilirubin, alkaline phosphatase, serum potassium.

Dosage: Capsules, Oral Solution. Adults and children, initial: 12–15 mg/kg/day given 4–12 hr prior to transplantation; **then,** 15 mg/kg/day postoperatively for 1–2 weeks followed by 5% decrease in dose per week to maintenance dose of 5–10 mg/kg/day. **IV (only in patients unable to take PO medication):** 2–6 mg/kg/day 4–12 hr prior to transplantation and postoperatively until patient can be switched to PO dosage. *Note:* Steroid therapy must be used concomitantly.

NURSING CONSIDERATIONS

Administration/Storage

1. The oral solution may be diluted with milk, chocolate milk, or juice immediately before being administered. The oral solutions should not be stored in the refrigerator.
2. Due to variable absorption of the oral solution, blood levels of cyclosporine should be monitored.
3. The IV concentration should be diluted 1 mL in 20–100 mL 0.9% sodium chloride injection or 5% dextrose injection. The IV solution is given by slow IV infusion over 2–6 hr.
4. Due to the possibility of anaphylaxis, clients receiving IV cyclosporine should be closely monitored for 30 min following the initiation of the infusion. Epinephrine (1:1,000) should be available at the bedside for treating anaphylaxis.
5. Clients with malabsorption from the GI tract may not achieve appropriate blood levels.

Assessment

1. List all drugs the client is currently taking and note the potential for any drug interactions.
2. Obtain baseline complete blood cell counts, white cell differential and platelet count.
3. Prior to administration, obtain a BUN and serum creatinine level.

Interventions

1. Monitor the client's blood pressure and pulse. Document and report to the physician any changes from the baseline data.
2. Observe the client for complaints of fatigue, malaise, unexplained bleeding or bruising, bleeding from the gums, nosebleeds or hematuria. Monitor CBC, white cell differential and platelet count. Document and report any deviation from baseline data.
3. If the client finds the oral medication unpalatable, mix with milk or juice. Mix the medication in a glass container to minimize adherence to the container. The medication should be taken immediately after mixing.
4. Monitor the client for jaundice, fever, and other signs of hepatotoxicity. Assess drug levels and monitor liver and renal function studies throughout drug therapy.
5. Routinely inspect the client's teeth and gums. Note any signs of changes in dentition.
6. Anticipate that clients will receive concomitant administration of adrenal corticosteroids.

Client/Family Teaching

1. Demonstrate and explain how to measure the dose of medication accurately.
2. Review the side effects of drug therapy. Because this drug is so important to transplant clients in preventing rejection, the client and family should be provided a written list of all possible side effects of drugs and know which side effects need to be reported to the physician.

3. Explain the importance of following the written guidelines for medication therapy explicitly. Call the physician with questions or if problems arise.

4. Advise the client to keep an account of daily weight. Discuss the importance of reporting any persistent diarrhea, nausea and vomiting and of recording the intake and output.

5. Advise client that taking the drug with food may reduce nausea and associated GI upset.

6. Instruct the client not to stop the drug abruptly. If the drug must be discontinued, it should be done gradually.

7. Stress the importance of using nystatin swish and swab as directed to prevent the development of thrush.

8. Warn clients that they may develop acne and hirsutism as a side effect. This should be reported to the physician as a dermatologist referral may be necessary.

DIMETHYLSULFOXIDE (DMSO)   (dye-METH-ill-sul-FOX-ide)

Rimso-50 (Rx)

Classification: Local anti-inflammatory agent.

Action/Kinetics: DMSO is a clear liquid miscible with both water and most organic solvents. It is widely used as an industrial solvent and has many pharmacologic effects, including nerve blockade, bacteriostasis, diuresis, inhibition of cholinesterase, muscle relaxation, and vasodilation. It also penetrates membranes readily. The drug is currently indicated only for symptomatic relief of interstitial cystitis (mechanism is unknown). Its use for musculoskeletal disorders is widely debated, and conclusive evidence for its efficacy in such disorders as well as for enhancing percutaneous absorption of other drugs is lacking. DMSO is used for these disorders on an investigational basis; the compound is distributed by certain clinics outside the United States, and is available through mail order houses in the United States.

Widely distributed after topical administration. **Onset:** rapid. DMSO is metabolized to dimethyl sulfide and dimethyl sulfone. DMSO and the sulfone are excreted through the urine and feces; DMSO is also excreted through the skin and lungs and gives off a garlic-type odor. **t½, DMSO:** 12–15 hr.

Uses: Symptomatic relief of interstitial cystitis. *Investigational:* Musculoskeletal disorders, scleroderma, arthritis, tendinitis, cancer of the breast and prostate, herpes infections, retinitis pigmentosa, head and spinal cord injury, and stroke. Also, as a carrier to increase the percutaneous absorption of other drugs.

Contraindications: Urinary tract cancer. Hypersensitivity to DMSO.

Special Concerns: Use during pregnancy only if benefits clearly outweigh risks (pregnancy category: C). Use with caution during lactation. Safety and effectiveness have not been determined in children.

Side Effects: *After topical use:* Nausea, vomiting, sedation, headache, rashes, burning or aching eyes. Garlic-like taste and breath. Transient chemical cystitis. Discomfort following administration (usually subsides with repeated use).

Drug Interaction: ↓ Effect of sulindac due to ↓ rate of conversion to active metabolite.

Dosage: Irrigation. *Cystitis:* **Adults,** Instillation of 50 mL of DMSO directly into the bladder for 15 min every 2 weeks until symptomatic relief is achieved. *Musculoskeletal disorders:* Application of 50%–90% solution or gel to skin.

NURSING CONSIDERATIONS

Administration/Storage

1. To prevent spasms, use an analgesic lubricant such as lidocaine jelly, in the urethra before inserting the catheter.
2. Dilute DMSO immediately before instillation in a glass vessel. Use 1 part DMSO to 1 part of sterile water.
3. Solution is to be retained by client for 15 min and then expelled by voiding.
4. If the client is not relieved by the usual treatment, the physician may order the following:
   - Distend the bladder gently by gravity instillation of 500 mL of 1 part DMSO and 1 part sterile water, mixed in a glass delivery container.
   - Then instill the standard 50 mL of undiluted DMSO.
   - Instruct the client to retain the fluid for 15 minutes, and then void.
5. To reduce bladder spasms, administer an oral analgesic or a suppository containing belladonna and opium prior to instillation.
6. If the client has a sensitive bladder, the first one to three instillations can be performed under saddle block anesthesia.
7. Instillations should be performed only by personnel specifically trained in the procedure.

Assessment

Determine that client has an ophthalmic examination performed prior to administration of the drug.

Interventions

1. Explain to the client that the instillation may cause moderate to severe discomfort. This will, however, lessen with repeated administrations.
2. Monitor the client closely during the procedure. Measure the amount of urine expelled.
3. If the client experiences an unusual amount of discomfort or increased discomfort, document and report so that the physician can order an analgesic or anesthesia.
4. Inform the client that there may be a garlic-like taste after the drug has been instilled and that there will be a garlic-like odor to the breath and skin for 72 hours after the treatment.
5. Ensure that ophthalmic examinations are done periodically during the course of therapy.
6. Liver and renal function studies should be performed at least every 6 months.

DISULFIRAM   (dye-SUL-fih-ram)

Antabuse (Rx)

Classification: Treatment of alcoholism.

Action/Kinetics: Disulfiram produces severe hypersensitivity to alcohol. It is used as an adjunct in the treatment of alcoholism. The toxic reaction to disulfiram appears to be due to the inhibition of liver enzymes that participate in the normal degradation of alcohol. When alcohol and disulfiram are both present, acetaldehyde accumulates in the blood. High levels of acetaldehyde produce a series of symptoms referred to as the disulfiram-alcohol reaction or syndrome. The specific symptoms are listed under *Side Effects*. The symptoms vary individually, are dose-dependent, with respect to both alcohol and disulfiram, and persist for periods ranging from 30 min to several hours. A single dose of disulfiram may be effective for 1–2 weeks. **Onset:** May be delayed up to 12 hr as disulfiram is initially localized in fat stores.

Uses: To prevent further ingestion of alcohol in chronic alcoholics. Disulfiram should be given only to cooperating patients fully aware of the consequences of alcohol ingestion.

Contraindications: Alcohol intoxication. Severe myocardial or occlusive coronary disease. Use of paraldehyde or alcohol-containing products such as cough syrups. If patient is exposed to ethylene dibromide.

Special Concerns: Use in pregnancy only if benefits outweigh risks. Use with caution in narcotic addicts or patients with diabetes, goiter, epilepsy, psychosis, hypothyroidism, hepatic cirrhosis, or nephritis.

Side Effects: In the absence of alcohol, the following symptoms have been reported: Drowsiness (most common), headache, restlessness, fatigue, psychoses, peripheral neuropathy, dermatoses, hepatotoxicity, metallic or garlic taste, arthropathy, impotence.

In the presence of alcohol, the following symptoms may be manifested. *CV:* Flushing, chest pain, palpitations, tachycardia, hypotension, syncope, arrhythmias, cardiovascular collapse, myocardial infarction, acute congestive heart failure. *CNS:* Throbbing headaches, vertigo, weakness, uneasiness, confusion, unconsciousness, seizures, death. *GI:* Nausea, severe vomiting, thirst. *Respiratory:* Respiratory difficulties, dyspnea, hyperventilation, respiratory depression. *Other:* Throbbing in head and neck, sweating.

In the event of an Antabuse-alcohol interaction, measures should be undertaken to maintain blood pressure and treat shock. Oxygen, antihistamines, ephedrine, and/or vitamin C may also be used.

Drug Interactions	
Anticoagulants, oral	↑ Effect of anticoagulants by ↑ hypoprothrombinemia
Barbiturates	↑ Effect of barbiturates due to ↓ breakdown by liver
Chlordiazepoxide, diazepam	↑ Effect of chlordiazepoxide or diazepam due to ↓ plasma clearance
Isoniazid	↑ Side effects of isoniazid (especially CNS)
Metronidazole	Acute toxic psychosis or confusional state
Paraldehyde	Concomitant use produces Antabuse-like effect
Phenytoin	↑ Effect of phenytoin due to ↓ breakdown by liver
Tricyclic antidepressants	Acute organic brain syndrome

Dosage: Tablets. Adults, initial (after alcohol-free interval of 12–48 hr): 500 mg daily for 1–2 weeks; **maintenance:** *usual,* 250 mg daily (range: 120–500 mg daily). Dose should not exceed 500 mg/day.

NURSING CONSIDERATIONS

Administration/Storage

1. Tablets can be crushed or mixed with liquid.
2. Clients should always carry appropriate identification indicating disulfiram is being taken.
3. Have oxygen, pressor agents, and antihistamines available to treat disulfiram-alcohol reactions.

Client/Family Teaching

1. Emphasize to the family that disulfiram should never be given to the client without client's knowledge.
2. Explain the effects of disulfiram and emphasize the need for close medical and psychiatric supervision.
3. If the client experiences CNS side effects, explain that these will lessen as the drug is continued.
4. Explain that ingesting as little as 30 mL of 100-proof alcohol (e.g., one shot) while on disulfiram therapy may cause severe symptoms and possibly death.
5. Advise the client to avoid alcohol in any form, in foods, sauces, or other medications, such as cough syrups, or tonics. Clients should also be advised to avoid vinegar, paregoric, liniments or lotions containing alcohol.
6. Instruct the client to read carefully all labels on foods before consuming them to avoid those that may contain alcohol.
7. Discuss with clients the fact that they may feel tired, experience drowsiness, headaches and develop a metallic or garlic-like taste. These side effects tend to subside after about 2 weeks of therapy.
8. Explain to male clients that they may have occasional impotence. This is usually transient. Remind clients that they should discuss this problem with the physician before discontinuing the medication.
9. If skin eruptions occur, advise the client to consult the physician since an antihistamine may be prescribed.
10. Advise clients to carry an identification card stating that they are taking disulfiram and describing the symptoms and treatment if clients have a disulfiram reaction. Included should be the name of the physician treating the client and a telephone number where the physician may be reached. (Cards may be obtained from the Ayerst Laboratories, 685 Third Avenue, New York, NY 10017).
11. Advise the client and family to attend meetings of local support groups such as Alcoholics Anonymous (AA) and Al-Anon to gain a better understanding of the disease. These groups offer the support, structure, referral and encouragement that may help the client in the quest for an alcohol free life.

EPOETIN ALFA, RECOMBINANT   (eh-poh-**EE**-tin)

Epogen (Rx)

Classification: Recombinant human erythropoietin.

Action/Kinetics: Epoetin alfa is a 165 amino acid glycoprotein made by recombinant DNA technology; it has the identical amino acid sequence and same biological effects as endogenous erythropoietin (which is normally synthesized in the kidney and stimulates red blood cell production). Epoetin alfa will elevate or maintain the red blood cell level decreasing the need for blood transfusions. $t^1/_2$: 4–13 hr in patients with chronic renal failure. **Peak serum levels after SC:** 5–24 hr.

Uses: Treatment of anemia associated with chronic renal failure, including patients on dialysis (end-stage renal disease) or not on dialysis.

Contraindications: Uncontrolled hypertension, hypersensitivity to mammalian cell-derived products, hypersensitivity to human albumin.

Special Concerns: Pregnancy category: C. Safety and efficacy have not been established in children. The safety and efficacy of epoetin alfa are not known in patients with a history of seizures or underlying hematologic disease (e.g., hypercoagulable disorders, myelodysplastic syndromes, sickle cell anemia). Use with caution in patients with porphyria, during lactation, and preexisting vascular disease.

Side Effects: *CV:* Hypertension, tachycardia, edema, clotted vascular access. Rarely, myocardial infarction, cerebrovascular accident, transient ischemic attacks. *GI:* Nausea, vomiting, diarrhea. *CNS:* Headache, dizziness, seizures. *Miscellaneous:* Arthralgias, fatigue, chest pain, skin reaction at administration site, asthenia, hyperkalemia, shortness of breath.

Dosage: IV, initial (dialysis or nondialysis patients), SC (non-dialysis patients): 50–100 units/kg 3 times weekly. The rate of increase of hematocrit depends on both dosage and patient variation. **Maintenance:** Individualize.

NURSING CONSIDERATIONS

Administration/Storage

1. During hemodialysis, clients treated with epoetin alfa may require increased anticoagulation with heparin to prevent clotting of the artificial kidney.
2. The hematocrit should be determined twice weekly until it has stabilized in the target range and the maintenance dose of epoetin alfa has been determined. Also, after any dosage adjustment, the hematocrit should be monitored twice weekly for 2–6 weeks.
3. The dose of epoetin alfa should be reduced by about 25 units/kg 3 times weekly when the target range (30–33%) is reached. Maintenance doses must then be individually determined.
4. If the hematocrit exceeds 36%, the drug should be withheld temporarily until the hematocrit decreases to 30–33%. Upon re-initiation of therapy, the dose should be reduced by about 25 units/kg 3 times weekly.
5. The dose of epoetin alfa should be reduced immediately if the hematocrit increases more than 4 points in any two-week period. After reduction, the hematocrit should be monitored twice a week for 2–6 weeks with maintenance doses individually determined.
6. The dose of epoetin alfa should be increased in increments of 25 units/kg 3 times weekly if the hematocrit does not increase by 5–6 points after 8 weeks of therapy. Further increases of 25 units/kg 3 times weekly may be made at 4–6 week intervals until a desired response is observed.
7. The preparation should not be shaken as shaking will denature the glycoprotein making it biologically inactive.
8. Vials showing particulate matter or discoloration should not be used.
9. Only one dose per vial should be withdrawn and any unused portion should be discarded. The product contains no preservative.
10. Epoetin alfa should not be given with any other drug solutions.

Assessment

1. During the nursing history, note if client has any history of hypersensitivity to mammalian cell-derived products or human albumin.
2. Determine client iron stores prior to initiating therapy. Transferrin saturation should be at least 20% and serum ferritin should be at least 200 ng/mL. It may be necessary to provide supplemental iron to increase or maintain transferrin saturation to levels required to support stimulation of erythropoiesis by epoetin alfa.

3. Obtain baseline CBC and platelet count before starting therapy.

4. Note history of hypertension and perform baseline readings.

Interventions

1. Monitor CBC and platelet count throughout therapy and report to the physician. Drug dose may need to be adjusted frequently.

2. Assess BP and monitor throughout epoetin alfa therapy. Hypertension should be controlled prior to initiation of drug therapy.

3. Monitor renal function studies, electrolytes, phosphorus and uric acid levels especially in clients with chronic renal failure.

Client/Family Teaching

1. Advise clients and family that over 95% of clients with chronic renal failure manifested significant increases in hematocrit and nearly all clients were transfusion-independent within 2 months after beginning epoetin alfa therapy.

2. Explain that the desired drug response may take as long as 6 weeks.

3. Stress the importance of reporting for scheduled lab studies as drug dose must be adjusted based on these results.

4. Provide a printed list of drug side effects. Instruct client to report any persistent and/or bothersome side effects of epoetin alfa therapy to the physician.

5. Explain the importance of the client continuing to follow the prescribed dietary and dialysis recommendations.

6. Caution client not to perform any tasks that require mental alertness during the first **90** days of therapy with epoetin alfa.

Evaluation

Assess hematocrit twice weekly. A clinically significant response to epoetin alfa may not be observed for 2 weeks and may require up to 6 weeks in some clients.

ETHANOLAMINE OLEATE INJECTION 5%   (eth-an-**OH**-lah-meen **OH**-lee-ayt)

Ethamolin (Rx)

Classification: Sclerosing agent.

Action/Kinetics: The oleic portion of the product induces an inflammatory reaction of the intimal endothelium of the vein, leading to fibrosis and occlusion. The drug may also diffuse through the venous wall producing an extravascular inflammatory response. Ethanolamine oleate disappears within 5 min from the injection site via the portal vein.

Use: To prevent rebleeding in patients with esophageal varices who have had a recent bleeding episode. *Note:* The drug has no effect on portal hypertension, the cause of esophageal varices; thus, retreatment may be necessary.

Contraindications: Patients with esophageal varices who have not bled. Known sensitivity to ethanolamine, oleic acid, or ethanolamine oleate. Not recommended for use in treating varicosities of the leg.

Special Concerns: Use during pregnancy only when clearly needed (pregnancy category: C). Use with caution during lactation. Safety and efficacy in children have not been determined.

Side Effects: *At site of varices:* Pleural effusion or infiltration, esophageal ulcer, esophageal stricture, retrosternal pain. Less commonly, esophagitis, necrosis, periesophageal abscess, tearing of the esophagus, sloughing of the mucosa overlying the injected varix, perforation. *Miscellaneous:* Pyrexia, pneumonia, aspiration pneumonia, anaphylaxis, acute renal failure.

Dosage: Local IV only: 1.5–5 mL/varix. **Maximum total dose/treatment:** 20 mL.

NURSING CONSIDERATIONS

Administration/Storage

1. Smaller doses should be used in clients with significant liver dysfunction (Child Class C) or accompanying cardiopulmonary disease.
2. Submucosal injections should not be used as they may result in ulceration at the site of injection.
3. The drug may be given at the time of acute bleeding and again after 1 week, 6 weeks, 3 months, and 6 months in order to obliterate the varix.
4. The drug should be stored at room temperature (15°–30°C or 59°–86°F) and protected from light.

Assessment

1. Note any client history of sensitivity to ethanolamine, oleic acid or ethanolamine oleate and document.
2. Determine if the client has any history of liver or cardiovascular disease.
3. Obtain baseline CBC, liver and renal function studies.
4. Determine when last bleed from esophageal varices occurred.

Interventions

1. Monitor CBC, liver and renal function studies throughout drug therapy.
2. Anticipate reduced dose in clients with impaired liver, cardiac and/or renal function.
3. Monitor vital signs, intake and output and record.
4. Observe client closely for any evidence of rebleeding from esophageal varices.
5. Observe client for any symptoms associated with pleural effusion and/or pneumonia such as chest pain, dyspnea, cough and pyrexia. Document and report to the physician as these are side effects related to drug therapy.

ETRETINATE   (eh-**TRET**-ih-nayt)

Tegison (Rx)

Classification: Systemic antipsoriatic.

Action/Kinetics: Etretinate is related to vitamin A; it acts to decrease the thickness, erythema, and scale of lesions in individuals with psoriasis. Significant first-pass metabolism occurs in the active acid form of the drug. The ingestion of milk or a high-lipid diet increases the absorption of etretinate. Has a long half-life due to storage in adipose tissue. The drug has been found in the blood of certain patients up to 3 years after therapy was terminated. Etretinate itself is bound more than 99% to plasma lipoproteins, whereas the active acid metabolite is bound to albumin.

Uses: Severe recalcitrant psoriasis unresponsive to psoralens plus UVA light, systemic corticosteroids, methotrexate, or topical tar plus UVB light. *Investigational:* Severe, intractable keratinization disorders; severe, intractable oral lichen planus.

Contraindications: Individuals who are pregnant, intend to become pregnant, or who are not using effective contraceptive measures while taking the drug (pregnancy category: X). Lactation. Use in children unless other alternatives have been exhausted.

Side Effects: The toxic effects of etretinate resemble those of hypervitaminosis A. They include benign intracranial hypertension (pseudotumor cerebri); the symptoms include headache, nausea, vomiting, papilledema, and visual disturbances. *CNS:* Fatigue, headache, fever, lethargy, pain, dizziness, rigors, amnesia, anxiety, abnormal thought processes, depression, emotional lability, flu-like symptoms, faint feeling. *CV:* Edema, thrombosis, fainting, postural hypotension, chest pain, atrial fibrillation, phlebitis. *GI:* GI pain, changes in appetite, nausea, constipation, flatulence, melena, diarrhea, alteration in taste, ulcers of mouth, tooth caries. *Hepatic:* Hepatitis. *Ophthalmic:* Decreased visual acuity, blurred vision, decrease in night vision, corneal erosion, irregular and punctate staining, abrasions, iritis, retinal hemorrhage, photophobia, eye irritation, eyeball pain, double vision, scotoma. *Dermatologic:* Peeling of soles, palms, fingertips; loss of hair, itching, rash, dry skin, skin fragility, red scaly face, bruising, sunburn, cold clammy skin, bullous eruptions, onycholysis, changes in perspiration, paronychia, pyogenic granuloma, impaired healing, herpes simplex, hirsutism, abnormal skin odor, urticaria, granulation tissue. Skin atrophy, infection, fissures, nodules or ulceration. *Musculoskeletal:* Joint and bone pain, myalgia, muscle cramps, gout, ossification of interosseous ligaments and tendons of extremities, hyperkinesia. *Hematologic:* Significant alterations of platelets, reticulocytes, hemoglobin, white blood cells, or prothrombin time. *Renal:* Kidney stones; white blood cells, proteins, glucose, acetone, blood, casts, or hemoglobin in the urine; dysuria, urinary retention, polyuria. *Other:* Dyspnea, coughing, changes in electrolytes (either increased or decreased potassium, sodium, chloride, calcium, phosphorus, carbon dioxide), abnormal menses, earache, otitis externa, changes in equilibrium, drainage or infection of ear.

Laboratory Test Interferences: ↑ Triglycerides, AST (SGOT), ALT (SGPT), globulin, cholesterol, alkaline phosphatase, bilirubin, BUN. ↑ or ↓ Total protein albumin.

Dosage: Capsules. Adults: initial, 0.75–1 mg/kg/day in divided doses, not to exceed 1.5 mg/kg/day. **Maintenance:** 0.5–0.75 mg/kg/day, usually after 8–16 weeks of therapy. *Erythrodermic psoriasis:* **initial,** 0.25 mg/kg/day; **then,** increase by 0.25 mg/kg/day each week until optimum response has been obtained.

NURSING CONSIDERATIONS

Administration/Storage

1. Individualization of dosage is required to achieve maximal therapeutic effects with a tolerable degree of side effects.
2. Lesions may require up to 9 months of therapy to be completely cleared.
3. The drug should be administered with food.
4. Since etretinate is similar to vitamin A, clients should not take vitamin A supplements during therapy.
5. Most clients have relapses within 2 months after therapy is terminated. Subsequent courses of therapy, up to 9 months, result in a response similar to that achieved during the initial course of therapy.

Assessment

1. Determine if female clients are sexually active and likely to be pregnant, prior to initiating therapy.
2. Ensure that women of childbearing age, who are to receive this medication, are using reliable forms of birth control.
3. Obtain pretreatment blood lipids under fasting conditions. The ingestion of milk or a high-lipid diet increases the absorption of drug.

Client/Family Teaching

1. Advise clients that they may experience a worsening of psoriasis at the beginning of therapy.
2. Instruct clients to take the medication with meals to avoid GI upset. Review dietary recommendations.
3. Discuss with clients who wear contact lenses the fact that they may experience a decreased tolerance to contact lenses during and following therapy.
4. Stress the importance of reporting for all laboratory tests.
5. Provide a printed list of drug side effects. Instruct the client to report any symptoms that may indicate toxicity, such as headaches, nausea and vomiting, dizziness, and visual disturbances to the physician.
6. Advise client not to donate blood during therapy and for several years thereafter due to the possible risks to a developing fetus if a pregnant client receives such blood.

HEMIN   (HEE-min)

Panhematin (Rx)

Classification: Iron-containing metalloporphyrin.

Action/Kinetics: This drug possibly inhibits biosynthesis of porphyrin by inhibition of the rate-limiting enzyme delta-aminolevulinic acid synthetase.

Uses: Acute intermittent porphyria (especially related temporally to the menstrual cycle), porphyria variegata, hereditary coproporphyria.

Contraindications: Porphyria cutanea tarda, hypersensitivity to hemin.

Special Concerns: Safe use in pregnancy (pregnancy category: C), lactation, and in children not established.

Side Effects: *Renal:* Oliguria, increased retention of nitrogen, renal shut down. *Other:* Phlebitis with or without leucocytosis, pyrexia.

Drug Interactions	
Anticoagulants	Additive anticoagulant effect
Barbiturates	↓ Effect of hemin
Estrogens	↓ Effect of hemin

Dosage: IV infusion only: 1–4 mg/kg daily over a period of 10–15 min for 3–14 days (determined by clinical response). In severe cases up to 6 mg/kg/day may be given.

NURSING CONSIDERATIONS

Administration/Storage

1. Before initiating hemin therapy, glucose, 400 g/day, should be tried first for 1–2 days.
2. Administer hemin over a period of 10–15 min using a large arm vein or central venous catheter to avoid phlebitis.
3. To reconstitute, add 43 mL of sterile water for injection and shake for 2–3 min. Use immediately.
4. A filtered IV system should be used, since reconstituted solution is not transparent and undissolved particles may not be visible.
5. Other drugs should not be added to the IV unless it has been determined they will not interfere with the chemical or physical stability of hemin.

Assessment

Obtain liver and renal function studies as baseline data against which to compare subsequent studies.

Interventions

Obtain complete blood cell count and urine porphyrins, and monitor routinely throughout drug therapy.

Client/Family Teaching

Explain that hemin is not a cure for porphyria, but that it offers symptomatic improvement.

HYALURONIDASE (hy-al-your-**ON**-ih-days)

Hyalase ✿, Wydase (Rx)

Classification: Enzyme, miscellaneous.

Action/Kinetics: Hyaluronidase, an enzyme that hydrolyzes hyaluronic acid, a constituent of connective tissue, acts to promote the diffusion of injected liquids. The purified enzyme has no effect on blood pressure, respiration, temperature, and kidney function. However, it is antigenic and repeated use may induce the formation of antibodies which neutralize the effect. It will not result in spread of localized infection as long as it is not injected into the infected area. The effects last 24–48 hr.

Uses: Adjunct to promote absorption and dispersion of liquids and drugs, for hypodermoclysis, adjunct in urography to improve resorption of radiopaque agents, administration of local anesthetics. (Hyaluronidase can be added to primary drug solution or injected prior to administration of primary drug solution.)

Contraindications: Do not inject into acutely infected or cancerous areas.

Special Concerns: Pregnancy category: C. Use with caution during lactation.

Side Effects: Rarely, sensitivity reactions, including urticaria and anaphylaxis.

Dosage: *Drug and fluid dispersion:* **Adults and older children, usual:** 150 units added to the injection solution. *Subcutaneous urography:* (when IV injection cannot be used) *with patient in prone position:* 75 units **SC** over each scapula, followed by contrast medium in same site.

Hypodermoclysis: 150 units which facilitates absorption of 1,000 mL fluid (give at a rate no faster than would be used for IV infusion); **pediatric, less than 3 years of age:** volume of single clysis should be limited to 200 mL; **premature infants, neonates:** volume should not exceed 25 mL/kg/day given at a rate no greater than 2 mL/min.

NURSING CONSIDERATIONS

See also *Nursing Considerations* for *Cholinergic Blocking Agents,* p. 949, and *Narcotic Analgesics,* p. 753.

Administration/Storage

1. Conduct a preliminary skin test for sensitivity by injecting 0.02 mL of the solution intradermally. A positive reaction occurs within 5 min when a wheal with pseudopods appears and persists for 20 to 30 min and is accompanied by localized itching. The appearance of erythema alone is not a positive reaction.
2. Methods for administering hyaluronidase during clysis therapy:
   • Inject hyaluronidase under the skin before clysis is started.
   • After the clysis has been started, inject solution of hyaluronidase into tubing close to the needle.
3. Control rate and volume of fluid for the older client so that they will not exceed those used for IV administration.
4. Do not inject hyaluronidase into an area that is malignant.
5. Check the physician's orders for dosage of hyaluronidase, type and amount of parenteral solution, the rate of flow, and the site of injection.
6. Hyaluronidase is incompatible with heparin and epinephrine.
7. Hyaluronidase solution must be refrigerated. The reconstituted sterile solution maintains potency for 2 weeks if stored below 30° C (86° F).

Interventions

1. Monitor the client's bleeding times (PT/PTT).
2. Monitor liver and renal function studies and compare with premedication studies.
3. Observe the area receiving clysis for pale color, coldness, hardness, and pain. If untoward signs occur, reduce the rate of flow and notify the physician.

HYDROXYPROPYL CELLULOSE OPHTHALMIC INSERT

Lacrisert (Rx)

Classification: Wetting agent, hydrophilic.

Action/Kinetics: Lacrisert contains 5 mg of hydroxypropyl cellulose in a rod-shaped (1.27 mm diameter; 3.5 mm long), water-soluble preparation. It contains no preservatives or other ingredients. This preparation stabilizes and thickens precorneal tear film and prolongs the breakup time for tear film. It also lubricates and protects the eye.

Use: Moderate to severe dry eye syndrome including keratoconjunctivitis sicca. Also exposure keratitis, decreased corneal sensitivity, and recurrent corneal lesions. *Investigational:* Ocular lubricant, neuroparalytic keratitis.

Contraindications: Hypersensitivity to hydroxypropyl cellulose.

Side Effects: Transient blurring of vision, ocular discomfort or irritation, photophobia, hypersensitivity, edema of eyelids, eyelids mat or become sticky, hyperemia.

Dosage: Ocular system. Adults and children: One 5 mg insert daily placed into the conjunctival sac of the eye. Some patients may require two inserts daily.

NURSING CONSIDERATIONS

Interventions

1. Review instructions in the package insert on how to insert and remove Lacrisert. Follow the instructions carefully.
2. Assess the client for signs and symptoms relieved from the medication. These include relief from dry eye syndrome, such as conjunctival hyperemia, exudation, itching, burning, a sensation of the presence of a foreign body, smarting, photophobia, dryness, and blurred or cloudy vision.

Client/Family Teaching

1. Instruct the client in how to insert and remove Lacrisert. Review the package insert with the client and advise to follow the instructions as written.
2. Instruct the client to avoid rubbing the eyes, thereby preventing a dislodging of Lacrisert.
3. Advise clients that if Lacrisert is accidentally expelled, they may insert another Lacrisert as needed.
4. Explain the need to report for regular ophthalmic examinations.
5. Discuss with the client the need to report any adverse reactions to the ophthalmologist.
6. Explain that the medication may retard, stop, or reverse progressive visual deterioration.
7. Advise the client to avoid operating a car or other hazardous machinery because the drug may cause transitory blurring of vision.

IMMUNE GLOBULIN IV (HUMAN)   (GLOB-you-lin)

Gamimune N, Gammagard, Sandoglobulin, Venoglobulin-I (Rx)

Classification: IgG antibody product. **Note:** The available products differ significantly with respect to the process by which they are made (e.g., donor pool and fractionation/purification) as well as isotonicity. Thus, information on each product should be carefully read before use.

Action/Kinetics: Immune globulin IV is a polyvalent antibody product derived from a human volunteer pool. It contains the various IgG antibodies which normally occur in humans. The products may also contain traces of IgA and IgM. Plasma in the manufacturing pool has been found nonreactive for hepatitis B antigen. Also, there have been no documented cases of viral transmission. The antibodies present in the products will cause both opsonization and neutralization of microbes and toxins. The reconstituted products may contain sucrose, maltose, protein, and/or small amounts of sodium chloride. Doses of immune globulin IV will restore abnormally low IgG levels to within the normal range with equilibrium reached between the intra- and extravascular compartments within 6 days. The percentage of IgG in the products is over 90%. **t½:** Gamimune N and Sandoglobulin, 3 weeks; Venoglobulin-I, 29 days.

Use: Severe combined immunodeficiency and primary immunoglobulin deficiency syndromes, including congenital agammaglobulinemia, X-linked agammaglobulinemia, and Wiskott-Aldrich syndrome. Acute and chronic idiopathic thrombocytopenic purpura in both children and adults. B-cell chronic lymphocytic leukemia (Gammagard).

Contraindications: Patients with selective IgA deficiency who have antibodies to IgA (the products contain IgA). Sensitivity to human immune globulin.

Special Concerns: Pregnancy category: C. The various products are used for different conditions and at different doses; thus, check information carefully.

Side Effects: Headache. Hypersensitivity or anaphylactic reactions. Agammaglobulinemic and hypogammaglobulinemic patients never having received immunoglobulin therapy or where the time from the last treatment is more than 8 weeks may manifest untoward reactions if the infusion rate exceeds 1 mL/min. Symptoms include flushing of the face, hypotension, tightness in chest, chills, fever, dizziness, diaphoresis, and nausea.

Dosage: IV only for all products.

Gamimune N. *Immunodeficiency syndrome:* 100–200 mg/kg given once a month; if response is satisfactory, dose can be increased to 400 mg/kg or infusion may be repeated more frequently than once a month. Rate of infusion: 0.01–0.02 mL/kg/min for 30 min; if no discomfort is experienced, the rate can be increased up to 0.08 mL/kg/min. *Idiopathic thrombocytopenic purpura:* 400 mg/kg for 5 consecutive days.

Gammagard. *Immunodeficiency syndrome:* 200–400 mg/kg (minimum of 100 mg/kg monthly). *B-cell lymphocytic leukemia:* 400 mg/kg q 3–4 weeks. *Idiopathic thrombocytopenic purpura:* 1,000 mg/kg; additional doses depend on platelet count (up to 3 doses can be given on alternate days). Rate of infusion: 0.5 mL/kg initially; may be increased gradually to 4 mL/kg/hr if there is no patient distress.

Sandoglobulin. *Immunodeficiency syndrome:* 200 mg/kg once monthly; increase to 300 mg/kg if patient response satisfactory (i.e., IgG serum level of 300 mg/dl). Rate of administration: 3% solution at an initial rate of 0.5–1 mL/min; after 15–30 min can increase to 1.5–2.5 mL/min (subsequent infusions at a rate of 2–2.5 mL/min). If the 6% solution is used, the initial infusion rate should be 1–1.5 mL/min and increased after 15–30 min to a maximum of 2.5 mL/min. *Idiopathic thrombocytopenic purpura:* 400 mg/kg for 2–5 consecutive days.

Venoglobulin-I. *Immunodeficiency disease:* 200 mg/kg monthly; can increase to 300–400 mg/kg if response is insufficient or can repeat infusion more frequently than once monthly. *Idiopathic thrombocytopenic purpura:* **Induction:** 500 mg/kg for 2–7 consecutive days; **maintenance:** 500–2,000 mg/kg as a single infusion q 2 weeks or less if platelet count falls to < 30,000/μL.

NURSING CONSIDERATIONS

Administration/Storage

1. Follow the administration guidelines explicitly and follow the manufacturer's directions carefully for reconstitution of either the 3% or 6% solution.
2. In agamma- or hypogammaglobulinemic clients, the 3% solution should be used. Initially, administer at a rate of 10–20 drops/min (0.5–1 mL/min). After 15–30 min the rate may be increased to 30–50 drops/min (1.5–2.5 mL/min). Subsequent infusions may be given at a rate of 40–50 drops/min (2–2.5 mL/min). If the first bottle of the 3% solution is given in these clients with good tolerance, subsequent infusions may be given using the 6% solution.
3. The solutions should not be shaken as excessive foaming will occur.
4. The solution should be infused only if it is clear and at room temperature.
5. These products should only be given IV as the IM and SC routes have not been evaluated.

6. Epinephrine should be readily available in the event of an acute anaphylactic reaction.

7. These products should be given by a separate IV line without mixing with other IV fluids or medications.

8. A rapid decrease in serum IgG level in the first week postinfusion will be observed; this is expected and is due to the equilibration of IgG between the plasma and extravascular space.

9. Utilize an electronic infusion device for administration.

Interventions

1. Monitor vital signs throughout the infusion.

2. If the client develops hypotension, decrease or interrupt the rate of infusion until the hypotension subsides.

3. Administer drug therapy in a closely monitored environment.

4. Monitor liver function studies, hematologic values, IgG levels and appropriate blood and urine chemistries.

Client/Family Teaching

1. Explain that drug may cause nausea, vomiting, fever, chills, flushing, lightheadedness, and tightness in the chest. These symptoms should be reported to the physician immediately because they may be related to the dosage and rate of drug administration.

2. Discuss the need to have drug therapy once a month to maintain appropriate IgG serum levels.

3. Explain that the drug is derived from human plasma and discuss the associated potential risks.

ISOTRETINOIN   (eye-soh-**TRET**-ih-noyn)

Accutane, Accutane Roche ✲ (Rx)

Classification: Vitamin A metabolite (antiacne, keratinization stabilizer).

Action/Kinetics: Isotretinoin reduces sebaceous gland size, decreases sebum secretion, and inhibits abnormal keratinization. Approximately 25% of the oral dosage form is bioavailable. **Peak plasma levels:** 3 hr. **Steady state blood levels following 80 mg daily:** 160 ng/mL. The drug is nearly 100% bound to plasma protein. $t\frac{1}{2}$: 10–20 hr. **Time to peak levels:** 3 hr. Metabolized in the liver to 4-oxo-isotretinoin which is also active. Approximately equal amounts are excreted through the urine and in the feces.

Uses: Severe recalcitrant cystic acne unresponsive to other therapy. *Investigational:* Cutaneous disorders of keratinization, leukoplakia, mycosis fungoides.

Contraindications: Due to the possibility of fetal abnormalities or spontaneous abortion, women who are pregnant or intend to become pregnant should not use the drug (pregnancy category: X). Certain conditions for use should be met in women with childbearing potential (see package insert). Use during lactation and in children.

Side Effects: *Skin:* Cheilitis, skin fragility, pruritus, dry skin, desquamation of facial skin, drying of mucous membranes, brittle nails, photosensitivity, rash, hypo- or hyperpigmentation, urticaria, erythema nodosum, hirsutism, excess granulation of tissues as a result of healing. *CNS:* Headache, fatigue, pseudotumor cerebri (i.e., headaches, papilledema, disturbances in vision), depression. *Ocular:* Conjunctivitis, optic neuritis, corneal opacities, dry eyes, decrease in acuity of night vision. *GI:* Dry mouth, nausea, vomiting, abdominal pain, inflammatory bowel disease, anorexia, weight loss, inflammation and bleeding of gums. *Neuromuscular:* Arthralgia, muscle pain, bone and joint pain and stiffness, skeletal hyperostosis. *Other:* Epistaxis, dry nose and mouth, respiratory infections, bruising, petechiae, disseminated herpes simplex, edema, transient chest pain, development of diabetes.

Drug Interactions	
Alcohol	Potentiation of ↑ in serum triglycerides
Benzoyl peroxide	↑ Drying effects of isotretinoin
Minocycline	↑ Risk of development of pseudotumor cerebri or papilledema
Tetracycline	↑ Risk of development of pseudotumor cerebri or papilledema
Tretinoin	↑ Drying effects of isotretinoin
Vitamin A	↑ Risk of toxicity

Laboratory Test Interferences: ↑ Plasma triglycerides, sedimentation rate, platelet counts, alkaline phosphatase, SGOT, SGPT, GGTP, LDH, fasting serum glucose, uric acid in blood, cholesterol, creatinine phosphokinase levels in patients who exercise vigorously. ↓ HDL, red blood cell parameters, white blood cell counts.

Dosage: Capsules. Adults, individualized, initial: 0.5–1 mg/kg daily (range: 0.5–2 mg/kg daily) divided in 2 doses for 15–20 weeks. Dose should be adjusted based on toxicity and clinical response; if cyst count decreases by 70% or more, drug may be discontinued. If necessary, a second course of therapy may be instituted after a rest period of 2 months. Doses of 0.05–0.5 mg/kg daily are effective but result in higher frequency of relapses. For keratinization disorders, doses up to 4 mg/kg daily have been used.

NURSING CONSIDERATIONS

Administration/Storage

1. Do not crush the drug.
2. Administer the drug with meals.
3. Before using the drug, the client should complete a client consent form included with the package insert. Follow appropriate institutional guidelines.
4. If a second course of drug therapy is needed, the client should have a rest period of 2 months before it begins.

Assessment

1. Note if the client is a female of childbearing age. Perform a pregnancy test on all sexually active women of childbearing age.
2. Take a complete drug history, noting those medications with which the drug interacts unfavorably.
3. Obtain baseline blood glucose levels and liver function studies, especially lipoprotein, cholesterol and triglycerides.

Interventions

1. Once a month perform pregnancy tests on sexually active women who are of childbearing age. The drug is teratogenic. Advise the client to practice contraception.

2. Monitor the client's cholesterol, triglycerides, and blood glucose levels throughout the drug therapy.

3. To ensure compliance, give the client only a 30-day prescription.

Client/Family Teaching

1. Advise clients who receive isotretinoin to avoid donating blood for 30 days after the drug therapy has been discontinued.

2. Instruct females of childbearing age to practice some reliable form of birth control while receiving this drug as severe fetal damage may occur.

3. Advise clients to report to the physician immediately if they develop a persistent headache, nausea and vomiting, or visual disturbances.

4. Instruct clients who wear contact lenses that they may develop sensitivity to contacts during and after therapy.

5. Discuss with the client that the condition may become worse before healing starts.

6. Advise clients to avoid taking OTC medications, especially vitamin A, without physician knowledge and approval.

7. Instruct client to eliminate or to markedly reduce consumption of alcohol.

8. Advise clients to avoid prolonged exposure to sunlight as the drug may cause photosensitivity.

LACTULOSE   (LAK-tyou-lohs)

Cholac, Chronulac, Constilac, Constulose, Duphalac, Enulose, Generlac, Lactulax✱, Portalac (Rx)

Classification: Ammonia detoxicant, laxative.

Action/Kinetics: Lactulose, a disaccharide containing both lactose and galactose, causes a decrease in the blood concentration of ammonia in patients suffering from portal-systemic encephalopathy. The mechanism involved is attributed to the bacteria-induced degradation of lactulose in the colon, resulting in an acid medium. Ammonia will then migrate from the blood to the colon to form ammonium ion, which is trapped and cannot be absorbed. A laxative action due to increased osmotic pressure from lactic, formic, and acetic acids then expels the trapped ammonium. The decrease in blood ammonia concentration improves the mental state, EEG tracing, and diet protein tolerance of patients. The increased osmotic pressure also results in a laxative effect, which may take up to 24 hr. The drug is partly absorbed from the GI tract.

Uses: Prevention and treatment of portal-systemic encephalopathy, including hepatic and prehepatic coma. Chronic constipation.

Contraindications: Patients on galactose-restricted diets.

Special Concerns: Safe use during pregnancy (pregnancy category: B) and lactation and in children has not been established. Use with caution in presence of diabetes mellitus.

Side Effects: *GI:* Nausea, vomiting, diarrhea, cramps, flatulence, gaseous distention, belching.

Drug Interaction: Neomycin may cause ↓ degradation of lactulose due to neomycin-induced ↑ in elimination of certain bacteria in the colon.

Dosage: Syrup. *Encephalopathy:* **Adults, initial,** 30–45 mL (20–30 g) t.i.d.–q.i.d.; adjust q 2–3 days to obtain 2 or 3 soft stools daily. Long-term therapy may be required in portal-systemic encephalopathy; **infants:** 2.5–10 mL/day (1.6–6.6 g/day) in divided doses; **older children and**

adolescents: 40–90 mL/day (26.6–60 g/day) in divided doses. *During acute episodes:* 30–45 mL (20–30 g) q 1–2 hr to induce rapid initial laxation. *Retention enema:* 300 mL (200 g), diluted to 1,000 mL with water or saline and retained for 30–60 min; may be repeated q 4–6 hr. *Chronic constipation:* **Adults and children,** 15–30 mL/day (10–20 g/day) as a single dose after breakfast (up to 60 mL/day may be required).

NURSING CONSIDERATIONS

Administration/Storage

1. To minimize sweet taste, dilute with water or fruit juice or add to desserts.
2. When given by gastric tube, dilute well to prevent vomiting and the possibility of aspiration pneumonia.
3. Store below 30°C (86°F). Avoid freezing.

Interventions

1. Report any client complaint of GI distress to the physician. The problem may subside as the therapy continues, or the dose of medication may need to be reduced.
2. Monitor the serum potassium levels of clients who have portal-systemic encephalopathy. This is to determine whether the drug is causing further potassium loss that will intensify symptoms of the disease.
3. The medication contains carbohydrate. Therefore observe clients who have diabetes for flushed, dry skin, complaints of dry mouth and intense thirst, a fruity odor to the breath, abdominal pain and low blood pressure. These are symptoms of hyperglycemia that are more likely to occur in clients with diabetes.
4. Keep the client clean and dry. Assess the client's skin condition frequently because skin breakdown may occur rapidly.

MINOXIDIL TOPICAL SOLUTION   (min-**OX**-ih-dill)

Rogaine (Rx)

Classification: Hair growth stimulant.

Action/Kinetics: Minoxidil topical solution stimulates vertex hair growth in patients with male pattern baldness. The mechanism is unknown, but may be related to the fact that minoxidil dilates arterioles and stimulates resting hair follicles into active growth. Oral minoxidil is used to treat hypertension and, when used systemically, is associated with a significant number of potential side effects. Following topical administration, approximately 1.4% is absorbed into the systemic circulation. **Onset:** 4 months but is variable. **Duration:** New hair growth may be lost 3–4 months after withdrawal of therapy. Minoxidil and its inactive metabolites are excreted in the urine.

Uses: To treat male pattern baldness (alopecia androgenetica) of the vertex of the scalp. The drug is less effective in frontal baldness.

Special Concerns: Pregnancy category: C. Use with caution in patients with hypertension, coronary heart disease, or predisposition to heart failure. Safety and efficacy in patients under 18 years of age have not been determined. Increased systemic absorption may occur if the scalp is irritated or there are abrasions.

Side Effects: *Dermatologic:* Allergic contact dermatitis, irritant dermatitis, itching. *Allergic:* Hives, facial swelling, allergic rhinitis. *CNS:* Dizziness, lightheadedness, headache.

Drug Interactions

Corticosteroids, topical	Enhance absorption of topical minoxidil
Guanethidine	Possible ↑ risk of orthostatic hypotension
Petrolatum	Enhances absorption of topical minoxidil
Retinoids	Enhance absorption of topical minoxidil

Dosage: Topical Solution. Adult, 1 mL of the 2% solution is applied to the affected area of the scalp in the morning and before bedtime. The total daily dose should not exceed 2 mL.

NURSING CONSIDERATIONS

Administration/Storage

1. Only clients with normal, healthy scalps should use topical minoxidil. Dermatitis, scalp abrasions, scalp psoriasis, or severe sunburn may increase the absorption of topical minoxidil and lead to systemic side effects (See *Minoxidil, oral,* p. 513).
2. The hair and scalp should be dry prior to application of topical minoxidil.
3. The product comes with a metered spray attachment (for application to large areas of the scalp), extender spray attachment (for application to small scalp areas or under the hair), and a rub-on applicator tip (to spread the solution on the scalp). The directions on the package insert should be carefully followed for each of these methods of application.
4. If the fingertips are used to apply the drug, the hands should be washed thoroughly after application.
5. At least 4 months of continuous therapy is necessary before evidence of hair growth can be expected. Further hair growth continues through one year of treatment.
6. The alcohol base in topical minoxidil will cause irritation and burning of the eyes, abraded skin, or mucous membranes. If there is contact with any of these areas, wash the site with copious amounts of water.

Interventions

Clients on topical minoxidil therapy should be monitored 1 month after starting therapy and every 6 months thereafter for any systemic effects. These should be documented and reported to the physician.

Client/Family Teaching

1. Advise the client that the new hair growth is not permanent. Cessation of therapy will lead to hair loss within a few months. Thus, the topical minoxidil must be used for an indefinite period of time.
2. Discuss the fact that the treatment has positive benefits for only approximately one-half the population. Assist the client to set realistic goals.
3. Explain that it may take up to 4 months of continuous therapy before any response is noted.
4. Instruct client to report any evidence of irritation or rash at the site of treatment.

MONOCTANOIN   (mahn-**OCK**-tah-noyn)

Moctanin (Rx)

Classification: Solubilizer for gallstones.

Action/Kinetics: Monoctanoin is a semisynthetic esterified glycerol which causes complete dissolution of gallstones in approximately one-third of treated patients, with an additional one-third manifesting a decrease in the size of stones. The decreased size may allow the stone to pass spontaneously.

Uses: To solubilize cholesterol gallstones located in the biliary tract, especially when other treatments have failed or can not be undertaken. Most effective if the stones are radiolucent.

Contraindications: Biliary tract infection, recent duodenal ulcer or jejunitis, clinical jaundice, impaired hepatic function, acute pancreatitis, porto-systemic shunting.

Special Concerns: Use with caution during pregnancy (pregnancy category: C) and lactation. Safety and effectiveness in children have not been established.

Side Effects: *GI:* Irritation of GI and biliary tracts, ascending cholangitis, erythema in antral and duodenal mucosa, ulceration or irritation of the mucosa of the common bile duct, duodenal erosion, abdominal pain or discomfort, nausea, vomiting, diarrhea, indigestion, anorexia, burning, bile shock. *CNS:* Fever, fatigue, lethargy, depression, headache. *Other:* Leukopenia, pruritus, chills, diaphoresis, hypokalemia, allergic symptoms.

Dosage: Infusion via catheter inserted into common bile duct. Perfuse at rate not to exceed 3–5 mL/hr at a pressure of 10 cm water (to minimize irritation) for 7–21 days.

NURSING CONSIDERATIONS

Administration/Storage

1. The drug should not be administered IM or IV.
2. The drug should be maintained at a temperature of 37°C for maximum effects.
3. To reduce viscosity and enhance the bathing effect on the stones, the drug should be diluted with 120 mL sterile water for injection.
4. Perfusion pressure should never exceed 15 cm water (use overflow manometer or peristaltic pump).
5. The perfusion should be continued for approximately 9–10 days after which x-ray or endoscopy studies should be conducted. If tests do not show a reduction in size or dissolution of stones, the drug should be discontinued.
6. Irritation of the GI and biliary tracts may occur. These usually disappear within 2–7 days after the termination of therapy.
7. The drug is intended only for direct biliary duct infusion.

Assessment

1. Note if the client has a history of biliary tract infection or recent duodenal ulcer.
2. If the client has a history of hepatic dysfunction, obtain baseline liver function studies.

Interventions

1. Note any client complaint of GI irritation.
2. Monitor stools for occult blood. Document and report to the physician.
3. Observe the client for fever, lethargy, depression, pruritus, diaphoresis and hypokalemia. Document and report these findings to the physician.

MORRHUATE SODIUM   (MOR-you-ayt)

(Rx)

Classification: Sclerosing agent.

Action/Kinetics: Morrhuate sodium is derived from cod liver oil. When injected into a vein, it initiates the formation of a thrombus, followed by fibrous tissue which then obliterates the particular blood vessel. After injection, 2 to 4 inches of the vein harden immediately. The entire vein becomes hard and firm within 24 hr. Injection is followed by a mild feeling of stiffness, which persists for 48 hr. The skin above the vein assumes a bronze discoloration that disappears gradually and which usually does not cause cramping pain.

Uses: Obliteration of small, uncomplicated varicose veins of the legs. *Investigational:* Treatment of internal hemorrhoids and esophageal varices.

Contraindications: Hypersensitivity to drug. Acute superficial thrombophlebitis, underlying arterial disease, varicosities resulting from pelvic or abdominal tumors, uncontrolled diabetes, asthma, bedridden patients, hyperthyroidism, tuberculosis, respiratory diseases, skin diseases, sepsis, blood dyscrasias, neoplasms, persistent occlusion of deep veins, incompetence of valves or deep veins.

Special Concerns: Use during pregnancy (pregnancy category: C) only if benefits clearly outweigh risks. Use with particular caution in patient previously treated with morrhuate sodium.

Side Effects: *GI:* Nausea, vomiting. *CNS:* Weakness, dizziness, headache, drowsiness. *Allergic:* Anaphylaxis. *Other:* Asthma, respiratory depression, postoperative sloughing, cardiovascular collapse, pulmonary embolism. *At site of injection:* Necrosis, burning, cramping feeling, urticaria.

Dosage: IV only. *Small or medium veins:* 50–100 mg (1–2 mL of 5% solution); *large veins:* 150–250 mg (3–5 mL of 5% solution). Treatment may be repeated after 5–7 days. No more than 5 mL should be administered during any one day.

NURSING CONSIDERATIONS

Administration/Storage

1. Injection of a test dose (0.25–1 mL of 5% solution) may be requested 24 hours before treatment, to test the client for sensitivity.
2. The normal color of the injection is yellow to light brown. Only use clear solution for injection.
3. If the ampule is cold, contains solid matter, or if the medication is to be injected into a small vein, submerge the ampule in hot water to warm the medication.
4. The solution froths easily. Use a large-gauge needle to fill the syringe, but change to a small-gauge needle for the actual injection.
5. Morrhuate sodium is usually administered by a physician familiar with the injection technique.
6. Assist in emptying the vein for injection by elevating the limb. After injection, assist by applying digital pressure or a tourniquet for *only 2–3 minutes* to prevent dilution of the drug by the backflow of blood.
7. Place a dry sterile dressing over the site of injection.
8. After administration, the vein quickly becomes swollen and hard for approximately 2–4 inches. After one day, the vein is hard and tender to the touch and for 48 hr there is an aching sensation and the area feels stiff.
9. Examine the site of injection before the client leaves the office for evidence of an allergic reaction, sloughing, bleeding, or other adverse reactions.

10. Have available epinephrine 1:1,000, antihistamines, corticosteroids, and oxygen in the event of an anaphylactic reaction.

Interventions

1. Observe the client for several hours after the sensitivity test for a hypersensitivity reaction.
2. If the client has received the therapy before, test for hypersensitivity because the client may have developed sensitivity to morrhuate sodium in the interim.

Client/Family Teaching

Explain to the client that they can expect a change in skin color, an aching, stiff sensation, and hardness of the vein following the treatment.

MUROMONAB-CD3   (myou-roh-MON-ab)

Orthoclone OKT3 (Rx)

Classification: Immunosuppressive agent.

Action/Kinetics: Muromonab-CD3 is a murine monoclonal antibody; the antibody is a purified IgG$_{2a}$ immunoglobulin. The antibody acts to prevent rejection of transplanted kidney tissue by blocking the action of T cells which play a significant role in acute rejection. Specifically, the CD3 molecule in the membrane of T cells is blocked; this molecule is necessary for signal transduction. The drug does not cause myelosuppression. Antibodies to muromonab-CD3 have been observed after approximately twenty days. **Average serum levels after three days:** 0.9 mcg/mL. **Time to steady-state trough levels:** 3 days. **Duration:** 1 week for return of circulating CD3 positive T cells to pretreatment levels.

Uses: To reverse acute allograft rejection in kidney transplant patients; used in combination with azathioprine, cyclosporine, corticosteroids. *Investigational:* Treat acute rejection of liver and heart transplants.

Contraindications: Hypersensitivity to drug (or any product of murine origin), patients with edema (fluid overload). Use during lactation.

Special Concerns: Use during pregnancy only if benefits outweigh risks (pregnancy category: C). Although used in children, safety and effectiveness have not been assessed.

Side Effects: Significant and serious side effects may occur within 0.5–6 hr following the first dose. Thus, therapy must be initiated in a hospital by physicians experienced in immunosuppressive therapy and where equipment is available to perform cardiopulmonary resuscitation. *First-dose symptoms:* Fever, chills (can be minimized by giving 1 mg/kg methylprednisolone sodium succinate; can be reversed by giving acetaminophen and/or by using a cooling blanket); dyspnea (can be minimized or reversed by giving 100 mg hydrocortisone sodium succinate injection within 30 min after muromonab-CD3 administration, with an additional 100 mg as needed); pulmonary edema (can be minimized by ensuring a clear chest, using x-ray within 24 hr of injection, or by ensuring that less than a 3% weight gain has occurred in the week prior to drug injection; can be reversed by prompt intubation and use of oxygen).

Within first two days of therapy: Fever, chills, dyspnea, wheezing, chest pain, nausea, vomiting, diarrhea, tremor, severe pulmonary edema. *Within 45 days of therapy:* Infections (which may be life-threatening) due to cytomegalovirus, herpes simplex virus, *Staphylococcus epidermidis, Pneumocystis carinii, Legionella, Cryptococcus, Serratia,* and other gram-negative bacteria.

Dosage: IV bolus. Adults: 5 mg daily for 10–14 days; **pediatric, less than 12 years:** 0.1 mg/kg daily for 10–14 days.

NURSING CONSIDERATIONS

Administration/Storage

1. Treatment should be initiated as soon as acute renal rejection is diagnosed.
2. The bolus should be given in less than one minute.
3. The drug is not to be given by IV infusion or with any other drug solutions.
4. If the body temperature of the client is 100°F (37.8°C), drug therapy should not be initiated.
5. The solution (which is a protein) should be drawn into a syringe through a 0.2- or 0.22-μm filter; the filter is then discarded and the needle attached.
6. The appearance of a few translucent particles of protein does not affect the potency of the preparation.
7. The dose of other immunosuppressant drugs should be decreased as follows during muromonab-CD3 use: prednisone, 0.5 mg/kg daily; azathioprine, 25 mg daily. Cyclosporine should be discontinued. Maintenance doses of these drugs can be resumed approximately 3 days prior to termination of muromonab-CD3 therapy.
8. The drug should be stored at 2°–8°C (36°–46°F) and should not be frozen or shaken.

Interventions

1. Monitor the client's intake and output.
2. Weigh the client daily and document and report any evidence of rapid weight gain.
3. Take the client's temperature every 4 hours. If the temperature goes above 100° F, withhold the drug until the temperature goes below 100° F.
4. Monitor the client's renal status for a decrease in urine volume and a decrease in creatinine clearance. These are signs of transplant rejection and should be reported to the physician immediately.

Client/Family Teaching

Explain to the client that chills, fever, shortness of breath, and malaise are first-dose symptoms that will diminish on consecutive treatment days.

NICOTINE POLACRILEX (NICOTIN RESIN COMPLEX)   (NIK-oh-teen)

Nicorette (Rx)

Classification: Smoking deterrent.

Action/Kinetics: Following chewing, nicotine is released from an ion exchange resin in the gum product, providing blood nicotine levels approximating those produced by smoking cigarettes. The amount of nicotine released is dependent on the rate and duration of chewing. Following repeated administration every 30 min, nicotine blood levels reach 25–50 ng/mL. If the gum is swallowed, only a minimum amount of nicotine is released. Nicotine is metabolized mainly by the liver, with about 10%–20% excreted unchanged in the urine.

Uses: Adjunct with behavioral modification in smokers wishing to give up the smoking habit. Is considered only as an initial aid, with the ultimate goal being abstention from all forms of nicotine. Most likely to benefit are individuals with the following characteristics:

1. Smoke brands of cigarettes containing > 0.9 mg nicotine;
2. smoke > 15 cigarettes daily;
3. inhale cigarette smoke deeply and frequently;
4. smoke most frequently during the morning;
5. smoke the first cigarette of the day within 30 min of arising;
6. indicate cigarettes smoked in the morning are the most difficult to give up;
7. smoke even if the individual is ill and confined to bed;
8. find it necessary to smoke in places where smoking is not allowed.

Contraindications: Pregnancy (category: X), lactation, nonsmokers, serious arrhythmias, angina, vasospastic disease, active temporomandibular joint disease.

Special Concerns: Safety and effectiveness in children and adolescents who smoke have not been determined. Use with caution in hypertension, peptic ulcer disease, oral or pharyngeal inflammation, gastritis, stomatitis, hyperthyroidism, insulin-dependent diabetes, and pheochromocytoma.

Side Effects: *CNS:* Dizziness, irritability, headache. *GI:* Nausea, vomiting, indigestion, GI upset, salivation, eructation. *Other:* Sore mouth or throat, hiccoughs, sore jaw muscles.

Overdosage may cause symptoms of nicotine poisoning including: *GI:* Nausea, vomiting, diarrhea, salivation, abdominal pain. *CNS:* Headache, dizziness, confusion, weakness, fainting, seizures. *Respiratory:* Labored breathing, respiratory paralysis (cause of death). *Other:* Cold sweat, disturbed hearing and vision, hypotension, and rapid, weak pulse.

Treatment of overdosage includes ipecac syrup if vomiting has not occurred, saline laxative, gastric lavage followed by activated charcoal (if patient is unconscious), maintenance of respiration, maintenance of cardiovascular function.

Drug Interactions	
Caffeine	Possibly ↓ blood levels of caffeine due to ↑ rate of breakdown by liver
Catecholamines	↑ Levels of catecholamines
Cortisol	↑ Levels of cortisol
Furosemide	Possible ↓ diuretic effect of furosemide
Glutethimide	Possible ↓ absorption of glutethimide
Imipramine	Possibly ↓ blood levels of imipramine due to ↑ rate of breakdown by liver
Pentazocine	Possibly ↓ blood levels of pentazocine due to ↑ rate of breakdown by liver
Theophylline	Possibly ↓ blood levels of theophylline due to ↑ rate of breakdown by liver

Dosage: Gum. Initial: one piece of gum chewed whenever the urge to smoke occurs; **maintenance:** about 10 pieces of gum daily during the first month, not to exceed 30 pieces daily.

NURSING CONSIDERATIONS

Administration/Storage

1. The individual must want to stop smoking and should do so immediately.
2. Each piece of gum should be chewed slowly for about 30 min.
3. Clients should be evaluated monthly and if the individual has not smoked for 3 months, the gum should be slowly withdrawn. Nicotine should not be used for longer than 6 months.

Client/Family Teaching

1. Advise the client to use the gum only as directed.
2. Provide a printed list of drug (gum) side effects. Instruct the client to report to the physician any bothersome side effects.
3. Discuss with the client the local support groups that can help the client to stop smoking and provide emotional and psychological support throughout the endeavor.

Evaluation

Evaluate for a positive clinical response such as a decrease in the number of cigarettes smoked per day or complete cessation.

OCTREOTIDE ACETATE   (ok-**TREE**-oh-tyd)

Sandostatin (Rx)

Classification: Antineoplastic.

Action/Kinetics: Octreotide exerts effects similar to the natural hormone somatostatin. It suppresses secretion of serotonin and GI peptides including gastrin, insulin, glucagon, secretin, motilin, vasoactive intestinal peptide, and pancreatic polypeptide. The drug stimulates fluid and electrolyte absorption from the GI tract. It also inhibits growth hormone. The drug is rapidly absorbed from injection sites. **Peak levels:** Approximately 25 min. **t½:** 1.5 hr. **Duration:** Up to 12 hr. About one-third of a dose is excreted unchanged in the urine.

Uses: Metastatic carcinoid tumors; vasoactive intestinal tumors (VIPomas). The drug inhibits severe diarrhea in both situations and causes improvement in hypokalemia in VIPomas. *Investigational:* Life-threatening hypotension, acromegaly.

Special Concerns: Use during pregnancy only if clearly needed (pregnancy category: B). Use with caution during lactation. Use with caution in diabetics, in patients with gallbladder disease, and in patients with severe renal failure requiring dialysis.

Side Effects: *GI:* Nausea, diarrhea or loose stools, abdominal pain, malabsorption of fat, vomiting; less commonly, constipation, anorexia, dry mouth, flatulence, rectal spasm, GI bleeding, swollen stomach, heartburn, cholelithiasis. *CNS:* Headache, dizziness, lightheadedness, fatigue; less commonly, anxiety, seizures, depression, vertigo, hyperesthesia, drowsiness, pounding in head, irritability, decrease in libido, malaise, forgetfulness, nervousness, syncope, tremor, shakiness, Bell's palsy. *CV:* Flushing, edema; less commonly, hypertension, thrombophlebitis, shortness of breath, congestive heart failure, ischemia, palpitations, orthostatic hypotension, chest pain. *Metabolic:* Hyperglycemia or hypoglycemia, hyperosmolarity of urine, increase in CPK. *Musculoskeletal:* Asthenia, weakness; less commonly, muscle pain or cramping, back pain; joint, shoulder, arm, and leg pain; leg cramps. *Dermatological:* Less commonly, thinning or flaking of skin, bruising, bleeding from superficial wounds, hair loss, rash, pruritus. *GU:* Prostatitis, oliguria, pollakiuria. *Other:* Pain, wheal, or erythema at injection site; less commonly, rhinorrhea, galactorrhea, hypothyroidism, numbness, hyperhidrosis, hyperdipsia, warm feeling or burning sensation, visual disturbance, chills, fever, throat discomfort, eyes burning.

Drug Interactions: Octreotide may interfere with drugs such as diazoxide, insulin, beta-adrenergic blocking agents, or sulfonylureas. Close monitoring is necessary.

Dosage: SC (recommended), IV bolus (emergencies). Initial, SC: 50 mcg 1–2 times daily. **Then,** *for carcinoid tumors:* 100–600 mcg daily in 2–4 divided doses for the first two weeks; **maintenance, usual:** 450 mcg daily (range: 50–1,500 mcg daily). *VIPomas:* 200–300 mcg daily in 2–4 divided doses for the first two weeks; **maintenance:** 150–750 mcg daily. **Pediatric, SC:** 1–10 mcg/kg daily.

NURSING CONSIDERATIONS

Administration/Storage

1. Experience is lacking for doses greater than 750 mcg daily.
2. Ampules should be inspected for particulate matter and discoloration; if present, the ampule must not be used.
3. Multiple injections at the same site should be avoided within a short period of time. Preferred sites for injection are the abdomen, hip, and the thigh.
4. Reactions at the site of injection can be minimized by letting the solution warm to room temperature before giving the injection and by giving the injection slowly.
5. GI side effects can be minimized by giving the drug between meals and at bedtime.
6. Ampules should be stored for long periods at 2°C–8°C (36°F–46°F) although they may be stored at room temperature the day they will be used.

Interventions

1. Monitor serum electrolyte and blood glucose levels. The drug alters serum glucose levels and may require an adjustment of antidiabetic drug dosage in clients with diabetes.
2. Obtain baseline thyroid function studies and monitor throughout therapy. The drug may cause biochemical hypothyroidism, necessitating replacement therapy.
3. Because the drug may alter fat absorption and gallbladder function, monitor the appropriate laboratory values and ultrasonography studies during long-term therapy.
4. Monitor the client's intake and output. Perform abdominal assessments routinely during therapy. Document and report any abnormal findings to the physician.

Client/Family Teaching

1. Provide printed information and advise the client of the more frequent side effects, such as nausea, vomiting, dizziness, headache, diarrhea, abdominal pain, and weakness. If any of these symptoms persist, advise the client to report them to the physician.
2. Explain that the drug is usually administered SC. There may be pain at the site of injection. Discuss the need to rotate administration sites and provide written guidelines for the administration, dose and site rotation.
3. Demonstrate the appropriate technique for SC injection and have the client do a return demonstration.
4. Explain that the dosage of drug is highly individualized. Therefore, it is important to take only as prescribed.
5. Advise the client to keep the medication refrigerated.

PENTOXIFYLLINE (pen-tox-**IF**-ih-lin)

Trental (Rx)

Classification: Agent affecting blood viscosity.

Action/Kinetics: Pentoxifylline and its active metabolites decrease the viscosity of blood. This results in increased blood flow to the microcirculation and an increase in tissue oxygen levels. Although not known with certainty, the mechanism may include (1) decreased synthesis of thromboxane A_2 thus decreasing platelet aggregation, (2) increased blood fibrinolytic activity (decreasing fibrinogen levels), and (3) decreased red blood cell aggregation and local hyperviscosity by increasing cellular ATP. **Peak plasma levels:** 1 hr. Significant first-pass effect. **t½:** pentoxifylline, 0.4–0.8 hr; metabolites, 1–1.6 hr. **Time to peak levels;** 2–4 hr. Excretion is via the urine.

Uses: Peripheral vascular disease including intermittent claudication. The drug is not intended to replace surgery. *Investigational:* To improve circulation in patients with cerebrovascular insufficiency, transient ischemic attacks, sickle cell thalassemia, diabetic angiopathies and neuropathies, high-altitude sickness, strokes, hearing disorders, circulation disorders of the eye, and Raynaud's phenomenon.

Contraindications: Intolerance to pentoxifylline, caffeine, theophylline, or theobromine.

Special Concerns: Pregnancy (pregnancy category: C). Use with caution in impaired renal function and during lactation. Safety and efficacy in children less than 18 years of age not established. Geriatric patients may be at greater risk for manifesting side effects.

Side Effects: *CV:* Angina, chest pain, hypotension, edema. *GI:* Abdominal pain, flatus/bloating, dyspepsia, salivation, bad taste in mouth, nausea/vomiting, anorexia, constipation, dry mouth and thirst. *CNS:* Dizziness, headache, tremor, malaise, anxiety, confusion. *Ophthalmologic:* Blurred vision, conjunctivitis, scotomata. *Dermatologic:* Pruritus, rash, urticaria, brittle fingernails. *Respiratory:* Dyspnea, laryngitis, nasal congestion, epistaxis. *Miscellaneous:* Flu-like symptoms, leukopenia, sore throat, swollen neck glands, change in weight.

Drug Interaction: Prothrombin times should be monitored carefully if the patient is on warfarin therapy.

Dosage: Extended-release Tablets. Adults: 400 mg t.i.d. with meals. Treatment should be continued for at least 8 weeks. If side effects occur, dosage can be reduced to 400 mg b.i.d.

NURSING CONSIDERATIONS

Assessment

1. Note any client history of sensitivity to caffeine, theophylline, or theobromine.
2. If client is female, sexually active and of childbearing age, determine if pregnant.
3. Obtain baseline CBC and renal function studies.

Client/Family Teaching

1. Provide the client with written instructions concerning adverse side effects such as angina and palpitations that should be reported to the physician.
2. Discuss with the client the need to continue the treatment for at least 8 weeks, even though effectiveness is not yet apparent.
3. Advise the client to take the medication with meals to minimize GI upset.
4. Explain the importance of follow-up visits and reporting for laboratory studies to evaluate the effectiveness of the drug.

PIGMENTING AGENTS—PSORALENS

Action/Kinetics: The appearance of areas of skin discoloration, characteristic of vitiligo, is associated with a defect in the formation of the dark pigment melanin from a precursor. Special drugs (pigmenting agents) can initiate the formation of melanin; the drugs also inhibit DNA synthesis, cell division, and epidermal turnover. The transformation is enhanced by ultraviolet radiation from natural or artificial sources.

Two substances, methoxsalen and trioxsalen, collectively referred to as psoralens, are used to promote color development and sun protection in affected skin areas. The agents are also useful for selected patients with unusually low tolerance to sun exposure. Methoxsalen is for both topical and systemic use; trioxsalen is for systemic use only. Methoxsalen is also used for the treatment of recalcitrant psoriasis.

The agents are more rapidly effective on fleshy areas, such as the face, abdomen and buttocks, than on bony areas, such as the dorsum of the hands and feet. The drugs are only effective in conjunction with functioning pigment-producing cells (melanocytes). Use of pigmenting agents is difficult. Excess exposure to ultraviolet radiation results in erythema and severe burns; overdosage results in blistering and serious burning.

Uses: See individual drugs.

Contraindications: Hepatic insufficiency, familial sun sensitivity, melanoma, aphakia, invasive squamous cell carcinoma, diseases associated with photosensitivity (porphyria, systemic lupus erythematosus, hydroa [a seasonally recurring rash triggered by exposure to sunlight], polymorphic light eruptions), leukoderma of infectious origin, albinism, cardiac disease or in patients unable to withstand heat stress.

Special Concerns: Use during pregnancy only if benefits clearly outweigh risks. Use with caution during lactation, in patients with tartrazine sensitivity, and in patients with hepatic insufficiency.

Side Effects: *Skin:* Burning, blistering, erythema. *GI:* Gastric discomfort, nausea. *Other:* Cataracts, premature aging of skin, basal cell epitheliomas. *When combined with ultraviolet light:* Pruritus, erythema.

Treatment of Overdosage: In acute oral overdosage, discontinue therapy, and empty stomach by inducing emesis. Place patient in dark room for 8 hours or until cutaneous reaction subsides. Supportive measures for treatment of burns should be instituted.

Drug Interactions: Use with care in patients receiving the following drugs or chemicals that cause photosensitivity: anthralin, bacteriostatic soaps containing halogenated salicylanilides, coal tar, griseofulvin, methylene blue, methyl orange dye, nalidixic acid, phenothiazines, rose bengal dye, sulfonamides, tetracyclines, thiazide diuretics, and toluidine blue dye.

Dosage: See individual agents.

NURSING CONSIDERATIONS

Administration

1. Read the package insert with the information supplied by the manufacturer before assisting the physician or instructing the client about psoralens.
2. Psoralens are to be administered to clients by an experienced physician, usually in the office.
3. Be prepared to provide burn therapy for clients who have had an overdose of drug or are overexposed to the sun.

Assessment

Ascertain that liver function tests have been performed before initiating therapy, and that these tests are performed routinely during the treatment.

Client/Family Teaching

1. Advise the client to maintain the dosage schedule.
2. To prevent severe burns, provide written guidelines and explain the following procedure for measured exposure to the sun, following treatment.
   - After oral therapy, the client should protect their skin from the sun for at least 8 hours. The physician may order a metered exposure time to be instituted 2 hours after taking the medication.
   - After topical therapy, advise the client to protect their skin from the sun for 12–48 hours, except for the metered exposure time ordered by the physician, 2 hours after application of the unguent.
   - To determine sun-exposure time, use the guide provided by the manufacturer of the medication.
3. Advise the client to wear UV sunglasses when exposed to the sun.
4. Advise the client to wear light-screening lipbalm to protect lips when exposed to the sun.
5. If the client is undergoing sunlamp exposure it should be done under the supervision and direction of a physician experienced in psoralen administration. Inform the physician as to the type of sunlamp the client has at home, so that appropriate recommendations may be made.
6. Explain that the results of the treatment may be delayed from a few weeks to 6–9 months after the treatment is initiated.
7. Advise the client that periodic treatments may be required to maintain pigmentation.
8. Explain the need to check with the physician about any medication to be taken concomitantly because these drugs may increase susceptibility to burns. Also, if the medication causes photosensitivity, the susceptibility to burns may be even greater.
9. Advise the client not to take the chemical substance furocoumarin. This is found in certain foods such as limes, figs, parsley, parsnips, mustard, carrots and celery. The result of combining these foods with the treatment is a more severe reaction to the sun.

METHOXSALEN ORAL (meth-OX-ah-len)

Hard Gelatin Capsules: 8-MOP, Oxsoralen✿. Soft Gelatin Capsules: Oxsoralen-Ultra, Ultra MOP✿. (Rx)

Classification: Pigmenting agent.

Action/Kinetics: *Oxsoralen-Ultra:* **Peak serum levels:** 0.5–1 hr (when taken with milk); **t½:** 2 hr. **Time for peak photosensitivity:** 1.5–2.1 hr. The mean dose to produce erythema is significantly less for Oxsoralen-Ultra than for Oxsoralen. *Oxsoralen:* **Peak serum levels:** Approximately 3 hr (when taken with milk). **t½:** 2 hr. **Time for peak photosensitivity:** 3.9–4.25 hr. Methoxsalen is rapidly metabolized in the liver with approximately 95% excreted through the urine within 24 hr; however, up to 10% may be excreted through the feces.

Uses: Repigmenting agent in idiopathic vitiligo. Severe, recalcitrant psoriasis. Mycosis fungoides. *Note:* Oxsoralen-Ultra is used only for psoriasis. *Investigational:* Alopecia areata, atopic dermatitis, inflammatory dermatoses, eczema, lichen planus, and to increase skin tolerance to sunlight.

Special Concerns: Pregnancy category: C. Safety and effectiveness have not been determined in children; however, children less than 12 years of age may be more sensitive to the effects of methoxsalen.

Additional Side Effects: *CNS:* Headache, dizziness, depression, malaise, nervousness, insomnia, malaise. *Dermatologic:* Hypopigmentation, rashes, vesicle formation, herpes simplex, miliaria, urticaria, folliculitis. *Other:* Edema, leg cramps, hypotension, cutaneous tenderness, GI upset, worsening of psoriasis.

When used with ultraviolet light: Pruritus, erythema.

Dosage: Hard Gelatin Capsules. *Vitiglio:* **Adults and children over 12 years,** 20 mg daily 2–4 hr before ultraviolet exposure given 2–3 times weekly (at least 48 hr apart). Initial exposure to sunlight should not exceed 15 min for light skin colors, 20 min for medium skin colors, and 25 min for dark skin colors; exposure may be increased 5 min each treatment determined by tenderness and erythema. Initial exposure to artificial light should not exceed one-half of that listed for sunlight. *Psoriasis, mycosis fungoides:* 0.6 mg/kg 2 hr before high-intensity ultraviolet light exposure, given 2–3 times a week (at least 48 hr apart).

Soft Gelatin Capsules. *Psoriasis:* **Adults and children over 12 years:** 0.4 mg/kg 1–1.5 hr before high-intensity ultraviolet light exposure (exposure time based on skin type—manufacturer's directions should be carefully consulted).

NURSING CONSIDERATIONS

See also *Nursing Considerations* for *Pigmenting Agents,* p. 1388.

Administration/Storage

1. The soft gelatin capsules provide greater bioavailability and earlier onset for photosensitization than the hard gelatin capsules.
2. Administer oral preparation with milk or meals to prevent gastric distress.
3. When used for psoriasis the client's weight changes to an adjacent weight range, no change in dose is necessary.
4. Follow light exposure times indicated in the guide provided by the manufacturer.
5. The client should not sunbathe for 24 hours prior to or for 48 hours after methoxsalen ingestion and ultraviolet light exposure.
6. Wrap-around sun glasses should be worn for 24 hours after methoxsalen ingestion.
7. Oxsoralen-Ultra should not be interchanged with Oxsoralen as Oxsoralen-Ultra has greater bioavailability and will cause earlier time for photosensitivity.

METHOXSALEN TOPICAL   (meth-OX-ah-len)

Oxsoralen Lotion, UltraMOP Lotion(Rx)

Classification: Pigmenting agent.

Action/Kinetics: Topical administration produces more intensive photosensitivity reactions than systemic administration. Topical usage is only indicated for small well-defined lesions (less than 10 sq cm). **Onset:** Up to 6 months for vitiligo; 1 hr for increased sensitivity of skin to sunlight.

Uses: Vitiligo as a repigmenting agent (used with ultraviolet light or sunlight). *Investigational:* Psoriasis, increase skin tolerance to sunlight, mycosis fungoides, alopecia areata, inflammatory dermatoses, eczema, lichen planus.

Special Concerns: Pregnancy category: C. Dosage has not been established in children less than 12 years of age.

Dosage: Topical Solution. Adults and children over 12 years: One percent suspension, applied to small well-defined lesions, allowed to dry for 1–2 min and then reapplied. This is undertaken 2–2.5 hr before ultraviolet light exposure. Treatment may be repeated either once weekly or q 3–5 days.

NURSING CONSIDERATIONS

See also *Nursing Considerations* for *Pigmenting Agents,* p. 1388.

Administration/Storage

1. Lotion is applied to well-defined vitiligous lesions only by the physician. Never give to a client for home application.
2. After application, expose to sunlight for no more than 1 min initially (can be increased). The duration of exposure to artificial light should be one-half the minimal erythema dose after exposure to sunlight or based on the minimal phototoxic dose (see manufacturer's directions).
3. Decrease the frequency of treatment if marked erythema is produced.
4. Keep treated areas protected from light with bandages or a sun screening agent. Client should not sunbathe for 48 hours after therapy.
5. Significant repigmentation may not occur for 6–9 months and occurs more rapidly on the face, abdomen and buttocks and less rapidly on the dorsa of the hands and feet.
6. In the event of overdosage, place the client in a darkened room until cutaneous reactions subside.

TRIOXSALEN   (try-**OX**-sah-len)

Trisoralen (Rx)

Classification: Pigmenting agent.

Action/Kinetics: Trioxsalen is more potent but produces fewer side effects than methoxsalen. The dosage of trioxsalen or exposure time following the drug should not be increased. **Onset:** Up to 6 months for vitiligo; 1 hr for increased sensitivity of skin to sunlight.

Uses: Repigmenting agent in idiopathic vitiligo. Increase tolerance to sunlight, enhance skin pigmentation. *Investigational:* Treatment of psoriasis.

Special Concerns: Pregnancy category: C. Safety and effectiveness have not been established in children less than 12 years of age.

Dosage: Tablets. *Vitiligo:* **Adults and children over 12 years,** 20–40 mg 2–4 hr before exposure to ultraviolet light 2–3 times a week with at least 48 hr between treatments. *To increase tolerance to sunlight and/or enhance pigmentation:* Same as vitiligo but not for longer than 14 days. Severe burning may occur if the dose is increased. For duration of exposure, see *Methoxsalen, oral.*

NURSING CONSIDERATIONS

See *Nursing Considerations* for *Pigmenting Agents,* p. 1388, and *Methoxsalen, oral* p. 1390.

PIMOZIDE   (PIH-moh-zyd)

Orap (Rx)

Classification: Neuroleptic agent.

Action/Kinetics: Pimozide blocks dopamine receptors at both the pre- and postsynaptic receptors in the CNS thus decreasing motor and phonic tics in Tourette's syndrome. **Peak serum levels:** 6–8 hr. **t½:** 55 hr in schizophrenic patients. **Time to peak levels:** 6–8 hr. Significant first-pass effect; excreted through the kidneys.

Uses: Gilles de la Tourette's syndrome to suppress motor and phonic tics. *Investigational:* Chronic schizophrenic patients who do not manifest excitement, agitation, or hyperactivity.

Contraindications: Tics other than Tourette's disorder. Cardiac arrhythmias, concomitantly with drugs which prolong the QT interval, severe CNS depression or coma.

Special Concerns: Safety in pregnancy (pregnancy category: C), lactation, and in children under 12 years has not been established. Use with caution in liver or kidney disease and in patients hypersensitive to antipsychotic drugs. Geriatric patients require a lower initial dose and are more likely to develop transient hypotension, increased anticholinergic and sedative effects, and extrapyramidal effects.

Side Effects: *CNS:* Headache, drowsiness, seizures, dizziness, insomnia, sedation, akinesia, akathisia, tremors, fainting, Parkinsonism-like symptoms, extrapyramidal symptoms, persistent tardive dyskinesia, transient dyskinetic symptoms after abrupt withdrawal, rigidity, speech disorders, changes in handwriting, depression, excitement, nervousness. *GI:* Nausea, vomiting, diarrhea, constipation, thirst, anorexia, increased appetite, increased salivation, belching, dry mouth. *CV:* Hypotension, hypertension, tachycardia, palpitations, chest pain. Prolongation of the QT interval with possible ventricular arrhythmias; flattening, notching, and inversion of the T-wave; appearance of U-waves. *Musculoskeletal:* Muscle cramps and tightness, asthenia, stooped posture. *GU:* Urinary frequency, nocturia, impotence. *Other:* Hyperpyrexia, visual disturbances, sensitivity of eyes to light, blurred vision, cataracts, changes in taste, loss of libido, rash or skin irritation, weight gain or loss, sweating, chest pain, periorbital edema, menstrual disorders, secretions from breast. Sudden death has been noted in patients taking high doses of pimozide. *Note:* Neuroleptic malignant syndrome has been observed with antipsychotic drugs. Symptoms include hyperpyrexia, catatonia, muscle rigidity, irregular pulse or blood pressure, tachycardia, diaphoresis, cardiac dysrhythmias, acute renal failure, and increased creatinine phosphokinase.

Drug Interactions	
Alcohol	↑ CNS depressant effect
Analgesics	↑ CNS depressant effect
Antianxiety agents	↑ CNS depressant effect
Antiarrhythmics	Additive effect on QT interval
Anticonvulsants	↑ Risk of seizures
Narcotics	↑ CNS depressant effect
Phenothiazines	Additive effect on QT interval
Sedative-hypnotics	↑ CNS depressant effect
Tricyclic antidepressants	Additive effect on QT interval

Dosage: Tablets. *Tourette's syndrome:* **Adults, initial,** 1–2 mg/day in divided doses; **then,** increase dose every other day to maintenance dose of the lesser of 10 mg/day or 0.2 mg/kg/day. Doses should not exceed 10 mg/day or 0.2 mg/kg/day. *Psychoses:* **Adults,** 2–4 mg once daily; dose can be increased at weekly intervals by 2–4 mg a day.

NURSING CONSIDERATIONS

Administration/Storage

1. The drug should be introduced slowly and gradually.
2. Periodically, gradually withdraw the drug to assess the need for continued therapy.

Assessment

1. Obtain a baseline ECG before initiating therapy. Repeat periodically throughout the therapy, noting if the drug causes a prolonged Q-T interval.
2. Perform a baseline assessment of all body systems prior to starting drug therapy.
3. List the drugs the client is taking and note any potential interactions.

Interventions

1. Routinely assess all body systems and compare with baseline data. Document findings and report any variations to the physician.
2. Be aware that the drug may lower the client's seizure threshold. Therefore, monitor the client closely for this phenomenon.

Client/Family Teaching

1. Advise the client to inspect the mouth at least once a week for fine vermiform movements of the tongue, an early sign of tardive dyskinesia. Advise the client to notify the physician and discontinue taking the medication under medical supervision.
2. Instruct the client not to stop taking the drug abruptly. The physician should be notified in order to provide the client with appropriate guidance for a gradual discontinuation of the drug.
3. Advise the client not to perform tasks that require mental alertness until the drug effects become apparent.

Evaluation

Assess for a positive clinical response as evidenced by suppression of motor and phonic tics.

POLYETHYLENE GLYCOL-ELECTROLYTE SOLUTION (pah-lee-ETH-ih-leen GLYE-kol)

Colyte, GoLYTELY (Rx)

Classification: Colonic lavage.

Action/Kinetics: Polyethylene glycol acts as an osmotic agent with little net absorption or secretion of ions. The preparation also contains sodium sulfate, sodium bicarbonate, and sodium and potassium chloride. This solution results in no net absorption of electrolytes. **Onset:** 30–60 min. **Duration:** 4 hr.

Uses: Prior to GI examination to clean the bowel.

Contraindications: Gastric retention, bowel perforation, toxic colitis, megacolon, GI obstruction.

Special Concerns: Use in pregnancy only if benefits clearly outweigh risks (pregnancy category: C). Safety and efficacy in children not established.

Side Effects: *GI:* Nausea, vomiting, bloating, cramps, abdominal fullness (transient).

Dosage: PO or nasogastric tube. Adults: 4 liters prior to GI exam (8 ounces consumed rapidly every 10 min).

NURSING CONSIDERATIONS

Administration/Storage

1. Have the client fast for 3–4 hours before taking the solution.
2. When preparing the solution, the container should be shaken several times to ensure a complete dissolution of the powder.
3. Administer the solution the night before the test, especially if the client is to receive a barium enema.
4. Reconstituted, the solution should be refrigerated and used within 48 hours. Refrigeration enhances palatability.
5. Once the solution is administered, the client can have only clear liquids prior to the examination.

Interventions

1. Assess the client for evidence of electrolyte imbalance.
2. Provide the client with specific written guidelines for the individual preparation.
3. Expect the client to protest the need to drink 4 liters of fluid. This is a large volume to consume in such a short period of time. Provide encouragement.

PRALIDOXIME CHLORIDE   (prah-lih-**DOX**-eem)

2-Pam Chloride, Protopam Chloride (Rx)

Classification: Cholinesterase inhibitor antidote.

Action/Kinetics: The enzyme cholinesterase is inhibited by phosphate esters such as insecticides (e.g., sarin, parathion). Pralidoxime, an antidote for cholinesterase inhibitors, is sometimes given prophylactically to persons exposed to insecticides or to correct overdosage with cholinergic drugs. Pralidoxime competes with cholinesterase for the carbamate or phosphorus group of the inhibitor. When displaced, the enzyme reassumes its physiologic role. Pralidoxime is less effective in antagonizing carbamate-type cholinesterase inhibitors (e.g., neostigmine); it may even aggravate symptoms of carbamate pesticide poisoning.

The drug should be administered immediately after poisoning. It is ineffective when given more than 36 hr after exposure. Administration as an antidote should be combined with gastric lavage (after PO ingestion) and (after skin contamination) thorough washing of skin with alcohol or sodium bicarbonate.

Since GI absorption of the poison is slow, and possible fatal relapses may occur, patient should be watched for 48 to 72 hr after poisoning. Variably absorbed from GI tract. **Peak plasma concentrations: PO,** 2–3 hr; **IM,** 10–20 min; **IV,** 5–15 min. **t½:** 0.8–2.7 hr. Partially metabolized in liver, excreted in urine.

Laboratory determinations of RBCs (depressed to 50% of normal), plasma cholinesterase, and urinary para-nitrophenol (parathion poisoning only) measurements are desirable to confirm diagnosis and follow progress of the patient.

Uses: Parathion and other organophosphate poisoning, prophylaxis of agricultural workers. Relieves paralysis of respiratory muscle. Overdosage in treatment of myasthenia gravis.

Special Concerns: Pregnancy category: C.

Side Effects: *CNS:* Dizziness, headache, drowsiness. *Ophthalmologic:* Diplopia, impaired accommodation. *CV:* Tachycardia, increased blood pressure. *Other:* Nausea, hyperventilation, muscle weakness. Use at reduced dosage in patients with impaired renal function.

Drug Interactions

Aminophylline, barbiturates, morphine	↑ Effect of these drugs
Phenothiazines, reserpine, succinylcholine, theophylline	**These drugs should be avoided in patients with organophosphate poisoning**

Dosage: IV, IV Infusion. *Organophosphate poisoning.* **Adults, IV infusion:** 1–2 g in 100 mL saline given over 15–30 min, or alternatively by slow IV injection, 5% solution in water over 5 min; if response is poor, repeat after 1 hr. **Pediatric:** 20–40 mg/kg/dose given as for adults. *Anticholinergic overdosage* (as with drugs used to treat myasthenia gravis): **IV,** 1–2 g followed by increments of 250 mg q 5 min. *Organophosphate poisoning with no severe GI symptoms:* **PO,** 1–3 g q 5 hr.

NURSING CONSIDERATIONS

Administration/Storage

1. In case of severe poisoning, establish a patent airway before initiating therapy.
2. Have atropine sulfate available to use in conjunction with pralidoxime.
3. Pretreat client with atropine sulfate (adults, **IV:** 2–4 mg atropine sulfate; pediatric, **IV or IM:** 0.5–1 mg atropine sulfate; these doses are repeated every 10–15 minutes until signs of atropine toxicity appear).
4. Pralidoxime is infused in adults in 100 mL NaCl injection over 30 min or injected at rate of 200 mg/min. Pediatric: Give as 5% solution.
5. If atropine is used together with pralidoxime, the symptoms of atropine toxicity will appear earlier than when atropine is used alone.
6. Have emergency drugs and equipment available when treating clients for insecticide poisoning.

Assessment

1. Obtain baseline laboratory studies, including a complete blood cell count.
2. Note any history of asthma or peptic ulcer and report to the physician. These conditions contraindicate the use of cholinergic drugs.
3. Make every effort to determine what insecticide the client was exposed to and when the poisoning occurred. Pralidoxime is not effective in the treatment of poisoning by carbamate insecticides.

Interventions

1. Observe the client for desired and undesired responses to therapy.
   - Desired responses are characterized by a reduction in muscle weakness, cramps, and paralysis.
   - Undesired responses include dizziness, headaches, hypertension, or drowsiness.
   - Assess client for 48–72 hr after the poisoning.
2. Observe the client for signs of atropine poisoning, such as flushing, tachycardia, a dry mouth, blurred vision or "atropine jag." The latter is characterized by excitement, delirium, and hallucinations.

3. If the poison was taken by mouth, administer pralidoxime as an antidote and be prepared to assist with gastric lavage.

4. If the poison was on the skin, thoroughly wash the skin with alcohol or sodium bicarbonate.

5. If the client has myasthenia gravis and is being treated for overdosage of cholinergic drugs, observe for a rapid change from cholinergic crisis to a myasthenic crisis. These clients will require more cholinergic drugs to treat the myasthenic crisis. Notify the physician immediately. Have edrophonium on hand to use to diagnose such a situation.

Client/Family Teaching

1. When provided with the opportunity, alert the public to the possible hazards of using insecticides.

2. Caution people to adhere to the instructions on the container.

3. Advise the client, who has been treated for poisoning, to avoid all contact with insecticides for several weeks.

RITODRINE HYDROCHLORIDE   (RYE-toe-dreen)

Yutopar (Rx)

Classification: Uterine relaxant.

Action/Kinetics: Stimulates beta$_2$ receptors of smooth muscle of the uterus, which results in inhibition of uterine contractility. It may also directly inhibit the actin-myosin interaction. The effects of the drug are inhibited by the beta-adrenergic blocking agents. Increased blood levels of insulin, glucose, and free fatty acids and decreased levels of potassium have been observed during IV infusion. **Onset, PO:** 30–60 min; **IV:** 5 min. **Peak plasma concentration, IV:** After a 9 mg infusion over 60 min, 32–50 ng/mL; **PO:** after a dose of 10 mg, 5–15 ng/mL. **Time to peak serum levels:** 20–60 min. **t½, after IV:** 15–17 hr; **after PO:** 12–20 hr. Ninety percent of drug excreted within 24 hr through the urine.

Uses: Preterm labor in selected patients after the twentieth week of gestation. When indicated, therapy with ritodrine should be initiated as early as possible after diagnosis. However, decision to use ritodrine should include determination of fetal maturity.

Contraindications: Before 20th week of pregnancy (pregnancy category: B) and when continuation of pregnancy is hazardous to mother (e.g., eclampsia, severe preeclampsia, intrauterine fetal death, antepartum hemorrhage, pulmonary hypertension, chorioamnionitis, and maternal hyperthyroidism, cardiac disease or uncontrolled diabetes mellitus). Also, medical conditions (e.g., uncontrolled hypertension, pheochromocytoma, bronchial asthma, hypovolemia, cardiac arrhythmias due to tachycardia or digitalis toxicity) that would be aggravated by beta-adrenergic agonists.

Side Effects: All effects are related to the stimulation of beta receptors by the drug. **IV.** *CV:* Increase in maternal and fetal heart rate, increase in maternal systolic and marked decrease in diastolic blood pressure (widening of pulse pressure), tachycardia, palpitations, arrhythmias, chest pain, angina, heart murmur, myocardial ischemia. Sinus bradycardia following drug withdrawal. *GI:* Nausea, vomiting, bloating, ileus, GI upset, diarrhea or constipation. *CNS:* Headache, tremors, malaise, nervousness, jitteriness, restlessness, anxiety, emotional changes, drowsiness, weakness. *Metabolic:* Transient increases in insulin and blood glucose, increases in cAMP and free fatty acids, decrease in potassium, glycosuria, lactic acidosis. *Respiratory:* Dyspnea, hyperventilation. *Other:* Erythema, anaphylaxis, rash, hemolytic icterus, sweating, chills.

   PO use. *CV:* Increase in heart rate of mother, palpitations, arrhythmias. *Other:* Tremors, nausea, rashes, restlessness. *In the neonate:* Hypoglycemia and ileus are infrequently observed; also hypocalcemia and hypotension in neonates whose mothers also received other beta-receptor agonists.

Drug Interactions	
Anesthetics, general	Additive hypotension or cardiac arrhythmias
Atropine	↑ Systemic hypertension
Beta-adrenergic blocking agents	↓ Effect of ritodrine
Corticosteroids	↑ Risk of pulmonary edema
Diazoxide	Additive hypotension or cardiac arrhythmias
Magnesium sulfate	Additive hypotension or cardiac arrhythmias
Meperidine	Additive hypotension or cardiac arrhythmias
Sympathomimetics	Additive effects of sympathomimetics

Laboratory Test Interferences: ↑ Plasma glucose and insulin; ↓ plasma potassium.

Dosage: IV: initial, 0.05–0.1 mg/min (20 drops/min using microdrip chamber); **then,** depending on response, increase by 0.05 mg/min (10 microdrops/min) q 10 min until desired response occurs. **Effective dose range:** 0.15–0.35 mg/min (30–70 drops/min). Continue infusion antepartum for a minimum of 12 hr after contractions cease. **PO therapy following initial IV treatment:** 10 mg 30 min before cessation of IV therapy; **then,** for first 24 hr, 10 mg q 2 hr; **maintenance:** 10–20 mg q 4–6 hr, not to exceed 120 mg/day. Dosage is determined by uterine activity and incidence of side effects.

NURSING CONSIDERATIONS

Administration/Storage

1. The drug should be reconstituted with dextrose solution. Solutions containing sodium chloride should be avoided, if possible, as their use increases the possibility of pulmonary edema. Final dilution will contain 0.3 mg/mL ritodrine.
2. To minimize hypotension, administer IV dose while the client is in the left lateral position.
3. Use a Y-set up, infusion pump, and microdrip tubing (60 microdrops/mL) for drug administration.
4. Do not use discolored solutions or those containing precipitate. Use diluted solution within 48 hr.
5. PO maintenance therapy is usually initiated 30 min before discontinuing IV therapy.

Assessment

1. Note any evidence or history of preeclampsia, hypertension, or diabetes before initiating drug therapy.
2. Determine that a sonogram and amniocentesis have been performed to establish fetal maturity. This determines whether ritodrine can be used.
3. Establish gestational age prior to initiating drug therapy. Ritodrine should not be used before the 20th week of pregnancy.

Interventions

1. Avoid concomitant administration of beta-adrenergic blocking drugs, such as propranolol, because these drugs inhibit the action of ritodrine.
2. Assess the response to IV therapy with ritodrine by evaluating the strength and frequency of contractions and monitoring the fetal heart rate. Document and report an increased fetal heart rate.

3. Monitor and record vital signs.
   • Maintain blood pressure by positioning the client in a left lateral position and evaluating level of hydration.
   • Report any increase in systolic blood pressure, decrease in diastolic blood pressure and tachycardia.
4. Monitor intake and output and auscultate lung sounds to assess fluid status.
5. Prevent circulatory overload. Closely monitor IV flow rate and infused volume during drug administration.
6. Assess for any respiratory dysfunction that may precede pulmonary edema, especially when the client is also receiving corticosteroids.
7. Assess for signs and symptoms of electrolyte imbalance. Be particularly alert to hypokalemia, hyperglycemia, and acidosis in clients with diabetes.
8. Assess the postpartum client who has received both ritodrine and general anesthesia for potentiation of hypotensive effects.
9. Neonates of mothers who have received ritodrine should be assessed for hyper- or hypoglycemia, hypocalcemia, hypotension, and ileus. Have emergency medication and equipment available to support the neonate.

SODIUM BENZOATE AND SODIUM PHENYLACETATE   (BEN-zoh-ayt, FEN-ill-AH-seh-tayt)
Ucephan (Rx)

Classification: Drug for hyperammonemia.

Action/Kinetics: In patients with urea cycle enzymopathies, there is a deficiency (either partial or complete) of argininosucciante synthetase, carbamylphosphate synthetase, and ornithine transcarbamylase. This leads to elevated blood ammonia levels which is fatal in nearly 80% of patients. Sodium benzoate and sodium phenylacetate lower elevated blood ammonia levels by decreasing ammonia formation, thus substituting for the defective enzymes in these individuals.

Uses: Prophylaxis and chronic treatment of hyperammonemia in patients with urea cycle enzymopathies.

Contraindications: Hypersensitivity to sodium benzoate or sodium phenylacetate. The sodium ions in this product should be used with care (if at all) in congestive heart failure, edema due to sodium retention, and renal insufficiency.

Special Concerns: Pregnancy category: C. Use with caution during lactation and in neonates with hyperbilirubinemia.

Side Effects: *GI:* Nausea, vomiting, worsening of peptic ulcers. *Respiratory:* Respiratory alkalosis and hyperventilation.

Drug Interactions	
Penicillin	↑ Renal tubular secretion due to competition from sodium benzoate and sodium phenylacetate
Probenecid	↓ Renal excretion of conjugation products of sodium benzoate and sodium phenylacetate

Dosage: Oral Solution. Adults: 2.5 mL/kg daily (250 mg each of sodium benzoate and sodium phenylacetate) in 3–6 equally divided doses. Total daily dose should not exceed 100 mL (i.e., 10 g each of sodium benzoate and sodium phenylacetate).

NURSING CONSIDERATIONS

Administration/Storage

1. This product must be diluted in 4–8 oz of milk (or infant formula) and given with meals. Acidic liquids should not be used since the drug may precipitate in an acid medium. The mixture should be visually inspected for compatibility before it is administered.
2. Sodium benzoate and sodium phenylacetate should be considered as adjunctive therapy for urea cycle enzymopathies.
3. For optimum results, combine with a low-protein diet and amino acid supplements.
4. Care should be exercised when mixing and administering sodium phenylacetate since contact with the skin and clothing will result in a lingering odor.
5. The product should be stored at room temperature; excess heat should be avoided.

Interventions

Monitor electrolyte levels, pH, and serum ammonia levels throughout therapy.

Client/Family Teaching

1. Instruct the client to follow a low-protein diet. Refer to a dietician for assistance with the diet and meal planning.
2. Provide written guidelines for the correct dilution and administration of the drug.
3. Instruct the client in keeping an accurate record of weight and advise him to report any significant changes to the physician.
4. Teach the client how to assess for edema and to report if evident.
5. Explain the importance of reporting for follow-up visits to the physician and for scheduled laboratory studies so that the effectiveness of the drug therapy can be evaluated.
6. Discuss with the client the importance of reporting to the physician any side effects and/or changes in mental attitude.

SODIUM TETRADECYL SULFATE   (teh-trah-**DEH**-sill)

Sotradecol, Trombovar✶ (Rx)

See also *Morrhuate Sodium,* p. 1381.

Classification: Sclerosing agent.

Action/Kinetics: On injection, this surface-active agent (detergent) causes sufficient irritation to the intima of the vein to result in a thrombus, followed by fibrous tissue which causes obliteration.

Uses: Obliteration of primary varicose veins of legs. *Investigational:* Esophageal varices.

Special Concerns: Pregnancy category: C.

Dosage: IV only, *small veins:* 5–20 mg (0.5–2 mL of 1% injection). *Medium-large veins:* 15–60 mg (0.5–2 mL of 3% injection). Treatment may be repeated after 5 to 7 days.

NURSING CONSIDERATIONS

See also *Nursing Considerations* for *Morrhuate Sodium,* p. 1381.

Administration/Storage

1. To test the client for sensitivity, inject a test dose of 0.5 mL of 1% injection. This may be requested by the physician several hours before treatment.
2. Sodium tetradecyl sulfate is usually administered by a physician familiar with the injection technique.
3. Inject only small amounts (2 mL maximum in a single varicose vein) and no more than 10 mL of the 3% injection during 1 treatment.
4. Inject slowly.
5. Avoid extravasation.
6. Do not use if the product is precipitated.
7. Have epinephrine 1:1,000 solution available to treat any allergic reaction.

Interventions

1. For several hours after administration of the test dose, inspect the injection site for an allergic reaction.
2. Explain to the client that a permanent discoloration may occur at the site of the injection. Encourage the client to select an area for injection that would be acceptable cosmetically.

TIOPRONIN   (tie-oh-**PROH**-nin)

Thiola (Rx)

Classification: Prevention of cystinuria.

Action/Kinetics: Tiopronin undergoes thiol-disulfide exchange with cystine to form a tiopronin-cystine complex thus reducing the levels of cystine which is only sparingly soluble. Reducing cystine levels maintains cystine concentrations below the solubility limit in the urine, thus preventing formation of stones. Up to 48% of the drug will appear in the urine in the first 4 hr following administration and up to 78% by 72 hr.

Uses: Prophylaxis of cystine stone formation. Usually reserved for patients with urinary cystine levels greater than 500 mg/day; those who are resistant to treatment with high fluid intake, alkali and diet modification; and, those who show adverse effects to d-penicillamine.

Contraindications: History of drug-induced agranulocytosis, aplastic anemia, or thrombocytopenia. Lactation.

Special Concerns: Use during pregnancy only if the benefits outweigh the potential risks (pregnancy category: C). Safety and efficacy have not been established in children less than 9 years of age.

Side Effects: *Dermatologic:* Generalized rash—erythematous, maculopapular, morabilliform—accompanied by pruritus. Wrinkling and friability of skin. *Miscellaneous:* Drug fever, lupus erythematosus-like reaction, hypogeusia, vitamin B_6 deficiency.

Dosage: Tablets. Adults, initial, 800 mg daily in patients with cystine stones; **children,** 15 mg/kg/day. **Maintenance:** Depends on urinary cystine levels and should be based on the dosage required to decrease urinary cystine levels to below its solubility limit (usually < 250 mg/L).

NURSING CONSIDERATIONS

Administration/Storage

1. A conservative program including large amounts of fluid and a modest amount of alkali (to maintain urinary pH from 6.5–7) in the diet should be tried prior to initiating tiopronin therapy.
2. Maintenance dosage should be given t.i.d. at least 1 hr before or 2 hr after meals.

Assessment

1. Note urinary pH and cystine level.
2. Obtain baseline CBC and liver function studies.

Interventions

1. Monitor and record urinary pH during drug therapy.
2. Measure intake and output and promote a high fluid intake.
3. Urinary cystine should be measured 1 month after initiation of therapy and every 3 months thereafter.

Client/Family Teaching

1. Advise the client to take tiopronin only as prescribed.
2. Stress the importance of reporting for follow-up lab studies as the dose of drug may need to be adjusted by the physician.
3. Provide a printed list and advise the client to report any adverse side effects. Symptoms such as fever, chills, sore throat, or excessive bleeding and bruising may necessitate the discontinuation of drug therapy.
4. Remind the client to drink plenty of fluids during drug therapy. Encourage client to maintain a record of her intake and output and daily urine pH levels to share with the physician.

TRETINOIN (RETINOIC ACID, VITAMIN A ACID)   (TRET-ih-noyn)

Retin A, StieV AA ✹ (Rx)

Classification: Antiacne drug.

Action/Kinetics: Topical tretinoin is believed to decrease micro-comedone formation by decreasing the cohesiveness of follicular epithelial cells. The drug is also believed to increase mitotic activity and increase turnover of follicular epithelial cells as well as decrease keratin synthesis. Some systemic absorption occurs (approximately 5% is recovered in the urine).

Uses: Acne vulgaris. *Investigational:* Lamellar ichthyosis, follicularis keratosis, verruca plana.

Contraindications: Eczema, sunburn.

Special Concerns: Use with caution during pregnancy (pregnancy category: B) and lactation. Safety and effectiveness have not been determined in children.

Side Effects: *Dermatologic:* Red, edematous, crusted, or blistered skin; hyperpigmentation or hypopigmentation, increased susceptibility to sunlight.

Dosage: Apply cream, gel, or liquid lightly over the affected areas once daily at bedtime. Beneficial effects many not be seen for 2–6 weeks.

NURSING CONSIDERATIONS

Administration/Storage

1. The liquid should be applied carefully with the fingertip, cotton swab, or gauze pad only to affected areas.
2. Excessive amounts of the gel will cause a "pilling" effect.

Assessment

Note if the client is of childbearing age and sexually active. Determine if she is pregnant prior to initiating therapy.

Client/Family Teaching

1. Advise the client to keep the medication away from mucous membranes, eyes, mouth, and the angles of the nose.
2. Explain to the client that upon application there will be a transitory feeling of warmth and stinging.
3. Explain that the client should expect dryness and peeling of skin from the affected areas.
4. Instruct the client to wash her hands thoroughly, immediately after applying tretinoin.
5. Advise client that during the early weeks of therapy, the lesions may worsen. This is caused by the effect of the drug on deep lesions that had been previously undetected. If the lesions become severe, the client should notify the physician and anticipate that the drug will be discontinued until the integrity of the skin has been restored.
6. Advise women of childbearing age to practice some form of birth control while they are receiving drug therapy.
7. Advise clients to avoid excessive exposure to sunlamps and to the sun. Persons who must be in sunlight while using the medication should be instructed to use a sunscreen or protective clothing over affected areas.

URSODIOL   (ur-so-**DYE**-ohl)

Actigall (Rx)

Classification: Gall stone solubilizer.

Action/Kinetics: Ursodiol is a naturally occurring bile acid which inhibits the hepatic synthesis and secretion of cholesterol; it also inhibits intestinal absorption of cholesterol. The drug acts to solubilize cholesterol in micelles and to cause dispersion of cholesterol as liquid crystals in aqueous media. The drug undergoes a significant first-pass effect where it is conjugated with either glycine or taurine and then secreted into hepatic bile ducts.

Uses: In patients with radiolucent, noncalcified gall stones (< 20 mm) in whom elective surgery would be risky.

Contraindications: Patients with calcified cholesterol stones, radio-opaque stones, or radiolucent bile pigment stones. Acute cholecystitis, cholangitis, biliary obstruction, gallstone pancreatitis, biliary-gastrointestinal fistula, allergy to bile acids, chronic liver disease.

Special Concerns: Pregnancy category: B. Use with caution during lactation. Safety and efficacy have not been determined in children. Safety for use beyond 24 months is not known.

Side Effects: *GI:* Diarrhea, nausea, vomiting, dyspepsia, metallic taste, abdominal pain, biliary pain, cholecystitis, constipation, stomatitis, flatulence. *Skin:* Pruritus, rash, dry skin, urticaria. *CNS:* Headache, fatigue, anxiety, depression, sleep disorders. *Other:* Sweating, thinning of hair, back pain, arthralgia, myalgia, rhinitis, cough.

Drug Interactions	
Antacids, aluminum-containing	↓ Effect of ursodiol due to ↓ absorption from GI tract
Cholestyramine	↓ Effect of ursodiol due to ↓ absorption from GI tract
Clofibrate	↓ Effect of ursodiol by ↑ hepatic cholesterol secretion
Colestipol	↓ Effect of ursodiol due to ↓ absorption from GI tract
Contraceptives, oral	↓ Effect of ursodiol by ↑ hepatic cholesterol secretion
Estrogens	↓ Effect of ursodiol by ↑ hepatic cholesterol secretion

Dosage: Capsules. Adults: 8–10 mg/kg daily in 2 or 3 divided doses, usually with meals.

NURSING CONSIDERATIONS

Administration/Storage

1. If partial stone dissolution is not observed within 12 months, the drug will probably not be effective.
2. For the first year of therapy, ultrasound of the gallbladder should be performed every 6 months to determine the response.

Assessment

1. Obtain a baseline ultrasound of the gallbladder and order liver function studies to serve as a baseline against which to measure subsequent studies and evaluate response throughout drug therapy.
2. List the drugs the client is taking, noting those with which ursodiol interacts unfavorably.
3. If the client is female, determine the possibility of pregnancy.
4. In screening the client, note that the drug is not indicated for calcified cholesterol stones, radiopaque stones or radiolucent bile pigment stones.

Interventions

1. Note any client complaints of nausea, vomiting, diarrhea, abdominal pain or the presence of a metallic taste in the mouth. Document and report to the physician.
2. Observe the client for complaints of headache, anxiety, depression and sleep disorders. Document and report these findings to the physician.

Client/Family Teaching

1. Explain that the ursodiol therapy may take up to 24 months, and that the drug will need to be taken 2–3 times per day.
2. Advise client to avoid taking antacids unless prescribed by the physician. Many antacids have an aluminum base which adsorbs the drug.

3. Discuss with the client the fact that stones may recur after the dissolution of the current stones.

4. Provide client with a printed list of drug side effects. Explain the importance of reporting to the physician symptoms such as persistent nausea and vomiting, abdominal pain, headaches, itching, rash or altered bowel function.

5. For women of childbearing age, discuss the need to practice birth control as pregnancy should be avoided during drug therapy. The use of estrogens and oral contraceptives may decrease the effectiveness of the drug, therefore other forms of birth control are advisable.

6. Stress the importance of reporting for follow-up visits to the physician and of reporting for routine laboratory studies and ultrasonography to evaluate the effectiveness of the drug therapy.

Evaluation

1. Evaluate for a positive clinical response to ursodiol therapy as demonstrated by the dissolution of gallstones.

2. If, on ultrasound, gallstones appear to have dissolved, ursodiol therapy should be continued for 1–3 months and dissolution confirmed again with ultrasound.

APPENDIX 1
Commonly Used Laboratory Test Values

Test	Range	Units	Conversion Factor	SI Range	Units
Alanine aminotransferase [ALT]	0–35	U/L	0.01667	0–0.58	ukat/L
Albumin, serum	4–6	g/dL	10	40–60	g/L
Alkaline phosphatase	30–120	U/L	0.01667	0.5–2	ukat/L
Aspartate aminotransferase [AST]	0–35	U/L	0.01667	0–0.58	ukat/L
Bilirubin, total (serum)	0.1–1	mg/dL	17.1	2–18	umol/L
Bilirubin, conjugated	0–0.2	mg/dL	17.1	0–4	umol/L
Calcium, serum	8.8–10.4	mg/dL	0.2495	2.2–2.58	mmol/L
				0–0	
Chloride, serum	95–110	mEq/L	1	95–110	mmol/L
Cholesterol					
< 29 years	< 200	mg/dL	0.02586	< 5.2	mmol/L
30–39 years	< 225	mg/dL	0.02586	< 5.85	mmol/L
40–49 years	< 245	mg/dL	0.02586	< 6.35	mmol/L
> 50 years	< 265	mg/dL	0.02586	< 6.85	mmol/L
Cortisol, serum					
0800 hours	4–19	ug/L	27.59	110–520	nmol/L
1600 hours	2–15	ug/L	27.59	50–410	nmol/L
2400 hours	5	ug/L	27.59	140	nmol/L
Creatine kinase (CK)					
Isoenzymes	0–130	U/L	0.01667	0–2.167	ukat/L
MB fraction	> 5 in MI	%	0.01	> 0.05	1
Creatinine, serum	0.6–1.2	mg/dL	88.4	50–110	umol/L
Creatinine clearance	75–125	mL/min	0.01667	1.24–2.08	mL/s
Erythrocyte count					
male	4.3–5.9	106/mm³	1	4.3–5.9	1012/L
female	3.5–5	106/mm³	1	3.5–5	1012/L
Erythrocyte sedimentation rate (ESR)					
male	0–20	mm/hr	1	0–20	mm/hr
female	0–30	mm/hr	1	0–30	mm/hr
Gases, arterial blood					
pO_2	75–105	mm Hg	0.1333	10–14	kPa
pCO_2	33–44	mm Hg	0.1333	4.4–5.9	kPa
Gamma-glutamyltransferase (GGT)	0–30	U/L	0.01667	0–0.5	ukat/L
Glucose, plasma (fasting)	70–110	mg/dL	0.05551	3.9–6.1	mmol/L
Hematocrit					
male	39–49	%	0.01	0.39–0.49	1
female	33–43	%	0.01	0.33–0.43	1
				0–0	

Test	Range	Units	Conversion Factor	SI Range	Units
Hemoglobin					
male	14–18	g/dL	10	140–180	g/L
female	11.5–15.5	g/dL	10	115–155	g/L
Iron, serum					
male	80–180	ug/dL	0.1791	14–32	umol/L
female	60–160	ug/dL	0.1791	11–29	umol/L
Iron binding capacity	250–460	ug/dL	0.1791	45–82	umol/L
Lactic dehydrogenase	50–150	U/L	0.01667	0.82–2.66	ukat/L
Lipoproteins					
low density (LDL)	50–190	mg/dL	0.02586	1.3–4.9	mmol/L
high density (HDL) male	30–70	mg/dL	0.02586	0.8–1.8	mmol/L
female	30–90	mg/dL	0.02586	0.8–2.35	mmol/L
Leukocyte count	3200–9800	mm³	0.001	3.2–9.8	109/L
differential		%	0.01		1
Magnesium, serum	1.8–3	mg/dL	0.4114	0.8–1.2	mmol/L
	1.6–2.4	mEq/L	0.5	0.8–1.2	mmol/L
Mean corpuscular hemoglobin (MCH)	27–33	pg	1	27–33	pg
Mean corpuscular					
hemoglobin concentration (MCHC)	33–37	g/dL	10	330–370	g/L
Mean corpuscular volume (MCV)	76–100	um³	1	76–100	fL
Osmolality, plasma	280–330	mOsm/kg	1	280–330	mmol/kg
Osmolality, urine	50–1200	mOsm/kg	1	50–1200	mmol/kg
Phosphate, serum	2.5–5	mg/dL	0.3229	0.8–1.6	mmol/L
Platelet count	130–400	103/mm³	1	130–400	109/L
Potassium, serum	3.5–5	mEq/L	1	3.5–5	mmol/L
Reticulocyte count	1–24	#/1000 RBC's	0.001	0.001–0.024	1
Sodium, serum	135–147	mEq/L	1	135–147	mmol/L
Thyroid stimulating hormone (TSH)	2–11	uU/mL	1	2–11	mU/L
Thyroxine (T_4)	4–11	ug/dL	12.87	51–142	nmol/L
Thyroid binding globulin (TBG)	12–28	ug/dL	12.87	150–360	nmol/L
Thyroxine, free serum	0.8–2.8	ng/dL	12.87	10–36	pmol/L
Triiodothyronine (T_3)	75–220	ng/dL	0.01536	1.2–3.4	nmol/L
T_3 uptake	25–35	%	0.01	0.25–0.35	1
Transferrin	170–370	mg/dL	0.01	1.7–3.7	g/L
Triglycerides	<160	mg/dL	0.01129	<1.8	mmol/L
Urea nitrogen	8–18	mg/dL	0.357	3–6.5	mmol/L
Zinc, serum	75–120	ug/dL	0.153	11.5–18.5	umol/L

"SI units" is the abbreviation of *Système International d'Unités*. It is a uniform system of reporting numerical values permitting interchangeability of information among nations and between disciplines.

(From Young DS: Implementation of SI units for clinical laboratory data. *Annals of Internal Medicine* 106:114–129, 1987.) Courtesy American College of Physicians.

ADDITIONAL PHYSIOLOGIC VALUES

HEMATOLOGY

White Blood Cells (leukocytes)	5,000–10,000/mm³
Neutrophils	50–70%
Segments	50–65%
Bands	0–5%
Basophils	0.25–0.5%
Eosinophils	1–3%
Lymphocytes	25–35%
Monocytes	2–6%

Bleeding Time	1–3 min (Duke)
	1–5 min (Ivy)
Coagulation Time (Lee White)	5–15 min
Prothrombin Time	10–15 sec (same as control)
Thrombin Time	Within 5 sec of control
Partial Thromboplastin Time (PTT)	60–70 sec
Activated Partial Thromboplastin time (APTT)	30–45 sec
Fibrinogen Split Products (FSP)	2–10 mcg/mL
Ceruloplasmin	27–37 mg/dL
Copper	100–200 mcg/dL

ENZYMES

Amylase	60–180 Somogyi U/dL
Creatine Phosphokinase (CPK)	5–35 mcg/dL; 15-120 IU/L
MB (+)	>5% of total CPK
Lipase	0–1.5 U/mL
Phosphatase, Acid	0.5–2.0 Bodansky units
Proteins	
Total	6–8 g/dL
Fibrinogen	0.2–0.4 g/dL
Globulin	1.5–3.0 g/dL

OTHER

Acetone	0.3–2.0 mg/dL
Alpha-1-antitrypsin	159–400 mg/dL
Ammonia	3.2–4.5 g/dL
Nonprotein Nitrogen (NPN)	15–35 mg/dL
Uric acid	Males: 3.5–7.8 mg/dL
	Females: 2.5–6.8 mg/dL

SEROLOGY

Antinuclear Antibodies (ANA)	Negative
Carcinoembryonic Antigen (CEA)	<2.5 ng/mL
Cold Agglutinins (CA)	1:8 antibody titer
Immunoglobulins (Ig)	900–2,200 mg/dL
IgG	600–1,900 mg/dL
IgA	60–330 mg/dL
IgM	45–145 mg/dL
IgD	0.5–3.0 mg/dL
IgE	10–506 units/mL
Rheumatoid Factor (RF)	<1:20 titer

CEREBROSPINAL FLUID (CSF)

Cell Count	0–8/mm^3
Chloride	118–132 mEq/L
Culture	No organisms
Glucose	40–80 mg/dL
Pressure	75–175 cm water
Protein	15–45 mg/dL
Sodium	145–150 mg/dL

BLOOD GASES

Whole Blood Oxygen, Capacity	17–24 vol %
Arterial	
Saturation	96–100% of capacity
pCO_2	35–45 mm Hg
pO_2	75–100 mm Hg
pH	7.38–7.44
Bicarbonate, Normal Range	24–28 mEq/L
Base Excess (BE)	+2 to −2 (± 2 mEq/L)
Venous	
Saturation	60–85% capacity
pCO_2	40–54 mm Hg
pO_2	20–50 mm Hg
pH	7.36–7.41
Bicarbonate, Normal Range	22–28 mEq/L

URINALYSIS

Casts	Occasional hyaline
Electrolytes	
Calcium	7.4 mEq/24 hr
Chloride	70–250 mEq/24 hr
Magnesium	15–300 mg/24 hr
Phosphorus, Inorganic	0.9–1.3 g/24 hr
Potassium	25–120 mEq/24 hr
Sodium	40–220 mEq/24 hr
Glucose	0
5-Hydroxyindoleacetic Acid (HIAA)	2–10 mg/24 hr
Ketones	0
Nitrogenous Constituents	
Ammonia	30–50 mEq/24 hr
Creatinine Clearance	100–200 mL/min
Creatinine	Males: 20–26 mg/kg/24 hr
	Females: 14–22 mg/kg/24 hr
Protein	10–50 mg/24 hr
Urea	6–17 g/24 hr
Uric Acid	0.25–0.75 g/24 hr
Osmolality	500–1,200 mOsm/L
pH	6.0 (average: 4.6–8.0)
Protein	0
Red Blood Cells	1–2/LPF (low power field)
Specific Gravity	1.005–1.030
Steroids	
17-Hydroxycorticosteroids	Males: 5–15 mg/24 hr
	Females: 3–13 mg/24 hr
17-Ketosteroids	Males: 8–25 mg/24 hr
	Females: 5–15 mg/24 hr
Urobilinogen	0–4 mg/24 hr
Vanillylmandelic Acid (VMA)	1.5–7.5 mg/24 hr
Volume	600–2,500 mL/24 hr
White Blood Cells	3–4

APPENDIX 2

Food-Drug Interactions and Nursing Considerations

I Drug	II Food Interactant	III Interaction (Effect and Mechanism)	IV Nursing Considerations Client/Family Teaching
Acetaminophen	High-carbohydrate foods, such as bread, cereal, and crackers	↓ Absorption rate of acetaminophen ↑ Onset of therapeutic effect by altering GI motility and emptying rate	1. Instruct client to restrict intake of foods high in CHO and/or administer medication 2 hr before or 2 hr after food ingestion. 2. Advise client to take on an empty stomach with a full glass of water.
Aminoglycosides	Urinary alkalinizers (See Table 2, p. 25) Urinary acidifiers (See Table 2, p. 25)	↓ Antibacterial activity of aminoglycosides ↑ Antibacterial activity of aminoglycosides	1. Restrict foods that are urinary alkalinizers (See Table 2, p. 25) 2. Maintain adequate intake of foods that are acidifiers (See Table 2, p. 25)
Acetylsalicylic acid	Acidic foods, such as coffee, cola drinks, citrus fruits, Food	↑ Gastric acidity that corrodes stomach lining and may cause ulcers ↓ Absorption rate	1. Instruct client to avoid acid foods (See Column II). 2. For rapid onset of action, advise client to take drug on an empty stomach with a full glass of water.
Barbiturates	Alcohol Protein-deficient diet Acidic foods (see above)	↑ Absorption ↑ Duration of action of drug by inhibiting cytochrome (P-450) enzymes which degrade barbiturates ↑ Activity through tubular reabsorption	1. Advise client not to drink alcohol when taking barbiturates. 2. Explain importance of eating a well–balanced diet to prevent protein deficiency. 3. Provide a printed list of signs and symptoms that are more likely to occur in clients with a protein deficiency. 4. Stress the importance of avoiding acidic foods.

1409

I Drug	II Food Interactant	III Interaction (Effect and Mechanism)	IV Nursing Considerations Client/Family Teaching
Bisacodyl	Dairy foods and antacids	Wears away enteric coating of drugs too early causing abdominal cramping	1. Advise client to avoid dairy foods and antacids at time of administration. 2. Instruct client not to use chewed or broken tablets.
Carbamazepine	Food	↑ Absorption of carbamazepine by increasing dissolution	Advise client to take drug with food.
Cephalosporins (oral)	Food	Delays absorption rate by altering GI motility and emptying rate	Instruct client it is preferable to take medication on an empty stomach 1 or 2 hr before or 2 hr after food ingestion.
Chlorpropamide	Alcoholic beverages, over-the-counter alcohol-containing	↑ Hypoglycemia by reducing activity of chlorpropamide, and by the additive hypoglycemic effect of alcohol. Possible Antabuse-like reaction (abdominal cramps) vomiting, flushing of skin)	Avoid alcohol including any over-the-counter products.
Cimetidine	Food	Delayed absorption helps maintain effective blood level between doses	Advise client to take drug with food.
Clindamycin	Pectin, found in the peel of citrus fruits and apple pulp	↓ Absorption by the formation insoluble compounds	Advise client to avoid the use of citrus fruits and peels, apple pulp, or any other pectin-containing foods.
Digoxin	Prune juice, bran cereals, and other foods high in fiber	↓ Cardiovascular activity of digoxin by delaying absorption rate	1. Instruct client to avoid taking prune juice, bran cereals, and other foods high in fiber. 2. Offer alternative methods for bowel regularity.
Diuretics	Monosodium glutamate (MSG) used in seasoned salts, meat tenderizers, frozen vegetables, and oriental cuisine	↑ Removal of excess water from tissue. In combination with diuretic, can deplete vitamin C and B complex and minerals, sodium, calcium, and potassium. Adverse effects of MSG can occur	1. Instruct client not to use MSG with diuretics. When dining out, advise client to ask if MSG was used in food preparation.

Drug	Food	Effect	Nursing Implications
Licorice (natural)		(tightening of chest, flushing of face.) ↑ Salt and water retention, ↑ Potassium excretion	2. Advise client to avoid natural licorice when on diuretic therapy.
Erythromycin	Acidic foods, such as coffee, cola drinks, citrus fruits, pickles, and tomatoes	↓ Antibacterial activity ↓ Absorption rate by altering GI motility and emptying rate	1. Instruct client to avoid acidic foods (See Column II). 2. Advise client to take on an empty stomach with a full glass of water.
Ethyl alcohol	Food	↓ Absorption by delaying gastric emptying	Explain to client to take with food to reduce degree of intoxication; milk is particularly effective.
Furazolidone	Food high in tyramine (See Nursing Considerations under Monoamine oxidase inhibitions, p. 659 for a list of foods high in tyramine)	Possible hypertensive reaction due to inhibition of metabolism of tyramine (6 mg of tyramine may cause hypertensive crisis)	1. Advise client not to eat foods high in tyramine. See Nursing Considerations under MAO inhibitors, p. 659.
	Alcohol	Possible Antabuse-like reaction (abdominal cramps, vomiting, flushing of skin)	2. Advise client to avoid alcoholic beverages.
Furosemide	Food	↓ Absorption of furosemide	
Griseofulvin	Food with a high fat content such as butter, margarine, oils, cream, lard, fat in meat	↑ Absorption due to greater solubilization by increased bile secretions	Instruct client to take with diet high in fats (usually breakfast) to ensure greater absorption of drug.
Hydralazine	Food	↑ Absorption because of bioavailability	1. Instruct client to take with foods. 2. Advise consistency of administration, preferably with meals.
Indomethacin	Food	↓ Absorption and ↑ time to reach peak serum levels	Despite interaction, instruct client to take drug with food to avoid GI irritation.
Iron sulfate	Dairy foods, eggs, cereals, starches, and clays	↓ Absorption by formation of insoluble salts	1. Advise client not to take or give to children with foods or substances listed in column II.
	Citrus juices	↑ Absorption of iron	2. Encourage client to take iron product with citrus juices.
Isoniazid	Food	↓ Absorption of isoniazid	Advise client to take on an empty stomach with a full glass of water.

1411

I Drug	II Food Interactant	III Interaction (Effect and Mechanism)	IV Nursing Considerations Client/Family Teaching
Levodopa	Foods high in protein such meat, fish, poultry, milk, cheese, dairy products, peanut butter, legumes, and nuts Foods high in pyridoxine (B_6)	↓ Absorption rate by competing for intestinal absorption, change in pH, or gastric emptying time. This results in ↓ peak plasma levels and therapeutic effect. ↓ Therapeutic effect by accelerating conversion of levodopa to dopamine	1. Instruct client to avoid high-protein diets or diets in which the protein intake fluctuates. 2. Advise clients that foods high in pyridoxine, such as yeast, whole grains (especially corn), brown rice, blackstrap molasses, salmon, tuna, lentils, beans, seeds, nuts, tomatoes, sweet potatoes, bananas, pears, cabbage, yams, walnuts. Smaller amounts of B_6 in milk, eggs, and vegetables should be avoided.
Lincomycin	Food Pectin found in the peel of citrus fruits and apple pulp	↓ Absorption and therapeutic effect by altering GI motility and emptying time. ↓ Absorption by formation of insoluble compounds	1. Advise client to take on an empty stomach with a full glass of water. 2. Instruct client to avoid citrus fruits, apples, or any other pectin-containing foods.
Lithium	Food Low-salt diets	↑ Absorption rate by delaying gastric emptying and transition ↓ Renal clearance of lithium	1. Advise client to take drug with food. 2. Provide a printed list of drug side effects. Instruct client to with-hold drug and notify the physician should diarrhea, vomiting, drows-iness, muscular weakness, and lack of coordination occur as these may be symptoms of lithium toxicity.
Methenamine mandelate	Urinary alkalinizers (See Table 2, p. 25) Urinary acidifiers (See Table 2, p. 25)	↓ Antibacterial activity ↑ Antibacterial activity	1. Advise client to restrict urinary alkalinizers (See Table 2, p. 25). 2. Instruct client to include urinary acidi-fiers in diet (see Table 2, p. 25). 3. Encourage client to increase intake of vitamin C to promote acid urine.

Metronidazole	Alcoholic beverages, wines, beers, tonics, cough formulas	Possible Antabuse-like reaction (abdominal cramps, vomiting, flushing of skin)	Advise client not to consume alcoholic beverages including alcohol-containing OTC preparations.
Monoamine oxidase inhibitors	Food high in tyramine	Hypertensive effect by inhibiting metabolism of tyramine and norepinephrine to toxic levels. Usually signaled by sudden, severe headaches; GET HELP. Note: 6 mg of tyramine may cause hypertensive crisis.	Instruct client that foods high in tyramine, such as beer, broad beans, aged cheeses (brie, cheddar, Camembert, Stilton), Chianti wine, sherry, beef and chicken liver, caffeine, cola drinks, figs, licorice, pickled or kippered herring, tea, cream, yogurt, yeast extract, chocolate, avocados, bananas, caviar, dried fish, bologna, salami, and sausage should be avoided.
Nitrofurantoin	Food	↑ Bioavailability due to greater dissolution in gastric juices and decreased gastric emptying time	1. Advise client to take with food to minimize gastric irritation.
	Low-protein diets, dairy products, and urinary alkalinizers (see Table 2, p. 25)	↑ Drug excretion due to alkalinization of urine	2. Instruct client to restrict intake of alkalinizers (see Table 2, p. 25).
			3. Provide proper dietary instructions and encourage adequate protein intake.
Penicillin (Amoxicillin and Penicillin V are less affected by food)	Food	↓ Therapeutic effect delayed or reduced by absorption or altering gastric motility and emptying rate	Advise client to take on an empty stomach with a full glass of water.
Phenytoin	Monosodium glutamate	↑ Absorption rate of MSG leading to generalized weakness, numbness at back of neck, and palpitations	Instruct client not to eat foods prepared with MSG. When dining out, instruct client to ask if MSG was used in the food preparation.
Propranolol	Food	↑ Absorption by reducing first-pass hepatic metabolism	Advise client to take drug with food.
Propantheline	Food	↓ Therapeutic effect by reducing rate of absorption	Instruct client to take on an empty stomach with a full glass of water.

1413

I Drug	II Food Interactant	III Interaction (Effect and Mechanism)	IV Nursing Considerations Client/Family Teaching
Quinidine	Urinary alkalinizers (see Table 2, p. 25)	↓ Excretion of drug; may cause quinidine intoxication manifested by cardiac, respiratory, and CNS alteration in function	1. Instruct client to restrict alkalinizers (see Table 2, p. 25). 2. Encourage client to take on an empty stomach with a full glass of water. 3. Advise client to take with food or milk, if necessary, to reduce gastric irritation.
Riboflavin	Food	↑ Absorption by food delays gastric emptying or transit time	Advise client to take with food.
Rifampin	Food	↓ Serum levels and decreases peak levels due to reduced rate of absorption	Instruct client to take with food.
Spironolactone	Food	↑ Bioavailability by increasing absorption	Instruct client to take on an empty stomach with a full glass of water.
Sulfadiazine, Sulfisoxazole	Food	Delays absorption rate by altering GI motility and emptying time	Instruct client to take on an empty stomach with a full glass of water.
Tetracycline	Milk, dairy products, foods high in iron	↓ Absorption by formation of insoluble salts with nutrients	1. Advise client not to take drug with dairy products and foods high in iron. 2. Advise client not to take iron supplements or antacids with tetracyclines.
Theophylline	Low-carbohydrate and high-protein diet	↓ Plasma half-life by increasing levels of cytochrome P-450 enzymes leading to more rapid oxidation	1. Advise client to eat a well-balanced diet, avoiding significant diet changes of carbohydrate and protein.
	Charcoal-broiled beef	↓ Therapeutic effect by ↑ drug metabolism	2. Advise client to take on an empty stomach and to use a liquid theophylline product if faster absorption is needed.

		3. Instruct client to take with food only if necessary to reduce gastric irritation.
Thiamine	Food	↓ Absorption rate by altering GI motility and transit time but extent of absorption is unchanged	Advise client to take with food.
Thyroid hormone	Kale, cabbage, carrots, cauliflower, spinach, peaches, brussel sprouts, turnips	↓ Thyroid hormone activity and interferes with drug activity	Instruct client to avoid excessive consumption of foods listed in Column II.
Tolbutamide	Alcohol (chronic intake or acute intoxication)	↑ Hypoglycemia by decreasing drug metabolism and additive effect of alcohol Possible Antabuse-like reaction (abdominal cramps, vomiting, flushing of skin)	Advise client to avoid the use of alcohol.
Warfarin	Foods high in vitamin K such as liver and leafy, green vegetables, potatoes, citrus juices, vegetable oil, egg yolk, green tea. Cooking oil with silicone additives	↓ Drug activity by presence of vitamin K that antagonizes warfarin ↓ Drug activity by formation of insoluble salts that are not absorbed	1. Advise client to consult with physician regarding appropriate diet while on anticoagulant therapy. 2. Instruct client to avoid excessive use of foods high in vitamin K and acidic foods, such as coffee, cola drinks, citrus fruits, pickles, and tomatoes. (see column II). 3. Instruct client not to use cooking oil with silicone additives.

APPENDIX 3

Controlled Substances in the U.S. and Canada

Controlled Substances Act–United States

The U.S. Federal Controlled Substances Act of 1970 placed drugs controlled by the Act into five categories or schedules based on their potential to cause psychological and/or physical dependence and their potential for abuse. Selected drugs in Schedules II, III, and IV are listed here.

Schedule I: Includes substances for which there is a high abuse potential and no current approved medical use. Substances in this category include heroin, marijuana, LSD, peyote, mescaline, psilocybin, other hallucinogens, certain opiates and opium derivatives.

Schedule II: Includes drugs that have a high abuse potential, high ability to produce physical and/or psychological dependence, and a current approved or acceptable medical use.

Schedule III: Includes drugs for which there is less potential for abuse than drugs in Schedule II and for which there is a current approved medical use. Certain drugs in this category are preparations containing limited quantities of codeine, such as Ascriptin with Codeine, Empirin with Codeine, Fiorinal with Codeine, Phenaphen with Codeine, Tylenol with Codeine, and others.

Schedule IV: Includes drugs for which there is a relatively low abuse potential and for which there is a current approved medical use.

Schedule V: Drugs in this category consist mainly of preparations containing limited amounts of certain narcotic drugs for use as antitussives and antidiarrheals. Federal law provides that limited quantities of these drugs (e.g., codeine) may be bought without a prescription by an individual at least 18 years of age. The product must be purchased from a pharmacist who, must keep appropriate records. However, state laws do vary and in certain states these products do require a prescription. Examples include Paregoric, Terpin Hydrate and Codeine, Robitussin A-C Syrup, Tussi-Organidin, and others.

Controlled Substances–Canada

In Canada, narcotics are governed by the Narcotics Control regulations and are designated by N. Drugs that are considered subject to abuse, which have an approved medical use, and are not narcotics are designated by C.

| | Drug Schedule | |
Drug	United States	Canada
Alfentanil	II	N
Alprazolam	IV	*
Amobarbital	II	C
Amphetamine	II	Not available
Aprobarbital	III	*

Drug	Drug Schedule	
	United States	Canada
Benzphetamine	III	Not available
Buprenorphine	V	*
Butabarbital	III	C
Butorphanol	*	C
Chloral hydrate	IV	*
Chlordiazepoxide	IV	*
Clonazepam	IV	*
Clorazepate	IV	*
Codeine	II	N
Dextroamphetamine	II	C
Diazepam	IV	*
Diethylpropion	IV	C
Ethchlorvynol	IV	*
Ethinamate	IV	*
Fenfluramine	IV	*
Fentanyl	II	N
Flurazepam	IV	*
Glutethimide	III	*
Halazepam	IV	*
Hydrocodone	Not available	N
Hydromorphone	II	N
Levorphanol	II	N
Lorazepam	IV	*
Mazindol	IV	*
Meperidine	II	N
Mephobarbital	IV	C
Meprobamate	IV	*
Methadone	II	N
Methamphetamine	II	Not available
Metharbital	III	C
Methylphenidate	II	C
Methyprylon	III	*
Morphine	II	N
Nalbuphine	*	C
Opium	II	N
Oxazepam	IV	*
Oxycodone	II	N
Oxymorphone	II	N
Paraldehyde	IV	*
Pemoline	IV	*
Pentazocine	IV	N
Pentobarbital,		
PO, parenteral	II	C
Rectal	III	C
Phendimetrazine	III	Not available
Phenmetrazine	II	Not available
Phenobarbital	IV	C
Phentermine	IV	C

| Drug | Drug Schedule | |
	United States	Canada
Prazepam	IV	*
Propoxyphene	IV	N
Secobarbital		
PO	II	C
Parenteral	II	*
Rectal	III	*
Talbutal	III	*
Temazepam	IV	*
Triazolam	IV	*

*Not controlled

Medic Alert Systems

WHO NEEDS MEDIC ALERT? Persons with any medical problem or condition that cannot be easily seen or recognized need the protection of Medic Alert. Heart conditions, diabetes, severe allergies and epilepsy are common problems. Others are listed on the application form under this page. About one in every five persons has some special medical problem.

WHY MEDIC ALERT? Tragic or even fatal mistakes can be made in emergency medical treatment unless the special problem of the person is known. A diabetic could be neglected and die because he was thought to be intoxicated. A shot of penicillin could end the life of one who is allergic to it. Persons dependent on medications must continue to receive them at all times.

WHEN IS MEDIC ALERT IMPORTANT? Whenever a person cannot speak for himself — because of unconsciousness, shock, delirium, hysteria, loss of speech, etc. — the Medic Alert emblem speaks for him.

HOW DOES MEDIC ALERT WORK? The Medic Alert emblem —worn on the wrist or neck — is recognized the world over. On the back of the emblem is engraved the medical problem and the file number of the wearer, and the telephone number of Medic Alert's Central File. Doctors, police, or anyone giving aid can immediately get vital information — addresses of the personal physician and nearest relative, etc. — via collect telephone call (24 hours a day) to the Central File.

WHAT IS MEDIC ALERT? It is a charitable, nonprofit organization. Its services are maintained by a one-time-only membership fee and by voluntary contributions from friends, corporations and foundations. Additional services such as replacement of lost emblems and up-dating of records are charged to members at cost. Membership is tax deductible as a medical expense, and contributions are always deductible on income tax returns.

WHERE IS MEDIC ALERT? Medic Alert Foundation International was founded in Turlock, California in 1956, after a doctor's daughter almost died from reaction to a sensitivity test for tetanus antitoxin. The Foundation is endorsed by over 100 organizations including the American Academy of General Practice (and many more national and state medical organizations) the International Associations of Fire Chiefs, Police Chiefs, the National Sheriffs' Association, and the National Association of Life Underwriters.

For further information, write to:

Medic Alert Foundation International
Turlock, CA 95380
Phone (209) 632-2371.

John D. McPherson, President

Produced internally by Medic Alert Foundation

MEDIC ALERT EMBLEMS ARE SHOWN IN ACTUAL SIZE

BRACELETS:

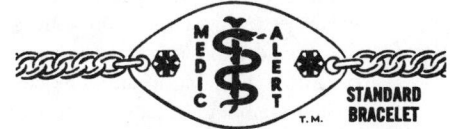

STANDARD BRACELET

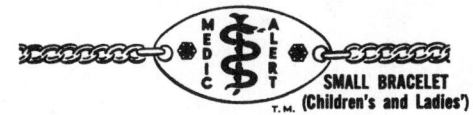

SMALL BRACELET
(Children's and Ladies')

DISC:

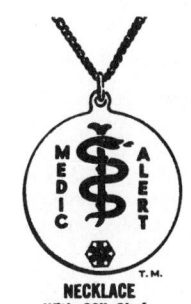

NECKLACE
With 26" Chain

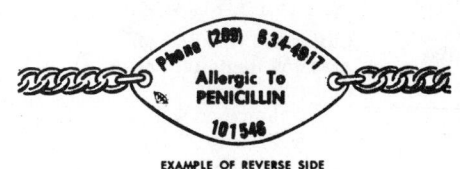

EXAMPLE OF REVERSE SIDE
OF MEDIC ALERT
EMBLEM

ALL MEMBERSHIP FEES AND DONATIONS ARE TAX-DEDUCTIBLE

APPENDIX 5
Certified Poison Control Centers

The poison control centers in the following list are certified by the American Association of Poison Control Centers. To receive certification, each center must meet certain criteria. It must, for example, serve a large geographic area; it must be open 24 hours a day and provide direct dialing or toll-free access; it must be supervised by a medical director; and it must have registered pharmacists or nurses available to answer questions from the public.

Staff members of these centers are trained to resolve toxicity situations in the home of the caller, but, in some instances, hospital referrals are given.

The centers have a wide variety of toxicology resources, including a computer capability covering some 350,000 substances that are updated quarterly. They also offer a range of educational services to the public as well as to the health-care professional. In some states, these large centers exist side by side with smaller poison control centers that provide more limited information.

American Association of Poison Control Centers

ALABAMA

Alabama Poison Center
Alabama Poison Center
809 University Boulevard East
Tuscaloosa, AL 35401
Emergency Numbers
  800/462-0800 AL only
  205/345-0600
FAX: 205/759-7994
Director: Richard W. Looser, B.S.;
  205/345-0938
Medical Director: Perry L.
Lovely, M.D.: 205/345-0600

Children's Hospital of Alabama Regional Poison Control Center
1600 7th Avenue South
Birmingham, AL 35233
Emergency Numbers
  205/939-9201 AL only
  800/292-6678
  205/933-4050
Director: William D. King,
R. Ph., M.P.H.: 205/939-9720
Medical Director: Edward C.
Kohaut, M.D.: 205/939-9100

ARIZONA

Arizona Poison and Drug Information Center
Health Sciences Center,
  Room 3204K
1501 North Campbell
Tucson, AZ 85724
Emergency Numbers
  602/626-6016 (Tucson)
  800/362-0101 (statewide)
FAX: 602/626-4063
Director: Theodore G. Tong,
Pharm. D.: 602/626-7899
Medical Director: John B.
Sullivan, Jr., M.D.:
  602/626-6312

Samaritan Regional Poison Center
Good Samaritan Medical
Center
1130 East McDowell, Suite A5
Phoenix AZ 85006
Emergency Numbers
  602/253-3334
FAX: 602/239-4138
Director: Joyce M. Bradley,
R.N., M.S.: 602/253-0813

Medical Director: Donald B.
Kunkel, M.D.: 602/253-2314

CALIFORNIA

Fresno Regional Poison Control Center
Fresno Community Hospital
and Medical Center
Fresno and R Streets
Fresno, CA 93715
Emergency Numbers
  209/445-1222
  800/346-5922
FAX: 209/442-6483
Director: Brent R. Ekins,
Pharm. D.: 209/442-6479
Medical Director: Rick Geller,
M.D.: 209/442-6408

Los Angeles County Medical Association
Regional Poison Center
1925 Wilshire Boulevard
Los Angeles, CA 90057
Emergency Numbers
  213/664-2121
  213/484-5151
  800/777-6476

FAX: 213/413-5255
Director: Corrine Ray, R.N.,
B.S.: 213/664-2121
Medical Director: Marc J.
Bayer, M.D.: 818/364-3107

San Diego Regional Poison Center
UCSD Medical Center
225 Dickinson Street
San Diego, CA 92103-1990
Emergency Numbers
  619/543-6000
  800/876-4766
FAX: 619/692-1667
Director: Anthony S.
Manoguerra, Pharm. D.
619/543-6010
Medical Director: George M.
Shumaik. M.D.: 619/543-3666

San Francisco Regional Poison Center
San Francisco General
Hospital
1001 Potrero Avenue,
Room IE86
San Francisco, CA 94110
Emergency Numbers
  415/476-6600
  800/523-2222
FAX: 415/821-8513
Director/Medical Director:
Kent R. Olson, M.D.:
415/821-5524

UC Davis Regional Poison Control Center
2315 Stockton Boulevard
Room 1511
Sacramento, CA 95817
Emergency Numbers
  916/453-3692
  800/342-9293 (Northern
  CA only)
FAX: 916/453-7796
Director: Judith Alsop,
Pharm, D.: 916/453-3414
Medical Director: Timothy
Albertson, M.D., Ph.D.:
916/453-5010

COLORADO

Rocky Mountain Poison and Drug Center
645 Bannock Street
Denver, CO 80204-4507
Emergency Numbers
  303/629-1123 (CO)

FAX: 303/623-1119
Director: Barry H Rumack,
M.D.: 303/893-7774
Medical Director: Kenneth
Kulig, M.D., F.A.C.E.P.:
303/893-7774

FLORIDA

Florida Poison Information Center
The Tampa General Hospital
Davis Islands
Post Office Box 1289
Tampa, FL 33601
Emergency Numbers
  813/253-444 (Tampa only)
  800/282-3171 (Florida)
Director: Sven A. Normann,
Pharm.D.: 813/251-7044
Co-Medical Directors: James
V. Hillman, M.D.: Gregory G.
Gaar, M.D.: 813/251-6911

GEORGIA

Georgia Regional Poison Control Center
80 Butler Street, S.E.
Atlanta, GA 30335-3801
Emergency Numbers
  404/589-4400
  800/282-5846 (GA only)
FAX: 404/525-2816
Director: Gaylord P. Lopez,
Pharm.D.: 404/589-4400
Medical Director: Robert J.
Geller, M.D.: 404/589-4400

KENTUCKY

Kentucky Regional Poison Center of Kosair Children's Hospital
224 East Broadway, Suite 305
Louisville, KY 40202
Emergency Numbers
  502/589-8222
  800/722-5725 (KY Toll Free)
Director: Nancy J. Matyunas,
Pharm.D.: 502/562-7263
Medical Director: George C.
Rodgers Jr., M.D., Ph.D.:
502/562-8837

MARYLAND

Maryland Poison Center
20 North Pine Street
Baltimore, MD 21201

Emergency Numbers
  301/528-7701
  800/492-2414 (MD only)
FAX: 301/328-7184
Director: Gary M. Oderda,
Pharm.D., M.P.H.: 301/328-7604
Medical Director: Richard L.
Gorman, M.D.: 301/328-7604

MASSACHUSETTS

Massachusetts Poison Control System
300 Longwood Avenue
Boston, MA 02115
Emergency Numbers
  617/232-2120 Boston Area
  800/682-9211 Toll Free in MA
Director/Medical Director:
Alan Woolf, M.D., M.P.H.:
617/735-6609

MICHIGAN

Blodgett Regional Poison Center
1840 Wealthy Street S.E.
Grand Rapids, MI 49506
Emergency Numbers
  800/632-2727 MI only
FAX: 616/774-7204
Director: Daniel J. McCoy,
Ph.D.: 616/774-7851
Medical Director: John R.
Mauer, M.D.: 616/774-7851

Poison Control Center
Children's Hospital of
Michigan
3901 Beaubien Boulevard
Detroit, MI 48201
Emergency Numbers
  313/745-5711 (Metro
  Detroit)
  800/462-6642 (Rest of MI)
FAX: 313/745-5602
Director/Medical Director:
Regine Aronow, M.D.:
313/745-5335
Administrative Manager:
Richard Dorsch, M.D.:
313/745-5329

MINNESOTA

Hennepin Regional Poison Center
Hennepin County Medical
Center
701 Park Avenue South
Minneapolis, MN 55415

Emergency Numbers
612/347-3141
FAX: 612/347-3968
Director: Michael J. Wieland,
R.Ph.: 612/347-3144
Medical Director: Louis J.
Ling, M.D.: 612/347-3174

**Minnesota Regional Poison
Center**
St. Paul-Ramsey Medical
Center
640 Jackson Street
St. Paul, MN 55101
Emergency Numbers
612/221-2113
800/222-1222 (MN only)
Director: Leo Sioris,
Pharm.,D.: 612/221-3192
Medical Director: Samuel
Hall, M.D., A.B.M.T.:
612/221-3470

MISSOURI

**Cardinal Glennon Children's
Hospital**
Regional Poison Center
1465 South Grand Boulevard
St. Louis, MO 63104
Emergency Numbers
800/392-9111 (MI only)
314/772-5200
800/366-8888
FAX: 314/557-5355
Director: Michael W.
Thompson, B.S. Pharm.:
314/772-8300
Medical Director: Anthony J.
Scalzo, M.D.: 314/772-8300

NEW JERSEY

**New Jersey Poison
Information and Education
System**
201 Lyons Avenue
Newark, NJ 07112
Emergency Numbers
800/962-1253 (NJ only)
201/923-0764 (Outside NJ)
FAX: 201/926-0013
Director/Medical Director:
Steven M. Marcus, M.D:
201/926-7443

NEW MEXICO

**New Mexico Poison and
Drug Information Center**
University of New Mexico
Albuquerque, NM 87131

Emergency Numbers
505/843-2551
800/432-6866 (NM only)
Director: William G.
Troutman, Pharm.D.:
505/277-4261
Medical Director: Dan
Tandberg, M.D.: 505/277-5064

NEW YORK

**Long Island Regional Poison
Control Center**
2201 Hempstead Turnpike
East Meadow, NY 11554
Emergency Numbers
516/542-2323
Director/Medical Director:
Howard C. Mofenson, M.D.:
516/542-3707

New York City Poison Center
455 First Avenue, Room 123
New York, NY 10016
Emergency Numbers
212/340-4494
212/764-7667
FAX: 212/340-4525
Director: Richard S.
Weisman, Pharm.D.:
212/340-4497
Medical Director: Lewis
Goldfrank, M.D.: 212/561-3346

NORTH CAROLINA

**Duke Regional Poison
Control Center**
Duke University Medical
Center
Box 3007
Durham, NC 27710
Emergency Numbers
800/672-1697 (NC only)
Medical Director: Shirley
Osterhout, M.D.: 919/684-4438
Assistant Director: Chris
Rudd, Pharm.D.:
919/681-4574

OHIO

Central Ohio Poison Center
700 Children's Drive
Columbus, OH 43205
Emergency Numbers
614/228-1323
800/682-7625
Director: Judith G. D'Orsi,
B.A.: 614/461-2717

Medical Director: Mary Ellen
Mortensen, M.D.:
614/461-2256

**Regional Poison Control
System and Cincinnati Drug
and Poison Information
Center**
231 Bethesda Avenue, M.L,
#144
Cincinnati, OH 45267-0144
Emergency Numbers
513/558-5111
FAX: 513/558-5301
Director: Leonard T. Sigell,
Ph.D.: 513/558-9182
Medical Director: Clifford G.
Grulee, Jr., M.D.:
513/558-7336

OREGON

Oregon Poison Center
Oregon Health Sciences
University
3181 SW Sam Jackson Park
Road
Portland, OR 97201
Emergency Numbers
503/279-8968;
800/452-7165 (OR only)
Director: Terry Putman, R.N.:
503/279-7799
Medical Director: Brent T.
Burton, M.D.: 503/279-7799

PENNSYLVANIA

**Delaware Valley Regional
Poison Control Center**
One Children's Center
34th & Civic Center
Boulevard
Philadelphia, PA 19104
Emergency Numbers
215/386-2100
FAX: 215/386-3692
Director: Thomas E.
Kearney, Pharm.D.:
215/823-7203
Medical Director: Fred M.
Henretig, M.D.: 215/596-8454

Pittsburgh Poison Center
One Children's Place
3705 5th Avenue at DeSoto
Pittsburgh, PA 15213
Emergency Numbers
412/681-6669
FAX: 412/692-5868

Director: Edward P.
Krenzelok, Pharm.D.:
412/692-5600
Assistant Director: Bonnie S.
Dean, R.N., B.S.N.:
412/692-5600
Medical Director: Sandra M.
Schneider, M.D.:
412/648-6000 ext. 3669

RHODE ISLAND

593 Eddy Street
Providence, RI 02903
Emergency Numbers
 401/277-5727
 401/277-8062 (TDD)
Director: Philip N. Johnson,
Ph.D.: 401/277-5906
Medical Director: William J.
Lewander, M.D.: 401/277-5906

TEXAS

North Texas Poison Center
5201 Harry Hines Boulevard
Dallas, TX 75235
Emergency Numbers
 214/590-5000
 800/441-0040 (TX only)
FAX: 214/590-8096
Attention: Poison Center
Director: Lena C. Day, R.N.,
B.S.N., C.S.P.I.: 214/590-5625

Medical Director: Gary Reed,
M.D.: 214/688-2992
Assistant Medical Director:
Tom Kurt, M.D.: 214/590-6625

Texas State Poison Center
University of Texas Medical
Branch
Galveston, TX 77550-2780
Emergency Numbers
 409/765-1420 (Galveston)
 800/392-8548 (TX only)
 713/654-1701 (Houston)
 512/478-4490 (Austin)
Director: Michael D. Ellis,
M.S.: 409/761-3332
Medical Director: Wayne R.
Snodgrass, M.D., Ph.D.:
409/761-1561

UTAH

Intermountain Regional Poison Control Center
50 North Medical Drive,
Building 528
Salt Lake City, UT 84132
Emergency Numbers
 801/581-2151
Director: Joseph C. Veltri,
Pharm. D.: 801/581-7504
Medical Director: Douglas
Rollins, M.D., Ph.D.:
801/581-5117

WASHINGTON, D.C.

National Capital Poison Center
Georgetown University
Hospital
3800 Reservoir Road, N.W.
Washington, DC 20007
Business/Emergency
Numbers
 202/625-3333
 202/784-4660 (TTY)
FAX: 202/784-2530
Director/Medical Director:
Toby Litovitz, M.D.:
202/784-2088

WEST VIRGINIA

West Virginia Poison Center
3110 MacCorkle Avenue, S.E.
Charleston, WV 25304
Emergency Numbers
 304/348-4211 (local)
 800/642-3625 (intrastate)
FAX: 304/348-9560
Director: Gregory P. Wedin,
Pharm. D.: 304/347-1212
Medical Director: David E.
Seidler, M.D.: 304/347-1212

APPENDIX 6
Computing Areas of Burns

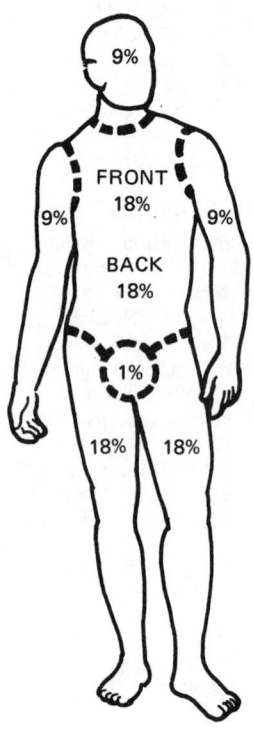

Diagram for use in calculating the extent of burns or other injuries for an adult

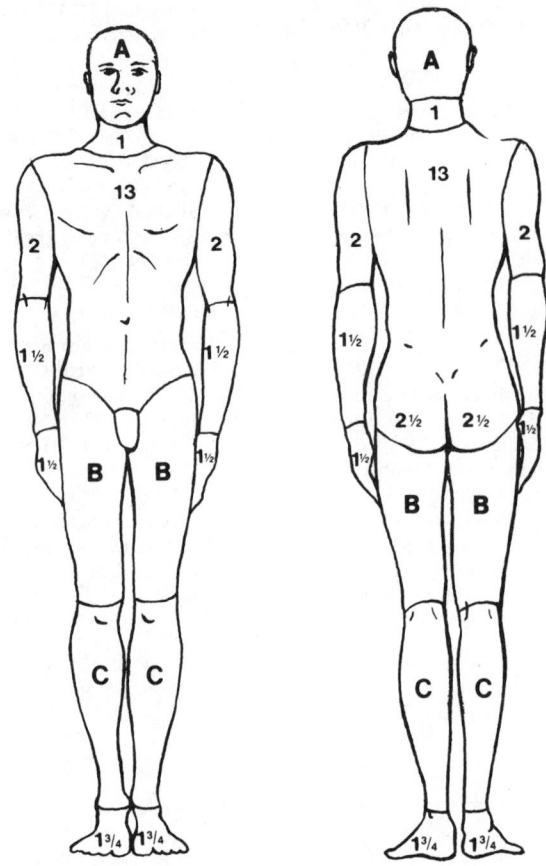

Relative percentages of areas affected by growth

	At birth	1 yr	5 yr	10 yr	15 yr	Adult
A: Half of head	9½%	8½%	6½%	5½%	4½%	3½%
B: Half of thigh	2¾%	3¼%	4%	4¼%	4½%	4¾%
C: Half of leg	2½%	2½%	2¾%	3%	3¾%	3½%

Lund and Browder chart for estimating the extent of burns. Because this chart takes proportional age-size differences into account, it can be used for infants and children, as well as for adults. (Adapted with permission from *Surgery, Gynecology, & Obstetrics* 79 [1944] 352.)

APPENDIX 7

Food and Drug Administration–Assigned Pregnancy Categories

A: Adequate and well-controlled studies have failed to demonstrate a risk to the fetus in the first trimester of pregnancy (and there is no evidence of risk in later trimesters).

B: Animal reproduction studies have failed to demonstrate a risk to the fetus and there are no adequate and well-controlled studies in pregnant women.

C: Animal reproduction studies have shown an adverse effect on the fetus and there are no adequate and well-controlled studies in humans, but potential benefits may warrant use of the drug in pregnant women despite potential risks.

D: There is positive evidence of human fetal risk based on adverse reaction data from investigational or marketing experience or studies in humans, but potential benefits may warrant use of the drug in pregnant women despite potential risks.

X: Studies in animals or humans have demonstrated fetal abnormalities and/or there is positive evidence of human fetal risk based on adverse reaction data from investigational or marketing experience and the risks involved in use of the drug in pregnant women clearly outweigh potential benefits.

Glossary

Achlorhydria. Absence of hydrochloric acid in the stomach.

Acidosis. Increased acidity of body fluids.

Acrocyanosis. Cyanosis (blueness) of the extremities.

Acromegaly. Overgrowth of bones of extremities and head in adults due to excess secretion of growth hormone.

Acroparesthesia. Tingling, prickling, or numbness of extremities.

Addison's disease. Condition due to deficiency of adrenal cortex.

Adrenergic. Pertaining to the sympathetic portion of the autonomic nervous system.

Agranulocytosis. Low white blood cell count especially neutropenia – characterized by fever, ulceration of mucous membranes, and prostration.

Akathisia. Extreme restlessness, increased motor movement.

Akinesia. Partial or complete loss of muscle movement.

Alopecia. Absence or loss of hair (especially on the head).

Amblyopia. Reduced or dimness of vision.

Amenorrhea. Absences of menses.

Anabolic, anabolism. The building up of body tissues.

Anaphylaxis. Allergic hypersensitivity reaction of the body due to a drug or foreign protein.

Androgenic. Causing masculine characteristics.

Angina, anginal. Usually refers to angina pectoris – severe pain in the heart usually due to insufficient oxygenation.

Angioedema. Allergic reaction resulting in edematous areas of the skin, viscera, or mucous membranes.

Anorexia. Loss of appetite.

Anuria. Absence of urine formation.

Aphakia. Absence of the crystalline lens of the eye.

Aphasia. Loss or impairment of speech.

Aplastic anemia. Anemia due to impairment of the bone marrow.

Apnea. Temporary cessation of breathing.

Arthralgia. Joint pain.

Ascites. Fluid accumulation in the peritoneal cavity.

Asthenia. Muscle weakness; decreased or loss of muscle strength.

Atopic. Out of place, displaced.

Azotemia. Increased urea or nitrogen in the blood.

Bactericidal. Agent that kills bacteria.

Bacteriostatic. Decreasing or inhibiting growth of bacteria.

Biologic half-life. The time it takes for one-half the drug to be excreted or removed from the blood.

Blepharospasm. Twitching of the eyelid(s).

Bradycardia. Slow heart rate.

Bruxism. Grinding of the teeth (usually during sleep).

Buerger's disease. Also called thromboangiitis obliterans. Chronic inflammatory disease especially the peripheral arteries and veins of the extremities – may cause paresthesia or gangrene.

Catabolism. Breakdown of complex body substances with the usual release of energy.

Cellulitis. Inflammation of cellular or connective tissue.

Cheilitis. Inflammation of the lip(s).

Cheilosis. Condition where lips become reddened with fissures at the angles – usually due to riboflavin deficiency.

Chloasma. Skin discoloration, usually yellow-brown in color.

Cholangitis. Inflammation of the bile ducts.

Cholecystitis. Inflammation of the gallbladder.

Cholelithiasis. Presence of stones or calculi in the gallbladder or bile ducts.

Cholestasia. Decrease or stoppage of bile excretion.

Cholinergic. Pertaining to the parasympathetic portion of the autonomic nervous system.

Chorea. Involuntary muscle twitches of the face or limbs.

Cirrhosis. A chronic, degenerative disease of the liver.

Claudication. Limping or lameness.

Colitis. Inflammation of the colon.

Conjunctivitis. Inflammation of the conjunctiva of the eye.

Cretinism. Congential deficiency of thyroid hormone resulting in arrested physical and mental development.

Cryptorchidism. Failure of the testicles to descend into the scrotum.

Crystalluria. Appearance of crystals in the urine.

Cyanosis. Abnormal amounts of reduced hemoglobin in the blood resulting in a blue-gray discoloration of the skin.

Cycloplegia. Paralysis of the ciliary muscles of the eye.

Diaphoresis. Heavy perspiration.

Diathesis. Predisposition to a certain condition or disease.

Diplopia. Double vision.

Dysarthria. Difficulty or deficiency of speech.

Dyscrasia. A synonym for disease – usually refers to an abnormal condition of the blood cells.

Dyskinesia. Impairment of voluntary muscle movement.

Dysmenorrhea. Painful or difficult menstruation.

Dyspareunia. Painful sexual intercourse.

Dyspepsia. Disturbed digestion.

Dysphagia. Difficulty or inability to swallow.

Dysphonia. Hoarseness. Difficulty in speaking.

Dyspnea. Labored or difficult breathing.

Dystonia. Impairment of muscle tone.

Dysuria. Painful or difficult urination.

Ecchymosis. Hemorrhagic areas of the skin producing discoloration ranging from blue-black to green-brown or yellow.

Ectopic. At a site other than normal. Often refers to pregnancy or heart beat.

Emesis. Vomiting.

Encephalopathy. Any dysfunction of the brain.

Endarteritis. Inflammation of the intima of an artery.

Enteritis. Inflammation of the intestines.

Enuresis. Urinary incontinence.

Eosinophilia. Increase in the number of circulating eosinophils.

Epistaxis. Bleeding from the nose.

Eructation. Belching.

Erythema. Redness of the skin.

Erythema multiforme. A skin rash characterized by dark red papules, vesicles, and bullae usually on the extremities.

Erythema nodosum. Red, painful nodules on the legs usually from arthritis.

Exanthema. Any skin eruption with inflammation.

Exfoliative dermatitis. Chronic imflammation of the skin characterized by itchy, scaling, and flaking skin.

Exophthalmus. Protrusion of the eyeball(s).

First-pass effect. When drugs administered orally are absorbed from the GI tract into the hepatic circulation, they may be rapidly metabolized by the liver, thereby losing much of their activity before reaching the general circulation.

Flatus. Gas in the GI tract. Expelling of gas from the body.

Florid. Bright red coloration of the skin.

Galactorrhea. Excessive flow of milk.

Gastritis. Inflammation of the stomach.

Gingivitis. Inflammation of the gums.

Glaucoma. Disease of the eye manifested by increased intraocular pressure.

Glossitis. Inflammation of the tongue.

Gluten-free. The elimination of gluten from the diet by avoiding all products containing wheat, rye, oats, or barley and vegetables such as beans, cabbage, dried peas, cucumbers, and turnips.

Glycosuria. Presence of glucose in the urine.

Gynecomastia. Enlargement of the mammary glands in the male.

Hematemesis. Vomiting of blood.

Hematinic. An agent that promotes hemoglobin formation by supplying factors essential for its synthesis.

Hematuria. Blood in the urine.

Hemoglobinemia. Presence of hemoglobin in the plasma.

Hemoglobinuria. Presence of hemoglobin in the urine.

Hemolytic. Destruction of red blood cells.

Hemoptysis. Coughing up or spitting of blood caused by bleeding in the respiratory tract.

Hepatotoxicity. Damage to the liver.

Hirsutism. Excessive growth or presence of hair.

Hypercalcemia. Excessive calcium in the blood.

Hypercapnia. Increased carbon dioxide in the blood.

Hyperglycemia. Increased blood sugar.

Hyperhidrosis. Excessive sweating.

Hyperkalemia. Increased potassium in the blood.

Hypernatremia. Increased sodium in the blood.

Hyperplasia. Excessive growth of normal cells of an organ.

Hyperpyrexia. Increased body temperature.

Hypersensitivity. Increased response to a drug or other substance.

Hypertrichosis. Excess growth of hair.

Hyperuricemia. Increased amount of uric acid in the blood.

Hypocapnia. Decrease in amount of carbon dioxide in the blood.

Hypochlorhydria. Decreased secretion of hydrochloric acid.

Hypoglycemia. Decrease in the amount of glucose in the blood.

Hypokalemia. Deficiency of potassium in the blood.

Hyponatremia. Decrease in the amount of sodium in the blood.

Hypoprothrombinemia. Deficiency of prothrombin in the blood.

Idiopathic. Disease state of unknown origin.

Ileus. Obstruction of the intestine.

Iodism. A condition related to prolonged, excessive accumulation of iodine or its components.

Ischemic. Reduction of blood supply to an organ or tissue.

Jaundice. Skin, mucous membranes, whites of eyes, and body fluids become yellow due to excess bilirubin.

Ketosis. Accumulation of ketone bodies.

Kraurosis. Drying and atrophy of any mucous membrane (usually refers to the vulva).

Lacrimation. Secretion of tears.

Lethargic, lethargy. Drowsiness, sluggishness, stupor.

Leukopenia. Abnormal decrease in white blood cells.

Leukorrhea. Mucous discharge from the vagina or cervical canal.

Libido. Sexual drive.

Lipodystrophy. Usually refers to atrophy of subcutaneous fat following insulin injections.

Lithiasis. Formation of calculi in the body.

Lochia. Blood, mucus, and tissue discharge from the uterus during the puerperal period.

Lupus erythematosus. Chronic inflammatory disease of connective tissue affecting nervous system, mucous membranes, skin, kidneys, and joints. Manifested by a characteristic rash, fever, joint pain, malaise. Occurs most often in young women.

Lymphadenopathy. Disease involving the lymph nodes.

Melasma. Discoloration or pigmentation of the skin.

Melena. Black, tarry stools due to presence of blood.

Menorrhagia. Excessive bleeding at time of menses.

Methemoglobinemia. Condition in which an excessive amount of hemoglobin is converted to methemoglobin causing cyanosis.

Miosis. Constriction of pupils of the eye.

Myalgia. Muscle pain or tenderness.

Mycosis. Any disease caused by a fungus.

Mydriasis. Dilation of the pupils of the eye.

Myopathy. Disease or abnormal condition of skeletal muscle.

Myxedema. Hypofunction of the thyroid gland in adults.

Narcolepsy. Uncontrollable attacks of desire to sleep.

Necrosis. Areas of tissue or bone which die.

Nephrotoxicity. Damage to the kidneys.

Neuritis. Inflammation of nerve(s).

Neuropathy. Any disease involving the nerves or nervous system.

Neutropenia. Abnormal decrease in the number of neutrophils in the blood.

Nocturia. Excessive urination during the night.

Nystagmus. Involuntary oscillatory movement of the eyeballs.

Obstructive jaundice. Jaundice due to a decrease in the flow of bile from the liver to duodenum (usually caused by mechanical obstruction).

Oligospermia. Deficiency in the number of spermatozoa in seminal fluid.

Oliguria. Decrease in the amount of urine formed.

Onchocerciasis. A condition or infestation produced by a genus of filarial worms that live in subcutaneous and connective tissues and are usually encapsulated.

Onycholysis. Detachment or loosening of nail from the nailbed.

Ophthalmic. Referring to the eye.

Opisthotonus. Body in the dorsal position becomes arched with head and feet touching the surface.

Orchitis. Inflammation of the testes.

Orthostatic hypotension. Drop in blood pressure when standing up quickly from a reclining or sitting position.

Osteitis. Inflammation of a bone.

Osteomalacia. Softening of the bones.

Osteoporosis. Bones become porous and may break more easily.

Otic. Pertaining to the ear.

Otitis. Inflammation of the ear.

Palpitations. Rapid or throbbing pulsation (often refers to the heart).

Pancreatitis. Inflammation of the pancreas.

Pancytopenia. Abnormal decrease in all formed cells in the blood.

Papilledema. Inflammation and edema of the optic nerve where it enters the eyeball.

Paraparesis. Partial paralysis of the legs.

Paresis. Partial paralysis.

Paresthesia. Sensation of numbness, tingling, or prickling.

Petachiae. Purplish red spot(s) on the skin, mucous membranes, or serous membranes caused by intradermal or submucosal bleeding.

Peyronie's disease. Hardening of the erectile tissue of the penis causing distortion.

Pharyngitis. Inflammation of the pharynx.

Phlebitis. Inflammation of a vein.

Photophobia. Intolerance of light.

Piloerection. Erection of hair – referred to as "hair standing on end."

Polydipsia. Excessive thirst.

Polyphagia. Excessive appetite.

Polyuria. Excessive formation and discharge of urine.

Porphyria. Disorder in which increased amounts of porphyrin are synthesized. Characterized by abdominal pain, psychological, GI, and neurologic disturbances.

Prepubescent. Before reaching puberty; characterized by the time when either males or females become functionally able to reproduce.

Presbyopia. Loss of accommodation of the eye with advancing age.

Priapism. Painful and continuous erection of the penis due to disease.

Proteinuria. Appearance of protein (usually albumin) in the urine.

Pruritus. Severe itching.

Psoriasis. Skin disease of genetic origin manifested by pink or light red lesions and scaling.

Purpura. Hemorrhage occurring in the skin and mucous membranes.

Rales. An abnormal sound of the chest due to passage of air through bronchi containing secretions or which are constricted.

Raynaud's phenomenon. Peripheral vascular disease manifested by cold, cyanotic, painful fingers and hands due to vasoconstriction.

Repository. An agent designed to exhibit its effect over an extended period of time.

Rhinitis. Inflammation of the mucosa of the nose.

Scleroderma. Disease characterized by induration of the skin in localized or diffuse areas.

Sclerosis. Hardening of a tissue or organ.

Seborrheic. Referring to glands that secrete sebaceous matter.

Sepsis. Febrile reaction due to microorganisms or their poisonous byproducts.

Sialorrhea. Excessive salivation.

Siderosis. Chronic inflammation of the lungs due to prolonged inhalation of dust of iron salts.

Splenomegaly. Enlargement of the spleen.

Steatorrhea. Fatty stools.

Stenosis. Narrowing of any duct or orifice.

Stevens-Johnson syndrome. Extreme inflammatory eruption of skin and mucosa of mouth, pharynx, anogenital region, and conjunctiva with high fever. May be fatal.

Stomatitis. Inflammation of the mouth.

Superinfection. Overgrowth of bacteria different from those causing the original infection.

Syncope. Fainting.

Synergy. When agents work together to achieve a result not attainable by only one agent.

Tachycardia. Abnormal increase in heart rate.

Tamponade. Usually refers to the heart where there is excess accumulation of fluid around the heart.

Tetany. Sudden, intermittent, tonic spasms most often involving the extremities.

Thalassemia. Hereditary anemia occurring in Mediterraneans and Southeast Asians.

Thrombocytopenia. Abnormal decrease in the number of circulating blood platelets.

Thromboplebitis. Inflammation of a vein with accompanying thrombus formation.

Thrombosis. Formation or existence of a blood clot within the vascular system.

Tinnitus. Ringing of the ears.

Torticollis. Spasms of the neck muscles causing a stiff neck and the head is drawn to one side with chin pointing to the other side.

Urticaria. Hives characterized by severe itching and rash.

Uveitis. Inflammation of the iris, choroid, and/or ciliary body of the eye.

Vasculitis. Inflammation of a lymph or blood vessel.

Venous Access Device (VAD). A type of catheter implanted into the venous circulation with a subcutaneous reservoir for long-term fluid and/or drug administration.

Vertigo. Term usually used to describe dizziness, lightheadedness, and/or giddiness.

Xerophthalmia. Dryness of the conjunctiva with epithelial keratinization. Usually due to vitamin A deficiency.

Xerostomia. Dryness of mouth resulting from lack of normal salivation.

Bibliography

AMA Drug Evaluations, ed 6. Chicago, American Medical Association, 1986.

American Hospital Formulary Service, Drug Information 90. Bethesda, MD, American Society of Hospital Pharmacists, 1990.

Becker T. *Cancer Chemotherapy, A Manual for Nurses.* Boston, Little, Brown, 1981.

Brunner LS, Suddarth DM. *Textbook of Medical-Surgical Nursing,* ed 6. Philadelphia, Lippincott, 1988.

Burns N. Cancer chemotherapy. A systemic approach, *Nursing '78,* pp. 39–47, May 1978.

Cape R. *Aging: Its Complex Management.* New York, Harper & Row, 1978.

Chemotherapy and You. U.S. Dept. of Health and Human Services, NIH Publication 81–1136. November 1980.

Coblio NA. *Nursing '81,* pp 48–49, 1981.

Craig CR, Stitzel RE. *Modern Pharmacology,* ed 3. Boston, Little, Brown, 1990.

Current Concepts in Chemotherapy Administration. *Seminars in Oncology Nursing.* May 3(2), 1987.

Daniels, L. How can you improve patient compliance? *Nursing '78,* pp 39–47, May 1978.

Drug Information For the Health Care Provider, ed 10. U.S. Pharmacopeia Drug Information, 1990.

Drug Therapy and Pregnancy: Maternal, Fetal and Neonatal Considerations. (Symposium) *Obstetrics and Gynecology* 58(5)(suppl), November 1981.

Eliopoulos C. *A Guide to the Nursing of the Aged.* Baltimore, Williams & Wilkins, 1987.

Facts and Comparisons. St. Louis, Lippincott, Facts and Comparisons Division. Current.

Falvo DR. *Effective Patient Education.* Rockville, MD, Aspen Publications, 1985.

Food and Drug Interactions. *FDA Consumer,* U.S. Dept. of Health Education and Welfare, U.S. Government Printing Office Publication 311–254/3, March 1978.

Fredette SL, et al. Nursing diagnosis in cancer chemotherapy: In theory. *Am J Nursing,* pp 2013–2020, November 1981.

Fredette SL, et al. Nursing diagnosis in cancer chemotherapy: In practice. *Am J Nursing,* pp 2021–2022, November 1981.

Geuer H. Brompton's mixture. *Nursing '80,* p 57, May 1980.

Gilman AG, Goodman LS, Gilman A. *Goodman and Gilman's The Pharmacological Basis of Therapeutics,* ed 7. New York, Macmillan, 1985.

Golbus M. Teratology for the Obstetrician: Current Status. *Obstetrics and Gynecology* 55(3), pp 269–277, 1979.

Gotch, P. Teaching patients about adrenal corticosteroids. *Am J Nursing,* pp 78–81, January 1981.

Govoni LE, Hayes JE. *Drugs and Nursing Implications,* ed 6. Norwalk, CT, Appleton & Lange, 1988.

Graef JW. *Manual of Pediatric Therapeutics.* Boston, Little Brown, 1974.

Hahn AB, Oestreich SJK, Barkin RL. *Mosby's Pharmacology in Nursing,* ed 16. Norwalk, CT, Appleton & Lange, 1986.

Hansen M, Woods S. Nitroglycerin ointment, where and how to apply it. *Am J Nursing,* pp 112–114, June 1980.

Hansten PD. *Drug Interactions,* ed 6. Philadelphia, Lea & Febiger, 1989.

Hill R, Stern L. Drugs in pregnancy: Effects on the fetus and newborn. *Drugs* 17, March 1979.

Howard F, Hill J. Drugs in pregnancy. *Obstetrical and Gynecological Survey* 34(9), pp 643–652, 1979.

Jensen M, Bobak I. *Handbook of Maternity Care*. St. Louis, Mosby, 1980.

Jones D, Dunbar C, Jirovec M. *Medical Surgical Nursing*, ed 2. New York, McGraw-Hill, 1982.

Kane, R.L., Ouslander, J.G., Abrass, I.B. *Essentials of Clinical Geriatrics*, ed 2. New York, McGraw-Hill, Health Division 1989.

Kee J. *Fluids and Electrolytes with Clinical Applications*, ed 3. New York, Wiley, 1982.

Kee J. *Laboratory and Diagnostic Tests with Nursing Implications*, ed 16. Norwalk, CT, Appleton-Century-Crofts, 1983.

King E, Wieck L, Dyer M. *Illustrated Manual of Nursing Techniques*. Philadelphia, Lippincott, 1986.

Kozier B, Erb B. *Fundamentals of Nursing*, ed 3. Menlo Park, CA, Addison-Wesley, 1987.

Lamy P. How your patient's diet can affect drug response. *Drug Therapy*, pp 82–88, August 1980.

Langslet J, Habel M. The aminoglycoside antibiotics. *Am J Nursing*, pp 1144–1146, June 1981.

Lewis LW. *Fundamental Skills in Patient Care*, ed 3. Philadelphia, Lippincott, 1984.

Levitt D. Cancer Chemotherapy. *RN*, pp 56–59, February 1981.

Luckmann J, Sorensen K. *Medical-Surgical Nursing*. Philadelphia, Saunders, 1980.

Mangini RJ (ed). *Drug Interaction Facts*. St. Louis, Lippincott, Facts and Comparisons Division. Current.

Martin EW. *Hazards of Medication*. Philadelphia, Lippincott, 1978.

Martin L. *Health Care of Women*. Philadelphia, Lippincott, 1978.

Matthewson, M. Intravenous Therapy. *Critical Care Nurse*, 9, pp 21–36, 1990.

Mehl B. Food-drug interactions. *Primary Cardiology*, pp 128–137, September 1981.

Niebyl, J. Teratology and Drugs in Pregnancy and Lactation. *Danforth's Obstetrics and Gynecology*, ed 6. Philadelphia, Lippincott, 1990.

Patient Lips. *Am. J. Nursing*, 3, pp 37–39, 1990.

Petrillo M, Sanger S. *Emotional Care of Hospitalized Children*, ed 2. Philadelphia, Lippincott, 1980.

Phipps WJ, Long BC, Woods NF. *Medical-Surgical Nursing*, ed 2. St. Louis, Mosby, 1983.

Pilliterri A. *Nursing Care of the Growing Family, A Maternal-Newborn Text*. Boston, Little, Brown, 1980.

Physicians' Desk Reference, ed 44. Oradell, NJ, Medical Economics Co., 1990.

Plummer AL. *Principles and Practices of Intravenous Therapy*, ed 3. Boston, Little, Brown, 1982.

Postotnik P. Drugs and pregnancy. *FDA Consumer*. U.S. Government Printing Office, October 1978.

Purcell JA, Holder CK. Intravenous nitroglycerin. *Am J Nursing*, pp 254–259, February 1982.

Rayburn WF, Zuspan FP. *Drug Therapy in Obstetrics and Gynecology*. Norwalk, CT, Appleton-Century-Crofts, 1982.

Redman BK. *The Process of Patient Education*. St. Louis, Mosby, 1988.

Sheridan E, Patterson HR, Gustafson EA. *Falconer's The Drug, The Nurse, The Patient*, ed 7. Philadelphia, Saunders, 1985.

Sherman, J.L., Fierds, S.K. *Guide To Patient Evaluation*, ed 5. Medical Examination Publishing Co., 1988.

Skitklorius C. Toward impeccable IV techniques. *RN*, pp 37–40, April 1981.

Spencer RT, Nichols NW, Waterhouse HP, West FW, Bankert EG. *Clinical Pharmacology and Nursing Management*. Philadelphia, Lippincott, 1983.

Steffl BM. *Handbook of Gerontological Nursing*. New York, Van Nostrand Reinhold Co., 1984.

Swonger, A.K., Matejski, M.P. *Nursing Pharmacology: An Integrated Approach To Drug Therapy and Nursing Practice*, Glenview, IL/Boston, Scott, Foresman, Little, Brown 1988.

Symposium on Drugs in Pregnancy. *Obstetrics and Gynecology 58* (suppl) 1981.

Wallach J. *Interpretation of Diagnostic Tests*, ed 4. Boston, Little, Brown, 1986.

Walters, P. Chemo: A nurse's guide to action, administration, and side effects. *R.N.* 53, pp 52–67, 1990.

Weeks J. Administering medication to children. *Maternal Child Nursing,* 5, pp 63–64, January/February 1980.

Whitson B, McFarlane J. *The Pediatric Nursing Skills Manual.* New York, Wiley, 1980.

Willis J. Drugs that take the joy out of sex. *FDA Consumer,* pp 31–32, July/August 1981.

Wolff L, Weitzel MH, Zornow RA, Zsohar H. *Fundamentals of Nursing.* Philadelphia, Lippincott, 1983.

Wong D, Whaley L. *Clinical Handbook of Pediatric Nursing.* St. Louis, Mosby, 1981.

Yaffe SJ (ed). *Pediatric Pharmacology.* New York, Grune & Stratton, 1980.

Yurick AG, et al. *The Aged Person and the Nursing Process,* ed 2. Norwalk, CT, Appleton-Century-Crofts, 1984.

Index

A

A20–Standard, 271
Abbokinase, 432
  Open-Cath, 432
Abbreviations, commonly used, xix
ABDIC, 299(t)
Abiplatin✦, 351
Abortifacients, 1220–1225
  nursing considerations, 1220
Absorption of drugs, defined, 9
ABVD, 299(t)
Accutane, 1375
  Roche✦, 1375
ACe, 299(t)
ACE, 299(t)
Acebutolol, 913
  hydrochloride, 486
Acephen, 794
Aceta, 793
Acetaminophen, 793, 1409(t)
  buffered, 794
Acetazolam✦, 734, 1255
Acetazolamide, 734, 1255
  sodium, 1255
Acetohexamide, 1074, 1112
Acetohydroxamic acid, 261
Acetophenazine maleate, 633
Acetylcarbromal, 597
Acetylcholine chloride,
  intraocular, 938(t)
Acetylcysteine, 1000
Acetylsalicylic acid, buffered, 783
Accurbron, 976
Aches-N-Pain, 807
Achromycin IM, 177
  IV, 177
  Ophthalmic, 177
  V, 177
Acidifying and alkalinizing agents, 1304–1310
Acidulin, 1088
Aclovate, 1154(t)
A-COPP, 299(t)
ACT, 290(t), 341
Actamin, 793
  Extra, 793
ACTH, 1164
  gel, 1164
Acthar, 1164
  Gel ✦, 1164
Acti-B12✦, 1322
Acticort 100, 1156(t), 1171
Actidil, 1017
ACTIFED, 986
Actigall, 1402

Actinomycin D, 290(t), 341
Activase, 425
  rt-PA✦, 425
ACU-Dyne, 258
Acutrim 16 Hour, 853, 905
  Late Day, 853, 905
  II Maximum Strength, 853, 905
Acycloguanosine, 273
Acyclovir, 273
Adalat, 460
  FT✦, 460
  P.A.✦, 460
Adapin, 672
Adenocard, 535
Adenosine, 535
  5-monophosphate, 1348
  phosphate, 1348
Adipex-P, 852
Administration of drugs, 7–9
  by oral route, 31
  by gastrostomy tube, 32
  by inhalation, 33
  by intra-arterial infusion, 53
  by nasal application, 37
  by nasogastric tube, 31
  by oral irrigations and gargles, 36
  by parenteral routes, 43
  by perfusion, 54
Adphen, 852
ADR, 291(t), 299(t), 344
Adrenalin Chloride, 895, 910(t)
  Solution, 894
Adrenergic blocking
  (sympatholytic) drugs, 912
Adrenergic drugs, see Symapthomimetics
Adrenocorticosteroids and analogs, 1148–1180
Adrenocorticotropic hormone, 1164
Adria, 299(t)
Adriamycin PFS, 344
  RDF, 344
Adrucil, 333
Adsorbocarpine, 939(t)
Adsorbonac Ophthalmic, 1292
Advil, 807
AeroBid, 1170
Aerolate, 976
  Jr, 976
  Sr, 976
Aerolone, 898
Aeroseb-Dex, 1155(t), 1167
  -HC, 1156(t), 1171
Aerosporin, 167
Afko-Lube, 1058

Afrin 12 Hour Nasal Spray, 910(t)
  12 hour nose drops, 910(t)
  children's strength 12 hour nose drops, 910(t)
  regular drops, 910(t)
  menthol nasal spray, 910(t)
  nasal spray, 910(t)
  nose drops, 910(t)
Afrinol, 907
Aftate for Athlete's Foot, 200
  for Jock Itch, 200
Agents for attention deficit disorders, 858–862
Agents that act directly on vascular smooth muscle, 514–519
Agents that depress the activity of the sympathetic nervous system, 478–514
Agoral Plain, 1059
AHA, 261
AHF, 408
A-hydroCort, 1171
Airbron✦, 1000
AK Chlor✦, 109
Akarpine, 940(t)
AK-Dex, 1168, 1169
  Ophthalmic, 1155(t)
AK-Dilate, 903
AK-Homatropine, 956(t)
Akineton Hydrochloride, 699
  Lactate, 699
AK-Mycin, 119
AK-NaCl, 1292
AK-Nefrin, 903
Akne-mycin, 119
AK-Pentolate, 955(t)
AK-Pred, 1157(t), 1174
AK-Sulf, 209
AK-Taine, 867(t)
AK-Tate, 1174
AK-Tracin, 124
AK-Zol, 734, 1255
Ala-Cort, 1156(t), 1171
Ala-Scalp HP, 1156(t), 1171
Ala-Tet, 177
Albalon Liquifilm✦, 910(t)
Albamycin, 132
Alba-Temp 300, 793
Albumin, normal human serum, 25%, 416
  25%, 416
Albuminar-25, 416
  -5, 416
Albutein 25%, 416
  5%, 416

Boldface = generic drug name   Regular type = trade names
italics = therapeutic drug class   CAPITALS = combination drugs

Boldface = generic drug name   Regular type = trade names
italics = therapeutic drug class   CAPITALS = combination drugs

Boldface = generic drug name   Regular type = trade names
italics = therapeutic drug class   CAPITALS = combination drugs

Boldface = generic drug name   Regular type = trade names
italics = therapeutic drug class   CAPITALS = combination drugs

---

Boldface = generic drug name   Regular type = trade names
italics = therapeutic drug class   CAPITALS = combination drugs

Boldface = generic drug name   Regular type = trade names
italics = therapeutic drug class   CAPITALS = combination drugs

Guanethidine, 504
Guanfacine hydrochloride,
500
Guanidine hydrochloride,
928
Guiatuss, 984
Gustalac, 1024
Gynecort, 1156(t), 1171
Gyne-Lotrimin, 184
Gynergen♣, 915
Gynogen, 1190
L.A. 10, 1190
20, 1190
40, 1190

H

H Cort, 1171
Halazepam, 619
Halcinoide, 1156(t)
Haldol, 647
Decanoate 50, 647
100, 647
Lactate, 647
Haldrone, 1173
Halenol, 794
Elixir, 793
Extra Strength, 794
Caplets, 794
Halofed, 907
Adult Strength, 907
Halog, 1156(t)
-E, 1156(t)
Haloperidol, 647
decanoate, 647
lactate, 647
Haloprogin, 190
Halotestin, 1227(t)
Halotex, 190
Halothane, 874(t)
Halotussin, 984
Halperon, 647
Haltran, 807
Harmonyl, 526(t)
HCG, 1208
Heavy metal antagonists,
1340–1347
Hemabate, 1222
Hemin, 1370
Hemocyte, 383
Hemofil M, 408
Hemostatics, 402–413
systemic agents, 406
topical, 402
Hepahydrin, 1087
Hepalean♣, 396
-Lok♣, 400
Heparin and protamine sulfate,
396–402
Heparin calcium, 396
lock flush, 400
sodium in dextrose, 396

sodium in sodium chloride,
396
sodium injection, 396
Heparin Leo♣, 396
HepatAmine, 1300
Hep-Lock, 400
Herplex Liquifilm, 279
HES, 422
Hespan, 422
Hetastarch, 422
Hexa-Betalin, 1326
Hexadrol, 1167
Hexadrol phosphate, 1168
Hexocyclium methylsulfate,
945(t)
Hi-Cor 1.0, 1156(t), 1171
2.5, 1156(t), 1171
Hip-Rex♣, 264
Hiprex, 264
Hismanil, 1009
Hispril, 1006(t)
Histaject Modified, 1009
Histamine and antihistamines,
1002–1017
Histerone 50, 1230
100, 1230
Hi-Vegi-Lip, 1089
HMS Liquifilm, 1157(t)
HN, 324
HN₂, 293(t)
H₁ blockers, 1003–1017
H₂Cort, 1156(t)
Hold, 982
Homatrine, 956(t)
Homatropine, 1071(t)
HBr, 956(t)
Honvol♣, 364, 1186
Hormonal and antihormonal
antineoplastic agents,
364–376
Hormones and hormone
antagonists, 1093–1247
abortifacients, 1220
adrenocorticosteroids and
analogs, 1149
androgens and anabolic
steroids, 1230
calcitonin, calcium salts, and
calcium regulators, 1135
estrogens, progestins, and oral
contraceptives, 1181
insulin, oral antidiabetics, and
insulin antagonists, 1093
posterior pituitary hormones
and related drugs/growth
hormone, 1234
thyroid and antithyroid drugs,
1120
8-Hour Bayer Timed-Release, 783
H.P. Acthar Gel, 1164
Human insulin, 1104
Humatin, 83, 258
Humatrope, 1246

Humibid L.A., 984
Sprinkle, 984
HuMIST Saline Nasal, 1292
Humorsol Ophthalmic, 938(t)
Humulin 70/30, 1104
BR, 1104
L, 1104
N, 1104
R, 1104
U Ultralente, 1104
Hurricaine, 864(t)
Hyalase♣, 1371
Hyaluronidase, 1371
Hybolin Decanoate, 1228(t)
improved, 1228(t)
HYCODAN SYRUP, 990
TABLETS, 990
HYD, 292(t), 335
Hydantoins, 722–729
Hydeltrasol, 1174
Hydeltra-T.B.A., 1174
Hydergine, 858
LC, 858
Hyderm♣, 1156(t), 1171
Hydralazine, 1411(t)
hydrochloride, 516
HYDRALAZINE, AND
HYDROCHLOROTHIAZIDE,
531
HYDRALAZINE AND ISONIAZID,
24(T)
Hydramine, 688, 983, 1014, 1078
Cough, 688, 983, 1014, 1078
Hydrate, 1013, 1078
Hydrea, 335
Hydrex, 1277(t)
Hydril, 688, 983, 1014, 1078
Hydrochloric acid, diluted,
1088
Hydrochlorides of opium
alkaloids, 763
Hydrochlorothiazide, 1282
Hydrocil Instant, 1057
Hydrocortisone, 1171
acetate cream, 1156(t)
lotion, 1156(t)
ointment, 1156(t)
rectal, 1156(t)
suppositories, 1156(t)
butyrate, 1157(t)
cream, rectal, 1156(t)
topical, 1156(t)
cypionate, 1171
lotion, 1156(t)
ointment, 1156(t)
sodium, 1171
phosphate, 1171
succinate, 1171
topical aerosol foam,
1156(t)
aerosol solution, 1156(t)
solution, 1156(t)
valerate, 1157(t)

Boldface = generic drug name   Regular type = trade names
italics = therapeutic drug class   CAPITALS = combination drugs

Boldface = generic drug name   Regular type = trade names
italics = therapeutic drug class   CAPITALS = combination drugs

Boldface = generic drug name   Regular type = trade names
italics = therapeutic drug class   CAPITALS = combination drugs

Boldface = generic drug name   Regular type = trade names
italics = therapeutic drug class   CAPITALS = combination drugs

Boldface = generic drug name   Regular type = trade names
italics = therapeutic drug class   CAPITALS = combination drugs

Boldface = generic drug name   Regular type = trade names
italics = therapeutic drug class   CAPITALS = combination drugs

Boldface = generic drug name   Regular type = trade names
italics = therapeutic drug class   CAPITALS = combination drugs

Boldface = generic drug name   Regular type = trade names
italics = therapeutic drug class   CAPITALS = combination drugs

Boldface = generic drug name   Regular type = trade names
italics = therapeutic drug class   CAPITALS = combination drugs